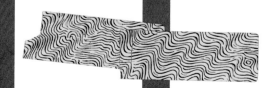

Clinical Pharmacology

And I will use regimens for the benefit of the ill in accordance with my ability and my judgement.
The Hippocratic Oath c.400 BC

But doctors are lucky: the sun shines on their successes and the earth hides their failures.
Michael de Montaigne 1533–1592

Morals do not forbid making experiments on one's neighbour or on one's self … among the experiments that may be tried on man, those that can only harm are forbidden, those that are innocent are permissible, and those that may do good are obligatory.
Claude Bernard 1813–1878

It may seem a strange principle to enunciate as the very first requirement in a Hospital that it should do the sick no harm.
Florence Nightingale 1820–1910

The ingenuity of man has ever been fond of exerting itself to varied forms and combinations of medicines.
William Withering 1741–1799

A desire to take medicine is, perhaps, the great feature which distinguishes man from other animals.
William Osler 1849–1920

All things are poisons and there is nothing that is harmless, the dose alone decides that something is no poison.
Paracelsus 1493–1541

Medical science aims at the truth and nothing but the truth.
William J Mayo 1861–1939

What we find in books is like the fire in our hearths. We fetch it from our neighbors, we kindle it at home, we communicate it to others, and it becomes the property of all.
Voltaire 1694–1778

Clinical Pharmacology

Twelfth edition

Morris J. Brown
MA MSc FRCP FAHA FBPharmacolS FMedSci

Professor of Endocrine Hypertension, William Harvey Research Institute of the Barts and the London School of Medicine and Dentistry, London, UK

Pankaj Sharma
MD PhD FRCP

Professor of Neurology and Director, Institute of Cardiovascular Research, Royal Holloway College, University of London; and Consultant Neurologist, Imperial College Healthcare NHS Trust, London, UK

Fraz A. Mir
MA, FRCP

Consultant Clinical Pharmacologist, Division of Experimental Medicine and Immunotherapeutics, Department of Medicine, University of Cambridge, Addenbrooke's Hospital, Cambridge, UK

Peter N. Bennett
MD FRCP

Formerly Reader in Clinical Pharmacology, University of Bath; and Consultant Physician, Royal United Hospital, Bath, UK

ELSEVIER   Edinburgh   London   New York   Oxford   Philadelphia   St Louis   Sydney   2019

ELSEVIER

ISBN: 978-0-7020-7328-1
IE: 978-0-7020-7329-8

Printed in China
Last digit is the print number: 9 8 7 6 5 4 3 2 1

Content Strategist: Pauline Graham
Content Development Specialist: Fiona Conn
Senior Project Manager: Manchu Mohan
Design: Amy Buxton
Illustration Manager: Teresa McBryan
Marketing Manager: Deborah Watkins

Contents

Contents

For your own satisfaction and for mine, please read this preface![1]

A preface should tell the prospective reader about the subject of a book, its purpose and its plan. This book is about the scientific basis and practice of drug therapy. It addresses medical students and doctors in particular, but also anyone concerned with evidence-based drug therapy and prescribing.

The scope and rate of drug innovation increase. Doctors now face a professional lifetime of handling drugs that are new to themselves – drugs that do new things as well as drugs that do old things better – and drugs that were familiar during medical training become redundant.

We write not only for readers who, like us, have a special interest in pharmacology. We try to make pharmacology understandable for those whose primary interests lie elsewhere but who recognise that they need some knowledge of pharmacology if they are to meet their moral and legal 'duty of care' to their patients. We are aware, too, of medical curricular pressures that would reduce the time devoted to teaching clinical pharmacology and therapeutics, and such diminution is surely a misguided policy for a subject that is so integral to the successful practice of medicine. Thus, we try to tell readers what they need to know without burdening them with irrelevant information, and we try to make the subject interesting. We are very serious, but seriousness does not always demand wearying solemnity.

All who prescribe drugs would be wise to keep in mind the changing and ever more exacting expectations of patients and of society in general. Doctors who prescribe casually or ignorantly now face not only increasing criticism but also civil (or even criminal) legal charges. The ability to handle new developments depends, now more than ever, on comprehension of the principles of pharmacology. These principles are not difficult to grasp and are not so many as to defeat even the busiest doctors who take upon themselves the responsibility of introducing manufactured medicines into the bodies of their patients. The exercise of prescribing calls for the meticulous selection of medicines and so the avoidance of polypharmacy, which now seems rampant.

The principles of pharmacology and drug therapy appear in Chapters 1–11 and their application in the subsequent specialist chapters, where we draw on the knowledge and authority of a range of experts, to whom we express our gratitude. The names of those who contributed to the present and previous editions appear on subsequent pages.

We seek to offer a reasonably brief solution to the problem of combining practical clinical utility with an account of the principles on which clinical practice rests.

The quantity of practical technical detail to include is a matter of judgment. In general, where therapeutic practices are complex, potentially dangerous or commonly updated, e.g. anaphylactic shock, we provide more detail, together with websites for the latest advice; we give less or even no detail on therapy that specialists undertake, e.g. anticancer drugs. Nevertheless, especially with modern drugs that are unfamiliar, prescribers should consult formularies, approved guidelines or the manufacturer's current literature, relevant to their country of practice.

---

[1] St Francis of Sales: Preface to *Introduction to the devout life* (1609).

Preface

Use of the book. Francis Bacon[2] wrote that 'Some books are to be tasted, others to be swallowed, and some few to be chewed and digested.' Perhaps elements of each activity can apply to parts of our text. Students and doctors are, or should be, concerned to understand and to develop a rational, critical attitude to drug therapy, and they should therefore chiefly address issues of how drugs act and interact in disease and how evidence of therapeutic effect is obtained and evaluated.

To this end, they should read selectively and should not impede themselves by attempts to memorise lists of alternative drugs and doses and minor differences among them, which should never be required of them in examinations. Thus, we do not encumber the text with exhaustive lists of preparations, which properly belong in a formulary, although we hope that enough has been mentioned to cover much routine prescribing, and many drugs have been included solely for identification.

The role and status of a textbook. In this computer age, a textbook still plays a coveted role. Unlike electronic search engines, a textbook allows one to browse and amble a route to the question posed, perhaps acquiring information along the way that one had never thought existed. We aspire to provide one such route.

A useful guide to drug use must offer clear conclusions and advice. If it is to be of reasonable size, it may often omit alternative acceptable courses of action. What it recommends should rest on sound evidence, where this exists, and on an assessment of the opinions of the experienced where it does not.

Increasingly, guidelines produced by specialist societies and national and international bodies have influenced the selection of drugs. We provide or refer to these as representing a consensus of best practice in particular situations. Similarly, we assume that the reader possesses a formulary, local or national, that will provide guidance on the availability, including doses, of a broad range of drugs. Yet the practice of medicinal therapeutics by properly educated and conscientious doctors working in settings complicated by intercurrent disease, metabolic differences or personality, involves challenges beyond the rigid adherence to published recommendations. The role of a textbook is to provide the satisfaction of understanding the basis for a recommended course of action and to achieve an optimal result by informed selection and use of drugs. In this our twelfth edition, we can but reassert our belief in this principle. The textbook is dead: long live the textbook.

MJB, PS, FAM, PNB

---

[2]Francis Bacon (1561–1626) *Essays* (1625) 'Of studies'. Philosopher and scientist, Bacon introduced the idea of the experimental or inductive method of reasoning for understanding nature.

Contributors

Mark Abrahams MB ChB DA FRCA FFPMRCA
Clinical Director,
Musculoskeletal Services,
Cambridge University Hospitals NHS
Foundation Trust,
Cambridge, UK
Chapter 18 Pain and analgesics

Graeme Alexander MB ChB, MA, MD, FRCP
UCL Professor, Institute for Liver and
Digestive Health, Royal Free Hospital
Pond St, Hampstead, London, UK.
Chapter 34 Liver and biliary tract

Sani Aliyu MBBS FRCP FRCPath
Consultant in Microbiology and
Infectious Diseases,
Cambridge University Hospitals NHS
Foundation Trust,
Cambridge, UK
*Chapter 15 Viral, fungal, protozoal and
helminthic infections*

John Louis-Auguste BA MB ChB MRCP
Specialist Registrar in Gastroenterology,
Charing Cross Hospital,
London, UK
*Chapter 32 Oesophagus, stomach and
duodenum, Chapter 33 Intestines*

Trevor Baglin MA MB Ch B PhD FRCP FRCPath
Consultant Haematologist,
Cambridge University Hospitals NHS
Foundation Trust,
Cambridge University Teaching Hospitals
NHS Trust,
Cambridge, UK
Chapter 29 Drugs and haemostasis

Devinder Singh Bansi BM DM FRCP
Consultant Gastroenterologist,
Imperial College Healthcare NHS Trust,
London, UK
*Chapter 32 Oesophagus, stomach and
duodenum, Chapter 33 Intestines*

Paul Bentley MA, MRCP, PhD
Clinical Senior Lecturer and Honorary
Consultant in Neurology and Stroke
Medicine,
Imperial College,
London, UK
*Chapter 21 Neurological disorders
– epilepsy, Parkinson's disease and
multiple sclerosis*

Blanca M. Bolea-Alamanac MD MSc (Affective Neuroscience) PhD
Assistant Professor,
Department of Psychiatry,
University of Toronto and Staff
Psychiatrist,
Centre for Addiction and Mental Health,
Toronto, Canada
Chapter 20 Psychotropic drugs

Chrysothemis Brown MA MBBS PhD MRCPCH
Wellcome Trust Post-doctoral Clinical
Research Fellow,
Institute of Child Health,
UCL,
London, UK
Chapter 39 Vitamins, calcium, bone

Diana C. Brown MD MSc FRCP
Consultant Endocrinologist,
BUPA Cromwell Hospital,
London, UK
*Chapter 35 Adrenal corticosteroids,
antagonists, corticotrophin, Chapter 37
Thyroid hormones, antithyroid drugs*

Simon Davies DM (Oxon) MBBS MRCPsych MSc (Epidemiol) MSc (Affective Neuroscience)
Associate Professor,
Department of Psychiatry,
University of Toronto and Staff
Psychiatrist,
Centre for Addiction and Mental Health,
Toronto, Canada
Chapter 20 Psychotropic drugs

David A. Enoch BSc MBBS MSc MRCP FRCPath DTM&H
Consultant Medical Microbiologist,
Clinical Microbiology & Public Health
Laboratory,
National Infection Service
Public Health England,
Cambridge University Hospitals NHS
Foundation Trust,
Cambridge, UK
*Chapter 12 Chemotherapy of infections,
Chapter 13 Antibacterial drugs, Chapter
14 Chemotherapy of bacterial infections*

Contributors

Wendy N. Erber MBBS MD DPhil FRCPath FRCPA FAHMS
Pro Vice-Chancellor & Executive Dean and Professor of Pathology and Laboratory Medicine,
Faculty of Health and Medical Sciences,
University of Western Australia,
Perth, Australia
Chapter 30 Red blood cell disorders

Mark Evans MD FRCP
University Lecturer,
University of Cambridge;
Honorary Consultant Physician,
Wellcome Trust/MRC Institute of Metabolic Science,
Cambridge University Hospitals Foundation Trust,
Cambridge, UK
Chapter 36 Diabetes mellitus, insulin, oral antidiabetes agents, obesity

Mark Farrington MA MB BChir FRCPath
Consultant Medical Microbiologist,
National Infection Service, Public Health England,
Cambridge University Hospitals NHS Foundation Trust,
Cambridge, UK
Chapter 12 Chemotherapy of infections, Chapter 13 Antibacterial drugs, Chapter 14 Chemotherapy of bacterial infections

Andrew Grace MB PhD FRCP FACC FESC FAHA
Research Group Head,
Department of Biochemistry,
University of Cambridge;
Consultant Cardiologist,
Cambridge University Health Partners,
Cambridge, UK
Chapter 25 Cardiac arrhythmia

Thomas K. K. Ha MD FRACP FRCP
Consultant Dermatologist,
Cambridge University Hospitals NHS Foundation Trust,
Cambridge, UK
Chapter 17 Drugs and the skin

Charlotte Hateley MBBS MRes MRCP (UK) DTM&H
ST3 Gastroenterology and Hepatology Registrar,
Imperial College Healthcare NHS Trust,
London, UK
Chapter 32 Oesophagus, stomach and duodenum, Chapter 33 Intestines

Stephen Haydock PhD FRCP
Consultant Physician,
Musgrove Park Hospital,
Taunton, UK
Chapter 10 Poisoning, overdose, antidotes, Chapter 11 Drug dependence

Thomas F. Hiemstra PhD FRCPE
University Lecturer in Trials,
University of Cambridge;
Honorary Consultant Nephrologist,
Cambridge University Hospitals NHS Foundation Trust,
Cambridge, UK
Chapter 27 Kidney and genitourinary tract

Ian Hudson BSc MBBS MD DCH DipPharmMed FFPM FRCP
Chief Executive,
Medicines and Healthcare Products Regulatory Agency
Chapter 4 Evaluation of drugs in humans, Chapter 6 Regulation of medicines

Lucinda Kennard BSc MBBS MRCP (UK) AFHEA
Specialist Registrar in Clinical Pharmacology & Allergy,
Cambridge University Hospitals NHS Foundation Trust,
Cambridge, UK
Chapter 28 Respiratory system

Mike Laffan DM FRCP FRCPath
Professor of Haemostasis and Thrombosis,
Centre for Haematology,
Imperial College,
London, UK
Chapter 29 Drugs and haemostasis

Michael C. Lee MBBS FRCA PhD FFPMRCA
Consultant and University Lecturer,
Department of Medicine,
Division of Anaesthesia,
University of Cambridge,
Cambridge, UK
Chapter 18 Pain and analgesics

Keith MacDonald MSc BSc (Hons) DipRadPharmSci FRPharmS
Deputy Director, Licensing Division,
Medicines and Healthcare Products Regulatory Agency, London, UK
Chapter 6 Regulation of medicines

Justin C. Mason PhD FRCP
Professor of Vascular Rheumatology,
Imperial College,
London, UK
Chapter 16 Drugs for inflammation and joint disease

Karim Meeran MD FRCP FRCPath
Professor of Endocrinology,
Faculty of Medicine,
Imperial College,
London, UK
Chapter 38 Hypothalamic, pituitary and sex hormones

Jerry P. Nolan FRCA FRCP FFICM FRCEM (Hon)
Honorary Professor of Resuscitation Medicine,
School of Clinical Sciences,
University of Bristol;
Consultant in Anaesthesia & Intensive Care Medicine,
Royal United Hospital,
Bath, UK
Chapter 19 Anaesthesia and neuromuscular block

David Nutt DM FRCP FRCPsych FMedSci
The Edmond J Safra Chair in Neuropsychopharmacology,
Imperial College,
London, UK
Chapter 20 Psychotropic drugs

Sir Munir Pirmohamed MB ChB (Hons) PhD FRCP FRCP(E) FBPhS FMedSci
David Weatherall Chair of Medicine and NHS Chair of Pharmacogenetics,
University of Liverpool;
Associate Executive Pro-Vice Chancellor for Clinical Research,
University of Liverpool;
Director,
MRC Centre for Drug Safety Science and Wolfson Centre for Personalised Medicine,
Liverpool, UK
Chapter 8 General pharmacology

June Raine BM BCh MSc FRCP
Director,
Vigilance and Risk Management of Medicines,
Medicines and Healthcare Products, Regulatory Agency,
London, UK
Chapter 4 Evaluation of drugs in humans, Chapter 6 Regulation of medicines

Sir Michael Rawlins GBE MD FRCP FMedSci
Chair,
Medicines and Healthcare Products Regulatory Agency (MHRA),
London, UK
Chapter 5 Health technology assessment

John P. D. Reckless DSc, MD, FRCP
Honorary Reader,
University of Bath,
Bath, UK
Chapter 26 Hyperlipidaemias

Mike Schachter MB BSc FRCP
Principal Teaching Fellow in Clinical Pharmacology,
Imperial College,
London, UK
*Chapter 1 Clinical pharmacology,
Chapter 2 Topics in drug therapy,
Chapter 8 General pharmacology,
Chapter 9 Unwanted effects and adverse drug reactions*

Surender K. Sharma MD PhD
Chief,
Division of Pulmonary,
Critical Care and Sleep Medicine;
Head,
Department of Medicine;
All India Institute of Medical Sciences,
New Delhi, India
Chapter 14 Chemotherapy of bacterial infections

M. Hasib Sidiqi MBBS FRACP FRCPA
Advance Hematology Fellow,
Mayo Clinic Rochester, MN, USA;
Clinical Lecturer,
University of Western Australia,
Perth, Australia
Chapter 30 Red blood cell disorders

Rahat Tauni BSc MBBS (Hons) MRCP CertMedEd
Specialist Registrar,
Diabetes and Endocrinology,
Cambridge University Hospitals NHS Foundation Trust,
Cambridge, UK
Chapter 36 Diabetes mellitus, insulin, oral antidiabetes agents, obesity

Clare Thornton PhD MRCP (Rheum)
Consultant Rheumatologist,
Homerton University Hospital,
London, UK
Chapter 16 Drugs for inflammation and joint disease

Patrick Vallance FRCP FMedSci FRS
President Research and Development,
GlaxoSmithKline,
Brentford, UK
Chapter 3 Discovery and development of drugs

Harpreet Wasan MBBS FRCP
Consultant & Reader in Medical Oncology,
Hammersmith Hospital,
Imperial College Healthcare NHS Trust,
London, UK
Chapter 31 Neoplastic disease and immunosuppression

Acknowledgements

The present work reflects our wide reuse of material by those who wrote chapters for previous editions of this book. The editors have pleasure in acknowledging their proficiency and take this opportunity of expressing to them our grateful thanks. Those who contributed to the tenth edition are:

Dr Nigel S Baber (Chapters 4, 5, 7, 8), Professor Sir Peter Rubin (Chapter 3), Dr Francis Hall (Chapter 16), Dr Charles R J Singer (Chapter 30), Dr Pippa G Corrie and Dr Charles R J Singer (Chapter 31), Dr Michael Davis (Chapters 33, 34, 35), Dr Gerard S Conway (Chapter 38).

MJB, PS, FAM, PNB

Section | 1 |

General

Chapter | 1 |

Clinical pharmacology

Mike Schachter

SYNOPSIS

Clinical pharmacology comprises all aspects of the scientific study of drugs in humans. Its objective is to optimise drug therapy and it is justified in so far as it is put to practical use.

The use of drugs[1] to increase human happiness by elimination or suppression of diseases and symptoms and to improve the quality of life in other ways is a serious matter and involves not only technical, but also psychosocial considerations. Overall, the major benefits of modern drugs are on *quality* of life (measured with difficulty), and exceed those on *quantity* of life (measured with ease).[2] In some situations we can attempt both objectives.

Medicines are part of our way of life from birth, when we may enter the world with the aid of drugs, to death, where drugs assist (most of) us to

depart with minimal distress and perhaps even with a remnant of dignity. In between these events we regulate our fertility, often, with drugs. We tend to take such usages for granted.

But during the intervals remaining, an average family experiences illness on 1 day in 4 and between the ages of 20 and 45 years a lower-middle-class man experiences approximately one life-endangering illness, 20 disabling (temporarily) illnesses, 200 non-disabling illnesses and 1000 symptomatic episodes: the average person in the USA can expect to have about 12 years of bad health in an average lifespan,[3] and medicines play a major role: 'At any time, 40–50% of adults [UK] are taking a prescribed medicine.'[4]

Over the centuries humans have sought relief from discomfort in 'remedies' concocted from parts of plants, animals and other sources; numerous formularies attest to their numbers and complexity. Gradually, a more critical view emerged, recognising the need for proper investigation of medications. In 1690, John Locke[5] was moved to write, 'we should be able to tell beforehand that rhubarb will purge, hemlock kill, and opium make a man sleep ...'.

Yet it was only in the early years of the 20th century that we began to see the use of specific chemical substances to achieve particular

---

[1]A World Health Organization scientific group has defined a drug as 'any substance or product that is used or intended to be used to modify or explore physiological systems or pathological states for the benefit of the recipient' (WHO 1966 Technical Report Series no. 341:7). A less restrictive definition is 'a substance that changes a biological system by interacting with it'. (Laurence DR, Carpenter J 1998 A dictionary of pharmacology and allied topics. Elsevier, Amsterdam, p 106)

A *drug* is a single chemical substance that forms the active ingredient of a *medicine* (a substance or mixture of substances used in restoring or preserving health). A medicine may contain many other substances to deliver the drug in a stable form, acceptable and convenient to the patient. The terms will be used more or less interchangeably in this book. To use the word 'drug' intending only a harmful, dangerous or addictive substance is to abuse a respectable and useful word.

[2]Consider, for example, the worldwide total of suffering relieved and prevented *each day* by anaesthetics (local and general) and by analgesics, not forgetting dentistry which, because of these drugs, no longer strikes terror into even the most stoical as it has done for centuries.

---

[3]Quoted in: USA Public Health Service 1995.

[4]George C F 1994 Prescribers' Journal 34:7. A moment's reflection will bring home to us that this is an astounding statistic which goes a long way to account for the aggressive promotional activities of the highly competitive international pharmaceutical industry; the markets for medicines are colossal.

[5]Locke J 1690 An Essay Concerning Human Understanding. Clarendon Press, Oxford, book iv, chapter iii, p. 556. The English philosopher John Locke (1632–1704) argued that all human knowledge came only from experience and sensations.

biological effects; that is, the exact science of drug action, which is pharmacology. Subsequently the discipline underwent a major expansion resulting from technology that allowed the understanding of molecular action and the capacity to exploit this. The potential consequences for drug therapy are enormous. All cellular mechanisms (normal and pathological), in their immense complexity, are, in principle, identifiable. What seems almost an infinite number of substances, transmitters, local hormones, cell growth factors, can be made, modified and tested to provide agonists, partial agonists, inverse agonists and antagonists. Moreover, the unravelling of the human genome opens the way for interference with disease processes in ways that were never thought possible before now.

Increasingly large numbers of substances will deserve to be investigated and used for altering physiology to the advantage of humans. With all these developments, and their potential for good, comes capacity for harm, whether inherent in the substances themselves or resulting from human misapplication. Successful use of the power conferred (by biotechnology in particular) requires understanding of the growing evidence base of *the true consequences of interference*. The temporary celebrity of new drugs is not a new phenomenon. Jean Nicholas Corvisart[6] (1755–1821) reputedly expressed the issue in the dictum: 'Here is a new remedy; take it fast, as long as it still works'.

Clinical pharmacology provides the scientific basis for:
- the general aspects of rational, safe and effective drug therapy
- drug therapy of individual diseases
- the safe introduction of new medicines.

The drug and information explosion of the past six decades, combined with medical need, has called into being a new discipline, clinical pharmacology.[7] The discipline finds recognition as both a health-care and an academic specialty; indeed, no medical school can be considered complete without a department or sub-department of clinical pharmacology.

A signal pioneer was Harry Gold[8] (1899–1972), of Cornell University, USA, whose influential studies in the 1930s showed the qualities needed to be a clinical pharmacologist. In 1952, he wrote in a seminal article:

> *a special kind of investigator is required, one whose training has equipped him not only with the principles and technics of laboratory pharmacology but also with knowledge of clinical medicine …*
>
> *Clinical scientists of all kinds do not differ fundamentally from other biologists; they are set apart only to the extent that there are special difficulties and limitations, ethical and practical, in seeking knowledge from man.*[9]

Willingness to learn the principles of pharmacology, and how to apply them in individual circumstances of infinite variety is vital to success without harm: to maximise benefit and minimise risk. All of these issues are the concern of clinical pharmacology and are the subject of this book.

More detailed aspects comprise:

1. Pharmacology
   - *Pharmacodynamics*: how drugs, alone and in combination, affect the body (young, old, well, sick).
   - *Pharmacokinetics*: absorption, distribution, metabolism, excretion or how the body – well or sick – affects drugs.
2. Therapeutic evaluation
   - Whether a drug is of value.
   - How it may best be used.
   - Formal therapeutic trials.

---

[6]He was Emperor Napoleon's favourite physician.

[7]The term was first used by Paul Martini (1889–1964). He addressed issues that are now integral parts of clinical trials, including the use of placebo, control groups, sample size, relationship between dose and response and probability of efficacy. His monograph *Methodology of Therapeutic Investigation* (Springer, Berlin, 1932), was published in German and went largely unnoticed by English speakers (Shelly J H, Baur M P 1999 Paul Martini: the first clinical pharmacologist? Lancet 353:1870–1873).

[8]Gold H 1952 The proper study of mankind is man. American Journal of Medicine 12:619. The title is taken from *An Essay on Man* by Alexander Pope (English poet, 1688–1744), which begins with the lines: 'Know then thyself, presume not God to scan,/The proper study of mankind is man'. Indeed, the whole passage is worth appraisal, for it reads as if it were relevant to modern clinical pharmacology and drug therapy.

[9]Self-experimentation has always been a feature of clinical pharmacology. A survey of 250 members of the Dutch Society of Clinical Pharmacology evoked 102 responders of whom 55 had carried out experiments on themselves (largely for convenience) (van Everdingen J J, Cohen A F 1990 Self-experimentation by doctors. Lancet 336:1448). A spectacular example occurred at the 1983 meeting of the American Urological Association at Las Vegas, USA, during a lecture on pharmacologically induced penile erection, when the lecturer stepped out from behind the lectern to demonstrate personally the efficacy of the technique (Zorgniotti A W 1990 Self-experimentation. Lancet 36:1200).

- Surveillance studies for both efficacy and safety (adverse effects) – pharmacoepidemiology and pharmacovigilance.
3. Control
   - Rational prescribing and formularies.
   - Official regulation of medicines.
   - Social aspects of the use and misuse of medicines.
   - Pharmacoeconomics.

Clinical pharmacology finds expression in concert with other clinical specialties. Therapeutic success with drugs is becoming more and more dependent on the user having at least an outline understanding of both pharmacodynamics and pharmacokinetics. This outline is quite simple and easy to acquire. However humane and caring doctors may be, they cannot dispense with scientific skill. Knowledge of clinical pharmacology underpins decisions in therapeutics, which is concerned with the prevention, suppression or cure of disease and, from the point of view of society, is the most vital aspect of medicine.

Pharmacology is the same science whether it investigates animals or humans. The need for it grows rapidly as not only scientists, but now the whole community, can see its promise of release from distress and premature death over yet wider fields. The concomitant dangers of drugs (fetal deformities, adverse reactions, dependence) only add to the need for the systematic and ethical application of science to drug development, evaluation and use, i.e. clinical pharmacology.

Guide to further reading

Baber, N.S., Ritter, J.M., Aronson, J.K., 2004. Medicines regulation and clinical pharmacology. Br. J. Clin. Pharmacol. 58 (6), 569–570 (and other articles in this issue).

Dollery, C.T., 2006. Clinical pharmacology – the first 75 years and a view of the future. Br. J. Clin. Pharmacol. 61, 650–665.

FitzGerald, G.A., 2007. Clinical pharmacology or translational medicine and therapeutics: reinvent or rebrand and expand? Clin. Pharmacol. Ther. 81 (1), 19–20.

Honig, P., 2007. The value and future of clinical pharmacology. Clin. Pharmacol. Ther. 81 (1), 17–18.

Laurence, D.R., 1989. Ethics and law in clinical pharmacology. Br. J. Clin. Pharmacol. 27, 715–722.

Rawlins, M.D., 2005. Pharmacopolitics and deliberative democracy. Clin. Med. (Northfield Il) 5, 471–475.

Rawlins, M.D., 2015. National Institute for Clinical Excellence: NICE works. J. R. Soc. Med. 108 (6), 211–219.

Reidenberg, M.M., 2008. A new look at the profession of clinical pharmacology. Clin. Pharmacol. Ther. 83 (2), 213–217 (and other articles in this issue).

Report. Pricewaterhouse Cooper 2016 Clinical Pharmacology and Therapeutics. The case for savings in the NHS 168:1–25.

Waldman, S.A., Christensen, N.B., Moore, J.E., Terzic, A., 2007. Clinical pharmacology: the science of therapeutics. Clin. Pharmacol. Ther. 81 (1), 3–6.

Chapter | 2 |

Topics in drug therapy

Mike Schachter

SYNOPSIS

Drug therapy involves considerations beyond the strictly scientific pharmacological aspects of medicines. These include numerous issues relating to prescribers and to patients:

- **The therapeutic situation.**
- **Treating patients with drugs.**
- **Iatrogenic disease.**
- **Benefits and risks.**
- **Public view of drugs and prescribers.**
- **Criticisms of modern drugs.**
- **Drug-induced injury.**
- **Complementary and alternative medicine.**
- **Placebo medicines.**
- **Guidelines, 'essential' drugs and prescribing.**
- **Compliance – patient and doctor.**
- **Pharmacoeconomics.**

The therapeutic situation

Some background

Alleviating effects of disease and trauma has been a major concern of human beings from the earliest times. Records of the ancient civilisations of Mesopotamia (modern Iraq), India, China, Mexico and Egypt, from about 3000 BC, describe practices of diagnosis and treatment predicated on differing, often complex, concepts of disease: the supernatural, religious theories (sin, punishment of sin, uncleanness), omens, deities and rites. Among many modes of therapy, a reliance on diet and use of herbs figured prominently (the Mexicans knew of 1200 medicinal plants).

From about 500 BC, the Greek system of humoural medicine began to replace the supernatural with thinking that was rational, scientific and naturalistic. Its core concept was that health was an equilibrium, and disease a disequilibrium, of the four constituent fluids or 'humours' of the body (yellow bile, phlegm, blood and black bile). It followed that the condition was correctable by evacuation techniques to re-establish the balance, and hence came blooding, leeching, cathartics, sweating and emetics. Here, the focus was on the *patient*, as the degree of humoural imbalance was specific to that individual.

Remarkably, this system persisted among 'learned and rational' (i.e. university-trained) physicians until it was challenged in the 17th century. Thomas Sydenham[1] (1624–1689) showed that during epidemics, many people could suffer the same disease, and different epidemics had distinct characteristics. Later, Giovanni Morgagni (1682–1771), by correlating clinical and autopsy findings, demonstrated that diseases related to particular organs. Now the study of *disease*, rather than the patient, became the centre of attention. Yet it was only in the 19th century that medicine developed as a science, when the microscope revealed the cell as the basic construction unit of the body and specific entities of pathology became recognisable, most notably in the case of infection with microorganisms ('germ theory').

The one major dimension of medicine that remained underdeveloped was therapeutics. An abundance of preparations in pharmacopoeias compared with a scarcity of genuinely effective therapies contributed to a state of 'therapeutic nihilism', expressed trenchantly by Oliver Wendell Holmes (1809–1894):

> *'Throw out opium …; throw out a few specifics …; throw out wine, which is a food, and the vapours*

---

[1] His work had such a profound influence on medicine that he was called the 'English Hippocrates'.

*which produce the miracle of anaesthesia, and I firmly
believe that if the whole materia medica, as now used,
could be sunk to the bottom of the sea, it would be all
the better for mankind, – and all the worse for the
fishes…'[2]*

The writer was exaggerating to emphasise his point, but
the position was to change throughout the 20th century as
understanding of human physiology and pathophysiology
deepened and agents that could be relied on to interfere
with these processes became available. Modern physicians
have at their disposal an array of medicines that empowers
them to intervene beneficially in disease but also carries
new responsibilities.

> Drug therapy involves a great deal more than matching
> the name of the drug to the name of a disease; it
> requires knowledge, judgement, skill and wisdom, but
> above all a sense of responsibility.

Treating patients with drugs

A book can provide knowledge and contribute to the formation of judgement, but it can do little to impart skill and
wisdom, which are the products of example of teachers and
colleagues, of experience and of innate and acquired capaci-
ties. But: 'It is evident that patients are not treated in a
vacuum and that they respond to a variety of subtle forces
around them in addition to the specific therapeutic agent.'[3]

When a patient receives a drug, the response can be the
result of numerous factors:

- The pharmacodynamic effect of the drug and
  interactions with any other drugs the patient may be
  taking.
- The pharmacokinetics of the drug and its
  modification in the individual by genetic influences,
  disease, other drugs.
- The act of medication, including the route of
  administration and the presence or absence of the
  doctor.
- What the doctor has told the patient.
- The patient's past experience of doctors.
- The patient's estimate of what has been received and
  of what ought to happen as a result.

---

[2]Medical Essays (1891). American physician and poet, and Dean of
Harvard Medical School; he introduced the term 'anaesthesia' instead
of 'suspended animation' or 'etherisation'. Address delivered before
the Massachusetts Medical Society, 30 May 1860 (Oliver Wendell
Holmes, Medical Essays. Kessinger Publishing, p. 140).
[3]Sherman L J 1959 The significant variables in psychopharmaceutic
research. American Journal of Psychiatry 116:208–214.

- The social environment, e.g. whether it is supportive
  or dispiriting.

The relative importance of these factors varies according
to circumstances. An unconscious patient with meningococcal
meningitis does not have a personal relationship with the
doctor, but patients sleepless with anxiety because they
cannot cope with their family responsibilities may respond
as much to the interaction of their own personality with
that of the doctor as to anxiolytics.

The physician may consciously use all of the factors listed
above in therapeutic practice. But it is still not enough that
patients get better: it is essential to know why they do so.
This is because potent drugs should be given only if their
pharmacodynamic effects are needed; many adverse reactions
have been shown to be due to drugs that are not needed,
including some severe enough to cause hospital admission.

Drugs can do good

Medically, this good may sometimes seem trivial, as in the
avoidance of a sleepless night in a noisy hotel or of social
embarrassment from a profusely running nose due to
seasonal pollen allergy (hay fever). Such benefits are not
necessarily trivial to recipients, concerned to be at their best
in important matters, whether of business, pleasure or
passion, i.e. with quality of life.

Or the good may be literally life-saving, as in serious
acute infections (pneumonia, septicaemia) or in the prevention of life-devastating disability from severe asthma, from
epilepsy or from blindness due to glaucoma.

Drugs can do harm

This harm may be relatively trivial, as in hangover from a
hypnotic or transient headache from glyceryl trinitrate used
for angina.

The harm may be life-destroying, as in the rare sudden
death following an injection of penicillin, rightly regarded
as one of the safest of antibiotics, or the destruction of the
quality of life that occasionally attends the use of drugs that
are effective in rheumatoid arthritis (adrenocortical steroids,
penicillamine) and Parkinson's disease (levodopa).

There are risks in taking medicines, just as there are risks
in food and transport. There are also risks in declining to
take medicines when they are needed, just as there are risks
in refusing food or transport when they are needed.

Efficacy and safety do not lie solely in the molecular
structure of the drug. Doctors must choose which drugs to
use and must apply them correctly in relation not only to
their properties, but also to those of the patients and their
disease. Then patients must use the prescribed medicine
correctly (see Compliance, p. 19).

Uses of drugs/medicines

> Drugs are used in three principal ways:
> - To cure disease: primary and auxiliary.
> - To suppress disease.
> - To prevent disease (prophylaxis): primary and secondary.

Cure implies *primary* therapy, as in bacterial and parasitic infections, that eliminates the disease and the drug is withdrawn; or *auxiliary* therapy, as with anaesthetics and with ergometrine and oxytocin in obstetrics.

Suppression of diseases or symptoms is used continuously or intermittently to avoid the effects of disease without attaining cure (as in hypertension, diabetes mellitus, epilepsy, asthma), or to control symptoms (such as pain and cough) while awaiting recovery from the causative disease.

Prevention (prophylaxis). In *primary prevention*, the person does not have the condition and avoids getting it. For malaria, vaccinations and contraception, the decision to treat healthy people is generally easy.

In *secondary prevention*, the patient has the disease and the objective is to reduce risk factors, so as to retard progression or avoid repetition of an event, e.g. aspirin and lipid-lowering drugs in atherosclerosis and after myocardial infarction, antihypertensives to prevent recurrence of stroke.

Taking account of the above, a doctor might ask the following questions before treating a patient with drugs:

1. Should I interfere with the patient at all?
2. If so, what alteration in the patient's condition do I hope to achieve?
3. Which drug is most likely to bring this about?
4. How can I administer the drug to attain the right concentration in the right place at the right time and for the right duration?
5. How will I know when I have achieved the objective?
6. What other effects might the drug produce, and are these harmful?
7. How will I decide to stop the drug?
8. Does the likelihood of benefit, and its importance, outweigh the likelihood of damage, and its importance (i.e. the benefit versus risk, or efficacy against safety)?

Physician-induced (iatrogenic) disease

They used to have a more equitable contract in Egypt: for the first three days the doctor took on the patient at the patient's risk and peril: when the three days were up, the risks and perils were the doctor's.

But doctors are lucky: the sun shines on their successes and the earth hides their failures.[4]

It is a salutary thought that each year medical errors kill an estimated 44 000–98 000 Americans (more than die in motor vehicle accidents) and injure 1 000 000.[5] Among inpatients in the USA and Australia, about one-half of the injuries caused by medical mismanagement result from surgery, but therapeutic mishaps and diagnostic errors are the next most common. In one survey of adverse drug events, 1% were fatal, 12% life-threatening, 30% serious and 57% significant.[6] About one-half of the life-threatening and serious events were preventable. Errors of prescribing account for one-half and those of administering drugs for one-quarter of these. Inevitably, a proportion of lapses result in litigation, and in the UK 20–25% of complaints received by the medical defence organisations about general practitioners follow medication errors.

The most shameful act in therapeutics, apart from actually killing a patient, is to injure a patient who is but little disabled or who is suffering from a self-limiting disorder. Such iatrogenic disease,[7] induced by misguided treatment, is far from rare.

Doctors who are temperamentally extremist will do less harm by therapeutic nihilism than by optimistically overwhelming patients with well-intentioned polypharmacy. If in doubt whether or not to give a drug to a person who will soon get better without it, *don't*.

In 1917 the famous pharmacologist Sollmann felt able to write:

> *Pharmacology comprises some broad conceptions and generalisations, and some detailed conclusions, of such great and practical importance that every student and practitioner should be absolutely familiar with them. It comprises also a large mass of minute details, which would constitute too great a tax on human memory, but which cannot safely be neglected.*[8]

The doctor's aim must be not merely to give the patient what will do good, but to give only what will do good – or

---

[4]Michel de Montaigne (1533–1592). French essayist.
[5]Kohn L, Corrigan J, Donaldson M (eds) for the Committee on Quality of Health Care in America, Institute of Medicine 2000 To Err is Human: Building a Safer Health System. National Academy Press, Washington, DC.
[6]Bates D W, Cullen D J, Laird N et al 1995 Incidence of adverse drug events and potential adverse drug events. Journal of the American Medical Association 274:29–34.
[7]Iatrogenic means 'physician-caused', i.e. disease consequent on following medical advice or intervention (from the Greek *iatros*, physician).
[8]Sollman T A 1917 Manual of Pharmacology. Saunders, Philadelphia.

at least more good than harm. The information explosion of recent decades is now under better control such that prescribers can, from their desktop computer terminals, enter the facts about their patient (age, sex, weight, principal and secondary diagnoses) and receive suggestions for which drugs should be considered, with proposed doses and precautions.

Benefits and risks of medicines

Modern technological medicine has been criticised, justly, for following the tradition of centuries by waiting for disease to occur and then trying to cure it rather than seeking to prevent it in the first place. Although many diseases are partly or wholly preventable by economic, social and behavioural means, these are too seldom adopted and are slow to take effect. In the meantime, people continue to fall sick, and to need and deserve treatment.

We all have eventually to die from something and, even after excessive practising of all the advice on how to live a healthy life, the likelihood that the mode of death for most of us will be free from pain, anxiety, cough, diarrhoea or paralysis (the list is endless) seems so small that it can be disregarded. Drugs already provide immeasurable solace in these situations, and the development of better drugs should be encouraged.

Doctors know the sick are thankful for drugs, just as even the most dedicated pedestrians and environmentalists struck down by a passing car are thankful for a motor ambulance to take them to hospital. The reader will find reference to the benefits of drugs in individual diseases throughout this book, and further expansion is unnecessary here. But a general discussion of the risk of adverse events is appropriate.

Unavoidable risks

Consider, for the sake of argument, the features that a completely risk-free drug would exhibit:

- The physician would know exactly what action is required and use the drug correctly.
- The drug would deliver its desired action and nothing else, either by true biological selectivity or by selective targeted delivery.
- The drug would achieve exactly the right amount of action – neither too little nor too much.

These criteria may be *completely* fulfilled, for example in a streptococcal infection sensitive to penicillin in patients whose genetic constitution does not render them liable to an allergic reaction to penicillin.

These criteria are *partially* fulfilled in insulin-deficient diabetes. But the natural modulation of insulin secretion in response to need (food, exercise) does not operate with injected insulin, and even sophisticated technology cannot yet exactly mimic the normal physiological responses. The criteria are still further from realisation, for example in some cancers and schizophrenia.

Some reasons why drugs fail to meet the criteria of being risk-free include the following:

- *Drugs may be insufficiently selective*. As the concentration rises, a drug that acts at only one site at low concentrations begins to affect other target sites (receptors, enzymes) and recruit new (unwanted) actions; or a disease process (cancer) is so close to normal cellular mechanisms that perfectly selective cell kill is impossible.
- *Drugs may be highly selective* for one pathway, but the mechanism affected has widespread functions, and interference with it cannot be limited to one site only, e.g. atenolol on the β-adrenoceptor, aspirin on cyclo-oxygenase.
- *Prolonged modification* of cellular mechanisms can lead to permanent change in structure and function, e.g. carcinogenicity.
- *Insufficient knowledge of disease processes* (some cardiac arrhythmias) and of drug action can lead to interventions that, although undertaken with the best intentions, are harmful.
- *Patients are genetically heterogeneous* to a high degree and may have unpredicted responses to drugs.
- *Dosage adjustment* according to need is often unavoidably imprecise, e.g. in depression.
- *Prescribing 'without due care and attention'*.[9]

Reduction of risk

Strategies that can limit risk include those directed at achieving:

- *Better knowledge of disease* (research) – as much as 40% of useful medical advances derive from basic research that was not funded towards a specific practical outcome.
- *Site-specific effect* – by molecular manipulation.
- *Site-specific delivery* – drug targeting:
  - by topical (local) application.
  - by target-selective carriers.
- Informed, careful and responsible prescribing.

Two broad categories of risk

1. *First are those that we accept by deliberate choice*. We do so even if we do not exactly know their magnitude, or

---

[9]This phrase is commonly used in the context of motor vehicle accidents, but applies equally well to the prescribing of drugs.

we know but wish they were smaller, or, especially when the likelihood of harm is sufficiently remote though the consequences may be grave, we do not even think about the matter. Such risks include transport and sports, both of which are inescapably subject to potent physical laws such as gravity and momentum, and surgery to rectify disorders that we could tolerate or treat in other ways, as with much cosmetic surgery.

2. *Second are those risks that cannot be significantly altered by individual action.* We experience risks imposed by food additives (preservatives, colouring), air pollution and some environmental radioactivity. But there are also risks imposed by nature, such as skin cancer due to excess ultraviolet radiation in sunny climes, as well as some radioactivity.

It seems an obvious course to avoid unnecessary risks, but there is disagreement on what risks are truly unnecessary and, on looking closely at the matter, it is plain that many people habitually take risks in their daily and recreational life that it would be a misuse of words to describe as necessary. Furthermore, some risks, although known to exist, are, in practice, ignored other than by conforming to ordinary prudent conduct. These risks are negligible in the sense that they do not influence behaviour, i.e. they are neglected.[10]

Elements of risk

Risk has two elements:
- The likelihood or probability of an adverse event.
- Its severity.

In medical practice in general, concern ceases when risks fall below about 1 in 100 000 instances, when the procedure then is regarded as 'safe'. In such cases, when disaster occurs, it can be difficult indeed for individuals to accept that they 'deliberately' accepted a risk; they feel 'it should not have happened to me', and in their distress they may seek to lay blame on others where there is no fault or negligence, only misfortune (see Warnings and consent).

The benefits of chemicals used to colour food verge on or even attain negligibility. Although some cause allergy in humans, our society permits their use.

There is general agreement that drugs prescribed for disease are themselves the cause of a significant amount of disease (adverse reactions), of death, of permanent disability, of recoverable illness and of minor inconvenience. In one major UK study the prevalence of adverse drug reactions as a cause of admission to hospital was 6.5% (see Chapter 9 for other examples).

Three major grades of risk

These are: *unacceptable, acceptable* and *negligible*. Where disease is life-threatening and there is reliable information on both the disease and the drug, then decisions, though they may be painful, present relatively obvious problems. But where the disease risk is remote, e.g. mild hypertension, or where drugs are to be used to increase comfort or to suppress symptoms that are, in fact, bearable, or for convenience rather than for need, then the issues of risk acceptance are less obvious.

Risks should not be weighed without reference to benefits any more than benefits should be weighed without reference to risks.

Risks are among the facts of life. In whatever we do and in whatever we refrain from doing, we are accepting risk. Some risks are obvious, some are unsuspected and some we conceal from ourselves. But risks are universally accepted, whether willingly or unwillingly, whether consciously or not.[11]

Whenever a drug is taken a risk is taken

The risk comprises the properties of the drug, the prescriber, the patient and the environment; it is often so small that second thoughts are hardly necessary, but sometimes it is substantial. The doctor must weigh the likelihood of gain for the patient against the likelihood of loss. There are often insufficient data for a rational decision to be reached, but a decision must yet be made, and this is one of the greatest difficulties of clinical practice. Its effect on the attitudes of doctors is often not appreciated by those who have never been in this situation. The patient's protection lies in the doctor's knowledge of the drug and of the disease, and experience of both, together with knowledge of the patient.

We continue to use drugs that are capable of killing or disabling patients at doses within the therapeutic range where the judgement of overall balance of benefit and risk is favourable. This can be very difficult for the patient who has suffered a rare severe adverse reaction to understand and to accept (see below).

In some chronic diseases that ultimately necessitate suppressive drugs, the patient may not experience benefit in the early stages. Patients with early Parkinson's disease may experience little inconvenience or hazard from the condition, and premature exposure to drugs can exact such a price in

---

[10]Sometimes the term 'minimal risk' is used to mean risk about equal to going about our ordinary daily lives; it includes travel on public transport, but not motor bicycling on a motorway.

[11]Pochin E 1975 The acceptance of risk. British Medical Bulletin 31:184–190.

unwanted effects that they prefer the untreated state. What patients will tolerate depends on their personality, their attitude to disease, their occupation, mode of life and relationship with their doctor (see Compliance, p. 19).

Public view of drugs and prescribers

The current public view of modern medicines, ably fuelled by the mass media, is a compound of vague expectation of 'miracle' cures and 'breakthroughs' (often with the complicity of doctors) with outrage when anything goes wrong. It is also unreasonable to expect the public to trust the medical profession (in collaboration with the pharmaceutical industry) to the extent of leaving to them all drug matters, and of course this is not the case.

The public wants benefits without risks and without having to alter their unhealthy ways of living; a deeply irrational position, but then humans are not perfectly rational. It is easy to understand that a person who has taken into his or her body a chemical with intent to relieve suffering, whether or not it is self-induced, can feel profound anger when harm ensues.

Expectations have been raised, and now, at the beginning of the 21st century, with the manifest achievements of technology all around us, the naïve expectation that happiness can be a part of the technological package is increasingly seen to be unrealisable.

Patients are aware that there is justifiable criticism of the standards of medical prescribing – indeed doctors are in the forefront of this – as well as justifiable criticism of promotional practices of the profitably rich, aggressive, transnational pharmaceutical industry.

There are obvious areas where some remedial action is possible:

- *Improvement of prescribing* by doctors, including better communication with patients, i.e. doctors must learn to feel that introduction of foreign chemicals into their patients' bodies is a serious matter, which many or most do not seem to at present.[12]
- Introduction of *no-fault compensation schemes* for serious drug injury (some countries already have these).

---

[12]Doctors who seek to exculpate themselves from serious, even fatal, prescribing errors by appealing to undoubted difficulties presented by the information explosion of modern times, allied to pressures of work, are unlikely to get sympathy, and increasingly are more likely to be told, 'If you can't stand the heat, get out of the kitchen' (a dictum attributed to Harry S Truman, US President 1948–1952, though he assigns it to US Army General Harry Vaughn). Pharmacists and nurses stand ready and willing to relieve doctors of the burden of prescribing.

- *Informed* public discussion of the issues between the medical profession, industrial drug developers, politicians and other 'opinion-formers' in society, and patients (the public).
- *Restraint* in promotion *by the pharmaceutical industry* including self-control by both industry and doctors in their necessarily close relationship, which the public is inclined to regard as a conspiracy, especially when the gifts and payments made to doctors get into the news. (This is much less prevalent than it was in the 1990s.)

If restraint by both parties is not forthcoming, and it may not be, then both doctor and industry can expect even more control to be exercised over them by politicians responding to public demand. If doctors do not want their prescribing to be restricted, they should prescribe better.

Criticisms of modern drugs

Extremist critics have attracted public attention for their view that modern drug therapy, indeed modern medicine in general, does more harm than good; others, while admitting some benefits from drugs, insist that this is medically marginal. These opinions rest on the undisputed fact that favourable trends in many diseases preceded the introduction of modern drugs and were due to economic and environmental changes, sanitation, nutrition and housing. They also rest on the claim that drugs have not changed *expectation of life or mortality* (as measured by national mortality statistics), or at least it is very difficult to show that they have, and that drugs indisputably can cause illness (adverse reactions).

If something is to be measured, then the correct criteria must be chosen. Overall mortality figures are an extremely crude and often an irrelevant measure of the effects of drugs whose major benefits are so often on quality of life rather than on its quantity.

Two examples of inappropriate measurements will suffice:

1. In the case of many infections, it is not disputed that environmental changes have had a greater beneficial effect on health than the subsequently introduced antimicrobials. But this does not mean that environmental improvements alone are sufficient in the fight against infections. When comparisons of illnesses in the pre- and post-antimicrobial eras are made, like is not compared with like. Environmental changes achieved their results when mortality from infections was high and antimicrobials were not available; antimicrobials were introduced later against

a background of low mortality as well as of environmental change; decades separate the two parts of the comparison, and observers, diagnostic criteria and data recording changed during this long period. It is evident that determining the value of antimicrobials is not simply a matter of looking at mortality rates.

2. About 1% of the UK population has diabetes mellitus, a figure which is increasing rapidly, and about 1% of death certificates mention diabetes. This is no surprise because all must die and insulin is no cure[13] for this lifelong disease. A standard medical textbook of 1907 stated that juvenile-onset 'diabetes is in all cases a grave disease, and the subjects are regarded by all assurance companies as uninsurable lives: life seems to hang by a thread, a thread often cut by a very trifling accident'. Most, if not all, life insurance companies now accept young people with diabetes with no or only modest financial penalty, the premium of a person 5–10 years older. Before insulin replacement therapy was available, few survived beyond 3 years[14] after diagnosis; they died for lack of insulin. It is unjustified to assert that a treatment is worthless just because its mention on death certificates (whether as a prime or as a contributory cause) has not declined. The relevant criteria for juvenile-onset diabetes are change in the age at which the subjects die and the quality of life between diagnosis and death, and both of these have changed enormously.

Drug-induced injury[15]
(see also Ch. 9)

Responsibility for drug-induced injury raises important issues affecting medical practice and development of needed new drugs, as well as of law and of social justice.

Negligence and strict and no-fault liability

All civilised legal systems provide for compensation to be paid to a person injured as a result of using a product of any kind that is defective due to negligence (fault: failure to exercise reasonable care).[16] But there is a growing opinion that special compensation for serious personal injury, beyond the modest sums that general social security systems provide, should be automatic and not dependent on fault and proof of fault of the producer, i.e. there should be 'liability irrespective of fault', 'no-fault liability' or 'strict liability'.[17] After all, victims need assistance (compensation) regardless of the cause of injury and whether or not the producer and, in the case of drugs, the prescriber deserves censure. The question why a person who has suffered injury due to the biological accident of disease should have to depend on social security payments while an identical injury due to a drug (in the absence of fault) should attract special added compensation receives no persuasive answer except that this is what society seems to want.

Many countries are now revising their laws on liability for personal injury due to manufactured products and are legislating Consumer Protection Acts (Statutes) which include medicines, for 'drugs represent the class of product in respect of which there has been the greatest pressure for surer compensation in cases of injury'.[18]

Issues that are central to the debate include:

- *Capacity to cause harm* is inherent in drugs in a way that sets them apart from other manufactured products; and harm often occurs in the absence of fault.
- *Safety*, i.e. the degree of safety that a person is entitled to expect, and adverse effects that should be accepted without complaint, must often be a matter of opinion and will vary with the disease being treated, e.g. cancer or insomnia.
- *Causation*, i.e. proof that the drug in fact caused the injury, is often impossible, particularly where it

---

[13]A cure eliminates a disease and may be withdrawn when this is achieved.
[14]Even if given the best treatment. 'Opium alone stands the test of experience as a remedy capable of limiting the progress of the disease', wrote the great Sir William Osler, successively Professor of Medicine in Pennsylvania, McGill, Johns Hopkins and Oxford universities, in 1918, only 3 years before the discovery of insulin.
[15]This discussion is about drugs that have been properly manufactured and meet proper standards, e.g. of purity, stability, as laid down by regulatory bodies or pharmacopoeias. A manufacturing defect would be dealt with in a way no different from manufacturing errors in other products.

[16]A plaintiff (person who believes he or she has been injured) seeking to obtain compensation from a defendant (via the law of negligence) must prove three things: (1) that the defendant owed a duty of care to the plaintiff; (2) that the defendant failed to exercise reasonable care; and (3) that the plaintiff has suffered an actual injury as a result.
[17]The following distinction is made in some discussions of product liability. *Strict liability*: compensation is provided by the producer/manufacturer. *No-fault liability* or scheme: compensation is provided by a central fund.
[18]Royal Commission on Civil Liability and Compensation for Personal Injury 1978. HMSO, London: Cmnd. 7054. Although the Commission considered compensation for death and personal injury suffered by any person through manufacture, supply or use of products, i.e. all goods whether natural or manufactured, and included drugs and even human blood and organs, it made no mention of tobacco and alcohol.

increases the incidence of a disease that occurs naturally.

- *Contributory negligence*. Should compensation be reduced in smokers and drinkers where there is evidence that these pleasure drugs increase liability to adverse reactions to therapeutic drugs?
- *The concept of defect*, i.e. whether the drug or the prescriber or indeed the patient can be said to be 'defective' so as to attract liability, is a highly complex matter and indeed is a curious concept as applied to medicine.

Nowhere has a scheme that meets all the major difficulties yet been implemented. This is not because there has been too little thought, it is because the subject is so difficult. Nevertheless, no-fault schemes operate in New Zealand, Scandinavia and France.[19] The following principles might form the basis of a workable compensation scheme for injury due to drugs:

- *New unlicensed drugs undergoing clinical trial in small numbers of subjects* (healthy or patient volunteers): the developer should be strictly liable for all adverse effects.
- *New unlicensed drugs undergoing extensive trials in patients who may reasonably expect benefit*: the producer should be strictly liable for any serious effect.
- *New drugs after licensing by an official body*: the manufacturer and the community should share liability for serious injury, as new drugs provide general benefit. An option might be to institute a defined period of formal prospective drug surveillance monitoring, in which both doctors and patients agree to participate.
- *Standard drugs in day-to-day therapeutics*: there should be a no-fault scheme, operated by or with the assent of government that has authority, through tribunals, to decide cases quickly and to make awards. This body would have authority to reimburse itself from others – manufacturer, supplier, prescriber – wherever that was appropriate. An award must not have to wait on the outcome of prolonged, vexatious, adversarial, expensive court proceedings. Patients would be compensated where:
    - causation was proven on 'balance of probability'[20]
    - the injury was serious
    - the event was rare and remote and not reasonably taken into account in making the decision to treat.

Complementary, alternative and traditional medicine

Practitioners of complementary and alternative medicine (CAM)[21] are severely critical of modern drugs, and use practices according to their own special beliefs. It is appropriate, therefore, to discuss such medical systems here.

The term 'complementary and alternative medicine' covers a broad range of heterogeneous systems of therapy (from acupuncture to herbalism to yoga), and diagnosis (from bioresonance to pulse and tongue diagnosis). The present discussion relates largely to CAM but recognises that traditional or indigenous medicinal therapeutics has developed since before history in all societies. This comprises a mass of practices varying from the worthless to highly effective remedies, such as digitalis (England), quinine (South America), reserpine (India) and atropine (various countries). It is the task of science to find the gems and to discard the dross,[22] and at the same time to leave intact socially valuable supportive aspects of traditional medicine.

There is no doubt that the domain of CAM has grown in popularity; a survey estimated that about 20% of the UK population had consulted a CAM practitioner in the previous year.[23] In Germany, the figure exceeds 60%, with $2.06 billion in over-the-counter sales in 2003.[24] Usage rises sharply among those with chronic, relapsing conditions such as cancer, multiple sclerosis, human immunodeficiency virus (HIV) infection, psoriasis and rheumatological diseases. It is difficult to resist the conclusion that when scientific medicine neither guarantees happiness nor wholly eliminates the disabilities of degenerative diseases in long-lived populations, and when drugs used in modern medicine cause serious harm, public

[19]Gaine W J 2003 No-fault compensation schemes. British Medical Journal 326:997–998.
[20]This is the criterion for (UK) civil law, rather than 'beyond reasonable doubt', which is the criterion of criminal law.

[21]The definition adopted by the Cochrane Collaboration is as follows: 'Complementary and alternative medicine (CAM) is a broad domain of healing resources that accompanies all health systems, modalities and practices and their accompanying theories and beliefs, other than those intrinsic to the politically dominant health system of a particular society or culture in a given historical period. CAM includes all such practices and ideas self-defined by their users as preventing or treating illness or promoting health and well-being. Boundaries within CAM and between the CAM domain and that of the dominant system are not always sharp or fixed.'
[22]Traditional medicine is fostered particularly in countries where scientific medicine is not accessible to large populations for economic reasons, and destruction of traditional medicine would leave unhappy and sick people with nothing. For this reason, governments are supporting traditional medicine and at the same time initiating scientific clinical evaluations of the numerous plants and other items employed, many of which contain biologically active substances. The World Health Organization is supportive of these programmes.
[23]Ernst E 2000 The role of complementary and alternative medicine. British Medical Journal 32:1133–1135.
[24]De Smet P A 2005 Herbal medicine in Europe – relaxing regulatory standards. New England Journal of Medicine 352:1176–1178.

disappointment naturally leads to a revival of interest in alternatives that alluringly promise efficacy with complete safety. These range from a revival of traditional medicine to adoption of the more modern cults.[25]

Features common to medical cults are: absence of scientific thinking, naïve acceptance of hypotheses, uncritical acceptance of causation, e.g. reliance on anecdote or opinion (as opposed to evidence), assumption that if recovery follows treatment it is due to the treatment, and close attention to the patient's personal feelings. Lack of understanding of how therapeutic effects may be measured is also a prominent feature. An extensive analysis of recommendations of CAM therapies for specific medical conditions from seven textbook sources revealed numerous treatments recommended for the same condition – for example, addictions (120 treatments recommended), arthritis (121), asthma (119) and cancer (133) – but there was lack of agreement between these authors as to the preferred therapies for specified conditions.[26] The question must arise that if numerous and heterogeneous treatments are effective for the same condition, could they not have some common feature, such as the ability of the practitioner to inspire confidence in the patient?

A proposition belongs to science if we can say what kind of event we would accept as refutation (and this is easy in therapeutics). A proposition (or theory) that cannot clash with any possible or even conceivable event (evidence) is outside science, and this in general applies to cults where everything is interpreted in terms of the theory of the cult;

the possibility that the basis of the cult is false is not entertained. This appears to be the case with medical cults, which join freudianism, and indeed religions, as outside science (after Karl Popper). Willingness to follow where the evidence leads is a distinctive feature of conventional scientific medicine.

> A scientific approach does not mean treating a patient as a mere biochemical machine. It does not mean the exclusion of spiritual, psychological and social dimensions of human beings. But it does mean treating these in a rational manner.

Some common false beliefs of CAM practitioners are that synthetic modern drugs are toxic, but products obtained in nature are not.[27] Scientific medicine is held to accept evidence that remedies are effective only where the mechanism is understood, that it depends on adherence to rigid and unalterable dogmas, and recognises no form of evaluation other than the strict randomised controlled trial. Traditional (pre-scientific) medicine is deemed to have special virtue, and the collection and formal analysis of data on therapeutic outcomes, failures as well as successes, is deemed inessential. There is also a tenet that if the patient gets better when treated in accordance with certain beliefs, this provides evidence for the truth of these beliefs (the *post hoc ergo propter hoc*[28] fallacy).

Exponents of CAM often state that comparative controlled trials of their medicines against conventional medicines are impracticable because the classic double-blind randomised controlled designs are inappropriate and in particular do not allow for the individual approach characteristic of

---

[25]A cult is a practice that follows a dogma, tenet or principle based on theories or beliefs of its promulgator to the exclusion of demonstrable scientific experience (definition of the American Medical Association). Scientific medicine changes in accord with evidence obtained by scientific enquiry applied with such intellectual rigour as is humanly possible. But this is not the case with cults, the claims for which are characterised by absence of rigorous intellectual evaluation and unchangeability of beliefs. The profusion of medical cults prompts the question why, if each cult has the efficacy claimed by its exponents, conventional medicine and indeed the other cults are not swept away. Some practitioners use conventional medicine and, where it fails, turn to cult practices. Where such complementary practices give comfort, they are not to be despised, but their role and validity should be clearly defined. No community can afford to take these cults at their own valuation; they must be tested, and tested with at least the rigour required to justify a therapeutic claim for a new drug. It is sometimes urged in extenuation that traditional and cult practices do no harm to patients, unlike synthetic drugs. But, even if that were true (which it is not), investment of scarce resources in delivering what may be ineffective, though sometimes pleasing, experiences, e.g. dance therapy, exaltation of flowers or the admittedly inexpensive urine therapy, means that resources are not available for other desirable social objectives, e.g. housing, art subsidies, medicine. We do not apologise for this diversion to consider medical cults and practices, for the world cannot afford unreason, and the antidote to unreason is reason and the rigorous pursuit of knowledge, i.e. evidence-based medicine.

[26]Ernst E (ed) 2001 The Desktop Guide to Complementary and Alternative Medicine. Harcourt, Edinburgh.

[27]Black cohosh (*Cimicifuga racemosa*), taken for hot flushes and other menopausal symptoms (but no better than placebo in clinical trial), can cause serious liver disorder. Herbal teas containing pyrrolizidine alkaloids (*Senecio, Crotalaria, Heliotropium*) cause serious hepatic veno-occlusive disease. Comfrey (*Symphytum*) is similar but also causes hepatocellular tumours and haemangiomas. Sassafras (carminative, antirheumatic) is hepatotoxic. Mistletoe (*Viscum*) contains cytotoxic alkaloids. Ginseng contains oestrogenic substances that have caused gynaecomastia; long-term users may show 'ginseng abuse syndrome' comprising central nervous system excitation; arterial hypertension can occur. Liquorice (*Glycyrrhiza*) has mineralocorticoid action. An amateur 'health food enthusiast' made himself a tea from 'an unfamiliar [*to him*] plant' in his garden; unfortunately this was the familiar foxglove (*Digitalis purpurea*) and as a result he became very ill, but happily recovered. Other toxic natural remedies include lily of the valley (*Convallaria*) and horse chestnut (*Aesculus*). 'The medical herbalist is at fault for clinging to outworn historical authority and for not assessing his drugs in terms of today's knowledge, and the orthodox physician is at fault for a cynical scepticism with regard to any healing discipline other than his own' (Penn R G 1983 Adverse reactions to herbal medicines. Adverse Drug Reaction Bulletin 102:376–379). The Medicines and Healthcare products Regulatory Agency provides advice at: http://www.mhra.gov.uk.

[28]Latin: after this; therefore on account of this.

complementary medicine. But modern therapeutic trial designs can cope with this. There remain extremists who contend that they understand scientific method, and reject it as invalid for what they do and believe, i.e. their beliefs are not, in principle, refutable. This is the position taken up by magic and religion where subordination of reason to faith is a virtue.

CAM particularly charges that conventional medicine seriously neglects patients as whole integrated human beings (body, mind, spirit) and treats them too much as machines. Conventional practitioners may well feel uneasily that there has been and still is truth in this, that with the development of specialisation some doctors have been seduced by the enormous successes of medical science and technology and have become liable to look too narrowly at their patients where a much broader (holistic) approach is required. It is evident that such an approach is likely to give particular satisfaction in psychological and psychosomatic conditions for which conventional doctors in a hurry have been all too ready to think that a prescription meets all the patients' needs.

CAM does not compete with the successful mainstream of scientific medicine. Users of CAM commonly have chronic conditions and have tried conventional medicine but found that it has not offered a satisfactory solution, or has caused adverse effects. The problems, when they occur, are often at the interface between CAM and mainstream medicine. A doctor prescribing a conventional medicine may be unaware that a patient is taking herbal medicine, and there is ample scope for unwanted herb–drug interaction by a variety of mechanisms.[29] These include the following:

- *CYP450 enzyme induction* – St John's wort (by reducing the plasma concentration or therapeutic efficacy of warfarin, ciclosporin, simvastatin, oral contraceptives).
- *CYP450 enzyme inhibition* – piperine (by increasing the plasma concentration of propranolol and theophylline).
- *Additive action* – St John's wort on serotonin-specific reuptake inhibitors (by increasing their unwanted effects).

More troubling is the issue of conflicting advice between CAM and mainstream drugs, as witnessed by the advice to travellers from some homoeopathic pharmacies to use their products for malaria prophylaxis in place of conventional drugs (an action that drew criticism from the Society of Homoeopaths). Regulations being introduced by European Union Directive (and voluntarily in the UK) will move towards formal registration of practitioners of some forms of CAM (notably herbal medicines), according to agreed standards of qualification.

The following will suffice to give the flavour of homoeopathy, the principal complementary medicine system involving medicines, and the kind of criticism with which it has to contend.

Homoeopathy

Homoeopathy[30] is a system of medicine founded by Samuel Hahnemann (German physician, 1755–1843) and expounded by him in the *Organon of the Rational Art of Healing*.[31] Hahnemann described his position:

> *After I had discovered the weakness and errors of my teachers and books I sank into a state of sorrowful indignation, which had nearly disgusted me with the study of medicine. I was on the point of concluding that the whole art was vain and incapable of improvement. I gave myself up to solitary reflection, and resolved not to terminate my train of thought until I had arrived at a definite conclusion on the subject.*[32]

By understandable revulsion at the medicine of his time, by experimentation on himself (a large dose of quinine made him feel as though he had a malarial attack) and by search of records he 'discovered' a 'law' that is central to *homoeopathy*,[33] and from which the name is derived:

> *Similar symptoms in the remedy remove similar symptoms in the disease. The eternal, universal law of Nature, that every disease is destroyed and cured through the similar artificial disease which the appropriate remedy has the tendency to excite, rests on the following proposition: that only one disease can exist in the body at any one time.*

In addition to the above, Hahnemann 'discovered' that dilution potentiates the effect of drugs, but not of trace impurities (provided the dilution is shaken correctly, i.e. by 'succussion'), even to the extent that an effective dose may not contain a single molecule of the drug. It has been pointed

---

[29]Hu Z, Yang X, Ho P C et al 2005 Herb–drug interactions: a literature review. Drugs 65:1239–1282.

[30]Greek: *homos* = same; *patheia* = suffering.
[31]1810: trans. Wheeler C E 1913 (Organon of the Rational Art of Healing.) Dent, London.
[32]Hahnemann S 1805 Aesculapius in the Balance. Leipzig.
[33]By contrast, *allopathy* was a system of medicine based on the principle that induction of a new disease would drive out an existing disease. It was practised by measures that included purging, bleeding and sweating. Use of the word to distinguish homoeopathy from conventional scientific medicine is clearly incorrect.

out[34] that the 'thirtieth potency' (1 in 10^{30}), recommended by Hahnemann, provided a solution in which there would be one molecule of drug in a volume of a sphere of literally astronomical circumference.

The therapeutic efficacy of a dilution at which no drug is present (including sodium chloride prepared in this way) is explained by the belief that a spiritual energy diffused throughout the medicine by the particular way in which the dilutions are shaken (succussion) during preparation, or that the active molecules leave behind some sort of 'imprint' on solvent or excipient.[35] The absence of potentiation of the inevitable contaminating impurities is attributed to the fact that they are not incorporated by serial dilution. Thus, writes a critic: 'We are asked to put aside the whole edifice of evidence concerning the physical nature of materials and the normal concentration–response relationships of biologically active substances in order to accommodate homoeopathic potency'.[36] But no hard evidence that tests the hypothesis is supplied to justify this, and we are invited, for instance, to accept that sodium chloride merely diluted is no remedy, but that 'it raises itself to the most wonderful power through a well prepared dynamisation process' and stimulates the defensive powers of the body against the disease.

Pharmacologists have felt, in the absence of conclusive evidence from empirical studies that homoeopathic medicines can reproducibly be shown to differ from placebo, that there is no point in discussing its hypotheses.[37] But empirical studies can be made without accepting any particular theory of causation; nor should the results of good studies be disregarded just because the proposed theory of action seems incredible or is unknown.

A meta-analysis of 186 double-blind and/or randomised placebo-controlled trials of homoeopathic remedies found that 89 had adequate data for analysis. The authors concluded that their results 'were not compatible with the hypothesis that the clinical effects are completely due to placebo', but also found 'insufficient evidence from these studies that homoeopathy is clearly efficacious for any single clinical condition'.[38] A subsequent analysis of 110 homoeopathic and 110 conventional medicine trials found that there was 'weak evidence for a specific effect of homeopathic remedies, but strong evidence for a specific effect of conventional interventions'. The authors concluded: 'This finding is compatible with the notion that the clinical effects of homeopathy are placebo effects'.[39] These studies evoked strong reactions from practitioners of homoeopathy and others, but they raise the possibility that patients' reactions to homoeopathy, and indeed some other forms of CAM, may rest within an understanding of the complex nature of the placebo response and, in particular, its biology (see below).

Conclusion

There is a single fundamental issue between conventional scientific medicine and traditional, complementary and alternative medicine (although it is often obscured by detailed debates on individual practices); the issue is: What constitutes acceptable evidence, i.e. what is the nature, quality and interpretation of evidence that can justify general adoption of modes of treatment and acceptance of hypotheses? When there is agreement that a CAM treatment works, it becomes conventional and, in respect of that treatment, there is no difference between CAM and orthodox scientific medicine.

In the meantime, we depend on the accumulation of evidence from empirical studies to justify the allocation of resources for future research.

Placebo medicines

A placebo[40] is any component of therapy that is without specific biological activity for the condition being treated.

Placebo medicines are used for two purposes:

- As a control in scientific evaluation of drugs (see Therapeutic trials, p. 45).

---

[34]Clark A J 1937 General pharmacology. In: Hefter's Handbuch. Springer, Berlin.

[35]Homoeopathic practitioners repeatedly express their irritation that critics give so much attention to dilution. They should not be surprised, considering the enormous implications of their claim.

[36]Cuthbert A W 1982 Pharmaceutical Journal (15 May):547.

[37]Editorial 1988 When to believe the unbelievable. Nature 333:787. A report of an investigation into experiments with antibodies in solutions that contained no antibody molecules (as in some homoeopathic medicines). The editor of *Nature* took a three-person team (one of whom was a professional magician, included to detect any trickery) on a week-long visit to the laboratory that claimed positive results. Despite the scientific seriousness of the operation, it developed comical aspects (codes of the contents of test tubes were taped to the laboratory ceiling); the *Nature* team, having reached an unfavourable view of the experiments, 'sped past the (*laboratory*) common-room filled with champagne bottles destined now not to be opened'. Full reports in this issue of *Nature* (28 July 1988), including an acrimonious response by the original scientist, are highly recommended reading, both for scientific logic and for entertainment. See also Nature (1994) 370:322.

[38]Linde K, Clausius N, Melchart D et al 1997 Are the clinical effects of homoeopathy placebo effects? A meta-analysis of placebo-controlled trials. Lancet 350:834–843.

[39]Shang A, Huwiler-Müntener K, Nartey L et al 2005 Are the clinical effects of homeopathy placebo effects? Comparative study of placebo-controlled trials of homeopathy and allopathy. Lancet 366:726–732.

[40]Latin: *placebo* = shall be pleasing or acceptable. For a comment on its historical use, see Edwards M 2005 Lancet 365:1023.

- To benefit or please a patient, not by any pharmacological actions, but for psychological reasons.

All treatments have a psychological component, whether to please (placebo effect) or, occasionally, to vex (negative placebo or *nocebo*[41] effect).

A placebo medicine is a vehicle for 'cure' by suggestion, and is surprisingly often successful, if only temporarily.[42] All treatments carry a placebo effect – physiotherapy, psychotherapy, surgery, entering a patient into a therapeutic trial, even the personality and style of the doctor – but the effect is most easily investigated with drugs, for the active and the inert can often be made to appear identical to allow comparisons.

The deliberate use of drugs as placebos is a confession of therapeutic failure by the doctor. Failures, however, are sometimes inevitable, and an absolute condemnation of the use of placebos on all occasions would be unrealistic.

> A placebo-reactor is an individual who reports changes of physical or mental state after taking a pharmacologically inert substance.

Placebo-reactors are suggestible people who are likely to respond favourably to any treatment. They have misled doctors into making false therapeutic claims.

Negative reactors, who develop adverse effects when given a placebo, exist but, fortunately, are fewer.

Some 30–80% of patients with chronic stable angina pectoris and 30–50% with depression respond to placebos. Placebo reaction is an inconstant attribute: a person may respond at one time in one situation and not at another time under different conditions. In one study on medical students, psychological tests revealed that those who reacted to a placebo tended to be extroverted, sociable, less dominant, less self-confident, more appreciative of their teaching, more aware of their autonomic functions and more neurotic than their colleagues who did not react to a placebo under the particular conditions of the experiment.

Modern brain-scanning techniques provide evidence that the placebo effect has a physiological basis. Positron emission tomography showed that both opioid and placebo analgesia were associated with increased activity in the same cortical area of the brain, the greatest responses occurring in high placebo responders.[43] Functional magnetic resonance imaging demonstrated that strong cortical activation correlated with greater placebo-induced pain relief.[44]

It is important that all who administer drugs should be aware that their attitudes to the treatment may greatly influence the outcome. Undue scepticism may prevent a drug from achieving its effect, and enthusiasm or confidence may potentiate the actions of drugs.

Tonics are placebos, often expensive multivitamin supplements. They may be defined as substances that aspire to strengthen and increase the appetite of those so weakened by disease, misery, overindulgence in play or work, or by physical or mental inadequacy, that they cannot face the stresses of life. The essential feature of this weakness is the absence of any definite recognisable defect for which there is a known remedy. As tonics are placebos, they must be harmless.[45]

Guidelines, 'essential' drugs and prescribing

Increasingly, doctors recognise that they need guidance through the bountiful menu (thousands of medicines) so seductively served to them by the pharmaceutical industry. Principal sources of guidance are the pharmaceutical industry ('prescribe my drug') and governments ('spend less'), and also the developing (profit-making) managed care/insurance bodies ('spend less') and the proliferating drug bulletins offering independent, and supposedly unbiased advice ('prescribe appropriately').

Even the pharmaceutical industry, in its more sober moments, recognises that their ideal world in which doctors, advised and informed by industry alone, were free to prescribe

---

[41]Latin: *nocebo* = shall injure; the term is little used.
[42]As the following account by a mountain rescue guide illustrates: 'The incident involved a 15-year-old boy who sustained head injuries and a very badly broken leg. Helicopter assistance was unavailable and therefore we had to carry him by stretcher to the nearest landrover (several miles away) and then on to a waiting ambulance. During this long evacuation, the boy was in considerable distress and we administered Entonox (a mixture of nitrous oxide and oxygen, 50% each) sparingly as we only had one small cylinder. He repeatedly remarked how much better he felt after each intake of Entonox (approximately every 20 minutes) and after 7 hours or so, we eventually got him safely into the ambulance and on his way to hospital. On going to replace the Extonox we discovered the cylinder was still full of gas due to the equipment being faulty. There was no doubt that the boy felt considerable pain relief because he thought he was receiving Entonox.'

[43]Petrovic P, Kalso E, Petersson K et al 2002 Placebo and opioid analgesia – imaging a shared neuronal network. Science 295:1737–1740.
[44]Wager T D, Rilling J K, Smith E S et al 2004 Placebo induced changes in fMRI in anticipation and experience of pain. Science 303:1162–1167.
[45]Tonics (licensed) available in the UK include: Gentian Mixture, acid (or alkaline) (gentian, a natural plant bitter substance, and dilute hydrochloric acid or sodium bicarbonate); Labiton (thiamine, caffeine, alcohol, all in low dose).

whatever they pleased,[46] to whomsoever they pleased, for as long as they pleased with someone other than the patient paying, is an unrealisable dream of a 'never-never land'.

The industry knows that it has to learn to live with restrictions of some kinds, and one of the means of restriction is the formulary, a list of formulations of medicines with varying amounts of added information. A formulary may list all nationally licensed medicines prescribable by health-care professionals, or list only preferred drugs.

It may be restricted to what a third-party payer will reimburse, or to the range of formulations stocked in a hospital (and chosen by a local drugs and therapeutics committee, which all hospitals or groups of hospitals should have), or the range agreed by a partnership of general practitioners or primary care health centre.

All restricted formularies are heavily motivated to keep costs down without impairing appropriate prescribing. They should make provision for prescribing outside their range in cases of special need with an 'escape clause'.

Thus, restricted formularies are in effect guidelines for prescribing. There is a profusion of these from national sources, hospitals, group practices and specialty organisations (e.g. epilepsy, diabetes mellitus).

'Essential' drugs

Economically disadvantaged countries may seek help to construct formularies. Technical help comes from the World Health Organization (WHO) with its 'Model List of Essential Medicines',[47] i.e. drugs (or representatives of classes of drugs) 'that satisfy the health care needs of the majority of the population; they should therefore be available at all times in adequate amounts and in the appropriate dosage forms'. Countries seeking such advice can use the list as a basis for their own choices (the WHO also publishes model prescribing information).[48] The list, updated regularly, contains about 300 items.

The pharmaceutical industry dislikes the concept of drugs classed as *essential*, as others, by implication, are therefore judged inessential. But the WHO programme has attracted

much interest and approval (see WHO Technical Report series: 'The use of essential drugs': current edition).

Cost-containment

Cost-containment in prescription drug therapy attracts increasing attention. It may involve two particularly contentious activities:

1. *Generic substitution*, where a generic formulation (see Ch. 7) is substituted (by a pharmacist) for the proprietary formulation prescribed by the doctor.
2. *Therapeutic substitution*, where a drug of different chemical structure is substituted for the drug prescribed by the doctor. The substitute is of the same chemical class and is deemed to have similar pharmacological properties and to give similar therapeutic benefit. Therapeutic substitution is a particularly controversial matter where it is done without consulting the prescriber, and legal issues may be raised in the event of adverse therapeutic outcome.

The following facts and opinions are worth some thought:

- UK National Health Service (NHS) spending on drugs has been 9–11% per year (of the total cost) for nearly 50 years.
- General practitioners (i.e. primary care) spend some 80% of the total cost of drugs.
- In the past 25 years, the number of NHS prescriptions has risen from 5.5 to over 13 per person.
- The average cost per head of medicines supplied to people older than 75 years of age is nearly five times that of medicines supplied to those below pensionable age (in the UK: women 62 years, men 65 years, but under revision).
- Under-prescribing can be just as harmful to the health of patients as over-prescribing.

It is crucially important that incentives and sanctions address quality of prescribing as well as quantity: 'it would be wrong if too great a preoccupation with the cost issue in isolation were to encourage under-prescribing or have an adverse effect on patient care' (Report).

Reasons for under-prescribing include: lack of information or lack of the will to use available information (in economically privileged countries there is, if anything, a surplus of information); fear of being blamed for adverse reactions (affecting doctors who lack the confidence that a knowledge of pharmacological principles confers); and fear of sanctions against over-costly prescribing. Prescription frequency and cost per prescription are lower for older than for younger doctors. There is no evidence that the patients of older doctors are worse off as a result.

---

[46]It is difficult for us now to appreciate the naïve fervour and trust in doctors that allowed them almost unlimited rights to prescribe in the early years of the UK National Health Service (founded in 1948). Beer was a prescription item in hospitals until, decades later, an audit revealed that only 1 in 10 bottles reached a patient. More recently (1992): 'There could be fewer Christmas puddings consumed this year. The puddings were recently struck off a bizarre list of items that doctors were able to prescribe for their patients. They were removed by Health Department officials without complaint from the medics, on the grounds they had "no therapeutic or clinical value".' (Lancet (1992) 340:1531).
[47]Available on the WHO website: http://www.who.org.
[48]There is an agency for WHO publications in all UN countries.

Taking a drug history

The reasons for taking a drug history from patients are as follows:

- Drugs are a *cause* of disease. Withdrawal of drugs, if abrupt, can also cause disease, e.g. benzodiazepines, antiepilepsy drugs.
- Drugs can *conceal* disease, e.g. adrenal steroid.
- Drugs can *interact,* producing a positive adverse effect or a negative adverse effect, i.e. therapeutic failure. This is an increasing problem with polypharmacy, especially in the elderly.
- Drugs can give *diagnostic clues,* e.g. ampicillin and amoxicillin causing rash in infectious mononucleosis – a diagnostic adverse effect, not a diagnostic test.
- Drugs can cause *false results* in clinical chemistry tests, e.g. plasma cortisol, urinary catecholamine, urinary glucose, serum renin and aldosterone.
- Drug history can assist *choice of drugs* in the future.
- Drugs can leave *residual effects* after administration has ceased, e.g. chloroquine, amiodarone.
- Drugs available for *independent patient self-medication* are increasing in range and importance.

(See also Appendix: the prescription.)
Prescribing should be appropriate:[49]

> *Appropriate [prescribing is that] which bases the choice of a drug on its effectiveness, safety and convenience relative to other drugs or treatments (e.g. surgery or psychotherapy), and considers cost only when those criteria for choice have been satisfied. In some circumstances appropriateness will require the use of more costly drugs. Only by giving appropriateness high priority will [health providers] be able to achieve their aim of ensuring that patients' clinical needs will be met. (Report)*

Prescribing that is *inappropriate* is the result of several factors:

- Giving in to patient pressure to write unnecessary prescriptions. The extra time spent in careful explanation will, in the long run, be rewarded.
- Continuing patients, especially the elderly, on courses of medicinal treatment over many months without proper review of their medication.

- Doctors may 'prescribe brand-name drugs rather than cheaper generic equivalents, even where there is no conceivable therapeutic advantage in so doing. The fact that the brand-name products often have shorter and more memorable names than their generic counterparts' contributes to this (Report). (See also Ch. 7.)
- 'Insufficient training in clinical pharmacology. Many of the drugs on the market may not have been available when a general practitioner was at medical school. The sheer quantity of new products may lead to a practitioner becoming over-reliant on drugs companies' promotional material, or sticking to "tried and tested" products out of caution based on ignorance' (Report).
- Failure of doctors to keep up to date (see below, Doctor compliance). Computerising prescribing addresses some of these issues, for example by prompting regular review of a patient's medication, by instantly providing generic names from brand names, by giving ready access to formularies and prescribing guidelines.

Repeat prescriptions

About two-thirds of general (family) practice prescriptions are for repeat medication (half issued by the doctor at a consultation and half via the practice nurse or receptionist without patient contact with the doctor). Some 95% of patients' requests are acceded to without further discussion; 25% of patients who receive repeat prescriptions have had 40 or more repeats; and 55% of patients older than 75 years of age are on repeat medication (with periodic review).

Many patients taking the same drug for years are doing so for the best reason, i.e. firm diagnosis for which effective therapy is available, such as epilepsy, diabetes, hypertension, but some are not.

Warnings and consent

Doctors have a professional duty to inform and to warn, so that patients, who are increasingly informed and educated, may make meaningful personal choices, which it is their right to do (unless they opt to leave the choice to the doctor, which it is also their right). Patients now have access to a potentially confusing quantity of detail about the unwanted effects of drugs (information sheet, the Internet, the media), but without the balancing influence of data on their frequency of occurrence. It would be prudent for doctors to draw attention at least to adverse effects that are common, serious (even if uncommon), or avoidable or mitigated if recognised.

---

[49]The text on appropriate prescribing and some quotations (designated 'Report') are based on a UK Parliamentary Report (The National Health Service Drugs Budget 1994 HMSO, London). Twelve members of Parliament took evidence from up to 100 organisations and individuals orally and/or in writing.

Warnings to patients are of two kinds:
- Warnings that will affect the patient's choice to accept or reject the treatment.
- Warnings that will affect the safety of the treatment once it has begun, e.g. risk of stopping treatment, occurrence of drug toxicity.

Just as engineers say that the only safe aeroplane is the one that stays on the ground in still air on a disused airfield or in a locked hangar, so the only safe drug is one that stays in its original package. If drugs are not safe, then plainly patients are entitled to be warned of their hazards, which should be explained to them, as to probability, nature and severity.

There is no formal legal or ethical obligation for doctors to warn all patients of all possible adverse consequences of treatment. It is their duty to adapt the information they give (not too little, and not so much as to cause confusion) so that the best interest of each patient is served. If there is a 'real' (say 1–2%) risk inherent in a procedure of some misfortune occurring, then doctors should warn patients of the possibility that the injury may occur, however well the treatment is performed. Doctors should take into account the personality of the patient, the likelihood of any misfortune arising and what warning was necessary for each particular patient's welfare.[50]

Doctors should consider what their particular individual patients would wish to know (i.e. would be likely to attach significance to) and not only what they think (paternalistically) the patients ought to know. It is part of the professionalism of doctors to tell what is appropriate to the individual patient's interest. If things go wrong, doctors must be prepared to defend what they did or, more important in the case of warnings, what they did not do, as being in their patient's best interest. Courts of law will look critically at doctors who seek to justify under-information by saying that they feared to confuse or frighten the patient (or that they left it to the patient to ask, as one doctor did). The increasing availability of patient information leaflets (PILs) prepared by the manufacturer indicates the increasing trend to give more information. Doctors should know what their patients have read (or not read, as is so often the case) when patients express dissatisfaction.

Evidence that extensive information on risks causes 'unnecessary' anxiety or frightens patients suggests that this is only a marginal issue and it does not justify a general policy of withholding of information.

Legal hazards for prescribers

Doctors would be less than human if, as well as trying to help their patients, they were not also concerned about protecting themselves from allegations of malpractice (negligence). A lawyer specialising in the field put the legal position regarding a doctor's duty pungently:

The provision of information to patients is treated by (English) law as but one part of the way a doctor discharges the obligation he owes to a patient to take reasonable care in all aspects of his treatment of that patient. The provision of information is a corollary of the patient's right to self-determination which is a right recognised by law. Failure to provide appropriate information will usually be a breach of duty and if that breach leads to the patient suffering injury then the basis for a claim for compensation exists.[51]

The keeping of appropriate medical records, written at the time of consultation (and which is so frequently neglected), is not only good medical practice; it is the best way of ensuring that there is an answer to unjustified allegations, made later, when memory has faded. At the very least, these should include records of warning about treatments that are potentially hazardous.

Compliance

Successful therapy, especially if it is long term, comprises a great deal more than choosing a standard medicine. It involves patient and doctor compliance.[52] The latter is liable to be overlooked (by doctors), for doctors prefer to dwell on the deficiencies of their patients rather than of themselves.

Patient compliance

Patient compliance is the extent to which the actual behaviour of the patient coincides with medical advice and instructions; it may be complete, partial, erratic, nil, or there may be over-compliance. To make a diagnosis and to prescribe evidence-based effective treatment is a satisfying experience

---

[50]Legal correspondent 1980 British Medical Journal 280:575.

[51]Ian Dodds-Smith.
[52]The term 'compliance' meets objection as having undertones of obsolete, authoritarian attitudes, implying 'obedience' to doctors' 'orders'. The words 'adherence or concordance' are preferred by some, the latter because it expresses the duality of drug prescribing (by the doctor) and taking (by the patient), i.e. a therapeutic alliance. We retain compliance, pointing out that it applies equally to those doctors who neither keep up to date, nor follow prescribing instructions, and to patients who fail, for whatever reason, to keep to a drug regimen.

for doctors, but too many assume that patients will gratefully or accurately do what they are told, i.e. obtain the medicine and consume it as instructed. This assumption is wrong.

The rate of non-presentation (or redemption) of prescriptions in the UK is around 5%, but is up to 20% or even more in the elderly (who pay no prescription charge). Where lack of money to pay for the medicine is not the cause, this is due to lack of motivation or apprehension about drugs.

Having obtained the medicine, some 25–50% (sometimes even more) of patients either fail to follow the instruction to a significant extent (taking 50–90% of the prescribed dose), or they do not take it at all.

Patient non-compliance or non-adherence is identified as a major factor in therapeutic failure in both routine practice and in scientific therapeutic trials; but, sad to say, doctors are too often non-compliant about remedying this. All patients are potential non-compliers;[53] clinical criteria cannot reliably predict good compliance, but non-compliance often can be predicted.

In addition to therapeutic failure, undetected non-compliance may lead to rejection of the best drug when it is effective, leading to substitution by second-rank medicines.

Non-compliance may occur because:

- the patient has not understood the instructions, so cannot comply,[54] or
- the patient understands the instructions, but fails to carry them out.

Prime factors for poor patient compliance are:

- *Frequency and complexity of the drug regimen.* Many studies attest to polypharmacy as an inhibitor of compliance, i.e. more than three drugs taken concurrently or more than three drug-taking occasions in the day (the ideal of one occasion only is often unattainable).

- *Unintentional non-compliance*, or forgetfulness,[55] may be addressed by associating drug-taking with cues in daily life (breakfast, bedtime), by special packaging (e.g. calendar packs) and by enlisting the aid of others (e.g. carers, teachers).
- *'Intelligent' or wilful non-compliance.*[56] Patients decide they do not need the drug (asymptomatic disease) or they do not like the drug (unwanted effects), or take 2–3-day 'drug holidays'.
- *Illness.* This includes cognitive impairment and psychological problems, with depression being a particular problem.
- *Lack of information.* Oral instructions alone are not enough; one-third of patients are unable to recount instructions immediately on leaving the consulting room. Lucid and legible labelling of containers is essential, as well as patient-friendly information leaflets, which are increasingly available via doctors and pharmacists, and as package inserts.
- *Poor patient–doctor relationship and lack of motivation* to take medicines as instructed offer a major challenge to the prescriber whose diagnosis and prescription may be perfect, yet loses efficacy by patient non-compliance. Unpleasant disease symptoms, particularly where these are recurrent and known by previous experience to be quickly relieved, provide the highest motivation (i.e. self-motivation) to comply. But particularly where the patient does not feel ill, adverse effects are immediate, and benefits are perceived to be remote, e.g. in hypertension, where they may be many years away in the future, doctors must consciously address themselves to motivating compliance. The best way to achieve compliance is to cultivate the patient–doctor relationship. Doctors cannot be expected actually to like all their patients,

---

[53]Even where the grave consequences of non-compliance are understood (glaucoma: blindness) (renal transplant: organ rejection), significant non-compliance has been reported in as many as 20% of patients; psychologists will be able to suggest explanations for this.
[54]Cautionary tales. (1) A 62-year-old man requiring a metered-dose inhaler (for the first time) was told to 'spray the medicine to the throat'. He was found to have been conscientiously aiming and firing the aerosol to his anterior neck around the thyroid cartilage, four times a day for 2 weeks (Chiang A, Lee J C 1994 New England Journal of Medicine 330:1690). (2) A patient thought that 'sublingual' meant able to speak two languages; (3) another that tablets cleared obstructed blood vessels by exploding inside them (E A Kay) – reference, no doubt, to colloquial use of the term 'clot-busting drugs' (for thrombolytics). These are extreme examples; most are more subtle and less detectable. Doctors may smile at the ignorant naïvety of patients, but the smile should give way to a blush of shame at their own deficiencies as communicators.

[55]Where non-compliance, whether intentional or unintentional, is medically serious, it becomes necessary to bypass self-administration (unsupervised) and to resort to directly observed (supervised) oral administration or to injection (e.g. in schizophrenia).
[56]Of the many causes of failure of patient compliance, the following case must be unique. On a transatlantic flight the father of an asthmatic boy was seated in the row behind two doctors. He overheard one of the doctors expressing doubt about the long-term safety in children of inhaled corticosteroids. He interrupted the conversation, explaining that his son took this treatment; he had a lengthy conversation with one of the doctors, who gave his name. Consequently, on arrival, he faxed his wife at home to stop the treatment of their son immediately. She did so, and 2 days later the well-controlled patient had a brisk relapse that responded to urgent treatment by the family doctor (who had been conscientiously following guidelines recently published in an authoritative journal). The family doctor later ascertained that the doctor in the plane was a member of the editorial team of the journal that had so recently published the guidelines that were favourable to inhaled corticosteroid (Cox S 1994 Is eavesdropping bad for your health? British Medical Journal 309:718).

but it is a great help (where liking does not come naturally) if they make a positive effort to understand how individual patients must feel about their illnesses and their treatments, i.e. to empathise with their patients. This is not always easy, but its achievement is the action of the true professional, and indeed is part of their professional duty of care.

Suggestions for doctors to enhance patient compliance/adherence

- Form a non-judgemental alliance or partnership with the patient, giving the patient an opportunity to ask questions.
- Plan a regimen with the minimum number of drugs and drug-taking occasions, adjusted to fit the patient's lifestyle. Use fixed-dose combinations, sustained-release (or injectable depot) formulations, or long $t_{1/2}$ drugs as appropriate; arrange direct observation of each dose in exceptional cases.
- Provide clear oral and written information adapted to the patient's understanding and medical and cultural needs.
- Use patient-friendly packaging, e.g. calendar packs, where appropriate; or monitored-dose systems, e.g. boxes compartmented and labelled (Dosette boxes).
- See the patient regularly and not so infrequently that the patient feels the doctor has lost interest.
- Enlist the help of family members, carers, friends.
- Use computer-generated reminders for repeat prescriptions.

Directly observed therapy (DOT) (where a reliable person supervises each dose). In addition to the areas where supervision is obviously in the interest of patients, e.g. a child, DOT is employed (even imposed) among free-living uncooperative patients who may be a menace to the community, such as those with multiple drug-resistant tuberculosis.

> **What every patient needs to know**[57]
> - An account of the disease and the reason for prescribing.

- The name of the medicine.
- The objective: to treat the disease and/or to relieve symptoms, i.e. how important the medicine is, whether the patient can judge its efficacy and when benefit can be expected to occur.
- How and when to take the medicine.
- Whether it matters if a dose is missed and what, if anything, to do about it (see p. 22).
- How long the medicine is likely to be needed.
- How to recognise adverse effects and any action that should be taken, including effects on car driving.
- Any interaction with alcohol or other medicines.

A remarkable instance of non-compliance, with hoarding, was that of a 71-year-old man who attempted suicide and was found to have in his home 46 bottles containing 10 685 tablets. Analysis of his prescriptions showed that over a period of 17 months he had been expected to take 27 tablets of several different kinds daily.[58]

From time to time there are campaigns to collect all unwanted drugs from homes in an area. Usually the public are asked to deliver the drugs to their local pharmacies. In one UK city (population 600 000), 500 000 'solid dose units' (tablets, capsules, etc.) were handed in (see below, Opportunity cost); such quantities have even caused local problems for safe waste disposal.

Factors that are *insignificant* for compliance are: age[59] (except at extremes), sex, intelligence (except at extreme deficiency) and educational level (probably).

Over-compliance. Patients (up to 20%) may take more drug than is prescribed, even increasing the dose by 50%. In diseases where precise compliance with frequent or complex regimens is important, for example in glaucoma where sight is at risk, there have been instances of obsessional patients responding to their doctors' overemphatic instructions by clock-watching in a state of anxiety to avoid the slightest deviance from timed administration of the correct dose, to the extent that their daily (and nightly) life becomes dominated by this single purpose.

Evaluation of patient compliance. Merely asking patients whether they have taken the drug as directed is not likely

---

[57]After: Drug and Therapeutics Bulletin 1981; 19:73. *Patient information leaflets*. In economically privileged countries, original or patient-pack dispensing is becoming the norm, i.e. patients receive an unopened pack just as it left the manufacturer. The pack contains a patient information leaflet (PIL) (which therefore accompanies each repeat prescription). Regulatory authorities increasingly determine its content. In this litigious age, requirements to be comprehensive and, to protect both manufacturer and regulatory authority, impair the patient-friendliness of PILs. But studies have shown that patients who receive leaflets are more satisfied than those who do not. Doctors need to have copies of these leaflets so that they can discuss with their patients what they are (or are not) reading.

---

[58]Smith S E, Stead K C 1974 Non-compliance or mis-prescribing? Lancet i:937 [letter].
[59]But the elderly are commonly taking several drugs – a major factor in non-compliance – and monitoring compliance in this age group becomes particularly important. The over-60s in the UK are, on average, each receiving two or three medications.

to provide reliable evidence.[60] It is safest to assume that any event that can impair compliance will sometimes happen.

Estimations of compliance come from a variety of measures. DOT (above) is the most accurate, and identification of the drug or metabolites in plasma (or an artificial biological marker in the case of a clinical trial) is persuasive at least of recent compliance.

Requiring patients to produce containers when they attend the doctor, who counts the tablets, seems to do little more than show the patient that the doctor cares about the matter (which is useful); a tablet absent from a container has not necessarily entered the patient's body. On the other hand, although patients are known to practise deliberate deception, to maintain effective deception successfully over long periods requires more effort than most patients are likely to make. Memory aids, such as drug diaries, monitored-dosage systems (e.g. compartmented boxes) and electronic containers that record times of opening are helpful.

Some pharmacodynamic effects, such as heart rate with a β-adrenoceptor blocker, provide a physiological marker as an indicator of the presence of drug in the body. Monitoring plasma drug concentrations is possible, but to do so without informing the patient raises ethical issues.

Doctor compliance

Doctor compliance is the extent to which the behaviour of doctors fulfils their professional duty:

- not to be ignorant
- to adopt new advances when they are sufficiently proved (which doctors are often slow to do)
- to prescribe accurately[61]
- to tell patients what they need to know
- to warn, i.e. to recognise the importance of the act of prescribing (see also p. 6).

In one study in a university hospital, where standards might be expected to be high, there was an error of drug use (dose, frequency, route) in 3% of prescriptions and an error of prescription writing (in relation to standard hospital instructions) in 30%. Many errors were trivial, but many could have resulted in overdose, serious interaction or under-treatment.

In other hospital studies, error rates in drug administration of 15–25% have been found, with rates rising rapidly where four or more drugs are being given concurrently, as is often the case; studies of hospital inpatients show that each receives about six drugs, and up to 20 during a stay is not rare. Merely providing information (on antimicrobials) did not influence prescribing, but gently asking physicians to justify their prescriptions caused a marked fall in inappropriate prescribing.

On a harsher note, in recent years doctors who gave drugs about which they later admitted ignorance (e.g. route of administration and/or dose) stood charged with manslaughter[62] and were convicted. Shocked by this, fellow doctors have written to the medical press offering understanding sympathy to these, sometimes junior, colleagues, in effect saying 'There, but for the grace of God, go I'.[63] The public response, however, is not sympathetic. Doctors put themselves forward as trained professionals who offer a service of responsible, competent provision of drugs that they have the legal right to prescribe. The public is increasingly inclined to hold them to that claim, and, where doctors seriously fail, to exact retribution.[64]

If you do not know about a drug, find out before you act, or take the personal consequences, which, increasingly, may be very serious indeed.

Underdosing

Use of suboptimal doses of drugs in serious disease occurs, sacrificing therapeutic efficacy to avoid serious adverse effects. Instances are commonest with drugs of low therapeutic index (see Index), i.e. where the effective and toxic dose ranges are close, or even overlap, e.g. heparin, anticancer drugs, aminoglycoside antimicrobials. In these cases, dose adjustment to obtain maximum benefit with minimum risk requires both knowledge and attentiveness.

The clinical importance of missed dose(s)

Even the most conscientious of patients will miss a dose or doses occasionally. Patients should therefore be told

---

[60]Hippocrates (460–377 BC) noted that patients are liars regarding compliance. The way the patient is questioned may be all important, e.g. 'Were you able to take the tablets?' may get a truthful reply, whereas 'Did you take the tablets?' may not, because the latter question may be understood by the patient as implying personal criticism (Pearson RM 1982 Who is taking their tablets? British Medical Journal 285:757).

[61]Accuracy includes legibility: a doctor wrote Intal (sodium cromoglicate) for an asthmatic patient; the pharmacist read it as Inderal (propranolol) – the patient died. See also, Names of drugs (Ch. 7).

[62]Unlawful killing in circumstances that do not amount to murder (which requires an intention to kill), e.g. causing death by negligence that is much more serious than mere carelessness; reckless breach of the legal duty of care.

[63]Attributed to John Bradford, an English preacher and martyr (16th century), on seeing a convicted criminal pass by.

[64]A doctor wrote a prescription for isosorbide dinitrate 20 mg 6-hourly, but because of the illegibility of the handwriting the pharmacist dispensed felodipine in the same dose (maximum daily dose 10 mg). The patient died, and a court ordered the doctor and pharmacist to pay compensation of $450 000 to the family. Charatan F 1999 Family compensated for death after illegible prescription. British Medical Journal 319:1456.

whether this matters and what they should do about it, if anything.

> Missed dose(s) may lead to:
> • Loss of therapeutic efficacy (acute disease).
> • Resurgence (chronic disease).
> • Rebound or withdrawal syndrome.

Loss of therapeutic efficacy involves the *pharmacokinetic properties* of drugs. With some drugs of short $t_{1/2}$, the issue is simply a transient drop in plasma concentration below a defined therapeutic concentration. The issues are more complex where therapeutic effect may not decline in parallel with plasma concentration, as with recovery of negative feedback homoeostatic mechanisms (adrenocortical steroids).

A single missed dose may be important with some drugs, e.g. oral contraceptives, but with others (long $t_{1/2}$), omission of several doses is tolerated without any serious decline in efficacy, e.g. levothyroxine.

These pharmacokinetic considerations are complex and important, and are, or should be, taken into account by drug manufacturers in devising dosage schedules and informative data sheets. Manufacturers should aim at one or two doses per day (not more), and this is generally best achieved with drugs with relatively long biological effect $t_{1/2}$ or, where the biological effect $t_{1/2}$ is short, by using sustained-release formulations.

Discontinuation syndrome (recurrence of disease, rebound, or withdrawal syndrome) may occur due to a variety of mechanisms (see Index).

Pharmacoeconomics (see also Ch. 5)

Even the richest societies cannot satisfy the appetite of their citizens for health care based on their real needs, on their wants and on their (often unrealistic) expectations.

Health-care resources are rationed[65] in one way or another, whether according to national social policies or to individual wealth. The debate on supply is not about whether there should be rationing, but about what form rationing should take; whether it should be explicit or concealed (from the public).

Doctors prescribe, patients consume and, increasingly throughout the world, third (purchasing) parties (government, insurance companies) pay the bill with money they have obtained from increasingly reluctant healthy members of the public.

The purchasers of health care are now engaged in serious exercises to contain drug costs in the short term without impairing the quality of medical care, or damaging the development of useful new drugs (which is an enormously expensive and long-term process). This can be achieved successfully only if reliable data are available on costs and benefits, both absolute and relative. The difficulties of generating such data, not only during development, but later under conditions of actual use, are enormous and are addressed by a special breed of professionals: the health economists.

> *Economics* is the science of the distribution of wealth and resources. Prescribing doctors, who have a duty to the community as well as to individual patients, cannot escape involvement with economics.

The economists' objective

The objective is to define needs, thereby enabling the deployment of resources according to priorities set by society, which has an interest in fairness between its members.

Resources can be distributed by the outcome of an unregulated power struggle between professionals and associations of patients and public pressure groups – all, no doubt, warm-hearted towards deserving cases of one kind or another, but none able to view the whole scene. Alternatively, distribution can occur by a planned evaluation that allows division of the resources based on some visible attempt at fairness.

A health economist[66] writes:

> *The economist's approach to evaluating drug therapies is to look at a group of patients with a particular disorder and the various drugs that could be used to treat them. The costs of the various treatments and some costs associated with their use (together with the costs of giving no treatment) are then considered in terms of impact on health status (survival and quality of life) and impact on other health care costs (e.g. admissions to hospital, need for other drugs, use of other procedures).*

Economists are often portrayed as people who want to focus on cost, whereas in reality they see everything in terms of a balance between costs and benefits.

---

[65]The term 'rationing' is used here to embrace the allocation of priorities as well as the actual withholding of resources (in this case, drugs).

[66]Professor Michael Drummond

A report on clinical pharmacologists in the UK National Health Service (NHS) by the international accountancy firm PricewaterhouseCoopers '…explores the costs and financial benefits of hiring … additional clinical pharmacologists for the UK and quantifies significant social, clinical and financial benefits as a result of this investment.' The key finding was '… each £1 spent to hire additional clinical pharmacologists has the potential to reduce NHS costs by almost £6.'[67]

Four economic concepts have particular importance to the thinking of every doctor who makes a decision to prescribe, i.e. to distribute resources:

- *Opportunity cost* means that which has to be sacrificed in order to carry out a certain course of action, i.e. costs are benefits foregone elsewhere. Money spent on prescribing is not available for another purpose; wasteful prescribing is as an affront to those who are in serious need, e.g. institutionalised mentally handicapped citizens who everywhere would benefit from increased resources, or patients requiring hip replacement.
- *Cost-effectiveness analysis* is concerned with how to attain a given objective at minimal financial cost, e.g. prevention of post-surgical venous thromboembolism by heparins, warfarin, aspirin or external pneumatic compression. Analysis includes the cost of materials, adverse effects, any tests, nursing and doctor time and duration of stay in hospital (which may greatly exceed the cost of the drug).
- *Cost-benefit analysis* is concerned with issues of whether (and to what extent) to pursue objectives and policies; it is thus a broader activity than cost-effectiveness analysis and puts monetary values on the quality as well as on the quantity (duration) of life.
- *Cost-utility analysis* is concerned with comparisons between programmes, such as an antenatal drug treatment which saves a young life, or a hip replacement operation which improves mobility in a man of 60 years. Such differing issues are also the basis for comparison by computing quality-adjusted life years (see below).
- An allied measure is the *cost-minimisation analysis*, which finds the least costly programme among those shown or assumed to be of equal benefit. Economic analysis requires that both quantity and quality of life be measured. The former is easy; the latter is hard to determine.

In the UK the National Institute for Health and Clinical Excellence (NICE) appraises the clinical effectiveness and cost-effectiveness of drugs, devices and diagnostic tools, and advises health-care professionals in the NHS on their use. The NHS is legally obliged to make resources available to implement NICE guidance, so avoiding differential treatment according to a patient's area of residence – so-called 'post-code prescribing'.

Quality of life

Everyone is familiar with the measurement of the benefit of treatment in saving or extending life, i.e. life expectancy: the measure is the *quantity* of life (in years). But it is evident that life may be extended and yet have a low quality, even to the point that it is not worth having at all. It is therefore useful to have a unit of health measurement that combines the quantity of life with its *quality*, to place individual and social decision-making on a sounder basis than mere intuition. Economists met this need by developing the *quality-adjusted life year* (QALY) whereby estimations of years of life expectancy are modified according to estimations of quality of life.

Quality of life has four principal dimensions:[68]

1. Physical mobility.
2. Freedom from pain and distress.
3. Capacity for self-care.
4. Ability to engage in normal work and social interactions.

The approach for determining quality of life is by questionnaire, to measure what the subject perceives as personal health. The assessments are refined to provide improved assessment of the benefits and risks of medicines to the individual and to society. The challenge is to ensure that these are sufficiently robust to make resource allocation decisions between, for example, the rich and the poor, the educated and the uneducated, the old and the young, as well as between groups of patients with very different diseases. Plainly, quality of life is a major aspect of what is called *outcomes research*.

---

[67]Report. PricewaterhouseCoopers 2016 Clinical Pharmacology and Therapeutics. The case for savings in the NHS 168:1–25.

[68]Williams A 1983 In: Smith G T (ed) Measuring the Social Benefits of Medicine. Office of Health Economics, London.

Guide to further reading

Buetow, S., Elwyn, G., 2007. Patient safety and patient error. Lancet 369, 158–161.

De Smet, P.A., 2004. Health risks of herbal remedies. Clin. Pharmacol. Ther. 76 (1), 1–17.

Ernst, E., 2008. A historical perspective on placebo. Clin. Med. (Northfield Il) 8 (1), 9–10.

Kandela, P., 1999. Sketches from *The Lancet*: doctors' handwriting. Lancet 353, 1109.

Ker, K., Edwards, P., Roberts, I., 2011. Misadventures to patients during surgical and medical care in England and Wales: an analysis of deaths and hospital episodes. J. R. Soc. Med. 104, 292–298.

Loudon, I., 2006. A brief history of homeopathy. J. R. Soc. Med. 99, 607–610.

Mason, S., Tovey, P., Long, A.F., 2002. Evaluating complementary medicine: methodological challenges of randomised controlled trials. Br. Med. J. 325, 832–834.

McGuffin, M., 2008. Should herbal medicines be regulated as drugs? Clin. Pharmacol. Ther. 83 (3), 393–395.

Maxwell, S.R., 2016. Rational prescribing: the principles of drug selection. Clin. Med. (Lond) 16 (5), 459–464.

Neale, G., Chapman, E.J., Hoare, J., Olsen, S., 2006. Recognising adverse events and critical incidents in medical practice in a district general hospital. Clin. Med. (Northfield Il) 6 (4), 157–162.

Osterberg, L., Blaschke, T., 2005. Adherence to medication. N. Engl. J. Med. 353 (5), 487–497.

Panesar, S.S., Cleary, K., Sheikh, A., 2009. Reflections on the National Patient Safety Agency's database of medical errors. J. R. Soc. Med. 102, 256–258.

Posadzki, P., Watson, L.K., Alotaibi, A., Ernst, E., 2013. Prevalence of use of complementary and alternative medicine. Clin. Med. (Lond.) 13 (2), 126–131.

Rawlins, M.D., 2004. NICE work—providing guidance to the British National Health Service. N. Engl. J. Med. 351 (3), 1381–1385.

Simpson, S.H., Eurich, D.T., Majumdar, S.R., et al., 2006. A meta-analysis of the association between adherence to drug therapy and mortality. Br. Med. J. 333, 15.

Appendix: the prescription

The prescription is the means by which patients receive medicines that are considered unsafe for sale directly to the public. Its format is officially regulated to ensure precision in the interests of safety and efficacy, and to prevent fraudulent misuse; full details appear in national formularies, and prescribers have a responsibility to comply with these.

Prescriptions of pure drugs or of formulations from the *British National Formulary* (BNF)[69] are satisfactory for almost all purposes. The composition of many of the preparations in the BNF is laid down in official pharmacopoeias, e.g. British Pharmacopoeia (BP). There are also many national and international pharmacopoeias.

Traditional extemporaneous prescription-writing art, defining drug, base, adjuvant, corrective, flavouring and vehicle, is obsolete, as is the use of the Latin language. Certain convenient Latin abbreviations do survive for lack of convenient English substitutes. They appear below, without approval or disapproval.

> The elementary requirements of a prescription (now usually viewed on-screen by a computer programme) are that it should state what is to be given to whom and by whom prescribed, and give instructions on how much should be taken, how often, by what route and for how long, or the total quantity to be supplied, as below.

1. Date.
2. Address of doctor.
3. Name and address of patient: date of birth is also desirable for safety reasons; in the UK it is a legal requirement for children younger than 12 years of age.
4. ℞. This is a traditional esoteric symbol[70] for 'Recipe—take thou', which is addressed to the pharmacist. It is pointless; but as many doctors gain a harmless pleasure from writing it with a flourish before the name of a proprietary preparation of whose exact nature they may be ignorant, it is likely to survive as a sentimental link with the past.
5. Name and dose of the medicine.
   Abbreviations. Only abbreviate where there is an official abbreviation. Never use unofficial abbreviations or invent your own; *it is not safe to do so.*

Quantities (after BNF):
- 1 gram or more: write 1 g, etc.
- less than 1 g: write as milligrams (e.g. 500 mg, not 0.5 g)
- less than 1 mg: write as micrograms (e.g. 100 µg, not 0.1 mg)
- for decimals, a zero should precede the decimal point where there is no other figure (e.g. 0.5 mL, not .5 mL; for a range, 0.5–1 g)
- do not abbreviate *microgram, nanogram,* or *unit*
- use millilitre (mL or ml), not cubic centimetre (cc)
- for home/domestic measures, see below. State dose and dose frequency; for 'as required', specify minimum dose interval or maximum dose per day.

6. **Directions to the pharmacist,** if any: 'mix', 'make a solution'. Write the total quantity to be dispensed (if this is not stated in 5 above) or duration of supply.
7. **Instruction for the patient,** to be written on container by the pharmacist. Here brevity, clarity and accuracy are especially important. It is dangerous to rely on the patient remembering oral instructions. The BNF provides a list of recommended 'cautionary and advisory labels for dispensed medicines', representing a balance between 'the unintelligibly short and the inconveniently long', for example: 'Do not stop taking this medicine except on your doctor's advice'.

   Pharmacists nowadays use their own initiative in giving advice to patients.
8. **Signature of doctor.**

Example of a prescription for a patient with an annoying unproductive cough:

1. 1., 2., 3., as above
2. ℞
3. Codeine Linctus, BNF, 5 mL
4. Send 60 mL
5. Label: Codeine Linctus (or NP). Take 5 mL twice a day and on retiring
6. Signature of doctor.

Computer-issued prescriptions must conform to recommendations of professional bodies. Computer-generated facsimile signatures do not meet the legal requirement.

If altered by hand (undesirable), the alteration must be signed.

Medicine containers. Reclosable child-resistant containers and blister packs are now standard, as is dispensing in manufacturers' original sealed packs containing a patient information leaflet. These add to immediate cost but may

---

[69]Supplied free to all doctors practising in the UK National Health Service.
[70]Derived from the eye of Horus, Ancient Egyptian sun god.

save money in the end (increased efficiency of use, and safety).

Unwanted medicines. Patients should be encouraged to return these to the original supplier for disposal.

Drugs liable to cause dependence or be the subject of misuse. Doctors have a particular responsibility to ensure that: (1) they do not create dependence, (2) the patient does not increase the dose and create dependence, (3) they do not become an unwitting source of supply to addicts. To many such drugs, special prescribing regulations apply (see BNF).

Abbreviations (see also Weights and measures, below)

b.d.: bis in die	twice a day (b.i.d. is also used)
BNF	British National Formulary
BP	British Pharmacopoeia
BPC	British Pharmaceutical Codex
i.m.: intramuscular	by intramuscular injection
IU	International Unit
i.v.: intravenous	by intravenous injection
NP: nomen proprium	proper name
o.d.: omni die	every day
o.m.: omni mane	every morning
o.n.: omni nocte	every night
p.o.: per os	by mouth
p.r.: per rectum	by the anal/rectal route
p.r.n.: pro re nata	as required. It is best to add the maximum frequency of repetition, e.g. aspirin and codeine tablets, 1 or 2 p.r.n., 4-hourly
p.v.: per vaginam	by the vaginal route
q.d.s.: quater die sumendus	four times a day (q.i.d. is also used)
rep.: repetatur	let it be repeated, as in rep. mist(ura), repeat the mixture
s.c.: subcutaneous	by subcutaneous injection
stat: statim	immediately
t.d.s.: ter (in) die sumendus	three times a day (t.i.d. is also used)

Weights and measures

In this book, doses are given in the metric system, or in international units (IU) when metric doses are impracticable.

Equivalents:

1 litre (L or l) = 1.76 pints
1 kilogram (kg) = 2.2 pounds (lb).

Abbreviations:

1 gram (g)
1 milligram (mg) (1×10^{-3} g)
1 microgram[71] (1×10^{-6} g)
1 nanogram[71] (1×10^{-9} g)
1 decilitre (dL) (1×10^{-1} L)
1 millilitre (mL) (1×10^{-3} L).

Home/domestic measures. A standard 5-mL spoon and a graduated oral syringe are available. Otherwise the following approximations will serve:

1 tablespoonful = 14 mL (or ml)
1 dessertspoonful = 7 mL (or ml)
1 teaspoonful = 5 mL (or ml).

Percentages, proportions, weight in volume

Some solutions of drugs (e.g. local anaesthetics, adrenaline/epinephrine) for parenteral use are labelled in a variety of ways: percentage, proportion, or weight in volume (e.g. 0.1%, 1:1000, 1 mg/mL). In addition, dilutions may have to be made by doctors at the time of use. Such drugs are commonly dangerous in overdose, and great precision is required, especially as any errors are liable to be by a factor of 10 and can be fatal. Doctors who do not feel confident with such calculations (because they do not do them frequently) should feel no embarrassment,[72] but should recognise that they have a responsibility to check their results with a competent colleague or pharmacist before proceeding.

---

[71]Spell out in full in prescriptions.
[72]Called to an emergency tension pneumothorax on an intercontinental flight, two surgeons, who chanced to be passengers, were provided with lidocaine 100 mg in 10 mL (in the aircraft medical kit). They were accustomed to thinking in percentages for this drug and 'in the heat of the moment' neither was able to make the conversion. Chest surgery was conducted successfully with an adapted wire coat-hanger as a trocar ('sterilised' in brandy), using a urinary catheter. The patient survived the flight and recovered in hospital. Wallace W A 1995 Managing in-flight emergencies: a personal account. British Medical Journal 311:374.

Chapter | 3 |

Discovery and development of drugs

Patrick Vallance

SYNOPSIS

- **Preclinical drug development. Discovery of new drugs in the laboratory is an exercise in prediction. Selecting the target for a drug is probably the key decision.**
- **Techniques of discovery. Several approaches, including using small molecules, large proteins and nucleic-based approaches, and cells broaden what we think of as a medicine.**
- **Studies in animals. Some are required by regulation (for safety), others give insight into the effect of the drug in the whole body, but none replaces the need for clinical testing.**
- **Experimental medicine. Getting the medicine into the clinic to test its properties and its effects on biological systems in humans is a key step.**
- **Ethical issues.**
- **Need for animal testing.**
- **Prediction. Failures of prediction occur, and a drug may be abandoned at any stage, including after marketing. New drug development is colossally expensive, and it is important to consider commercial return to fund drug discovery and development.**
- **Orphan drugs and diseases.**

Making a new medicine

Discovering and developing a new medicine requires combining the skills of biology, chemistry, clinical medicine and, of course, pharmacology. There are four key decision points along the way:

1. Selecting the molecular target you want the drug to act on to produce the desired effect.
2. Choosing the right chemical as the drug candidate. All the promise and all the faults become fixed at this point.
3. Designing the right clinical experiment to show that the medicine will really do what you want it to do.
4. Showing how the medicine improves health and benefits health-care systems.

Medicinal therapeutics rests on the two great supporting pillars of pharmacology:

1. *Selectivity* – the desired effect alone is obtained: 'We must learn to aim, learn to aim with chemical substances' (Paul Ehrlich).[1]
2. *Dose* – 'The dose alone decides that something is no poison' (Paracelsus).[2]

Once a target has been selected, the process of finding the right chemical to act as an antagonist, agonist, inhibitor, activator or modulator of the protein function depends on a process of screening. For decades, the rational discovery of new medicines depended on modifications of the structures of natural chemical mediators. This may still be the route to find the drug, but more often now large libraries

---

[1]Paul Ehrlich (1845–1915), a German scientist, who pioneered the scientific approach to drug discovery. The 606th organic arsenical that he tested against spirochaetes (in animals) became a successful medicine (Salvarsan 1910); it and a minor variant were used against syphilis until superseded by penicillin in 1945.
[2]Paracelsus (1493–1541) was a controversial figure who has been portrayed as both ignorant and superstitious. He had no medical degree; he burned the classical medical works (Galen, Avicenna) before his lectures in Basle (Switzerland) and had to leave the city following a dispute about fees with a prominent churchman. He died in Salzburg (Austria), either as a result of a drunken debauch or because he was thrown down a steep incline by 'hitmen' employed by jealous local physicians. But he was right about the dose.

of compounds are screened against the target in robotic high-throughput screens. However, it is worth remembering that the exact molecular basis of drug action may remain unknown, and this book contains frequent examples of old drugs whose mechanism of action remains mysterious. The evolution of *molecular medicine* (including recombinant DNA technology) in the past 30 years has led to identification of many thousands of potential drug targets, but the function of many of these genes remains unknown. The hope was that the identification of targets identified by genetics coupled with high throughout screening would lead to a great increase in the productivity of drug discovery. This has turned out not to be the case since it is clearly important to understand both the function of the target and the nature of the interaction of the chemical drug with the target in order to make a selective and safe medicine. However, the advent of modern clinical genetics means that it is increasingly possible to identify causal pathways of human diseases. This leads to a much more certain starting point for drug discovery.

Of discovering a truly novel medicine, i.e. one that does something valuable for patients that had previously not been possible (or that does safely what could previously have been achieved only with substantial risk), are increased when the discovery and development programme is founded on precise knowledge of the biological processes it is desired to change. The commercial rewards of a successful product are potentially enormous and provide a great incentive for developers to invest and risk huge sums of money. Most projects in drug discovery and development fail. Indeed the chances of making it through from target selection to having a medicine on the market are in order of 2–3 in 100.

The huge increase in understanding of molecular signalling – both between cells and within cells – has opened many new opportunities to develop medicines that can target discrete steps in the body's elaborate pathways of chemical reactions.[3] The challenge, of course, is to do so in a way that produces benefit without harm. The more fundamental the pathway targeted, the more likely there is to be a big effect, whether beneficial, harmful or both. No benefit comes without some risk.

The molecular, industrialised and automated approach to drug discovery that followed sequencing of the genome and application of high-throughput chemical approaches led to two consequences:

1. More potential drugs and therapeutic targets were identified that could be experimentally validated in animals and humans. This 'production line' approach also led to a loss of integration of the established specialties (chemistry, biochemistry, pharmacology)

and to an overall lack of understanding of how physiological and pathophysiological processes contribute to the interaction of drug and disease.

2. Theoretically, new drugs could be targeted at selected groups of patients based on their genetic make-up. This concept of 'the right medicine for the right patient' is the basis of *pharmacogenetics* (see p. 106), the genetically determined variability in drug response.

Pharmacogenetics has gained momentum from recent advances in molecular genetics and genome sequencing, due to:

- rapid screening for gene variants
- knowledge of the genetic sequences of target genes such as those coding for enzymes, ion channels and other receptor types involved in drug response.

These opportunities have been enhanced by the recent advent of gene editing techniques that allow precise manipulation of genetic sequences and subsequent testing of the phenotypic consequences of such changes. These techniques can now be applied at industrial scale and can lead to much more rapid identification of promising drug targets.

Expectations of pharmacogenetics and its progeny, pharmacoproteomics (understanding of and drug effects on protein variants) remain high, but the applicability will not be universal. They include the following:

- The identification of subgroups of patients with a disease or syndrome based on their genotype. The most extreme of obvious examples of this are diseases caused by single gene defects. The ability accurately to subclassify based on common genetic variation is less clear.
- Targeting of specific drugs for patients with specific gene variants. This is most advanced in the field of cancer (usually targeting somatic changes in cancers) and increasingly in the field of the pharmacogenetics of safety (i.e. unwanted drug effects).

Consequences of these expectations include: smaller clinical trial programmes with well-defined patient groups (based on phenotypic and genotypic characterisation), better understanding of the pharmacokinetics and dynamics according to genetic variation, and improved monitoring of adverse events after marketing.

New drug development proceeds thus:

- Idea or hypothesis. 'This protein causes this disease/ these effects which I could stop by affecting protein function (drugs usually affect protein function as a primary mechanism).'
- Design and synthesis of substances. 'This molecule produces the wanted effect on protein function and has the physico-chemical characteristics that make it a

---

[3]Culliton B J 1994 Nature Medicine 1:1 [editorial].

potential medicine.' This is true for traditional small molecules, for antibody therapies and for nucleic acid-based approaches.

- Studies on tissues and whole animal (preclinical studies). 'When I test it in appropriate models it does what I expect and that allows me to believe it would do the same in humans.'
- Studies in humans (clinical studies) (see Ch. 4). 'Initially I want to know whether the molecule has drug-like properties in terms of its kinetics. I then want to know that it does what I need it to do in terms of the effect on disease.'
- Granting of an official licence to make therapeutic claims and to sell (see Ch. 6). 'Is my medicine better than placebo? Does it do more than existing medicines and is it well tolerated? What effect does it have on populations as used in practice?'
- Post-licensing (marketing) studies of safety and comparisons with other medicines. 'Now many thousands of patients have taken it, am I still sure that it is safe?'

The (critical) phase of progress from the laboratory to humans is often termed 'translational science' or 'experimental medicine'. It was defined as 'the application of biomedical research (pre-clinical and clinical), conducted to support drug development, which aids in the identification of the appropriate patient for treatment (patient selection), the correct dose and schedule to be tested in the clinic (dosing regimen) and the best disease in which to test a potential agent'.[4]

It will be obvious from the account that follows that drug development is an extremely arduous, highly technical and enormously expensive operation. Successful developments (1% of compounds that proceed to full test eventually become licensed medicines) must carry the cost of the failures (99%).[5] It is also obvious that such programmes are likely

to be carried to completion only when the organisations and the individuals within them are motivated overall by the challenge to succeed and to serve society, as well as to make the company profitable. A previous edition of this chapter included a quote from a paper I wrote from my time in academia, and I leave it here:

Let us get one thing straight: the drug industry works within a system that demands it makes a profit to satisfy shareholders. Indeed, it has a fiduciary[6] duty to do so. The best way to make a lot of money is to invent a drug that produces a dramatically beneficial clinical effect, is far more effective than existing options, and has few unwanted effects. Unfortunately most drugs fall short of this ideal.[7]

Techniques of discovery

(See Fig. 3.1)

The *newer technologies*, the impact of which has yet to be fully felt, include the following:

Molecular modelling and structural biology aided by three-dimensional computer graphics (including virtual reality) allows the design of structures based on new and known molecules to enhance their desired, and to eliminate their undesired, properties to create highly selective targeted compounds. In principle all molecular structures capable of binding to a single high-affinity site can be modelled. The advent of really high power computing is likely to lead to significant advances 'in *silico* drug discovery'.

High throughput screening allows the screening of millions of compounds against a single target or a cell-based screen to determine activity against the target. Traditionally these are large robotic screens but newer technologies, including use of small molecules using coding tags, allow miniaturisation of the process. The quality of the 'hit' which is the starting point for medicinal chemistry 'lead optimisation', depends on the quality of the molecules in the compound collection and the nature of the biochemical target used for the screen.

Fragments. If the crystal structure of the protein target is known, it is possible to screen small fragments of potential drugs to find those that bind and where they bind. It is then possible to construct a drug by adding fragments.

Proteins as medicines: biotechnology. The targets of most drugs are proteins (cell receptors, enzymes), and it

---

[4]Johnstone D 2006 pA₂ online (E-journal of the British Pharmacological Society) 4(2). Available at: http://www.pa2online.org/articles/article.jsp?volume=5&issue=13&article=54.
[5]The cost of development of a new chemical entity (NCE) (a novel molecule not previously tested in humans) from synthesis to market (general clinical use) is estimated at over $1.6 billion; the process may take as long as 15 years (including up to 10 years for clinical studies), which is relevant to duration of patent life and so to ultimate profitability; if the developer does not see profit at the end of the process, the investment will not be made. The drug may fail at any stage, including the ultimate, i.e. at the official regulatory body, after all the development costs have been incurred. It may also fail (due to adverse effects) within the first year after marketing, which constitutes a catastrophe (in reputation and finance) for the developer as well as for some of the patients. Pirated copies of full regulatory dossiers have substantial black market value to competitor companies, who have used them to leapfrog the original developer to obtain a licence for their unresearched copied molecule. Dossiers may be enormous, even a million pages or the electronic equivalent, the latter being very convenient as it allows instant searching.

---

[6]Held or given in trust (OED).
[7]Vallance P 2005 Developing an open relationship with the drug industry. Lancet 366:1062–1064.

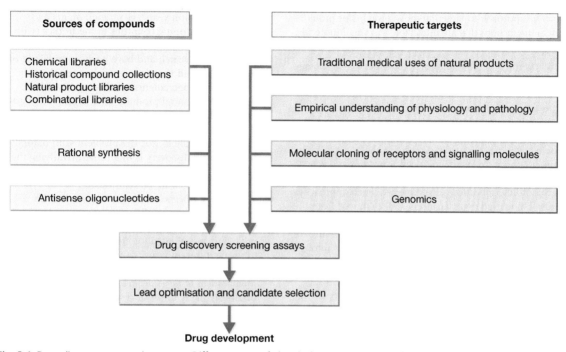

Fig. 3.1 Drug discovery sources in context. Different types of chemical compounds *(top left)* are tested against bioassays that are relevant to therapeutic targets, which are derived from several possible sources of information *(right)*. The initial lead compounds discovered by the screening process are optimised by analogue synthesis and tested for appropriate pharmacokinetic properties. The candidate compounds then enter the development process involving regulatory toxicology studies and clinical trials.

is only lack of technology that has hitherto prevented the exploitation of proteins (and peptides) as medicines. This technology is now available, and some of the most successful new medicines of the last few years have been biological – antibodies or peptides. The practical limitations are that (1) they need to be injected, as they are digested when swallowed and (2) they target soluble factors and targets on the cell membrane but are generally unable to target intracellular proteins. However, these limitations are offset by their high degree of specificity, their often very long half-life (for antibodies) that means that the medicine may be given by monthly injections, and the more predictable toxicity when compared to the rather unpredictable effect of classical small-molecule drugs (the usual 'white pills'). Biotechnology involves the use of recombinant DNA technology/genetic engineering to clone and express human genes, for example in microbial (*Escherichia coli* or yeast) cells so that they manufacture proteins. Such techniques can deliver hormones and autacoids in commercial amounts (such as insulin and growth hormone, erythropoietins, cell growth factors and plasminogen activators, interferons, vaccines and – probably most important – antibodies, for example for the treatment of cancers and inflammatory diseases).

Transgenic animals (that breed true for the gene) are also used as models for human disease as well as for production of medicines.

Human cell systems – increasingly human cells systems are used for drug discovery. This approach is particularly valuable when specific genetic changes can be made to mimic disease change. Cells can also be grown in 'organoids' that mimic some of the features of specific organs. Phenotypic screening, the process of screening molecules in cell models and then working backwards to find the molecular target, is becoming a much more common approach.

Antisense approaches. Nucleic acid approaches are being developed to silence gene expression and therefore reduce the expression of culprit proteins. There are various ways of achieving this including antisense, locked nucleic acids, small interfering RNAs and interfering with microRNAs. The problems are (1) delivery – they are injectables, (2) the distribution in the body – mainly liver and kidney, and (3) the difficulty in getting the nucleic acid into cells. Nonetheless, where the treatment aim is local (intraocular injection or inhalation to the lung), or where a liver effect is desired, it is clear that this approach works and provides a potentially attractive approach to targeting those proteins or protein–protein interactions that are intractable to a small molecule, peptide or antibody approach.

Gene therapy of human genetic disorders is 'a strategy in which nucleic acid, usually in the form of DNA, is administered to modify the genetic repertoire for therapeutic purposes', e.g. in diseases caused by single gene defects. Once again significant problems remain, in particular the methods of delivery and the safety and efficiency of the vectors used to deliver the genes. So far success has been seen in the treatment of certain rare haemopoetic disorders and genetic immunodeficiency states where the gene transfer can be done ex vivo and the modified cells reinjected. Such approaches are also being used to treat cancers. Cells removed from the body can be manipulated either to express a new gene or to modify expression of a gene and then the cells re-infused. Successful treatment of some haematological cancers through use of genetically modified T lymphocytes suggests that this will become a new type of 'drug treatment'.

Stem cells. Stem cells are impacting drug discovery as they potentially provide a source of human cells, or even disease-specific human cells that can be used for screening and safety testing. Stem cell therapy is a reality in the form of bone marrow transplants, but in other areas is still at a very early stage. However, the promise is of regenerative treatments based either on stem cell replacement or chemical stimulation of endogenous stem cells.

Immunopharmacology. Understanding of the molecular basis of immune responses has allowed the definition of mechanisms by which cellular function is altered by a legion of local hormones or autacoids in, for example, infections, cancer, autoimmune diseases, or organ transplant rejection. These processes present targets for therapeutic intervention – hence the rise of immunopharmacology. Stimulation of the immune system has become an important way to treat certain types of cancer. So manipulation of specific parts of the immune system to achieve activation or suppression is an important therapeutic approach.

Older approaches to the discovery of new medicines that continue in use include:

- *Animal models of human disease* or an aspect of it of varying relevance to humans. It is always the case that the animal model is never a true model of human disease and can only model parts of the disease process. The trend in industry is to use more human tissue and cell approaches, move fast to the clinic and not to rely too heavily on animal models.
- *Natural products*: modern technology for screening has revived interest and intensified the search. Companies look across the world for leads from microorganisms (in soil or sewage or even from insects entombed in amber 40 million years ago), fungi, plants and animals. Developing countries in the tropics (with their luxuriant natural resources) are prominent targets in this search and have justly complained of exploitation and many now require formal profit-sharing agreements to allow such searches. Historically, natural products have been particularly successful for finding antibiotics, as evolution has done over a much longer time period what medicinal chemists struggle to do. The problem with natural product drug discovery is often that identifying the precise active ingredient is hard and the molecules usually cannot easily be synthesised.
- *Traditional medicine,* which is being studied for possible leads to usefully active compounds. This is particularly true in China where traditional medicines are being re-evaluated for effects. The most notable example in recent years is the rediscovery of artemisinin for malaria treatment.
- *Modifications of the structures of known drugs*: these are obviously likely to produce more agents with similar basic properties, but may deliver worthwhile improvements. It is in this area that the 'me too' and 'me again' drugs are developed. However, such approaches are very unlikely to be commercially successful in a world that rightly demands true advances in patient care as a prerequisite for making profits and charging high costs to cover the price of innovative discovery.
- New *uses for drugs already in general use* as a result of intelligent observation and serendipity,[8] or advancing knowledge of molecular mechanisms, e.g. aspirin for antithrombotic effect. Once a good drug is on the market, new uses are often discovered. A recent example is rituximab, a monoclonal antibody that kills B cells. Initially developed for the treatment of B cell lymphoma, it was found to be effective for suppressing B cell autoimmunity in diseases such as rheumatoid arthritis.

Drug quality

It is easy for an investigator or prescriber, interested in pharmacology, toxicology and therapeutics, to forget the fundamental importance of chemical and pharmaceutical aspects. An impure, unstable drug or formulation is useless. Pure drugs that remain pure drugs after 5 years of storage

---

[8]Serendipity is the faculty of making fortunate discoveries by general sagacity or by accident; the word derives from a fairytale about three princes of Serendip (Sri Lanka) who had this happy faculty.

in hot, damp climates are vital to therapeutics. The record of manufacturers in providing this is impressive. Much of the early work in drug discovery is spent trying to identify the right molecule with the appropriate physical and chemical properties to make it reliable as a medicine.

Studies in animals[9]

Generally, the following are undertaken:

Pharmacodynamics – to investigate the *actions* relating to the proposed therapeutic use. In addition, there is a need to investigate potential undesirable pharmacodynamic effects of the substance on physiological functions.

Pharmacokinetics – the study of the *fate* of the active substance and its metabolites within the organism (absorption, distribution, metabolism and excretion of these substances). The programme should be designed to allow comparison and extrapolation between animal and human.

Toxicology – to reveal physiological and/or histopathological changes induced by the drug, and to determine how these changes relate to dose.[10] These involve:

- Acute toxicity: single-dose studies that allow qualitative and quantitative assessment of toxic reactions.
- Chronic and subchronic toxicity: repeat-dose studies to characterise the toxicological profile of a drug following repeated administration. This includes the identification of potential target organs and exposure–response relationships, and may include the potential for reversibility of effects.

Generally, it is desirable that tests be performed in two relevant species, based on the pharmacokinetic profile, one a rodent and one a non-rodent. The duration of the studies depends on the conditions of clinical use and is defined by Regulatory Agencies (Tables 3.1 and 3.2).

---

[9]Mouse, rat, hamster, guinea-pig, rabbit, cat, dog, and sometimes monkey are used (but not all for any one drug). Non-clinical (pharmacotoxicological) studies must be carried out in conformity with the provisions of internationally agreed standards known as Good Laboratory Practice (GLP). In Europe, regulations ensure that all tests on animals are conducted in accordance with Council Directive 86/609/EEC. Certain studies in animals can be substituted by validated in vitro tests provided that the test results are of comparable quality and usefulness for the purpose of safety evaluation. The pharmacological and toxicological tests must demonstrate the potential toxicity of the product and any dangerous or undesirable toxic effects that may occur under the proposed conditions of use in human beings; these should be evaluated in relation to the pathological condition concerned. The studies must also demonstrate the pharmacological properties of the product, in both qualitative and quantitative relationship to the proposed use in human beings.
[10]Details can be found at: http://www.ema.europa.eu/.

Table 3.1 Single and repeated dose toxicity requirements to support studies in healthy normal volunteers (Phase 1) and in patients (Phase 2) in the European Union (EU), and Phases 1, 2 and 3 in the USA and Japan[1]

Duration of clinical trial	Minimum duration of repeated-dose toxicity studies	
	Rodents	Non-rodents
Single dose	2 weeks[2]	2 weeks
Up to 2 weeks	2 weeks	2 weeks
Up to 1 month	1 month	1 month
Up to 3 months	3 months	3 months
Up to 6 months	6 months	6 months
>6 months	6 months	Chronic[3]

[1]In Japan, if there are no Phase 2 clinical trials of equivalent duration to the planned Phase 3 trials, conduct of longer-duration toxicity studies is recommended as given in Table 3.2.
[2]In the USA, specially designed single-dose studies with extended examinations can support single-dose clinical studies.
[3]Regulatory authorities may request a 12-month study or accept a 6-month study, determined on a case-by-case basis.

Table 3.2 Repeated-dose toxicity requirements to support Phase 3 studies in the EU, and marketing in all regions[1]

Duration of clinical trial	Minimum duration of repeated-dose toxicity studies	
	Rodents	Non-rodents
Up to 2 weeks	1 month	1 month
Up to 1 month	3 months	3 months
Up to 3 months	6 months	3 months
>3 months	6 months	Chronic[2]

[1]When a chronic non-rodent study is recommended if clinical use more than 1 month.
[2]Regulatory authorities may request a 12-month study or accept a 6-month study, determined on a case-by-case basis.

Genotoxicity – to reveal the changes that a drug may cause in the genetic material of individuals or cells. Mutagenic substances present a hazard to health because exposure carries the risk of inducing germline mutation (with the possibility of inherited disorders) and somatic mutations (including those leading to cancer). A standard battery of investigations includes: a test for gene mutation in bacteria (e.g. the Ames test); an in vitro test with cytogenetic evaluation of chromosomal damage with mammalian cells *or* an in vitro mouse lymphoma thymidine kinase (tk) assay; an in vivo test for chromosomal damage using rodent haematopoietic cells (e.g. the mouse micronucleus test).

Carcinogenicity – to reveal carcinogenic effects. These studies are performed for any medicinal product if its expected clinical use is prolonged (about 6 months), either continuously or repeatedly. These studies are also recommended if there is concern about their carcinogenic potential, e.g. from a product of the same class or similar structure, or from evidence in repeated-dose toxicity studies. Studies with unequivocally genotoxic compounds are not needed, as they are presumed to be trans-species carcinogens, implying a hazard to humans.

Reproductive and developmental toxicity – these tests study effects on adult male or female reproductive function, toxic and teratogenic effects at all stages of development from conception to sexual maturity and latent effects, when the medicinal product under investigation has been administered to the female during pregnancy. Embryo/fetal toxicity studies are normally conducted on two mammalian species, one a non-rodent. If the metabolism of a drug in a particular species is known to be similar to that in humans, it is usual to include this species. Studies in juvenile animals may also be required prior to developing drugs for use in children.

Local tolerance – to ascertain whether drugs are tolerated at sites in the body at which they may come into contact in clinical use. The testing strategy is such that any mechanical effects of administration or purely physicochemical actions of the product can be distinguished from toxicological or pharmacodynamic ones.

Biotechnology-derived pharmaceuticals – present a special case, and the standard regimen of toxicology studies is not appropriate. The choice of species used depends on the expression of the relevant receptor. If no suitable species exists, homologous proteins or transgenic animals expressing the human receptor may be studied and additional immunological studies are required. The study of biopharmaceutical safety provides challenges different from small molecules. Whereas the promiscuity of small molecules can lead to unexpected scaffold-related toxicity, this is usually not the case for biopharmaceuticals. But biopharmaceuticals may produce very different kinetics, binding and immunological effects in different species and therefore predictions of receptor occupancy and detailed analysis of immunological differences between species become of key importance. Sometimes antibody treatments need to be tested in primates as rodents and other species may not respond to the agent.

A new challenge in toxicology is how to consider effects of nucleic acid and gene therapies. The latter present a particular challenge as gene insertion may cause disruption of normal genes and can increase the chance of inducing cancer-promoting mutations.

Ethics and legislation

Controversy surrounding the use of animals in scientific research is not new. The renowned Islamic physician Avicenna (980–1037) was aware of the issues for he held that 'the experimentation must be done with the human body, for testing a drug on a lion or a horse might not prove anything about its effect on man'.[11] Leonardo da Vinci (1452–1519) predicted that one day experimentation on animals would be judged a crime, but Descartes[12] asserted that 'Animals do not speak, therefore they do not think, therefore they do not feel'. Later, Jeremy Bentham (1748–1832), the founding father of utilitarian philosophy, asked of animals: 'The question is not, Can they reason? nor Can they talk? but Can they suffer?'.

In our present world, billions of animals are raised to provide food and many to be used for scientific experiments. The arguments that evolve from this activity centre on the extent to which non-human animals can be respected as sentient beings of moral worth, albeit with differences among species. In recent years, a boisterous animal rights movement, asserting the moral status of animals, has challenged their use as experimental subjects.[13] Mainstream medical and scientific opinion around the world accepts that animal research continues to be justified, subject to important protections. This position is based on the insight that research involving animals has contributed hugely to advances in biological knowledge that have in turn allowed modern therapeutics to improve human morbidity and mortality. However, each experiment must be justified and its results must be expected to deliver insight into safety or efficacy. Animal models do contribute to the understanding of human physiology and disease because we share so many biological

---

[11]Bull J P 1959 The historical development of clinical therapeutic trials. Journal of Chronic Diseases 10:218–248.
[12]René Descartes (1596–1650), French philosopher, mathematician and scientist, acknowledged as one of the chief architects of the modern age.
[13]The publication of *Animal Liberation* (New York: New York Review/ Random House) by Peter Singer in 1975 is widely regarded as having provided its moral foundation.

characteristics, and a medicine when introduced into the organism is exposed to a vast array of conditions that we do not fully understand and are unable to reproduce outside the living body. The study of a drug in the whole organism remains an essential step in the process of discovery and development of medicines.

Safety testing in animals is at present the only reliable way to evaluate risks before undertaking clinical trials of potentially useful medicines in humans. The investigation of reproductive effects and potential carcinogenicity would not be undertaken in humans for both ethical and practical reasons. Animal testing eliminates many unsafe test materials before clinical testing on humans and minimises the risk of possible adverse effects when people are exposed to potential new medicines. In other words, experiments in animal models provide a critical safety check on candidate drugs; potentially hazardous or ineffective drugs can be eliminated, and for those drugs that do progress to clinical trials, target organs identified in animal studies can be monitored.

Animal research has contributed to virtually every area of medical research, and almost all best known drug and surgical treatments of the past and present owe their origins in some way to evidence from animals. The antibacterial effectiveness of penicillin was proved in tests on mice. Insulin came about because of research on rabbits and dogs in the 1920s. Polio-myelitis epidemics, which until the 1950s killed and paralysed millions of children, were consigned to history by vaccines resulting from studies on a range of laboratory animals, including monkeys. Major heart surgery, such as coronary artery bypass grafts and heart transplants, was developed through research on dogs and pigs. The BCG vaccine for tuberculosis was developed through research on rats and mice. Meningitis due to *Haemophilus influenzae* type b, formerly common especially in children, is now almost unknown in the UK because of a vaccine developed through work on mice and rabbits. Almost all of the highly effective drug treatments we currently use were developed using animals: β-adrenoceptor blockers, angiotensin-converting enzyme inhibitors, cytotoxics, analgesics, psychotropics and so on.

Given this evidence, there is broad public support for the position that experiments on animals are a regrettable necessity that should be limited to what is deemed essential while alternatives are developed. In the UK, for example, this reservation is expressed in progressively more stringent legislation. The Animals (Scientific Procedures) Act 1986 makes it an offence to carry out any scientific procedure on animals except under licence, the requirements of which include that:

- animals are only used as a last resort.
- every practical step is taken to avoid distress or suffering.

- the smallest possible number of animals is used.
- the potential benefits have to be weighed against the cost to the animals; the simplest or least sentient species is used.
- the work is realistic and achievable, and the programme designed in the way most likely to produce satisfactory results.
- the results must impact the decision-making process for discovery or development of the medicine.

Despite the continued necessity of animal studies in drug discovery and development, there is now a very clear aim to move medicines into the clinic as soon as safely possible. Detailed clinical experimentation is often a better way to sort out questions related to effects on human biology and pharmacokinetics.

Safety prediction

Knowledge of the *mode of action* of a potential new drug obviously greatly enhances prediction from animal studies of what will happen in humans. Whenever practicable, such knowledge should be obtained; sometimes this is quite easy, but sometimes it is impossible. Many drugs have been introduced safely without such knowledge, the later acquisition of which has not always made an important difference to their use (e.g. antimicrobials). Pharmacological studies are integrated with those of the toxicologist to build up a picture of the undesired as well as the desired drug effects.

In *pharmacological testing*, the investigators know what they are looking for and choose the experiments to gain their objectives.

In *toxicological testing*, the investigators have a less clear idea of what they are looking for; they are screening for risk, unexpected as well as predicted, and certain major routines must be done. Toxicity testing is therefore liable to become a routine to meet regulatory requirements to a greater extent than the pharmacological studies. The predictive value of special toxicology (above) is particularly controversial. All drugs are poisons if enough is given, and the task of the toxicologist is to find out whether, where and how a compound acts as a poison to animals, and to give an opinion on the significance of the data in relation to risks likely to be run by human beings. This will remain a nearly impossible task until molecular explanations of all effects can be provided.

Toxicologists are in an unenviable position. When a useful drug is safely introduced, they are considered to have done no more than their duty. When an accident occurs, they are invited to explain how this failure of prediction came about. When they predict that a chemical is unsafe in a major way for humans, this prediction is never tested. The easiest decision to make in drug discovery is to stop a project, and it is the only decision that can never be shown to be wrong. However, it is also a decision that may deny the world a new and effective medicine.

Orphan drugs and diseases

A free-market economy is liable to leave untreated both rare diseases, e.g. some cancers (in all countries), and some common diseases, e.g. parasitic infections (in poor countries).

In order to stimulate drug discovery and development in rare diseases, legislation in some countries has provided specific incentives to industry to develop medicines for 'orphan diseases'. Interestingly, many rare diseases are monogenic and the cause is clear. This, unlike most common diseases, means that the drug target is absolutely clear. In view of the greater certainty around cause, the smaller clinical trials and the more receptive regulatory environment, several pharmaceutical companies are working assiduously in this area. It is also the case that some rare diseases give significant insights into common diseases and how to approach them. The natural accidents of nature that cause a rare disease through a genetic change will often give an insight into a pathway or phenotype that has relevance to understanding common diseases. Many of the new approaches such as gene therapy also tend to be applied first in severe rare diseases.

Guide to further reading

Dollery, C.T., 2007. Beyond genomics. Clin. Pharmacol. Ther. 82 (2), 366–370.

Evans, W.E., Relling, M.V., 2004. Moving towards individualized medicine with pharmacogenomics. Nature 429, 464–468.

Garattini, S., Chalmers, I., 2009. Patients and the public deserve big changes in the evaluation of drugs. Br. Med. J. 338, 804–806.

Lean, M.E.J., Mann, J.I., Hoek, J.A., et al., 2008. Translational research. Br. Med. J. 337, 705–706.

Lesko, L.J., 2007. Personalized medicine: elusive dream or imminent reality? Clin. Pharmacol. Ther. 81 (6), 807–816.

MacPherson, R., 2015. The curious stories of drugs with two lives: a new paradigm in drug development. J. Roy. Soc. Med. 108 (7), 255–258.

Meyer, U.A., 2004. Pharmacogenetics – five decades of therapeutic lessons from genetic diversity. Nat. Rev. Genet. 5 (9), 669–676.

Pound, P., Ebrahim, S., Sandercock, P., et al., 2004. Where is the evidence that animal research benefits humans? Br. Med. J. 328, 514–517.

Vallance, P., Levick, M., 2007. Drug discovery and development in the age of molecular medicine. Clin. Pharmacol. Ther. 82 (2), 363–365.

Weinshilboum, R., Wang, L., 2004. Pharmacogenomics: bench to bedside. Nat. Rev. Drug Discov. 3 (9), 739–748.

Chapter | 4 |

Evaluation of drugs in humans

Ian Hudson, June Raine

SYNOPSIS

This chapter is about evidence-based drug therapy.

New drugs are progressively introduced by clinical pharmacological studies in rising numbers of healthy and/or patient volunteers until sufficient information has been gained to justify formal therapeutic studies. Each of these is usually a randomised controlled trial (RCT), in which a precisely framed question is posed and answered by treating equivalent groups of patients in different ways.

The key to the ethics of such studies is informed consent from patients, efficient scientific design and review by an independent research ethics committee. In an age of transparency, regulation and publication are key interpretative factors in the analysis of trial results as are calculations of confidence intervals and statistical significance. Potential clinical significance develops within the confines of controlled clinical trials. This is best expressed by stating not only the percentage differences, but also the absolute difference or its reciprocal, the number of patients who have to be treated to obtain one desired outcome.

Surveillance studies and the reporting of spontaneous adverse reactions respectively determine the clinical profile of the drug and detect rare adverse events. Further trials to compare new medicines with existing medicines are also required. These form the basis of cost-effectiveness comparisons.

Topics include:

- **Experimental therapeutics.**
- **Ethics of research.**
- **Rational introduction of a new drug.**
- **Need for statistics.**
- **Types of trial: design, size.**
- **Meta-analysis.**
- **Pharmacoepidemiology.**

Experimental therapeutics

After preclinical evidence of efficacy and safety have been obtained in animals, potential medicines are tested in healthy volunteers and volunteer patients. Studies in healthy normal volunteers can help to determine the safety, tolerability, pharmacokinetics and, for some drugs (e.g. anticoagulants and anaesthetic agents), their dynamic effect and likely dose range. For many drugs, the dynamic effect and hence therapeutic potential can be investigated only in patients, e.g. drugs for parkinsonism will have no measurable efficacy in subjects without the relevant movement disorder.

Modern medicine is sometimes accused of dispassionate application of science to human problems and of subordinating the interest of the individual to those of the group (society).[1] Official regulatory bodies rightly require scientific

---

[1] Guidance to researchers in this matter is clear. The World Medical Association Declaration of Helsinki (Edinburgh revision 2000) states that 'considerations related to the well-being of the human subject should take precedence over the interests of science and society'. The General Assembly of the United Nations adopted in 1966 the International Covenant on Civil and Political Rights, of which Article 7 states, 'In particular, no one shall be subjected without his free consent to medical or scientific experimentation'. This means that subjects are entitled to know that they are being entered into research even though the research is thought to be 'harmless'. But there are people who cannot give (informed) consent, e.g. the demented. The need for special procedures for such is now recognised, for there is a consensus that, without research, they and the diseases from which they suffer will become therapeutic 'orphans'.

evaluation of drugs. Drug developers need to satisfy the official regulators, and they also seek to persuade the medical profession to prescribe their products. Patients, too, are more aware of the comparative advantages and limitations of their medicines than they used to be. To some extent, this helps encourage patients to participate in trials so that future patients can benefit, as they do now, from the knowledge gained from such trials. An ethical framework is required to ensure that the interests of the individual participant are protected (and, more obviously, those of an individual or corporate investigator).

Research involving human subjects

The definition of research continues to present difficulties. The distinction between medical research and innovative medical practice derives from the intent. In medical practice the sole intention is to benefit the individual patient consulting the clinician, not to gain knowledge of general benefit, though such knowledge may incidentally emerge from the clinical experience gained. In medical research the primary intention is to advance knowledge so that patients in general may benefit; the individual patient may or may not benefit directly.[2]

Consider also the process of *audit*, which is used extensively to assess performance, e.g. by individual health-care workers, by departments within hospitals or between hospitals. Audit is a systematic examination designed to determine the degree to which an action or set of actions achieves predetermined standards. Research seeks to address 'known unknowns' and often discovers 'unknown unknowns,[3] audit is limited to the monitoring of 'known knowns': maybe important, but clearly limited.

Ethics of research in humans[4]

Some dislike the word 'experiment' in relation to humans, in what is done. It is better that all should recognise from the true meaning of the word, 'to ascertain or establish by trial',[5] that the benefits of modern medicine derive almost wholly from experimentation and that some risk is inseparable from much medical advance.

The issue of (adequately informed) *consent* is a principal concern for Research Ethics Committees (also called Institutional Review Boards). People have the right to choose for themselves whether or not they will participate in research, i.e. they have the right to self-determination (the ethical principle of *autonomy*). They should be given whatever information is necessary for making an adequately informed choice (consent) with the right to withdraw at any stage. Consent procedures, especially information on risks, are of central importance in research. This is appropriate given that in research, patients may be submitting themselves to extra risks, or simply to extra inconvenience (e.g. more or longer visits). It is a moot point whether more consent in routine practice might not go amiss. It is also likely that patients participating in well-conducted trials receive more, and sometimes better, care and attention than might otherwise be available. Sometimes the unintended consequences of ethical procedures include causing unnecessary apprehension to patients with long, legalistic documents, and creating a false impression of clinical researchers as people from whom patients need protection.

The moral obligation of all doctors lies in ensuring that in their desire to help patients (the ethical principle of *beneficence*) they should never allow themselves to put the individual who has sought their aid at any disadvantage (the ethical principle of *non-maleficence*).[6]

In principle, it may be thought proper to perform a therapeutic trial only when doctors (and patients) have genuine uncertainty as to which treatment is best.[7] Not all trials are comparisons of different treatments. Some, especially early-phase trials of new drugs, are comparisons of different doses. Comparisons of new with old should usually offer patients the chance of receiving current best treatment with one which might be better. Since this is often rather more than is offered in resource-constrained routine care, the obligatory patient information sheet mantra that 'the decision whether to take part has no bearing on your usual care' may be an over-simplification. But it is also simplistic to view the main purpose of all trials with medicines as comparative.

---

[2]Report: Royal College of Physicians of London 1996 Guidelines on the Practice of Ethics Committees in Medical Research Involving Human Subjects. Royal College of Physicians, London.
[3]American Defence Secretary Donald Rumsfeld, on 12 February 2002, at a press briefing where he addressed the absence of evidence linking the government of Iraq with the supply of weapons of mass destruction to terrorist groups.
[4]For extensive practical detail, see Council for International Organisations of Medical Sciences (CIOMS) in collaboration with the World Health Organization (WHO) 2002 International Ethical Guidelines for Biomedical Research Involving Human Subjects. CIOMS, Geneva. (WHO publications are available in all UN member countries.) See also: Guideline for Good Clinical Practice, International Conference on Harmonisation Tripartite Guideline. EU Committee on Proprietary Medicinal Products (CPMP/ICH/135/95). Smith T 1999 Ethics in Medical Research: A Handbook of Good Practice. Cambridge University Press, Cambridge.

[5]*Oxford English Dictionary*. See also: Edwards M 2004 Historical keywords: Trial. Lancet 364:1659.
[6]Kety S. Quoted by Beecher H K 1959 Journal of the American Medical Association 169:461.
[7]This is the uncertainty principle: the concept that patients entering a randomised therapeutic trial will have equal potential for benefit and risk is referred to as *equipoise*.

The past decade has seen the pharmaceutical industry make great efforts to match the pace of new understanding about disease pathogenesis, and models of research are being adapted to the complexity of common disease that is now apparent. In diseases where many good medicines already exist, the industry spent much time developing minor modifications which were broadly equivalent to current therapy with possible advantages for some patients. With many of the standard blockbusters now off patent, new drugs for such diseases are unattractive, and the industry is concentrating more on harder therapeutic targets where no satisfactory treatment yet exists. Just as in basic science, non–hypothesis-led 'fishing expedition' research – genome wide association studies, microarrays – is no longer frowned upon, so the imaginative clinical investigator must throw his stone – a new medicine – into the pond, and be able to make sense of the ripples. One such approach is to move away from trial design in which the average response of the group is of interest towards the design in which the investigator attempts to match differences in response to differences – ethnic, gender, genetic – among the patients. Matches at a molecular level give clues both to how the drug may best be used, and who will benefit most. Other types of new approach are referred to as 'umbrella and basket trials', 'real world trials' and 'novel endpoints'.

The ethics of the randomised and placebo-controlled trial

Providing that ethical surveillance is rooted in the ethical principles of *justice*,[8] there should be no difficulty in clinical research adapting to current needs. And even if the nature of early phase research is changing, the randomised controlled trial (RCT) will remain the cornerstone of how cause and effect is proven in clinical practice, and how drugs demonstrate the required degree of efficacy and safety to obtain a licence for their marketing.

The use of a placebo (or dummy) raises both ethical and scientific issues (see *placebo medicines* and the *placebo effect*, Ch. 2). There are clear-cut cases when placebo use would be ethically unacceptable and scientifically unnecessary, e.g. drug trials in epilepsy and tuberculosis, when control groups comprise patients receiving the best available therapy.

The pharmacologically inert (placebo) treatment arm of a trial is useful:

---

[8]The 'four principles' approach (above) is widely utilised in biomedical ethics. A full description and an analysis of the contribution of this and other ethical theories to decision making in clinical, including research, practice can be found in: Beauchamp T L, Childress J F 2013 Principles of Biomedical Ethics, 7th edn. Oxford University Press, Oxford.

- To distinguish the *pharmacodynamic effects* of a drug from the psychological effects of the act of medication and the circumstances surrounding it, e.g. increased interest by the doctor, more frequent visits, for these latter may have their placebo effect. Placebo responses have been reported in 30–50% of patients with depression and in 30–80% with chronic stable angina pectoris.
- To distinguish *drug effects* from natural fluctuations in disease that occur with time, e.g. with asthma or hay fever, and other external factors, provided active treatment, if any, can be ethically withheld. This is also called the 'assay sensitivity' of the trial.
- To avoid *false conclusions*. The use of placebos is valuable in Phase 1 healthy volunteer studies of novel drugs to help determine whether minor but frequently reported adverse events are drug related or not. Although a placebo treatment can pose ethical problems, it is often preferable to the continued use of treatments of unproven efficacy or safety. The ethical dilemma of subjects suffering as a result of receiving a placebo (or ineffective drug) can be overcome by designing clinical trials that provide mechanisms to allow them to be withdrawn ('escape') when defined criteria are reached, e.g. blood pressure above levels that represent treatment failure. Similarly, placebo (or new drug) can be added against a background of established therapy; this is called the 'add on' design.
- To provide a result using *fewer research subjects*. The difference in response when a test drug is compared with a placebo is likely to be greater than that when a test drug is compared with the best current, i.e. active, therapy (see later).

Investigators who propose to use a placebo, or otherwise withhold effective treatment, should justify their intention. The variables to consider are:

- The severity of the disease.
- The effectiveness of standard therapy.
- Whether the novel drug under test aims to give only symptomatic relief, or has the potential to prevent or slow up an irreversible event, e.g. stroke or myocardial infarction.
- The length of treatment.
- The objective of the trial (equivalence, superiority or non-inferiority; see p. 45). Thus it may be quite ethical to compare a novel analgesic against placebo for 2 weeks in the treatment of osteoarthritis of the hip (with escape analgesics available). It would not be ethical to use a placebo alone as comparator in a 6-month trial of a novel drug in active rheumatoid arthritis, even with escape analgesia.

The precise use of the placebo will depend on the study design, e.g. whether crossover, when all patients receive placebo at some point in the trial, or parallel group, when only one cohort receives placebo. Generally, patients easily understand the concept of distinguishing between the imagined effects of treatment and those due to a direct action on the body. Provided research subjects are properly informed and give consent freely, they are not the subject of deception in any ethical sense; but a patient given a placebo in the absence of consent is deceived, and research ethics committees will, rightly, decline to agree to this. (See also: Lewis et al (2002) in Guide to further reading, at the end of this chapter.)

Injury to research subjects[9]

The question of compensation for accidental (physical) injury due to participation in research is a vexed one. Plainly there are substantial differences between the position of healthy volunteers (whether or not they are paid) and that of patients who may benefit and, in some cases, who may be prepared to accept even serious risk for the chance of gain. There is no simple answer. But the topic must always be addressed in any research carrying risk, including the risk of withholding known effective treatment. The CIOMS/WHO Guidelines[4] state:

> *Research subjects who suffer physical injury as a result of their participation are entitled to such financial or other assistance as would compensate them equitably for any temporary or permanent impairment or disability. In the case of death, their dependants are entitled to material compensation. The right to compensation may not be waived.*
> *Therefore, when giving their informed consent to participate, research subjects should be told whether there is provision for compensation in case of physical injury, and the circumstances in which they or their dependants would receive it.*

---

[9]Injury to participants in clinical trials is uncommon, and serious injury is rare. In March 2006, eight healthy young men entered a trial of a humanised monoclonal antibody designed to be an agonist of a particular receptor on T lymphocytes that stimulates their production and activation. This was the first administration to humans; preclinical testing in rabbits and monkeys at doses up to 500 times those received by the volunteers apparently showed no ill effect. Six of the volunteers quickly became seriously ill and required admission to an intensive care facility with multi-organ failure due to a 'cytokine release syndrome', in effect a massive attack on the body's own tissues. All the volunteers recovered but some with disability. This toxicity in humans, despite apparent safety in animals, may be due to the specifically humanised nature of the monoclonal antibody. Testing of perceived high-risk new medicines is likely to be subject to particularly stringent regulation in future. See Wood A J, Darbyshire J 2006 Injury to research volunteers – the clinical research nightmare. New England Journal of Medicine 354:1869–1871.

Payment of subjects in clinical trials

Healthy volunteers are usually paid to take part in a clinical trial. The rationale is that they will not benefit from treatment received and should be compensated for discomfort and inconvenience. There is a fine dividing line between this and a financial inducement, but it is unlikely that more than a small minority of healthy volunteer studies would now take place without a 'fee for service' provision, including 'out of pocket' expenses. It is all the more important that the sums involved are commensurate with the invasiveness of the investigations and the length of the studies. The monies should be declared and agreed by the ethics committee.

There is an intuitive abreaction by physicians to pay patients (compared with healthy volunteers), because they feel the accusation of inducement or persuasion could be levelled at them, and because they assuage any feeling of taking advantage of the doctor–patient relationship by the hope that the medicines under test may be of benefit to the individual. This is not an entirely comfortable position.[10]

Rational introduction of a new drug to humans

When pre-clinical laboratory studies, in vitro and in animals, predict that a new molecule may be a useful medicine, i.e. effective and safe in relation to its benefits, then the time has come to put it to the test in humans. When a new chemical entity offers a possibility of doing something that has not been done before or of doing something familiar in a different or better way, it can be seen to be worth testing. But where it is a new member of a familiar class of drug, potential advantage may be harder to detect. Yet these 'me too' drugs are often worth testing. Prediction from animal studies of modest but useful clinical advantage is particularly uncertain and, therefore, if the new drug seems reasonably effective and safe in animals it is rational to test it in humans. From the commercial standpoint, the investment in the development of a new drug can currently be over £500 million, but will be substantially less for a 'me too' drug entering an already developed and profitable market.

Phases of clinical development

Human experiments progress in a commonsense manner that is conventionally divided into four phases (Fig. 4.1).

---

[10]Freedman B 1987 Equipoise and the ethics of clinical research. New England Journal of Medicine 317:141–145.

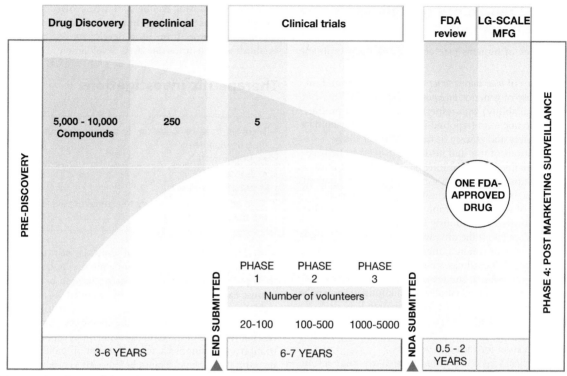

Fig. 4.1 The phases of drug discovery and development. *(With permission of Pharmaceutical Research and Manufacturers of America.)*

These phases are divisions of convenience in what is a continuous expanding process. It begins with a small number of subjects (healthy subjects and volunteer patients) closely observed in laboratory settings, and proceeds through hundreds of patients, to thousands before the drug is agreed to be a medicine by a national or international regulatory authority. It is then licensed for either general or restricted licensable prescribing (though this is by no means the end of the evaluation). The process may be abandoned at any stage for a variety of reasons, including poor tolerability or safety, inadequate efficacy and commercial pressures. The phases are:

* *Phase 1. Human pharmacology* (20–50 subjects): healthy volunteers or volunteer patients, according to the class of drug and its safety:
  * pharmacokinetics (absorption, distribution, metabolism, excretion)
  * pharmacodynamics (biological effects) where practicable, tolerability, safety, efficacy.
* *Phase 2. Therapeutic exploration* (50–300 subjects):
  * patients

* pharmacokinetics and pharmacodynamic dose ranging, in carefully controlled studies for efficacy and safety,[11] which may involve comparison with placebo.
* *Phase 3. Therapeutic confirmation* (RCTs; 250–1000+ subjects):
  * patients
  * efficacy on a substantial scale; safety; comparison either with placebo of current standard of care. with.
* *Phase 4. Therapeutic use* (pharmacovigilance, post-licensing studies) (2000–10 000 + subjects):
  * surveillance for safety and efficacy: further formal therapeutic trials, especially comparisons with other drugs, marketing studies and pharmacoeconomic studies.

---

[11]Moderate to severe adverse events have occurred in about 0.5% of healthy subjects. See Orme M, Harry J, Routledge P, Hobson S 1989 British Journal of Clinical Pharmacology 27:125; Sibille M et al 1992 European Journal of Clinical Pharmacology 42:393.

Official regulatory guidelines and requirements[12]

For studies in humans (see also Ch. 6) these ordinarily include:

- Studies of *pharmacokinetics* and *bioavailability* and, in the case of generics, *bioequivalence* (equal bioavailability) with respect to the reference product.
- *Therapeutic trials* (reported in detail) that substantiate the safety and efficacy of the drug under likely conditions of use, and justify the dose(s) to be used in patients. A drug for long-term use in a common condition will require a total of at least 1000 patients (preferably more), depending on the therapeutic class, of which (for chronic diseases) at least 100 have been treated continuously for about 1 year.
- *Special groups*. If the drug will be used in, for example, the elderly or children, then these populations should be studied. New drugs are not normally studied in pregnant women. Studies in patients having disease that affects drug metabolism and elimination may be needed, such as patients with impaired liver or kidney function.
- *Fixed-dose combination* products will require explicit justification for each component.
- *Interaction studies* with other drugs likely to be taken simultaneously. Plainly, all possible combinations cannot be evaluated; a rational choice, based on knowledge of pharmacodynamics, metabolic route and pharmacokinetics, is made.
- The application for a licence for general use (marketing application) should include a draft Summary of Product Characteristics for prescribers. A Patient Information Leaflet must be submitted. These should include information on the form of the product (e.g. tablet, capsule, sustained-release, liquid), its uses, efficacy, dosage (adults, children, elderly where appropriate), contraindications, warnings and precautions (less strong), side effects/adverse reactions, overdose and how to treat it.

The emerging discipline of *pharmacogenomics* seeks to identify patients who will respond beneficially or adversely to a new drug by defining certain genotypic profiles.

---

[12]Guidelines for the conduct and analysis of a range of clinical trials in different therapeutic categories are released from time to time by the Committee on Medicinal Products for Human Use (CHMP) of the European Commission. These guidelines apply to drug development in the European Union. Other regulatory authorities issue guidance, e.g. the Food and Drug Administration in the USA, the Ministry of Health, Labour and Welfare in Japan. There has been considerable success in aligning different guidelines across the world through the International Conferences on Harmonisation (ICH). The source for CHMP guidelines is https://www.gov.uk/government/news/welcome-to-our-new-mhra-website.

Individualised dosing regimens may be evolved as a result (see p. 103). This tailoring of drugs to individuals is consuming huge resources from drug developers but has yet to establish a place in routine drug development.

Therapeutic investigations

There are three key questions to be answered during drug development:
- Does it work?
- Is it safe?
- What is the dose?

In addition, it is necessary to ascertain how best to use the drug, and in whom.

With few exceptions, none of these is easy to answer definitively within the confines of a pre-registration clinical trials programme. Efficacy and safety have to be balanced against each other. What may be regarded as acceptably 'safe' for a new oncology drug in advanced lung cancer would not be so regarded in the treatment of childhood eczema. The use of the term 'dose', without explanation, is irrational as it implies a single dose for all patients. Pharmaceutical companies cannot be expected to produce a large array of different doses for each medicine, but the maxim to use the smallest effective dose that results in the desired effect holds true. Some drugs require titration; others have a wide safety margin so that one 'high' dose may achieve optimal efficacy with acceptable safety. There are two classes of endpoint or outcome of a therapeutic investigation:

- The *therapeutic* effect itself (sleep, eradication of infection), i.e. the outcome.
- A *surrogate* effect, an early effect that can be reliably correlated with long-term therapeutic benefit, e.g. blood lipids or glucose or blood pressure, where improvement (usually reduction) predicts reduced risk of cardiovascular morbidity. A surrogate endpoint might also be a pharmacokinetic parameter, if it is indicative of the therapeutic effect, e.g. plasma concentration of an antiepileptic drug.

Use of surrogate effects presupposes that the disease process is fully understood. They are best justified in diseases for which the true therapeutic effect can be measured only by studies which involve large numbers of patients, and/or take many years. Such long-term outcome studies are indeed always preferable but may be impracticable on organisational, financial and sometimes ethical grounds prior to releasing new drugs for general prescription. It is in areas such as these that the techniques of large-scale surveillance for efficacy, as well as for safety, under conditions of ordinary

Table 4.1 Process of therapeutic evaluation

	Pre-registration		Post-registration	
	Pharmaceutical company	**Regulatory authority**	**Pharmaceutical company**	**Regulatory authority**
Purpose of therapeutic evaluation	To select best candidate for development and registration	To satisfy the regulatory authority on efficacy, safety and quality	To promote drug to expand the market	To add to indications (by variation to licence) and to add evolving safety information

use (below), would be needed to supplement the necessarily smaller and shorter formal therapeutic trials employing surrogate effects. Surrogate endpoints are of particular value in early drug development to select candidate drugs from a range of agents. In cases of unmet need, conditional approval may be provided for drugs on the basis of surrogate endpoints, pending results from larger or longer trials.

Therapeutic evaluation

The *aims* of therapeutic evaluation are three-fold:

1. To assess the efficacy, safety and quality of new drugs, either to meet clinical needs, or to supplement the existing drugs for a condition.[13]
2. To expand the indications for the use of current drugs (or generic drugs[14]) in clinical and marketing terms.
3. To protect public health over the lifetime of a given drug.

The *process* of therapeutic evaluation may be divided into pre- and post-registration phases (Table 4.1), the purposes of which are set out below.

When a new drug is being developed, the first therapeutic trials are devised to find out the best that the drug can do under conditions ideal for showing efficacy, e.g. uncomplicated disease of mild to moderate severity in patients taking no other drugs, with carefully supervised administration by specialist doctors. Interest lies particularly in patients who complete a full course of treatment. If the drug is ineffective in these circumstances, there is no point in proceeding with an expensive development programme. Such studies are sometimes called *explanatory trials* as they attempt to 'explain' why a drug works (or fails to work) in ideal conditions.

If the drug is found useful in these trials, it becomes desirable next to find out how closely the ideal may be approached in the uncontrolled environment of routine medical practice: in patients of all ages, at all stages of disease, with complications, taking other drugs and relatively unsupervised. Interest continues in all patients from the moment they are entered into the trial and it is maintained if they fail to complete, or even to start, the treatment; the need is to know the outcome in all patients deemed suitable for therapy, not only in those who successfully complete therapy.[15]

The reason some drop out may be related to aspects of the treatment, and it is usual to analyse these according to the clinicians' *initial* intention (*intention-to-treat analysis*), i.e. investigators are not allowed to risk introducing bias by exercising their own judgement as to who should or should not be excluded from the analysis. In these real-life, or 'naturalistic', conditions the drug may not perform so well, e.g. minor adverse effects may now cause patient non-compliance, which had been avoided by supervision and enthusiasm in the early trials. These naturalistic studies are sometimes called '*pragmatic*' trials.

The *methods* used to test the therapeutic value depend on the stage of development, who is conducting the study (a pharmaceutical company, or an academic body or health service at the behest of a regulatory authority), and the *primary endpoint* or *outcome* of the trial. The methods include:

- Formal therapeutic trials.
- Superiority, equivalence and non-inferiority trials.
- Safety surveillance methods.

Formal therapeutic trials are conducted during Phase 2 and Phase 3 of pre-registration development, and in the post-registration phase to test the drug in new indications. *Equivalence* trials aim to show the therapeutic equivalence of two treatments, usually the new drug under development

---

[13]The latter are often considered 'me-too' drugs, but can prove invaluable either in individual patients who do not tolerate the alternatives, or because of an apparently minor difference which subsequently proves of importance.

[14]A drug for which the original patent has expired, so that any pharmaceutical company may market it in competition with the inventor. The term 'generic' has come to be synonymous with the non-proprietary or approved name (see Ch. 7).

[15]Information on both categories (method effectiveness and use effectiveness) is valuable (Sheiner L B, Rubin D B 1995 Intention-to-treat analysis and the goals of clinical trials. Clinical Pharmacology and Therapeutics 57(1):6–15).

and an existing drug used as a standard active comparator. Equivalence trials may be conducted before or after registration for the first therapeutic indication of the new drug (see p. 47 below for further discussion). *Safety surveillance methods* use the principles of pharmacoepidemiology (see p. 52) and are concerned mainly with evaluating adverse events and especially rare events, which formal therapeutic trials are unlikely to detect.

Need for statistics

In order truly to know whether patients treated in one way are benefited more than those treated in another, it is essential to use statistical methods. *Statistics* has been defined as 'a body of methods for making wise decisions in the face of uncertainty'.[16] Used properly, they are tools of great value for promoting efficient therapy. More than 100 years ago Francis Galton saw this clearly:

> *The human mind is … a most imperfect apparatus for the elaboration of general ideas … In our general impressions far too great weight is attached to what is marvellous … Experience warns us against it, and the scientific man takes care to base his conclusions upon actual numbers … to devise tests by which the value of beliefs may be ascertained.*[17]

Concepts and terms

Hypothesis of no difference

When it is suspected that treatment A may be superior to treatment B, and the truth is sought, it is convenient to start with the proposition that the treatments are equally effective – the 'no difference' hypothesis *(null hypothesis)*. After two groups of patients have been treated and it has been found that improvement has occurred more often with one treatment than with the other, it is necessary to decide how likely it is that this difference is due to a real superiority of one treatment over the other.

To make this decision, we need to understand two major concepts, *statistical significance* and *confidence intervals*.

A statistical significance test[18] such as the Student's *t*-test or the chi-squared (χ^2) test will tell how often an observed difference would occur due to chance (random influences)

if there is, in reality, no difference between the treatments. Where the statistical significance test shows that an observed difference would occur only five times if the experiment were repeated 100 times, this is often taken as sufficient evidence that the null hypothesis is *unlikely* to be true. Therefore, the conclusion is that there is (probably) a real difference between the treatments. This level of probability is generally expressed in therapeutic trials as: 'the difference was statistically significant', or 'significant at the 5% level' or '*P* = 0.05' (*P* is the probability based on chance alone). Statistical significance simply means that the result is *unlikely* to have occurred if there was *no* genuine treatment difference, i.e. there probably *is* a difference.

If the analysis reveals that the observed difference, or greater, would occur only once if the experiment were repeated 100 times, the results are generally said to be 'statistically highly significant', or 'significant at the 1% level' or '*P* = 0.01'.

Confidence intervals. The problem with the *P* value is that it conveys no information on the *amount* of the differences observed or on the *range* of possible differences between treatments. A result that a drug produces a uniform 2% reduction in heart rate may well be statistically significant, but it is clinically meaningless. What doctors are interested to know is the *size* of the difference, and what degree of assurance (confidence) they may have in the *precision* (reproducibility) of this estimate. To obtain this, it is necessary to calculate a confidence interval (see Figs 4.2 and 4.3).[19]

A confidence interval expresses a range of values that contains the true value with 95% (or other chosen percentage) certainty. The range may be broad, indicating uncertainty, or narrow, indicating (relative) certainty. A wide confidence interval occurs when numbers are small or differences observed are variable and points to a lack of information, whether the difference is statistically significant or not; it is a warning against placing much weight on (or confidence in) the results of small or variable studies. Confidence intervals are extremely helpful in interpretation, particularly of small studies, as they show the degree of uncertainty related to a result. Their use in conjunction with non-significant results may be especially enlightening.[20]

A finding of 'not statistically significant' can be interpreted as meaning there is no clinically useful difference only if the confidence intervals for the results are also stated in the report and are narrow. If the confidence intervals are wide, a real difference may be missed in a trial with a small number of subjects, i.e. the absence of evidence that there is a

---

[16]Wallis W A, Roberts H V 1957 Statistics, A New Approach. Methuen, London.
[17]Galton F 1879 Generic images. Proceedings of the Royal Institution.
[18]Altman D G, Gore S M, Gardner M J, Pocock S J 1983 Statistical guidelines for contributors to medical journals. British Medical Journal 286:1489–1493.

[19]Gardner M J, Altman D G 1986 Confidence intervals rather than P values: estimation rather than hypothesis testing. British Medical Journal 292:746–750.
[20]Altman D G, Gore S M, Gardner M J, Pocock S J 1983 Statistical guidelines for contributors to medical journals. British Medical Journal 286:1489–1493.

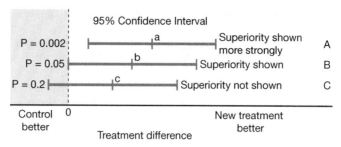

Fig. 4.2 Relationship between significance tests and confidence intervals for the comparisons between a new treatment and control. The treatment differences a, b, c are all in favour of 'New treatment', but superiority is shown only in A and B. In C, superiority has not been shown. This may be because the effect is small and not detected. The result, nevertheless, is compatible with equivalence or non-inferiority. Adequate precision and power are assumed for all the trials.

difference is not the same as showing that there is no difference. Small numbers of patients inevitably give low precision and low power to detect differences.

Types of error

The above discussion provides us with information on the likelihood of falling into one of the two principal kinds of error in therapeutic experiments, for the hypothesis that there is no difference between treatments may either be accepted incorrectly or rejected incorrectly.

Type I error (α) is the finding of a difference between treatments when in reality they do not differ, i.e. *rejecting* the null hypothesis incorrectly. Investigators decide the degree of this error which they are prepared to tolerate on a scale in which 0 indicates complete rejection of the null hypothesis and 1 indicates its complete acceptance; clearly the level for α must be set near to 0. This is the same as the significance level of the statistical test used to detect a difference between treatments. Thus α (or $P = 0.05$) indicates that the investigators will accept a 5% chance that an observed difference is not a real difference.

Type II error (β) is the finding of no difference between treatments when in reality they do differ, i.e. *accepting* the null hypothesis incorrectly. The probability of detecting this error is often given wider limits, e.g. $\beta = 0.1$–0.2, which indicates that the investigators are willing to accept a 10–20% chance of missing a real effect. Conversely, the *power* of the study ($1 - \beta$) is the probability of avoiding this error and detecting a real difference, in this case 80–90%.

It is up to the investigators to decide the target difference[21] and what probability level (for either type of error) they will accept if they are to use the result as a guide to action.

Plainly, trials should be devised to have adequate *precision* and *power*, both of which are consequences of the size of study. It is also necessary to make an estimate of the likely size of the difference between treatments, i.e. the target difference. Adequate power is often defined as giving an 80–90% chance of detecting (at 1–5% statistical significance, $P = 0.01$–0.05) the defined useful target difference (say 15%). It is rarely worth starting a trial that has a less than 50% chance of achieving the set objective, because the power of the trial is too low.

Types of therapeutic trial

A therapeutic trial is:

a carefully, and ethically, designed experiment with the aim of answering some precisely framed question. In its most rigorous form it demands equivalent groups of patients concurrently treated in different ways or in randomised sequential order in crossover designs. These groups are constructed by the random allocation of patients to one or other treatment … In principle the method has application with any disease and any treatment. It may also be applied on any scale; it does not necessarily demand large numbers of patients.[22]

This is the classical RCT, the most secure method for drawing a causal inference about the effects of treatments. Randomisation attempts to control biases of various kinds when assessing the effects of treatments. RCTs are employed at all phases of drug development and in the various types

---

[21]The target difference. Differences in trial outcomes fall into three grades: (1) that the doctor will ignore, (2) that will make the doctor wonder what to do (more research needed), and (3) that will make the doctor act, i.e. change prescribing practice.

[22]Bradford Hill A 1977 Principles of Medical Statistics. Hodder and Stoughton, London. If there is a 'father' of the modern scientific therapeutic trial, it is he.

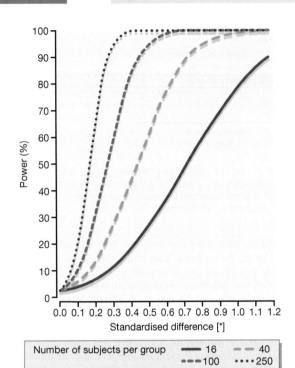

Number of subjects per group ⎯ 16 – – 40 ═══ 100 •••• 250

*Difference between treatments/standard deviation
(based on a two-sided test at the 0.05 level)

Fig. 4.3 Power curves – an illustrative method of defining the number of subjects required in a given study. In practice, the actual number would be calculated from standard equations. In this example, the curves are constructed for 16, 40, 100 and 250 subjects per group in a two-limb comparative trial. The graphs can provide three pieces of information: (1) the number of subjects that need to be studied, given the power of the trial and the difference expected between the two treatments; (2) the power of a trial, given the number of subjects included and the difference expected; and (3) the difference that can be detected between two groups of subjects of given number, with varying degrees of power. Also see p. 48. *(With permission from Baber N, Smith R N, Griffin J P, O'Grady J, D'Arcy P F (eds) 1998 Textbook of Pharmaceutical Medicine, 3rd edn. Queen's University of Belfast Press, Belfast.)*

and designs of trials discussed below. Fundamental to any trial are:

- A hypothesis.
- The definition of the primary endpoint.
- The method of analysis.
- A protocol.

Other factors to consider when designing or critically appraising a trial are:

- The characteristics of the patients.

- The general applicability of the results.
- The size of the trial.
- The method of monitoring.
- The use of interim analyses.[23]
- The interpretation of subgroup comparisons.

The aims of a therapeutic trial, not all of which can be attempted at any one occasion, are to decide:

- Whether a treatment is effective.
- The magnitude of that effect (compared with other remedies – or doses, or placebo).
- The types of patients in whom it is effective.
- The best method of applying the treatment (how often, and in what dosage if it is a drug).
- The disadvantages and dangers of the treatment.

Dose–response trials. Response in relation to the dose of a new investigational drug may be explored in all phases of drug development. Dose–response trials serve a number of objectives, of which the following are of particular importance:

- Confirmation of efficacy (hence a therapeutic trial).
- Investigation of the shape and location of the dose–response curve.
- The estimation of an appropriate starting dose.
- The identification of optimal strategies for individual dose adjustments.
- The determination of a maximal dose beyond which additional benefit is unlikely to occur.
- Defining the upper limit of dosing from a safety viewpoint.

Superiority, equivalence and non-inferiority in clinical trials. The therapeutic efficacy of a novel drug is most convincingly established by demonstrating superiority to placebo, or to an active control treatment, or by demonstrating a dose–response relationship (as above).

In some cases the purpose of a comparison is to show not necessarily superiority, but either equivalence or non-inferiority. Such trials avoid the use of placebo, explore possible advantages of safety, dosing convenience and cost, and present an alternative or 'second-line' therapy. Examples of a possible outcome in a 'head to head' comparison of two active treatments appear in Fig. 4.2.

There are in general, two types of equivalence trials in clinical development: *bio*-equivalence and *clinical* equivalence. In the former, certain pharmacokinetic variables of a new formulation have to fall within specified (and regulated)

---

[23]Particularly in large-scale outcome trials, an independent data monitoring committee is given access to the results as these are accumulated; the committee is empowered to discontinue a trial if the results show significant advantage or disadvantage to one or other treatment.

margins of the standard formulation of the same active entity. The advantage of this type of trial is that, if bio-equivalence is 'proven', then proof of clinical equivalence is not required.

Design of trials

Techniques to avoid bias

The two most important techniques are:

- randomisation.
- blinding.

Randomisation introduces a deliberate element of chance into the assignment of treatments to the subjects in a clinical trial. It provides a sound statistical basis for the evaluation of the evidence relating to treatment effects, and tends to produce treatment groups that have a balanced distribution of prognostic factors, both known and unknown. Together with blinding, it helps to avoid possible bias in the selection and allocation of subjects.

Randomisation may be accomplished in simple or more complex ways, such as:

- Sequential assignments of treatments (or sequences in crossover trials).
- Randomising subjects in blocks. This helps to increase comparability of the treatment groups when subject characteristics change over time or there is a change in recruitment policy. It also gives a better guarantee that the treatment groups will be of nearly equal size.
- By dynamic allocation, in which treatment allocation is influenced by the current balance of allocated treatments.[24]

Blinding. The fact that both doctors and patients are subject to bias due to their beliefs and feelings has led to the invention of the double-blind technique, which is a control device to prevent bias from influencing results. On the one hand, it rules out the effects of hopes and anxieties of the patient by giving both the drug under investigation and a placebo (dummy) of identical appearance in such a way that the subject (the first 'blind' person) does not know which he or she is receiving. On the other hand, it also rules out the influence of preconceived hopes of, and unconscious communication by, the investigator or observer by keeping him or her (the second 'blind' person) ignorant of whether he or she is prescribing a placebo or an active drug. At the same time, the technique provides another control, a means of comparison with the magnitude of placebo effects. The device is both philosophically and practically sound.[25]

A non-blind trial is called an *open trial*.

The double-blind technique should be used wherever possible, and especially for occasions when it might at first sight seem that criteria of clinical improvement are objective when in fact they are not. For example, the range of voluntary joint movement in rheumatoid arthritis has been shown to be influenced greatly by psychological factors, since the amount of pain patients will put up with is influenced by their mental state.

Blinding should go beyond the observer and the observed. None of the investigators should be aware of treatment allocation, including those who evaluate endpoints, assess compliance with the protocol and monitor adverse events. Breaking the blind (for a single subject) should be considered only when the subject's physician deems knowledge of the treatment assignment essential in the subject's best interests.

Sometimes the double-blind technique is not possible, because, for example, side effects of an active drug reveal which patients are taking it or tablets look or taste different. In principle, it never carries a disadvantage ('only protection against biased data'), but can add substantially to the cost of doing trials, and an unblinded (or, partially blinded) trial might be considered preferable to a trial which is prohibited by cost. This is most likely to be a dilemma for late-phase studies of licensed medicines, and blinding of the medication should at the least be replaced by blinding of the measurements: that is, the measurers are unaware of treatment allocation. Blinding is not, of course, used with new chemical entities fresh from the animal laboratory, whose dose and effects in humans are unknown, although the subject may legitimately be kept in ignorance (single blind) of the time of administration.

Some (e.g. ophthalmologists) are understandably disinclined to refer to the 'double-blind' technique; they call it 'double-masked'.

---

[24]Note also *patient preference trials*. Conventionally, patients are invited to participate in a clinical trial, give consent and are then randomised to a particular treatment group. In special circumstances, randomisation takes place first; the patients are informed of the treatment to be offered and are allowed to opt for this or another treatment. This is called 'pre-consent randomisation' or 'pre-randomisation'. In a trial of simple mastectomy versus lumpectomy with or without radiotherapy for early breast cancer, recruitment was slow because of the disfiguring nature of the mastectomy option. A policy of pre-randomisation was then adopted, letting women know the group to which they would be allocated should they consent. Recruitment increased sixfold and the trial was completed, providing sound evidence that survival was as long with the less disfiguring option (Fisher B, Bauer M, Margolese R et al 1985 Five-year results of a randomised clinical trial comparing total mastectomy and segmental mastectomy with and without radiotherapy in the treatment of breast cancer. New England Journal of Medicine 312:665–673). However, the benefit of enhanced recruitment may be limited by potential for introducing bias.

[25]Modell W, Houde R W 1958 Factors influencing clinical evaluation of drugs; with special reference to the double-blind technique. Journal of the American Medical Association 167:2190–2199.

Some common design configurations

Parallel group design

This is the most common clinical trial design for confirmatory therapeutic (Phase 3) trials. Subjects are randomised to one of two or more treatment 'arms'. These treatments will include the investigational drug at one or more doses, and one or more control treatments such as placebo and/or an active comparator. Parallel group designs are particularly useful in conditions that fluctuate over a short term, e.g. migraine or irritable bowel syndrome, but are also used for chronic stable diseases such as Parkinson's disease and some types of cancer. The particular advantages of the parallel group design are simplicity, the ability to approximate more closely the likely conditions of use, and the avoidance of 'carry-over effects' (see below).

Crossover design

In this design, each subject is randomised to a sequence of two or more treatments, and hence acts as his or her own control for treatment comparisons. The advantage of this design is that subject-to-subject variation is eliminated from treatment comparison so that the number of subjects is reduced. Larger crossover studies have been used to study factors contributing to subject-to-subject variation in response, permitting recognition of 'stratification variables' which can help future groups of patients to be selected (or excluded) as more or less likely to respond to the drug.

In the basic crossover design, each subject receives each of the two treatments in a randomised order. There are variations to this in which each subject receives a subset of treatments or ones in which treatments are repeated within the same subject (to explore the reproducibility of effects).

The potential disadvantage of the crossover design is carry-over, i.e. the residual influence of treatments on subsequent treatment periods. This can often be avoided either by separating treatments with a 'wash-out' period or by selecting treatment lengths based on a knowledge of the disease and the new medication. The crossover design is best suited for chronic stable diseases, e.g. hypertension, chronic stable angina pectoris, where the baseline conditions are attained at the start of each treatment arm. The pharmacokinetic characteristics of the new medication are also important, the principle being that the plasma concentration at the start of the next dosing period is zero and no dynamic effect can be detected. The crossover design is often used for pharmacokinetic studies.

Factorial designs

In the factorial design, two or more treatments are evaluated simultaneously through the use of varying combinations of the treatments. The simplest example is the 2×2 factorial design in which subjects are randomly allocated to one of four possible combinations of two treatments A and B. These are: A alone, B alone, A + B, neither A nor B (placebo). The main uses of the factorial design are to:

- Make efficient use of clinical trial subjects by evaluating two treatments with the same number of individuals.
- Examine the interaction of A with B.
- Establish dose–response characteristics of the combination of A and B when the efficacy of each has been previously established.

Multicentre trials

Multicentre trials are carried out for two main reasons. First, they are an efficient way of evaluating a new medication, by accruing sufficient subjects in a reasonable time to satisfy trial objectives. Second, multicentre trials may be designed to provide a better basis for the subsequent generalisation of their findings. Thus they provide the possibility of recruiting subjects from a wide population and of administering the medication in a broad range of clinical settings. Multicentre trials can be used at any phase in clinical development, but are especially valuable when used to confirm therapeutic value in Phase 3. Large-scale multicentre trials using minimised data collection techniques and simple endpoints have been of immense value in establishing modest but real treatment effects that apply to a large number of patients, e.g. drugs that improve survival after myocardial infarction.

N-of-1 trials

Patients give varied treatment responses, and the average effect derived from a population sample may not be helpful in expressing the size of benefit or harm for an individual. The best way to settle doubt as to whether a test drug is effective for an individual patient might be the N-of-1 trial. This is a crossover design in which each patient receives two or more administrations of drug or placebo in random manner; the results from individuals can then be displayed. Two conditions apply. First, the disease in which the drug is being tested must be chronic and stable. Second, the treatment effect must wear off rapidly. N-of-1 trials are not used routinely in drug development and, if so, only at the Phase 3 stage.[26,27] In some instances, such trials can now be replaced, or supplemented, by genomic (or other

[26]Senn S 1997 N-of-1 Trials: Statistical Issues in Drug Development. John Wiley, Chichester, pp. 249–255.
[27]Jull A, Bennet D 2005 Do N-of-1 trials really tailor treatment? Lancet 365:1992–1994.

'omic') measurements (cross-refer to Prof Pirmohamed's pharmacogenetics section). In drug development, however, enthusiasm for finding the right drug for the right patient can be offset by potential difficulties or delays in finding the right patients for the right drug. In other words, it may prove quicker to recruit a larger number of unselected patients, and retrospectively analyse predictors of response, than to wait until enough 'ideal' patients have been found for a smaller study of likely responders. Where, however, a previously characterised subset of a chronic disease is available, development can be streamlined. An example is the rapid testing and approval of ivacaftor for the 5% of patients with cystic fibrosis with a G551D mutation of the *CFTR* gene.[28]

Historical controls

Any temptation simply to give a new treatment to all patients and to compare the results with the past (historical controls) is almost always unacceptable, even with a disease such as leukaemia. The reasons are that standards of diagnosis and treatment change with time, and the severity of some diseases (infections) fluctuates. The general provision stands that controls must be concurrent and concomitant. Exceptions exist, such as some exploratory studies, and drugs for unmet need with large effects. Insulin therapy for type 1 diabetes mellitus has never been tested in a prospective study.

Size of trials

Before the start of any controlled trial it is necessary to decide the number of patients that will be needed to deliver an answer, for ethical as well as practical reasons. This is determined by four factors:

1. The *magnitude* of the difference sought or expected on the primary efficacy endpoint (the target difference). For between-group studies, the focus of interest is the mean difference that constitutes a clinically significant effect.
2. The *variability* of the measurement of the primary endpoint as reflected by the standard deviation of this primary outcome measure. The magnitude of the expected difference (above) divided by the standard deviation of the difference gives the *standardised difference* (see Fig. 4.3).
3. The defined *significance* level, i.e. the level of chance for accepting a Type I (α) error. Levels of 0.05 (5%) and 0.01 (1%) are common targets.

4. The *power* or desired probability of detecting the required mean treatment difference, i.e. the level of chance for accepting a Type II (β) error. For most controlled trials, a power of 80–90% (0.8–0.9) is frequently chosen as adequate, although higher power is chosen for some studies.

It will be intuitively obvious that a *small* difference in the effect that can be detected between two treatment groups, or a *large* variability in the measurement of the primary endpoint, or a *high* significance level (low *P* value) or a large power requirement, all act to increase the required sample size. Fig. 4.3 gives a graphical representation of how the power of a clinical trial relates to values of clinically relevant standardised difference for varying numbers of trial subjects (shown by the individual curves). It is clear that the larger the number of subjects in a trial, the smaller is the difference that can be detected for any given power value.

The aim of any clinical trial is to have small Type I and II errors, and consequently sufficient power to detect a difference between treatments, if it exists. Of the four factors that determine sample size, the power and significance level are chosen to suit the level of risk felt to be appropriate. The magnitude of the effect can be estimated from previous experience with drugs of the same or similar action; the variability of the measurements is often known from published experiments on the primary endpoint, with or without drug. These data will not be available for novel substances in a new class, and frequently the sample size in the early phase of development is chosen on a more arbitrary basis. Numbers required to detect the difference in frequency of a categorical outcome, e.g. fractures in a trial of osteoporosis or remissions in a cancer trial, are generally larger than numbers required to detect differences in a continuous quantitative variable. As an example, a trial that would detect, at the 5% level of statistical significance, a treatment that raised a cure rate from 75% to 85% would require 500 patients for 80% power.

Fixed sample size and sequential designs

Defining when a clinical trial should end is not as simple as it first appears. In the standard clinical trial, the end is defined by the passage of all of the recruited subjects through the complete design. However, it is results and decisions based on the results that matter, not the number of subjects. The result of the trial may be that one treatment is superior to another or that there is no difference. These trials are of *fixed sample size*. In fact, patients are recruited sequentially, but the results are analysed either at a fixed time-point, or (if the primary outcome is number of events), after a fixed number of events have occurred.

The results of this type of trial may be disappointing if they miss the agreed and accepted level of significance, either

---

[28]Ramsey B W, Davies J, McElvaney N G, et al. A CFTR potentiator in patients with cystic fibrosis and the G551D mutation. New Engl and Journal of Medicine 2011;365:1663–1672.

because of greater than predicted variability, or because of too few events.

It is not legitimate, having just failed to reach the agreed level (say, $P = 0.05$), to take in a few more patients in the hope that they will bring P value down to 0.05 or less, for this is deliberately not allowing chance and the treatment to be the sole factors involved in the outcome, as they should be.

An alternative (or addition) to repeating the fixed sample size trial is to use a *sequential design* in which the trial is run until a useful result is reached.[29] These adaptive designs, in which decisions are taken on the basis of results to date, can assess results on a continuous basis as data for each subject become available or, more commonly, on groups of subjects (group sequential design). The essential feature of these designs is that the trial is terminated when a *pre-determined* result is attained and not when the investigator looking at the results thinks it appropriate. Reviewing results in a continuous or interim basis requires *formal interim analysis,* and there are specific statistical methods for handling the data, which need to be agreed in advance. Group sequential designs are especially successful in large long-term trials of mortality or major non-fatal endpoints when safety must be monitored closely.

Such sequential designs recognise the reality of medical practice and provide a reasonable balance between statistical, medical and ethical needs. Interim analyses, however, reduce the power of statistical significance tests each time that they are performed, and carry a risk of a false positive results if chance differences between groups are encountered before the scheduled end of a trial.

Sensitivity of trials

Definitive therapeutic trials are expensive and on occasion may be so prolonged that aspects of treatment have been superseded by the time a result is obtained. A single trial, however well designed, executed and analysed, can answer only the question addressed. The regulatory authorities give guidance as to the number and design of trials that, if successful, would lead to a therapeutic claim. But changing clinical practice in the longer term depends on many other factors, of which confirmatory trials in other centres by different investigators under different conditions are an important part.

Meta-analysis

The two main outcomes for therapeutic trials are to influence clinical practice and, where appropriate, to make a successful

claim for a drug with the regulatory authorities. Investigators tend to be optimistic and frequently plan their trials to look for large effects. Reality is different. The results of a planned (or unplanned) series of clinical trials may vary considerably for several reasons, but most significantly because the studies are too small to detect a treatment effect. In common but serious diseases such as cancer or heart disease, however, even small treatment effects can be important in terms of their total impact on public health. It may be unreasonable to expect dramatic advances in these diseases; we should be looking for small effects. Drug developers, too, should be interested not only in whether a treatment works, but also how well, and for whom.

The collecting together of a number of trials with the same objective in a *systematic review*[30] and analysing the accumulated results using appropriate statistical methods is termed *meta-analysis*. The principles of a meta-analysis are that:

- It should be comprehensive, i.e. include data from all trials, published and unpublished.
- Only RCT should be analysed, with patients entered on the basis of 'intention to treat'.[31]
- The results should be determined using clearly defined, disease-specific endpoints (this may involve a re-analysis of original trials).

There are strong advocates and critics of the concept, its execution and interpretation. Arguments that have been advanced against meta-analysis are:

- An effect of reasonable size ought to be demonstrable in a single trial.
- Different study designs cannot be pooled.
- Lack of accessibility of all relevant studies.
- Publication bias ('positive' trials are more likely to be published).

In practice, the analysis involves calculating an *odds ratio* for each trial included in the meta-analysis. This is the ratio of the number of patients experiencing a particular endpoint, e.g. death, and the number who do not, compared with the equivalent figures for the control group. The number of deaths *observed* in the treatment group is then compared with the number to be *expected* if it is assumed that the treatment is ineffective, to give the *observed minus expected* statistic. The treatment effects for all trials in the analysis

[30]A review that strives comprehensively to identify and synthesise all the literature on a given subject (sometimes called an 'overview'). The unit of analysis is the primary study, and the same scientific principles and rigour apply as for any study. If a review does not state clearly whether and how all relevant studies were identified and synthesised, it is not a systematic review (Cochrane Library 1998).
[31]Reports of therapeutic trials should contain an analysis of all patients entered, regardless of whether they dropped out or failed to complete, or even started the treatment for any reason. Omission of these subjects can lead to serious bias (Laurence D R, Carpenter J 1998 A Dictionary of Pharmacological and Allied Topics. Elsevier, Amsterdam).

[29]Whitehead J 1992 The Design Analysis of Sequential Clinical Trials, 2nd edn. Ellis Horwood, Chester.

are then obtained by summing all the 'observed minus expected' values of the individual trials to obtain the overall odds ratio. An odds ratio of 1.0 indicates that the treatment has no effect, an odds ratio of 0.5 indicates a halving and an odds ratio of 2.0 indicates a doubling of the risk that patients will experience the chosen endpoint.

From the position of drug development, the general requirement that scientific results have to be repeatable has been interpreted in the past by the Food and Drug Administration (the regulatory agency in the USA) to mean that two well controlled studies are required to support a claim. But this requirement is itself controversial and its relation to a meta-analysis in the context of drug development is unclear.

In clinical practice, and in the era of cost-effectiveness, the use of meta-analysis as a tool to aid medical decision-making and underpinning 'evidence-based medicine' is well established.

Fig. 4.4 shows detailed results from 11 trials in which antiplatelet therapy after myocardial infarction was compared with a control group. The number of vascular events per treatment group is shown in the second and third columns, and the odds ratios with the point estimates (the value most likely to have resulted from the study) are represented by black squares and their 95% confidence intervals (CI) in the fourth column.

The size of the square is proportional to the number of events. The diamond gives the point estimate and CI for overall effect.

Results: implementation

The way in which data from therapeutic trials are presented can influence doctors' perceptions of the advisability of adopting a treatment in their routine practice.

Relative and absolute risk

The results of therapeutic trials are commonly expressed as the percentage reduction of an unfavourable (or percentage

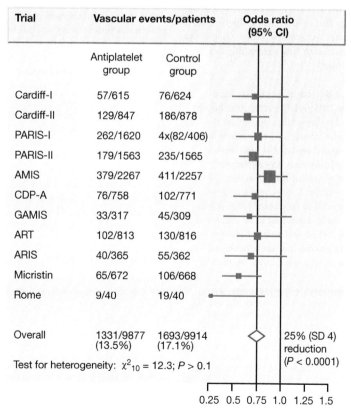

Fig. 4.4 A clear demonstration of benefits from meta-analysis of available trial data, when individual trials failed to provide convincing evidence (see text). *(With permission of Collins R 2001 Lancet 357:373–380.)*

increase in a favourable) outcome, i.e. as the *relative risk*, and this can be very impressive indeed until the figures are presented as the number of individuals actually affected per 100 people treated, i.e. as the *absolute risk*.

Where a baseline risk is *low*, a statement of relative risk alone is particularly misleading as it implies large benefit where the actual benefit is small. Thus a reduction of risk from 2% to 1% is a 50% relative risk reduction, but it saves only one patient for every 100 patients treated. But where the baseline is high, say 40%, a 50% reduction in relative risk saves 20 patients for every 100 treated.

> To make clinical decisions, readers of therapeutic studies need to know: how many patients must be treated[32] (and for how long) to obtain one desired result *(number needed to treat)*. This is the inverse (or reciprocal) of absolute risk reduction.

Relative risk reductions can remain high (and thus make treatments seem attractive) even when susceptibility to the events being prevented is low (and the corresponding numbers needed to be treated are large). As a result, restricting the reporting of efficacy to just relative risk reductions can lead to great – and at times excessive – zeal in decisions about treatment for patients with low susceptibilities.[33]

A real-life example follows:

> *Antiplatelet drugs reduce the risk of future non-fatal myocardial infarction by 30% [relative risk] in trials of both primary and secondary prevention. But when the results are presented as the number of patients who need to be treated for one nonfatal myocardial infarction to be avoided [absolute risk] they look very different.*
> *In secondary prevention of myocardial infarction, 50 patients need to be treated for 2 years, while in primary prevention 200 patients need to be treated for 5 years, for one non-fatal myocardial infarction to be prevented. In other words, it takes 100 patient-years of treatment in primary prevention to produce the same beneficial outcome of one fewer non-fatal myocardial infarction.[34]*

---

[32]See Cooke R J, Sackett D L 1995 The number needed to treat: a clinically useful treatment effect. British Medical Journal 310:452.
[33]Sackett D L, Cooke R J 1994 Understanding clinical trials: what measures of efficacy should journal articles provide busy clinicians? British Medical Journal 309:755.
[34]For example, drug therapy for high blood pressure carries risks, but the risks of the disease vary enormously according to severity of disease: 'Depending on the initial absolute risk, the benefits of lowering blood pressure range from preventing one cardiovascular event a year for about every 20 people treated, to preventing one event for about every 5000–10000 people treated. The level of risk at which treatment should be started is debatable' (Jackson R, Barham P, Bills J et al 1993 Management of raised blood pressure in New Zealand: a discussion document. British Medical Journal 307:107–110).

Whether a low incidence of adverse drug effects is acceptable becomes a serious issue in the context of absolute risk. Non-specialist doctors, particularly those in primary care, need and deserve clear and informative presentation of therapeutic trial results that measure the overall impact of a treatment on the patient's life, i.e. on clinically important outcomes such as morbidity, mortality, quality of life, working capacity or fewer days in hospital. Without it, they cannot adequately advise patients, who may themselves be misled by inappropriate use of statistical data in advertisements or on Internet sites.

> **Important aspects of therapeutic trial reports**
> - Statistical significance and its clinical importance.
> - Confidence intervals.
> - Number needed to treat, or absolute risk.

Pharmacoepidemiology

Pharmacoepidemiology is the study of the use and effects of drugs in large numbers of people. Some of the principles of pharmacoepidemiology are used to gain further insight into the efficacy, and especially the safety, of new drugs once they have passed from limited exposure in controlled therapeutic pre-registration trials to the looser conditions of their use in the community. Trials in this setting are described as *observational* because the groups to be compared are assembled from subjects who are, or who are not (the controls), taking the treatment in the ordinary way of medical care. These (Phase 4) trials are subject to greater risk for selection bias[35] and confounding[36] than *experimental* studies (RCTs), where entry and allocation of treatment are strictly controlled (increasing internal validity). Observational studies, nevertheless, come into their own when sufficiently large randomised trials are logistically and financially impracticable. The following approaches are used.

Observational cohort[37] studies

Patients receiving a drug are followed up to determine the outcomes (therapeutic or adverse). This is usually

---

[35]A systematic error in the selection or randomisation of patients on admission to a trial such that they differ in prognosis, i.e. the outcome is weighted one way or another by the selection, not by the trial.
[36]When the interpretation of an observed association between two variables may be affected by a strong influence from a third variable (which may be hidden or unknown). Examples of confounders would be concomitant drug therapy or differences in known risk factors, e.g. smoking, age, sex.
[37]Used here for a group of people having a common attribute, e.g. they have all taken the same drug.

forward-looking (prospective) research. A cohort study does not require a suspicion of causality; subjects can be followed 'to see what happens' (event recording). *Prescription event monitoring* (below) is an example, and there is an increasing tendency to recognise that most new drugs should be monitored in this way when prescribing becomes general. Major difficulties include the selection of an appropriate control group, and the need for large numbers of subjects and for prolonged surveillance. This sort of study is scientifically inferior to the *experimental* cohort study (the RCT) and is cumbersome for research on drugs.

Investigation of the question of thromboembolism and the combined oestrogen–progestogen contraceptive pill by means of an observational cohort study required enormous numbers of subjects[38] (the adverse effect is, fortunately, uncommon) followed over years. An investigation into cancer and the contraceptive pill by an observational cohort would require follow-up for 10–15 years. Happily, epidemiologists have devised a partial alternative: the case–control study.

Case–control studies

This reverses the direction of scientific logic from a forward-looking, 'what happens next' (*prospective*) to a backward-looking, 'what has happened in the past' (*retrospective*)[39] investigation. The case–control study requires a definite hypothesis or suspicion of causality, such as an adverse reaction to a drug. The investigator assembles a group of patients who have the condition. A control group of people who have not had the reaction is then assembled (matched, e.g. for sex, age, smoking habits) from hospital admissions for other reasons, primary care records or electoral rolls. A complete drug history is taken from each group, i.e. the two groups are 'followed up' backwards to determine the proportion in each group that has taken the suspect agent. Case–control studies do not prove causation.[40] They reveal associations, and it is up to investigators and critical readers to decide the most plausible explanation.

A case–control study has the advantage that it requires a much smaller number of cases (hundreds) of disease and can thus be done quickly and cheaply. It has the disadvantage

that it follows up subjects backwards, and there is always suspicion of the intrusion of unknown and so unavoidable biases in the selection of both patients and controls. Here again, independent repetition of the studies, if the results are the same, greatly enhances confidence in the outcome.

Surveillance systems: pharmacovigilance

When a drug reaches the market, a good deal is known about its therapeutic activity but rather less about its safety when used in large numbers of patients with a variety of diseases, for which they are taking other drugs. The term *pharmacovigilance* refers to the process of identifying and responding to issues of drug safety through the detection in the population of drug effects, usually adverse, taking action to minimise risk and monitoring the effectiveness of that action. Over a number of years, increasingly sophisticated systems have been developed to provide surveillance of drugs in the post-marketing phase. For understandable reasons, they are strongly supported by authorities.

Four kinds of logic can be applied to drug safety monitoring:

- To gain experience from regular reporting of suspected adverse drug reactions from health professionals during the regular clinical use of the drug.
- To attempt to follow a complete cohort of (new) drug users for as long as it is deemed necessary to have adequate information.
- To perform special studies in areas which may be predicted to give useful information.
- To examine disease trends for drug-related causality.[41]

Drug safety surveillance relies heavily on the techniques of pharmacoepidemiology, which include the following:

Voluntary reporting. Health-care professionals and patients may report suspected adverse reaction to drugs. In the UK, this is called the 'Yellow Card' system, and the Commission on Human Medicines advises the Medicines and Healthcare products Regulatory Agency of the government on trends and signals. It is recommended that for:

- newer drugs: all suspected reactions should be reported, i.e. any adverse or any unexpected event, however minor, that could conceivably be attributed to the drug
- established drugs: all serious suspected reactions should be reported, even if the effect is well recognised.

---

[38]The Royal College of General Practitioners (UK) recruited 23 000 women takers of the pill and 23 000 controls in 1968 and issued a report in 1973. It found an approximately doubled incidence of venous thrombosis in combined-pill takers (the dose of oestrogen was reduced because of this study).

[39]For this reason, such studies have been named *trohoc* (cohort spelled backwards) studies (Feinstein A 1981 Journal of Chronic Diseases 34:375).

[40]Experimental cohort studies (i.e. randomised controlled trials) are on firmer ground with regard to causation as there should be only one systematic difference between the groups (i.e. the treatment being studied). In case–control studies, the groups may differ systematically in several ways.

[41]Edwards I R 1998 A perspective on drug safety. In: Edwards I R (ed) Drug Safety. Adis International, Auckland, p. xii.

Inevitably the system depends on the intuitions and willingness of those called on to respond. Surveys suggest that no more than 10% of serious reactions are reported. Voluntary reporting is effective for identifying reactions that develop shortly after starting therapy, i.e. at providing early warnings of drug toxicity, particularly rare adverse reactions. Thus, it is the first line in post-marketing surveillance. Reporting is particularly low, however, for reactions with long latency, such as tardive dyskinesia from chronic neuroleptic use. As the system has no limit of quantitative sensitivity, it may detect the rarest events, e.g. those with an incidence of 1:5000 to 1:10 000. Voluntary systems are, however, unreliable for estimating the *incidence* of adverse reactions as this requires both a high rate of reporting (the numerator) and a knowledge of the rate of drug usage (the denominator).

Prescription event monitoring. This is a form of observational cohort study. Prescriptions for a drug (say, 20 000) are collected (in the UK this was made practicable by the existence of a National Health Service in which prescriptions are sent to a single central authority for pricing and payment of the pharmacist). The prescriber is sent a questionnaire and asked to report all events that have occurred (not only suspected adverse reactions) with judgement regarding causality.[42] However, the monitoring requires resource and is not currently undertaken in the UK.

Medical record linkage allows computer correlation in a population of life and health events (birth, marriage, death, hospital admission) with history of drug use. It is being developed as far as resources permit. It includes prescription event monitoring (above). The largest UK medical record linkage is the Clinical Practice Research Datalink (CPRD) at the Medicines and Healthcare products Regulatory Agency. Containing more than 20 million records, this type of resource is a more practical mode of detecting events associated with a particular drug than individual prescription monitoring. Indeed, it is a very valuable resource for pharmacoepidemiological-type studies, answering some key public health questions and serving as a very valuable resource for evaluating drug safety signals.

Population statistics, e.g. birth defect registers and cancer registers. These are insensitive unless a drug-induced event is highly remarkable or very frequent. If suspicions are aroused, then case–control and observational cohort studies will be initiated.

Strength of evidence

A number of types of clinical investigation are described in this chapter, and elsewhere in the book. When making clinical decisions about a course of therapeutic action, it is obviously relevant to judge the strength of evidence generated by different types of study. This has been summarised as follows, in rank order:[43]

1. Systematic reviews and meta-analyses, for which a prospective RCT is a now a preferred condition of inclusion.
2. RCTs with definitive results (confidence intervals that do not overlap the threshold of the clinically significant effect).[44]
3. RCTs with non-definitive results (a difference that suggests a clinically significant effect but with confidence intervals overlapping the threshold of this effect).
4. Cohort studies.
5. Case–control studies.
6. Cross-sectional surveys.
7. Case reports.

In conclusion[45]

Drug development is a high risk business. Early hopes and expectations can later be substantially modified by the realities of clinical practice, when the risks as well as the benefits of a medicine emerge with the passage of time. Only 1 in 10 drugs entering humans, subsequently enters the clinic and use in the wider clinical population, and more than half (60%) fail at phase 2 (see Ch. 3).

---

[42]Inman W H W, Rawson N S B, Wilton L V 1986 Prescription-event monitoring. In: Inman W H W (ed) Monitoring for Drug Safety, 2nd edn. MTP, Lancaster, p. 217.

[43]Guyatt G H, Sackett D L, Sinclair J C et al 1995 Users' guides to the medical literature. IX. A method for grading health care recommendations. Evidence-Based Medicine Working Group. Journal of the American Medical Association 274:1800–1804.
[44]The reporting of randomised controlled trials has been systemised so that only high-quality studies will be considered. See Moher D, Schulz K F, Altman D G 2001 CONSORT Group. The CONSORT statement: revised recommendations for improving the quality of reports of parallel group randomised trials. Lancet 357:1191–1194.
[45]'Quick, let us prescribe this new drug while it remains effective'. Richard Asher.

Guide to further reading

Biomarkers Definitions Working Group, 2001. Biomarkers and surrogate endpoints: preferred definitions and conceptual framework. Clin. Pharmacol. Ther. 69 (3), 89–95.

Bland, J.M., Altman, D.G., 2000. Statistical notes: the odds ratio. BMJ 320, 1468.

Bracken, M.B., 2008. Why animal studies are often poor indicators of human reactions to exposure. J. R. Soc. Med. 101, 120–122.

Chatellier, G., Zapletal, E., Lemaitre, D., et al., 1996. The number needed to treat: a clinically useful nomogram in its proper context. BMJ 312, 426–429.

Doll, R., 1998. Controlled trials: the 1948 watershed. BMJ 317, 1217–1220 (and following articles).

Egger, M., Smith, G.D., Phillips, A.N., 1997. Meta-analysis: principles and procedures. Br. Med. J. 315, 1533–1537 (see also other articles in the series entitled 'Meta-analysis').

Emanuel, E.J., Miller, F.G., 2001. The ethics of placebo-controlled trials – a middle ground. N. Engl. J. Med. 345, 915–919.

Garattini, S., Chalmers, I., 2009. Patients and the public deserve big changes in the evaluation of drugs. BMJ 338, 804–806.

GRADE Working Group, 2008. GRADE: what is 'quality of evidence' and why is it important to clinicians? BMJ 336, 924–929 (and the other papers of this series).

Greenhalgh, T., 1997. Papers that report drug trials. Br. Med. J. 315, 480–483 (see also other articles in the series entitled 'How to read a paper').

Kaptchuk, T.J., 1998. Powerful placebo: the dark side of the randomised controlled trial. Lancet 351, 1722–1725.

Khan, K.S., Kunz, R., Kleijnen, J., Antes, G., 2003. Five steps to conducting a systematic review. J. R. Soc. Med. 96, 118–121.

Lewis, J.A., Jonsson, B., Kreutz, G., et al., 2002. Placebo-controlled trials and the Declaration of Helsinki. Lancet 359, 1337–1340.

Miller, F.G., Rosenstein, D.L., 2003. The therapeutic orientation to clinical trials. N. Engl. J. Med. 348, 1383–1386.

Ramsey, B.W., Nepom, G.T., Lonial, S., 2017. Academic, Foundation, and Industry Collaboration in Finding New Therapies. N. Engl. J. Med. 376, 1762–1769.

Rochon, P.A., Gurwitz, J.H., Sykora, K., et al., 2005. Reader's guide to critical appraisal of cohort studies: 1. Role and design. BMJ 330, 895–897.

Rothwell, P.M., 2005. External validity of randomised controlled trials: 'to whom do the results of this trial apply? Lancet 365, 82–93.

Rothwell, P.M., 2005. Treating individuals 2. Subgroup analysis in randomised controlled trials: importance, indications, and interpretation. Lancet 365, 176–186.

Sackett, D., Rosenberg, W., Gray, J., et al., 2009. Evidence based medicine: what it is and what it isn't [editorial]. Can. Med. Assoc. J. 312, 1–8.

Silverman, W.A., Altman, D.G., 1996. Patients' preferences and randomised trials. Lancet 347, 171–174.

Vlahakes, G.J., 2006. Editorial. The value of phase 4 clinical testing. N. Engl. J. Med. 354, 413–415.

Waller, P.C., Jackson, P.R., Tucker, G.T., Ramsay, L.E., 1994. Clinical pharmacology with confidence [intervals]. Br. J. Clin. Pharmacol. 37, 309.

Williams, R.L., Chen, M.L., Hauck, W.W., 2002. Equivalence approaches. Clin. Pharmacol. Ther. 72, 229–237.

Woodcock, J., Ware, J.H., Miller, P.W., 2016. Clinical Trial Series. N. Engl. J. Med. 374, 2167.

Zwarenstein, M., Treweek, S., Gagnier, J.J., et al., 2008. CONSORT group: Pragmatic Trials in Healthcare (Practihc) group. Improving the reporting of pragmatic trials: an extension of the CONSORT statement. BMJ 337, a2390.

Chapter | 5 |

Health technology assessment

Michael Rawlins

SYNOPSIS

For pharmaceuticals, health technology assessment bridges the gap between licensing of pharmaceuticals and everyday clinical practice.

It involves:

- **Defining the scope of the assessment.**
- **Assessing the overall clinical effectiveness of the product (or products).**
- **Assessing their cost-effectiveness.**

The critical steps comprise:

- **A systematic review of the evidence.**
- **Estimating cost-effectiveness.**
- **Drawing appropriate conclusions on which decision-makers can act.**

A cost-effectiveness analysis attempts to provide a rational basis for decision-making in the face of resource constraints. It is used to estimate the extra cost to the health-care system of adopting a product, in relation to the additional benefit the product might bring. It therefore goes further than the criteria for licensing (quality, safety and efficacy), and health technology assessment has therefore sometimes been called 'the fourth hurdle'.

A health technology assessment may be used by a variety of agencies. It may inform the decisions of individual practitioners in the treatment of their own patients, or it may be used by a hospital to develop their treatment policies. Health technology assessment is critical for those involved in developing clinical guidelines for the management of specific conditions, and they may be used by policy makers for an entire health-care system.

The scope

The term *health technology* encompasses all approaches to the prevention, screening, diagnosis and treatment of disease. Treatments, in health technology assessments, not only encompass pharmaceuticals (including vaccines) but can include devices and interventional (surgical) procedures as well as techniques such as physiotherapy, speech therapy or cognitive behavioural therapy. Although this chapter is concerned with health technology assessment as it relates to pharmaceuticals, a similar approach is used in other therapeutic areas.

Before embarking on the health technology assessment of a pharmaceutical product, the scope of the enquiry needs to be carefully defined:

1. Obviously the product, or group of products, under investigation needs to be characterised.
2. The nature of the comparator health technology (or technologies) also requires definition. Depending on the circumstances, the comparator might be another pharmaceutical product indicated for the same condition; it might be a device or procedure used for the same or similar purposes; or it might be 'best supportive care'. In any event, the comparator should reflect current clinical practice.
3. Difficulties arise when a potential comparator is not licensed for a particular indication but is, nevertheless, widely used in routine clinical practice. This is a particular problem in the health technology assessment of products for use in children and for whom potential comparators reflect 'custom and practice' even though unlicensed. The wise course of action, in such circumstances, is to include comparators that reflect current clinical practice.

4. At the start of any health technology assessment, the clinical outcome(s) of interest should be decided. The most desirable, of course, is the 'ultimate outcome', such as dead versus alive or recovered versus not recovered. There are circumstances, however, when an assessment is focused on an 'intermediate' (or surrogate) outcome where there is confidence that this reflects the ultimate outcome. For example, in the assessment of statins for the treatment of hypercholesterolaemia, a decision would need to be taken as to whether the long-term 'ultimate' outcome (i.e. reduction in coronary artery disease) should be used or whether the assessment should be concerned with an 'intermediate' outcome (i.e. a reduction in LDL cholesterol).

5. The type of evidence required to demonstrate the effectiveness of a product must also be determined. In many instances this may be restricted to the results of randomised controlled trials. There may be circumstances, however, where other study designs are more appropriate. In the assessment of a vaccine, for example, evidence from randomised controlled trials may usefully be supplemented by the results of observational studies that have examined its efficacy under circumstances that more closely reflect its performance in the 'real world'. Sometimes historical controlled trials may be appropriate when the outcome is clear and unambiguous, particularly in the case of rare diseases.

6. Decisions must also be made about the form any economic evaluation should take. These include the economic perspective and the type of analysis that is most appropriate. Such matters are discussed later.

Clinical effectiveness

An assessment of the clinical effectiveness of a product requires a full 'systematic review' of the available evidence. A systematic review involves four steps:

1. Developing the protocol

The development of a protocol for a systematic review is just as important in secondary research as it is for primary research. The objectives of the review will usually have been defined by the scope (as above). The protocol will, in addition, include the relevant:

- pharmacological product or therapeutic class
- comparator(s), which may include a non-pharmacological procedure

- study designs for assessing the effectiveness of the product
- clinical endpoints used in the studies that are to be included in the review.

2. Defining the methods

The literature search will, at a minimum, involve a comprehensive search of the three major electronic databases (MEDLINE, EMBASE and CENTRAL). Although there is some overlap between each database, one alone is inadequate. The usual approach is to start the search in a broad manner by looking at the abstracts of all the studies that appear to be relevant and then only include those that match the criteria that have been established for the review. In a review of the clinical effectiveness of statins, for example, the review criteria may have required the assessment to be restricted to randomised controlled trials where the outcome is the secondary prevention of vascular death or disability. All other study designs, involving different patient populations or surrogate outcomes, would be excluded. The search will also include any relevant references gleaned from scrutiny of the list of publications in the included studies.

One of the major problems in identifying appropriate studies in any systematic review is so-called 'publication bias'. There is a tendency for negative studies, or those demonstrating only very modest benefits, to either remain unpublished or to be published in a non–English language journal. The inclusion of such studies is extremely important if a reliable indication of a product's 'effect size' is to be made. Common techniques to avoid publication bias include enquiry of both the particular manufacturer as well as of known experts in the particular field. The assessment team must also decide whether to attempt to identify articles in non–English language journals and get them translated. This step substantially increases the cost of the review and is not invariably undertaken.

3. Analysing the data

After extracting the relevant data from each of the studies that meet the review inclusion criteria, an 'evidence table' is constructed. In such a table, the relevant data for each study are summarised and usually include:

- The study's bibliographic reference.
- The type of study (e.g. randomised controlled trial, case–control study).
- Number of patients in each arm.
- Patient characteristics (e.g. age, gender).
- Study setting (e.g. hospital inpatients, GPs' surgeries).
- Intervention(s) including dose(s) and route(s) of administration.

Table 5.1 Jadad score calculation

Item	Score
Was the study described as randomised?	0/1
Was the method of randomisation described and appropriate?	0/1
Was the study described as double blind?	0/1
Was the method of double blinding described and appropriate?	0/1
Was there a description of withdrawals and dropouts?	0/1
Deduct 1 point if the method of randomisation was described and was inappropriate?	0/–1
Deduct 1 point if the study was described as double blind but the method of blinding was described and inappropriate?	0/–1

- Comparator interventions (e.g. placebo, active comparator).
- Length of follow-up.
- Outcome measure(s) and effect size(s).
- Additional comments.

The evidence table may also include some attempt to assess the quality of each study. There is no generally accepted approach to doing this, but one of the more common methods is to use the Jadad score (Table 5.1). This itemises those elements in the design and conduct of a study (i.e. randomisation and blinding) that contribute most to a study's internal validity. A score of 5 would indicate that the particular study appeared to have avoided both selection and ascertainment biases. A score of 0 would cast considerable doubt on a study's internal validity.

Qualitative synthesis

Almost all systematic reviews include an element of narrative or 'qualitative' synthesis outlining, or expanding on, aspects of the included studies. Narrative syntheses become a more significant component in systematic reviews of complex interventions (such as a comparison between an antidepressant and cognitive behavioural therapy in the treatment of mild depression). The defining characteristic of a formal narrative synthesis is the use of a textual approach that provides an analysis of the relationships within and between studies, and an overall assessment of the robustness of the evidence. It is a more subjective process than meta-analysis and, when used, needs to be rigorous and transparent to reduce the potential for bias.

Quantitative synthesis (meta-analysis)

A qualitative synthesis of the results in a systematic review may itself be sufficient. It is very common, however, to attempt a quantitative synthesis – or meta-analysis – of the individual outcomes from each study so as to provide the most reliable estimate of the overall size of a product's effects.

A meta-analysis (see also, Ch. 4, p. 50) involves, at its most simple level, extracting the summary statistical data for each study. The relevant data are the mean differences in outcomes at the end of the study with their 95% confidence intervals. Estimates of the effect size of the included studies, and the pooled estimate from all the studies, are often depicted as a 'forest plot'[1]; an example is shown in Fig. 5.1.

This forest plot summarises the results of each of five placebo-controlled trials, designed to assess the effect of anticoagulation with warfarin on the frequency of ischaemic stroke in patients with non-valvular atrial fibrillation.[2] In a typical forest plot, there is an abbreviated reference to each trial on the left. The point estimate (mean) of the results of each study is represented as a square; and the horizontal line running through the square is its 95% confidence interval. The size of each square is proportional to the size of the study compared to the others. The column on the right shows the individual odds ratios (the expression of benefit used in this meta-analysis), and their 95% confidence intervals, for each study. By convention, improvement (a decrease in the frequency of ischaemic stroke) is shown to the left of the vertical 'no effect' line; a worsening (an increase in the frequency of ischaemic stroke) is shown to the right.

In the forest plot in Fig. 5.1, the outcome is expressed as odds ratios. In each of five studies, the frequency of ischaemic stroke is reduced by treatment with warfarin, and all five 'squares' are to the left of the 'no effect' (odds ratio = 1) vertical line. In three of the studies, the 95% confidence interval does not cross the 'no effect' line, and the results would be statistically significant with P values of less than 0.05. In the other two studies, the upper boundaries of the 95% confidence interval cross the 'no effect' line and would not reach conventional levels of statistical significance (i.e. the P value is more than 0.05). The overall pooled mean effect size, taking account of the results of all five studies, is shown as a diamond in Fig. 5.1; and the horizontal line again represents its 95% confidence interval. The value of a forest plot is that the results can be seen and interpreted

---

[1]The 'forest plot' is so called because (to some – though not to the author's – eyes) the 'plot' resembles a forest!
[2]Aguilar M I, Hart R 2005 Oral anticoagulants for preventing stroke in patients with non-valvular atrial fibrillation and no previous history of stroke or transient ischemic attacks. Cochrane Database of Systematic Reviews Issue 3, Art. No.: CD001927. DOI: 10.1002/14651858. CD001927.pub2.

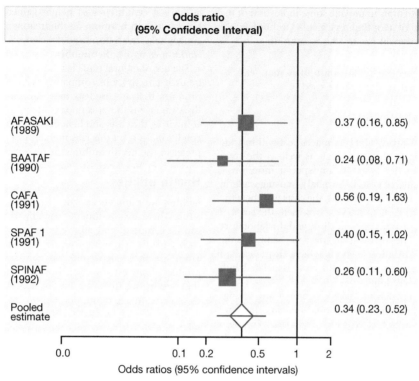

Fig. 5.1 Forest plot of five placebo-controlled trials of warfarin's efficacy in preventing ischaemic stroke in patients with non-valvular atrial fibrillation. (Odds ratios with 95% confidence intervals.)

almost at a glance. Although not all the studies in Fig. 5.1 were statistically significant, the mean effects of each study showed benefit, and the pooled estimate is highly significant.

4. Drawing conclusions

The final step in a systematic review is to discuss its strengths and weaknesses, and to draw conclusions. Both strengths and weaknesses will depend in large part on the range and quality of the included studies. The veracity of any conclusions will also depend on the extent to which there might have been publication bias so that important trials with negative results were never published. There are statistical techniques that can sometimes be helpful in establishing probable publication bias.

Scrutiny of Fig. 5.1 suggests that it would be reasonable, by any standards, to regard warfarin as effective in the prevention of ischaemic stroke in patients with non-valvular atrial fibrillation. Moreover, the authors were able to estimate that about 25 strokes and about 12 disabling or fatal strokes would be prevented yearly for every 1000 patients with atrial fibrillation treated with warfarin.

Cost-effectiveness

No health-care system is able to meet all the demands of its patients. The resources used to provide health care, in any individual country, are directly proportional to its wealth, so that wealthier nations with higher gross domestic products are able to devote more resources to health care than poorer ones. The manner in which health-care priorities are decided varies between countries, but rationing decisions are necessary – explicitly or implicitly – in all countries because resources are finite and demand is (almost) infinite.

A cost-effectiveness analysis attempts to provide a health-care system with a rational basis for decision-making in the face of resource constraints. In pharmacoeconomics, this involves trying to estimate the extra cost to the health-care system of adopting a product in relation to the additional benefit the product might bring. If a health-care system devotes very large sums of money to a product that gives only modest benefits, other people, with other conditions, will be denied the opportunity of cost-effective care. The cost-effectiveness component of a health technology assessment thus attempts to provide some indication of the 'opportunity cost' of adopting a particular technology. In doing so, the assessment has to take account of:

1. The relevant costs.
2. The benefits expressed in an appropriate manner.
3. The type of analysis that will be used.

1. Costs

The costs of using a particular pharmaceutical will include the acquisition costs of the product, as well as the costs associated with its use (such as any special monitoring requirements, additional visits to hospital). In using warfarin for the prevention of ischaemic stroke, the costs will therefore have to include the costs of the warfarin itself, the costs of attending a hospital anticoagulant clinic and the laboratory monitoring costs. The costs will also have to encompass the consequences of any adverse effects which, in the case of warfarin, would need to comprise the costs associated with warfarin-induced bleeding.

The costs will also have to take account of any savings from which a health-care system would benefit. These are sometimes known as 'cost offsets' which, in the case of warfarin to prevent ischaemic stroke, would include the savings made by the reduction in strokes among treated patients.

The costs might also include the wider costs and savings to society as a whole. In this case, the costs (and cost offsets) would be extended to include any reduction in time off work; or, continuing the warfarin example, the savings resulting from fewer strokes that would reduce the costs associated with unemployment or disability.

Whether the economic *perspective* (as economists describe it) should be based on the costs and savings to the health-care system alone, or whether it should be societal, is a complicated and controversial issue. It is a political, fiscal (relating to government revenue, especially taxes) and governmental problem rather than an economic one. For this reason, there is considerable variation between countries as to the economic perspective taken. A societal perspective is adopted in Sweden, for example, but in the UK the perspective is limited to the National Health Service.

2. Benefits

For the purposes of an economic analysis, the benefits of a health technology can, broadly, be expressed either in 'natural units' (e.g. life years gained), or as 'health utility' gained.

Natural units

The number of life years saved as a result of using a product is a commonly used natural unit for products that extend life. Other natural units might include the number of additional centimetres of height gained from the use of human growth hormone in the treatment of children with congenital growth hormone deficiency; or, again using the warfarin example, the number of strokes prevented.

The use of natural units is relatively simple, and they can be used effectively in comparing the costs and benefits of products that are used to treat the same condition. The disadvantage is that it is impossible to use natural units for comparing the costs and benefits of treatments for different conditions. It is for this reason that most economic analyses prefer to use health 'utilities' as the measure of benefit.

Health utilities

Utilities are numbers assigned to preferences according to a rule. There are a number of ways by which health utilities can be captured, and all are based on an assessment, by each person, of the improvement in their quality of life. These are then aggregated across the patients using the product of interest as well as those using the comparator(s). If the study itself did not collect health-related quality-of-life data, there are techniques that allow it to be imputed.

The most widely used technique for capturing health-related quality-of-life data is the so-called 'EuroQol EQ-5D questionnaire'. It is not disease-specific and captures patients' preferences for particular health states.

The health utility measure provided by the EQ-5D ranges from 0 (dead) to 1 (perfect health). When patients benefit from a particular treatment, their health state might move from (say) 0.5 to 0.8 with a corresponding utility gain of 0.3. This is multiplied by the number of years for which it is enjoyed to yield the 'quality-adjusted life years' (QALY). If patients could on average expect to enjoy a utility gain of 0.3 for 10 years, the number of quality-adjusted life years gained would be 3.0 (0.3 times 10).

3. Type of analysis

Two types of analysis are possible depending on whether the benefits are expressed in natural units or as utilities. Both require calculating an 'incremental cost-effectiveness ratio' (ICER) by dividing the incremental costs by the incremental benefits. Treatment pathways, however, can be extraordinarily complicated; and in arriving at an ICER, health economists must of necessity construct an economic model. There is a great variety of these, and they vary in their complexity. No attempt is made to discuss them further here, and their interpretation requires considerable expertise.

Cost-effectiveness analysis

In a cost-effectiveness analysis, the ICER is expressed as the incremental cost (£) per incremental gain in some natural unit. In the case of a product that, in advanced cancer, results

Table 5.2 Incremental cost-effectiveness ratios for some anti-cancer drugs appraised by the National Institute for Health and Clinical Excellence

Treatment	Condition	Incremental cost-effectiveness ratio (£/QALY)
Rituximab	Aggressive non-Hodgkin's lymphoma	6100
Paclitaxel	Metastatic ovarian cancer	8500
Gemcitabine	Metastatic pancreatic cancer	12 500
Vinorelbine	Metastatic breast cancer	14 500
Trastuzumab	Early breast cancer	18 000
Pertuzumab	Neoadjuvant treatment of HER2-positive breast cancer	23 467
Imatinib	Inoperable or metastatic gastrointestinal stromal tumour	32 000
Crizotumab	Advanced non–small cell lung cancer	50 200
Bevacizumab	Metastatic colorectal cancer	62 860
Necitumumab	Metastatic non–small cell lung cancer	110 248

in (say) a 6-month extension of life at a total cost of (say) £10 000, the ICER would be £20 000 per life year gained.

As already discussed, although this measure is sometimes used, it is impossible to make comparisons across conditions. How would a decision-maker make a 'value for money' comparison between £20 000 per life year gained for treating advanced cancer, with £20 000 per centimetre height gained from the use of growth hormone in a child with congenital growth hormone deficiency?

Cost-utility analysis

In this form of analysis, the ICER is expressed as the ratio of the incremental costs to the incremental utility gain. The most common expression of this form of ICER is as cost (£) per incremental gain in the quality adjusted life years (£ per QALY). Examples of ICERs for some cancer drugs are shown in Table 5.2. A health technology assessment may also include economic evaluations in subgroups of patients, such as those older than 65 years of age, or those with other identifiable prognostic characteristics. This is usually undertaken when the overall ICER for the product is likely to represent poor value for money, but when there may be subgroups who might gain greater benefit.

In conclusion

A health technology assessment is concerned with analysing the totality of the available clinical and economic evidence.

Bodies undertaking health technology assessments are not usually, however, decision-makers. Health technology assessments should provide decision-makers with a sophisticated analysis of the available data, together with a critical evaluation of the strengths and weaknesses of the assessment as well as the limitations in the economic analyses.

One of the most critical issues, in the assessment of the clinical data, is the extent to which the benefits in trials can be extrapolated beyond the data. In the trials depicted in Fig. 5.1, the average duration of follow-up was 1.5 years. Does this mean that treatment should be stopped after this? The mean age of participants was 69 years of age, with very few younger than 50 years or older than 80 years of age. Does this mean that treatment should be denied to younger people? Or to the very elderly? These are the decisions that decision-makers themselves must make. A reasonable decision-maker could reasonably conclude that to stop warfarin treatment after 1.5 years would be wrong, and that denying the very likely benefits to those younger and older than those in the trials would be equally wrong. These decisions are ones, though, that require judgements to be made rather than strict adherence to the tenets of health technology assessment. Health technology assessment plays a crucial role in underpinning evidence-based clinical practice, but it does not supplant the place of judgement![3]

[3]Rawlins M D 2010 The evaluation and provision of effective medicines. In: Warrell D A, Cox T M, Firth J D, Benz E J (eds) Oxford Textbook of Medicine, 5th edn. Oxford University Press, Oxford

Guide to further reading

Higgins, J.P.T., Green, S. (Eds.), 2011. Cochrane Handbook for Systematic Reviews of Interventions Version 5.1.0. The Cochrane Collaboration, Oxford.

Matthews, J.N.S., 2006. An Introduction to Randomized Controlled Trials. Chapman and Hall, London.

Morris, S., Devlin, N., Parkin, D., 2007. Economic Analysis in Health Care. John Wiley, Chichester.

Rawlins, M.D., 2011. Therapeutics, Evidence and Decision-Making. Hodder, London.

Rawlins, M.D., 2016. Cost, Effectiveness and Value: How to Judge. J. Am. Med. Assoc. 316, 1447–1448.

Chapter | 6 |

Regulation of medicines

Ian Hudson, Keith MacDonald, June Raine

SYNOPSIS

This chapter describes the background to why it became necessary to regulate the use and supply of drugs, and the ways in which these processes are managed:

- **Basis for regulation: safety, efficacy, quality.**
- **Present medicines regulatory system.**
- **Present-day requirements.**
- **Counterfeit drugs.**
- **Complementary and alternative medicine.**
- **Medicines regulation: the future.**

Basis for regulation

Neither patients nor doctors are in a position to decide for themselves, across the range of medicines that they use, which ones are well manufactured, free of contamination, and stable, effective and safe. They need assurance that the medicines they are offered fulfil these requirements and are supported by information that permits optimal use. The information about, the benefit risk of medicines continually evolves during use, and there is an obligation on licence holders continually to review their licence with particular regard to safety. Marketing Authorisation Holders (MAHs), i.e. pharmaceutical companies, can also change the efficacy claims to their licence (e.g. new indications, extension of age groups) or change the safety information (e.g. add new warnings, or contraindications). The quality aspects may also need to be revised as manufacturing practices change. MAHs operate in a market economy and have strong profit motives for making claims about their drugs. Only independent regulators can provide the assurance about all those aspects in the lifecycle of a medicine (insofar as it can be provided).

The principles of official (statutory) medicines regulation are that:

- Clinical trials of investigational medicinal products require prior approval by the medicines' regulator and a positive opinion from a research ethics committee.
- No medicines will be marketed without prior licensing by the independent regulator. A licence will be granted on the basis of scientific evaluation of:
  - *Safety*, in relation to its use: evaluation at the point of marketing is provisional in the sense that it is followed in the community by a pharmacovigilance programme.
  - *Efficacy* (now often including quality of life).
  - *Quality*, e.g., purity, stability (shelf-life).
  - *Supply*, i.e. whether the drug is suitable to be unrestrictedly available to the public or whether it should be confined to sales through pharmacies or on doctors' prescriptions; and what printed information should accompany its sale (labelling, leaflets).
- A licence shall specify the clinical indications that may be promoted and shall be for a limited period (5 years), which is renewable on application, with further 5-year renewals depending on risk. A regulatory authority may review the risk:benefit balance or safety of a drug at any time and restrict the licence, or remove the drug from the market for good cause.[1]

---

[1]As from 2006, the European Community regulations require one renewal at 5 years and a second at 10 years only if safety issues demand it, with safety update reviews every 3 years after licensing.

- A licence may be varied (altered) by an application from the pharmaceutical company to update efficacy, safety and quality sections; safety variations may be initiated by the regulatory authority, and/or restrictions on indication or claims for efficacy. The regulatory authority can insist on safety additions or can require restrictions in efficacy indications but cannot force additional efficacy indications.

Plainly manufacturers and developers are entitled to be provided with guidance on what substances are regulated and what are not,[2] and what kinds and amounts of data are likely to persuade a regulatory authority to grant a marketing authorisation (licence) and for what medical purpose. In summary, medicines regulation aims to provide an objective, rigorous and transparent assessment of efficacy, safety and quality in order to protect and promote public health but not to impede the pharmaceutical industry. Inevitably, an interesting tension exists between the regulators and the regulated depending on the circumstances; increasingly regulators feel it is part of their role to support innovation.[3]

Historical background

The beginning of substantial government intervention in the field of medicines paralleled the proliferation of synthetic drugs in the early 20th century when the traditional and familiar pharmacopoeia[4] expanded slowly and then, in mid-century, with enormous rapidity. The first comprehensive regulatory law that required pre-marketing testing was passed in the USA in 1938, following the death of about 107 people due to the use of diethylene glycol (a constituent of anti-freeze) as a solvent for a stable liquid formulation of sulphanilamide for treating common infections.[5]

---

[2]It is obviously impossible to list substances that will be regulated if anybody should choose 1 day to synthesise them. Therefore regulation is based on the supply of 'medicinal products', i.e. substances are regulated according to their proposed use; and they must be defined in a way that will resist legal challenge (hence the stilted regulatory language). The following terms have gained informal acceptance for 'borderline substances' (which may or may not be regulated): nutriceutical – a food or part of a food that provides medicinal benefits; cosmeceutical – a cosmetic that also has medicinal use.
[3]However much doctors may mock the bureaucratic 'regulatory mind', regulation provides an important service, and it is expedient that doctors should have some insight into its working and some of the very real problems faced by public servants and their advisory committees who are trying to do good without risking losing their jobs and reputations.
[4]Pharmacopoeia: a book (often official) listing drugs and, for example, their standards of purity, manufacture, assay and directions for use.
[5]Report of the Secretary of Agriculture submitted in response to resolutions in the House of Representatives and Senate (USA) 1937 Journal of the American Medical Association 111:583, 919. Recommended reading. A similar episode occurred as recently as 1990–1992 (Hanif M, Mobarak M R, Ronan A et al 1995 Fatal renal failure caused by diethylene glycol in paracetamol elixir: the Bangladesh epidemic. British Medical Journal 311:88–91). Note: diethylene glycol is cheap.

Other countries did not take on board the lesson provided by the USA, and it took the thalidomide disaster[6,7] to make governments all over the world initiate comprehensive control over all aspects of drug introduction, therapeutic claims and supply. In 1960–1961 in (West) Germany, the incidence of phocomelia in newborns was noted. The term means 'seal extremities' and is a deformity in which the long bones of the limbs are defective and substantially normal or rudimentary hands and feet arise on, or nearly on, the trunk, like the flippers of a seal; other abnormalities may occur. Phocomelia is ordinarily exceedingly rare. Case–control and prospective observational cohort studies in antenatal clinics where women had yet to give birth provided evidence incriminating a sedative and hypnotic called thalidomide; it was recommended for use in pregnant women, although it had not been tested in the appropriate animal model. The worst had happened: a trivial new drug was the cause of the greatest disaster in the short history of modern scientific drug therapy. Many thalidomide babies died, but many live on with deformed limbs, eyes, ears, heart and alimentary and urinary tracts. The world total of survivors was probably about 10 000.

In the UK, two direct consequences were the development of a spontaneous adverse drug reaction reporting scheme (the Yellow Card system) and legislation to provide regulatory control on the safety, quality and efficacy of medicines through the systems of standards, authorisation, pharmacovigilance (see p. 53) and inspection (Medicines Act 1968). A further landmark was the establishment of the Committee on Safety of Medicines in 1971 (from 2006 renamed the Commission on Human Medicines) to advise the Licensing Authority in the UK. In 1995, the new European regulatory system was introduced (see below).

Despite these protective systems, other drug disasters occurred. In 1974 the β-blocking agent practolol was withdrawn because of a rare but severe syndrome affecting the eyes and other mucocutaneous regions in the body (not detected by animal tests), and in 1982 benoxaprofen, a non-steroidal anti-inflammatory drug, was found to cause serious adverse effects including onycholysis and photosensitivity in elderly patients. More recent examples that have gained wide public notice include the association of serotonin-specific reuptake inhibitors with increased risk of suicidal behaviour in children and young people, and that of cyclo-oxygenase I and II inhibitors with an increased risk of cardiovascular disease (see p. 251).

---

[6]Mellin G W, Katzenstein M 1962 The saga of thalidomide. Neuropathy to embryopathy, with case reports of congenital anomalies. New England Journal of Medicine 267:1184–1192, 1238–1244.
[7]Dally A 1998 Thalidomide: was the tragedy preventable? Lancet 351:1197–1199.

Current medicines regulatory systems

All countries where medicines are licensed have a regulatory framework. When a pharmaceutical company seeks worldwide marketing rights, its programmes *must* satisfy each jurisdiction including: the Food and Drug Administration (FDA) of the USA; the European regulations and guidance issued by the European Commission and overseen by the European Medicines Agency[8] (EMA); and the Japanese Pharmaceuticals and Medical Devices Agency (PMDA). The national regulatory bodies of the individual European Union members remain in place but work with the EMA, which acts as a single source of authority. National licences for medicines that fall within the scope of the 'centralised authorisation procedure' can still be granted through individual member states other than for medicines within the scope of the centralised authorisation procedure which maintain particular responsibility for their own public health issues. Significant harmonisation of practices and procedures at a global level was also achieved through the International Conference on Harmonisation (ICH) involving Europe, Japan and the USA and recently extended to include Canada, Switzerland, Brazil and South Korea.

In the European Union, drugs can be licensed in three ways:

1. The *centralised procedure* allows applications to be made directly to the EMA; applications are allocated for assessment to one member state (the rapporteur) assisted by a second member state (co-rapporteur). Approval of the licence is then binding on all member states. This approach is mandatory for biotechnology products and for certain new medicinal products.
2. The *mutual recognition* and *decentralised procedure* allows applicants to nominate one member state (known as a 'reference member state') which assesses the application and seeks opinion from the other (concerned) member states. Granting the licence will ensure simultaneous mutual recognition in these other states, provided agreement is reached among them. There is an arbitration procedure for both MRP and DCP. The significant difference between MRP and DCP is that MRP is based on an MA that has already been approved in a MS. In DCP the application is submitted in RMS and CMS simultaneously.
3. A product to be marketed in a single country, which does not require the centralised procedure, can have its licence applied for through the national route.

The European systems are conducted according to strict timelines and written procedures. Once a medicine has been licensed for sale by one of the above procedures, its future regulatory life remains within that procedure. Periodic risk:benefit updates must be reviewed every 6 months for the first 2 years, and then annually until 5 years. Thereafter, there may be a second renewal at 10 years, if safety issues demand.[1] The renewal of a licence is primarily the responsibility of the pharmaceutical company, but requires approval from the regulatory authority. This provides the opportunity for companies to review, in particular, the safety aspects to keep the licence in line with current clinical practice. Any major changes to licences must be made by variation of the original licence (safety, efficacy or quality; see below) and supported by data, which for a major indication can be substantial.

Rare diseases

Since the pharmaceutical industry has little interest, under normal market conditions, in developing and marketing medicines intended for small numbers of patients (orphan medicinal products), the European Union offers a range of incentives to encourage the development of medicines for conditions affecting no more than 5 in 10 000 people.

These incentives include a period of 10 years market exclusivity, the provision of protocol assistance (scientific advice specifically tailored for orphan medicinal products) and fee reductions and waivers for regulatory procedures.

Requirements

Authorisation for clinical trials in the UK

The EU Clinical Trial Directive 2001/20/EC harmonised the laws and administrative procedures relating to the regulation of clinical trials across Europe and replaced the previous legislation in each of the separate member states. It is implemented in the UK through the Medicines for Human Use (Clinical Trials) Regulations.[9] All interventional clinical trials of an investigational medical product (so-called 'CTIMPs'), including human volunteer trials, require regulatory approval through a Clinical Trial Authorisation (CTA) application that must include summaries of preclinical, clinical and pharmaceutical data. For most trials, a response must be provided by the regulatory authority within 30 days, with a maximum of up to 60 days. There is a complementary process to allow for amendments to the original

---

[8]Formerly the European Medicines Evaluation Agency (EMEA).

[9]2004 Statutory Instrument No. 1031. The Stationery Office, UK.

application, and there is a requirement to notify each involved regulatory agency when the trial is completed. In contrast to the procedures for licensing medicines, CT authorisation is a national competence. A trial to be conducted in five countries currently requires five separate submissions and approvals. A new CT regulation is expected to come into effect during 2018 and introduces a single submission portal (for EU studies) and coordinated assessment among concerned member states.

Regulatory review of a new drug marketing application

A drug regulatory authority requires the following:

- *Quality checks:* full information on manufacturing process including purity, stability, formulation and analytical testing. It is necessary to provide this information both for the drug substance and the finished medicinal product.
- *Preclinical tests:* tests carried out in animals to allow some prediction of potential efficacy and safety in humans (see Ch. 4).
- Clinical (human) tests (Phases 1, 2, 3).
- Knowledge of the environmental impact of pharmaceuticals. Regulatory authorities expect manufacturers to address this concern in their application to market new chemical entities. Aspects include manufacture (chemical pollution), packaging (waste disposal), pollution in immediate use, e.g. antimicrobials and, more remotely, drugs or metabolites entering the food chain or water e.g. hormones.

The full process of regulatory review of a truly novel drug (new chemical entity) may take months.

Regulatory review

Using one of the regulatory systems described above, an authority normally conducts a review in three stages:

1. Examination of preclinical data to determine the mode of action of the agent, biodistribution and safety.[10]
2. Examination of the clinical studies to assess quality of data and to determine whether the drug has been

shown to be therapeutically efficacious with safety appropriate to its use.[11]
3. Quality in addition to non-clinical and clinical review. These are conducted concurrently.

If the decision is favourable, the drug is granted a marketing authorisation (for 5 years: renewable), which allows it to be marketed for *specified therapeutic uses*. The authority must satisfy itself of the adequacy of the information to be provided to prescribers in a Summary of Product Characteristics (SPC) and also a Patient Information Leaflet (PIL).

The PIL must also be approved by the licensing authority, be deemed fairly to represent the SPC, and be comprehensive and understandable to patients and carers. Where a drug has special advantage, but also has special risk, restrictions on its promotion and use can be imposed, e.g. isotretinoin and clozapine (see Index).

Central to the decision to grant a marketing authorisation is the assessment procedure undertaken by professional medical, scientific, statistical and pharmaceutical staff at one of the national agencies. In the UK these are employed as civil servants within the Medicines and Healthcare products Regulatory Agency (MHRA) and are advised by various independent expert committees.[12]

When a novel drug is granted a marketing authorisation a positive benefit risk is endorsed in the authorised indication. But the testing is not over: the most stringent test of all is about to begin. It will be used in all sorts of people of all ages and sizes, and having all sorts of other conditions. Its use can no longer be supervised so closely as hitherto. Doctors will prescribe it, and patients will use it correctly and incorrectly. It will have effects that have not been anticipated. It will be taken in overdose. It has to find its place in therapeutics, through extended comparisons with other drugs available for the same diseases.

Drugs used to prevent a long-term morbidity, e.g. stroke in hypertensive patients, can be proven effective only in *outcome* trials that are usually considered too expensive even to start until marketing of the drug is guaranteed. The effect of a drug at preventing rare occurrences requires many thousands of patients, more than are usually studied during development. Similarly, rare adverse events cannot be detected prior to marketing, and it would be unethical to expose large numbers of trial patients to a novel drug for purely safety reasons.[13]

---

[10]The licensing authority in England is the health minister, though in practice the Medicines and Healthcare products Regulatory Agency (MHRA) is the executive arm within the Department of Health.
[11]Common sense dictates that what, in regulatory terms, is 'safe' for leukaemia would not be 'safe' for anxiety.

[12]Breckenridge A M 2004 The changing scene of the regulation of medicines in the UK. British Journal of Clinical Pharmacology 58:571–574.
[13]After marketing, doctors should use a new drug only when they believe it an improvement (in efficacy, safety, convenience or cost) on the older alternatives.

Post-licensing responsibilities

It is in the pharmaceutical company's interest to promote the rapid uptake in use of the product in the patient population in whom benefit has been demonstrated. The regulatory authorities are more concerned with the safety profile of the drug and protection of public health. The most important source of safety data once the drug is in clinical use is spontaneous reporting of adverse events, which will generate 'signals' and raise suspicion of infrequent but potentially serious adverse events caused by the drug.[14] Proving the causal link from sporadic signals can be extremely difficult, and is entirely dependent on the number and quality of these spontaneous reports, as well as other data sources such as pharmacoepidemiological studies. In the UK, reports of suspected adverse reactions are captured through the Yellow Card system (see p. 53) and may be completed by doctors, nurses or pharmacists and, most recently, by patients. Other countries have their own systems. The importance of encouraging prompt and accurate spontaneous reporting of suspected adverse reactions cannot be overemphasised.

Since 2005, companies are required to submit at the time of licence application the details of subsequent review and management systems in the form of a risk management plan. This may include a post-authorisation surveillance study (PASS). Other studies investigating the safety of a medicine that are not directly sponsored by the manufacturer may be identified from various organisations. These include the Drug Safety Research Unit (Southampton, UK), the Medicines Monitoring Unit (MEMO) (Tayside, UK), and the use of computerised record linkage schemes (in place in the USA for many years for medical claims) such as the UK Clinical Practice Research Datalink (CPRD) at the MHRA. All these systems have the important capacity to obtain information on very large numbers of patients (many millions in the database itself, and 10 000–20 000 in *observational cohort* studies and *case–control* studies), complementing the spontaneous reporting system (see Ch. 4).

In the EU, many new drugs are highlighted as being under special consideration by the regulatory authorities, by marking the product information with a symbol, the inverted black triangle (▾). The regulatory authority communicates emerging data on safety of drugs to doctors through letters or papers in journals, through specialist bulletins, e.g. Drug Safety Update in the UK, and for very significant issues by direct letters ('Direct Healthcare Professional Communication') and an electronic cascade system (the Central Alerting System) in the UK.

Two other important regulatory activities that affect marketed drugs are:

- variations to licences.
- reclassifications.

Variations are substantial changes instigated usually by pharmaceutical companies, but sometimes by the regulatory authority, to the efficacy, safety or quality aspects of the medicine. Most significant variations involve additions to indications or dosing regimens, or to the warnings and contraindication sections of the SPC. They need to be supported by evidence and undergo formal assessment and approval by regulators.

Reclassification means change in the legal status of a medicine and is the process by which a prescription-only medicine can be converted to one that is available directly to the public through pharmacies and general retail outlets. It follows a rigorous assessment process with a particular stress on safety aspects of the medicine; it involves advice from the Commission on Human Medicines and public consultation. The purpose of reclassification is to allow easier access of the general public to effective and safe medicines for self-medication. In the UK, emergency contraception ('morning after' pill), simvastatin and omeprazole have been reclassified to be available from pharmacies without a prescription, under supervision of a pharmacist.

Discussion

Common sense would seem to dictate that safety and efficacy of a drug should be fully defined before it is granted marketing authorisation. For practical and ethical reasons, pre-licensing trials with very close supervision are limited to hundreds, sometimes thousands, of patients and are powered to detect efficacy. Post-licensing studies are increasingly regarded as essential to complete the evaluation of drugs under conditions of ordinary use on a large scale, these programmes being preferable to attempts to enlarge and prolong formal therapeutic trials.

It has been proposed by some that a *risk:benefit* assessment of new (candidate) medicines against old medicines should be part of a regulatory application.[15,16] It is argued that a novel drug finds its place only after several, sometimes many,

[14]Waller P C, Bahri P 2002 Regulatory pharmacovigilance in the EU. In: Mann R, Andrews E (eds) Pharmacovigilance. John Wiley, Chichester, pp. 183–194.

[15]Garratini S, Bertile V 2004 Risk:benefit assessment of old medicines. British Journal of Clinical Pharmacology 58:581–586.
[16]Motola D, De Ponti F, Rossi P et al 2005 Therapeutic innovation in the European Union: analysis of the drugs approved by the EMEA between 1995 and 2003. British Journal of Clinical Pharmacology 59:457–478.

years, and to delay licensing is simply impracticable on financial grounds. Thus a 'need clause' in licensing is not generally practicable or supported. This is why *comparative* therapeutic studies of a new drug with existing drugs are not required for licensing in countries having a research-based pharmaceutical industry. A need clause is, however, appropriate for low- and middle-income countries (see World Health Organization Essential Drugs Programme); indeed, such countries have no alternative.

The licensing authority in the UK is not concerned with the pricing of drugs or their cost-effectiveness. The cost of medicines does, however, concern all governments, as part of the rising costs of national health services. A serious attempt to control costs on drug usage by the introduction of national guidelines on disease management (including the use of individual drugs) and the appraisal of new and established medicines for cost-effectiveness now operate through a government-funded body called the National Institute for Health and Clinical Excellence (NICE). The present text includes a section on what is called health technology assessment by the former Chairman of NICE (see Ch. 5). In addition, elements of guidance notes issued by NICE appear throughout the book.

Licensed medicines for unlicensed indications

Doctors may generally prescribe any medicine for any legitimate medical purpose, when they judge it to be in the best interest of the patient.[17] But if they use a drug for an indication that is not formally included in the product licence ('off-label' use), they would be wise to think carefully and to keep particularly good records, for, if a patient is dissatisfied, prescribers may find themselves having to justify the use in a court of law. (Written records made at the time of a decision carry substantial weight, but records made later, when trouble is already brewing, lose much of their power to convince, and records that have been altered later are will undermine any defence.) Manufacturers are not always willing to go to the trouble and expense of the rigorous clinical studies required to extend their licence unless a new use is likely to generate significant profits. They are prohibited by law from promoting an unlicensed use. Much prescribing for children is in fact 'off label' because clinical trials are usually conducted in adults and information sufficient for regulatory purposes in children does not exist. Paediatricians have to use adult data, scaled by body-weight or surface

area, together with their clinical experience. To address this issue, companies are now required to conduct trials in children if a new medicine is likely to be used in the paediatric population.

Unlicensed medicines and accelerated licensing

Regulatory systems make provision for the supply of an unlicensed medicine, e.g. one that has not yet completed its full programme of clinical trials, for patients who, on the judgement of their doctors, have no alternative among licensed drugs. The doctor must apply to the manufacturer, who may supply the drug for that particular patient and at the doctor's own responsibility. Various terms are used, e.g. supply on a 'named patient' basis (UK); 'compassionate' drug use (USA). It is illegal to exploit this sensible loophole in supply laws to conduct research. Precise record-keeping of such use is essential. But there can be desperate needs involving large numbers of patients, e.g. tuberculosis, and regulatory authorities may respond by licensing a drug before completion of the usual range of studies (making it clear that patients must understand the risks they are taking). Unfortunately such well-intentioned practice discourages patients from entering formal trials and may, in the long run, actually delay the definition of life-saving therapies. Recognising the need to allow use of unlicensed drugs in areas of unmet medical need, the MHRA introduced an Earlier Access to Medicines Scheme, which gives a regulatory opinion on an unlicensed drug to support such use.

Decision-taking

> It must be remembered always that, although there are risks in taking drugs, there are also risks in not taking drugs, and there are risks in not developing new drugs.

The responsibility to protect public health on the one hand, yet to allow timely access to novel medicines on the other, is one shared by drug regulators, expert advisory bodies and developers. It is complicated by an ever-increasing awareness of the risks and benefits (real or perceived) of medicines by the general public. Some new medicines are registered with the high expectation of effectiveness and with very little safety information; rare and unpredictable adverse events may take years to appear with sufficient conviction that causality is accepted. In taking decisions

---

[17]In many countries, this excludes supply of drugs such as heroin or cocaine for controlled/supervised maintenance of drug addicts. In the UK such supply is permitted to doctors.

about drug regulation, it has been pointed out that there is uncertainty in three areas:[18]

- Facts.
- Public reaction to the facts.
- Future consequences of decisions.

Regulatory authorities need to plough a fine furrow between being too cautious and responsible, at least in part, for the stagnation in new drug development and being too permissive, allowing safety lapses.

It is self-evident that it is much harder to detect and quantify a good that is not done than it is to detect and quantify a harm that is done. Therefore, although it is part of the decision-taker's job to facilitate the doing of good, the avoidance of harm looms larger. Regulators do have a responsibility to encourage and facilitate innovation to enable public health gains. Indeed, there are regulatory tools that allow approval either in an accelerated way, or conditional approvals based on early data or validation of new biomarkers, or in rare diseases where it is impossible to generate significant clinical data. Also, there is a much more permissive approach to licensing emerging, with schemes such as adaptive licensing, promising innovative medicines initiative in UK or the accelerated review and breakthrough designations in the USA.

Counterfeit drugs

Fraudulent medicines make up as much as 6% of pharmaceutical sales worldwide. They present a serious health (and economic) problem in countries with weak regulatory authorities and lacking money to police drug quality. In these countries, counterfeit medicines may make up 20–50% of available products. The trade may involve: false labelling of legally manufactured products, in order to play one national market against another; also, low-quality manufacture of correct ingredients; wrong ingredients, including added ingredients (such as corticosteroids added to herbal medicine for arthritis); no active ingredient; or false packaging. The trail from raw material to appearance on a pharmacy shelf may involve as many as four countries, with the final stages (importer, wholesaler) quite innocent, so well has the process been obscured. Developed countries have inspection and enforcement procedures to detect and take appropriate action on illegal activities.

The public has a role to play. A patient with obsessive-compulsive disorder was receiving treatment with olanzapine. His custom was rigorously to polish the tablets each day before consumption. After one of his repeat prescriptions, his polishing became ever more thorough until the blue colour started to wear off the tablets. He rang the company to complain. Instead of being dismissed as a touch eccentric, the company investigated and found the tablets to be – well, not true blue.[19]

Complementary and alternative medicine

(See also p. 12)

The broad term complementary and alternative medicine (CAM) covers a range of widely varied diagnostic and therapeutic practices; it includes herbal and traditional (mainly Chinese) medicines, homoeopathic remedies and dietary supplements.[20] The public demand for these substances is substantial, and the financial interests are huge: annual global sales of complementary medicines have reached an estimated $83 billion. The efficacy, safety and quality of herbal[21] and homoeopathic[22] preparations have been critically reviewed. Physicians need to be aware that their patients may be taking CAM preparations, not least because of the risk for adverse reactions and drug–drug interactions, e.g. enzyme induction with St John's wort (Hypericum perforatum).[23]

In the UK, largely for historical reasons, the regulation of CAM has developed in a piecemeal way. Some herbal medicines are licensed via the traditional herbals medicines regulations; some are exempt from licensing; some are sold as food supplements; and some products are available in all three categories. Herbal products were granted a Product Licence of Right (PLR) when the licensing system was introduced in the 1970s. Proof of efficacy, safety and quality (mandatory for conventional chemical and biologically developed medicinal products) is usually absent. From 2011, European legislation requires registration of certain CAM based on quality, safety and traditional use. Manufacturers are obliged to report adverse reactions. The rules are different for herbals and homeopathics (as in the legislation, and timings of introduction are different), but the principles of ensuring safety and quality and restricting use to minor self-limiting conditions apply to both.

[18]Lord Ashby 1976 Proceedings of the Royal Society of Medicine 69:721.

[19]The term may originate from the blue cloth made in the English city of Coventry in the late Middle Ages; it resisted fading on washing and thus remained 'true', i.e. reliable.
[20]Baber N S 2003 Complementary medicine, clinical pharmacology and therapeutics [editorial]. British Journal of Clinical Pharmacology 55:225.
[21]Barnes J 2003 Quality, efficacy and safety of complementary medicines; fashions, facts and the future. British Journal of Clinical Pharmacology Part I: Regulation and Quality 55:226–233; Part II: Efficacy and Safety 55:331–340.
[22]Ernst E 2002 A systematic review of systematic reviews of homeopathy. British Journal of Clinical Pharmacology 54:577–582.
[23]Henderson L, Yue Q Y, Bergquist C et al 2002 St John's wort (Hypericum perforatum): drug interactions and clinical outcomes. British Journal of Clinical Pharmacology 54:349–356.

Medicines regulation: the future

In the UK, the principal responsibilities of medicine regulation, i.e. for safe and effective medicines of high quality, will remain the same, but the following themes will provide special attention:

- The promotion and protection of public health: the obligations to ministers, the public and industry are unchanged, but regulators will operate in an environment in which the public increasingly expects more effective medicines without sacrifice of safety. Some results of this are already apparent.
- A wider and more rapid international pharmacovigilance.[24]
- A much more flexible approach to licensing and an increased emphasis on lifecycle.

- Greater transparency in regulatory decision-making.
- New generations of advanced therapies – e.g. gene therapy, cell therapy, tissue therapy – and biosimilars.
- Pharmacogenetics (see Ch. 8).
- The results of assessed applications for new medicines will see a shift from complex technical to patient-oriented documents with clear expressions of risk and benefit.
- A widening of the availability of medicines for chronic disorders through pharmacies, by nurses and other non-medical professionals, and directly to the public.
- Attention to the regulation of medicines for special populations, e.g. the licensing of old and new medicines for children.
- Risk:benefit management throughout product lifecycle.
- Precision medicine, combination products (with devices), companion diagnostics, links with data/algorithms; use of electronic health-care records for trials and vigilance; real-world trials on databases.

---

[24]Waller P C, Evan S J W 2003 A model for the future conduct of pharmacovigilance. Pharmacoepidemiology and Drug Safety 12:17–19.

Guide to further reading

Giezen, T.J., Mantel-Teeuwisse, A.K., Straus, S.M., et al., 2008. Safety-related regulatory actions for biologicals approved in the United States and the European Union. J. Am. Med. Assoc. 300, 1887–1896.

Permanand, G., Mossialos, E., McKee, M., 2006. Regulating medicines in Europe: the European Medicines Agency, marketing authorisation, transparency and

pharmacovigilance. Clin. Med. (Northfield Il) 6 (1), 87–90.

Raine, J., Wise, L., Blackburn, S., et al., 2011. European perspective on risk management and drug safety. Clin. Pharmacol. Ther. 89, 650–654.

Report, 2009. The licensing of medicines in the UK. Drug Ther. Bull. 47 (4), 45–48.

Rudolf, P.M., Bernstein, I.B.G., 2004. Counterfeit drugs. N. Engl. J. Med. 350, 1384–1386.

Zarin, D.A., Tse, T., Ide, N.C., 2005. Trial registration at ClinicalTrials. gov between May and October 2005. N. Engl. J. Med. 353, 2779–2787.

Chapter | 7 |

Classification and naming of drugs

Morris J. Brown

SYNOPSIS

In any science there are two basic requirements, classification and nomenclature (names):

- **Classification – drugs cannot be classified and named according to a single rational system because the requirements of chemists, pharmacologists and doctors differ.**
- **Nomenclature – nor is it practicable always to present each drug under a single name because the formulations in which they are presented as prescribable medicines may vary widely and be influenced by commercial considerations.**

  Generic (non-proprietary) names should be used as far as possible when prescribing except where pharmaceutical bioavailability differences have overriding importance.

  The wider availability of proprietary medicines through pharmacy sale and direct to the public has the potential for greater confusion to consumers (patients) and doctors.

Classification

It is evident from the way this book is organised that there is no homogeneous system for classifying drugs that suits the purpose of every user. Drugs are commonly categorised according to the convenience of whoever is discussing them: clinicians, pharmacologists or medicinal chemists. Drugs may be classified by:

- *Body system*, e.g. alimentary, cardiovascular.
- *Therapeutic use*, e.g. receptor blockers, enzyme inhibitors, carrier molecules, ion channels.

- Mode or site of action: *molecular interaction*, e.g. glucoside, alkaloid, steroid.
  - *Cellular site*, e.g. loop diuretic, catecholamine uptake inhibitor (imipramine).
  - *Molecular structure*, e.g. glycoside, alkaloid, steroid.[1]

Nomenclature (names)

Any drug may have names in all three of the following classes:

1. The full chemical name.
2. A non-proprietary (official, approved, generic) name used in pharmacopoeias and chosen by official bodies; the World Health Organization (WHO) chooses recommended International Nonproprietary Names (rINNs). The harmonisation of names began 50 years ago, and most countries have used rINNs for many years. The USA is an exception, but even here most US National Names are the same as their rINN counterparts. In the UK, there are two exceptions to the policy: adrenaline (rINN epinephrine) and noradrenaline (rINN norepinephrine). Manufacturers are advised to use both names on the product packaging and information literature.

   In general we use rINNs in this book and aim to minimise some unavoidable differences with, where appropriate, alternative names in the text and index (in brackets).

---

[1]The ATC classification system developed by the Nordic countries and widely used in Europe meets most classification requirements. Drugs are classified according to their anatomical, therapeutic and chemical characteristics into five levels of specificity, the fifth being that for the single chemical substance.

3. A proprietary (brand) name that is the commercial property of a pharmaceutical company or companies. In this book proprietary names are distinguished by an initial capital letter.

Example: one drug – three names
1. 3-(10,11-dihydro-5H-dibenz[b.f]-azepin-5-yl) propyldimethylamine
2. Imipramine
3. Tofranil (UK), Melipramine, Novopramine, Pryleugan, Surplix, etc. (various countries).

The *full chemical name* describes the compound for chemists. It is obviously unsuitable for prescribing.

A non-proprietary (generic,[2] approved) name is given by an official (pharmacopoeia) agency, e.g. WHO.

Three principles remain supreme and unchallenged in importance: the need for distinction in sound and spelling, especially when the name is handwritten; the need for freedom from confusion with existing names, both non-proprietary and proprietary, and the desirability of indicating relationships between similar substances.[3]

The generic names *diazepam*, *nitrazepam* and *flurazepam* are all of benzodiazepines. Their proprietary names are Valium, Mogadon and Dalmane respectively. Names ending in *-olol* are adrenoceptor blockers; those ending in *-pril* are angiotensin-converting enzyme (ACE) inhibitors; and those in *-floxacin* are quinolone antimicrobials. Any pharmaceutical company may manufacture a drug that has a well-established use and is no longer under patent restriction, in accordance with official pharmacopoeial quality criteria, and may apply to the regulatory authority for a licence to market. The task of authority is to ensure that these *generic* or *multi-source pharmaceuticals* are interchangeable, i.e. they are pharmaceutically and biologically equivalent, so that a formulation from one source will be absorbed and give the same blood concentrations and have the same therapeutic efficacy as that from another. (Further formal therapeutic trials are not demanded for these well-established drugs.) A prescription for a generic drug formulation may be written for any

officially licensed product that the dispensing pharmacy has chosen to purchase (on economic criteria; see 'generic substitution' below).[4]

The *proprietary name* is a trademark applied to particular formulation(s) of a particular substance by a particular manufacturer. Manufacture is confined to the owner of the trademark or to others licensed by the owner. It is designed to maximise the difference between the names of similar drugs marketed by rivals for obvious commercial reasons. To add confusion, some companies give their proprietary products the same names as their generic products in an attempt to capture the prescription market, both proprietary and generic, and some market lower-priced generics of their own proprietaries. When a prescription is written for a proprietary product, pharmacists under UK law must dispense that product only. But, by agreement with the prescribing doctor, they may substitute an approved generic product *(generic substitution)*. What is not permitted is the substitution of a different molecular structure deemed to be pharmacologically and therapeutically equivalent *(therapeutic substitution)*.

Non-proprietary names

The principal reasons for advocating the habitual use of non-proprietary (generic) names in prescribing are described below.

Clarity. Non-proprietary names give information on the class of drug; for example, nortriptyline and amitriptyline are plainly related, but their proprietary names, Allegron and Triptafen, are not. It is not unknown for prescribers, when one drug has failed, unwittingly to add or substitute another drug of the same group (or even the same drug), thinking that different proprietary names must mean different classes of drugs. Such occurrences underline the wisdom of prescribing generically, so that group similarities are immediately apparent, but highlight the requirement for brand names to be as distinct from one another as possible. Relationships cannot, and should not, be shown by brand names.

Economy. Drugs sold under non-proprietary names are usually, but not always, cheaper than those sold under proprietary names.

Convenience. Pharmacists may supply whatever version they stock,[5] whereas if a proprietary name is used they are

---

[2]The generic name is now widely accepted as being synonymous with the non-proprietary name. Strictly 'generic' (L. *genus*, race, a class of objects) should refer to a group or class of drug, e.g. benzodiazepines, but by common usage the word is now taken to mean the non-proprietary name of individual members of a group, e.g. diazepam.
[3]Trigg R B 1998 Chemical nomenclature. Kluwer Academic, Dordrecht, pp. 208–234.

[4]European Medicines Agency and US Food and Drug Administration guidelines are available and give pharmacokinetic limits that must be met.
[5]This can result in supply of a formulation of appearance different from that previously used. Patients naturally find this disturbing.

obliged to supply that preparation alone. They may have to buy in the preparation named even though they have an equivalent in stock. Mixtures of drugs are sometimes given non-proprietary names, having the prefix *co-* to indicate more than one active ingredient, e.g. co-amoxiclav for Augmentin.[6] No prescriber can be expected to write out the ingredients, so proprietary names are used in many cases, there being no alternative. International travellers with chronic illnesses will be grateful for rINNs (see above), as proprietary names often differ from country to country. The reasons are linguistic as well as commercial (see below).

Proprietary names

The principal non-commercial reason for advocating the use of proprietary names in prescribing is consistency of the product, so that problems of quality, especially of bioavailability, are reduced. There is substance in this argument, though it is often exaggerated.

It is reasonable to use proprietary names when dosage, and therefore pharmaceutical bioavailability, is critical, so that small variations in the amount of drug available for absorption may have a big effect on the patient, e.g. drugs with a low therapeutic ratio, digoxin, hormone replacement therapy, adrenocortical steroids (oral), antiepileptics, cardiac antiarrhythmics, warfarin. In addition, with the introduction of complex formulations, e.g. sustained release, it is important clearly to identify these, and the use of proprietary names has a role.

The prescription and provision of proprietary drugs increases profits for the company who first invented the drug, and costs for the purchaser – variably the patient, insurer or national health-care system. There are no absolute rights or wrongs in this. Society rewards the inventer, because it requires inventions, but wishes a healthy generic market in order to restrain costs. The now widespread use of computer programmes for prescribing, which prompt the doctor to use non-proprietary names, has tilted the balance in favour of generics.

Generic names are intentionally longer than trade names to minimise the risk of confusion, but the use of accepted prefixes and stems for generic names works well and the average name length is four syllables, which is manageable. The search for proprietary names is a 'major problem' for pharmaceutical companies, increasing, as they are, their output of new preparations. A company may average 30 new preparations (not new chemical entities) a year, another warning of the urgent necessity for the doctor to cultivate a sceptical habit of mind. Names that 'look and sound medically seductive' are being picked out. 'Words that survive scrutiny will go into a stock-pile and await inexorable proliferation of new drugs'.[7] One firm (in the USA) commissioned a computer to produce a dictionary of 42 000 nonsense words of an appropriately scientific look and sound.

A more recent cause for confusion for patients (consumers) in purchasing proprietary medicines is the use by manufacturers of a well-established 'brand' name that is associated in the mind of the purchaser with a particular therapeutic effect, e.g. analgesia, when in fact the product may contain a quite different pharmacological entity. By a subtle change or addition to the brand name of the original medicine, the manufacturer aims to establish 'brand loyalty'. This unsavoury practice is called 'umbrella branding'. It is also important to doctors to be aware of what over-the-counter (OTC) medicines their patients are taking, as proprietary products that were at one time familiar to them may contain other ingredients, with the increased risk of adverse events and drug interactions.

For the practising doctor (in the UK) the *British National Formulary* provides a regularly updated and comprehensive list of drugs in their non-proprietary (generic) and proprietary names. 'The range of drugs prescribed by any individual is remarkably narrow, and once the decision is taken to "think generic" surely the effort required is small'.[8] And, we would add, worthwhile.

Confusing names. The need for both clear thought and clear handwriting is shown by medicines of totally different class that have similar names. Serious events have occurred as a result of the confusion of names and dispensing the wrong drug, e.g. Lasix (furosemide) for Losec (omeprazole) (death); AZT (intending zidovudine) was misinterpreted in the pharmacy and azathioprine was dispensed (do not use abbreviations for drug names); Daonil (glibenclamide) for De-nol (bismuth chelate) and for Danol (danazol). It will be noted that non-proprietary names are less likely to be confused with other classes of drugs.

---

[6]This is a practice confined largely to the UK. It is unknown in Europe, and not widely practised in the USA.

[7]Pharmaceutical companies increasingly operate worldwide and are liable to find themselves embarrassed by unanticipated verbal associations. For example, names marketed (in some countries), such as Bumaflex, Kriplex, Nokhel and Snootie, conjure up in the minds of native English speakers associations that may inhibit both doctors and patients from using them (see Jack & Soppitt 1991 in Guide to further reading).

[8]Editorial 1977 British Medical Journal 4:980 (and subsequent correspondence).

Guide to further reading

Aronson, J.K., 2000. Where name and image meet – the argument for adrenaline. Br. Med. J. 320, 506–509.

Chief Medical Officer, Department of Health, Medicines and Healthcare products Regulatory Agency, 2004. Change in names of certain medicinal substances. Professional letter of 17 March 2004, pp. 1–6 (available to download as PL CMO (2004)1: change in names of certain medicinal substances from http://www.dh.gov.uk (Accessed 20 October 2011).

Furberg, C.D., Herrington, D.M., Psaty, B.M., 1999. Are drugs within a class interchangeable? Lancet 354, 1201–1204. (and correspondence: are drugs interchangeable? Lancet 2000 355: 316–317).

George, C.F., 1996. Naming of drugs: pass the epinephrine please. Br. Med. J. 312, 1315 (and correspondence in Br. Med. J. 1996 313, 688–689).

Jack, D.B., Soppitt, A.L., 1991. Give a drug a bad name. Br. Med. J. 303, 1606–1608.

Section | 2 |

From pharmacology to toxicology

Chapter | 8 |

General pharmacology

Mike Schachter, Munir Pirmohamed

SYNOPSIS

How drugs act and interact; how they enter the body; what happens to them inside the body; how they are eliminated from it; the effects of genetics, age and disease on drug action – these topics are important even if they are not prominent in the mind of the prescriber, since an understanding of them will enhance rational decision taking.

Knowledge of the requirements for success and the explanations for failure and for adverse events will enable the doctor to maximise the benefits and minimise the risks of drug therapy.

Pharmacodynamics

- Qualitative aspects: receptors, enzymes, selectivity.
- Quantitative aspects: dose response, potency, therapeutic efficacy, tolerance.

Pharmacokinetics

- Time course of drug concentration: drug passage across cell membranes; order of reaction; plasma half-life and steady-state concentration; therapeutic drug monitoring.
- Individual processes: absorption, distribution, metabolism, elimination.
- Drug dosage: dosing schedules.
- Chronic pharmacology: the consequences of prolonged drug administration and drug discontinuation syndromes.

Individual or biological variation

- Pharmacogenomics: variability due to inherited influences.
- Variability due to environmental and host influences.
- Drug interactions: outside the body, at site of absorption, during distribution, directly on receptors, during metabolism, during excretion.

> Pharmacodynamics is what drugs do to the body; pharmacokinetics is what the body does to drugs.

The practice of drug therapy entails more than remembering an apparently arbitrary list of actions or indications. Scientific incompetence in the modern doctor is inexcusable and, contrary to some assertions, scientific competence is wholly compatible with a humane approach.

Pharmacodynamics

> Understanding how drugs act is not only an objective of the pharmacologist who seeks to develop new and better therapies, it is also the basis of intelligent use of medicines.

Qualitative aspects

The starting point is to consider what drugs do and how they do it, i.e. the nature of drug action. The body functions through control systems that involve chemotransmitters or local hormones, receptors, enzymes, carrier molecules and other specialised macromolecules such as DNA.

Most medicinal drugs act by altering the body's control systems and, in general, they do so by binding to some specialised constituent of the cell, selectively to alter its function and consequently that of the physiological or pathological system to which it contributes. Such drugs are structurally specific in that small modifications to their chemical structure may profoundly alter their effect.

Mechanisms

An overview of the mechanisms of drug action shows that drugs act on *specific receptors* in the cell membrane and interior by:

- *Ligand-gated ion channels*, i.e. receptors coupled directly to membrane ion channels; neurotransmitters act on such receptors in the postsynaptic membrane of a nerve or muscle cell and give a response within milliseconds.
- *G-protein–coupled receptor systems*, i.e. receptors bound to the cell membrane and coupled to intracellular effector systems by a *G-protein*. For instance, catecholamines *(the first messenger)* activate β-adrenoceptors through a coupled G-protein system. This increases the activity of intracellular adenylyl cyclase, increasing the rate of formation of cyclic AMP *(the second messenger)*, a modulator of the activity of several enzyme systems that cause the cell to act. The process takes seconds.
- *Protein kinase receptors*, so called because the structure incorporates a protein kinase, are targets for peptide hormones involved in the control of cell growth and differentiation, and the release of inflammatory mediators over a course of hours.
- *Cytosolic (nuclear) receptors*, i.e. within the cell itself, regulate DNA transcription and, thereby, protein synthesis, e.g. by steroid and thyroid hormones, a process that takes hours or days.

Drugs also act on processes within or near the cell by:

- *Enzyme inhibition*, e.g. platelet cyclo-oxygenase by aspirin, cholinesterase by pyridostigmine, xanthine oxidase by allopurinol.
- Inhibition or induction of *transporter processes* that carry substances into, across and out of cells, e.g. blockade of anion transport in the renal tubule cell by probenecid is used to protect against the nephrotoxic effects of cidofovir (used for cytomegalovirus retinitis).
- *Incorporation into larger molecules*, e.g. 5-fluorouracil, an anticancer drug, is incorporated into messenger RNA in place of uracil.
- In the case of successful antimicrobial agents, *altering metabolic processes* unique to microorganisms, e.g. penicillin interferes with formation of the bacterial cell wall; or by showing enormous quantitative differences in affecting a process common to both humans and microbes, e.g. inhibition of folic acid synthesis by trimethoprim.

Outside the cell drugs act by:

- Direct *chemical interaction*, e.g. chelating agents, antacids.
- *Osmosis*, as with purgatives, e.g. magnesium sulphate, and diuretics, e.g. mannitol, which are active because neither they nor the water in which they are dissolved is absorbed by the cells lining the gut and kidney tubules, respectively.

Receptors

Most receptors are protein macromolecules. When the agonist binds to the receptor, the proteins undergo an alteration in conformation, which induces changes in systems within the cell that in turn bring about the response to the drug over differing time courses. Many kinds of effector response exist, but those indicated above are the four basic types.

Radioligand binding studies have shown that the receptor numbers do not remain constant but change according to circumstances. When tissues are continuously exposed to an agonist, the number of receptors decreases *(down-regulation)*, and this may be a cause of *tachyphylaxis* (loss of efficacy with frequently repeated doses), e.g. in asthmatics who use adrenoceptor agonist bronchodilators excessively. Prolonged contact with an antagonist leads to formation of new receptors *(up-regulation)*. Indeed, one explanation for the worsening of angina pectoris or cardiac ventricular arrhythmia in some patients following abrupt withdrawal of a β-adrenoceptor blocker is that normal concentrations of circulating catecholamines now have access to an increased (up-regulated) population of β-adrenoceptors (see Chronic pharmacology, p. 100).

Agonists. Drugs that activate receptors do so because they resemble the natural transmitter or hormone, but their value in clinical practice often rests on their greater capacity to resist degradation and so to act for longer than the natural substances (endogenous ligands) they mimic; for this reason, bronchodilatation produced by salbutamol lasts longer than that induced by adrenaline/epinephrine.

Antagonists (blockers) of receptors are sufficiently similar to the natural agonist to be 'recognised' by the receptor and to occupy it without activating a response, thereby preventing (blocking) the natural agonist from exerting its effect. Drugs that have no activating effect whatever on the receptor are termed *pure antagonists*. A receptor occupied by a low-efficacy agonist is inaccessible to a subsequent dose of a high-efficacy agonist, so that, in this specific situation, a low-efficacy agonist acts as an antagonist. This can happen with opioids.

Partial agonists. Some drugs, in addition to blocking access of the natural agonist to the receptor, are capable of a low degree of activation, i.e. they have both antagonist and agonist action. Such substances show *partial agonist activity* (PAA). The β-adrenoceptor antagonists pindolol and oxprenolol have partial agonist activity (in their case it is often called *intrinsic sympathomimetic activity*, ISA), while propranolol is devoid of agonist activity, i.e. it is a pure antagonist.

A patient may be as extensively 'β-blocked' by propranolol as by pindolol, i.e. with eradication of exercise tachycardia, but the resting heart rate is lower on propranolol; such differences can have clinical importance.

Inverse agonists. Some substances produce effects that are specifically opposed to those of the agonist. The agonist action of benzodiazepines on the benzodiazepine receptor in the central nervous system produces sedation, anxiolysis and muscle relaxation, and controls convulsions; substances called β-carbolines, which also bind to this receptor, cause stimulation, anxiety, increased muscle tone and convulsions – they are *inverse agonists*. Both types of drug act by modulating the effects of the neurotransmitter γ-aminobutyric acid (GABA).

Receptor binding (and vice versa). If the forces that bind drug to receptor are weak (hydrogen bonds, van der Waals bonds, electrostatic bonds), the binding will be easily and rapidly reversible; if the forces involved are strong (covalent bonds), then binding will be effectively irreversible.

An antagonist that binds *reversibly* to a receptor can by definition be displaced from the receptor by mass action (see p. 83) of the agonist (and vice versa). A sufficient increase of the concentration of agonist above that of the antagonist restores the response. β-blocked patients who increase their low heart rate with exercise are demonstrating a rise in sympathetic drive and releasing enough catecholamine (agonist) to overcome the prevailing degree of receptor blockade.

Raising the dose of β-adrenoceptor blocker will limit or abolish exercise-induced tachycardia, showing that the degree of blockade is enhanced, as more drug becomes available to compete with the endogenous transmitter.

As agonist and antagonist compete to occupy the receptor according to the law of mass action, this type of drug action is termed *competitive antagonism*.

When receptor-mediated responses are studied either in isolated tissues or in intact humans, a graph of the logarithm of the dose given (horizontal axis) plotted against the response obtained (vertical axis) commonly gives an S-shaped (sigmoid) curve, the central part of which is a straight line. If the measurements are repeated in the presence of an antagonist, and the curve obtained is parallel to the original but displaced to the right, then antagonism is said to be competitive and the agonist to be *surmountable*.

Drugs that bind irreversibly to receptors include phenoxybenzamine (to the α-adrenoceptor). Because the drug fixes to the receptor, increasing the concentration of agonist does not fully restore the response, and antagonism of this type is described as insurmountable.

The log dose–response curves for the agonist in the absence of, and in the presence of, a non-competitive antagonist are not parallel. Some toxins act in this way; for example, α-bungarotoxin, a constituent of some snake and spider venoms, binds irreversibly to the acetylcholine receptor and is used as a tool to study it.

Restoration of the response after irreversible binding requires elimination of the drug from the body and synthesis of new receptor, and for this reason the effect may persist long after drug administration has ceased. Irreversible agents find little place in clinical practice.

Physiological (functional) antagonism

An action on the same receptor is not the only mechanism by which one drug may oppose the effect of another. Extreme bradycardia following overdose of a β-adrenoceptor blocker can be relieved by atropine, which accelerates the heart by blockade of the parasympathetic branch of the autonomic nervous system, the cholinergic tone of which (vagal tone) operates continuously to slow it.

Adrenaline/epinephrine and theophylline counteract bronchoconstriction produced by histamine released from mast cells in anaphylactic shock by relaxing bronchial smooth muscle (β₂-adrenoceptor effect). In both cases, a second drug overcomes the pharmacological effect, by a different physiological mechanism, i.e. there is *physiological* or *functional* antagonism.

Enzymes

Interaction between drug and enzyme is in many respects similar to that between drug and receptor. Drugs may alter enzyme activity because they resemble a natural substrate and hence compete with it for the enzyme. For example, enalapril is effective in hypertension because it is structurally similar to the part of angiotensin I that is attacked by angiotensin-converting enzyme (ACE); enalapril prevents formation of the pressor angiotensin II by occupying the active site of the enzyme and so inhibiting its action.

Carbidopa competes with levodopa for dopa decarboxylase, and the benefit of this combination in Parkinson's disease is reduced metabolism of levodopa to dopamine in the blood (but not in the brain because carbidopa does not cross the blood–brain barrier).

Ethanol prevents metabolism of methanol to its toxic metabolite, formic acid, by competing for occupancy of the enzyme alcohol dehydrogenase; this is the rationale for using ethanol in methanol poisoning. The above are examples of competitive *(reversible)* inhibition of enzyme activity.

Irreversible inhibition occurs with organophosphorus insecticides and chemical warfare agents (see Ch. 10), which combine covalently with the active site of acetylcholinesterase; recovery of cholinesterase activity depends on the formation of new enzyme. Covalent binding of aspirin to cyclo-oxygenase (COX) inhibits the enzyme in platelets for their entire lifespan because platelets have no system for synthesising new protein; this is why low doses of aspirin are sufficient for antiplatelet action.

Selectivity

The pharmacologist who produces a new drug and the doctor who gives it to a patient share the desire that it should possess a selective action so that additional and unwanted (adverse) effects do not complicate the management of the patient. Approaches to obtaining selectivity of drug action include the following.

Modification of drug structure. Many drugs have in their design a structural similarity to some natural constituent of the body, e.g. a neurotransmitter, a hormone, a substrate for an enzyme; replacing or competing with that natural constituent achieves selectivity of action. Enormous scientific effort and expertise go into the synthesis and testing of analogues of natural substances in order to create drugs capable of obtaining a specified effect, and that alone (see Therapeutic index, below). The approach is the basis of modern drug design and it has led to the production of adrenoceptor antagonists, histamine receptor antagonists and many other important medicines.

But there are biological constraints to selectivity. Anticancer drugs that act against rapidly dividing cells lack selectivity because they also damage other tissues with a high cell replication rate, such as bone marrow and gut epithelium.

Selective delivery (drug targeting). Simple topical application, e.g. skin and eye, and special drug delivery systems, e.g. intrabronchial administration of β_2-adrenoceptor agonist or corticosteroid (inhaled, pressurised, metered aerosol for asthma) can achieve the objective of target tissue selectivity. Selective targeting of drugs to less accessible sites of disease offers considerable scope for therapy as technology develops, e.g. attaching drugs to antibodies selective for cancer cells.

Stereoselectivity. Drug molecules are three-dimensional, and many drugs contain one or more *asymmetrical* or *chiral*[1] centres in their structures, i.e. a single drug can be, in effect, a mixture of two non-identical mirror images (like a mixture of left- and right-handed gloves). The two forms, which are known as *enantiomorphs,* can exhibit very different pharmacodynamic, pharmacokinetic and toxicological properties.

For example, (1) the S form of warfarin is four times more active than the R form,[2] (2) the peak plasma concentration of S fenoprofen is four times that of R fenoprofen after oral administration of RS fenoprofen, and (3) the S, but not the R, enantiomorph of thalidomide is metabolised to primary toxins.

Many other drugs are available as mixtures of enantiomorphs (racemates). Pharmaceutical development of drugs as single enantiomers rather than as racemic mixtures offers the prospect of greater selectivity of action and lessens the risk of toxicity.

Quantitative aspects

That a drug has a desired qualitative action is obviously all important, but is not by itself enough. There are also quantitative aspects, i.e. the right amount of action is required, and with some drugs the dose has to be adjusted very precisely to deliver this, neither too little nor too much, to escape both inefficacy and toxicity, e.g. digoxin, lithium, gentamicin. While the general correlation between dose and response may evoke no surprise, certain characteristics of the relation are fundamental to the way drugs are used, as described below.

Dose–response relationships

Conventionally, the horizontal axis shows the dose and the response appears on the vertical axis. The slope of the dose–response curve defines the extent to which a desired response alters as the dose is changed. A steeply rising and prolonged curve indicates that a small change in dose produces a large change in drug effect over a wide dose range, e.g. with the loop diuretic furosemide (used in doses from 20 mg to over 250 mg/day). By contrast, the dose–response curve for thiazide diuretics soon reaches a plateau, and the clinically useful dose range for bendroflumethiazide, for example, extends from 5 to 10 mg; increasing the dose beyond this produces no added diuretic effect, although it adds to toxicity.

Dose–response curves for wanted and unwanted effects can illustrate and quantify selective and non-selective drug action (Fig. 8.1).

Potency and efficacy

A clear distinction between potency and efficacy is pertinent, particularly in relation to claims made for usefulness in therapeutics.

Potency is the amount (weight) of drug in relation to its effect, e.g. if weight-for-weight drug A has a greater effect than drug B, then drug A is more potent than drug B, although the maximum therapeutic effect obtainable may be similar with both drugs.

---

[1]Greek: *cheir* = a hand.
[2]R (rectus) and S (sinister) refer to the sequential arrangement of the constituent parts of the molecule around the chiral centre.

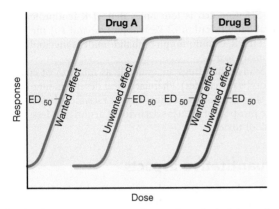

Fig. 8.1 Dose–response curves for two hypothetical drugs. For drug A, the dose that brings about the maximum wanted effect is less than the lowest dose that produces the unwanted effect. The ratio ED_{50} (unwanted effect)/ED_{50} (wanted effect) indicates that drug A has a large therapeutic index; it is thus highly *selective* in its wanted action. Drug B causes unwanted effects at doses well below producing its maximum benefit. The ratio ED_{50} (unwanted effect)/ED_{50} (wanted effect) indicates that the drug has a small therapeutic index: it is thus *non-selective*.

The diuretic effect of bumetanide 1 mg is equivalent to that of furosemide 50 mg; thus bumetanide is more potent than furosemide, but both drugs achieve about the same maximum effect. The difference in weight of drug administered is of no clinical significance unless it is great.

Pharmacological efficacy refers to the strength of response induced by occupancy of a receptor by an agonist (intrinsic activity); it is a specialised pharmacological concept. But clinicians are concerned with therapeutic efficacy, as follows.

Therapeutic efficacy or effectiveness, is the capacity of a drug to produce an effect and refers to the maximum such effect. For example, if drug A can produce a therapeutic effect that cannot be obtained with drug B, however much of drug B is given, then drug A has the higher *therapeutic efficacy*. Differences in therapeutic efficacy are of great clinical importance, usually more than potency.

Amiloride (*low* efficacy) can at best effect excretion of no more than 5% of the sodium load filtered by the glomeruli; there is no point in increasing the dose beyond that which achieves this, as this is its maximum diuretic effect. Bendroflumethiazide (*moderate* efficacy) can effect excretion of no more than 10% of the filtered sodium load no matter how large the dose. Furosemide can effect excretion of 25% and more of filtered sodium; it is a *high*-efficacy diuretic.

Therapeutic index. With progressive increases in dose, the desired response in the patient usually rises to a maximum beyond which further increases elicit no greater benefit but

induce unwanted effects. This is because most drugs do not have a single dose–response curve, but a different curve for each action, wanted as well as unwanted. Increases in dose beyond that which gives the maximum wanted response recruit only new and unwanted actions.

A sympathomimetic bronchodilator might exhibit one dose–response relation for decreasing airway resistance (wanted) and another for increase in heart rate (unwanted). Clearly, the usefulness of any drug relates closely to the extent to which such dose–response relations overlap.

Ehrlich (see p. 166) introduced the concept of the *therapeutic index* or ratio as the maximum tolerated dose divided by the minimum curative dose, but the index is never calculated thus as such single doses cannot be determined accurately in humans. More realistically, a dose that has some unwanted effect in 50% of humans, e.g. in the case of an adrenoceptor agonist bronchodilator a specified increase in heart rate, is compared with that which is therapeutic in 50% (ED_{50}), e.g. a specified decrease in airways resistance.

In practice, such information is not available for many drugs, but the therapeutic index does embody a concept that is fundamental in comparing the usefulness of one drug with another, namely, *safety in relation to efficacy*. Fig. 8.1 expresses the concept diagrammatically.

Tolerance

Continuous or repeated administration of a drug is often accompanied by a gradual diminution of the effect it produces. A state of *tolerance* exists when it becomes necessary to increase the dose of a drug to get an effect previously obtained with a smaller dose, i.e. reduced sensitivity. By contrast, the term *tachyphylaxis* describes the phenomenon of progressive lessening of effect (refractoriness) in response to frequently administered doses (see Receptors, p. 77); it tends to develop more rapidly than tolerance.

The use of opioids readily illustrates tolerance, as witnessed by the huge doses of morphine that may be necessary to maintain pain relief in terminal care; the effect is due to reduced pharmacological efficacy (see above) at receptor sites or to down-regulation of receptors. Tolerance is acquired rapidly with nitrates used to prevent angina, possibly mediated by the generation of oxygen free radicals from nitric oxide; it can be avoided by removing transdermal nitrate patches for 4–8 h, e.g. at night, to allow the plasma concentration to fall.

Accelerated metabolism by enzyme induction (see p. 95) also leads to tolerance, as experience shows with alcohol, taken regularly as opposed to sporadically. There is commonly cross-tolerance between drugs of similar structure.

Failure of certain individuals to respond to normal doses of a drug, e.g. resistance to warfarin, vitamin D, constitutes a form of natural tolerance (see Pharmacogenetics, p. 103).

Bioassay and standardisation

Biological assay (bioassay) is the process by which the activity of a substance (identified or unidentified) is measured on living material: e.g. contraction of bronchial, uterine or vascular muscle. It is used only when chemical or physical methods are not practicable as in the case of a mixture of active substances, or of an incompletely purified preparation, or where no chemical method has been developed. The activity of a preparation is expressed relative to that of a standard preparation of the same substance.

Biological standardisation is a specialised form of bioassay. It involves matching of material of unknown potency with an international or national standard with the objective of providing a preparation for use in therapeutics and research. The results are expressed as *units* of a substance rather than its weight, e.g. insulin, vaccines.

Pharmacokinetics

> To initiate a desired drug action is a *qualitative* choice but, when the qualitative choice is made, considerations of *quantity* immediately arise; it is possible to have too much or too little of a good thing. To obtain the right effect at the right intensity, at the right time, for the right duration, with minimal risk of unpleasantness or harm, is what pharmacokinetics is about.

Dosage regimens of long-established drugs grew from trial and error. Doctors learned by experience the dose, the frequency of dosing and the route of administration that was most likely to benefit and least likely to harm. But this empirical ('suck it and see') approach is no longer tenable. We now have an understanding of how drugs cross membranes to enter the body, how they are distributed round it in the blood and other body fluids, how they are bound to plasma proteins and tissues (which act as stores), and how they are eliminated from the body. Quantification of these processes paves the way for efficient development of dosing regimens.

> **Pharmacokinetics**[3] is concerned with the rate at which drug molecules cross cell membranes to enter the body, to distribute within it and to leave the body, as well as with the structural changes (metabolism) to which they are subject within it.

---

[3]Greek: *pharmacon* = drug; *kinein* = to move.

The discussion covers the following topics:

- Drug passage across cell membranes.
- Order of reaction or process (first and zero order).
- Time course of drug concentration and effect:
  - plasma half-life and steady-state concentration
  - therapeutic monitoring.
- The individual processes: absorption, distribution, metabolism (biotransformation), elimination.

Drug passage across cell membranes

Certain concepts are fundamental to understanding how drug molecules make their way around the body to achieve their effect. The first concerns the modes by which drugs cross cell membranes and cells.

Our bodies are labyrinths of fluid-filled spaces. Some, such as the lumina of the kidney tubules or intestine, connect to the outside world; the blood, lymph and cerebrospinal fluid are enclosed. Sheets of cells line these spaces, and the extent to which a drug can cross epithelia or endothelia is fundamental to its clinical use, determining whether a drug can be taken orally for systemic effect, and whether within the glomerular filtrate it will be reabsorbed or excreted in the urine.

Cell membranes are essentially bilayers of lipid molecules with 'islands' of protein, and they preserve and regulate the internal environment. *Lipid-soluble* substances diffuse readily into cells and therefore throughout body tissues. Adjacent epithelial or endothelial cells are linked by tight junctions, some of which are traversed by water-filled channels that allow the passage of water-soluble substances of small molecular size.

The jejunum and proximal renal tubule contain many such channels and are *leaky epithelia*, whereas the tight junctions in the stomach and urinary bladder do not have these channels and water cannot pass; they are termed *tight epithelia*. Special protein molecules within the lipid bilayer allow specific substances to enter or leave the cell preferentially, i.e. *energy-utilising transporter processes*, described later. The natural processes of passive diffusion, filtration and carrier-mediated transport determine the passage of drugs across membranes and cells, and their distribution round the body.

Passive diffusion

This is the most important means by which a drug enters the tissues and distributes through them. It refers simply to the natural tendency of any substance to move passively from an area of high concentration to one of low concentration. In the context of an individual cell, the drug moves at a rate proportional to the concentration difference across the cell membrane, i.e. it shows first-order kinetics (see p. 84); cellular energy is not required, which means that the process does not become saturated and is not inhibited by other substances.

The extent to which drugs are soluble in *water* or *lipid* is central to their capacity to cross cell membranes and depends on environmental pH and the structural properties of the molecule.

> Lipid solubility is promoted by the presence of a benzene ring, a hydrocarbon chain, a steroid nucleus or halogen (-Br, -Cl, -F) groups. Water solubility is promoted by the presence of alcoholic (-OH), amide (-CO·NH$_2$) or carboxylic (-COOH) groups, or the formation of glucuronide and sulphate conjugates.

It is useful to classify drugs in a physicochemical sense into:

- Those that are *variably* ionised according to environmental pH (electrolytes) (lipid soluble or water soluble).
- Those that are *incapable* of becoming ionised whatever the environmental pH (un-ionised, non-polar substances) (lipid soluble).
- Those that are *permanently* ionised whatever the environmental pH (ionised, polar substances) (water soluble).

Drugs that ionise according to environmental pH

Many drugs are *weak electrolytes*, i.e. their structural groups ionise to a greater or lesser extent, according to environmental pH. Most such molecules are present partly in the ionised and partly in the un-ionised state. The degree of ionisation influences lipid solubility (and hence diffusibility) and so affects absorption, distribution and elimination.

Ionisable groups in a drug molecule tend either to lose a hydrogen ion (acidic groups) or to add a hydrogen ion (basic groups). The extent to which a molecule has this tendency to ionise is given by the dissociation (or ionisation) constant (K_a), expressed as the pK_a, i.e. the negative logarithm of the K_a (just as pH is the negative logarithm of the hydrogen ion concentration). In an acidic environment, i.e. one already containing many free hydrogen ions, an acidic group tends to retain a hydrogen ion and remains un-ionised; a relative deficit of free hydrogen ions, i.e. a basic environment, favours loss of the hydrogen ion from an acidic group, which thus becomes ionised. The opposite is the case for a base. The issue may be summarised:

- Acidic groups become less ionised in an acidic environment.

- Basic groups become less ionised in a basic (alkaline) environment and vice versa.

This in turn influences *diffusibility* because:

- Un-ionised drug is lipid soluble and diffusible.
- Ionised drug is lipid insoluble and non-diffusible.

Quantifying the degree of ionisation helps to express the profound effect of environmental pH. Recall that when the pH of the environment is the same as the pK_a of a drug within it, then the ratio of un-ionised to ionised molecules is $1:1$. But for every unit by which pH is changed, the ratio of un-ionised to ionised molecules changes 10-fold. Thus, when the pH is 2 units less than the pK_a, molecules of an acid become 100 times more un-ionised, and when the pH is 2 units more than the pK_a, molecules of an acid become 100 times more ionised. Such pH change profoundly affect drug kinetics.

pH variation and drug kinetics. The *pH partition hypothesis* expresses the separation of a drug across a lipid membrane according to differences in environmental pH. There is a wide range of pH in the gut (pH 1.5 in the stomach, 6.8 in the upper and 7.6 in the lower intestine). But the pH inside the body is maintained within a limited range (pH 7.46 ± 0.04), so that only drugs that are substantially un-ionised at this pH will be lipid soluble, diffuse across tissue boundaries and so be widely distributed, e.g. into the central nervous system (CNS). Urine pH varies between the extremes of 4.6 and 8.2, and the prevailing pH affects the amount of drug reabsorbed from the renal tubular lumen by passive diffusion.

In the stomach, aspirin (acetylsalicylic acid, pK_a 3.5) is un-ionised and thus lipid soluble and diffusible. When aspirin enters the gastric epithelial cells (pH 7.4), it will ionise, become less diffusible and so will localise there. This *ion trapping* is one mechanism whereby aspirin is concentrated in, and so harms, the gastric mucosa. In the body, aspirin is metabolised to salicylic acid (pK_a 3.0), which at pH 7.4 is highly ionised and thus remains in the extracellular fluid. Eventually the molecules of salicylic acid in the plasma are filtered by the glomeruli and pass into the tubular fluid, which is generally more acidic than plasma and causes a proportion of salicylic acid to become un-ionised and lipid soluble so that it diffuses back into the tubular cells. Alkalinising the urine with an intravenous infusion of sodium bicarbonate causes more salicylic acid to become ionised and lipid insoluble so that it remains in the tubular fluid, and passes into the urine. Treatment for salicylate (aspirin) overdose utilises this effect.

Conversely, acidifying the urine increases the elimination of the base amfetamine (pK_a 9.9) (see Acidification of urine, p. 129).

Drugs that are incapable of becoming ionised

These include digoxin and steroid hormones such as prednisolone. Effectively lacking any ionisable groups, they are unaffected by environmental pH, are lipid soluble and so diffuse readily across tissue boundaries. These drugs are also referred to as *non-polar*.

Permanently ionised drugs

Drugs that are permanently ionised contain groups that dissociate so strongly that they remain ionised over the range of the body pH. Such compounds are termed *polar*, for their groups are either negatively charged (acidic, e.g. heparin) or positively charged (basic, e.g. ipratropium, tubocurarine, suxamethonium) and all have a very limited capacity to cross cell membranes. This is a disadvantage with heparin, which the gut does not absorb, so that it is given parenterally. Conversely, heparin is a useful anticoagulant in pregnancy because it does not cross the placenta (which the orally effective warfarin does and is liable to cause fetal haemorrhage as well as being teratogenic).

The following are particular examples of the relevance of drug passage across membranes.

Brain and cerebrospinal fluid (CSF). The capillaries of the cerebral circulation differ from those in most other parts of the body in that they lack the filtration channels between endothelial cells through which substances in the blood normally gain access to the extracellular fluid. Tight junctions between adjacent capillary endothelial cells, together with their basement membrane and a thin covering from the processes of astrocytes, separate the blood from the brain tissue, forming the *blood–brain barrier*. Compounds that are *lipid insoluble* do not cross it readily, e.g. atenolol, compared with propranolol (lipid soluble), and unwanted CNS effects are more prominent with the latter. Therapy with methotrexate (lipid insoluble) may fail to eliminate leukaemic deposits in the CNS.

Conversely *lipid-soluble* substances enter brain tissue with ease; thus diazepam (lipid soluble) given intravenously is effective within 1 min for status epilepticus, and effects of alcohol (ethanol) by mouth are noted within minutes; the level of general anaesthesia can be controlled closely by altering the concentration of inhaled anaesthetic gas (lipid soluble).

Placenta. Maternal blood bathes the chorionic villi, which consist of a layer of trophoblastic cells that enclose fetal capillaries. Their large surface area and the high placental blood flow (500 mL/min) are essential for gas exchange, uptake of nutrients and elimination of waste products. Thus a lipid barrier separates the fetal and maternal bloodstreams, allowing the passage of lipid-soluble substances but excluding water-soluble compounds, especially those with a molecular weight exceeding 600.[4]

This exclusion is of particular importance with short-term use, e.g. tubocurarine (mol. wt. 772) (lipid insoluble) or gallamine (mol. wt. 891) used as a muscle relaxant during caesarean section do not affect the infant; with prolonged use, however, all compounds will eventually enter the fetus to some extent (see Index).

Filtration

Aqueous channels in the tight junctions between adjacent epithelial cells allow the passage of some water-soluble substances. Neutral or uncharged, i.e. non-polar, molecules pass most readily because the pores are electrically charged. Within the alimentary tract, channels are largest and most numerous in jejunal epithelium, and filtration allows for rapid equilibration of concentrations and consequently of osmotic pressures across the mucosa. Ions such as sodium enter the body through the aqueous channels, the size of which probably limits passage to substances of low molecular weight, e.g. ethanol (mol. wt. 46). Filtration seems to play at most a minor role in drug transfer within the body except for glomerular filtration, which is an important mechanism of drug excretion.

Carrier-mediated transport

The membranes of many cells incorporate carrier-mediated transporter processes that control the entry and exit of endogenous molecules, and show a high degree of specificity for particular compounds because they have evolved from biological needs for the uptake of essential nutrients or elimination of metabolic products. Drugs that bear some structural resemblance to natural constituents of the body are likely to utilise these mechanisms.

Some carrier-mediated transport processes operate passively, i.e. do not require cellular energy, and this is *facilitated diffusion*, e.g. vitamin B_{12} absorption. Other, energy-requiring processes move substrates into or out of cells against a concentration gradient very effectively, i.e. by *active transport*; they are subject to saturation, inhibition and induction (see p. 93).

The order of reaction or process

In the body, drug molecules reach their sites of action after crossing cell membranes and cells, and many are metabolised in the process. The rate at which these movements or

---

[4]Most drugs have a molecular weight of less than 600 (e.g. diazepam 284, morphine 303), but some have more (erythromycin 733, digoxin 780).

changes take place is subject to important influences called the *order of reaction* or process. In biology generally, two orders of such reactions are recognised, and are summarised as follows:

- First-order processes by which a constant *fraction* of drug is transported/metabolised in unit time.
- Zero-order processes by which a constant *amount* of drug is transported/metabolised in unit time.

First-order (exponential) processes

In the majority of instances, the rates at which absorption, distribution, metabolism and excretion of a drug occur are directly proportional to its concentration in the body. In other words, transfer of drug across a cell membrane or formation of a metabolite is high at high concentrations and falls in direct proportion to be low at low concentrations (an exponential relationship).

This is because the processes follow the Law of Mass Action, which states that the rate of reaction is directly proportional to the active filtration masses of reacting substances. In other words, at high concentrations there are more opportunities for crowded molecules to interact with one another or to cross cell membranes than at low, uncrowded concentrations. Processes for which the rate of reaction is proportional to the concentration of participating molecules are *first-order processes*.

In doses used clinically, most drugs are subject to first-order processes of absorption, distribution, metabolism and elimination, and this knowledge is useful. The current chapter later describes how the rate of elimination of a drug from the plasma falls as the concentration in plasma falls, and the time for any plasma concentration to fall by 50% ($t_{1/2}$, the plasma half-life) is always the same. Thus, it becomes possible to quote a constant value for the $t_{1/2}$ of the drug. This occurs because rate and concentration are in proportion, i.e. the process obeys first-order kinetics.

Knowing that first-order conditions apply to a drug allows accurate calculations that depend on its $t_{1/2}$, i.e. time to achieve steady-state plasma concentration, time to elimination, and the construction of dosing schedules.

Zero-order processes (saturation kinetics)

As the amount of drug in the body rises, metabolic reactions or processes that have limited capacity become saturated. In other words, the rate of the process reaches a maximum amount at which it stays constant, e.g. due to limited activity of an enzyme, and any further increase in rate is impossible despite an increase in the dose of drug. In these circumstances, the rate of reaction is no longer proportional to dose, and exhibits *rate-limited* or *dose-dependent*[5] or *zero-order*

or *saturation* kinetics. In practice, enzyme-mediated metabolic reactions are the most likely to show rate limitation because the amount of enzyme present is finite and can become saturated. Passive diffusion does not become saturated. There are some important consequences of zero-order kinetics.

Alcohol (ethanol) (see also p. 146) is a drug whose kinetics has considerable implications for society as well as for the individual, as follows:

Alcohol is subject to first-order kinetics with a $t_{1/2}$ of about 1 h at plasma concentrations below 10 mg/dL (attained after drinking about two-thirds of a unit (glass) of wine or beer). Above this concentration the main enzyme (alcohol dehydrogenase) that converts the alcohol into acetaldehyde approaches and then reaches saturation, at which point alcohol metabolism cannot proceed any faster than about 10 mL or 8 g/h for a 70-kg man. If the subject continues to drink, the blood alcohol concentration rises disproportionately, for the rate of metabolism remains the same, as alcohol shows zero-order kinetics.

An illustration. Consider a man of average size who drinks about half (375 mL) a standard bottle of whisky (40% alcohol), i.e. 150 mL alcohol, over a short period, absorbs it and goes drunk to bed at midnight with a blood alcohol concentration of about 250 mg/dL. *If alcohol metabolism were subject to first-order kinetics, with a $t_{1/2}$ of 1 h throughout the whole range of social consumption, the subject would halve his blood alcohol concentration each hour* (Fig. 8.2). It is easy to calculate that, when he drives his car to work at 08.00 hours the next morning, he has a negligible blood alcohol concentration (less than 1 mg/dL) though, no doubt, a hangover might reduce his driving skill.

But at these high concentrations, alcohol is in fact subject to *zero-order* kinetics and so, metabolising about 10 mL alcohol per hour, after 8 h the subject has eliminated only 80 mL, leaving 70 mL in his body and giving a blood concentration of about 120 mg/dL. At this level, his driving skill is seriously impaired. The subject has an accident on his way to work and is breathalysed despite his indignant protests that he last touched a drop before midnight. Banned from the road, on his train journey to work he will have leisure to reflect on the difference between first-order and zero-order kinetics (though this is unlikely!).

In practice. The example above describes an imagined event, but similar cases occur in everyday therapeutics. Phenytoin, at low dose, exhibits a first-order elimination process, and there is a directly proportional increase in the

---

[5]We quote all of these terms since they appear in the relevant literature. *Note:* because the *rate* of a reaction is constant when it is zero order, it is dose *independent*, but as zero order is approached, with increasing dose the *kinetics* alter, and thus are called dose *dependent*.

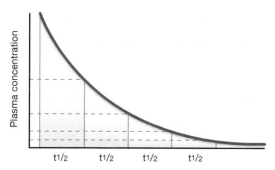

Fig. 8.2 Changes in plasma concentration following an intravenous bolus injection of a drug in the elimination phase (the distribution phase is not shown; see text). As elimination is a first-order process, the time for any concentration point to fall by 50% ($t_{1/2}$) is always the same.

steady-state plasma concentration with increase in dose. But gradually the enzymatic elimination process approaches and reaches saturation, the process becoming constant and zero order. While the dosing rate can be increased, the metabolism rate cannot, and the plasma concentration rises steeply and *disproportionately*, with danger of toxicity. Salicylate metabolism also exhibits saturation kinetics but at high therapeutic doses. Clearly saturation kinetics is a significant factor in delay of recovery from drug overdose, e.g. with aspirin or phenytoin.

Order of reaction and $t_{1/2}$**.** When a drug is subject to first-order kinetics, the $t_{1/2}$ is a constant characteristic, i.e. a constant value can be quoted throughout the plasma concentration range (accepting that there will be variation in $t_{1/2}$ between individuals), and this is convenient. But if the rate of a process is not directly proportional to plasma concentration, then the $t_{1/2}$ cannot be constant. Consequently, no single value for $t_{1/2}$ describes overall elimination when a drug exhibits zero-order kinetics. In fact, $t_{1/2}$ decreases as plasma concentration falls and the calculations on elimination and dosing that are so easy with first-order elimination (see below) become more complicated.

Zero-order absorption processes apply to iron, to depot intramuscular formulations and to drug implants, e.g. antipsychotics and sex hormones.

Time course of drug concentration and effect

Plasma half-life and steady-state concentration

The manner in which plasma drug concentration rises or falls when dosing begins, alters or ceases follows certain simple rules, which provide a means for rational control of

drug effect. Central to understanding these is the concept of *half-life* ($t_{1/2}$) or half-time.

Decrease in plasma concentration after an intravenous bolus injection

Following an intravenous bolus injection (a single dose injected in a period of seconds as distinct from a continuous infusion), plasma concentration rises quickly as drug enters the blood to reach a peak. There is then a sharp drop as the drug distributes round the body (distribution phase), followed by a steady decline as drug is removed from the blood by the liver or kidneys (elimination phase). If the elimination processes are first order, the time taken for any concentration point in the elimination phase to fall to half its value (the $t_{1/2}$) is always the same; see Fig. 8.2. Note that the drug is virtually eliminated from the plasma in five $t_{1/2}$ periods.

> The $t_{1/2}$ *is* the one pharmacokinetic value of a drug that it is most useful to know.

Increase in plasma concentration with constant dosing

With a constant rate infusion, the amount of drug in the body and with it the plasma concentration rise until a state is reached at which the rate of administration to the body is exactly equal to the rate of elimination from it: this is called the *steady state*. The plasma concentration is then on a plateau, and the drug effect is stable. Fig. 8.3 depicts the smooth changes in plasma concentration that result from a constant intravenous infusion. Clearly, giving a drug by regularly spaced oral or intravenous doses will result in plasma concentrations that fluctuate between peaks and troughs, but in time all of the peaks will be of equal height and all of the troughs will be of equal depth; this is also called a steady-state concentration, as the mean concentration is constant.[6]

Time to reach steady state

It is important to know *when* a drug administered at a constant rate achieves a steady-state plasma concentration, for maintaining the same dosing schedule then ensures a constant amount of drug in the body, and the patient will experience neither acute toxicity nor decline of effect. The $t_{1/2}$ provides the answer. Taking *ultimate* steady state attained as 100%:

in $1 \times t_{1/2}$ the concentration will be (100/2) 50%
in $2 \times t_{1/2}$ (50 + 50/2) 75%

---

[6]The peaks and troughs can be of practical importance with drugs of low therapeutic index, e.g. aminoglycoside antibiotics; it may be necessary to monitor for both safe and effective therapy.

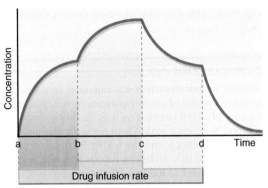

Fig. 8.3 Changes in plasma concentration during the course of a constant-rate intravenous infusion. (a) The infusion commences and plasma concentration rises to reach a steady state (plateau) in about $5 \times t_{1/2}$ periods. (b) The infusion rate is increased by 50%, and the plasma concentration rises further to reach a new steady state that is 50% higher than the original steady state; the process takes another $5 \times t_{1/2}$ periods. (c) The infusion is decreased to the original rate, and the plasma concentration returns to the original steady state in $5 \times t_{1/2}$ periods. (d) The infusion is discontinued, and the plasma concentration falls to virtually zero in $5 \times t_{1/2}$ periods.

in $3 \times t_{1/2}$ $(75 + 25/2)$ 87.5%
in $4 \times t_{1/2}$ $(87.5 + 12.5/2)$ 93.75%
in $5 \times t_{1/2}$ $(93.75 + 6.25/2)$ 96.875%

of the ultimate steady state.

> When a drug is given at a constant rate (continuous or repeated administration), the time to reach steady state depends *only* on the $t_{1/2}$ and, for all practical purposes, after $5 \times t_{1/2}$ periods the amount of drug in the body is constant and the plasma concentration is at a plateau (a and b in Fig. 8.3).

Change in plasma concentration with change or cessation of dosing

The same principle holds for *change* from any steady-state plasma concentration to a *new* steady state brought about by increase or decrease in the rate of drug administration. Provided the kinetics remain first order, increasing or decreasing the rate of drug administration (b and c in Fig. 8.3) gives rise to a new steady-state concentration in a time equal to $5 \times t_{1/2}$ periods.

Similarly, starting at any steady-state plasma concentration (100%), discontinuing the dose (d in Fig. 8.3) will cause the plasma concentration to fall to virtually zero in $5 \times t_{1/2}$ periods, as described in Fig. 8.2.

Note that the difference between the rate of drug administration (input) and the rate of elimination (output)

determines the actual *level* of any steady-state plasma concentration (as opposed to the *time taken* to reach it). If drug elimination remains constant and administration increases by 50%, in time the plasma concentration will reach a new steady-state concentration, which will be 50% greater than the original.

The relation between $t_{1/2}$ and time to reach steady-state plasma concentration applies to all drugs that obey first-order kinetics. This holds as much to dobutamine ($t_{1/2}$ 2 min), when it is useful to know that an alteration of infusion rate will reach a plateau within 10 min, as to digoxin ($t_{1/2}$ 36 h), when a constant daily oral dose will give a steady-state plasma concentration only after 7.5 days. This book quotes plasma $t_{1/2}$ values where they are relevant. Inevitably, natural variation within the population produces a range in $t_{1/2}$ values for any drug, and the text quotes only single average $t_{1/2}$ values while recognising that the population range may be as much as 50% from the stated figure in either direction.

Some $t_{1/2}$ values appear in Table 8.1 to illustrate their range and implications for dosing in clinical practice.

Biological effect $t_{1/2}$ is the time in which the biological effect of a drug declines by one-half. With drugs that act competitively on receptors (α- and β-adrenoceptor agonists and antagonists) the biological effect $t_{1/2}$ can be estimated with reasonable accuracy. Sometimes the biological effect $t_{1/2}$ cannot be provided, e.g. with antimicrobials when the number of infecting organisms and their sensitivity determine the outcome.

Therapeutic drug monitoring

Patients differ greatly in the dose of drug required to achieve the same response. The dose of warfarin that maintains a therapeutic concentration may vary as much as five-fold between individuals. This is a consequence of variation in rates of drug metabolism, disposition and tissue responsiveness, and it raises the question of how optimal drug effect can be achieved quickly for the individual patient.

In principle, drug effect relates to free (unbound) concentration at the tissue receptor site, which in turn reflects (but is not necessarily the same as) the concentration in the plasma. For many drugs, correlation between plasma concentration and effect is indeed better than that between dose and effect. Yet monitoring therapy by measuring drug in plasma is of practical use only in selected instances. The underlying reasons repay some thought.

Plasma concentration may not be worth measuring where dose can be titrated against a quickly and easily measured effect such as blood pressure (antihypertensives), body-weight (diuretics), INR (oral anticoagulants) or blood sugar (hypoglycaemics).

Plasma concentration has no correlation with effect with drugs that act irreversibly (named 'hit and run drugs' because

Table 8.1 Plasma $t_{1/2}$ of some drugs

Drug	$t_{1/2}$
Adenosine	<2 s
Dobutamine	2 min
Benzylpenicillin	30 min
Amoxicillin	1 h
Paracetamol	2 h
Midazolam	3 h
Tolbutamide	6 h
Atenolol	7 h
Dosulepin	25 h
Diazepam	40 h
Piroxicam	45 h
Ethosuximide	54 h

their effect persists long after the drug has left the plasma). Such drugs inactivate targets (enzyme, receptor) and restoration of effect occurs only after days or weeks, when resynthesis takes place, e.g. some monoamine oxidase inhibitors, aspirin (on platelets), some anticholinesterases and anticancer drugs.

Plasma concentration may correlate poorly with effect. When a drug is metabolised to several products, active to a varying degree or inactive, the assay of the parent drug alone is unlikely to reflect its activity, e.g. some benzodiazepines. Similarly, binding of basic drugs, e.g. lidocaine, to acute phase proteins, e.g. α_1-acid glycoprotein, spuriously increases the total concentration in plasma. The best correlation is likely to be achieved by measurement of free (active) drug in plasma water, but this is technically more difficult, and total drug in plasma is usually monitored in routine clinical practice. Saliva is sometimes used.

Plasma concentration may correlate well with effect. Plasma concentration monitoring has proved useful:

- As a guide to the effectiveness of therapy, e.g. plasma gentamicin and other antimicrobials against sensitive bacteria, plasma theophylline for asthma, plasma ciclosporin to avoid transplant rejection, lithium for mood disorder.
- To reduce the risk of adverse drug effects when therapeutic doses are close to toxic doses (low therapeutic index), e.g. otic damage with aminoglycoside antibiotics; adverse CNS effects of lithium, nephrotoxicity with ciclosporin.

- When the desired effect is suppression of infrequent sporadic events such as epileptic seizures or episodes of cardiac arrhythmia.
- To check patient compliance on a drug regimen, when there is failure of therapeutic effect at a known effective dose, e.g. anti-epilepsy drugs.
- To diagnose and manage drug overdose.
- When lack of therapeutic effect and toxicity may be difficult to distinguish. Digoxin is both a treatment for, and sometimes the cause of, cardiac supraventricular tachycardia; a plasma digoxin measurement will help to distinguish whether an arrhythmia is due to too little or too much digoxin.

Interpreting plasma concentration measurements. Recommended plasma concentrations for drugs appear throughout this book where these are relevant, but the following points ought to be kept in mind:

- The target therapeutic concentration range for a drug is a guide to optimise dosing together with other clinical indicators of progress.
- Take account of the time needed to reach steady-state dosing conditions (see above). Additionally, some drugs alter their own rates of metabolism by enzyme induction, e.g. carbamazepine and phenytoin, and it is best to allow 2–4 weeks between change in dose and meaningful plasma concentration measurement.
- As a general rule, when a drug has a short $t_{1/2}$ it is desirable to know both peak (15 min after an intravenous dose) and trough (just before the next dose) concentrations to provide efficacy without toxicity, as with gentamicin ($t_{1/2}$ 2.5 h). For a drug with a long $t_{1/2}$, it is usually best to sample just before a dose is due; effective immunosuppression with ciclosporin ($t_{1/2}$ 27 h) is obtained with trough concentrations of 50–200 μg/L when the drug is given by mouth.

Individual pharmacokinetic processes

Drug absorption into, distribution around, metabolism by and elimination from the body are reviewed.

Absorption

Commonsense considerations of anatomy, physiology, pathology, pharmacology, therapeutics and convenience determine the routes by which drugs are administered. Usually these are:

- *Enteral*: by mouth (swallowed) or by sublingual or buccal absorption; by rectum.
- *Parenteral*: by intravenous injection or infusion, intramuscular injection, subcutaneous injection or infusion, inhalation, topical application for local (skin, eye, lung) or for systemic (transdermal) effect.
- *Other routes*, e.g. intrathecal, intradermal, intranasal, intratracheal, intrapleural, are used when appropriate.

The features of the various routes, their advantages and disadvantages are relevant.

Absorption from the gastrointestinal tract

The *small intestine* is the principal site for absorption of nutrients, and it is also where most orally administered drugs enter the body. This part of the gut has an enormous surface area due to the intestinal villi, and an epithelium through which fluid readily filters in response to osmotic differences caused by the presence of food. Disturbed alimentary motility can reduce drug absorption, i.e. if food slows gastric emptying, or gut infection accelerates intestinal transit. Additionally, it is becoming apparent that uptake and efflux transporters in enterocytes (see p. 95) play a substantial role in controlling the absorption of certain drugs, e.g. digoxin, ciclosporin. Many sustained-release formulations probably depend on absorption from the colon.

Absorption of ionisable drugs from the *buccal mucosa* responds to the prevailing pH, which is 6.2–7.2. Lipid-soluble drugs are rapidly effective by this route because blood flow through the mucosa is abundant; these drugs enter directly into the systemic circulation, avoiding the possibility of first-pass (presystemic) inactivation by the liver and gut (see below).

The *stomach* does not play a major role in absorbing drugs, even those that are acidic and thus un-ionised and lipid soluble at gastric pH, because its surface area is much smaller than that of the small intestine and gastric emptying is speedy ($t_{1/2}$ 30 min).

Enterohepatic circulation

This system is illustrated by the bile salts which are formed in the liver, then conserved by circulating round liver, intestine and portal blood about eight times a day. Several drugs form conjugates with glucuronic acid in the liver and enter the bile. Too polar (ionised) to be reabsorbed, the glucuronides remain in the gut, are hydrolysed by intestinal enzymes and bacteria, and the parent drug, thus released, is reabsorbed and reconjugated in the liver. Enterohepatic recycling appears to help sustain the plasma concentration and so the effect of sulindac, pentaerithrityl tetranitrate and ethinylestradiol (in many oral contraceptives).

Systemic availability and bioavailability

A drug injected intravenously enters the systemic circulation and thence gains access to the tissues and to receptors, i.e. 100% is available to exert its therapeutic effect. If the same quantity of the drug is swallowed, it does not follow that the entire amount will reach first the portal blood and then the systemic blood, i.e. its availability for therapeutic effect via the systemic circulation may be less than 100%. The anticipated response to a drug must take account of its availability to the systemic circulation.

While considerations of reduced availability attach to any drug given by any route other than intravenously, and intended for systemic effect, in practice the issue concerns enteral administration. The extent of systemic availability is usually calculated by relating the area under the plasma concentration–time curve (AUC) after a single oral dose to that obtained after intravenous administration of the same amount (by which route a drug is 100% systemically available). Calculation of AUCs after oral doses also allows a comparison of the bioavailability of different pharmaceutical formulations of the same drug. Factors influencing systemic availability present in three main ways, as described below.

Pharmaceutical factors[7]

The amount of drug released from a dose form (and so becoming available for absorption) is referred to as its *bioavailability*. This is highly dependent on its pharmaceutical formulation. With tablets, for example, particle size (surface area exposed to solution), diluting substances, tablet size and pressure used in the tabletting process can affect disintegration and dissolution and so the bioavailability of the drug. Manufacturers must test their products to ensure that their formulations release the same amount of drug at the same speed from whatever manufactured batch or brand the patient may be taking.

Differences in bioavailability are prone to occur with *modified-release* (m/r) formulations, i.e. where the rate or place of release of the active ingredients has been modified (also called *sustained, controlled* or *delayed* release)

---

[7]Some definitions of enteral dose forms. *Tablet:* a solid dose form in which the drug is compressed or moulded with pharmacologically inert substances (excipients); variants include sustained-release and coated tablets. *Capsule:* the drug is provided in a gelatin shell or container. *Mixture:* a liquid formulation of a drug for oral administration. *Suppository:* a solid dose form shaped for insertion into rectum (or vagina, when it may be called a 'pessary'); it may be designed to dissolve, or it may melt at body temperature (in which case there is a storage problem in countries where the environmental temperature may exceed 37°C); the vehicle in which the drug is carried may be fat, glycerol with gelatin, or macrogols (polycondensation products of ethylene oxide) with gelatin. *Syrup:* the drug is provided in a concentrated sugar (fructose or other) solution. *Linctus:* a viscous liquid formulation, traditional for cough.

(see p. 99). Modified-release preparations from different manufacturers may differ in their bioavailability profiles despite containing the same amount of drug, i.e. there is neither *bioequivalence* nor *therapeutic equivalence*, and the problem is particularly acute where the therapeutic ratio is narrow. In this case, 'brand name prescribing', i.e. using only a particular brand name for a particular patient is justified, e.g. for m/r preparations of theophylline, lithium, nifedipine and diltiazem.

Physicians tend to ignore pharmaceutical formulation as a factor in variable or unexpected responses because they do not understand it and feel entitled to rely on reputable manufacturers and official regulatory authorities to ensure provision of reliable formulations. Good pharmaceutical companies reasonably point out that, having a reputation to lose, they take much trouble to make their preparations consistently reliable. This is a matter of great importance when dosage must be precise (anticoagulants, antidiabetics, adrenal corticosteroids).

Biological factors

Biological factors related to the gut include limitation of drug absorption by drug transporter systems (see p. 95), destruction of drug by gastric acid, e.g. benzylpenicillin, and impaired absorption due to rapid intestinal transit, which is important for all drugs that are absorbed slowly. Drugs may also bind to food constituents, e.g. tetracyclines to calcium (in milk), and to iron, or to other drugs (e.g. acidic drugs to colestyramine), and the resulting complex is not absorbed.

Presystemic (first-pass) elimination

Some drugs readily enter gut mucosal cells, but appear in low concentration in the systemic circulation. The reason lies in the considerable extent to which such drugs are metabolised in a single passage through the gut mucosa and (principally) the liver. As little as 10–20% of the parent drug may reach the systemic circulation unchanged. By contrast, after intravenous administration, 100% becomes systemically available and the patient experiences higher concentrations with greater, but more predictable, effect. Dosing, particularly *initial* doses, must take account of discrepancy in anticipated plasma concentrations between the intravenous and oral routes. The difference is usually less if a drug produces active metabolites.

Once a drug is in the systemic circulation, irrespective of which route is used, about 20% is subject to the hepatic metabolic processes in each circulation time because that proportion of cardiac output passes to the liver.

As the degree of presystemic elimination differs much between drugs and individuals, the phenomenon of first-pass elimination adds to variation in systemic plasma concentrations, and thus particularly in initial response to the drugs that are subject to this process. In drug overdose, decreased presystemic elimination with increased bioavailability may account for the rapid onset of toxicity with antipsychotic drugs.

Drugs for which *presystemic elimination* is significant include:[8]

Analgesics	Adrenoceptor blockers	Others
morphine	labetalol	chlorpromazine
	propranolol	isosorbide dinitrate
	metoprolol	nortriptyline

In severe hepatic cirrhosis with both impaired liver cell function and well-developed vessels shunting blood into the systemic circulation without passing through the liver, first-pass elimination reduces and systemic availability is increased. The result of these changes is an increased likelihood of exaggerated response to normal doses of drugs having high hepatic clearance and, on occasion, frank toxicity.

Drugs that exhibit the hepatic first-pass phenomenon do so because of the rapidity with which they are metabolised. The rate of delivery to the liver, i.e. blood flow, is then the main determinant of its rate of metabolism. Many other drugs are completely metabolised by the liver but at a slower rate, and consequently loss in the first pass through the liver is unimportant. Dose adjustment to account for presystemic elimination is unnecessary, e.g. for diazepam, phenytoin, theophylline, warfarin.

Advantages and disadvantages of enteral administration

By swallowing

For systemic effect. *Advantages* are convenience and acceptability.

Disadvantages are that absorption may be delayed, reduced or even enhanced after food, or slow or irregular after drugs that inhibit gut motility (antimuscarinic, opioid). Differences in presystemic elimination are a cause of variation in drug effect among patients. Some drugs are not absorbed (gentamicin), and others are destroyed in the gut (insulin, oxytocin, some penicillins). Tablets taken with too small a quantity of liquid and in the supine position, can lodge

---

[8]For a more detailed list, see Wilkinson G R 2005 Drug metabolism and variability among patients in drug response. New England Journal of Medicine 352:2211–2221.

in the oesophagus with delayed absorption[9] and may even cause ulceration (sustained-release potassium chloride and doxycycline tablets), especially in the elderly and those with an enlarged left atrium which impinges on the oesophagus.[10]

For effect in the gut. *Advantages* are that the drug is placed at the site of action (neomycin, anthelminthics), and with non-absorbed drugs the local concentration can be higher than would be safe in the blood.

Disadvantages are that drug distribution may be uneven, and in some diseases of the gut the whole thickness of the wall is affected (severe bacillary dysentery, typhoid) and effective blood concentrations (as well as luminal concentrations) may be needed.

Sublingual or buccal for systemic effect

Advantages are that the effect is quick, e.g. with glyceryl trinitrate as an aerosol spray, or as sublingual tablets that are chewed, giving greater surface area for solution. Spitting out the tablet will terminate the effect.

Disadvantages are the inconvenience if use has to be frequent, irritation of the mucous membrane and excessive salivation, which promotes swallowing, so losing the advantages of bypassing presystemic elimination.

Rectal administration

For systemic effect (suppositories or solutions). The rectal mucosa has a rich blood and lymph supply and, in general, dose requirements are either the same or slightly greater than those needed for oral use. Drugs chiefly enter the portal system, but those that are subject to hepatic first-pass elimination may escape this if they are absorbed from the lower rectum, which drains directly to the systemic circulation. The degree of presystemic elimination thus depends on distribution within the rectum, and this is somewhat unpredictable.

Advantages are that a suppository can replace a drug that irritates the stomach (aminophylline, indometacin); the route is suitable in vomiting, motion sickness, migraine or when a patient cannot swallow, and when cooperation is lacking (sedation in children).

Disadvantages are psychological in that the patient may be embarrassed or may even like the route too much; rectal

inflammation may occur with repeated use, and absorption can be unreliable, especially if the rectum is full of faeces.

For local effect, e.g. in proctitis or colitis, is an obvious use. A survey in the UK showed that a substantial proportion of patients did not remove the wrapper before inserting the suppository!

Advantages and disadvantages of parenteral administration

(for systemic and local effect)

Intravenous (bolus or infusion)

An intravenous bolus, i.e. rapid injection, passes round the circulation being progressively diluted each time; it is delivered principally to the organs with high blood flow (brain, liver, heart, lung, kidneys).

Advantages are that the intravenous route gives swift, effective and highly predictable blood concentration and allows rapid modification of dose, i.e. immediate cessation of administration is possible if unwanted effects occur during administration. The route is suitable for administration of drugs that are not absorbed from the gut or are too irritant (anticancer agents) to be given by other routes.

Disadvantages are the hazard if drug administration is too rapid, as plasma concentration may rise at a rate such that normal mechanisms of distribution and elimination are outpaced. Some drugs will act within one arm-to-tongue (brain) circulation time, which is 13 ± 3 s; with most drugs an injection given over four or five circulation times seems sufficient to avoid excessive plasma concentrations. Local venous thrombosis is liable to occur with prolonged infusion and with bolus doses of irritant formulations, e.g. diazepam, or microparticulate components of infusion fluids, especially if small veins are used, and extravasation may be very painful and damaging. Infection of the intravenous catheter and the small thrombi on its tip is also a risk during prolonged infusions.

Intramuscular injection

Blood flow is greater in the muscles of the upper arm than in the gluteal mass and thigh, and increases with physical exercise.

Advantages are that the route is reliable, it is suitable for some irritant drugs, and depot preparations (neuroleptics, hormonal contraceptives) are suitable for administration at monthly or longer intervals. Absorption is more rapid than following subcutaneous injection (soluble preparations are absorbed within 10–30 min).

Disadvantages are that the route is not acceptable for self-administration, it may be painful, and if any adverse effects occur with a depot formulation, it may not be removable.

---

[9]A woman's failure to respond to antihypertensive medication was explained when she was observed to choke on drinking. Investigation revealed a large pharyngeal pouch that was full of tablets and capsules. Her blood pressure became easy to control when the pouch was removed. Birch D J, Dehn T C B 1993 British Medical Journal 306:1012.

[10]Ideally solid dose forms should be taken while standing up, and washed down with 150 mL (a teacup) of water; even sitting (higher intra-abdominal pressure) impairs passage. At least, patients should be told to sit and take three or four mouthfuls of water (a mouthful = 30 mL) or a cupful. Some patients do not even know they should take water.

Subcutaneous injection

Advantages are that the route is reliable and is acceptable for self-administration.

Disadvantages are poor absorption in peripheral circulatory failure. Repeated injections at one site can cause lipoatrophy, resulting in erratic absorption (see Insulin, Ch. 36).

By inhalation

As a gas, e.g. volatile anaesthetics.

As an aerosol, e.g. β_2-adrenoceptor agonist bronchodilators. Aerosols are particles dispersed in a gas, the particles being small enough to remain in suspension for a long time instead of sedimenting rapidly under the influence of gravity; the particles may be liquid (fog) or solid (smoke). A nebuliser allows larger doses (see p. 507).

As a powder, e.g. sodium cromoglicate. Particle size and air-flow velocity are important. Most particles greater than 5 micrometres in diameter impact in the upper respiratory areas; particles of about 2 micrometres reach the terminal bronchioles; a large proportion of particles less than 1 micrometre are exhaled. Air-flow velocity diminishes considerably as the bronchi progressively divide, promoting drug deposition peripherally.

Advantages are the rapid uptake or elimination of drugs as gases, giving the close control that has marked the use of this route in general anaesthesia from its earliest days. Self-administration is practicable. Aerosols and powders provide high local concentration for action on bronchi, minimising systemic effects.

Disadvantages are that special apparatus is needed (some patients find pressurised aerosols difficult to use to best effect) and a drug must be non-irritant if the patient is conscious. Obstructed bronchi (mucus plugs in asthma) may cause therapy to fail.

Topical application

For local effect, e.g. to skin, eye, lung, anal canal, rectum, vagina.

Advantage is the provision of high local concentration without systemic effect (usually[11]).

Disadvantage is that absorption can occur, especially when there is tissue destruction so that systemic effects result, e.g. adrenal corticosteroids and neomycin to the skin, atropine to the eye. Ocular administration of a β-adrenoceptor blocker may cause systemic effects (bypassing first-pass elimination), and such eye drops are contraindicated in asthma or chronic lung disease.[12] There is extensive literature on this subject characterised by expressions of astonishment that serious effects, even death, can occur.

For systemic effect. Transdermal delivery systems release drug through a rate-controlling membrane into the skin and so into the systemic circulation. This avoids the fluctuations in plasma concentration associated with other routes of administration, as is first-pass elimination in the liver. Glyceryl trinitrate and postmenopausal hormone replacement therapy are available in the form of a sticking plaster attached to the skin or as an ointment (glyceryl trinitrate). One treatment for migraine is a nasal spray containing sumatriptan.

Distribution

If a drug is required to act throughout the body or to reach an organ inaccessible to topical administration, it must get into the blood and other body compartments. Most drugs distribute widely, in part dissolved in body water, in part bound to plasma proteins, in part to tissues. Distribution is often uneven, for drugs may bind selectively to plasma or tissue proteins or be localised within particular organs. Clearly, the site of localisation of a drug is likely to influence its action, e.g. whether it crosses the blood–brain barrier to enter the brain; the extent (amount) and strength (tenacity) of protein or tissue binding (stored drug) will affect the time it spends in the body and thereby its duration of action.

Distribution volume

The pattern of distribution from plasma to other body fluids and tissues is a characteristic of each drug that enters the circulation, and it varies among drugs. Precise information on the concentration of drug attained in various tissues and fluids is usually not available for humans.[13] But *blood plasma* is sampled readily in humans, the drug concentration in which, taking account of the dose given, is a measure of

---

[11]*A cautionary tale.* A 70-year-old man reported left breast enlargement and underwent mastectomy; histological examination revealed benign gynaecomastia. Ten months later the right breast enlarged. Tests of endocrine function were normal, but the patient himself was struck by the fact that his wife had been using a vaginal cream (containing 0.01% dienestrol), initially for atrophic vaginitis but latterly the cream had been used to facilitate sexual intercourse which took place two or three times per week. On the assumption that penile absorption of oestrogen was responsible for the disorder, exposure to the cream was terminated. The gynaecomastia in the remaining breast then resolved (DiRaimondo C V, Roach A C, Meador C K 1980 Gynecomastia from exposure to vaginal estrogen cream. New England Journal of Medicine 302:1089–1090).

---

[12]Two drops of 0.5% timolol solution, one to each eye, can equate to 10 mg by mouth.

[13]But positive emission tomography (PET) offers a prospect of obtaining similar information. With PET, a positron emitting isotope, e.g.15O, is substituted for a stable atom without altering the chemical behaviour of the molecule. The radiation dose is very low but can be imaged tomographically using photomultiplier–scintillator detectors. PET can be used to monitor effects of drugs on metabolism in the brain, e.g. 'on' and 'off' phases in parkinsonism. There are many other applications.

Table 8.2 Apparent distribution volume of some drugs (values are in litres for a 70-kg person who would displace about 70 L)*

Drug	Distribution volume	Drug	Distribution volume
Evans blue	3 (plasma volume)	Atenolol	77
Heparin	5	Diazepam	140
Salicylate	9	Pethidine	280
Inulin	15 (extracellular water)	Digoxin	420
Gentamicin	18	Nortriptyline	1000
Furosemide	21	Dosulepin	4900
Amoxicillin	28	Chloroquine	13 000
Antipyrine	43 (total body water)		

*Litres per kilogram are commonly used, but give a less vivid image of the implication of the term 'apparent', e.g. chloroquine.

whether a drug tends to remain in the circulation or to distribute from the plasma into the tissues. In other words:

- If a drug remains mostly in the plasma, its distribution volume will be small.
- If a drug is present mainly in other tissues, the distribution volume will be large.

Such information can be useful. In drug overdose, if a major proportion of the total body load is known to be in the plasma, i.e. the distribution volume is small, then haemodialysis/filtration is likely to be a useful option (as is the case with severe salicylate poisoning), but it is an inappropriate treatment for overdose with dosulepin (Table 8.2).

The principle for measuring the distribution volume is essentially that of using a dye to find the volume of a container filled with liquid. The weight of added dye divided by the concentration of dye once mixing is complete gives the distribution volume of the dye, which is the volume of the container. Similarly, the distribution volume of a drug in the body may be determined after a single intravenous bolus dose by dividing the dose given by the concentration achieved in plasma.[14]

---

[14]Clearly a problem arises in that the plasma concentration is not constant but falls after the bolus has been injected. To get round this, use is made of the fact that the relation between the logarithm of plasma concentration and the time after a single intravenous dose is a straight line. The log concentration–timeline extended back to zero time gives the theoretical plasma concentration at the time the drug was given. In effect, the assumption is made that drug distributes instantaneously and uniformly through a single compartment, the distribution volume. This mechanism, although rather theoretical, does usefully characterise drugs according to the extent to which they remain in or distribute out from the circulation.

The result of this calculation, the distribution volume, in fact only rarely corresponds with a physiological body space such as extracellular water or total body water, for it is a measure of the volume a drug would apparently occupy knowing the dose given and the plasma concentration achieved, and assuming the entire volume is at that concentration. For this reason, the term *apparent* distribution volume is often preferred. Indeed, the apparent distribution volume of some drugs that bind extensively to extravascular tissues, which is based on the resulting low plasma concentration, is many times total body volume.

> The distribution volume of a drug is the volume in which it appears to distribute (or which it would require) if the concentration throughout the body were equal to that in plasma, i.e. as if the body were a single compartment.

The list in Table 8.2 illustrates a range of apparent distribution volumes. The names of those substances that distribute within (and have been used to measure) physiological spaces are printed in italics.

Selective distribution within the body occurs because of special affinity between particular drugs and particular body constituents. Many drugs bind to proteins in the plasma; phenothiazines and chloroquine bind to melanin-containing tissues, including the retina, which may explain the occurrence of retinopathy. Drugs may also concentrate selectively in a particular tissue because of specialised transport mechanisms, e.g. iodine in the thyroid.

Plasma protein and tissue binding

Many natural substances circulate around the body partly free in plasma water and partly bound to plasma proteins; these include cortisol, thyroxine, iron, copper and, in hepatic or renal failure, by-products of physiological intermediary metabolism.

Drugs, too, circulate in the protein-bound and free states, and the significance is that the free fraction is pharmacologically active whereas the protein-bound component is a reservoir of drug that is inactive because of this binding. Free and bound fractions are in equilibrium, and free drug removed from the plasma by metabolism, renal function or dialysis is replaced by drug released from the bound fraction.

Albumin is the main binding protein for many natural substances and drugs. Its complex structure has a net negative charge at blood pH and a high *capacity* but low (weak) *affinity* for many basic drugs, i.e. a lot is bound, but it is readily released. Two particular sites on the albumin molecule bind acidic drugs with high affinity (strongly), but these sites have low capacity. Saturation of binding sites on plasma proteins in general is unlikely in the doses in which most drugs are used.

Other binding proteins in the blood include lipoprotein and α_1-acid glycoprotein, both of which carry basic drugs such as quinidine, chlorpromazine and imipramine. Thyroxine and sex hormones are bound in the plasma to specific globulins.

Disease may modify protein binding of drugs to an extent that is clinically relevant, as Table 8.3 shows. In *chronic renal failure*, hypoalbuminaemia and retention of products of metabolism that compete for binding sites on protein are both responsible for the decrease in protein binding of drugs. Most affected are acidic drugs that are highly protein bound, e.g. phenytoin, and initiating or modifying the dose of such drugs for patients with renal failure requires special attention (see also Prescribing in renal disease, p. 490).

Chronic liver disease also leads to hypoalbuminaemia and an increase of endogenous substances such as bilirubin that may compete for binding sites on protein. Drugs that are normally extensively protein bound should be used with special caution, for increased free concentration of diazepam, tolbutamide and phenytoin have been demonstrated in patients with this condition (see also Prescribing for patients with liver disease, p. 582).

The free, unbound, and therefore pharmacologically active percentages of some drugs appear in Table 8.3 to illustrate the range and, in some cases, changes recorded in disease.

Tissue binding. Some drugs distribute readily to regions of the body other than plasma, as a glance at Table 8.2 will show. These include many lipid-soluble drugs, which may

Table 8.3 Examples of plasma protein binding of drugs and effects of disease

Drug	% Unbound (free)
Warfarin	1
Diazepam	2 (6% in liver disease)
Furosemide	2 (6% in nephrotic syndrome)
Tolbutamide	2
Amitriptyline	5
Phenytoin	9 (19% in renal disease)
Triamterene	19 (40% in renal disease)
Trimethoprim	30
Theophylline	35 (71% in liver disease)
Morphine	65
Digoxin	75 (82% in renal disease)
Amoxicillin	82
Ethosuximide	100

enter fat stores, e.g. most benzodiazepines, verapamil and lidocaine. There is less information about other tissues, e.g. muscle, than about plasma protein binding because solid tissue samples require invasive biopsy. Extensive binding to tissues delays elimination from the body and accounts for the long $t_{1/2}$ of chloroquine and amiodarone.

Metabolism

The body treats most drugs as foreign substances (xenobiotics) and subjects them to various mechanisms for eliminating chemical intruders.

'Metabolism' is a general term for chemical transformations that occur within the body, and its processes change drugs in two major ways by:

* reducing lipid solubility
* altering biological activity.

Reducing lipid solubility

> Metabolic reactions tend to make a drug molecule progressively more water soluble and so favour its elimination in the urine.

Drug-metabolising enzymes developed during evolution to enable the body to dispose of lipid-soluble substances such as hydrocarbons, steroids and alkaloids that are ingested with food. Some environmental chemicals may persist indefinitely in our fat deposits, e.g. dicophane (DDT), with consequences that are currently unknown.

Altering biological activity

The end-result of metabolism usually is the abolition of biological activity, but various steps in between may have the following consequences:

1. Conversion of a pharmacologically *active* to an *inactive* substance – this applies to most drugs.
2. Conversion of one pharmacologically *active* to another *active* substance – this has the effect of prolonging drug action, as shown below.

Active drug	Active metabolite
amitriptyline	nortriptyline
codeine	morphine
chloroquine	hydroxychloroquine
diazepam	oxazepam
spironolactone	canrenone

3. Conversion of a pharmacologically *inactive* to an *active* substance (then called a 'prodrug'). The process then follows 1 or 2, above.

Inactive substance	Active metabolite(s)	Comment
aciclovir	aciclovir triphosphate	see p. 221
colecalciferol	calcitriol and alfacalcidol	highly active metabolites of vitamin D_3
cyclophosphamide	phosphoramide mustard	another metabolite, acrolein, causes the bladder toxicity; see p. 552

Inactive substance	Active metabolite(s)	Comment
perindopril	perindoprilat	less risk of first-dose hypotension (applies to all ACE inhibitors except captopril)
levodopa	dopamine	levodopa, but not dopamine, can cross the blood–brain barrier
sulindac	sulindac sulphide	possibly reduced gastric toxicity
sulfasalazine	5-aminosalicylic acid	see p. 576
zidovudine	zidovudine triphosphate	see p. 225

The metabolic processes

The liver is by far the most important drug-metabolising organ, although a number of tissues, including the kidney, gut mucosa, lung and skin, also contribute. It is useful to think of drug metabolism in two broad phases.

Phase I metabolism brings about a change in the drug molecule by oxidation, reduction or hydrolysis and usually introduces or exposes a chemically active site on it. The new metabolite often has reduced biological activity and different pharmacokinetic properties, e.g. a shorter $t_{1/2}$.

The principal group of reactions is the *oxidations*, in particular those undertaken by the (microsomal) *mixed-function oxidases* which, as the name indicates, are capable of metabolising a wide variety of compounds. The most important of these is a large 'superfamily' of haem proteins, the *cytochrome P450 enzymes*, which metabolise chemicals from the environment, the diet and drugs. By a complex process, the drug molecule incorporates one atom of molecular oxygen (O_2) to form a (chemically active) hydroxyl group, and the other oxygen atom converts to water.

The following explanation provides a background to the P450 nomenclature that accompanies accounts of the metabolism of several individual drugs in this book. The many cytochrome P450 isoenzymes[15] are indicated by the letters CYP (from cytochrome P450) followed by a

---

[15]An isoenzyme is one of a group of enzymes that catalyse the same reaction but differ in protein structure.

number denoting a family group, then a subfamily letter, and then a number for the individual enzyme within the family: for example, CYP2E1 is an isoenzyme that catalyses a reaction involved in the metabolism of alcohol, paracetamol, estradiol and ethinylestradiol.

The enzymes of families CYP1, 2 and 3 metabolise 70–80% of clinically used drugs as well as many other foreign chemicals and, within these, CYP3A, CYP2D and CYP2C are the most important. The very size and variety of the P450 superfamily ensures that we do not need new enzymes for every existing or yet-to-be synthesised drug. Induction and inhibition of P450 enzymes is a fruitful source of drug–drug interactions.[16]

Each P450 enzyme protein is encoded by a separate gene (57 have been identified in humans), and variation in genes leads to differences between individuals, and sometimes between ethnic groups, in the ability to metabolise drugs. Persons who exhibit *polymorphisms* (see p. 109) inherit diminished or increased ability to metabolise substrate drugs, predisposing to toxicity or lack of efficacy.

Phase I oxidation of some drugs results in the formation of *epoxides*, which are short-lived and highly reactive metabolites that bind irreversibly through covalent bonds to cell constituents and are toxic to body tissues. Glutathione is a tripeptide that combines with epoxides, rendering them inactive, and its presence in the liver is part of an important defence mechanism against hepatic damage by halothane and paracetamol.

Note that some drug oxidation reactions do not involve the P450 system: several biologically active amines are inactivated by monoamine oxidase (see p. 334) and methylxanthines (see p. 157); mercaptopurine by xanthine oxidase (see p. 258); and ethanol by alcohol dehydrogenase (see p. 146).

Hydrolysis (Phase I) reactions create active sites for subsequent conjugation of, e.g., aspirin or lidocaine, but this does not occur with all drugs.

Phase II metabolism involves combination of the drug with one of several polar (water-soluble) endogenous molecules (products of intermediary metabolism), often at the active site (hydroxyl, amino, thiol) created by Phase I metabolism. The kidney readily eliminates the resulting water-soluble conjugate, or the bile if the molecular weight exceeds 300. Morphine, paracetamol and salicylates form conjugates with glucuronic acid (derived from glucose); oral contraceptive steroids form sulphates; isoniazid, phenelzine and dapsone are acetylated. Conjugation with a more polar molecule is also an elimination mechanism for natural substances, e.g. bilirubin as glucuronide, oestrogens as sulphates.

Phase II metabolism almost invariably terminates biological activity.

Transporters[17]. It is convenient here to introduce the subject of *carrier-mediated transporter processes* whose physiological functions include the passage of amino acids, lipids, sugars, hormones and bile acids across cell membranes, and the protection of cells against environmental toxins.

There is an emerging understanding that membrane transporters have a key role in the overall disposition of drugs to their targeted organs. There are broadly two types: *uptake transporters*, which facilitate, for example, the passage of organic anions and cations into cells, and *efflux transporters*, which transport substances out of cells, often against high concentration gradients. Some transporters possess both influx and efflux properties.

Most efflux transporters are members of the ATP-binding cassette (ABC) superfamily that utilises energy derived from the hydrolysis of ATP; they include the P-glycoprotein family that expresses multidrug resistance protein 1 (MDR1) (see p. 551).

Their varied locations illustrate the potential for transporters widely to affect the distribution of drugs, namely in:

- Enterocytes of the small intestine, controlling absorption and thus bioavailability, e.g. of ciclosporin, digoxin.
- Liver cells, controlling uptake from the blood and excretion into the bile, e.g. of pravastatin.
- Renal tubular cells, controlling uptake from the blood, secretion into tubular fluid (and thus excretion) of organic anions, e.g. β-lactam antibiotics, diuretics, non-steroidal anti-inflammatory drugs.
- Brain capillary endothelial cells, controlling passage across the blood–brain barrier, e.g. of levodopa (but not dopamine) for benefit in Parkinson's disease (see p. 380).

In time, it is likely that drug occupancy of transporter processes will provide explanations for some drug-induced toxicities and for a number of drug–drug interactions.

Enzyme induction

The mechanisms that the body evolved over millions of years to metabolise foreign substances now enable it to meet the modern environmental challenges of tobacco smoke, hydrocarbon pollutants, insecticides and drugs. At times of high exposure, our enzyme systems respond by increasing

---

[16]In this expanding field, useful lists of substrate drugs for P450 enzymes with inducers and inhibitors can be found in reviews, e.g. Wilkinson G R 2005 Drug metabolism and variability among patients in drug response. New England Journal of Medicine 352:2211–2221, already cited.

[17]Parts of this section are based on the review by Ho R H, Kim R B 2005 Transporters and drug therapy: implications for drug disposition and disease. Clinical Pharmacology and Therapeutics 78:260–277.

in amount and so in activity, i.e. they become *induced*; when exposure falls off, enzyme production gradually lessens.

A first alcoholic drink taken after a period of abstinence from alcohol may have a noticeable effect on behaviour, but the same drink taken at the end of 2 weeks of regular drinking may pass almost unnoticed because the individual's liver enzyme activity is increased (induced), and alcohol is metabolised more rapidly, having less effect, i.e. tolerance is acquired. There is, nevertheless, a ceiling above which alcohol metabolising enzymes are not further induced.

Inducing substances in general share some important properties: they tend to be lipid soluble, are substrates, though sometimes only minor ones, e.g. DDT, for the enzymes they induce, and generally have a long $t_{1/2}$. The time for onset and offset of induction depends on the rate of enzyme turnover, but significant induction generally occurs within a few days, and it passes off over 2–3 weeks following withdrawal of the inducer.

Thus, certain drugs can alter the capacity of the body to metabolise other substances including drugs, especially in long-term use; this phenomenon has implications for drug therapy. More than 200 substances induce enzymes in animals but the list of proven enzyme inducers in humans is more restricted, as set out below.

Substances that cause enzyme induction in humans	
• barbecued meats	• nevirapine
• barbiturates	• phenobarbital
• Brussels sprouts	• phenytoin
• carbamazepine	• primidone
• DDT (dicophane, and other insecticides)	• rifampicin
• ethanol (chronic use)	• St John's wort
• glutethimide	• sulfinpyrazone
• griseofulvin	• tobacco smoke
• meprobamate	

Enzyme induction is relevant to drug therapy because:

- Clinically important drug–drug (and drug–herb[18]) *interactions* may result, for example, in failure of oral contraceptives, loss of anticoagulant control, failure of cytotoxic chemotherapy.

- *Disease* may result. Anti-epilepsy drugs accelerate the breakdown of dietary and endogenously formed vitamin D, producing an inactive metabolite – in effect a vitamin D deficiency state, which can result in osteomalacia. The accompanying hypocalcaemia can increase the tendency to fits and a convulsion may lead to fracture of the demineralised bones.
- *Tolerance* to drug therapy may result in and provide an explanation for suboptimal treatment, e.g. with an anti-epilepsy drug.
- *Variability* in response to drugs is increased. Enzyme induction caused by heavy alcohol drinking or heavy smoking may be an unrecognised cause for failure of an individual to achieve the expected response to a normal dose of a drug, e.g. warfarin, theophylline.
- *Drug toxicity* may occur. A patient who becomes enzyme induced by taking rifampicin is more likely to develop liver toxicity after paracetamol overdose by increased production of a hepatotoxic metabolite. (Such a patient will also present with a deceptively low plasma concentration of paracetamol due to accelerated metabolism; see p. 254).

Enzyme inhibition

The consequences of inhibiting drug metabolism can be more profound and more selective than enzyme induction because the outcome is prolongation of action of a drug or metabolite. Consequently, enzyme inhibition offers more scope for therapy (Table 8.4). Enzyme inhibition by drugs is also the basis of a number of clinically important drug interactions (see p. 109).

Elimination

The body eliminates drugs following their partial or complete conversion to water-soluble metabolites or, in some cases, without their being metabolised. To avoid repetition, the following account refers to the drug whereas the processes deal with both drug and metabolites.

Renal elimination

The following mechanisms are involved.

Glomerular filtration. The rate at which a drug enters the glomerular filtrate depends on the concentration of free drug in plasma water and on its molecular weight. Substances having a molecular weight in excess of 50 000 do not cross into the glomerular filtrate, whereas those of molecular weight less than 10 000 (which includes almost all drugs)[19] pass easily through the pores of the glomerular membrane.

---

[18]Tirona R G, Bailey D G 2006 Herbal product–drug interactions mediated by induction. British Journal of Clinical Pharmacology 61:677–681.

[19]Most drugs have a molecular weight of less than 1000.

Table 8.4 Some drugs that act by enzyme inhibition

Drug	Enzyme inhibited	In treatment of
Acetazolamide	Carbonic anhydrase	Glaucoma
Allopurinol	Xanthine oxidase	Gout
Benserazide	DOPA decarboxylase	Parkinson's disease
Disulfiram	Aldehyde dehydrogenase	Alcoholism
Enalapril	Angiotensin-converting enzyme	Hypertension, cardiac failure
Moclobemide	Monoamine oxidase, A type	Depression
Non-steroidal anti-inflammatory drugs	Cyclo-oxygenase	Pain, inflammation
Selegiline	Monoamine oxidase, B type	Parkinson's disease

Renal tubular transport. Uptake and efflux transporters in proximal renal tubule cells transfer organic anions and cations between the plasma and the tubular fluid (see p. 480).

Renal tubular diffusion. The glomerular filtrate contains drug at the same concentration as it is free in the plasma, but the fluid is concentrated progressively as it flows down the nephron so that a gradient develops, drug in the tubular fluid becoming more concentrated than in the blood perfusing the nephron. As the tubular epithelium has the properties of a lipid membrane, the extent to which a drug diffuses back into the blood will depend on its lipid solubility, i.e. on its pK_a in the case of an electrolyte, and on the pH of tubular fluid. If the fluid becomes more alkaline, an acidic drug ionises, becomes less lipid soluble and its reabsorption diminishes, but a basic drug becomes un-ionised (and therefore more lipid soluble) and its reabsorption increases. Manipulation of urine pH gains useful expression with sodium bicarbonate given to alkalinise the urine for salicylate overdose.

Faecal elimination

When any drug intended for systemic effect is taken by mouth, a proportion may remain in the bowel and be excreted in the faeces. Some drugs are intended not to be absorbed from the gut, as an objective of therapy, e.g. neomycin. The cells of the intestinal epithelium contain several carrier-mediated transporters that control the absorption of drugs. The efflux transporter MDR1, for example, drives drug from the enterocyte into the gut lumen, limiting its bioavailability (see p. 95). Drug in the blood may also diffuse passively into the gut lumen, depending on its pK_a and the pH difference between blood and gut contents. The effectiveness of activated charcoal by mouth for drug overdose depends partly on its adsorption of such diffused drug, and subsequent elimination in the faeces (see p. 128).

Biliary excretion. Transporters regulate the uptake of organic cations and anions from portal blood to hepatocyte, and thence to the bile (see p. 88). The bile canaliculi tend to reabsorb small molecules, and in general, only compounds having a molecular weight greater than 300 pass into bile. (See also Enterohepatic circulation, p. 88.)

Pulmonary elimination

The lungs are the main route of elimination (and of uptake) of volatile anaesthetics. Apart from this, they play only a trivial role in drug elimination. The route, however, acquires notable medicolegal significance when ethanol concentration is measured in the air expired by vehicle drivers involved in road traffic accidents (via the breathalyser).

Clearance

Elimination of a drug from the plasma is quantified in terms of its clearance. The term has the same meaning as the familiar renal creatinine clearance, which is a measure of removal of endogenous creatinine from the plasma. Clearance values can provide useful information about the biological fate of a drug. There are pharmacokinetic methods for calculating *total body* and *renal* clearance, and the difference between these represents *hepatic* clearance. The renal clearance of a drug eliminated only by filtration by the kidney obviously cannot exceed the glomerular filtration rate (adult male 124 mL/min, female 109 mL/min). If a drug has a renal clearance in excess of this, then the kidney tubules must actively secrete it, e.g. benzylpenicillin (renal clearance 480 mL/min).

Breast milk

Most drugs that are present in a mother's plasma appear to some extent in her milk, although the amounts are so small that loss of drug in milk is of no significance as a mechanism of elimination. Even small amounts, however, may sometimes be of significance for the suckling child, whose drug metabolic and eliminating mechanisms are immature.

While most drugs taken by the mother pose no hazard to the child, exceptions to this observation occur because some drugs are inherently toxic, or transfer to milk in significant amounts, or there are known adverse effects, as described below.

Drugs and breast feeding[20]

- *Alimentary tract.* Sulfasalazine may cause adverse effects, and mesalazine appears preferable.
- *Anti-asthma.* The neonate eliminates theophylline and diprophylline slowly; observe the infant for irritability or disturbed sleep.
- *Anticancer.* Regard all as unsafe because of inherent toxicity.
- *Antidepressants.* Avoid doxepin, a metabolite of which may cause respiratory depression.
- *Anti-arrhythmics (cardiac).* Amiodarone is present in high and disopyramide in moderate amounts.
- *Anti-epilepsy.* General note of caution: observe the infant for sedation and poor suckling. Primidone, ethosuximide and phenobarbital are present in milk in high amounts; phenytoin and sodium valproate less so.
- *Anti-inflammatory.* Regard aspirin (salicylates) as unsafe (possible association with Reye's syndrome).
- *Antimicrobials.* Metronidazole is present in milk in moderate amounts; avoid prolonged exposure (though no harm recorded). Avoid nalidixic acid and nitrofurantoin where glucose-6-phosphate dehydrogenase deficiency is prevalent. Avoid clindamycin, dapsone, lincomycin, sulphonamides. Regard chloramphenicol as unsafe.
- *Antipsychotics.* Phenothiazines, butyrophenones and thioxanthenes are best avoided unless the indications are compelling: amounts in milk are small but animal studies suggest adverse effects on the developing nervous system. In particular, moderate amounts of sulpiride enter milk. Avoid lithium if possible.
- *Anxiolytics and sedatives.* Benzodiazepines are safe if use is brief, but prolonged use may cause somnolence or poor suckling.

- β-*Adrenoceptor blockers.* Neonatal hypoglycaemia may occur. Sotalol and atenolol are present in the highest amounts in this group.
- *Hormones.* Oestrogens, progestogens and androgens suppress lactation in high dose. Oestrogen–progestogen oral contraceptives are present in amounts too small to be harmful, but may suppress lactation if it is not well established.
- *Miscellaneous.* Bromocriptine suppresses lactation. Caffeine may cause infant irritability in high doses.

Drug dosage

Drug dosage can be of five main kinds:

Fixed dose. The effect that is desired can be obtained at well below the toxic dose (many mydriatics, analgesics, oral contraceptives, antimicrobials), and enough drug can be given to render individual variation clinically insignificant.

Variable dose – with crude adjustments. Here fine adjustments make comparatively insignificant differences, and the therapeutic endpoint may be hard to measure (depression, anxiety), may change only slowly (thyrotoxicosis), or may vary because of pathophysiological factors (analgesics, adrenal corticosteroids for suppressing disease).

Variable dose – with fine adjustments. Here a vital function (blood pressure, blood sugar level), which often changes rapidly in response to dose changes and can easily be measured repeatedly, provides the endpoint. Adjustment of dose must be accurate. Adrenocortical *replacement* therapy falls into this group, whereas adrenocortical *pharmacotherapy* falls into the group above.

Maximum tolerated dose is used when the ideal therapeutic effect cannot be achieved because of the occurrence of unwanted effects (anticancer drugs; some antimicrobials). The usual way of finding this is to increase the dose until unwanted effects begin to appear and then to reduce it slightly, or to monitor the plasma concentration.

Minimum tolerated dose. This concept is less common than the one above, but it applies to long-term adrenocortical steroid therapy against inflammatory or immunological conditions, e.g. in asthma and some cases of rheumatoid arthritis, when the dose that provides symptomatic relief may be so high that serious adverse effects are inevitable if it is continued indefinitely. The compromise is incomplete relief on the grounds of safety. This can be difficult to achieve.

Dosing schedules

Dosing schedules are simply schemes aimed at achieving a desired effect while avoiding toxicity. The following discussion

---

[20]Bennett P N (ed) 1996 Drugs and Human Lactation. Elsevier, Amsterdam.

assumes that drug effect relates closely to plasma concentration, which in turn relates closely to the amount of drug in the body. The objectives of a dosing regimen where continuing effect is required are:

To specify an initial dose that attains the desired effect rapidly without causing toxicity. Often the dose that is capable of initiating drug effect is the same as that which maintains it. On repeated dosing, however, it takes $5 \times t_{1/2}$ periods to reach steady-state concentration in the plasma, and this lapse of time may be undesirable. The effect may be achieved earlier by giving an initial dose that is larger than the maintenance dose; the initial dose is then called the *priming* or *loading* dose, i.e. the dose that will achieve a therapeutic effect in an individual whose body does not already contain the drug.

To specify a maintenance dose: amount and frequency. Intuitively the maintenance dose might be half of the initial/priming dose at intervals equal to its plasma $t_{1/2}$, for this is the time by which the plasma concentration that achieves the desired effect, declines by half. Whether or not this approach is satisfactory or practicable, however, depends very much on the $t_{1/2}$ itself, as is illustrated by the following cases:

1. *Half-life 6–12 h.* In this instance, replacing one-half the initial dose at intervals equal to the $t_{1/2}$ can indeed be a satisfactory solution because dosing every 6–12 h is acceptable.
2. *Half-life greater than 24 h.* With once-daily dosing (which is desirable for compliance), giving half the priming dose every day means that more drug is entering the body than is leaving it each day, and the drug will accumulate to give unwanted effects. The solution is to replace only the amount of drug that leaves the body in 24 h, calculated from the initial dose, dose interval, and $t_{1/2}$.
3. *Half-life less than 3 h.* Dosing at intervals equal to the $t_{1/2}$ would be so frequent as to be unacceptable. The answer is to use continuous intravenous infusion if the $t_{1/2}$ is very short, e.g. dopamine $t_{1/2}$ 2 min (steady-state plasma concentration will be reached in $5 \times t_{1/2} = 10$ min), or, if the $t_{1/2}$ is longer, e.g. lidocaine ($t_{1/2}$ 90 min), to use a priming dose as an intravenous bolus followed by a constant intravenous infusion. Intermittent administration of a drug with short $t_{1/2}$ is nevertheless reasonable provided large fluctuations in plasma concentration are acceptable, i.e. that the drug has a large therapeutic index. Benzylpenicillin has a $t_{1/2}$ of 30 min but is effective in a 6-hourly regimen because the drug is so non-toxic that it is possible safely to give a dose that achieves a plasma concentration many times in excess of the minimum inhibitory concentration for sensitive organisms.

Dose calculation by body-weight and surface area

A uniform, fixed drug dose is likely to be ineffective or toxic in several circumstances, e.g. cytotoxic chemotherapy, aminoglycoside antibiotics. It is usual then to calculate the dose according to body-weight. Adjustment according to body surface area is also used and may be more appropriate, for this correlates better with many physiological phenomena, e.g. metabolic rate.

The relationship between body surface area and weight is curvilinear, but a reasonable approximation is that a 70-kg human has a body surface area of 1.8 m². A combination of body-weight and height gives a more precise value for surface area (obtained from standard nomograms) and other more sophisticated methods.[21]

The issue takes on special significance for children, if the only dose known is that for the adult; adjustment is then commonly made by body-weight, or body surface area, among other factors (see p. 105).

Prolongation of drug action

Giving a larger dose is the most obvious way to prolong a drug action, but this is not always feasible, and other mechanisms are used:

- *Vasoconstriction* will reduce local blood flow so that distribution of drug away from an injection site is retarded, e.g. combination with adrenaline/epinephrine prolongs local anaesthetic action.
- *Slowing of metabolism* may usefully extend drug action, as when a dopa decarboxylase inhibitor, e.g. carbidopa, is combined with levodopa (as co-careldopa) for parkinsonism.
- *Delayed excretion* is seldom practicable, the only important example being the use of probenecid to block renal tubular excretion of penicillin for single-dose treatment of gonorrhoea.
- *Altered molecular structure* can prolong effect, e.g. the various benzodiazepines.
- *Pharmaceutical formulation.* Manipulating the form in which a drug is presented by modified-release[22] systems can achieve the objective of an even as well as a prolonged effect.

---

[21]For example, Livingston E H, Lee S 2001 Body surface area prediction in normal-weight and obese patients. American Journal of Physiology Endocrinology and Metabolism 281:586–591.

[22]The term *modified* covers several drug delivery systems. *Delayed release*: available other than immediately after administration (mesalazine in the colon); *sustained release*: slow release as governed by the delivery system (iron, potassium); *controlled release*: at a constant rate to maintain unvarying plasma concentration (nitrate, hormone replacement therapy).

Sustained-release (oral) preparations can reduce the frequency of medication to once a day, and compliance becomes easier for the patient. The elderly can now receive most long-term medication as a single morning dose. In addition, sustained-release preparations may avoid bowel toxicity due to high local concentrations, e.g. ulceration of the small intestine with potassium chloride tablets; they may also avoid the toxic peak plasma concentrations that can occur when dissolution of the formulation, and so absorption of the drug, is rapid. Some sustained-release formulations also contain an immediate-release component to provide rapid, as well as sustained, effect.

Depot (injectable) preparations are more reliable because the environment in which they are deposited is more constant than can ever be the case in the alimentary tract, and medication can be given at longer intervals, even weeks. In general, such preparations are pharmaceutical variants, e.g. microcrystals, or the original drug in oil, wax, gelatin or synthetic media. They include phenothiazine neuroleptics, the various insulins and penicillins, preparations of vasopressin, and medroxyprogesterone (intramuscular, subcutaneous). Tablets of hormones can be implanted subcutaneously. The advantages of infrequent administration and better patient adherence in a variety of situations are obvious.

Reduction of absorption time

A soluble salt of the drug may be effective by being rapidly absorbed from the site of administration. In the case of subcutaneous or intramuscular injections, the same objective may be obtained with hyaluronidase, an enzyme that depolymerises hyaluronic acid, a constituent of connective tissue that prevents the spread of foreign substances, e.g. bacteria, drugs. Hyaluronidase combined with an intramuscular injection, e.g. a local anaesthetic, or a subcutaneous infusion leads to increased permeation with more rapid absorption. Hyaluronidase also promotes resorption of tissue accumulation of blood and fluid.

Fixed-dose drug combinations

This refers to combinations of drugs in a single pharmaceutical formulation. It does not mean concomitant drug therapy, e.g. in infections, hypertension and in cancer, when several drugs are given separately. Therapeutic aims should be clear. Combinations are logical if there is good reason to consider that the patient needs all the drugs in the formulation and that the doses are appropriate and will not need adjustment separately. Fixed-dose drug combinations are appropriate for:

- *Convenience*, with improved patient compliance, is appropriate with two drugs used at constant dose, long term, for an asymptomatic condition, e.g. a thiazide plus an ACE inhibitor in mild or moderate hypertension, and other antihypertensive drug combinations.
- *Enhanced effect*. Single-drug treatment of tuberculosis leads to the emergence of resistant mycobacteria and is prevented or delayed by using two or more drugs simultaneously. Combining isoniazid with rifampicin (Rifinah, Rimactazid) ensures that single-drug treatment cannot occur; treatment has to be two drugs or no drug at all. An oestrogen and progestogen combination provides effective oral contraception, for the same reason.
- *Minimisation of unwanted effects*. Levodopa combined with benserazide (Madopar) or with carbidopa (Sinemet) slows its metabolism outside the CNS so that smaller amounts of levodopa can be used, reducing its adverse effects.

Chronic pharmacology

The pharmacodynamics and pharmacokinetics of many drugs differ according to whether their use is in a single dose, or over a brief period (acute pharmacology), or long term (chronic pharmacology). An increasing proportion of the population take drugs continuously for large portions of their lives, as tolerable suppressive and prophylactic remedies for chronic or recurrent conditions are developed; e.g. for arterial hypertension, diabetes mellitus, psychiatric diseases, epilepsies. In general, the dangers of a drug therapy are not markedly greater if therapy lasts for years rather than months, but long-term treatment can introduce significant hazard into patients' lives unless management is skilful.

Interference with self-regulating systems

When self-regulating physiological systems (generally controlled by negative feedback systems, e.g. endocrine, cardiovascular) are subject to interference, their control mechanisms respond to minimise the effects of the interference and to restore the previous steady state or rhythm; this is *homeostasis*. The previous state may be a normal function, e.g. ovulation (a rare example of a positive feedback mechanism), or an abnormal function, e.g. high blood pressure. If the body successfully restores the previous steady state or rhythm, then the subject has become tolerant to the drug, i.e. needs a higher dose to produce the desired previous effect.

In the case of hormonal contraceptives, persistence of suppression of ovulation occurs and is desired, but persistence of other effects, e.g. on blood coagulation and metabolism, is not desired.

In the case of arterial hypertension, tolerance to a single drug commonly occurs, e.g. reduction of peripheral resistance by a vasodilator is compensated by an increase in blood volume that restores the blood pressure; this is why a diuretic is commonly used together with a vasodilator in therapy.

Feedback systems. The endocrine system serves fluctuating body needs. Glands are therefore capable either of increasing or decreasing their output by means of negative (usually) feedback systems. An administered hormone or hormone analogue activates the receptors of the feedback system so that high doses cause suppression of natural production of the hormone. On withdrawal of the administered hormone, restoration of the normal control mechanism takes time, e.g. the hypothalamic–pituitary–adrenal cortex system can take months to recover full sensitivity, and sudden withdrawal of administered corticosteroid can result in an acute deficiency state that may be life endangering.

Regulation of receptors. The number (density) of receptors on cells (for hormones, autacoids or local hormones, and drugs), the number occupied (receptor occupancy) and the capacity of the receptor to respond (affinity, efficacy) can change in response to the concentration of the specific binding molecule or ligand,[23] whether this be agonist or antagonist (blocker). The effects always tend to restore cell function to its normal or usual state. Prolonged high concentrations of agonist (whether administered as a drug or over-produced in the body by a tumour) cause a reduction in the number of receptors available for activation *(down-regulation)*; changes in receptor occupancy and affinity and the prolonged occupation of receptor antagonists lead to an increase in the number of receptors *(up-regulation)*. At least some of this may be achieved by receptors moving inside the cell and out again (internalisation and externalisation).

Down-regulation, and the accompanying receptor changes, may explain the 'on–off' phenomenon in Parkinson's disease (see p. 379) and the action of luteinising hormone releasing hormone (LHRH) super-agonists in reducing follicle stimulating hormone (FSH) concentrations for treating endocrine-sensitive prostate cancer.

Up-regulation. The occasional exacerbation of ischaemic cardiac disease on sudden withdrawal of a β-adrenoceptor blocker may be explained by up-regulation during its administration, so that, on withdrawal, an above-normal number of receptors suddenly become accessible to the normal transmitter, i.e. noradrenaline/norepinephrine.

Up-regulation with rebound sympathomimetic effects may be innocuous to a moderately healthy cardiovascular system, but the increased oxygen demand of these effects

can have serious consequences where ischaemic disease is present and increased oxygen need cannot be met (angina pectoris, arrhythmia, myocardial infarction). Unmasking of a disease process that has worsened during prolonged suppressive use of the drug, i.e. resurgence, may also contribute to such exacerbations.

The rebound phenomenon is plainly a potential hazard, and the use of a β-adrenoceptor blocker in the presence of ischaemic heart disease would be safer if rebound is eliminated. β-Adrenoceptor blockers that are not pure antagonists but have some agonist (sympathomimetic ischaemic) activity, i.e. partial agonists, may prevent the generation of additional adrenoceptors (up-regulation). Indeed, there is evidence that rebound is less or is absent with pindolol, a partial agonist β-adrenoceptor blocker.

Sometimes a distinction is made between *rebound* (recurrence at intensified degree of the symptoms for which the drug was given) and *withdrawal syndrome* (appearance of new additional symptoms). The distinction is quantitative and does not imply different mechanisms.

Rebound and withdrawal phenomena occur erratically. In general, they are more likely with drugs having a short $t_{1/2}$ (abrupt drop in plasma concentration) and pure agonist or antagonist action. They are less likely to occur with drugs having a long $t_{1/2}$ and (probably) with those having a mixed agonist–antagonist (partial agonist) action on receptors.

Abrupt withdrawal

Clinically important consequences occur, and might occur for a variety of reasons, e.g. a patient interrupting drug therapy to undergo surgery. The following are examples:

- *Cardiovascular system*: β-adrenoceptor blockers, antihypertensives (especially clonidine).
- *Nervous system*: all depressants (hypnotics, sedatives, alcohol, opioids), anti-epileptics, antiparkinsonian agents, tricyclic antidepressants.
- *Endocrine system*: adrenal corticosteroids.
- *Immune inflammation*: adrenal corticosteroids.

Resurgence of chronic disease, which has progressed in severity, although its consequences have been wholly or partly suppressed, i.e. a catching-up phenomenon, is a possible outcome of discontinuing effective therapy, e.g. levodopa in Parkinson's disease. Corticosteroid withdrawal in autoimmune disease may cause both resurgence and rebound.

Drug discontinuation syndromes, i.e. rebound, withdrawal and resurgence (defined above) are phenomena that are to be expected. The exact mechanisms may remain obscure, but clinicians have no reason to be surprised when they occur, and in the case of rebound they may wish to use gradual withdrawal wherever drugs are used to modify complex self-adjusting systems, and to suppress (without cure) chronic diseases.

---

[23]Latin: *ligare* = to bind.

Other aspects of chronic drug use

Metabolic changes over a long period may induce disease, e.g. thiazide diuretics (diabetes mellitus), adrenocortical hormones (osteoporosis), phenytoin (osteomalacia). Drugs may also enhance their own metabolism, and that of other drugs (enzyme induction).

Specific cell injury or cell functional disorder occurs with individual drugs or drug classes, e.g. tardive dyskinesia (dopamine receptor blockers), retinal damage (chloroquine, phenothiazines), retroperitoneal fibrosis (methysergide), non-steroidal anti-inflammatory drugs (nephropathy). Cancer may occur, e.g. with oestrogens (endometrium) and with immunosuppressive (anticancer) drugs.

Drug holidays. The term means the deliberate interruption of long-term therapy in order to restore sensitivity (which has been lost) or to reduce the risk of toxicity. Plainly, the need for holidays is a substantial disadvantage for any drug. Patients sometimes initiate their own drug holidays (see Patient compliance, p. 19).

Dangers of intercurrent illness are particularly notable with anticoagulants, adrenal corticosteroids and immunosuppressants.

Dangers of interactions with other drugs, herbs or food. See Index for individual drugs.

Conclusions

> Drugs not only induce their known listed primary actions, but may:
> - evoke compensatory responses in the complex interrelated physiological systems they affect, and these systems need time to recover on withdrawal of the drug (gradual withdrawal is sometimes mandatory and never harmful)
> - induce metabolic changes that may be trivial in the short term, but serious if they persist for a long time
> - produce localised effects in specially susceptible tissues and induce serious cell damage or malfunction
> - increase susceptibility to intercurrent illness and to interaction with other drugs that may be taken for new indications.

That such consequences occur with prolonged drug use need evoke no surprise. But a knowledge of physiology, pathology and pharmacology, combined with awareness that the unexpected can occur, will allow patients who require long-term therapy to be managed safely, or at least with minimum risk of harm.

Individual or biological variation

Prescribing for special risk groups

That individuals respond differently to drugs, both from time to time and from other individuals, is a matter of everyday experience. Doctors need to accommodate for individual variation, as it may explain both adverse response to a drug and failure of therapy. Sometimes there are obvious physical characteristics such as age, ethnicity (genetics) or disease that warn the prescriber to adjust drug dose, but there are no external features that signify, e.g. pseudocholinesterase deficiency, which causes prolonged paralysis after suxamethonium. An understanding of the reasons for individual variation in response to drugs is relevant to all who prescribe. Both pharmacodynamic and pharmacokinetic effects are involved, and the issues fall in two general categories: inherited influences and environmental and host influences.

Pharmacogenomics

Munir Pirmohamed

We are grateful to Professor Munir Pirmohamed, NHS Chair of at the University of Liverpool, UK, for providing the following account.

> 'Variability is the law of life, and as no two faces are the same, so no two bodies are alike, and no two individuals react alike, and behave alike ...' (Sir William Osler, 1849–1919).

Introduction

The response to drugs varies widely among patients – for example, it has been estimated that only about 30% of patients respond to antidepressants. Adverse drug reactions are also common, accounting for 6.5% of admissions to hospital. Part of this variability is due to patient-related factors (non-compliance, smoking, alcohol, co-morbidities) and poor prescribing. However, a significant proportion of the variability, which varies from drug to drug, is due to genetic factors. This area of study is termed *pharmacogenomics*.

> Pharmacogenomics can be defined as the study of the genomic basis of why individuals vary in their response (efficacy and/or toxicity) to drugs. This term is used interchangeably with pharmacogenetics. The first example can be traced back to the time of Pythagoras (born 569 BC, died between 500 and 475 BC), who described the phenomenon ascribed to red cell haemolysis in some Mediterranean populations eating fava beans (favism), which we now know to be due to glucose-6-phosphate dehydrogenase deficiency, the most common enzyme deficiency in man.

Sources of variability

In general, variability in drug response can be due to pharmacokinetic and/or pharmacodynamic factors (Fig. 8.4). Variability in the expression of the cytochrome P450 enzymes, which are responsible for Phase I drug metabolism, has been the focus of most of the work in pharmacokinetics. Cytochrome P450 2D6 (CYP2D6), for example, is one of the most variable P450 enzymes in man, is absent in 8% of the UK population, and is responsible for the metabolism of 25% of drugs, including CNS drugs (antidepressants and antipsychotics) and cardiovascular drugs (β-blockers and anti-arrhythmics). A recently approved drug eliglustat, used in the treatment of Gaucher's disease, requires determination of the *CYP2D6* status prior to drug use, with dose reduction in patients who are poor metabolisers.

Much less work has been done on pharmacodynamic factors causing variation in drug response, but as drugs can affect almost any protein in the body, almost every gene may have an effect on how individual drugs vary in their response. It is important to note, however, that for most drugs variability in response is due to a combination of pharmacokinetic and pharmacodynamic factors, both of which can be affected by environmental or genetic factors. Specific examples are provided below.

Identifying genetic variation. Much of the work in pharmacogenomics has been based on a study of candidate genes, i.e. a study of genes known to be involved in the

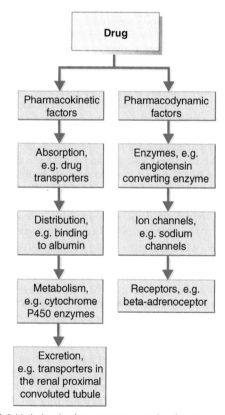

Fig. 8.4 Variation in drug response can be due to genetically determined factors in pharmacokinetic and pharmacodynamic processes in the body. Some examples are given in each box.

pharmacokinetics of the drug and its mechanism of action. Specifically the focus has been on single nucleotide polymorphisms (SNPs), which are base substitutions occurring with a frequency of at least 1% in the human population. With the advances in technologies, more recent work has focused on genome-wide association studies (GWAS), i.e. a study of all genes in the human genome without any prior knowledge of the pharmacokinetic and pharmacodynamic parameters of the drug. GWAS is already being surpassed by next-generation sequencing technologies, which provides an evaluation of common and rare variants in the human genome. The challenge with next-generation sequencing will be the determination of whether rare variants have a functional effect, and whether this will affect drug response.

Examples of pharmacogenomic variation

Drug efficacy

Cancer therapy. Cancer is essentially a genetic disease with approximately 30–80 mutations per cancer. These mutations within the cancer genome (the somatic genome) also change the responsiveness of the cancer to therapy. The best example is that of trastuzumab (Herceptin) in breast cancer; this drug improves disease-free and overall survival in patients with *HER2* gene amplification or over-expression of the protein on breast cancer cells. This adverse prognostic factor occurs in 20% of newly diagnosed breast cancers. In patients with metastatic malignant melanoma, approximately 50% of patients have the V600E somatic mutation in the proto-oncogene *BRAF*; in such cases, patients can be treated with the inhibitors, vemurafenib or dabrafenib. These patients often have a dramatic initial response, but unfortunately, there is recurrence of the tumour within a few months because of the occurrence of other somatic mutations.

Warfarin. Warfarin is a narrow therapeutic index drug where individual daily dose requirements vary by at least 40-fold. Inability to maintain an INR between 2 and 3 can predispose to either thrombosis (INR<2) or haemorrhage (INR>3). Warfarin is metabolised by various P450 enzymes, the most important being CYP2C9. Two variants in the *CYP2C9* gene (termed *CYP2C9*2* and *CYP2C9*3*) reduce the activity of the enzyme and overall rate of the metabolic turnover of warfarin. The mode of action of warfarin is through interruption of the vitamin K cycle specifically by inhibiting the enzyme vitamin K epoxide reductase complex 1 (VKORC1) – variation in this gene can affect the daily requirements for warfarin. In most global populations, it has now been shown that age and body mass index, together with genetic variation in *CYP2C9* and *VKORC1*, can account for at least 50% of the variation in daily dose requirements for warfarin. This resulted in the development of dosing algorithms to improve the prediction of individual dose requirements for warfarin. The utility of such dosing algorithms has been shown in randomized controlled trials where genotype-guided dosing was able significantly to improve the time within the therapeutic INR range compared with standard dosing.

Drug toxicity

Immune-mediated adverse drug reactions. Many type B or idiosyncratic adverse drug reactions are immunologically mediated. Immune response to antigens, including those derived from drugs, is partly under control of the HLA genes on chromosome 6, which is the polymorphic region of the human genome. Not surprisingly, HLA genes have also been found to be important determinants of susceptibility to these immune-mediated adverse reactions. The best example of this is with abacavir, a drug used to treat HIV, which causes hypersensitivity (skin rash, fever, gastrointestinal and respiratory manifestations) in 5% of patients. A strong association of abacavir hypersensitivity with the HLA allele, *HLA-B*57:01*, has now been shown in several populations. Furthermore, genotyping for *HLA-B*57:01* before prescribing abacavir has been shown to reduce the frequency of hypersensitivity, and is a cost-effective approach. In Europe, it is now mandatory to undertake *HLA-B*57:01* testing before the prescription of abacavir. Very strong genetic associations between the HLA genes and different forms of hypersensitivity, including those affecting the skin and liver, occur with a number of drugs (Table 8.5).

Statin myopathy. Statins are among the most widely used drugs in the world, with marked benefits in terms of reduction of cardiovascular morbidity and mortality. Although generally well tolerated, statins can occasionally cause muscle damage, which can range from muscle pains to rhabdomyolysis (associated with renal failure, which can be fatal). A genome-wide approach in patients on simvastatin showed that a variant in an influx drug transporter called *SLCO1B1* (also known as OATP1B1) increased the risk of statin-related myopathy. This transporter is highly expressed in the liver and is responsible for the transport of some statins from the blood into the hepatocyte. In patients expressing this variant, the activity of the transporter is reduced, which leads to a decrease in hepatocyte uptake and an increase in plasma concentrations of the statin. However, the mechanism by which the statin leads to muscle damage is unknown.

Summary

There are many genetic variations identified to be risk factors for lack of efficacy or predisposition to toxicity (Table 8.6).

Table 8.5 HLA alleles predisposing to immune-mediated adverse drug reactions

Drug	Therapeutic use	Adverse effect	HLA association
Abacavir	Anti-HIV	Hypersensitivity reaction	HLA-B*57:01
Allopurinol	Gout	Severe cutaneous adverse drug reaction	HLA-B*58:01
Carbamazepine	Anticonvulsant	Hypersensitivity reaction	HLA-B*15:02, HLA-A*31:01
Flucloxacillin	Antibiotic	Cholestatic hepatitis	HLA-B*57:01
Co-amoxiclav	Antibiotic	Cholestatic hepatitis	HLA-DRB1*15:01-DQB1*06:02
Lumiracoxib	Non-steroidal anti-inflammatory drug	Drug-induced liver injury	HLA-DRB1*15:01-DQB1*06:02
Dapsone	Antimicrobial	Hypersensitivity syndrome	HLA-B*13:01
Lapatinib	Breast cancer	Drug-induced liver injury	HLA-DQA1*02:01

As the technologies to interrogate the human genome improve, it is likely that more genetic tests that can be used before the prescription of the drug will be introduced. Although most studies have so far focused on the use of genetic tests to predict individual responses and thereby reduce variability through better drug choice and/or drug dose, it is important to note that genetic tests can also be used to aid diagnosis of serious adverse drug reactions, to identify patients who require more stringent monitoring while undergoing therapy (as we currently use liver and renal function tests).

Environmental and host influences

A multitude of factors related to both individuals and their environment contribute to differences in drug response. Some of the more relevant influences are the following:

Age

The neonate, infant and child[24]

Young human beings differ greatly from adults, not merely in size but also in the proportions and constituents of their bodies and the functioning of their physiological systems. These differences influence the way the body handles and responds to drugs:

- Rectal absorption is efficient with an appropriate formulation, e.g. of diazepam and theophyllines; this route may be preferred with an uncooperative infant.

- The intramuscular or subcutaneous routes tend to give unpredictable plasma concentrations, e.g. of digoxin or gentamicin, because of the relatively low proportion of skeletal muscle and fat. Intravenous administration is preferred in the seriously ill newborn.
- Drugs or other substances that come in contact with the skin are readily absorbed as the skin is well hydrated and the stratum corneum is thin; overdose toxicity may result, e.g. with hexachlorophene used in dusting powders and emulsions to prevent infection.
- An understandable reluctance to test drugs extensively in children means that reliable information is often lacking. Many drugs do not have a licence to be used for children, and their prescription must be 'off-licence', a practice that is recognised as necessary, if not actually promoted, by the UK drug regulatory authorities.[25] Attempts to correct this are underway across Europe.

Distribution. Total body water in the neonate amounts to 80%, compared with 65% of body-weight in older children. Consequently:

- Weight-related loading doses of aminoglycosides, aminophylline, digoxin and furosemide need to be larger for neonates than for older children.
- Less extensive binding of drugs to plasma proteins is generally without clinical importance, but there is a risk of kernicterus in the jaundiced neonate following displacement of bilirubin from protein-binding sites by vitamin K, X-ray contrast media or indometacin.

---

[24]A neonate is younger than 1 month of age, and an infant is 1–12 months of age.

[25]Stephenson T 2006 The medicines for children agenda in the UK. British Journal of Clinical Pharmacology 61:716–719.

Table 8.6 Examples of drugs which contain pharmacogenetic information in their product labels

Drug	Drug class	Genomic variation
Maraviroc	Antiretroviral, antagonist of the CC chemokine receptor 5 (CCR5)	CCR5 promoter and coding sequence polymorphisms
Trastuzumab (Herceptin)	Anticancer drug, anti-HER-2/neu monoclonal antibody used where there is over-expression of the human epidermal growth factor receptor-2 (HER2)	HER2/neu
Abacavir	Antiretroviral, nucleoside reverse transcriptase inhibitor	Human leucocyte antigen HLA-B*57:01 allele
Carbamazepine	Anti-epileptic	HLA-B*15:02 in patients of Asian ancestry
Warfarin	Anticoagulant, vitamin K epoxide reductase complex 1 inhibitor	CYP 2 C9*2 and 2 C9*3 and VKORC1 variants
Azathioprine	Antiproliferative immunosuppressant	Thiopurine methyltransferase (TPMT) deficiency
Valproic acid	Anti-epileptic and antimanic drug	Urea cycle disorder (UCD) deficiency
Hydralazine	Vasodilator antihypertensive drug	*N*-acetyl transferase (NAT)
Isoniazid	Antituberculous drug	*N*-acetyl transferase (NAT)
Voriconazole	Antifungal	CYP2C19 variants poor and extensive metabolisers
Diazepam	Anxiolytic	CYP2C19 variants poor and extensive metabolisers
Fluoxetine	Selective serotonin reuptake inhibitor	Cytochrome P450 CYP2D6, substrate and inhibitor
Tramadol	Analgesic	CYP2D6
Metoprolol	β-Adrenoceptor blocking drug	CYP2D6
Tamoxifen	Oestrogen-receptor antagonist	CYP2D6
Tretinoin	Acid form of vitamin A used in acute promyelocytic leukaemia	Presence of the t(15;17) translocation and/or PML/RARα gene fusion
Celecoxib	Non-steroidal anti-inflamatory drug, selective COX-2 inhibitor	CYP2C9 variants with poor metaboliser status
Primaquine Chloroquine	Antimalarials	Glucose-6-phosphate dehydrogenase (G6PD) deficiency
Suxamethonium	Anaesthetics	Butyrylcholinesterase deficiency
Eliglustat	Glucosylceramide synthetase inhibitor used in Gaucher's disease	CYP2D6 variants and poor metaboliser status

Metabolism. Drug-inactivating enzyme systems are present at birth but are functionally immature (particularly in the preterm baby), especially for oxidation and for conjugation with glucuronic acid. Inadequate conjugation and thus inactivation of chloramphenicol by neonates causes the fatal 'grey' syndrome, but this is not a widely used antibiotic.

After the initial weeks of life, because their drug metabolic capacity increases rapidly, young children may require a higher weight-related dose than adults.

Elimination. Glomerular filtration, tubular secretion and reabsorption are low in the neonate (even lower in preterm babies), reaching adult values in relation to body surface area only at 2–5 months. Drugs that the kidney excretes, e.g. aminoglycosides, penicillins, diuretics, require reduced dose; after about 6 months, body-weight– or surface area–related daily doses are the same for all ages.

Pharmacodynamic responses. There is scant information about developmental effects of interaction between drugs and receptors. Other sources suggest possible effects: e.g. thalidomide causes phocomelia only in the forming limb (see Index); tetracyclines stain only developing enamel; young children are particularly sensitive to liver toxicity from valproate.

Dosage in the young. No single rule or formula is suitable for all cases. Computation by body-weight may overdose an obese child, for whom calculation of ideal weight from age and height is preferred. Doses based on body surface area are generally more accurate and preferably should take into account both body-weight and height.[26] The fact that the surface area of a 70-kg adult human is 1.8 m² (see p. 99) then allows adjustment, as follows:

$$\text{Approximate dose} = \text{Surface area of child } (m^2)/1.8 \times \text{adult dose}$$

General guidance is available from formularies, e.g. the *British National Formulary*, and specialist publications.[27,28]

The elderly

The incidence of adverse drug reactions rises with age in the adult, especially after 65 years, because of:

- The increasing number of drugs that the elderly need because they tend to have multiple diseases.
- Poor compliance with dosing regimens.
- Bodily changes of ageing that require modified dosage regimens.

Absorption of drugs administered orally may be slightly slower because of reduced gastrointestinal blood flow and motility, but the effect is rarely important.

Distribution reflects the following changes:

- Lean body mass is less, and standard adult doses provide a greater amount of drug per kilogram.
- Body fat increases and may act as a reservoir for lipid-soluble drugs.

- Total body water is less and, in general, water-soluble drugs have a lower distribution volume. Standard doses of drugs, especially the loading doses of those that are water soluble, may thus exceed the requirement.
- Plasma albumin concentration is well maintained in the healthy elderly but may fall with chronic disease, giving scope for a greater proportion of unbound (free) drug, which may be important when priming doses are given.

Metabolism reduces as liver mass and liver blood flow decline. Consequently:

- Metabolic inactivation of drugs is slower, mostly for Phase I (oxidation) reactions; the capacity for Phase II (conjugation) is better preserved.
- Drugs normally extensively eliminated in first pass through the liver appear in higher concentration in the systemic circulation and persist in it for longer. There is, therefore, particular need initially to use lower doses of most neuroleptics, tricyclic antidepressants and cardiac anti-arrhythmic agents.
- Capacity for hepatic enzyme induction appears less.

Elimination. Renal blood flow, glomerular filtration and tubular secretion decrease with age above 55 years, a decline that raised serum creatinine concentration does not signal because production of this metabolite is diminished by the age-associated diminution of muscle mass. Indeed, in the elderly, serum creatinine may be within the concentration range for normal young adults even when the creatinine clearance is 50 mL/min (compared with 127 mL/min in adult males). Particular risk of adverse effects arises with drugs that are eliminated mainly by the kidney and that have a small therapeutic ratio, e.g. aminoglycosides, digoxin, lithium.

Pharmacodynamic response may alter with age, to produce either a greater or a lesser effect than is anticipated in younger adults, for example:

- Drugs that act on the CNS appear to produce an exaggerated response in relation to that expected from the plasma concentration, and sedatives and hypnotics may have a pronounced hangover effect. These drugs are also more likely to depress respiration because of reduced vital capacity and maximum breathing capacity in the elderly.
- Response to β-adrenoceptor agonists and antagonists may diminish in old age, possibly through reduced affinity for adrenoceptors, or smaller number of receptors.
- Baroreceptor sensitivity reduces, leading to greater potential for orthostatic hypotension with drugs that reduce blood pressure.

---

[26]For example, Insley J 1996 A Paediatric Vade-Mecum, 13th edn. Arnold, London.
[27]Neonatal and Paediatric Pharmacists Group, Royal College of Paediatrics and Child Health 2001 Pocket Medicines for Children. Royal College of Paediatrics and Child Health Publications, London.
[28]For practical advice, see World Health Organization 2005 Pocket Book of Hospital Care for Children. WHO, Geneva.

These pharmacokinetic and pharmacodynamic differences, together with broader issues particular to the elderly, influence the choice and use of drugs for this age group, as follows:

Rules of prescribing for the elderly[29]

1. Think about the necessity for drugs. Is the diagnosis correct and complete? Is the drug really necessary? Is there a better alternative?
2. Do not prescribe drugs that are not useful. Think carefully before giving an older adult a drug that may have major side-effects, and consider alternatives, including prescribing nothing.
3. Think about the dose. Is it appropriate to possible alterations in the patient's physiological state? Is it appropriate to the patient's renal and hepatic function at the time?
4. Think about drug formulation. Is a tablet the most appropriate form of drug, or would an injection, a suppository or a syrup be better? Is the drug suitably packaged for the elderly patient, bearing in mind any disabilities?
5. Assume any new symptoms may be due to drug side-effects or, more rarely, to drug withdrawal, unless shown to be otherwise. Rarely (if ever) treat a side-effect of one drug with another.
6. Take a careful drug history. Bear in mind the possibility of interaction with substances the patient may be taking without your knowledge, such as herbal or other non-prescribed remedies, old drugs taken from the medicine cabinet or drugs obtained from friends.
7. Use fixed combinations of drugs only when they are logical and well studied, and they either aid compliance or improve tolerance or efficacy. Few fixed combinations meet this standard.
8. When adding a new drug to the therapeutic regimen, see whether another can be withdrawn.
9. Attempt to check whether the patient's compliance is adequate, e.g. by counting remaining tablets. Has the patient (or relatives) been properly instructed?
10. Remember that stopping a drug is as important as starting it.

Older adults (80+ years) are particularly intolerant of neuroleptics (given for confusion) and of diuretics (given for ankle swelling that is postural and not due to heart failure), which cause adverse electrolyte changes. Both classes of drug may result in admission to hospital of semi-comatose 'senior citizens' who deserve better treatment from their juniors.

---

[29]By permission from Caird F I (ed) 1985 Drugs for the elderly. WHO (Europe), Copenhagen.

Pregnancy

As pregnancy evolves, profound changes occur in physiology, including fluid and tissue composition.

Absorption. Despite reduced gastrointestinal motility, there appears to be no major defect in drug absorption except that slow gastric emptying delays the appearance in the plasma of orally administered drugs, especially during labour. Absorption from an intramuscular site is likely to be efficient because vasodilatation increases tissue perfusion.

Distribution. Total body water increases by up to 8 L, creating a larger space within which water-soluble drugs may distribute. Plasma albumin (normal 33–55 g/L) declines by some 10 g/L from haemodilution. While this gives scope for increased free concentration of drugs that normally bind to albumin, unbound drug is also available to distribute, be metabolised and excreted. With phenytoin, for example, the free (and pharmacologically active) concentration does not alter, despite the dilutional fall in the total plasma concentration.

Thus therapeutic drug monitoring interpreted by concentrations appropriate for non-pregnant women may mislead. A useful general guide during pregnancy is to maintain concentrations at the lower end of the recommended range. Body fat increases by about 4 kg and provides a reservoir for lipid-soluble drugs.

Hepatic metabolism increases, although not blood flow to the liver. There is increased clearance of drugs such as phenytoin and theophylline, whose elimination depends on liver enzyme activity. Drugs that are so rapidly metabolised that elimination depends on delivery to the liver, i.e. on hepatic blood flow, have unaltered clearance, e.g. pethidine.

Elimination. Renal plasma flow almost doubles, and there is more rapid loss of renally excreted drugs, e.g. amoxicillin, the dose of which should be doubled for systemic infections (but not for urinary tract infections as penicillins are highly concentrated in the urine).

Placenta – see p. 83.

Disease

Pharmacokinetic changes

Absorption. Resection and reconstruction of the gut may lead to malabsorption, e.g. of iron, folic acid and fat-soluble vitamins after partial gastrectomy, and of vitamin B_{12} after ileal resection. Delayed gastric emptying and intestinal stasis during an attack of migraine interfere with drug absorption. Severe low-output cardiac failure or shock (with peripheral vasoconstriction) delays absorption from subcutaneous or intramuscular sites; reduced hepatic blood flow prolongs the presence in the plasma of drugs that are so rapidly extracted by the liver that removal depends on their rate of presentation to it, e.g. lidocaine.

Distribution. Hypoalbuminaemia from any cause, e.g. burns, malnutrition, sepsis, allows a higher proportion of free (unbound) drug in plasma. Although free drug is available for metabolism and excretion, there remains a risk of enhanced or adverse responses especially with initial doses of those that are highly protein bound, e.g. phenytoin.

Metabolism. Acute inflammatory disease of the liver (viral, alcoholic) and cirrhosis affect both the functioning of the hepatocytes and blood flow through the liver. Reduced extraction from the plasma of drugs that are normally highly cleared in first pass through the liver results in increased systemic availability of drugs such as metoprolol, labetalol and clomethiazole. Many other drugs exhibit prolonged $t_{1/2}$ and reduced clearance in patients with chronic liver disease, e.g. diazepam, tolbutamide, rifampicin (see p. 89). Thyroid disease has the expected effects, i.e. drug metabolism accelerates in hyperthyroidism and decelerates in hypothyroidism.

Elimination. Renal disease has profound effects on the elimination and hence duration of action of drugs eliminated by the kidney (see p. 490).

Pharmacodynamic changes

- *Asthmatic attacks* can be precipitated by β-adrenoceptor blockers.
- *Malfunctioning of the respiratory centre* (raised intracranial pressure, severe pulmonary insufficiency) causes patients to be intolerant of opioids, and indeed any sedative may precipitate respiratory failure.
- *Myocardial infarction* predisposes to cardiac arrhythmia with digitalis glycosides or sympathomimetics.
- *Myasthenia gravis* is aggravated by quinine and quinidine, and myasthenics are intolerant of competitive neuromuscular blocking agents and aminoglycoside antibiotics.

Food

- The presence of food in the stomach, especially if it is fatty, delays gastric emptying and the absorption of certain drugs, e.g. ampicillin and rifampicin. More specifically, calcium, for instance in milk, interferes with absorption of tetracyclines and iron (by chelation).
- Substituting protein for fat or carbohydrate in the diet is associated with an increase in drug oxidation rates. Some specific dietary factors induce drug metabolising enzymes, e.g. alcohol, charcoal grilled (broiled) beef, cabbage and Brussels sprouts.

Protein malnutrition causes changes that are likely to influence pharmacokinetics, e.g. loss of body-weight, reduced hepatic metabolising capacity, hypoproteinaemia.

Citrus flavinoids in grapefruit (but not orange) juice decrease hepatic metabolism and may lead to toxicity from amiodarone, terfenadine (cardiac arrhythmia), benzodiazepines (increased sedation), ciclosporin, felodipine (reduced blood pressure).

Drug interactions

When a drug is administered, a response occurs; if a second drug is given and the response to the first drug is altered, a drug–drug interaction is said to have occurred.

Dramatic *unintended* interactions excite most notice but they should not distract attention from the many *intended* interactions that are the basis of rational polypharmacy, e.g. multi-drug treatment of tuberculosis, naloxone for morphine overdose.

For completeness, alterations in drug action caused by diet (above) are termed *drug–food* interactions, and those by herbs *drug–herb* interactions.[30]

Clinical importance of drug interactions

The quantity of drugs listed in any national formulary provides ample scope for possible alteration in the disposition or effect of one drug by another drug. But, in practice, *clinically important adverse drug–drug interactions* become likely with:

- Drugs that have a steep dose–response curve and a small therapeutic index (see p. 79) because small quantitative changes at the target site, e.g. receptor or enzyme, lead to substantial changes in effect, e.g. digoxin or lithium.
- Drugs that are known enzyme inducers or inhibitors (see pp. 95–96).
- Drugs that exhibit saturable metabolism (zero-order kinetics), when small interference with kinetics may lead to large alteration of plasma concentration, e.g. phenytoin, theophylline.
- Drugs that are used long term, where precise plasma concentrations are required, e.g. oral contraceptives, anti-epilepsy drugs, cardiac anti-arrhythmia drugs, lithium.
- Severely ill patients, for they may be receiving several drugs; signs of iatrogenic disease may be difficult to

---

[30]Hu Z, Yang X, Ho P C et al 2005 Herb–drug interactions: a literature review. Drugs 65:1239–1282.

distinguish from those of existing disease, and the patient's condition may be such that he or she cannot tolerate further adversity.

- Patients who have significantly impaired liver or kidney function, for these are the principal organs that terminate drug action.
- The elderly, for they tend to have multiple pathology, and may receive several drugs concurrently (see p. 107).

Pharmacological basis of drug interactions

Listings of recognised or possible adverse drug–drug interactions are now readily available in national formularies, on compact disk or as part of standard prescribing software. We provide here an overview of the pharmacological basis for wanted and unwanted, expected and unexpected effects when drug combinations are used.

Drug interactions are of two principal kinds:

- *Pharmacodynamic interaction*: both drugs act on the target site of clinical effect, exerting synergism (below) or antagonism. The drugs may act on the same or different receptors or processes, mediating similar biological consequences. Examples include: alcohol + benzodiazepine (to produce enhanced sedation), atropine + β-adrenoceptor blocker (to indirectly reverse β-adrenoceptor blocker overdose).
- *Pharmacokinetic interaction*: the drugs interact remotely from the target site to alter plasma (and other tissue) concentrations so that the amount of the drug at the target site of clinical effect is altered, e.g. enzyme induction by rifampicin reduces the plasma concentration of warfarin; enzyme inhibition by ciprofloxacin increases the concentration of theophylline.

Interaction may result in antagonism or synergism.

Antagonism occurs when the action of one drug opposes that of another. The two drugs simply have opposite pharmacodynamic effects, e.g. histamine and adrenaline/ epinephrine on the bronchi exhibit physiological or functional antagonism; or they compete reversibly for the same drug receptor, e.g. flumazenil and benzodiazepines exhibit competitive antagonism.

Synergism[31] is of two sorts:

1. *Summation* or addition occurs when the effects of two drugs having the same action are additive, i.e. 2 + 2 = 4 (a β-adrenoceptor blocker plus a thiazide diuretic have an additive antihypertensive effect).

2. *Potentiation* (to make more powerful) occurs when one drug increases the action of another, i.e. 2 + 2 = 5. Sometimes the two drugs both have the action concerned (trimethoprim plus sulfonamide), and sometimes one drug lacks the action concerned (benserazide plus levodopa), i.e. 0 + 2 = 3.

Strictly, the term 'synergism' applies only to the second condition, but it is now commonly applied to both.

In broad terms, it is useful to distinguish the drug–drug interactions that occur:

- before drugs enter the body
- at important points during their disposition and metabolism
- at receptor sites.

Before administration. Intravenous fluids offer special scope for interactions (incompatibilities). Drugs commonly are weak organic acids or bases, produced as salts to improve their solubility. Plainly, the mixing of solutions of salts can result in instability, which may or may not be visible in the solution, i.e. precipitation. While specific sources of information are available in manufacturers' package inserts and formularies, issues of compatibility are complex and lie within the professional competence of the hospital pharmacy, which should prepare drug additions to infused solutions. In any situation involving unfamiliar drugs, their help and advice should be sought.

At the site of absorption. The complex environment of the gut provides opportunity for drugs to interfere with one another, both directly and indirectly, by altering gut physiology. Usually the result is to impair absorption.

By direct chemical interaction in the gut. Antacids that contain aluminium and magnesium form insoluble and non-absorbable complexes with tetracyclines, iron and prednisolone. Milk contains sufficient calcium to warrant its avoidance as a major article of diet with tetracyclines. Colestyramine interferes with the absorption of levothyroxine, digoxin and some acidic drugs, e.g. warfarin. Separating the dosing of interacting drugs by at least 2 h should largely avoid the problem.

By altering gut motility. Slowing of gastric emptying, e.g. opioid analgesics, tricyclic antidepressants (antimuscarinic effect), may delay and reduce the absorption of other drugs. Purgatives reduce the time spent in the small intestine and give less opportunity for the absorption of poorly soluble substances such as adrenal corticosteroids and digoxin.

By altering gut flora. Antimicrobials potentiate oral anticoagulants by reducing bacterial synthesis of vitamin K (usually only after antimicrobials are given orally in high dose, e.g. to treat *Helicobacter pylori*).

Interactions other than in the gut. Hyaluronidase promotes dissipation of a subcutaneous injection, and vasoconstrictors, e.g. adrenaline/epinephrine, felypressin,

---

[31]**Greek:** *syn* = **together;** *ergos* = **work.**

delay absorption of local anaesthetics, usefully to prolong local anaesthesia.

During distribution. Carrier-mediated transporters control processes such as bioavailability, passage into the CNS, hepatic uptake and entry into bile, and renal tubular excretion (see Index). Inhibitors and inducers of drug transporters can profoundly influence the disposition of drugs. The transporter MDR1 controls the entry of digoxin into cells; quinidine, verapamil and ciclosporin inhibit this transporter and increase the plasma concentration of digoxin (with potentially toxic effects). Probenecid inhibits the organic anion renal transporter, which decreases the renal clearance of penicillin (usefully prolonging its effect) but also that of methotrexate (with danger of toxicity). Elucidation of the location and function of transport systems will give the explanation for, and allow the prediction of, many more drug–drug interactions.

During metabolism. Enzyme induction (see p. 95) and, even more powerfully, enzyme inhibition (see p. 96) are important sources of drug–drug interaction.

At receptor sites. There are numerous examples. Beneficial interactions are sought in overdose, as with naloxone for morphine overdose (opioid receptor), atropine for anticholinesterase, i.e. insecticide poisoning (acetylcholine receptor), phentolamine for the monoamine oxidase inhibitor–sympathomimetic interaction (α-adrenoceptor). Unwanted interactions include loss of the antihypertensive effect of β-blockers with common cold remedies containing ephedrine, phenylpropanolamine or phenylephrine, usually taken unknown to the doctor (their α-adrenoceptor agonist action is unrestrained in the β-blocked patient).

Guide to further reading

Alfirevic, A., Pirmohamed, M., 2010. Drug-induced hypersensitivity reactions and pharmacogenomics: past, present and future. Pharmacogenomics 11, 497–499.

Callellini, M.D., Fiorelli, G., 2008. Glucose-6-phosphate dehydrogenase deficiency. Lancet 371, 64–72.

Daly, A.K., 2010. Genome-wide association studies in pharmacogenomics. Nat. Rev. Genet. 11, 241–246.

Davies, K., 2013. The era of genomic medicine. J. R. Coll. Physicians 13, 594–601.

Han, P.Y., Duffull, S.B., Kirkpatrick, C.M.J., Green, B., 2007. Dosing in obesity: a simple answer to a big problem. Clin. Pharmacol. Ther. 82, 505–508.

Ito, S., 2000. Drug therapy for breast-feeding women. N. Engl. J. Med. 343, 118–126.

Link, E., Parish, S., Armitage, J., et al., 2008. SLCO1B1 variants and statin-induced myopathy – a genome wide study. N. Engl. J. Med. 359, 789–799.

Maxwell, S.R., 2016. Rational prescribing: the principles of drug selection. J. R. Coll. Physicians 16, 459–464.

Peck, C.C., Cross, J.T., 2007. 'Getting the dose right': facts, a blueprint, and encouragements. Clin. Pharmacol. Ther. 82, 12–14.

Phillips, E.J., Mallal, S.A., 2010. Pharmacogenetics of drug hypersensitivity. Pharmacogenomics 11, 973–987.

Ping, P., 2009. Getting to the heart of proteomics. N. Engl. J. Med. 360, 532–534.

Pirmohamed, M., James, S., Meakin, S., et al., 2004. Adverse drug reactions as cause of admission to hospital: prospective analysis of 18820 patients. Br. Med. J. 329, 15–19.

Sim, S.C., Ingelman-Sundberg, M., 2011. Pharmacogenomic biomarkers: new tools in current and future drug therapy. Trends Pharmacol. Sci. 32, 72–81.

Strauss, S.E., 2001. Geriatric medicine. Br. Med. J. 322, 86–88.

Tucker, G.T., 2000. Chiral switches. Lancet 355, 1085–1087.

Wadelius, M., Pirmohamed, M., 2007. Pharmacogenetics of warfarin: current status and future challenges. Pharmacogenomics J. 7, 99–111.

Chapter | 9 |

Unwanted effects and adverse drug reactions

Mike Schachter

SYNOPSIS

As drugs are intended to relieve suffering, patients find it peculiarly offensive that they can also cause disease (especially if they are not forewarned). Therefore, it is important to know how much disease drugs do cause and why they cause it, so that preventive measures can be taken. The chapter will examine:

- **Background.**
- **Definitions.**
- **Attribution and degrees of certainty.**
- **Pharmacovigilance and pharmacoepidemiology.**
- **Sources of adverse drug reactions.**
- **Allergy in response to drugs.**
- **Effects of prolonged administration: chronic organ toxicity.**
- **Adverse effects on reproduction.**

Background

> *Cured yesterday of my disease, I died last night of my physician.*[1]

Nature is neutral, i.e. it has no 'intentions' towards humans, though it is often unfavourable to them. It is humans, in their desire to avoid suffering and death, who decide that some of the biological effects of drugs are desirable (therapeutic) and others undesirable (adverse). In addition to this arbitrary division, which has no fundamental biological basis, numerous non-drug factors promote or even cause unwanted effects. Because of the variety of these factors, attempts to make a simple account of the unwanted effects of drugs must be imperfect.

There is general agreement that drugs prescribed for disease are themselves the cause of a serious amount of disease (adverse reactions), ranging from mere inconvenience to permanent disability and death.

It is not enough to measure the incidence of adverse reactions to drugs, their nature and their severity, although accurate data are obviously useful. It is necessary to take, or to try to take, into account which effects are avoidable (by skilled choice and use) and which unavoidable (inherent in drug or patient).

As there can be no hope of eliminating all adverse effects of drugs, it is necessary to evaluate patterns of adverse reaction against one another. One drug may frequently cause minor ill-effects but pose no threat to life, though patients do not like it and may take it irregularly, to their own long-term harm. Another drug may be pleasant to take, so that patients take it consistently, with benefit, but on rare occasions it may kill someone. It is not obvious which drug is to be preferred.

Some patients, e.g. those with a history of allergy or previous reactions to drugs, are up to four times more likely to have another adverse reaction, so that the incidence does not fall evenly. It is also useful to discover the causes of adverse reactions (e.g. individuals who lack certain enzymes), for use of such knowledge can render avoidable what are at present unavoidable reactions.

More skilful prescribing will reduce avoidable adverse effects and this means that doctors, among all the other claims on their time, must find time better to understand drugs, as well as understanding patients and their diseases.

---

[1]From: The remedy worse than the disease. Matthew Prior (1664–1721).

Definitions

Many unwanted effects of drugs are medically trivial and, in order to avoid inflating the figures of drug-induced disease, it is convenient to retain the widely used term *side-effects* for minor reactions that occur at normal therapeutic doses, and that are predictable and usually dose related.

The term *adverse drug reaction* (ADR) should be confined to harmful or seriously unpleasant effects occurring at doses intended for therapeutic (including prophylactic or diagnostic) effect and which call for reduction of dose or withdrawal of the drug and/or forecast hazard from future administration; it is effects of this order that are of importance in evaluating drug-induced disease in the community. The term adverse 'reaction' is almost synonymous with adverse 'effect', except that an 'effect' relates to the drug and a 'reaction' to the patient. Both terms should be distinguished from an adverse 'event', which is an adverse happening that occurs during exposure to a drug without any assumption being made about its cause (see Prescription event monitoring, p. 53).

Toxicity implies a direct action of the drug, often at high dose, damaging cells, e.g. liver damage from paracetamol overdose, eighth cranial nerve damage from gentamicin. All drugs, for practical purposes, are toxic in overdose[2] and overdose can be absolute or relative; in the latter case an ordinary dose may be administered but may be toxic due to an underlying abnormality in the patient, e.g. disease of the kidney. *Mutagenicity, carcinogenicity* and *teratogenicity* (see Index) are special cases of toxicity.

Secondary effects are the indirect consequences of a primary drug action. Examples are: vitamin deficiency or opportunistic infection in patients whose normal bowel flora has been altered by antimicrobials; diuretic-induced hypokalaemia causing digoxin toxicity.

Intolerance means a low threshold to the normal pharmacodynamic action of a drug. Individuals vary greatly in their susceptibility to drugs, those at one extreme of the normal distribution curve being intolerant of the drugs, those at the other, tolerant.

Idiosyncrasy (see also Pharmacogenomics, p. 103) implies an inherent qualitative abnormal reaction to a drug, usually due to genetic abnormality, e.g. porphyria.

[2]A principle appreciated by Paracelsus 500 years ago, who stated that 'All things are poisons and there is nothing that is harmless; the dose alone decides that something is no poison'. The physician, alchemist and philosopher is regarded as the founder of chemical therapeutics; he was the first to use carefully measured doses of mercury to treat syphilis.

Attribution and degrees of certainty

When an unexpected event, for which there is no obvious cause, occurs in a patient already taking a drug, the possibility that it is drug attributable must always be considered. Distinguishing between natural progression of a disease and drug-induced deterioration is particularly challenging, e.g. sodium in antacid formulations may aggravate cardiac failure, tricyclic antidepressants may provoke epileptic seizures, and aspirin may cause bronchospasm in some asthmatics.

The following elements are useful in attributing the cause of an adverse event to a drug:

1. The *time sequence* in relation to taking the drug. The majority of reactions develop soon after exposure. Anaphylactic reactions (within minutes or hours) and hypersensitivity reactions (within weeks) may readily suggest an association, but delayed effects such as carcinogenesis or tardive dyskinesia (after years or even decades) present more difficulty.
2. The effects of *withdrawing* or *reintroducing* the drug. Most reactions subside when the drug is discontinued, unless an autoimmune reaction is established, when effects persist. Planned re-exposing a patient to a drug is rarely indicated unless treatment with it is essential and there is no reliable alternative.
3. The relationship to what is *already known* about the drug. This of course invites questions about consistency with the established pharmacology and toxicology of the drug or related substances.

Degrees of conviction for attributing adverse reactions to drugs may be ascribed as[3]:

- *Definite*: time sequence from taking the drug is reasonable; event corresponds to what is known of the drug and is not explicable by concurrent disease or drugs; event ceases on stopping the drug; event returns on restarting the drug (rarely advisable).
- *Probable*: time sequence is reasonable; event corresponds to what is known of the drug; event ceases on stopping the drug; event not reasonably explained by patient's disease or other drugs.
- *Possible*: time sequence is reasonable; event corresponds to what is known of the drug; uncertain relationship to effect of stopping the drug; event could readily have been result of the patient's disease or other therapy.
- *Conditional*: time sequence is reasonable; event does not correspond to what is known of the drug; event

[3]Journal of the American Medical Association 1975 234:1236.

Table 9.1 Detecting rare adverse drug reactions

Expected incidence of adverse reaction	Required number of patients for event		
	1 event	2 events	3 events
1 in 100	300	480	650
1 in 200	600	960	1300
1 in 1000	3000	4800	6500
1 in 2000	6000	9600	13 000
1 in 10 000	30 000	48 000	65 000

(From: Dollery C D, Bankowski Z (eds) 1983 Safety requirements for the first use of new drugs and diagnostic agents in man. CIOMS (WHO), Geneva, with permission)

could not reasonably be explained by the patient's disease or other drugs.

• *Doubtful*: event not meeting the above criteria.

Caution. About 80% of well people not taking any drugs admit on questioning to symptoms (often several) such as are commonly experienced as lesser adverse reactions to drugs. Administration of a placebo intensifies (or diminishes) these symptoms. Thus, many (minor) symptoms may be wrongly attributed to drugs. Similarly, minor and possibly transient abnormalities in laboratory results, e.g. liver function tests, occur in apparently healthy people.

Practicalities of detecting rare adverse reactions

For reactions with no background incidence, the number of patients required to give a good (95%) chance of detecting the effect appears in Table 9.1. Assuming that three events are required before any regulatory or other action should be taken, it shows the large number of patients that must be monitored to detect even a relatively high-incidence adverse effect. The problem can be many orders of magnitude worse if the adverse reactions closely resemble spontaneous disease with a background incidence in the population.

Pharmacovigilance and pharmacoepidemiology

The principal methods of collecting data on ADRs (pharmacovigilance) are:

• *Experimental studies*, i.e. formal therapeutic trials of Phases 1–3. These provide reliable data on only the

commoner events as they involve relatively small numbers of patients (hundreds); they detect an incidence of up to about 1 in 200.

• *Observational studies*, where the drug is observed epidemiologically under conditions of normal use in the community, i.e. pharmacoepidemiology and pharmacovigilance. Techniques used for post-marketing (Phase 4) studies include the observational cohort study and the case–control study. The surveillance systems are described on pages 53–54.

Drug-induced illness

The discovery of drug-induced illness can be analysed as follows[4]:

• *A drug commonly induces an otherwise rare illness*: this effect is likely to be discovered by clinical observation in the licensing (pre-marketing) formal therapeutic trials and the drug will almost always be abandoned; but some patients are normally excluded from such trials, e.g. pregnant women, and detection will then occur later.

• *A drug rarely or uncommonly induces an otherwise common illness*: this effect is likely to remain undiscovered. Cardiovascular risk from coxibs (e.g. rofecoxib, Vioxx) approximates as an example, but the degree of increased risk did become apparent after meta-analysis of several clinical trials and observational studies.

• *A drug rarely induces an otherwise rare illness*: this effect is likely to remain undiscovered before the drug is released for general prescribing. The effect could be detected by informal clinical observation or during any special post-registration surveillance and confirmed by a case–control study (see p. 53); aplastic anaemia with chloramphenicol[5] and the oculomucocutaneous syndrome with practolol were uncovered in this way.

• *A drug commonly induces an otherwise common illness*: this effect will not be discovered by informal clinical observation. If very common, it may be discovered in formal therapeutic trials and in case–control studies, but if only moderately common it may require observational cohort studies, e.g. pro-arrhythmic effects of anti-arrhythmic drugs.

---

[4]After Jick H 1977 The discovery of drug-induced illness. New England Journal of Medicine 296:481–485.
[5]Scott J L, Finegold S M, Belkin G A, Lawrence J S 1965 A controlled double-blind study of the hematologic toxicity of chloramphenicol. New England Journal of Medicine 272:1137–1142.

- *Drug adverse effects and illness incidence in an intermediate range*: both case–control and cohort studies may be needed.

Some impression of the features of drug-induced illness can be gained from the following statistics:

- In a large UK study, the prevalence of ADRs as a cause of admission to hospital was 6.5%, with a median bed stay of 8 days (4% of hospital bed capacity); most reactions were definitely or possibly avoidable; the commonest drugs were: low-dose aspirin, diuretics, warfarin, non-steroidal anti-inflammatory drugs (other than aspirin); the commonest adverse reaction was gastrointestinal bleeding.[6]
- Overall incidence in hospital inpatients is 10–20%, with possible prolongation of hospital stay in 2–10% of patients in acute medical wards.
- ADRs cause 2–3% of consultations in general practice.
- A study of 661 ambulatory patients found that 25% experienced adverse events, of which 13% were serious and 11% were preventable.[7]
- Predisposing factors for ADRs are: age over 60 years or under 1 month, female sex, previous history of adverse reaction, hepatic or renal disease, number of medications taken.
- A review of records of coroner's inquests for a (UK) district with a population of 1.19 million during the period 1986–1991 found that, of 3277 inquests on deaths, 10 were due to errors of prescribing and 36 were caused by adverse drug reactions.[8] Nevertheless, 17 doctors in the UK were charged with manslaughter in the 1990s, compared with two in each of the preceding decades, a reflection of 'a greater readiness to call the police or to prosecute'.[9]

It is important to avoid alarmist or defeatist reactions. Many treatments are dangerous, e.g. surgery, electroshock, drugs, and it is irrational to accept the risks of surgery for biliary stones or hernia and to refuse to accept any risk at all from drugs for conditions of comparable severity.

Many patients whose death is deemed to be partly or wholly caused by drugs, are dangerously ill already; justifiable risks may be taken in the hope of helping them; ill-informed criticism in such cases can act against the interest of the sick. On the other hand, there is no doubt that some of these accidents are avoidable. This is often more obvious when reviewing the conduct of treatment after the event, i.e. with the benefit of hindsight.

Sir Anthony Carlisle,[10] in the first half of the 19th century, said that 'medicine is an art founded on conjecture and improved by murder'. Although medicine has advanced rapidly, there is still a ring of truth in that statement, as witness anyone who follows the introduction of new drugs and observes how, after the early enthusiasm, there follow reports of serious toxic effects, and withdrawal of the drug may then follow. The challenge is to find and avoid these, and, indeed, the present systems for detecting adverse reactions came into being largely in the wake of the thalidomide, practolol and benoxaprofen disasters (see p. 64); they are now an increasingly sophisticated and effective part of medicines development.

> It is an absolute obligation on doctors to use only drugs about which they have troubled to inform themselves.

Drugs and skilled tasks

Many medicines affect performance, and it is relevant to review here some examples with their mechanisms of action. As might be expected, centrally acting and psychotropic drugs are prominent, e.g. the sedative antidepressants, benzodiazepines, non-benzodiazepine and other hypnotics, and antipsychotics (the 'classical' type more so than the 'atypicals'; see p. 336). Many drugs possess anticholinergic activity either directly (atropine, oxybutynin) or indirectly (tricyclic antidepressants, antipsychotics), the central effects of which cause confusion and impaired ability to process information. The first-generation H_1-receptor antihistamines (chlorphenamine, diphenhydramine) are notably sedating and impair alertness and concentration, which are features the recipient may not recognise. Drugs may also affect performance through cerebral depression (anti-epileptics, opioids), hypoglycaemia (antidiabetics) and hypotension (antihypertensives). For alcohol and cannabis, see pp. 145 and 159.

Car driving is a complex multifunction task that includes: visual search and recognition, vigilance, information processing under variable demand, decision-making and risk-taking, and sensorimotor control. It is plain that prescribers have a major responsibility here, both to warn patients and, in the case of those who need to drive for their work, to choose medicines with a minimal liability to cause impairment.[11]

[6]Pirmohamed M, James S, Meakin S et al 2004 Adverse drug reactions as a cause of admission to hospital: prospective analysis of 18 820 patients. British Medical Journal 329:15–19.
[7]Gandhi T K, Weingart S N, Borus J et al 2003 Adverse events in ambulatory care. New England Journal of Medicine 348:1556–1564.
[8]Ferner R E, Whittington R M 1994 Coroner's cases of death due to errors in prescribing or giving medicines or to adverse drug reactions: Birmingham 1986–1991. Journal of the Royal Society of Medicine 87:145–148.
[9]Ferner R E 2000 Medication errors that have led to manslaughter charges. British Medical Journal 321:1212–1216.

[10]Noted for his advocacy of the use of 'the simple carpenter's saw' in surgery.
[11]Gull D G, Langford N J 2006 Drugs and driving. Adverse Drug Reactions Bulletin 238:911–914.

Patients who must drive when taking a drug of known risk, e.g. benzodiazepine, should be specially warned of times of peak impairment.[12]

A patient who has an accident and was not warned of drug hazard, whether orally or by labelling, may successfully sue the doctor. It is also essential that patients be advised of the additive effect of alcohol with prescribed medicines.

How the patient feels is not a reliable guide to recovery of skills, and drivers may be more than usually accident prone without any subjective feeling of sedation or dysphoria. The criteria for safety in aircrew are much more stringent than are those for car drivers.

Resumption of car driving or other skilled activity after anaesthesia is a special case, and an extremely variable one, but where a sedative, e.g. intravenous benzodiazepine, opioid or neuroleptic, or any general anaesthetic, has been used it seems reasonable not to drive for 24 h at least.

The emphasis on psychomotor and physical aspects (injury) should not distract from the possibility that those who live by their intellect and imagination (politicians and even journalists may be included here) may suffer cognitive disability from thoughtless prescribing.

Sources of adverse drug reactions

The reasons why patients experience ADRs are varied and numerous, but reflection on the following may help a prescriber to anticipate and avoid unwelcome events:

- *The patient may be predisposed to an ADR* by age, sex, genetic constitution, known tendency to allergy, disease of drug eliminating organs (see Ch. 8), or social habits, e.g. use of tobacco, alcohol, other recreational drugs (see Ch. 11).
- *The known nature of the drug may forewarn.* Some drugs, e.g. digoxin, have steep dose–response curves and small increments of dose are more likely to induce adverse or toxic reactions (see p. 94). The capacity of the body to eliminate certain drugs, e.g. phenytoin, may saturate within the therapeutic dose range so that standard increases cause a disproportionate rise in plasma concentration, risking toxic effects (see p. 373). Some drugs, e.g. antimicrobials and particularly penicillins, have a tendency to cause

allergy. Anticancer agents warrant special care as they are by their nature cytotoxic (see Ch. 31). Use of these and other drugs may raise longer-term issues of mutagenicity, carcinogenicity and teratogenicity. Ingredients of a formulation, rather than the active drug, may also cause adverse reactions. Examples include the high sodium content of some antacids, and colouring and flavouring agents. The latter are designated in the list of contents by E numbers; tartrazine (E102) may cause allergic reactions.

- *The prescriber* needs to be aware that adverse reactions may occur after a drug has been used for a long time, at a critical phase in pregnancy, is abruptly discontinued (see p. 101) or given with other drugs (see Drug interactions, Ch. 8).

Aspects of the above appear throughout the book as is indicated. Selected topics are:

Age

The very old and the very young are liable to be intolerant of many drugs, largely because the mechanisms for disposing of them in the body are less efficient. The young are not simply 'small adults' and 'respect for their pharmacokinetic variability should be added to the list of our senior citizens' rights'.[13] Multiple drug therapy is commonly found in the old, which further predisposes to adverse effects (see Prescribing for the elderly, p. 107).

Sex

Females are more likely to experience adverse reactions to certain drugs, e.g. mefloquine (neuropsychiatric effects).

Genetic constitution

Inherited factors that influence response to drugs appear in general under Pharmacogenomics (see p. 103). For convenience, we describe here the *porphyrias*,[14] a specific group of disorders for which careful prescribing in a subgroup, the acute porphyrias, is vital.

Healthy people need to produce *haem*, e.g. for erythrocytes and haem-dependent enzymes. Haem is synthesised by a sequence of enzymes and in nonerythroid cells (including the liver) the *rate* of the synthetic process is controlled by the first of these, D-aminolaevulinic acid (ALA) synthase, on which haem provides a negative feedback.

---

[12]Nordic countries require that medicines liable to impair ability to drive or to operate machinery be labelled with a red triangle on a white background. The scheme covers antidepressants, benzodiazepines, hypnotics, drugs for motion sickness and allergy, cerebral stimulants, antiepileptics and antihypertensive agents. In the UK there are some standard labels that pharmacists are recommended to apply, e.g. 'Warning. May cause drowsiness. If affected do not drive or operate machinery. Avoid alcoholic drink'.

[13]Fogel B S 1983 New England Journal of Medicine 308:1600.
[14]The view that King George III suffered from acute porphyria is widely expressed but erroneous: his illness was probably bipolar disorder (Peters T 2011 King George III, bipolar disorder, porphyria and lessons for historians. Clinical Medicine 11:261–264).

The *porphyrias* comprise a number of rare, genetically determined, single-enzyme defects in haem biosynthesis and give rise to two main clinical manifestations: acute neurovisceral attacks and/or skin lesions. *Non-acute porphyrias* (porphyria cutanea tarda, erythropoietic protoporphyria and congenital erythropoietic porphyria) present with cutaneous photosensitivity that results from the overproduction of porphyrins, which are photosensitising. In porphyria cutanea tarda, a mainly acquired disorder of hepatic enzyme function, one of the main provoking agents is alcohol (and prescribed oestrogens in women).

The *acute hepatic porphyrias* (acute intermittent porphyria, variegate porphyria and hereditary co-proporphyria) are characterised by severe attacks of neurovisceral dysfunction precipitated principally by a wide variety of drugs (also by alcohol, fasting and infection). Clinical effects arise from the accumulation of the precursors of haem synthesis, D-ALA, porphobilinogen, though the exact mechanism remains obscure.

The exact *precipitating mechanisms* are uncertain. Induction of the haem-containing hepatic oxidising enzymes of the cytochrome P450 group causes an increased demand for haem. Therefore drugs that induce these enzymes would be expected to precipitate acute attacks of porphyria, and they do so: tobacco smoking and alcohol excess may also act via this mechanism. Apparently unexplained attacks of porphyria should be an indication for close enquiry into all possible chemical intake, including recreational substances such as marijuana, cocaine, amfetamines and ecstasy. Patients must be educated to understand their condition, to possess a list of safe and unsafe drugs, and to protect themselves from themselves and from others, including, especially, prescribing doctors.

Great care in prescribing for these patients is required if serious illness is to be avoided and it is therefore essential that patients and their clinicians have access to information concerning the safe use of prescription medication. Drug lists should be reviewed regularly, and a recent initiative in Europe has made a consensus-based list of safe drugs (available at http://www.porphyria-europe.org) as well as details of common prescribing problems and a link to a searchable drug safety database (http://www.drugs-porphyria.org).

If no recognised safe option is available, use of a drug about which there is uncertainty may be justified. Dr M. Badminton[15] writes: 'Essential treatment should never be withheld, especially for a condition that is serious or life threatening. The clinician should assess the severity of the condition and the activity of the porphyria and make a risk versus benefit assessment.' In these circumstances the clinician may wish to contact an expert centre for advice (see the list at http://www.porphyria-europe.com), which is likely to recommend that the patient be monitored as follows:

1. Measure porphyrin and porphobilinogen before starting treatment.
2. Repeat the measurement at regular intervals or if the patient has symptoms in keeping with an acute attack. If there is an increase in the precursor levels, stop the treatment and consider giving haem arginate for acute attack (see below).

In treatment of the acute attack the rationale is to use means of reducing D-ALA synthase activity. *Haem arginate* (human haematin) infusion, by replenishing haem and so removing the stimulus to D-ALA synthase, is effective if given early, and may prevent chronic neuropathy. Additionally, attention to nutrition, particularly the supply of carbohydrate, relief of pain (with an opioid), and of hypertension and tachycardia (with a β-adrenoceptor blocker) are important. Hyponatraemia is a frequent complication, and plasma electrolytes should be monitored.

The environment and social habits

Drug metabolism may be increased by hepatic enzyme induction from insecticide accumulation, e.g. dicophane (DDT), and from alcohol use and the tobacco habit, e.g. smokers require a higher dose of theophylline. Antimicrobials used in feeds of animals for human consumption have given rise to concern in relation to the spread of resistant bacteria that may affect man. Penicillin in the air of hospitals or in milk (see below) may cause allergy.

Allergy in response to drugs

Allergic reactions to drugs are the result of the interaction of drug or metabolite (or a non-drug element in the formulation) with patient and disease, and subsequent re-exposure.

Lack of previous exposure is not the same as lack of history of previous exposure, and 'first dose reactions' are among the most dramatic. Exposure is not necessarily medical, e.g. penicillins may occur in dairy products following treatment of mastitis in cows (despite laws to prevent this), and penicillin antibodies are commonly present in those who deny ever having received the drug. Immune responses to drugs may be harmful in varying degrees (allergy) or harmless; the fact that antibodies are produced does not mean a patient will necessarily respond to re-exposure with clinical manifestations; most of the UK population has antibodies to penicillins but, fortunately, comparatively few react clinically to penicillin administration.

---

[15]Department of Medical Biochemistry, University Hospital of Wales, Cardiff, UK. We are grateful to Dr Badminton for contributing the section on porphyria.

While macromolecules (proteins, peptides, dextran polysaccharides) can act as complete antigens, most drugs are simple chemicals (mol. wt. less than 1000) and act as incomplete antigens or haptens, which become complete antigens in combination with a body protein.

The chief target organs of drug allergy are the skin, respiratory tract, gastrointestinal tract, blood and blood vessels.

Allergic reactions in general may be classified according to four types of hypersensitivity, and drugs can elicit reactions of all types.

Type I reactions: immediate or anaphylactic type. The drug causes formation of tissue-sensitising immunoglobulin (Ig) E antibodies that are fixed to mast cells or leucocytes. On subsequent administration the allergen (conjugate of drug or metabolite with tissue protein) reacts with these antibodies, activating but not damaging the cell to which they are fixed and causing release of pharmacologically active substances, e.g. histamine, leukotrienes, prostaglandins, platelet activating factor, and causing effects such as urticaria, anaphylactic shock and asthma. Allergy develops within minutes and lasts for 1–2 h: it may of course be fatal.

Type II reactions: antibody-dependent cytotoxic type. The drug or metabolite combines with a protein in the body so that the body no longer recognises the protein as self, treats it as a foreign protein and forms antibodies (IgG, IgM) that combine with the antigen and activate complement which damages cells, e.g. penicillin- or methyldopa-induced haemolytic anaemia.

Type III reactions: immune complex-mediated type. Antigen and antibody form large complexes and activate complement. Small blood vessels are damaged or blocked. Leucocytes attracted to the site of reaction engulf the immune complexes and release pharmacologically active substances (including lysosomal enzymes), starting an inflammatory process.

These reactions include serum sickness, glomerulonephritis, vasculitis and pulmonary disease.

Type IV reactions: lymphocyte-mediated type. Antigen-specific receptors develop on T lymphocytes. Subsequent administration leads to a local or tissue allergic reaction, e.g. contact dermatitis.

Cross-allergy within a group of drugs is usual, e.g. the penicillins. (The extent of cross-reaction with cephalosporins is highly controversial.) When allergy to a particular drug is established, select a substitute from a chemically different group. Patients with allergic diseases (atopy), e.g. eczema, are more likely to develop allergy to drugs.

The distinctive features of allergic reactions are[16]:

- Lack of correlation with known pharmacological properties of the drug.
- Lack of linear relation with drug dose (very small doses may cause very severe effects).
- Rashes, angioedema, serum sickness syndrome, anaphylaxis or asthma; characteristics of classic protein allergy.
- Requirement of an induction period on primary exposure, but not on re-exposure.
- Disappearance on cessation of administration and reappearance on re-exposure to a small dose.
- Occurrence in a minority of patients receiving the drug.
- Possible response to desensitisation.

Principal clinical manifestations and treatment

1. Urticarial rashes and angioedema (types I, III). These are probably the commonest type of drug allergy. Reactions may be generalised, but frequently are worst in and around the external area of administration of the drug. The eyelids, lips and face are usually most affected and itching is usual; oedema of the larynx is rare but may be fatal. They respond to adrenaline/epinephrine, ephedrine, H_1-receptor antihistamine and adrenal steroid (see below).

2a. Non-urticarial rashes (types I, II, IV). These occur in great variety; frequently they are weeping exudative lesions. It is often difficult to be sure when a rash is due to a drug. Apart from stopping the drug, treatment is non-specific; in severe cases an adrenal steroid should be used. Skin sensitisation to antimicrobials may be very troublesome, especially among those who handle them (see Ch. 17 for more detail).

2b. Diseases of the lymphoid system. Infectious mononucleosis (and lymphoma, leukaemia) is associated with an increased incidence (> 40%) of a characteristic maculopapular, sometimes purpuric, rash which is probably allergic, when an aminopenicillin (ampicillin, amoxicillin) is taken; patients may not be allergic to other penicillins. Erythromycin may cause a similar reaction.

3. Anaphylactic shock (type I) occurs with penicillin, anaesthetics (intravenous), iodine-containing radio-contrast media and a huge variety of other drugs. A severe fall in blood pressure occurs, with bronchoconstriction, angioedema (including larynx) and sometimes death due to loss of fluid from the intravascular compartment and respiratory obstruction. Anaphylactic shock usually occurs suddenly, in less than an hour after the drug, but within minutes if it has been given intravenously.

---

[16]Assem E-S K 1998 Drug allergy and tests for its detection. In: Davies D M (ed) Davies's textbook of adverse drug reactions. Chapman and Hall, London, p. 790.

Treatment is urgent. The following account combines advice from the UK Resuscitation Council with comment on the action of the drugs used. Advice on the management of anaphylactic shock is altered periodically and the reader should check the relevant website (http://www.resus.org.uk) for the latest information.

- In adults, 500 µg of *adrenaline/epinephrine* injection (0.5 mL of the 1 in 1000 solution) should be given intramuscularly to raise the blood pressure and dilate the bronchi (vasoconstriction renders the subcutaneous route less effective). If there is no clinical improvement, further intramuscular injections of adrenaline/epinephrine 500 µg should be given at 5-min intervals according to blood pressure, pulse and respiration. (See website for doses in those <12 years.)
- If shock is profound, cardiopulmonary resuscitation/advanced life support are necessary. Consider also giving adrenaline/epinephrine 1: 10 000 by slow intravenous infusion, at a rate of 100 µg/min (1 mL/min of the dilute 1 in 10 000 solution over 5 min), preferably with continuous ECG monitoring, stopping when a response has been obtained. This procedure is hazardous and should be undertaken only by an experienced practitioner who can obtain immediate intravenous access and where other resuscitation facilities are available.
- The adrenaline/epinephrine should be accompanied by an H_1-receptor antihistamine, e.g. *chlorphenamine* 10–20 mg intramuscularly or by slow intravenous injection, and by *hydrocortisone* 200–500 mg intramuscularly or by slow intravenous injection. The adrenal steroid acts by reducing vascular permeability and by suppressing further response to the antigen–antibody reaction. Benefit from an adrenal steroid is not immediate; it is unlikely to begin for 30 min and takes hours to reach its maximum.
- In severe anaphylaxis, hypotension is due to vasodilatation and loss of circulating volume through leaky capillaries. Thus, when there is no response to drug treatment, 1–2 L of plasma substitute should be infused rapidly. Crystalloid may be safer than colloid, which causes more allergic reactions.
- Where bronchospasm is severe and does not respond rapidly to other treatment, a β_2-adrenoceptor agonist is a useful adjunctive measure. Noradrenaline/norepinephrine lacks any useful bronchodilator action (β effect) (see Adrenaline, Ch. 24).
- Where susceptibility to anaphylaxis is known, e.g. in patients with allergy to bee or wasp stings, preventive self-management is feasible. The patient is taught to administer adrenaline/epinephrine intramuscularly from a pre-filled syringe (EpiPen Auto-injector, delivering adrenaline/epinephrine 300 µg per dose).
- Half of the above doses of adrenaline/epinephrine may be safer for patients who are receiving amitriptyline or imipramine (increased effect; see p. 332).

Any hospital ward or other place where anaphylaxis may be anticipated should have all the drugs and equipment necessary to deal with it in one convenient kit, for when they are needed there is little time to think and none to run about from place to place (see also Pseudo-allergic reactions, p. 121).

4a. Pulmonary reactions: asthma (type I). Aspirin and other non-steroidal anti-inflammatory drugs may cause bronchoconstriction, and not only in asthmatic patients. Abnormal levels of leukotrienes synthesis following blockade of cyclo-oxygenase may be causal; this is a *pseudo-allergic reaction* (see below). Another such reaction is the well-known occurrence of cough due to angiotensin-converting enzyme inhibitors: in this case, pro-inflammatory peptides such as bradykinin accumulate and trigger cough.

4b. Other types of pulmonary reaction (type III) include syndromes resembling acute and chronic lung infections, pneumonitis, fibrosis and eosinophilia.

5. The serum sickness syndrome (type III). This occurs about 1–3 weeks after administration. Treatment is by an adrenal steroid, and as above if there is urticaria.

6. Blood disorders[17]

6a. Thrombocytopenia (type II, but also pseudo-allergic) may occur after exposure to any of a large number of drugs, including: gold, quinine, quinidine, rifampicin, heparin, thionamide derivatives, thiazide diuretics, sulphonamides, oestrogens, indometacin. Adrenal steroid may help.

6b. Granulocytopenia (type II, but also pseudo-allergic), sometimes leading to agranulocytosis, is a very serious reaction which may occur with many drugs, e.g. clozapine, carbamazepine, carbimazole, chloramphenicol, sulphonamides (including diuretic and hypoglycaemic derivatives), colchicine.

The value of precautionary leucocyte counts for drugs having special risk remains uncertain.[18] Weekly counts may

---

[17]Where cells are being destroyed in the periphery and production is normal, transfusion is useless or nearly so, as the transfused cells will be destroyed, though in an emergency even a short cell life (platelets, erythrocytes) may tip the balance usefully. Where the bone marrow is depressed, transfusion is useful and the transfused cells will survive normally.
[18]In contrast to the case of a drug causing bone marrow depression as a pharmacodynamic dose-related effect, when blood counts are part of the essential routine monitoring of therapy, e.g. cytotoxics.

detect presymptomatic granulocytopenia from antithyroid drugs, but onset can be sudden and an alternative view is to monitor only with drugs having special risk, e.g. clozapine, where it is mandatory. The chief clinical manifestation of agranulocytosis is sore throat or mouth ulcers, and patients should be warned to report such events immediately and to stop taking the drug, but they should not be frightened into non-compliance with essential therapy. Treatment of the agranulocytosis involves both stopping the drug responsible and giving a bactericidal drug, e.g. a penicillin, to prevent or treat infection.

6c. **Aplastic anaemia (type II, but not always allergic).** Causal agents include chloramphenicol, sulphonamides and derivatives (diuretics, antidiabetics), gold, penicillamine, allopurinol, felbamate, phenothiazines and some insecticides, e.g. dicophane (DDT). In the case of chloramphenicol, bone marrow depression is a normal pharmacodynamic effect, although aplastic anaemia may also be due to idiosyncrasy or allergy.

Death occurs in about 50% of cases, and treatment is as for agranulocytosis, with, obviously, blood transfusion.

6d. **Haemolysis of all kinds** is included here for convenience. There are three principal categories:

- *Allergy (type II)* occurs with penicillins, methyldopa, levodopa, quinine, quinidine, sulfasalazine and organic antimony. In some of these cases a drug–protein–antigen/antibody interaction may involve erythrocytes only casually, i.e. a true 'innocent bystander' phenomenon.
- *Dose-related pharmacodynamic action on normal cells,* e.g. lead, benzene, phenylhydrazine, chlorates (weed-killer), methyl chloride (refrigerant), some snake venoms.
- *Idiosyncrasy* (see Pharmacogenetics). Precipitation of a haemolytic crisis may also occur with the above drugs in the rare genetic haemoglobinopathies. Treatment is to withdraw the drug, and an adrenal steroid is useful in severe cases if the mechanism is immunological. Blood transfusion may be needed.

7. **Fever** is common; a mechanism is the release of interleukin-1 by leucocytes into the circulation; this acts on receptors in the hypothalamic thermoregulatory centre, releasing prostaglandin E_1.

8. **Collagen diseases (type II)** and syndromes resembling them. Systemic lupus erythematosus is sometimes caused by drugs, e.g. hydralazine, procainamide, isoniazid, sulphonamides. Adrenal steroid is useful.

9. **Hepatitis and cholestatic jaundice** are sometimes allergic (see Drugs and the liver, Ch. 34). Adrenal steroid may be useful.

10. **Nephropathy** of various kinds (types II, III) occurs, as does damage to other organs, e.g. myocarditis. Adrenal steroid may be useful.

Diagnosis of drug allergy

This still depends largely on clinical criteria, history, type of reaction, response to withdrawal and systemic re-challenge (if thought safe to do so).

Simple patch skin testing is naturally most useful in diagnosing contact dermatitis, but it is unreliable for other allergies. Skin prick tests are helpful in specialist hands for diagnosing IgE-dependent drug reactions, notably due to penicillin, cephalosporins, muscle relaxants, thiopental, streptokinase, cisplatin, insulin and latex. They can cause anaphylactic shock. False-positive results occur.

Development of reliable in vitro predictive tests, e.g. employing serum or lymphocytes, is a matter of considerable importance, not merely to remove hazard but also to avoid depriving patients of a drug that may be useful. Detection of drug-specific circulating IgE antibodies by the radioallergosorbent test (RAST) is best developed for many drugs and other allergens.

Drug allergy, once it has occurred, is not necessarily permanent, e.g. less than 50% of patients giving a history of allergy to penicillin have a reaction if it is given again, but re-challenging is best avoided if possible!

Desensitisation

Once patients become allergic to a drug, it is better that they should never again receive it. Desensitisation may be considered (in hospital) where a patient has suffered an IgE-mediated reaction to penicillin and requires the drug for serious infection, e.g. meningitis or endocarditis. Such people can be desensitised by giving very small amounts of allergen, which are then gradually increased (usually every few hours) until a normal dose is tolerated.

The procedure may necessitate cover with a corticosteroid and a β-adrenoceptor agonist (both of which inhibit mediator synthesis and release), and an H_1-receptor antihistamine may be added if an adverse reaction occurs. A full kit for treating anaphylactic shock should be at hand. Desensitisation may also be carried out for other antimicrobials, e.g. antituberculous drugs.

The mechanism underlying desensitisation may involve the production by the patient of blocking antibodies that compete successfully for the allergen but whose combination with it is innocuous; or the threshold of cells to the triggering antibodies may be raised. Sometimes allergy is to an ingredient of the preparation other than the essential drug, and merely changing the preparation is sufficient. Impurities are sometimes responsible, and purified penicillins and insulins reduce the incidence of reactions.

Prevention of allergic reactions

Prevention is important because these reactions are unpleasant and may be fatal; it provides good reason for taking a drug history. Patients should always be told if there is reason to believe they are allergic to a drug.

When looking for an alternative drug to avoid an adverse reaction, it is important not to select one from the same chemical group, as may inadvertently occur because the proprietary name gives no indication of the nature of the drug. This is another good reason for using the non-proprietary (generic) names as a matter of course.

> If a patient claims to be allergic to a drug then that drug should not be given without careful enquiry that may include testing (above). **Neglect of this has caused death.**

Pseudo-allergic reactions

These are effects that mimic allergic reactions but have no immunological basis and are largely genetically determined. They are due to release of endogenous, biologically active substances, e.g. histamine and leukotrienes, by the drug. A variety of mechanisms is probably involved, direct and indirect, including complement activation leading to formation of polypeptides that affect mast cells, as in true immunological reactions. Some drugs may produce both allergic and pseudo-allergic reactions.

Pseudo-allergic effects mimicking type I reactions (above) are called *anaphylactoid*; they occur with aspirin and other non-steroidal anti-inflammatory drugs and with *N*-acetylcysteine (indirect action as above) (see also Pulmonary reactions, above); corticotropin (direct histamine release); intravenous anaesthetics and a variety of other drugs given intravenously (morphine, tubocurarine, dextran, radiographic contrast media) and inhaled (cromoglicate). Severe cases are treated as for true allergic anaphylactic shock (above), from which, at the time, they are not distinguishable.

Type II reactions are mimicked by the haemolysis induced by drugs (some antimalarials, sulphonamides and oxidising agents) and food (broad beans) in subjects with inherited abnormalities of erythrocyte enzymes or haemoglobin.

Type III reactions are mimicked by nitrofurantoin (pneumonitis) and penicillamine (nephropathy). Lupus erythematosus due to drugs (procainamide, isoniazid, phenytoin) may be pseudo-allergic.

Miscellaneous adverse reactions

Transient reactions to intravenous injections are fairly common, resulting in hypotension, renal pain, fever or rigors, especially if the injection is very rapid.

Effects of prolonged administration: chronic organ toxicity

Although the majority of adverse events occur within days or weeks after a drug is administered, some reactions develop only after months or years of exposure. In general, pharmacovigilance programmes reveal such effects; once recognised, they demand careful monitoring during chronic drug therapy for their occurrence may carry serious consequences for the patient (and the non-vigilant doctor, medicolegally). Descriptions of such reactions appear with the accounts of relevant drugs; some examples are given.

Eye Toxic cataract can be due to chloroquine and related drugs, adrenal steroids (topical and systemic), phenothiazines and alkylating agents. Corneal opacities occur with phenothiazines and chloroquine. Retinal injury develops with thioridazine (particularly, of the antipsychotics), chloroquine and indometacin, and visual field defects with vigabatrin.

Nervous system. Tardive dyskinesias occur with neuroleptics; polyneuritis with metronidazole; optic neuritis with ethambutol.

Lung. Amiodarone may cause pulmonary fibrosis. Sulfasalazine is associated with fibrosing alveolitis.

Kidney. Gold salts caused nephropathy (rendering them obsolete for rheumatoid arthritis); see also analgesic nephropathy (p. 479).

Liver. Methotrexate may cause liver damage and hepatic fibrosis; amiodarone may induce steatohepatitis (fatty liver) (see also alcohol, p. 145).

Carcinogenesis: see also Preclinical testing (Ch. 3). Mechanisms of carcinogenesis are complex; prediction from animal tests is uncertain and causal attribution in humans has finally to be based on epidemiological studies. The principal mechanisms are:

- *Alteration of DNA* (genotoxicity, mutagenicity). Many chemicals or their metabolites act by causing mutations, activating oncogenes; those substances that are used as medicines include griseofulvin and alkylating cytotoxics. Leukaemias and lymphomas are the most common malignancies.

- *Immunosuppression.* Malignancies develop in immunosuppressed patients, e.g. after organ transplantation and cancer chemotherapy. There is a high incidence of lymphoid neoplasm. Chlorambucil, melphalan and thiotepa present particular high relative risks. The use of immunosuppression in, e.g., rheumatoid arthritis, also increases the incidence of neoplasms.

- *Hormonal.* Long-term use of oestrogen replacement in postmenopausal women induces endometrial cancer. Combined oestrogen/progestogen oral contraceptives may both suppress and enhance cancers (see Ch. 38). Diethylstilbestrol caused vaginal adenosis and cancer in the *offspring* of mothers who took it during pregnancy in the hope of preventing miscarriage. It was used for this purpose for decades after its introduction in the 1940s, on purely theoretical grounds. Controlled therapeutic trials were not done and there was no valid evidence of therapeutic efficacy. Male fetuses developed non-malignant genital abnormalities.[19]

Carcinogenesis due to medicines follows prolonged drug exposure,[20] i.e. months or years; the cancers develop most commonly over 3–5 years, but sometimes years after treatment has ceased. There is a higher incidence of secondary cancers in patients treated for a primary cancer.

Adverse effects on reproduction

The medical profession has a grave duty to refrain from all unessential prescribing for women of child-bearing potential of drugs with, say, less than 10–15 years of widespread use behind them. It is not sufficient safeguard merely to ask a woman if she is, or may be, pregnant, for it is also necessary to consider the possibility that a woman who is not pregnant at the time of prescribing may become so while taking the drug.

Testing of new drugs on animals for reproductive effects has been mandatory since the thalidomide disaster, even though the extrapolation of the findings to humans is uncertain (see Preclinical testing, Ch. 3). The placental transfer of drugs from the mother to the fetus is considered on page 86.

Drugs may act on the embryo and fetus:

- *Directly* (thalidomide, cytotoxic drugs, antithyroid drugs, aromatic retinoids, e.g. isotretinoin): any drug affecting cell division, enzymes, protein synthesis or DNA synthesis is a potential teratogen, e.g. many antimicrobials.

- *Indirectly*:
  - on the uterus (vasoconstrictors reduce blood supply and cause fetal anoxia, misoprostol causes uterine contraction leading to abortion)
  - on the mother's hormone balance.

Early pregnancy. During the first week after fertilisation, exposure to antimetabolites, misoprostol, ergot alkaloids or diethylstilbestrol can cause abortion, which may not be recognised as such. The most vulnerable period for major anatomical abnormality is that of organogenesis which occurs during weeks 2–8 of intrauterine life (4–10 weeks after the first day of the last menstruation). After the organs are formed, abnormalities are less anatomically dramatic. Thus, the activity of a teratogen (*teratos,* monster) is most devastating soon after implantation, at doses that may not harm the mother and at a time when she may not know she is pregnant.

Drugs known to be teratogenic include cytotoxics, warfarin, alcohol, lithium, methotrexate, phenytoin, sodium valproate, angiotensin-converting enzyme (ACE) inhibitors and isotretinoin. Selective interference can produce characteristic anatomical abnormalities; the phocomelia (flipper-like) limb defect was one factor that caused the effects of thalidomide to be recognised so readily (see p. 64).

Innumerable drugs have come under suspicion. Those subsequently found to be safe include diazepam (but see below), oral contraceptives, spermicides and salicylates. Naturally, the subject is a highly emotional one for prospective parents. A definitive list of unsafe drugs is not practicable. Much depends on the dose taken and at what stage of pregnancy. The best advice is to follow current literature.

Late pregnancy. Because the important organs are well formed, drugs will not cause the gross anatomical defects that can occur following exposure in early pregnancy. Administration of hormones, androgens or progestogens can cause fetal masculinisation; iodide and antithyroid drugs in high dose can cause fetal goitre, as can lithium; tetracyclines can interfere with tooth and bone development; ACE inhibitors are associated with renal tubular dysgenesis and a skull ossification defect. Tobacco smoking retards fetal growth; it does not cause anatomical abnormalities in humans as far as is known.

Inhibitors of prostaglandin synthesis (aspirin, indometacin) may delay onset of labour and, in the fetus, cause closure of the ductus arteriosus, patency of which is dependent on prostaglandins.

The suggestion that congenital cataract (due to denaturation of lens protein) might be due to drugs has some support in humans. Chloroquine and chlorpromazine are

---

[19]Herbst A L 1984 Diethylstilboestrol exposure – 1984 [effects of exposure during pregnancy on mother and daughters]. New England Journal of Medicine 311:1433–1435.
[20]Carcinogens that are effective as a single dose in animals are known, e.g. nitrosamines.

concentrated in the fetal eye. As both can cause retinopathy, it would seem wise to avoid them in pregnancy if possible.

For a discussion of anticoagulants in pregnancy, see Chapter 29.

Drugs given to the mother just prior to labour can cause postnatal effects. CNS depressants may persist in and affect the baby for days after birth; vasoconstrictors can cause fetal distress by reducing uterine blood supply; β-adrenoceptor blockers may impair fetal response to hypoxia; sulphonamides displace bilirubin from plasma protein (risk of kernicterus).

Babies born to mothers dependent on opioids may show a physical withdrawal syndrome.

Drugs given during labour. Any drug that acts to depress respiration in the mother can cause respiratory depression in the newborn; opioid analgesics are notorious in this respect, but there can also be difficulty with any sedatives and general anaesthetics; they may also cause fetal distress by reducing uterine blood flow, and prolong labour by depressing uterine muscle.

Diazepam (and other depressants) in high doses may cause hypotonia in the baby and possibly interfere with suckling. There remains the possibility of later behavioural effects due to impaired development of the central nervous system from psychotropic drugs use during pregnancy; such effects are known in animals.

Detection of teratogens. Anatomical abnormalities are the easiest to detect. Non-anatomical (functional) effects can also occur; they include effects on brain biochemistry that may have late behavioural consequences.

There is a substantial spontaneous background incidence of birth defect in the community (up to 2%), so the detection of a low-grade teratogen that increases the incidence of one of the commoner abnormalities presents an intimidating task. In addition, most teratogenic effects are probably multifactorial. In this emotionally charged area it is indeed hard for the public, and especially for parents of an affected child, to grasp that:

The concept of absolute safety of drugs needs to be demolished … In real life it can never be shown that a drug (or anything else) has no teratogenic activity at all, in the sense of never being a contributory factor in anybody under any circumstances. This concept can neither be tested nor proved.

Let us suppose for example, that some agent doubles the incidence of a condition that has natural incidence of 1 in 10 000 births. If the hypothesis is true, then studying 20 000 pregnant women who have taken the drug and 20 000 who have not may yield respectively two cases and one case of the abnormality. It does not take a statistician to realise that this signifies nothing,

and it may need ten times as many pregnant women (almost half a million) to produce a statistically significant result. This would involve such an extensive multicentre study that hundreds of doctors and hospitals have to participate. The participants then each tend to bend the protocol to fit in with their clinical customs and in the end it is difficult to assess the validity of the data.

Alternatively, a limited geographical basis may be used, with the trial going on for many years. During this time other things in the environment change, so again the results would not command our confidence. If it were to be suggested that there was something slightly teratogenic in milk, the hypothesis would be virtually untestable.

In practice we have to make up our minds which drugs may reasonably be given to pregnant women. Do we start from a position of presumed guilt or from one of presumed innocence? If the former course is chosen then we cannot give any drugs to pregnant women because we can never prove that they are completely free of teratogenic influence. It therefore seems that we must start from a position of presumed innocence and then take all possible steps to find out if the presumption is correct.

Finally, we must put things in perspective by considering the benefit/risk ratio. The problem of prescription in pregnancy cannot be considered from the point of view of only one side of the equation. Drugs are primarily designed to do good, and if a pregnant woman is ill it is in the best interests of her baby and herself that she gets better as quickly as possible. This often means giving her drugs. We can argue about the necessity of giving drugs to prevent vomiting, but there is no argument about the need for treatment of women with meningitis, septicaemia or HIV.

What we must try to avoid is medication by the media or prescription by politicians. A public scare about a well-tried drug will lead to wider use of less-tried alternatives. We do not want to be forced to practise the kind of defensive medicine that is primarily designed to avoid litigation.[21]

Male reproductive function

Impotence may occur with drugs affecting autonomic sympathetic function, e.g. many antihypertensives.

---

[21]*By permission from Smithells R W 1983 In: Hawkins D F (ed) Drugs and pregnancy. Churchill Livingstone, Edinburgh.*

Spermatogenesis is reduced by a number of drugs including sulfasalazine and mesalazine (reversible), cytotoxic anticancer drugs (reversible and irreversible) and nitrofurantoin. There has been a global decline in sperm concentration and an environmental cause, e.g. chemicals that possess oestrogenic activity, seems likely.

Causation of birth defects due to abnormal sperm remains uncertain.

Guide to further reading

Aronson, J.K., 2008. Routes of drug administration: uses and adverse effects. Part 1: intramuscular and subcutaneous injection. Drug Ther. Bull. 253, 971–974 (also Part 2: sublingual, buccal, rectal, and some other routes. 254, 975–978).

Aronson, J.K., Ferner, R.E., 2003. Joining the DoTS: new approach to classifying adverse drug reactions. Br. Med. J. 327, 1222–1225.

Baxter, K., Sharp, J.M., 2008. Adverse drug interactions. Drug Ther. Bull. 248, 952–954.

Eigenmann, P.A., Haenggeli, C.A., 2004. Food colourings and preservatives – allergy and hyperactivity. Lancet 364, 823–824.

Ferner, R.E., McDowell, S.E., 2006. Doctors charged with manslaughter in the course of medical practice, 1795–2005: a literature review. J. R. Soc. Med. 99, 309–314.

Gray, J., 2007. Why can't a woman be more like a man? Clin. Pharmacol. Ther. 82, 15–17.

Greenhalgh, T., Kostopoulou, O., Harries, C., 2004. Making decisions about benefits and harms of medicines. Br. Med. J. 329, 47–50.

Peters, T.J., Sarkany, R., 2005. Porphyria for the general physician. Clin. Med. (Northfield Il) 5, 275–281.

Strickler, B.H.C., Psaty, B.M., 2004. Detection, verification, and quantification of adverse drug reactions. Br. Med. J. 329, 44–47.

Trontell, A., 2004. Expecting the unexpected – drug safety, pharmacovigilance and the prepared mind. N. Engl. J. Med. 351, 1385–1387.

Woosley, R.L., 2004. Discovering adverse reactions: why does it take so long? Clin. Pharmacol. Ther. 76, 287–289.

Chapter | 10 |

Poisoning, overdose, antidotes

Stephen Haydock

SYNOPSIS

Deliberate overdose with drugs is a common clinical problem. Poisoning may also occur as a result of accidental ingestion, occupational exposure and in the context of recreational substance use. The effective management of poisoning is based upon the use of general supportive measures, reduction of drug absorption or increase in elimination and the use of specific pharmacological agents ('antidotes'). This chapter will examine:

- Background.
- Initial assessment.
- Resuscitation.
- Supportive treatment.
- Prevention of further absorption of the poison.
- Acceleration of elimination of the poison.
- Specific antidotes.
- Psychiatric and social assessment.
- Poisoning by non-drug chemicals: heavy metals, cyanide, methanol, ethylene glycol, hydrocarbons, volatile solvents, heavy metals, herbicides and pesticides.
- Poisoning by biological substances.

Introduction

The UK has one of the highest rates of deliberate self-harm in Europe but not of completed suicide. Deliberate self-harm involves intentional self-poisoning or self-injury irrespective of the intended purpose of that act. Self-poisoning is the commonest form of deliberate self-harm after self-mutilation. Poisoning, usually by medicines taken in overdose, is currently responsible for over 150 000 hospital attendances per annum in England and Wales (population 54 million). Prescribed drugs are involved in more than 75% of episodes, but teenagers tend to favour non-prescribed analgesics available by direct sale. In particular, over half of these involve ingestion of paracetamol, with the associated risk of serious toxicity. In order to address this problem, the pack size of paracetamol was reduced to 8 g for non-prescription purchase and 16 g for prescription in the UK in 1998. Recent evidence suggests that these changes have led to a significant reduction in deaths from paracetamol poisoning. The total number of deaths related to drug poisoning in England and Wales increased each year from 1993 to a peak in 1999, and then began to decline. Subsequent data have however shown a worrying upward trend, particularly in middle-aged men.

Most patients who die from deliberate ingestion of drugs do so before reaching medical assistance; overall only 11–28% of those who die following the deliberate ingestion of drugs reach hospital alive. The drugs most frequently implicated in hospital deaths of such individuals in the UK are paracetamol, tricyclic antidepressants and benzodiazepines. In India, deliberate self-harm is seen with similar prescribed agents, together with frequent deliberate self-harm with the antimalarial chloroquine and accidental or deliberate injury from pesticides such as the organophosphates or aluminium phosphide. In Sri Lanka, deliberate pesticide ingestion is also a serious public health issue.

Accidental self-poisoning, causing admission to hospital, occurs predominantly among children younger than 5 years of age, usually from medicines left within their reach or with commonly available domestic chemicals, e.g. bleach, detergents.

> Most patients who die from deliberate ingestion of drugs do so before reaching medical assistance. For those reaching hospital, the overall mortality is very low.

125

Initial assessment

It is important to obtain information on the poison taken. The key pieces of information are:

- the identity of the substance(s) taken.
- the dose(s).
- the time that has elapsed since ingestion.
- whether alcohol was also taken.
- whether the subject has vomited since ingestion.

Adults may be sufficiently conscious to give some indication of the poison or may have referred to it in a suicide note, or there may be other circumstantial evidence, e.g. knowledge of the prescribed drugs that the patient had access to, empty drug containers in pocket or at the scene. The ambulance crew attending to the patient at home may have very valuable information and may offer clues to the ingested drug as should any family or friends attending with the patient.

The response to a specific antidote may provide a diagnosis, e.g. dilatation of constricted pupils and increased respiratory rate after intravenous naloxone (opioid poisoning) or arousal from unconsciousness in response to intravenous flumazenil (benzodiazepine poisoning). Such agents should however be used with caution. Inappropriate use of naloxone can cause acute opiate withdrawal, and flumazenil may precipitate seizures.

Many substances used in accidental or self-poisoning produce recognisable symptoms and signs. Some arise from dysfunction of the central or autonomic nervous systems; other agents produce individual effects. They can be useful diagnostically and provide characteristic toxic syndromes or 'toxidromes' (Table 10.1). The utility of such toxidromes is limited by the overlap between drug classes and the common situation of ingestion of multiple drug classes.

In addition, sedatives, opioids and ethanol cause signs that may include respiratory depression, miosis, hyporeflexia, coma, hypotension and hypothermia. Other drugs and non-drug chemicals that produce characteristic effects include: salicylates, methanol and ethylene glycol, iron, selective serotonin reuptake inhibitors. Effects of overdose (and treatment) with other individual drugs or drug groups appear in the relevant accounts throughout the book.

Table 10.1 Characteristic drug 'toxidromes'

Toxidrome	Clinical features	Causative agents
Antimuscarinic	Tachycardia Dilated pupils Dry, flushed skin Urinary retention Decreased bowel sounds Mild increase in body temperature Confusion Cardiac arrhythmias Seizures	Antipsychotics Tricyclic antidepressants Antihistamines Antispasmodics Many plant toxins
Muscarinic	Salivation Lachrymation Abdominal cramps Urinary and faecal incontinence Vomiting Sweating Miosis Muscle fasciculation and weakness Bradycardia Pulmonary oedema Confusion CNS depression Seizures	Anticholinesterases Organophosphorus insecticides Carbamate insecticides Galantamine Donepezil
Sympatho-mimetic	Tachycardia Hypertension Hyperthermia Sweating Mydriasis Hyperreflexia Agitation Delusions Paranoia Seizures Cardiac arrhythmias	

Resuscitation

In concert with attempts to define the nature of the overdose, it is essential to carry out standard resuscitation methods. Maintenance of an adequate oxygen supply is the first priority, and the airway must be sucked clear of oropharyngeal secretions or regurgitated matter. Shock in acute poisoning is usually due to expansion of the venous capacitance bed, and placing the patient in the head-down position to encourage venous return to the heart, or a colloid plasma expander administered intravenously restores blood pressure. External cardiac compression may be necessary and should be continued until the cardiac output is self-sustaining, which may be a long time when the patient is hypothermic or poisoned with a cardiodepressant drug, e.g. tricyclic antidepressant, β-adrenoceptor blocker.

External cardiac compression may be required for prolonged periods of cardiac arrest, up to several hours. In young patients, the heart is anatomically and physiologically normal and will recover when the poison has been eliminated from the body.

Investigations may include arterial blood gas analysis and examination of plasma for specific substances that would require treatment with an antidote, e.g. with paracetamol, iron and digoxin.

Plasma concentration measurement may help to quantify the risk. Particular treatments such as haemodialysis or urine alkalinisation may be indicated for overdose with salicylate, lithium and some sedative drugs, e.g. trichloroethanol derivatives, phenobarbital.

Rapid biochemical drug screens of urine are widely available in hospital emergency departments (Box 10.1).

Supportive treatment

The majority of patients admitted to hospital will require only observation combined with medical and nursing supportive measures while they metabolise and eliminate the poison. Some will require specific measures to reduce absorption or to increase elimination. A few will require administration of a specific antidote. A very few will need intensive care facilities. In the event of serious overdose, always obtain the latest advice on management. In the UK, the National Poisons Information Service provides 24-hour specialist advice for discussion of complex cases via 0344 892 0111. The equivalent number in Ireland is (01) 809 2566. General advice is available on the Internet to registered users at http://www.toxbase.org.

The most efficient eliminating mechanisms are the patient's own physiological processes, which, given time, will inactivate and eliminate all the poison. Most patients recover from acute poisonings provided they are adequately oxygenated, hydrated and perfused.

Special problems introduced by poisoning are as follows:

- *Airway* maintenance is essential; some patients require a cuffed endotracheal tube but seldom for more than 24 h.
- *Ventilation*: a mixed respiratory and metabolic acidosis is common; the inspired air is supplemented with oxygen to correct the hypoxia. Mechanical ventilation is necessary if adequate oxygenation cannot be obtained or hypercapnia ensues.

Box 10.1 **Drugs that can be readily detected in urine in the emergency department**

Drugs detectable on rapid urine testing

Amfetamine
Methamfetamine
Cannabis
Methadone
Benzodiazepines
Barbiturates
Phencyclidine (angel dust)
Opiates

- *Hypotension*: this is common in poisoning and, in addition to the resuscitative measures indicated above, conventional inotropic support may be required.
- *In addition*: there is recent interest in the use of high-dose insulin infusions with euglycaemic clamping as a positive inotrope in the context of overdose with myocardial depressant agents. The very high insulin doses given (0.5–2 units/kg/h) have so far deterred physicians from the routine use of such therapy. There are, however, a number of case reports that support such an approach. Many of these are in the context of overdosage with non-dihydropyridine calcium channel blockers and beta (adrenoceptor) blockers that are often resistant to conventional inotropic agents. High-dose insulin therapy may therefore be appropriate in cases that fail to respond to conventional therapies.
- *Convulsions* should be treated if they are persistent or protracted. Intravenous benzodiazepine (diazepam or lorazepam) is the first choice.
- *Cardiac arrhythmia* frequently accompanies poisoning, e.g. with tricyclic antidepressants, theophylline, β-adrenoceptor blockers.
- *Acidosis, hypoxia and electrolyte disturbance* are often important contributory factors to cardiac rhythm disturbance, and it is preferable to observe the effect of correcting these before considering resort to an antiarrhythmic drug. If arrhythmia does lead to persistent peripheral circulatory failure, an appropriate drug may be cautiously justified, e.g. a β-adrenoceptor blocker for poisoning with a sympathomimetic drug.
- *Hypothermia* may occur if CNS depression impairs temperature regulation. A low-reading rectal thermometer is used to monitor core temperature, and the patient is nursed in a heat-retaining 'space blanket'.

- *Immobility* may lead to pressure lesions of peripheral nerves, cutaneous blisters, necrosis over bony prominences, and increased risk of thromboembolism that warrants prophylaxis.
- *Rhabdomyolysis* may result from prolonged pressure on muscles from agents that cause muscle spasm or convulsions (phencyclidine, theophylline); may be aggravated by hyperthermia due to muscle contraction, e.g. with MDMA ('ecstasy'). Aggressive volume repletion and correction of acid–base abnormality are needed; urine alkalinisation and/or diuretic therapy may be helpful in preventing acute tubular necrosis, but evidence is not conclusive.

Patients die from overdose:
- *Early* – from direct respiratory depression, fatal cardiac arrhythmias, fatal convulsions.
- *Delayed* – from organ damage consequent upon poorly managed cardiorespiratory support.
- *Late* – from delayed toxicity of the drug causing severe direct end organ damage, e.g. liver failure or from a subsequent fatal self-poisoning.

Preventing further absorption of the poison

From the environment

When a poison has been inhaled or absorbed through the skin, the patient should be taken from the toxic environment, the contaminated clothing removed and the skin cleansed.

From the alimentary tract ('gut decontamination')[1]

Gastric lavage should not be employed routinely, if ever, in the management of poisoned patients. Serious risks of the procedure include hypoxia, cardiac arrhythmias, laryngospasm, perforation of the GI tract or pharynx, fluid and electrolyte abnormalities and aspiration pneumonitis. Clinical studies show no beneficial effect. The procedure may be considered in very extraordinary circumstances for the hospitalised adult who is believed to have ingested a potentially life-threatening amount of a poison within the previous hour, and provided the airways are protected by a cuffed endotracheal tube. It is *contraindicated* for corrosive substances, hydrocarbons with high aspiration potential and where there is risk of haemorrhage from an underlying gastrointestinal condition.

Emesis using syrup of ipecacuanha is obsolete, as there is no clinical trial evidence that the procedure improves outcome.

Oral adsorbents. Activated charcoal (Carbomix) consists of a very fine black powder prepared from vegetable matter, e.g. wood pulp, coconut shell, which is 'activated' by an oxidising gas flow at high temperature to create a network of small (10–20 nm) pores with an enormous surface area in relation to weight (1000 m^2/g). This binds to, and thus inactivates, a wide variety of compounds in the gut. Indeed, activated charcoal comes nearest to fulfilling the long-sought notion of a 'universal antidote'.[2] Thus it is simpler to list the exceptions to its use, i.e. substances that are poorly adsorbed by charcoal:

- Metal salts (iron, lithium).
- Cyanide.
- Alcohols (ethanol, methanol, ethylene glycol).
- Petroleum distillates.
- Clofenotane (dicophane, DDT).
- Malathion.
- Strong acids and alkalis.
- Corrosive agents.

To be most effective, five to ten times as much charcoal as poison, weight for weight, is needed. In the adult, an initial dose of 50 g is usual, repeated if necessary. If the patient is vomiting, give the charcoal through a nasogastric tube. Unless a patient has an intact or protected airway, its administration is contraindicated.

Activated charcoal is most effective when given soon after ingestion of a potentially toxic amount of a poison and while a significant amount remains yet unabsorbed. Volunteer studies suggest that administration within 1 h prevents up to 40–50% of absorption. There are no satisfactorily designed clinical trials in patients to assess the benefit of single-dose activated charcoal. Benefit after 1 h cannot be excluded and may sometimes be justified. Charcoal in repeated doses accelerates the elimination of poison that has been absorbed (see later). Activated charcoal, although unpalatable, appears to be relatively safe, but constipation or mechanical bowel obstruction may follow repeated use. In the drowsy or

---

[1] Joint position statements and guidelines agreed by the American Academy of Clinical Toxicology and the European Association of Poison Centres and Clinical Toxicologists review the therapeutic usefulness of various procedures for gut decontamination. These appear in the *Journal of Toxicology, Clinical Toxicology* from 1997 onwards, the latest position statements being in 2004 and 2005.

[2] For centuries it was supposed not only that there could be, but that there actually was, a single antidote to all poisons. This was Theriaca Andromachi, a formulation of 72 (a magical number) ingredients among which particular importance was attached to the flesh of a snake (viper). The antidote was devised by Andromachus, whose son was physician to the Roman Emperor Nero (AD 37–68).

comatose patient, there is particular risk of aspiration into the lungs causing hypoxia through obstruction and arterio-venous shunting. Methionine, used orally for paracetamol poisoning, is absorbed by the charcoal.

Other oral adsorbents have specific uses. Fuller's earth (a natural form of aluminium silicate) binds and inactivates the herbicides paraquat (activated charcoal is superior) and diquat; colestyramine and colestipol will adsorb warfarin.

Whole-bowel irrigation[3] has no routine place in the management of the poisoned patient. While volunteer studies have shown marked reductions in the bioavailability of ingested drugs, there is no evidence of benefit from controlled clinical trials in patients. It should be used for the removal of sustained-release or enteric-coated formulations from patients who present more than 2 h after ingestion, e.g. iron, theophylline, aspirin. Evidence of benefit is conflicting. Activated charcoal in frequent (50 g) doses is generally preferred. Sustained-release formulations are common, and patients have died from failure to recognise the danger of continued release of drug from such products. Whole-bowel irrigation is also an option for the removal of ingested packets of illicit drugs. Contraindications include patients with bowel obstruction, perforation or ileus, with haemodynamic instability and with compromised unprotected airways.

Whole bowel irrigation demands special care in patients who are debilitated or who have significant concurrent medical conditions.

Cathartics have no routine role in gut decontamination, but a single dose of an osmotic agent (sorbitol, magnesium sulphate) may be justified on occasion.

Accelerating elimination of the poison

Techniques for eliminating absorbed poisons have a role that is limited, but important when applicable. Each method depends, directly or indirectly, on removing drug from the circulation, and successful use requires that:

* the poison should be present in high concentration in the plasma relative to that in the rest of the body, i.e. it should have a small volume of distribution.
* the poison should dissociate readily from any plasma protein binding sites.
* the effects of the poison should relate to its plasma concentration.

Methods used are:

---

[3]Irrigation with large volumes of a polyethylene glycol–electrolyte solution, e.g. Klean-Prep, by mouth causes minimal fluid and electrolyte disturbance (developed for preparation for colonoscopy). Magnesium sulphate may also be used.

Repeated doses of activated charcoal

Activated charcoal by mouth not only adsorbs ingested drug in the gut, preventing absorption into the body (see above), it also adsorbs drug that diffuses from the blood into the gut lumen when the concentration there is lower. As binding is irreversible, the concentration gradient is maintained and drug is continuously removed; this has been called 'intestinal dialysis'. Charcoal may also adsorb drugs that secrete into the bile, i.e. by interrupting an enterohepatic cycle. The procedure is effective for overdose of carbamazepine, dapsone, phenobarbital, quinine, salicylate and theophylline.

Repeated-dose activated charcoal is increasingly preferred to alkalinisation of urine (below) for phenobarbital and salicylate poisoning. In adults, activated charcoal 50 g is given initially, then 50 g every 4 h. Vomiting should be treated with an antiemetic drug because it reduces the efficacy of charcoal treatment. Where there is intolerance, the dose may be reduced and the frequency increased, e.g. 25 g every 2 h or 12.5 g every hour, but efficacy may be compromised.

Alteration of urine pH and diuresis

It is useful to alter the pH of the glomerular filtrate such that a drug that is a weak electrolyte will ionise, become less lipid soluble, remain in the renal tubular fluid, and leave the body in the urine (see p. 82).

Maintenance of a good urine flow (e.g. 100 mL/h) helps this process, but the alteration of tubular fluid pH is the important determinant. The practice of forcing diuresis with furosemide and large volumes of intravenous fluid does not add significantly to drug clearance but may cause fluid overload; it is obsolete.

The objective is to maintain a urine pH of 7.5–8.5 by an intravenous infusion of sodium bicarbonate. Available preparations of sodium bicarbonate vary between 1.2% and 8.4% (1 mL of the 8.4% preparation contains 1 mmol sodium bicarbonate), and the concentration given will depend on the patient's fluid needs.

Alkalinisation[4] may be used for: salicylate (>500 mg/L + metabolic acidosis, or in any case >750 mg/L); phenobarbital (75–150 mg/L); phenoxy herbicides, e.g. 2,4-D, mecoprop, dichlorprop; moderately severe salicylate poisoning that does not meet the criteria for haemodialysis.

Acidification may be considered for severe, acute poisoning with: amfetamine; dexfenfluramine; phencyclidine. The objective is to maintain a urine pH of 5.5–6.5 by giving an intravenous infusion of arginine hydrochloride (10 g) over 30 min, followed by ammonium chloride (4 g) every 2 h by mouth. It is very rarely indicated. Hypertension due to

---

[4]Proudfoot A T, Krenzelok E P, Vale J A 2004 Position paper on urine alkalinisation. Journal of Toxicology, Clinical Toxicology 42:1–26.

amfetamine-like drugs, for example, will respond to phenoxybenzamine (by α-adrenoceptor block).

Haemodialysis

The system requires a temporary extracorporeal circulation, e.g. from an artery to a vein in the arm. A semipermeable membrane separates blood from dialysis fluid; the poison passes passively from the blood, where it is present in high concentration, to enter the dialysis fluid, which is flowing and thus constantly replaced.

Haemodialysis significantly increases the elimination of: salicylate (>750 mg/L + renal failure, or in any case >900 mg/L); isopropanol (present in aftershave lotions and window-cleaning solutions); lithium; methanol; ethylene glycol; ethanol.

Haemofiltration

An extracorporeal circulation brings blood into contact with a highly permeable membrane. Water is lost by ultrafiltration (the rate being dependent on the hydrostatic pressure gradient across membrane) and solutes by convection; the main change in plasma concentrations results from replacement of ultrafiltrate with an appropriate solution.

Haemofiltration is effective for: phenobarbital (>100–150 mg/L, but repeat-dose activated charcoal by mouth appears to be as effective; see above) and other barbiturates; ethchlorvynol; glutethimide; meprobamate; methaqualone; theophylline; trichloroethanol derivatives.

Peritoneal dialysis

This involves instilling appropriate fluid into the peritoneal cavity. Poison in the blood diffuses down the concentration gradient into the dialysis fluid, which undergoes repeated drainage and replacement. The technique requires little equipment; it may be worth using for lithium and methanol poisoning. Its use is commonly confined to centres with specialist renal services.

Haemofiltration and peritoneal dialysis are more readily available but are less efficient (one-half to one-third) than haemodialysis.

> Haemodialysis is invasive, demands skill and experience on the part of the operator, and is costly in terms of staffing. It is reserved for cases of severe, prolonged or progressive clinical intoxication, when high plasma concentration indicates a dangerous degree of poisoning, and its effect constitutes a significant addition to natural methods of elimination.

Specific antidotes[5]

Specific antidotes reduce or abolish the effects of poisons through a variety of general mechanisms, as indicated in Table 10.2.

Table 10.3 illustrates these mechanisms with antidotes that are of therapeutic value.

Psychiatric and social assessment

Patients require a psychosocial assessment when they have recovered from the medical aspects of the overdose. The immediate risk and subsequent risk of suicide should be assessed. Do not dismiss even 'minor' cases of deliberate self-harm, as 20–25% of patients who die from deliberate self-harm will have presented to hospital with an episode of self-harm in the previous year. Interpersonal or social problems precipitate most cases of self-poisoning and require attention. Identify and treat any significant psychiatric illness. Consider the impact of any associated medical problems and their symptom control. Obtain information on associated alcohol and substance abuse. The detention of patients in order to treat the complications of self-poisoning when the patients seek to leave hospital is a complex one. Such decisions involve consideration of three important pieces of legislation, namely the Mental Health Act of 1983, the Human Rights Act of 1998 and the Mental Capacity Act of 2005. In UK hospitals, mental health assessments are usually performed prior to discharge by the hospital psychiatric liaison service. Most patients can be discharged without further psychiatric follow-up. Rarely, patients with a high suicide risk and/or an underlying severe psychiatric illness may require transfer to an inpatient psychiatric facility, either voluntarily or under the appropriate section of the 1983 Mental Health Act. More commonly, patients may benefit from community psychiatric support as outpatients. It is important to appreciate that a very significant number of patients who die from completed suicide will have previously attended hospital with apparently trivial self-harm.

[5]Mithridates the Great (?132 BC – 63 BC), king of Pontus (in Asia Minor), was noted for 'ambition, cruelty and artifice'. 'He murdered his own mother … and fortified his constitution by drinking antidotes' to the poisons with which his domestic enemies sought to kill him (Lemprière). When his son also sought to kill him, Mithridates was so disappointed that he compelled his wife to poison herself. He then tried to poison himself, but in vain; the frequent antidotes that he had taken in the early part of his life had so strengthened his constitution that he was immune. He was obliged to stab himself, but had to seek the help of a slave to complete his task. Modern physicians have to be content with less comprehensively effective antidotes, some of which are listed in Table 10.1.

Table 10.2 General mechanisms of the action of antidotes

Mechanism	Examples
Removal of circulating poison from plasma	• Chelating agents for heavy metal poisoning, e.g. desferrioxamine for iron poisoning • Chemical binding or precipitation, e.g. calcium gluconate for fluoride poisoning, binding to specific antibody, e.g. digoxin-specific antibody fragments in cardiac glycoside poisoning
Receptor agonism	• Direct agonism, e.g. isoprenaline in β-adrenoceptor antagonist poisoning • Indirect agonism, e.g. glucagon in β-adrenoceptor poisoning
Receptor antagonism	• Direct antagonism, e.g. atropine in organophosphate poisoning and many other examples
Replenish depleted natural 'protective' compound	• Replenish protective species, e.g. N-acetylcysteine in paracetamol poisoning • Bypass block in metabolism, e.g. folinic acid in methotrexate poisoning, vitamin K in warfarin poisoning
Prevent conversion to toxic metabolite	• Ethanol in methanol poisoning
Protective action on target enzyme	• Pralidoxime competitively reactivates cholinesterase

Poisoning by (non-drug) chemicals

Heavy metal poisoning and use of chelating agents

Acute or chronic exposure to heavy metals can harm the body.[6] Treatment is with chelating agents which incorporate the metal ions into an inner ring structure in the molecule (Greek: *chele*, claw) by means of structural groups called ligands (Latin: *ligare*, to bind). Effective agents form stable, biologically inert complexes that pass into the urine.

Dimercaprol (British Anti-Lewisite, BAL). Arsenic and other metal ions are toxic in low concentration because they combine with the SH-groups of essential enzymes, thus inactivating them. Dimercaprol provides SH-groups, which combine with the metal ions to form relatively harmless ring compounds that pass from the body, mainly in the urine. As dimercaprol itself is oxidised in the body and excreted renally, repeated administration is necessary to ensure that an excess is available to eliminate all of the metal.

Dimercaprol may be used in cases of poisoning by antimony, arsenic, bismuth, gold and mercury (inorganic, e.g. $HgCl_2$).

Adverse effects are common, particularly with larger doses, and include nausea, vomiting, lachrymation, salivation, paraesthesiae, muscular aches and pains, urticarial rashes, tachycardia and raised blood pressure. Gross overdosage may cause over-breathing, muscular tremors, convulsions and coma.

Unithiol (dimercaptopropanesulphonate, DMPS) effectively chelates lead and mercury; it is well tolerated.

Sodium calcium edetate is the calcium chelate of the disodium salt of ethylenediaminetetra-acetic acid (calcium EDTA). It is effective in acute lead poisoning because of its capacity to exchange calcium for lead: the kidney excretes the lead chelate, leaving behind a harmless amount of calcium. Dimercaprol may usefully be combined with sodium calcium edetate when lead poisoning is severe, e.g. with encephalopathy.

Adverse effects are fairly common, and include hypotension, lachrymation, nasal stuffiness, sneezing, muscle pains and possible nephrotoxicity.

Dicobalt edetate. Cobalt forms stable, non-toxic complexes with cyanide (see p. 133). It is toxic (especially if the wrong diagnosis is made and no cyanide is present), causing hypertension, tachycardia and chest pain. Cobalt poisoning is treated by giving sodium calcium edetate and intravenous glucose.

Penicillamine (dimethylcysteine) is a metabolite of penicillin that contains SH-groups; it may be used to chelate lead and copper (see Wilson's disease, p. 385). Its principal use is for rheumatoid arthritis (see Index).

Desferrioxamine (see Iron, p. 533).

Cyanide poisoning results in tissue anoxia by chelating the ferric part of the intracellular respiratory enzyme, cytochrome oxidase. It thus uncouples mitochondrial oxidative phosphorylation and inhibits cellular respiration in the presence of adequate oxygenation. Poisoning may occur as a result of: self-administration of hydrocyanic (prussic) acid; accidental exposure in industry; inhaling smoke from burning polyurethane foams in furniture; ingesting amygdalin which

---

[6]Sometimes in unexpected ways; an initiation custom in an artillery regiment involved pouring wine through the barrel of a gun after several shots had been fired. A healthy 19-year-old soldier drank 250 mL of the wine and within 15 min convulsed and became unconscious. His plasma, urine and the wine contained high concentrations of tungsten. He received haemodialysis and recovered. Investigation revealed that the gun barrels had recently been hardened by the addition of tungsten to the steel. Marquet P, François B, Vignon P, Lachâtre G 1996 A soldier who had seizures after drinking a quarter of a litre of wine. Lancet 348:1070.

Table 10.3 Specific antidotes useful in clinical practice

Some specific antidotes, indications and modes of action (see index for a fuller account of individual drugs)

Antidote	Indication	Mode of action
Acetylcysteine	Paracetamol, chloroform, carbon tetrachloride, radiocontrast nephropathy	Replenishes depleted glutathione stores
Atropine	Cholinesterase inhibitors, e.g. organophosphorus insecticides	Blocks muscarinic cholinoceptors
	β-Blocker poisoning	Vagal block accelerates heart rate
Benzatropine	Drug-induced movement disorders	Blocks muscarinic cholinoceptors
Calcium gluconate	Hydrofluoric acid, fluorides	Binds or precipitates fluoride ions
Desferrioxamine	Iron	Chelates ferrous ions
Dicobalt edetate	Cyanide and derivatives, e.g. acrylonitrile	Chelates to form non-toxic cobalti- and cobalto-cyanides
Digoxin-specific antibody fragments (FAB)	Digitalis glycosides	Binds free glycoside in plasma, complex excreted in urine
Dimercaprol (BAL)	Arsenic, copper, gold, lead, inorganic mercury	Chelates metal ions
Ethanol (or fomepizole)	Ethylene glycol, methanol	Competes for alcohol and acetaldehyde dehydrogenases, preventing formation of toxic metabolites
Flumazenil	Benzodiazepines	Competes for benzodiazepine receptors
Folinic acid	Folic acid antagonists, e.g. methotrexate, trimethoprim	Bypasses block in folate metabolism
Glucagon	β-Adrenoceptor antagonists	Bypasses blockade of the β-adrenoceptor; stimulates cyclic AMP formation with positive cardiac inotropic effect
Isoprenaline	β-Adrenoceptor antagonists	Competes for and activates β-adrenoceptors
Methionine	Paracetamol	Replenishes depleted glutathione stores
Naloxone	Opioids	Competes for opioid receptors
Neostigmine	Antimuscarinic drugs	Inhibits acetylcholinesterase, causing acetylcholine to accumulate at cholinoceptors
Oxygen	Carbon monoxide	Competitively displaces carbon monoxide from binding sites on haemoglobin
Penicillamine	Copper, gold, lead, elemental mercury (vapour), zinc	Chelates metal ions
Phenoxybenzamine	Hypertension due to α-adrenoceptor agonists, e.g. with MAOI, clonidine, ergotamine	Competes for and blocks α-adrenoceptors (long acting)
Phentolamine	As above	Competes for and blocks α-adrenoceptors (short acting)

Table 10.3 Specific antidotes useful in clinical practice—cont'd

Some specific antidotes, indications and modes of action (see index for a fuller account of individual drugs)

Antidote	Indication	Mode of action
Phytomenadione (vitamin K$_1$)	Coumarin (warfarin) and indanedione anticoagulants	Replenishes vitamin K
Pralidoxime	Cholinesterase inhibitors, e.g. organophosphorus insecticides	Competitively reactivates cholinesterase
Propranolol	β-Adrenoceptor agonists, ephedrine, theophylline, thyroxine	Blocks β-adrenoceptors
Protamine	Heparin	Binds ionically to neutralise
Prussian blue (potassium ferric hexacyanoferrate)	Thallium (in rodenticides)	Potassium exchanges for thallium
Sodium calcium edetate	Lead	Chelates lead ions
Unithiol	Lead, elemental and organic mercury	Chelates metal ions

is present in the kernels of several fruits including apricots, almonds and peaches (constituents of the unlicensed anticancer agent, laetrile); excessive use of sodium nitroprusside for severe hypertension.[7]

The symptoms of acute poisoning are due to tissue anoxia, with dizziness, palpitations, a feeling of chest constriction and anxiety. Characteristically the breath smells of bitter almonds. In more severe cases, there is acidosis and coma. Inhaled hydrogen cyanide may lead to death within minutes, but with the ingested salt several hours may elapse before the patient is seriously ill.

Cyanide toxicity causes a metabolic acidosis, reduced arterial/venous oxygen saturation difference and markedly elevated plasma lactate. The presence of these findings in the context of smoke inhalation should alert the physician to the possibility that cyanide poisoning has occurred and needs urgent treatment.

---

[7]Or in other more bizarre ways. 'A 23-year-old medical student saw his dog (a puppy) suddenly collapse. He started external cardiac massage and a mouth-to-nose ventilation effort. Moments later the dog died, and the student felt nauseated, vomited and lost consciousness. On the victim's arrival at hospital, an alert medical officer detected a bitter almonds odour on his breath and administered the accepted treatment for cyanide poisoning after which he recovered. It turned out that the dog had accidentally swallowed cyanide, and the poison eliminated through the lungs had been inhaled by the master during the mouth-to-nose resuscitation.' Journal of the American Medical Association 1983 249:353.

The principles of specific therapy are as follows:

Hydroxocobalamin (5 g for an adult) combines with cyanide to form cyanocobalamin and is excreted by the kidney. Adverse effects include transient hypertension (may be beneficial) and rare anaphylactic and anaphylactoid reactions. Co-administration with sodium thiosulphate (through a separate intravenous line or sequentially) may have added benefit. The use of hydroxocobalamin has largely superseded that of the alternative, dicobalt edetate.

- *Dicobalt edetate.* The dose is 300 mg given intravenously over 1 min (5 min if condition is less serious), followed immediately by a 50 mL intravenous infusion of 50% glucose; a further 300 mg of dicobalt edetate should be given if recovery is not evident within 1 min.
- Alternatively, a two-stage procedure may be followed by intravenous administration of:
  - *Sodium nitrite,* which rapidly converts haemoglobin to methaemoglobin, the ferric ion of which takes up cyanide as cyanmethaemoglobin (up to 40% methaemoglobin can be tolerated).
  - *Sodium thiosulphate,* which more slowly detoxifies the cyanide by permitting the formation of thiocyanate. When the diagnosis is uncertain, administration of thiosulphate plus oxygen is a safe course.

The increasing use of hydroxocobalamin as a first-line treatment is based upon animal studies that have shown a faster improvement of arterial blood pressure compared to sodium nitrate. No benefit in terms of mortality was seen in these studies.

There is evidence that *oxygen*, especially if at high pressure (hyperbaric), overcomes the cellular anoxia in cyanide poisoning; the mechanism is uncertain, but it is reasonable to administer high-flow oxygen.

Carbon monoxide (CO) is a colourless, odourless gas formed by the incomplete combustion of hydrocarbons, and poisoning results from its inhalation. The concentration (% saturation) of CO in the blood may confirm exposure (cigarette smoking alone may account for up to 10%) but is no guide to the severity of poisoning. CO binds reversibly to haemoglobin with about 250 times greater affinity than oxygen. Binding to one of the four oxygen-binding sites on the haemoglobin molecule significantly increases the affinity of the other three binding sites for oxygen which further reduces the delivery of oxygen to hypoxic tissues. In addition, CO has an even higher affinity for cardiac myoglobin, further worsening cardiac output and tissue oxygenation. Poor correlation between carboxyhaemoglobin in the blood and observed toxicity suggests that other mechanisms are involved.

Symptoms commence at about 10% carboxyhaemoglobin with a characteristic headache. Death may occur from myocardial and neurological injury at levels of 50–70%. Severe breathlessness is not a feature typical of severe intoxication. Delayed symptoms (2–4 weeks) include parkinsonism, cerebellar signs and psychiatric disturbances.

Investigations should include direct estimation of carboxyhaemoglobin in the blood. Consider the diagnosis even if the level is low and some time has passed since exposure or high-flow oxygen has been given. PaO_2 levels should be normal. Oxygen saturation is accurate only if directly measured (see above) and not calculated from the PaO_2. Administer oxygen through a tight-fitting mask, and continue for at least 12 h. Evidence for the efficacy of hyperbaric oxygen is conflicting, and transport to hyperbaric chambers may present logistic problems. It is advocated when the blood carboxyhaemoglobin concentration exceeds 40%, there is unconsciousness, neurological defect, ischaemic change on the ECG, pregnancy, or the clinical condition does not improve after 4 h of normobaric therapy.

Lead poisoning arises from a variety of occupational (house renovation and stripping old paint), and recreational sources. Environmental exposure has been a matter of great concern, as witnessed by the protective legislation introduced by many countries to reduce pollution, e.g. by removing lead from petrol. Lead in the body comprises a rapidly exchangeable component in blood (2%, biological $t_{1/2}$ 35 days) and a stable pool in dentine and the skeleton (95%, biological $t_{1/2}$ 25 years). Lead binds to sulfhydryl groups and interferes

with haem production. Since haem-containing proteins play a vital role in cellular oxidation, lead poisoning has wide-ranging effects, particularly in young children. With mild poisoning, there is lethargy and abdominal discomfort; severe abdominal symptoms and peripheral neuropathy and CNS disturbances indicate more serious toxicity. Serum lead values over 100 µg/mL are associated with impaired cognitive development in children; levels above 1000 µg/mL are potentially fatal.

Mild lead poisoning (<450 µg/mL) responds to removal from exposure and monitoring. Moderate poisoning requires oral chelation therapy such as *D*-penicillamine (unlicensed) or more recently with *succimer* (2,3-dimercaptosuccinic acid, DMSA), a water-soluble analogue of dimercaprol with a high affinity for lead. Severe lead poisoning calls for parenteral therapy with *sodium calcium edetate* to chelate lead from bone and the extracellular space; urinary lead excretion diminishes over 5 days as the extracellular store is exhausted. Redistribution of lead from bone to brain may account for subsequent worsening of symptoms (colic and encephalopathy).

Dimercaprol is more effective than sodium calcium edetate at chelating lead from the soft tissues such as brain, which is the rationale for *combined therapy with sodium calcium edetate*.

Methanol is widely available as a solvent and in paints and antifreezes, and constitutes a cheap substitute for ethanol. Methanol itself has low toxicity, but its metabolites are highly toxic. As little as 10 mL may cause permanent blindness, and 30 mL may kill. Methanol, like ethanol, is metabolised by zero-order processes that involve the hepatic alcohol and aldehyde dehydrogenases, but, whereas ethanol forms ethanal and ethanoic acid (partly responsible for the unpleasant effects of 'hangover'), methanol forms methanal and methanoic acid. Blindness may occur because aldehyde dehydrogenase present in the retina (for the interconversion of retinol and retinene) allows the local formation of methanal. Acidosis is due to the methanoic acid, which itself enhances pH-dependent hepatic lactate production, adding the problems of lactic acidosis.

The clinical features include severe malaise, vomiting, abdominal pain and tachypnoea (due to the acidosis). Loss of visual acuity and scotomata indicate ocular damage and, if the pupils are dilated and non-reactive, permanent loss of sight is probable. Coma and circulatory collapse may follow. The key laboratory finding is a high anion gap acidosis. Blood methanol concentrations do not correlate closely with the clinical picture.

Therapy is directed at:

- *Correcting the metabolic acidosis*. Achieving this largely determines the outcome; sodium bicarbonate is given intravenously in doses up to 2 mol in a few hours, carrying an excess of sodium which must be managed.

Methanol is metabolised slowly, and relapse may accompany too early discontinuation of bicarbonate.

- *Inhibiting methanol metabolism.* Ethanol, which occupies the dehydrogenase enzymes in preference to methanol, competitively prevents metabolism of methanol to its toxic products. A single oral dose of ethanol 1 mL/kg (as a 50% solution or as the equivalent in gin or whisky) is followed by 0.25 mL/kg/h orally or intravenously, aiming to maintain the blood ethanol at about 100 mg/100 mL until no methanol is detectable in the blood. Fomepizole (4-methylpyrazole), another competitive inhibitor of alcohol dehydrogenase, is effective in severe methanol poisoning and is less likely to cause cerebral depression (it is available in the UK on a named-patient basis).
- *Eliminating methanol and its metabolites.* Haemodialysis is two to three times more effective than peritoneal dialysis and is indicated in severe cases.
- Folinic acid 30 mg intravenously 6-hourly may protect against retinal damage by enhancing formate metabolism.

Ethylene glycol is readily accessible as a constituent of antifreezes for car radiators (available as a 95% concentration). Its use to give 'body' and sweetness to white table wines was criminal. Metabolism to glycolate and oxalate causes acidosis and renal damage, a situation that is further complicated by lactic acidosis. The lethal dose for an adult is around 100 mL.

In the first 12 h after ingestion, the patient appears as though intoxicated with alcohol but without the characteristic odour. Subsequently there is increasing acidosis, pulmonary oedema and cardiac failure. In 2–3 days, renal pain and tubular necrosis develop because calcium oxalate crystals form in the glomerular filtrate. Intravenous sodium bicarbonate corrects the acidosis, and with calcium gluconate, the hypocalcaemia. As with methanol (above), ethanol or fomepizole competitively inhibit the metabolism of ethylene glycol and haemodialysis eliminates the poison.

Hydrocarbons. Common hydrocarbons include paraffin oil (kerosene), petrol (gasoline) and benzene. The specific toxic effects depend upon the chemical structure of the hydrocarbon, the dose and route of administration. In general, they cause CNS depression and pulmonary damage from inhalation. It is vital to avoid aspiration into the lungs with spontaneous vomiting.

Volatile solvent abuse. Solvent abuse or 'glue sniffing' is common among teenagers, especially males, although the prevalence has probably declined over the last 35 years. Data from 2004 suggested that 6% of 15-year-olds had engaged in the practice in the previous year. The success of the modern chemical industry provides easy access to these substances as adhesives, dry cleaners, air fresheners, deodorants, aerosols and other products. Viscous products are inhaled from a plastic bag, liquids from a handkerchief or plastic bottle.

The immediate euphoriant and excitatory effects give way to confusion, hallucinations and delusions as the dose is increased. Chronic abusers, notably of toluene, develop peripheral neuropathy, cerebellar disease and dementia; damage to the kidney, liver, heart and lungs also occurs with solvents. Evidence from 2006 suggested that one person per week dies in the UK from this practice, and in 60% of these there was no previous history of abuse, suggesting that death commonly occurs on the first use. Over 50% of deaths from the practice follow cardiac arrhythmia, probably caused by sensitisation of the myocardium to catecholamines and by vagal inhibition from laryngeal stimulation due to aerosol propellants sprayed into the throat. Most deaths follow butane lighter fuel inhalation due to its particular tendency to induce cardiac arrhythmias. Death may also occur from acute intoxication impairing judgment, leading to injury.

Acute solvent poisoning requires immediate cardiorespiratory resuscitation and anti-arrhythmia treatment. Toxicity from carbon tetrachloride and chloroform involves the generation of phosgene, a First World War gas, which is inactivated by cysteine and by glutathione, formed from cysteine. Recommended treatment is therefore with *N*-acetylcysteine, as for poisoning with paracetamol.

Herbicides and pesticides

Organophosphorus pesticides are anticholinesterases; an account of poisoning and its management is given later. Organic carbamates are similar.

Dinitro-compounds. Dinitro-ortho-cresol (DNOC) and dinitrobutylphenol (DNBP) are selective weedkillers and insecticides, and cases of poisoning occur accidentally, e.g. by ignoring safety precautions. These substances can be absorbed through the skin and the hands, resulting in yellow staining of face or hair. Symptoms and signs indicate a very high metabolic rate (due to uncoupling of oxidative phosphorylation); copious sweating and thirst proceed to dehydration and vomiting, weakness, restlessness, tachycardia and deep, rapid breathing, convulsions and coma. Treatment is urgent and consists of cooling the patient and attention to fluid and electrolyte balance. It is essential to differentiate this type of poisoning from that due to anticholinesterases (see p. 396), because atropine given to patients poisoned with dinitro-compound will stop sweating and may cause death from hyperthermia.

Phenoxy herbicides (2,4-D, mecoprop, dichlorprop) are used to control broad-leaved weeds. Ingestion causes nausea, vomiting, pyrexia (due to uncoupling of oxidative phosphorylation), hyperventilation, hypoxia and coma. Urine alkalinisation accelerates elimination. Organochlorine pesticides, e.g. dicophane (DDT), may cause convulsions in acute overdose. Treat as for status epilepticus.

Rodenticides include warfarin and thallium (see Table 10.3); for strychnine, which causes convulsions, give diazepam.

Paraquat is a widely used herbicide that is extremely toxic if ingested; a mouthful of the commercial solution taken and spat out may be sufficient to kill. It is highly corrosive and can be absorbed through the skin. A common sequence is: ulceration and sloughing of the oral and oesophageal mucosa, renal tubular necrosis (5–10 days later), pulmonary oedema and pulmonary fibrosis. Whether the patient lives or dies depends largely on the condition of the lung. Treatment is urgent and includes activated charcoal or aluminium silicate (Fuller's earth) by mouth as adsorbents. Haemodialysis may have a role in the first 24 h, the rationale being to reduce the plasma concentration and protect the kidney, failure of which allows the slow but relentless accumulation of paraquat in the lung.

Diquat is similar to paraquat, but the late pulmonary changes may not occur.

Incapacitating agents

CS (chlorobenzylidene malononitrile, a tear 'gas'). It is possible that a physician will be called upon to treat individuals who have been exposed to incapacitating agents. Such agents are designed to cause a disablement that lasts for little longer than the period of exposure. CS is a solid that is disseminated as an aerosol (particles of 1 micron in diameter) by including it in a pyrotechnic mixture. It is an aerosol or smoke, not a gas. The particles aggregate and settle to the ground in minutes, so that the risk of prolonged exposure out of doors is not great. The onset of symptoms occurs immediately on exposure, and they disappear dramatically.

According to the concentration of CS to which a person is exposed, the effects vary from a slight pricking or peppery sensation in the eyes and nasal passages up to the maximal symptoms of streaming from the eyes and nose, spasm of the eyelids, profuse lachrymation and salivation, retching and sometimes vomiting, burning of the mouth and throat, cough and gripping pain in the chest.[8] Exposed subjects absorb small amounts only, and the plasma $t_{1/2}$ is about 5 s. There appear to be no long-lasting sequelae but, plainly, it would be prudent to assume that patients with asthma or chronic bronchitis could suffer an exacerbation from high concentrations.

CN (chloroacetophenone, a tear gas) is generally used as a solid aerosol or smoke; solutions (Mace) are used at close quarters.

CR (dibenzoxazepine) entered production in 1973 after testing on army volunteers. In addition to the usual properties (above), it may induce a transient rise in intraocular pressure. Its solubility allows use in water 'cannons'.

Poisoning by biological substances

Many plants form substances that are important for their survival either by enticing animals, which disperse their spores, or by repelling potential predators. Poisoning occurs when children eat berries or chew flowers, attracted by their colour; adults may mistake non-edible for edible varieties of salad plants and fungi (mushrooms), for they may resemble one another closely and some are greatly prized by epicures. Ingestion of plants is responsible for a significant number of calls to poison information services (10% in US and German surveys), but serious poisonings are rare. Deaths from plant poisoning are thus very rare in industrialised societies. A study from the USA covering the period 1983–2000 identified only 30 fatalities over this 18-year period. Plant poisoning is, however, a significant problem in the developing world. Such deaths are almost exclusively deliberate suicide or homicide.[9]

The range of toxic substances that these plants produce is exhibited in a diversity of symptoms that may be grouped broadly, as shown in Table 10.4.

In addition, many plants may cause cutaneous irritation, e.g. directly with nettle (*Urtica*), or dermatitis following sensitisation with *Primula*. Gastrointestinal symptoms, nausea, vomiting, diarrhoea and abdominal pain occur with numerous plants.

The treatment of plant poisonings consists mainly of giving activated charcoal to adsorb toxin in the gastrointestinal tract, supportive measures to maintain cardiorespiratory function, and control of convulsions with diazepam.

Specific measures. In 'death cap' (*Amanita phalloides*) mushroom poisoning, high-dose penicillin or silibinin (an extract of milk thistle) are used to inhibit amatoxin uptake by the liver and its enterohepatic circulation. Antitoxins, e.g. Digibind, are used for poisoning with plants that produce toxic cardiac glycosides.

---

[8]Home Office Report (1971) of the enquiry into the medical and toxicological aspects of CS. Part II. HMSO, London: Cmnd 4775.

[9]Eddleston M, Rezvi Sheriff M H, Hawton K 1998 Deliberate self-harm in Sri Lanka: an overlooked tragedy in the developing world. British Medical Journal 317:133–135.

Table 10.4 Commonly encountered plant poisonings

Symptom complex	Causative agent	Active ingredient
Atropenic • dilated pupils • blurred vision • dried mouth • flushing • confusion and delirium	• *Atropa belladonna* (deadly nightshade) • *Datura* (thorn apple)	Tropane alkaloids such as • atropine • hyoscine (scopolamine) • hyoscyamine
Nicotinic • hypersalivation • pupil dilatation • vomiting • convulsions • respiratory paralysis	• *Conium* (hemlock) • Laburnum	• coniine • cytisine
Muscarinic • salivation • lachrymation • meiosis • perspiration • bradycardia • bronchoconstriction • hallucinations	• *Inocybe* mushrooms • *Clitocybe* mushrooms	• muscarine • several rare species have hallucinogenic properties and produce psilocybin
Hallucinogenic • (so called 'magic mushrooms')	• *Psilocybe* mushrooms	• psilocybin
Cardiovascular • cardiac arrhythmias • vomiting • diarrhoea	• *Digitalis* (foxglove) • *Viscum album* (mistletoe) • *Convallaria* (lily of the valley) • *Thevetia peruviana* (yellow oleander) • *Strophanthus* (twisted corn flower) • *Aconitum* opens tetrodotoxin sensitive sodium channels in heart and nervous system	Cardenolide cardiac glycosides such as • digoxin • digitoxin • ouabain • oleandrin
Hepatotoxic	• *Amanita phalloides* (death cap mushroom) • *Senecio* (ragwort) • *Crotalaria* (common ingredient in bush teas)	• alpha amatin in mushrooms • pyrollizidine alkaloids in plants
Convulsant	• *Oenanthe* (water dropwort) • *Cicuta* (cowbane)	GABA antagonists • oenanthotoxin and closely related • cicutoxin

Guide to further reading

Bateman, N.D., 2015. Paracetamol poisoning; beyond the nomogram. Br. J. Clin. Pharmacol. 80 (1), 45–50.

Body, R., Bartram, T., Azam, F., Mackway-Jones, K., 2011. Guidelines in Emergency Medicine Network (GeMNet): guideline for the management of tricyclic antidepressant overdose. Emergency Med. J. 28, 347–368.

Bradbury, S., Vale, A., 2008. Poisons: epidemiology and clinical presentation. Clin. Med. (Northfield Il) 8 (1), 86–88 (and subsequent papers in this issue).

Buckley, N.A., Juurlink, D.N., Isbister, G., et al., 2011. Hyperbaric oxygen for carbon monoxide poisoning. Cochrane Database Syst. Rev. 13, (4).

Budnitz, D.S., Lovegrove, M.C., Crosby, A.E., 2011. Emergency department visits for acetaminophen-containing products. Am. J. Prev. Med. 40, 585–592.

Chyka, P.A., Erdman, A.R., Christianson, G., et al., 2007. Salicylate poisoning: an evidence-based consensus guideline for out-of-hospital management. Clin. Toxicol. 45, 95–131.

Diaz, J.H., 2016. Poisoning by herbs and plants: Rapid Toxidromic Classification and Diagnosis. Wilderness Environ. Med. 27 (1), 136–152.

Evison, D., Hinsley, D., Rice, P., 2002. Chemical weapons. Br. Med. J. 324, 332–335.

Gawande, A., 2006. When law and ethics collide – why physicians participate in executions. N. Engl. J. Med. 354 (12), 1221–1229.

Gosselin, S., Hoeqberg, L.C., Hoffman, R.S., et al., 2016. Evidence-based recommendations on the use of intravenous lipid emulsion therapy in poisoning. Clin. Toxicol. 54 (10), 899–923.

Holger, J.S., Engebretson, K.M., Marini, J.J., 2009. High dose insulin in toxic cardiogenic shock. Clin. Toxicol. 47 (4), 303–307.

Holstege, C.P., 2012. Toxidromes. Crit. Care Clin. 28 (4), 479–498.

Kales, S.N., Christiani, D.C., 2004. Acute chemical emergencies. N. Engl. J. Med. 350 (8), 800–808.

Kerins, M., Dargan, P.I., Jones, A.L., 2003. Pitfalls in the management of the poisoned patient. J. R. Coll. Physicians Edinb. 33, 90–103.

Ruben Thanacoody, H.K., Thomas, S.H.L., 2003. Antidepressant poisoning. Clin. Med. (Northfield Il) 3 (2), 114–118.

Skegg, K., 2005. Self-harm. Lancet 366, 1471–1483.

Thanacoody, R., Caravati, E.M., Troutman, B., Hojer, J., et al., 2015. Position paper update: Whole bowel irrigation for gastrointestinal decontamination of overdose patients. Clin. Toxicol. 53 (1), 5–12.

Volans, G., Hartley, V., McCrea, S., Monaghan, J., 2003. Non-opioid analgesic poisoning. Clin. Med. (Northfield Il) 3 (2), 119–123.

Wolf, A.D., Erdman, A.R., Nelson, L.S., et al., 2007. Tricyclic antidepressant poisoning: an evidence-based consensus guideline for out-of-hospital management. Clin. Toxicol. 45, 203–233.

Chapter 11

Drug dependence

Stephen Haydock

SYNOPSIS

Drugs used for non-medical purposes (abused, misused, used for recreational purposes) present a range of social problems, all of which have important pharmacological dimensions. General topics include:

- Introduction.
- Definitions.
- General patterns of use.
- Sites and mechanisms of action.
- Routes of administration and effect.
- Prescribing for drug dependence.
- Treatment of dependence.
- Mortality.
- Escalation.
- Novel psychoactive substances.
- Drugs and sport.

Individual substances are discussed:

- Opioids (see pp. 293–296).
- Ethyl alcohol and other cerebral depressants (benzodlazepines, GHB).
- Tobacco.
- Psychodysleptics (LSD, mescaline, tenamfetamine, phencyclidine, cannabis).
- Psychostimulants (cocaine, amfetamines, methylxanthines, khat).
- Volatile substances.

Introduction

The dividing line between legitimate use of drugs for social purposes and their abuse is indistinct, for it is not only a matter of which drug, but of the amount of drug and of whether the effect is antisocial or not. In the UK and elsewhere, the classification of drugs of abuse continues to be subject to controversy.[1]

'Normal' people seem to be able to use alcohol for their occasional purposes without harm, but, given the appropriate personality and/or environmental adversity, many may turn to it for relief and become dependent on it, both psychologically and physically. But drug abuse is not primarily a pharmacological problem; it is a social problem with important pharmacological aspects.

Abuse of drugs to improve performance in sport stems from a distinct and different motivation, namely, the obtaining of advantage in competition, but the practice yet has major implications for the health of the individual and for the participating and spectating sporting community.

---

[1]MacDonald R, Das A 2006 UK classification of drugs of abuse: an un-evidence-based mess. Lancet 368:559–561.

Definitions

Substance dependence is defined as:

when an individual persists in use of alcohol or other drugs despite problems related to use of the substance, substance dependence may be diagnosed. Compulsive and repetitive use may result in tolerance to the effect of the drug and withdrawal symptoms when use is reduced or stopped.[2]

Substance abuse is a term that is less clearly defined and becoming less used, in favour of the term 'substance dependence'. Nevertheless, the terms 'addict' or 'addiction' have not been completely abandoned in this book because they remain convenient. The WHO Expert Committee on Addiction Producing Drugs 1957 defined substance abuse in the context of two components:

Substance addiction *is a state of periodic or chronic intoxication produced by the repeated consumption of a drug (natural or synthetic). Its characteristics include: (i) an overpowering desire or need (compulsion) to continue taking the drug and to obtain it by any means; (ii) a tendency to increase the dose; (iii) a psychic (psychological) and generally a physical dependence on the effects of the drug; and (iv) detrimental effects on the individual and on society.*

Substance habituation is a condition resulting from the repeated consumption of a drug. Its characteristics include (i) a desire (but not a compulsion) to continue taking the drug for the sense of improved well-being which it engenders; (ii) little or no tendency to increase the dose; (iii) some degree of psychic dependence on the effect of the drug, but absence of physical dependence and hence of an abstinence syndrome (withdrawal), and (iv) detrimental effects, if any, primarily on the individual.

Psychological dependence is characterised by emotional distress if the drug of dependence is withdrawn. The subject may develop craving for the drug with anxiety, insomnia and dysphoria. It develops before physical dependence.

Physical (physiological) dependence implies that continued exposure to a drug induces adaptive changes in body tissues so that *tolerance* occurs, and that abrupt withdrawal of the drug leaves these changes unopposed, resulting generally in a *discontinuation (withdrawal) syndrome*, usually of rebound overactivity.

Tolerance follows the operation of homeostatic adaptation, e.g. to continued high occupancy of opioid receptors. Changes of similar type may occur with γ-aminobutyric acid (GABA) transmission, involving benzodiazepines. It also results from metabolic changes (enzyme induction) and physiological or behavioural adaptation to drug effects, e.g. opioids. Physiological adaptation develops to a substantial degree with cerebral depressants, but is minor or absent with excitant drugs. There is commonly cross-tolerance between drugs of similar, and sometimes even of dissimilar, chemical groups, e.g. alcohol and benzodiazepines. A general account of tolerance appears on page 80.

A *discontinuation (withdrawal) syndrome* occurs, for example, when administration of an opioid is suddenly stopped. Morphine-like substances (endomorphins, dynorphins) act as CNS neurotransmitters, and exogenously administered opioid suppresses their endogenous production by a feedback mechanism. Abrupt discontinuation results in an immediate deficiency of endogenous opioid, which thus causes the withdrawal syndrome. A general discussion of abrupt withdrawal of drug therapy appears on page 101.

Drugs of dependence are often divided into two groups, hard and soft. There are again no absolute definitions of these categories.

Hard drugs are those that are liable seriously to disable the individual as a functioning member of society by inducing severe psychological and, in the case of cerebral depressants, physical dependence. The group includes heroin and cocaine.

Soft drugs are less dependence producing. There may be psychological dependence, but there is little or no physical dependence except with heavy doses of depressants (alcohol). The group includes sedatives and tranquillisers, amfetamines, cannabis, hallucinogens, alcohol, tobacco and caffeine.

This classification fails to recognise individual variation in drug use. Alcohol can be used in heavy doses that are gravely disabling and induce severe physical dependence with convulsions on sudden withdrawal; i.e. for the individual the drug is 'hard'. But there are many people mildly psychologically dependent on it who retain their position in the home and society.

Hard use, where the drug is central in the user's life, and soft use, where it is merely incidental, are terms of assistance in making this distinction, i.e. what is classified is not the drug but the effect it has on, or the way it is used by, the individual. The term 'recreational' is often applied to such use, conferring an apparent sanction that relates more to the latter category.

Dependence/abuse liability of a drug is related to its capacity to produce immediate gratification, which may be a feature of the drug itself (amfetamine and heroin give rapid effect, whereas tricyclic antidepressants do not), and its route of administration, in descending order: inhalation/

---

[2]*Diagnostic and Statistical Manual of Mental Disorders,* American Psychiatric Association 2007.

Table 11.1 Current list of UK proscribed drugs

Class	Drug	Penalty for possession	Penalty for possession with intent to supply
Class A	Ecstasy, LSD, heroin, cocaine, crack, magic mushrooms, amfetamines (if prepared for injection)	Up to 7 years in prison or an unlimited fine or both	Up to life in prison or an unlimited fine or both
Class B	Amfetamines, cannabis, methylphenidate (Ritalin), pholcodine	Up to 5 years in prison or an unlimited fine or both	Up to 14 years in prison or an unlimited fine or both
Class C	Tranquillisers, some painkillers, γ-hydroxybutyrate (GHB), ketamine, anabolic steroids	Up to 2 years in prison or an unlimited fine or both	Up to 14 years in prison or an unlimited fine or both

Amyl nitrate and glues (including solvents, gases and aerosols) are not classified. Possession of these substances is not illegal; however, it is an offence to supply such a substance if it likely to be abused.

intravenous, intramuscular/subcutaneous. Those drugs with high dependence/abuse liability are subject to regulation, and non-medicinal use may be a criminal offence. The current UK list of controlled substances as proscribed by the Misuse of Drugs Act 1971 is shown in Table 11.1. Readers will be aware that the list is subject to change according to social factors and political expediency.

Drug abuse use has two principal forms: *continuous use* describes a true dependence, e.g. opioids, alcohol, benzodiazepines; *intermittent or occasional use* describes either a recreational experience, e.g. 'ecstasy' (tenamfetamine), LSD, cocaine, cannabis, solvents, or use to relieve stress, e.g. alcohol. Some drugs, e.g. alcohol, are used in both ways, but others, e.g. ecstasy, LSD, cannabis, are virtually confined to intermittent use.

Drives to drug abuse can be grouped as follows:

1. Relief of anxiety, tension and depression; escape from personal psychological problems; detachment from harsh reality; ease of social intercourse.
2. Rebellion against or despair about orthodox social values and the environment. Fear of missing something, and conformity with own social subgroup (the young, especially).
3. Fun, amusement, recreation, excitement, curiosity (the young, especially).
4. Improvement of performance in competitive sport (a distinct motivation, see below).

General patterns of use

Patterns of drug dependence differ with age. Men are more commonly involved than women. Patterns change

Table 11.2 Use of drugs of dependence by age in the UK

Age group

Younger than 14 years of age	Volatile inhalants, e.g. solvents of glues, aerosol sprays, vaporised (by heat) paints, 'solvent or substance' abuse, 'glue sniffing'
14–16 years of age	Cannabis, ecstasy, cocaine
16–35 years of age	Hard-use drugs, chiefly heroin, cocaine and amfetamines (including 'ecstasy'). Surviving users tend to reduce or relinquish heavy use as they enter middle age Also cannabis, magic mushrooms
Any age	Alcohol, tobacco, mild dependence on hypnotics and tranquillisers, occasional use of LSD and cannabis

as drugs come in and out of vogue. The general picture in the UK is shown in Table 11.2. Data on illicit drug use in the UK are provided from a number of sources, but up-to-date information on prevalence and patterns of usage can be obtained from the annual *British Crime Survey*. Data from the 2008/2009 survey indicate that one in three people between 16 and 59 years of age had ever used illicit drugs, while 1 in 10 had used an illicit substance in the previous year. The survey also allows observations on the trends in illicit drug use over time, as shown in Table 11.3.

Table 11.3 Trends in drug use in the UK (information derived from 2008/2009 British crime survey)

Increased use	Decreased use	Stable use
Between 1996 and 2008/2009		
• Any Class A drug	• Hallucinogens	• Any stimulant drug
• Cocaine powder	• LSD	• Opiates
• Tranquillisers	• Amphetamines	• Crack cocaine
	• Anabolic steroids	• Ecstasy
		• Magic mushrooms
		• Heroin
		• Amyl nitrate
		• Glues
Between 2007/8 and 2008/9		
• Any Class A drug	None	• Hallucinogens
• Any stimulant drug		• Opiates
• Cocaine powder		• Crack cocaine
• Ecstasy		• LSD
• Tranquillisers		• Magic mushrooms
• Anabolic steroids		• Heroin
• Ketamine		• Methadone
		• Amfetamines
		• Cannabis
		• Amyl nitrate
		• Glues

Sites and mechanisms of action

Drugs of abuse are extremely diverse in their chemical structures, mechanisms of action and anatomical and cellular targets. Nevertheless, there is an emerging consensus that addictive drugs possess a parallel ability to modulate the brain reward system that is key to activities that are vital for survival (e.g. eating and sexual behaviour). Of particular relevance is the medial forebrain bundle (MFB) that connects the ventral tegmental area and the nucleus accumbens. Natural and artificial rewards (including drugs of abuse) have been shown to activate the dopaminergic

neurones within the MFB. It seems that drugs of abuse can converge on common neural mechanisms in these areas to produce acute reward and chronic alterations in reward systems that lead to addiction. This is summarised in Fig. 11.1.

> Increasing evidence suggests that drugs of addiction all act by modulating dopaminergic transmission in the medial forebrain bundle.

Route of administration and effect

With the intravenous route or inhalation, much higher peak plasma concentrations can be reached than with oral administration. This accounts for the 'kick' or 'flash' that abusers report and which many seek, likening it to sexual orgasm or better. As an addict said, 'The ultimate high is death', and it has been reported that, when hearing of someone dying from an overdose, some addicts will seek out the vendor as it is evident he is selling 'really good stuff'.[3]

Prescribing for drug dependence

In the UK, supply of certain drugs for the purpose of sustaining addiction or managing withdrawal is permitted under strict legal limitations, usually by designated doctors. Guidance about the responsibilities and management of addiction is available.[4] By such procedures, it is hoped to limit the expansion of the illicit market, and its accompanying crime and dangers to health, e.g. from infected needles and syringes. The object is to sustain young (usually) addicts, who cannot be weaned from drug use, in reasonable health until they relinquish their dependence (often over about 10 years).

When injectable drugs are prescribed, there is currently no way of assessing the truth of an addict's statement that he or she needs x mg of heroin (or other drug), and the dose has to be assessed intuitively by the doctor. This has resulted in addicts obtaining more than they need and selling it, sometimes to initiate new users. The use of oral methadone or other opioid for maintenance by prescription is devised to mitigate this problem.

---

[3]Bourne P 1976 Acute Drug Abuse Emergencies. Academic Press, New York.
[4]See Department of Health 1999 Drug Misuse and Dependence – Guidelines on Clinical Management. The Stationery Office, London (3rd impression 2005).

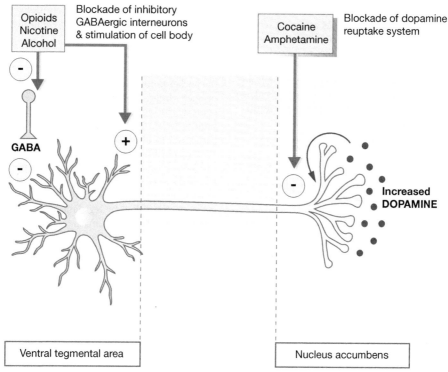

Fig. 11.1 Common pathway of drugs of addiction on the dopaminergic neurones.

Treatment of dependence

About £1.4 billion is spent per year in England alone on the management of drug dependence. This is directed at an estimated one-third of a million subjects. The majority are dependent on heroin. These are managed by either abstinence or, more commonly, maintenance on prescribed alternatives such as methadone.

Withdrawal of the drug. While obviously important, this is only a step on what can be a long and often disappointing journey to psychological and social rehabilitation, e.g. in 'therapeutic communities'. A heroin addict may be given methadone as part of a gradual withdrawal programme (see p. 297), for this drug has a long duration of action and blocks access of injected opioid to the opioid receptor so that if, in a moment of weakness, the subject takes heroin, the 'kick' is reduced. More acutely, the physical features associated with discontinuing high alcohol use may be alleviated by chlordiazepoxide given in decreasing doses for 7–14 days. Sympathetic autonomic overactivity can be treated with a β-adrenoceptor blocker.

Maintenance and relapse. Relapsed addicts who live a fairly normal life are sometimes best treated by supplying drugs under supervision. There is no legal objection to doing this in the UK. A less harmful drug by a less harmful route may be substituted, e.g. oral methadone for intravenous heroin. Addicts are often particularly reluctant to abandon the intravenous route, which provides the 'immediate high' that they find, or originally found, so desirable.

Severe pain in an opioid addict presents a special problem. High-efficacy opioid may be ineffective (tolerance), or overdose may result; low-efficacy opioids will not only be ineffective but may induce withdrawal symptoms, especially if they have some antagonist effect, e.g. pentazocine. This leaves as drugs of choice non-steroidal anti-inflammatory drugs (NSAIDs), e.g. indometacin, and nefopam (which is neither opioid nor NSAID).

Mortality

Young illicit users by intravenous injection (heroin, benzodiazepines, amfetamine) have a high mortality rate.

Death follows either overdose or the occurrence of septi-caemia, endocarditis, hepatitis, AIDS, gas gangrene, tetanus or pulmonary embolism from the contaminated materials used without aseptic precautions (schemes to provide clean equipment mitigate this). Smugglers of illicit cocaine or heroin sometimes carry the drug in plastic bags concealed by swallowing or in the rectum ('body packing'). Leakage of the packages, not surprisingly, may have a fatal result.[5]

Escalation

A variable proportion of subjects who start with cannabis eventually take heroin. This disposition to progress from occasional to frequent soft use of drugs through to hard drug use, when it occurs, is less likely to be due to pharmacological actions than to psychosocial factors, although increased suggestibility induced by cannabis may contribute.

De-escalation also occurs as users become disillusioned with drugs over about 10 years.

Novel psychoactive substances

Increasingly in recent years the worldwide drug scene includ-ing the UK has experienced an influx of 'designer drugs' that result from specific chemical modifications of active pharmacophore structures that modify central nervous system activity. Most such agents are produced in the Far East and have increased in use as that of conventional drugs of abuse has fallen. Such agents have conventionally been referred to as 'legal highs' and have been available through 'Head Shops' in most towns or via Internet web sites. They can be considered as being of three principle groups namely:

- Central nervous system stimulants or 'uppers' such as amphetamine, cocaine and ecstasy derivatives
- Central nervous system depressants or 'downers' such as benzodiazepine derivatives and gamma hydroxybutyrate

- Hallucinogens or 'all arounders' derived from LSD, mescaline, cannabinoids and ketamine.

The increasing popularity of such drugs and their ease of availability has prompted the UK government to take legal action to limit their availability and use. This has been on the background of considerable press concern over the risks of such drugs. However, the hazards should be seen in context. During 2004–2014, such novel psychoactive sub-stances were only contributory to 76 deaths in the UK compared to almost 8000 for heroin and morphine and 1750 deaths from cocaine. The regulation of novel psychoac-tive substances is via the 2016 Psychoactive Substances Act that seeks to get round the frequent new chemical modifica-tions that appear by restricting the sale of any agent not currently controlled by legislation that is deemed to exert a psychoactive effect in any person that consumes it. The law is therefore essentially a ban on the action and not the chemical structure. The law has been the subject of consider-able criticism, but it has had a significant impact in terms of preventing open sale of such agents and restricting availability of on-line purchase. Nicotine, alcohol and caffeine are exempt from the act.

Globalisation and the use of the Internet have spawned a large market for the development and sale of new designer drugs based upon older drugs of abuse.

Drugs and sport

Drugs are frequently used to enhance performance in sport, although efficacy is largely undocumented. Detection can be difficult when the drugs or metabolites are closely related to or identical to endogenous substances, and when the drug can be stopped well before the event without apparent loss of efficacy. In order to get round this problem, regulatory bodies set 'benchmarks'. Detection of levels of the naturally occurring compound above this level indicates potential doping. There remain unresolved issues at where exactly these benchmarks should be set. Research continues for improved methods of detecting drugs used in sport. The use of mass spectrometry[6] to detect the isotope content of compounds might enable natural and synthetic steroids to be differentiated. Other indirect methods are employed. Testosterone and its related compound, epitestosterone, are both eliminated in urine. The ratio of testosterone to

---

[5]A 49-year-old man became ill after an international flight. An abdominal radiograph showed a large number of spherical packages in his gastrointestinal tract, and body-packing was suspected. As he had not defaecated, he was given liquid paraffin. He developed ventricular fibrillation and died. Post-mortem examination showed that he had ingested more than 150 latex packets, each containing 5 g cocaine, making a total of almost 1 kg (lethal oral dose 1–3 g). The liquid paraffin may have contributed to his death as the mineral oil dissolves latex. Sorbitol or lactulose with activated charcoal should be used to remove ingested packages, or surgery if there are signs of intoxication. (Visser L, Stricker B, Hoogendoorn M, Vinks A 1998 Do not give paraffin to packers. Lancet 352:1352.)

[6]A highly sensitive technique that can identify minor differences between molecules. It is based on the principle that ions passing at high velocity through an electrical field at right angles to their motion will deviate from a straight line according to their mass and charge; the heaviest will deviate least, the lightest most.

epitestosterone increases with use of anabolic steroids and can be used to detect anabolic steroid use.

Performance enhancement

Table 11.4 summarises the mechanisms by which drugs can enhance performance in various sports; naturally, these are proscribed by the authorities (International Olympic Committee (IOC) Medical Commission, and the governing bodies of individual sports).

In addition, owing to the recognition of natural biological differences, most competitive events are sex segregated. In many events men have a natural physical biological advantage, and the (inevitable) consequence has been that women have been deliberately virilised (by administration of androgens) so that they may outperform their sisters.

It seems safe to assume that anything that can be thought up to gain advantage will be tried by competitors eager for immediate fame. Reliable data are difficult to obtain in these areas. No doubt placebo effects are important, i.e. beliefs as to what has been taken and what effects ought to follow.

For any minor injuries sustained during athletic training, NSAIDs and corticosteroids (topical, intra-articular) suppress symptoms and allow the training to proceed maximally. Their use is allowed subject to restrictions about route of administration, but strong opioids are disallowed. Similarly, the IOC Medical Code defines acceptable and unacceptable treatments for relief of cough, hay fever, diarrhoea, vomiting, pain and asthma. Doctors should remember that they may get their athlete patients into trouble with sports authorities by inadvertent prescribing of banned substances. The *British National Formulary* provides general advice for UK prescribers

Table 11.4 Use of illicit drugs in sport

Desirable property	Typical events	Drug of abuse	Comments
Strength	• Weightlifting • Rowing • Wrestling	Anabolic steroids	• Androstenedione, methandienone, nandrolone, stanozolol, testosterone • Said to increase muscle mass with high-protein diet • May permit more intensive training regimens • May precipitate episodes of violent behaviour ('roid rage') • Risk of liver damage (cholestasis and tumours) • Suppress pituitary gonadotrophins and hence testosterone production • Chorionic gonadotrophin may be taken to boost testosterone and tamoxifen to ameliorate other effects of anabolic steroids
		Clenbuterol	• β-Adrenoceptor agonist that may have similar effects on muscle as steroids
		Growth hormone	• Somatrem, somatropin, corticotropin • May be combined with anabolic steroids
Explosive energy	• 100 m sprint	Stimulants	• Amfetamine, bromantan, carphendon, cocaine, ephedrine and caffeine • Deaths reported in bicycle racing* due to hyperthermia, cardiac arrhythmia in subjects vasoconstricted under hot sun *Requires continuous hard exercise with periodic sprints*
Endurance	• Bicycling • Marathon running	Stimulants of erythropoiesis	• Erythropoitin • Enhances oxygen-carrying capacity of blood • 'Blood doping' involves transfusing athletes' previously donated and stored blood prior to competition
Steadiness of hand	• Pistol shooting	β-Blockers	• Propranolol and others reduce β-adrenoceptor–mediated tremor • May also reduce somatic symptoms of anxiety
Body pliancy	• Gymnastics	GRH antagonists	• Delay puberty
Weight reduction	• Boxing • Horse racing	Diuretics	• Loss of fluid to reduce weight prior to 'weigh in' • Sometimes used to 'flush out' other drugs of abuse • Increases risk of thromboembolism

(further information and advice, including the status of specific drugs in sport, can be obtained at http://www.uksport.gov.uk).

Types of drug dependence

The World Health Organization recommends that drug dependence be specified by type for purposes of detailed discussion. The subject can be treated according to the following principal types:

- Opioids (see pp. 293–296)
- Alcohol and other cerebral depressants (benzodiazepines, γ-hydroxybutyrate)
- Tobacco
- Psychodysleptics (LSD, mescaline, tenamfetamine, phencyclidine, cannabis)
- Psychostimulants (cocaine, amfetamines, methylxanthines, khat)
- Volatile substances.

Ethyl alcohol (ethanol)

Alcohol is important in medicine chiefly because of the consequences of its misuse/abuse. Alcohol-related mortality has increased steadily since the 1990s, with over 9000 deaths attributed to alcohol in 2008. Alcohol-related deaths are over twice as common in men as in women.

Pharmacokinetics

Absorption. The gastrointestinal absorption of alcohol taken orally is rapid, as it is highly lipid soluble and dif-fusible. The major site of absorption is the small intestine; solutions above 20% are absorbed more slowly because high concentrations of alcohol inhibit gastric peristalsis, thus delaying the arrival of the alcohol in the small intestine. Absorption is delayed by food, especially milk, the effect of which is probably due to the fat it contains. Carbohydrate also delays absorption of alcohol.

Distribution. It is distributed rapidly and throughout the body water (dist. vol. 0.7 L/kg men; 0.6 L/kg women) with no selective tissue storage. Maximum blood concentrations after oral alcohol therefore depend on numerous factors including: the total dose; sex; the strength of the solution; the time over which it is taken; the presence or absence of food in the stomach; the time relations of taking food and alcohol, and the kind of food eaten; the speed of metabolism and excretion.

Alcoholic drinks taken on an empty stomach will probably produce maximal blood concentration at 30–90 min and will not all be disposed of for 6–8 h or even more. There are very great individual variations.

Metabolism. About 95% of absorbed alcohol is metabolised by the liver, the remainder being excreted in the breath, urine and sweat; convenient methods of estimation of alcohol in all these media are available (Fig. 11.2).

Alcohol metabolism by alcohol dehydrogenase follows first-order kinetics after the smallest doses. Once the blood concentration exceeds about 10 mg/100 mL, the enzymatic processes are saturated, and the elimination rate no longer increases with increasing concentration but becomes steady at 10–15 mL/h in occasional drinkers. Thus alcohol is subject to dose-dependent kinetics, i.e. saturation or zero-order kinetics, with potentially major consequences for the individual.

Induction of hepatic drug-metabolising enzymes occurs with repeated exposure to alcohol. This contributes to tolerance in habitual users, and to toxicity. Increased formation of metabolites causes organ damage in chronic over-consumption (acetaldehyde in the liver and probably fatty ethyl esters in other organs) and increases susceptibility to

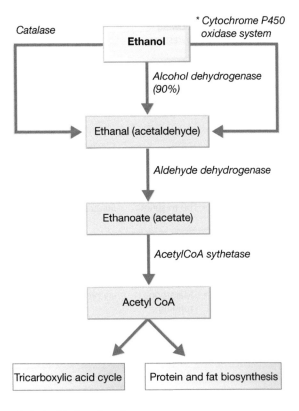

*Is inducible by ethanol

Fig. 11.2 Metabolism of ethanol by the liver.

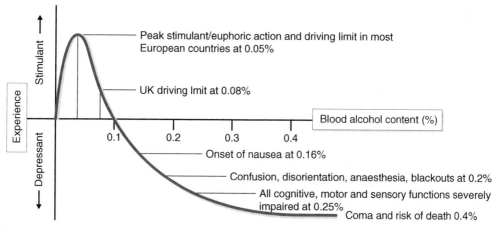

Fig. 11.3 Stimulatory and depressant effects of acute alcohol ingestion.

liver injury when heavy drinkers are exposed to anaesthetics, industrial solvents and drugs. But chronic use of large amounts reduces hepatic metabolic capacity by causing cellular damage. An acute substantial dose of alcohol (binge drinking) inhibits hepatic drug metabolism.

Inter-ethnic variation is recognised in the ability to metabolise alcohol (see p. 148).

The blood concentration of alcohol (Fig. 11.3) has great medicolegal importance. Alcohol in alveolar air is in equilibrium with that in pulmonary capillary blood, and reliable, easily handled measurement devices (breathalysers) are used by police at the roadside on both drivers and pedestrians.[7]

Pharmacodynamics

Alcohol exerts on cells in the CNS a generally depressant effect that is probably mediated through particular membrane ion channels and receptors. It seems likely that acetaldehyde acts synergistically with alcohol to determine the range of neurochemical and behavioural effects of alcohol consumption. There is considerable evidence that ethanol affects neurotransmitter release and activity. Alcohol enhances dopamine release, inhibits the reuptake of brain amines and enhances (inhibitory) $GABA_A$-stimulated flux of chloride through receptor-gated membrane ion channels, a receptor subtype effect that may be involved in the motor impairment

caused by alcohol (see p. 148). Other possible modes of action include inhibition of the (excitatory) *N*-methyl-D-aspartate (NMDA) receptor and inhibition of calcium entry via voltage-gated (L type) calcium channels.

Alcohol is not a stimulant; hyperactivity, when it occurs, is due to removal of inhibitory effects. Psychic effects are the most important socially, and it is to obtain these that the drug is habitually used in so many societies, to make social intercourse not merely easy but even pleasant. Environment, personality, mood and dose of alcohol are all relevant to the final effect on the individual.

Alcohol in ordinary doses may act chiefly on the arousal mechanisms of the brainstem reticular formation, inhibiting polysynaptic function and enhancing presynaptic inhibition. Direct cortical depression probably occurs only with large amounts. With increasing doses, the subject passes through all the stages of general anaesthesia and may die from respiratory depression. Loss of consciousness occurs at blood concentrations around 300 mg/100 mL, death at about 400 mg/100 mL. The usual cause of death in acute alcohol poisoning is inhalation of vomit.

Innumerable tests of physical and mental performance have been used to demonstrate the effects of alcohol. Results show that alcohol reduces visual acuity and delays recovery from visual dazzle; impairs taste, smell, hearing, muscular coordination and steadiness; and prolongs reaction time. It also causes nystagmus and vertigo. It commonly increases subjects' confidence in their ability to perform well when tested and tendency to underestimate their errors, even after quite low doses. There is a decline in attentiveness and ability to assimilate, sort and take quick decisions on continuously changing information input; an example is inattentiveness to the periphery of the visual field, which is important in motoring.

---

[7]An arrested man was told, in a police station by a doctor, that he was drunk. The man asked, 'Doctor, could a drunk man stand up in the middle of this room, jump into the air, turn a complete somersault, and land down on his feet?' The doctor was injudicious enough to say, 'Certainly not' – and was then and there proved wrong (Worthing C L 1957 British Medical Journal i:643). The introduction of the breathalyser, which has a statutory role only in road traffic situations, has largely eliminated such professional humiliations.

Table 11.5 Other physiological, pathological and metabolic effects of acute alcohol ingestion

Effect	Comments
Vomiting	• Partly a central effect (similar effects for oral and i.v. dose) • Also a local gastric effect • May cause death from inhalation of vomit
Diuresis	• Inhibition of pituitary ADH secretion
Gastric irritation	• Ethanol permits back diffusion of acid into the gastric mucosa • Acute binge produces erosions and petechial haemorrhages that can take 3 weeks to recover • 60% of chronic alcoholics have chronic gastritis
Impaired glucose tolerance	• Initially increases blood glucose by blocking glucose uptake • Inhibits gluconeogenesis • In presence of low glycogen stores can precipitate severe hypoglycaemia causing permanent neurological damage • Hypoglycaemia may be difficult to recognise in an intoxicated patient
Hyperuricaemia	• Gout may be precipitated due to increased uric acid levels due to degradation of adenine nucleotides • At high alcohol levels, generated lactate also competes for renal tubular elimination of urate
Abnormal lipid profile	• Large dose may precipitate hyperlipidaemia in some individuals
Sexual function	• Acute intoxication may result in impotence • Chronic consumption in addition lowers plasma testosterone
Calorific affect	• May be a useful source of energy in debilitated patients • Rapid absorption from GI tract without need for digestion • Supplies 7 calories per gram (fat supplies 9 calories per gram and carbohydrate/protein 4 calories per gram)
Acute hepatitis	• May occur with large alcohol binge and be extremely severe
Acute pancreatititis	• Usually a feature of long-term chronic alcohol usage • Less commonly can occur in 'weekend binge drinkers' • Has been described for a sole large alcohol load precipitating a first attack
Inter-ethnic intolerance	• Inter-ethnic variation in acute alcohol tolerance is well described • People of Asian origin (particularly Japanese) develop flushing, headache and nausea after what are small doses • May be due to slow metabolism of toxic acetaldehyde by variant forms of alcohol dehydrogenase

All of these are clearly highly undesirable effects when a person is in a position where failure to perform well may be dangerous. Some other important physiological and metabolic effects of acute alcohol ingestion are described in Table 11.5.

Acute alcohol poisoning is characterised by behaviour changes, excitement, mental confusion (including 'blackouts'), incoordination and even coma. Numerous other conditions can mimic this presentation, and diagnosis can be difficult if a sick or injured patient happens to have taken alcohol as well. Alcohol can cause severe hypoglycaemia; measurement of blood alcohol may clarify the situation. If sedation is essential, diazepam in low dose is least hazardous. Alcohol dialyses well, but dialysis is used only in extreme cases.

Chronic consumption

Tolerance to alcohol can be acquired, and the point has been made that it costs the regular heavy drinker 2.5 times as much to get visibly drunk as it would cost the average abstainer. This is probably due both to enzyme induction and to adaptation of the CNS.

Table 11.6 Physiological, pathological and metabolic effects of chronic alcohol ingestion

Effect	Comments

Organ damage	• Hepatic cirrhosis
	• CNS dysfunction
	  – seizures
	  – Korsakoff's syndrome
	  – dementia
	  – Wernicke's encephalopathy
	  – episodic memory loss
	• Peripheral neuropathy
	• Myopathy including cardiomyopathy
	• Cancer especially of the upper alimentary tract and lungs
	• Chronic pancreatitis

Malnutrition	• In heavy drinkers all calorie requirement comes from ethanol • They cease to eat adequately and develop nutritional deficiencies, especially of B-group vitamins and folate • Megalobastosis occurs
Hypertension	• Heavy chronic alcohol consumption is a common cause of hypertension • Hypertension is difficult to control in this circumstance
Abnormal lipid profile	• Moderate alcohol intake improves the HDL/LDL ratio • This may explain the protective effect on heart disease • Severe hypertriglyceridaemia may occur

Hyponatraemia	• Chronic alcoholism is frequently associated with significant hyponatraemia
	• Several mechanisms are important
	  – hypovolaemia
	  – severe hypotriglyceridaemia (pseudohyponatraemia)
	  – cerebral salt wasting
	  – reset osmostat syndrome
	  – beer potomania (large volume of beer and very little dietary sodium)

Psychosocial	• The effects of chronic alcohol use on family and personal life are profound, though outside the scope of this book
Reduced fertility	• Male fertility is reduced (lower testosterone, reduced sperm count and function) • Pregnancy is unlikely in alcoholic women with amenorrheoa due to liver injury • The spontaneous miscarriage rate doubles in second trimester by consumption of 1–2 units per day • The profound effects on developing fetus and baby are discussed in the text

The effects of chronic alcohol usage are summarised in Table 11.6. Reversal of all or most of the above effects is usual in early cases if alcohol is abandoned. In more advanced cases, the disease may be halted (except cancer), but in severe cases it may continue to progress. When wine rationing was introduced in Paris during the Second World War, deaths from hepatic cirrhosis dropped to about one-sixth of the previous level; 5 years after the war, they had regained their former level.

Car driving and alcohol

The effects of alcohol and psychotropic drugs on motor car driving have been the subject of well-deserved attention, and many countries have passed laws designed to prevent motor accidents caused by alcohol.

Alcohol is a factor in as many as 50% of motor accidents. For this reason, the compulsory use of a roadside breath test is acknowledged to be in the public interest. In the UK, having a blood concentration exceeding 80 mg alcohol per 100 mL blood (17.4 mmol/L)[8] while in charge of a car is a statutory offence. At this concentration, the liability to accident is about twice normal. Other countries set lower limits, e.g. Nordic countries,[9] some states of the USA, Australia, and Greece.

Where blood or breath analysis is not immediately available after an accident, it may be measured hours later and 'back calculated' to what it would have been at the time of the accident. It is usual to assume that the blood concentration falls at about 15 mg/100 mL/h. Naturally, the validity of such calculations leads to acrimonious disputes in the courts of law. (See also: Drugs and skilled tasks, p. 115.)

Alcohol-dependence syndrome

Alcohol dependence is a complex disorder with environmental, drug-induced and genetic components with multiple genes probably contributing to vulnerability to the condition. The major factors determining physical dependence are dose, frequency of dosing, and duration of abuse. Development involves alterations in CNS neurotransmission:

- *Acute* effect of alcohol appears to be blockade of NMDA receptors for which the normal agonist is glutamate, the main excitatory transmitter in the brain.
- *Chronic* exposure increases the number of (excitatory) NMDA receptors and also 'L type' calcium channels, while the action of the (inhibitory) GABA$_A$ neurotransmitter is reduced.
- *The resulting excitatory effects* may explain the anxiety, insomnia and craving that accompanies sudden withdrawal of alcohol (and may explain why resumption of drinking brings about relief, perpetuating dependence).

Withdrawal of alcohol

Abrupt withdrawal of alcohol from a person who has developed physical dependence, such as may occur when an ill or injured alcoholic is admitted to hospital, can precipitate withdrawal syndrome (agitation, anxiety and excess sympathetic autonomic activity) in 6–12 h. This may be followed by: alcohol withdrawal seizures (rum fits) in 6–48 h; alcoholic

hallucinosis (commonly visual) in 10–72 h; and delirium tremens in 3–7 days. Mortality from the last is high.

Generally, withdrawal should be supervised in hospital. Fixed-dose regimens have been traditionally used where patients received *chlordiazepoxide* by mouth, 10–50 mg four times daily, gradually reducing over 7–14 days. Due to the risk of over- or under-prescribing, increasingly symptom-triggered prescribing is used to facilitate the inpatient detoxification. Longer exposure to chlordiazepoxide should be avoided as it has the potential to induce dependence. A β-adrenoceptor blocker may be given to attenuate symptoms of sympathetic overactivity. General aspects of care, e.g. attention to fluid and electrolyte balance, are important.

It is usual to administer vitamins, especially thiamine, in which alcoholics are commonly deficient, and intravenous glucose unaccompanied by thiamine may precipitate Wernicke's encephalopathy.

Clomethiazole is an alternative, also for inpatient use, but it carries significant risk of dependence and should not be given if the patient is likely to persist in drinking alcohol. It is now rarely used in the UK. Anticonvulsants, e.g. carbamazepine, topiramate, have also been used to alleviate symptoms of alcohol withdrawal.

Acute alcohol withdrawal with tremors, sweating and restlessness is common after abstinence in heavy habitual drinkers. Delirium tremens is less common and needs to be recognised early due to very high mortality if not correctly managed.

Treatment of alcohol dependence

Psychosocial support is more important than drugs, which nevertheless may help.

Acamprosate chemically similar to both glutamate and GABA$_A$ appears to reduce the effect of excitatory amino acids such as glutamate, and modifies GABA$_A$ neurotransmission during withdrawal. If taken for 1 year (accompanied by counselling and psychosocial support), acamprosate increases the number of alcohol-free days and also the chance of subsequent complete abstinence. The benefit may last for 1 year after stopping treatment.

Acamprosate may cause diarrhoea, and cutaneous eruptions.

Disulfiram (Antabuse) discourages drinking by inducing immediate unpleasantness. It is an aldehyde dehydrogenase inhibitor, so that acetaldehyde (a toxic metabolite of alcohol) accumulates. It should be administered only under specialist supervision. A typical reaction of medium severity comes on about 5 min after taking alcohol and consists of generalised vasodilatation and fall in blood pressure, sweating, dyspnoea, headache, chest pain, nausea and vomiting. These

---

[8]Approximately equivalent to 35 μg alcohol in 100 mL expired air (or 107 mg in 100 mL urine). In practice, prosecutions are undertaken only when the concentration is significantly higher to avoid arguments about biological variability and instrumental error. Urine concentrations are little used, as the urine is accumulated over time and does not provide the immediacy of blood and breath.

[9]In 1990, Sweden lowered the limit to 20 mg/100 mL, which has been approached by ingestion of glucose which becomes fermented by gut flora in some people – the 'autobrewery' syndrome.

features may result from even small amounts of alcohol (such as may be present in some oral medicines or mouthwashes).

Severe reactions include convulsions and circulatory collapse, and may last several hours. Some advocate the use of a test dose of alcohol under supervision (after the fifth day of taking), so that patients can be taught what to expect, and also to induce an aversion to alcohol.

There is clinical trial evidence for other drugs to assist with alcohol withdrawal. In particular, naltrexone (an opioid antagonist) is registered by the US Food and Drug Administration (FDA) for this indication, but not in the UK. This remains an extremely active area of research.

Safe limits for chronic consumption

These cannot be defined accurately. But both patients and non-patients justifiably expect some guidance, and doctors and government departments will wish to be helpful. They may reasonably advise, as a 'safe' or prudent maximum (there being no particular individual contraindication). The current guidelines by the UK Chief Medical officer (2016) recommends no more than 14 units per week for men and women.[10]

Consistent drinking of more than these amounts carries a progressive risk to health. In other societies, recommended maxima are higher or lower. Alcoholics with established cirrhosis have usually consumed about 23 units (230 mL; 184 g) daily for 10 years. Heavy drinkers may develop hepatic cirrhosis at a rate of about 2% per annum. The type of drink (beer, wine, spirits) is not particularly relevant to the adverse health consequences; a standard bottle of spirits (750 mL) contains 300 mL (240 g) of alcohol (i.e. 40% by volume). Most people cannot metabolise more than about 170 g/day. On the other hand, regular low alcohol consumption may confer benefit: up to one drink per day appears not to impair cognitive function in women and may actually decrease the risk of cognitive decline,[11] and light-to-moderate alcohol consumption may reduce risk of dementia in people 55 years of age or older.[12]

The curve that relates mortality (vertical axis) to alcoholic drink consumption (horizontal axis) is J-shaped. As consumption rises above zero the all-cause mortality declines, then levels off, and then progressively rises. The benefit is largely a reduction of deaths due to cardiovascular and cerebrovascular disease for regular drinkers of 1–2 units per day for men older than 40 years of age and postmenopausal women. Consuming more than 2 units per day does not provide any major additional health benefit. The mechanism may be an improvement in lipoprotein (HDL/LDL) profiles and changes in haemostatic factors.[13] The effect appears to be due mainly to ethanol itself, but non-ethanol ingredients (antioxidants, phenols, flavinoids) may contribute. The rising (adverse) arm of the curve is associated with known harmful effects of alcohol (already described), but also, for example, with pneumonia (which may be secondary to direct alcohol effects, or with the increased smoking of alcohol users).

Alcohol in pregnancy and breast feeding

There is no level of maternal consumption that can be guaranteed safe for the fetus, and fetal injury can occur early in pregnancy (4–10 weeks), often before the pregnancy has been diagnosed (usually 3–8 weeks). The current advice in the UK is therefore that women should abstain from alcohol if they are pregnant or intending to become pregnant. The mechanisms by which alcohol exerts its toxicity on the fetus are complex and involve both ethanol and its metabolite acetaldehyde.

In addition to the fetal alcohol syndrome, there is general fetal/embryonic growth retardation (1% for every 10 g alcohol per day), and this is not 'caught up' later.

Fetal alcohol syndrome is a term that covers a spectrum of disorders;[14] it includes the following characteristics: microcephaly, mental retardation, low body-weight, poor coordination, hypotonia, small eyeballs and short palpebral fissures, lack of nasal bridge.[15]

Children of about 10% of alcohol abusers may show the syndrome. In women consuming 12 units of alcohol per day, the incidence may be as high as 30%.

Lactation. Even small amounts of alcohol taken by the mother delay motor development in the child; an effect on mental development is uncertain.

There is no 'safe' level of alcohol consumption in pregnancy.

---

[10]Report of an Inter-Departmental Working Group 1995 Sensible Drinking. Department of Health, London.
[11]Stampfer M J, Kang J H, Chen J et al 2005 Effects of moderate alcohol consumption on cognitive function in women. New England Journal of Medicine 352:245–253.
[12]Ruitenberg A, van Swieten J C, Witteman J C M et al 2002 Alcohol consumption and the risk of dementia: the Rotterdam study. Lancet 359:281–286.

[13]Rimm E B, Williams P, Fosher K et al 1999 Moderate alcohol intake and lower risk of coronary heart disease: meta-analysis of effects on lipids and haemostatic factors. British Medical Journal 319:1523–1528.
[14]Mukherjee R A S, Hollins A, Turk J 2006 Fetal alcohol spectrum disorder: an overview. Journal of the Royal Society of Medicine 99:298–302.
[15]For pictures see Streissguth A P, Clarren S K, Jones K L 1985 Natural history of the fetal alcohol syndrome: a 10-year follow-up of eleven patients. Lancet ii:85–91.

Table 11.7 Important interactions of alcohol with other drugs

Drug class	Example	Comments
Antibiotics	Metronidazole, trimethoprim, cephalosporins	Disulfuram-like action resulting in facial flushing, headaches, tachycardia and feinting
Vasodilators	GTN	Increased adverse effects with risk of hypotension and falls
Opioid analgesics	Morphine	Exacerbation of adverse effects with increased sedation
Non-steroidal anti-inflammatory agents	Ibuprofen, naproxen	Increased risk of GI ulceration and bleeding
Hypoglycaemic agents	Insulin, sulphonylureas	Increased hypoglycaemic risk
Anticoagulants	Warfarin	Acute alcohol ingestion inhibits metabolism and increases bleeding risk Chronic administration induces metabolism and reduces efficacy
Anticonvulsants	Phenytoin	Acute alcohol ingestion increases availability and side-effect profile Chronic administration induces metabolism and can increase seizure frequency
Anaesthetics	Propofol	Chronic alcohol ingestion results in resistance to effects of anaesthetic agents such that increased doses are required. Chronic consumption may increase risk of liver damage from halothane and enflurane
Tricyclic antidepressants	Amitriptyline	Acute and chronic ingestion can increase availability and worsen sedation and side effects

Alcohol and other drugs

The important interactions of alcohol with other drugs are shown in Table 11.7.

Miscellaneous uses of alcohol

- Used as a skin antiseptic, 70% by weight (76% by volume) is most effective. Stronger solutions are less effective.
- Alcohol injections are sometimes used to destroy nervous tissue in cases of intractable pain (trigeminal neuralgia, carcinoma involving nerves).
- As a treatment in ethylene glycol (antifreeze) poisoning.

Other cerebral depressants

Alcohol, benzodiazepines, clomethiazole and barbiturates broadly possess the common action of influencing GABA neurotransmission through the $GABA_A$–benzodiazepine receptor complex (see p. 353 and Fig. 20.5) and all readily induce tolerance and dependence.

γ-Hydroxybutyrate (GHB) is a metabolite of GABA, the major inhibitory transmitter in the CNS. It acts by binding to GABA receptors but additionally affects dopamine, serotonin and endogenous systems. It has euphoric and sedative effects and is popular at dance parties where it has achieved notoriety as a 'date-rape drug'. It is highly addictive, and frequent ingestion may induce dependency and a severe withdrawal state.

Benzodiazepine dependence is discussed on page 353.

Clomethiazole and barbiturate are now rarely used, and accordingly opportunity for abuse is limited.

Tobacco

In 1492, the explorer Christopher Columbus observed Native Americans using the dried leaves of the tobacco plant (later named *Nicotiana*[16]) for pleasure and also to treat ailments.

---

[16]After the French diplomat, Jean Nicot de Villemain, who introduced tobacco to Europe.

Following its introduction to Europe in the 16th century, tobacco enjoyed popularity to the extent of being considered a panacea, being called 'holy herb' and 'God's remedy'.[17] Only relatively recently have the harmful effects of tobacco come to light, notably from mortality studies among British doctors.[18] Current estimates hold that there are more than 1 billion smokers worldwide. In 1990 there were 3 million smoking-related deaths per year, projected to reach 10 million by 2030.[19]

Composition

Tobacco smoke is complex (over 4000 compounds have been identified) and varies with the type of tobacco and the way it is smoked. The chief pharmacologically active ingredients are nicotine, responsible for acute effects (1–2 mg per cigarette); tars, responsible for chronic effects (10–15 mg per cigarette). Amounts of both can vary greatly (even for the same brand) depending on the country in which cigarettes are sold.

Smoke of cigars and pipes is alkaline (pH 8.5). Nicotine is relatively un-ionised at this pH, and is readily absorbed in the mouth. Cigar and pipe smokers thus obtain nicotine without inhaling, and thus have a lower death rate from lung cancer, which is caused by non-nicotine constituents.

Smoke of cigarettes is acidic (pH 5.3). Nicotine is relatively ionised and insoluble in lipids. Desired amounts are absorbed only if nicotine is taken into the lungs, where the enormous surface area for absorption compensates for the lower lipid solubility. Cigarette smokers therefore inhale (and have a high rate of death from tar-induced lung cancer). The amount of nicotine absorbed from tobacco smoke varies from 90% in those who inhale to 10% in those who do not. Smoke drawn through the tobacco and taken in by the smoker is known as main-stream smoke; smoke that arises from smouldering tobacco and passes directly into the surrounding air is known as side-stream smoke. These differ in composition, partly because of the different temperatures at which they are produced. Side-stream smoke constitutes about 85% of smoke generated in an average room during cigarette smoking.

Environmental tobacco smoke has been classified as a known human carcinogen in the USA since 1992.[20] Although the risks of such 'passive' smoking are naturally smaller, the number of people affected is large. One study estimated that breathing other people's smoke increases a person's risk of ischaemic heart disease by one-quarter.[21] Tobacco smoke contains 1–5% carbon monoxide, and habitual smokers have 3–7% (heavy smokers as much as 15%) of their haemoglobin as carboxyhaemoglobin, which cannot carry oxygen. This is sufficient to reduce exercise capacity in patients with angina pectoris. Chronic carboxyhaemoglobinaemia causes polycythaemia (which increases the viscosity of the blood). Substances carcinogenic to animals (polycyclic hydrocarbons and nicotine-derived N-nitrosamines) have been identified in tobacco smoke condensates from cigarettes, cigars and pipes. Polycyclic hydrocarbons are responsible for the hepatic enzyme induction that occurs in smokers.

Tobacco dependence

The immediate satisfaction of smoking is due to nicotine and also to tars, which provide flavour. Initially the factors are psychosocial; pharmacodynamic effects are unpleasant. But under the psychosocial pressures the subject continues, learns to limit and adjust nicotine intake, so that the pleasant pharmacological effects of nicotine develop and tolerance to the adverse effects occurs. Thus to the psychosocial pressure is now added pharmacological pleasure.

Nicotine possesses all the characteristics of a drug of dependence:

- It modulates dopamine activity in the midbrain, particularly in the mesolimbic system, which promotes the development and maintenance of reward behaviour.
- Nicotine inhaled in cigarette smoke reaches the brain in 10–19 s.
- Short elimination $t_{1/2}$ requires regular smoking to maintain the effect.
- Inhaling cigarette smoke is thus an ideal drug delivery system to institute behavioural reinforcement and then dependence.

A report on the subject concludes that most smokers do not do so from choice but because they are addicted to nicotine.[22]

Tolerance and some physical dependence occur. Transient withdrawal effects include EEG and sleep changes, impaired performance in some psychomotor tests, disturbance of mood and increased appetite (with weight gain). It is, however, difficult to disentangle psychological from physical effects in these last effects.

[17]Dickson S A 1954 Panacea or Precious Bane. Tobacco in 16th Century Literature. New York Public Library, New York. Quoted in: Charlton A 2004 Medicinal uses of tobacco in history. Journal of the Royal Society of Medicine 97:292–296.
[18]Doll R, Hill A B 1954 The mortality of doctors in relation to their smoking habits. British Medical Journal i:1451–1455.
[19]Peto R, Lopez A D, Boreham A et al 1996 Mortality from smoking worldwide. British Medical Bulletin 52:12–21.
[20]Environmental Protection Agency (EPA 1992A/600/6–90/006 F).

[21]Law M R, Morris J K, Wald N J 1997 Environmental tobacco smoke exposure and ischaemic heart disease: an evaluation of the evidence. British Medical Journal 315:973–988.
[22]Tobacco Advisory Group, Royal College of Physicians 2000 Nicotine Addiction in Britain. Royal College of Physicians, London.

Nicotine shows all the characteristics of a drug of dependence with both tolerance and some physical dependence.

Acute effects of smoking tobacco

- Increased airways resistance occurs due to the non-specific effects of submicronic particles, e.g. carbon particles less than 1 micrometre across. The effect is reflex: even inert particles of this size cause bronchial narrowing sufficient to double airways resistance; this is insufficient to cause dyspnoea, though it might affect athletic performance. Pure nicotine inhalations of concentration comparable to that reached in smoking do not increase airways resistance.
- Ciliary activity, after transient stimulation, is depressed, and particles are removed from the lungs more slowly.
- Carbon monoxide absorption may be clinically important in the presence of coronary heart disease (see above), although it is physiologically insignificant in healthy young adults.

Nicotine pharmacology

Pharmacokinetics

Nicotine is absorbed through mucous membranes in a highly pH-dependent fashion. The $t_{1/2}$ is 2 h. It is metabolised largely by P450 (CYP) 2A6 to inert substances, e.g. cotinine, although some is excreted unchanged in the urine (pH dependent, it is un-ionised at acid pH). Cotinine is used as a marker for nicotine intake in smoking surveys because of its conveniently long $t_{1/2}$ (20 h).

Pharmacodynamics

Large doses[23]. Nicotine is an agonist to receptors at the ends of peripheral cholinergic nerves whose cell bodies lie

in the CNS: i.e. it acts at autonomic ganglia and at the voluntary neuromuscular junction (see Fig. 22.1). This is what is meant by the term 'nicotine-like' or 'nicotinic' effect. Higher doses paralyse at the same points. The CNS is stimulated, including the vomiting centre, both directly and via chemoreceptors in the carotid body. Tremors and convulsions may occur. As with the peripheral actions, depression follows stimulation.

Doses from/with smoking. Nicotine causes release of CNS catecholamines, serotonin, antidiuretic hormone, corticotropin and growth hormone. The effects of nicotine on viscera are probably largely reflex, from stimulation of sensory receptors (chemoreceptors) in the carotid and aortic bodies, pulmonary circulation and left ventricle. Some of the results are mutually antagonistic.

The following account tells what generally happens after one cigarette, from which about 1 mg of nicotine is absorbed, although much depends on the amount and depth of inhalation and on the duration of end-inspiratory breath-holding.

On the *cardiovascular system* the effects are those of sympathetic autonomic stimulation. There is vasoconstriction in the skin and vasodilatation in the muscles, tachycardia and a rise in blood pressure of about 15 mmHg systolic and 10 mmHg diastolic, and increased plasma noradrenaline/ norepinephrine. Ventricular extrasystoles may occur. Cardiac output, work and oxygen consumption rise. Nicotine increases platelet adhesiveness, an effect that may be clinically significant in the development of atheroma and thrombosis.

Metabolic rate. Nicotine increases the metabolic rate only slightly at rest,[24] but approximately doubles it during light exercise (occupational tasks, housework). This may be due to increase in autonomic sympathetic activity. The effect declines over 24 h on stopping smoking and accounts for the characteristic weight gain that is so disliked and which is sometimes given as a reason for continuing or resuming smoking. Smokers weigh 2–4 kg less than non-smokers (not enough to be a health issue).

Tolerance develops to some of the effects of nicotine, taken repeatedly over a few hours; a first experience commonly causes nausea and vomiting, which quickly ceases with repetition of smoking. Tolerance is usually rapidly lost; the first cigarette of the day has a greater effect on the cardiovascular system than do subsequent cigarettes.

Conclusion. The pleasurable effects of smoking are derived from a complex mixture of multiple pharmacological and non-pharmacological factors.

In this account, nicotine is represented as being the major (but not the sole) determinant of tobacco dependence after the smoker has adapted to the usual initial unpleasant effects.

---

[23]Fatal nicotine poisoning has been reported from smoking, from swallowing tobacco, from tobacco enemas, from topical application to the skin and from accidental drinking of nicotine insecticide preparations. In 1932 a florist sat down on a chair, on the seat of which a 40% free nicotine insecticide solution had been spilled. Fifteen minutes later he felt ill (vomiting, sweating, faintness and respiratory difficulty, followed by loss of consciousness and cardiac irregularity). He recovered in hospital over about 24 h. On the fourth day he was deemed well enough to leave hospital and was given his clothes, which had been kept in a paper bag. He noticed the trousers were still damp. Within 1 h of leaving hospital he had to be readmitted, suffering again from poisoning due to nicotine absorbed transdermally from his still contaminated trousers. He recovered over 3 weeks, apart from persistent ventricular extrasystoles (Faulkner J M 1933 Journal of the American Medical Association 100:1663).

---

[24]The metabolic rate at rest accounts for about 70% of daily energy expenditure.

But there remains some uncertainty as to its role, e.g. intravenous nicotine fails adequately to substitute the effects of smoking. An understanding of the full function of nicotine is important if less harmful alternatives to smoking, such as nicotine chewing gum, are to be exploited.

Effects of chronic smoking

Bronchogenic carcinoma

- The risk of death from lung cancer is related to the number of cigarettes smoked and the age of starting.
- It is similar between smokers of medium (15–21 mg), low (8–14 mg) and very low (<0.5 mg) tar cigarettes.
- Giving up smoking reduces the risk of death progressively from the time of cessation.[25]

Other cancers. The risk of smokers developing cancer of the mouth, throat and oesophagus is 5–10 times greater than that of non-smokers. It is as great for pipe and cigar smokers as it is for cigarette smokers. Cancer of the pancreas, kidney and urinary tract is also commoner in smokers.

Coronary heart disease (CHD). In the UK about 30% of CHD deaths can be attributed to smoking. Sudden death may be the first manifestation of CHD and, especially in young men, is related to cigarette smoking. Smoking is especially dangerous for people in whom other risk factors (raised blood cholesterol, high blood pressure) are present. Atherosclerotic narrowing of the smallest coronary arteries is enormously increased in heavy and even in moderate smokers; the increased platelet adhesiveness caused by smoking increases the readiness with which thrombi form. Stopping smoking reduces the excess risk of CHD in people younger than 65 years of age, and after about 4 years of abstinence the risk approximates to that of non-smokers.

Chronic lung disease. The adverse effects of cigarette smoke on the lungs may be separated into two distinct conditions:

- *Chronic mucus hypersecretion*, which causes persistent cough with sputum and fits with the original definition of simple chronic bronchitis. This condition arises chiefly in the large airways, usually clears up when the subject stops smoking and does not on its own carry any substantial risk of death.
- *Chronic obstructive lung disease*, which causes difficulty in breathing chiefly due to narrowing of the small airways, includes a variable element of destruction of peripheral lung units (emphysema), is progressive and largely irreversible and may ultimately lead to disability and death.

Both conditions can coexist in one person, and they predispose to recurrent acute infective illnesses.

Other effects. About 120 000 men in the UK 30–50 years of age are impotent because of smoking.[26]

Interactions with drug therapy. Induction of hepatic drug metabolising enzymes by non-nicotine constituents of smoke causes increased metabolism of a range of drugs, including oestrogens, theophylline and warfarin.

Women and smoking

Fertility. Women who smoke are more likely to be infertile or take longer to conceive than women who do not smoke:

- Smokers are more liable to have an earlier menopause than are non-smokers.
- Increased metabolism of oestrogens may not be the whole explanation.

Complications of pregnancy

- The risks of spontaneous abortion, stillbirth and neonatal death are approximately doubled.
- The placenta is heavier in smoking than non-smoking women, and its diameter larger, possibly from adaptations to lack of oxygen due to smoking, secondary to raised concentrations of circulating carboxyhaemoglobin.

The child

- The babies of women who smoke are approximately 200 g lighter than those of women who do not smoke.
- They have an increased risk of death in the perinatal period which is independent of other variables such as social class, level of education, age of mother, race or extent of antenatal care.
- The increased risk rises two-fold or more in heavy smokers and appears to be accounted for entirely by the placental abnormalities and the consequences of low birth-weight.
- Ex-smokers and women who give up smoking in the first 20 weeks of pregnancy have offspring whose birth-weight is similar to that of the children of women who have never smoked.

Starting and stopping use

Contrary to popular belief, it is not generally difficult to stop, with only 14% finding it 'very difficult'. But ex-smoker

---

[25]Peto R, Darby S, Deo H et al 2000 Smoking, smoking cessation and lung cancer in the UK since 1950: combination of national statistics with two case–control studies. British Medical Journal 321:323–329.

[26]Smoking and Reproductive Life: The Impact of Smoking on Sexual, Reproductive and Child Health. Available at: http://www.bma.org.uk (accessed 27 October 2011).

status is unstable, and the long-term success rate of a smoking withdrawal clinic is rarely above 30%. The situation is summed up by the witticism, 'Giving up smoking is easy, I've done it many times'.

Though they are as aware of the risks of smoking as men, women find it harder to stop; they have consistently lower success rates. This trend crosses every age group and occupation. Women particularly dislike the weight gain.

Aids to giving up

For those smoking more than 10 cigarettes per day, nicotine replacement and bupropion can provide effective therapy, particularly if supported by access to a smoking cessation clinic for behavioural support. Ideally, smoking should stop completely before embarking on a cessation regimen.

Nicotine is principally responsible for the addictive effects of tobacco smoking, and is therefore a logical pharmacological aid to quitting. It is available in a number of formulations, including chewing gum, transdermal patch, oral and nasal spray. When used casually without special attention to technique, nicotine formulations have proved no better than other aids, but if used carefully and withdrawn as recommended, the accumulated results are almost two times better than in smokers who try to stop without this assistance.[27]

Restlessness during terminal illness may be due to nicotine withdrawal and go unrecognised; a nicotine patch may benefit a (deprived) heavy smoker. Nicotine transdermal patches may cause nightmares and abnormal dreaming, and skin reactions (rash, pruritus and 'burning' at the application site).

Bupropion may provide an alternative, or addition, to nicotine. When the drug was being investigated as an antidepressant, researchers noticed that patients gave up smoking, and it was developed as an aid to smoking cessation. Bupropion selectively inhibits neuronal uptake of noradrenaline/norepinephrine and dopamine, and may reduce nicotine craving by an action on the mesolimbic system. Evidence suggests that bupropion may be at least as effective as the nicotine patch, with which it may usefully be combined. It may cause dry mouth and insomnia. It is contraindicated in patients with a history of eating disorder or epilepsy or who are experiencing acute symptoms of alcohol or benzodiazepine withdrawal; where potential for seizure exists, e.g. use of drugs that lower the seizure threshold, this hazard must be weighed against the possible benefits of smoking cessation.

---

[27]Lancaster T, Stead L, Silagy C, Sowden A 2000 Effectiveness of interventions to help people to stop smoking: findings from the Cochrane Library. British Medical Journal 321:355–358.

If the patient is heavily tobacco-dependent and severe anxiety, irritability, headache, insomnia and weight gain (about 3 kg) and tension are concomitants of attempts to stop smoking, an anxiolytic sedative (or β-adrenoceptor blocker) may be useful for a short time, but it is important to avoid substituting one drug dependence for another.

Electronic cigarettes are devices that electrically heat a liquid to produce an aerosol that is then inhaled. The liquid is principally propylene glycol and glycerol to which a flavouring is added with or without nicotine. Their use has increased significantly in recent years by those seeking to stop smoking. There is an emerging consensus that these devices are less detrimental to health than cigarette smoking. They have not been rigorously evaluated in terms of their effectiveness in large clinical trials, but limited evidence does indicate that they reduce smoking rates. Some groups remain opposed to their use on the basis of safety and the risk of such 'e-cigarettes' acting as a bridge to smoking in young people.

Psychodysleptics or hallucinogens

These substances produce mental changes that resemble those of some psychotic states in which the subject experiences hallucinations or illusions, i.e. disturbance of perception with the apparent awareness of sights, sounds and smells that are not actually present.

Experiences with these drugs vary greatly with the subject's expectations, existing frame of mind and personality and environment. Subjects can be prepared so that they are more likely to have a good 'trip' than a bad one.

Experiences with psychodysleptics

The following brief account of experiences with LSD (lysergic acid diethylamide, lysergide) in normal subjects will serve as a model. Experiences with mescaline and psilocybin are similar.

Vision may become blurred, and there may be hallucinations; these generally do not occur in the blind and are fewer if the subject is blindfolded. Objects appear distorted, and trivial things, e.g. a mark on a wall, may change shape and acquire special significance. Auditory acuity increases, but hallucinations are uncommon. Subjects who do not ordinarily appreciate music may suddenly come to do so. Foods may feel coarse and gritty in the mouth. Limbs may be left in uncomfortable positions. Time may seem to stop or to pass slowly, but usually it gets faster and thousands of years may seem suddenly to go by. The subject may feel relaxed and supremely happy, or may become fearful or depressed. Feelings of depersonalisation and dreamy states occur.

The experience lasts for a few hours, depending on the dose; intervals of normality then occur and become progressively longer.

Somatic symptoms and signs include nausea, dizziness, paraesthesiae, weakness, drowsiness, tremors, dilated pupils, ataxia. Effects on the cardiovascular system and respiration vary and probably reflect fluctuating anxiety.

Lysergide (LSD)

Lysergic acid is a semi-synthetic drug belonging to the ergoline family. An effective oral dose is about 30 µg. The $t_{1/2}$ is 3 h. (See description of experience, above.) Its mechanisms of action are complex and include agonist effect at pre-synaptic 5-HT receptors in the CNS. Tachyphylaxis (acute tolerance) occurs to LSD. Psychological dependence may occur, but physical dependence does not occur. Serious adverse effects include psychotic reactions (which can be delayed in onset) with suicide.

Mescaline is an alkaloid from the Mexican peyote cactus. It does not induce serious dependence, and the drug has little importance except to members of some North and Central American societies and to psychiatrists and biochemists who are interested in the mechanism of induced psychotic states.

Psilocybin is derived from varieties of the fungus *Psilocybe* ('magic mushrooms') that grow in many countries. It is related to LSD.

Tenamfetamine (ecstasy, MDMA: methylenedioxymethamfetamine) is structurally related to both mescaline and amfetamine. It has a $t_{1/2}$ of about 8 h. It is popular as a dance drug at 'rave' parties. An estimated 5% of the American adult population have used tenamfetamine at least once.[28] Popular names reflect the appearance of the tablets and capsules and include White Dove, White Burger, Red and Black, Denis the Menace. Tenamfetamine stimulates central and peripheral α- and β-adrenoceptors; thus the pharmacological effects are compounded by those of physical exertion, dehydration and heat.

In susceptible individuals (poor metabolisers who exhibit the CYP450 2D6 polymorphism), a severe and fatal idiosyncratic reaction may occur with fulminant hyperthermia, convulsions, disseminated intravascular coagulation, rhabdomyolysis, and acute renal and hepatic failure. Treatment includes activated charcoal, diazepam for convulsions, β-blockade (atenolol) for tachycardia, α-blockade (phentolamine) for hypertension, and dantrolene if the rectal temperature exceeds 39°C. In chronic users, positive emission tomographic (PET) brain scans show selective dysfunction of serotonergic neurones, raising concerns that neurodegenerative changes accompany long-term use of MDMA.[29]

Phencyclidine ('angel dust') is structurally related to pethidine. It induces analgesia without unconsciousness, but with amnesia, in humans (dissociative anaesthesia, see p. 314). It acts as an antagonist at NMDA glutamate receptors. It can be insufflated as a dry powder or smoked (cigarettes are dipped in phencyclidine dissolved in an organics solvent). Phencyclidine overdose can cause agitation, abreactions, hallucinations and psychosis, and if severe can result in seizures, coma, hyperthermia, muscular rigidity and rhabdomyolysis.

Ketamine (K, special K) has similar effects to those of phencyclidine. It is used as a short-acting general anaesthetic. It can be injected as liquid or inhaled as powder or swallowed as tablet. It is an NMDA antagonist. It induces perceptual changes and hallucinations similar to LSD, and in addition induces dissociative analgesia, with consequent risk of serious injury. Nausea, vomiting and risk of death can result from inhalation of vomitus. It has been used as a date-rape drug. There is increasing evidence that it can cause serious long-term bladder damage.

Methylxanthines (xanthines)

The three xanthines, *caffeine, theophylline* and *theobromine*, occur in plants. They are qualitatively similar but differ markedly in potency:

* Tea contains caffeine and theophylline.
* Coffee contains caffeine.
* Cocoa and chocolate contain caffeine and theobromine.
* The cola nut ('cola' drinks) contains caffeine.
* Theobromine is weak and of no clinical importance (although responsible for the toxicity of chocolate when ingested by dogs).

Pharmacokinetics. Absorption of xanthines after oral or rectal administration varies with the preparation used. It is generally extensive (>95%). Caffeine metabolism varies much among individuals ($t_{1/2}$ 2–12 h). Xanthines are metabolised (>90%) by numerous mixed-function oxidase enzymes, and xanthine oxidase. (For further details on theophylline, see Asthma.)

---

[28]Roehr B 2005 Half a million Americans use methamfetamine every week. British Medical Journal 332:476.

[29]In an extreme usage, a man was estimated to have taken about 40 000 tablets of ecstasy between the ages of 21 and 30 years. At maximum he took 25 pills per day for 4 years. At age 37 years, and after 7 years off the drug, he was experiencing paranoia, hallucinations, depression, severe short-term memory loss, and painful muscle rigidity around the neck and jaw. Several of these features were thought to be permanent. (Kouimtsidis C 2006 Neurological and psychopathological sequelae associated with a lifetime intake of 40 000 ecstasy tablets. Psychosomatics 47:86–87.)

Pharmacodynamics. Caffeine and theophylline have complex and incompletely elucidated actions, which include inhibition of phosphodiesterase (the enzyme that breaks down cyclic AMP, see pp. 494, 502), effects on intracellular calcium distribution, and on noradrenergic function.

Actions on mental performance. Caffeine is more potent than theophylline, but both drugs stimulate mental activity where it is below normal. Thought is more rapid and fatigue is removed or its onset delayed. The effects on mental and physical performance vary according to the mental state and personality of the subject. Reaction time is decreased. Performance that is inferior because of excessive anxiety may become worse. Caffeine can also improve physical performance, both in tasks requiring more physical effort than skill (athletics) and in tasks requiring more skill than physical effort (monitoring instruments and taking corrective action in an aircraft flight simulator). In general, caffeine induces feelings of alertness and well-being, euphoria or exhilaration. Onset of boredom, fatigue, inattentiveness and sleepiness is postponed.

Overdose will certainly reduce performance (see Chronic overdose, below). Acute overdose, e.g. intravenous aminophylline, can cause convulsions, hypotension, cardiac arrhythmia and sudden death.

Other effects

Respiratory stimulation occurs with substantial doses.

Sleep. Caffeine affects sleep of older people more than it does that of younger people. Onset of sleep (sleep latency) is delayed, bodily movements are increased, total sleep time is reduced and there are increased awakenings. Tolerance to this effect does not occur, as is shown by the provision of decaffeinated coffee.[30]

Skeletal muscle. Metabolism is increased, and this may play a part in the enhanced athletic performance mentioned above. There is significant improvement of diaphragmatic function in chronic obstructive pulmonary disease.

Cardiovascular system. Both caffeine and theophylline directly stimulate the myocardium and cause increased cardiac output, tachycardia, and sometimes ectopic beats and palpitations. This effect occurs almost at once after intravenous injection and lasts for half an hour. Theophylline contributes usefully to the relief of acute left ventricular failure. There is peripheral (but not cerebral) vasodilatation due to a direct action of the drugs on the blood vessels, but stimulation of the vasomotor centre tends to counter this.

Changes in the blood pressure are therefore somewhat unpredictable, but caffeine 250 mg (single dose) usually causes a transient rise of blood pressure of about 14/10 mmHg in occasional coffee drinkers (but has no additional effect in habitual drinkers); this effect can be used advantageously in patients with autonomic nervous system failure who experience postprandial hypotension (two cups of coffee with breakfast may suffice for the day). In occasional coffee drinkers two cups of coffee (about 160 mg caffeine) per day raise blood pressure by 5/4 mmHg. Increased coronary artery blood flow may occur but increased cardiac work counterbalances this in angina pectoris.

When theophylline (aminophylline) is given intravenously, slow injection is essential in order to avoid transient peak concentrations which are equivalent to administering an overdose (below).

Smooth muscle (other than vascular muscle, which is discussed above) is relaxed. The only important clinical use for this action is in reversible airways obstruction (asthma), when the action of theophylline can be a very valuable addition to therapy.

Kidney. Diuresis occurs in normal people chiefly due to reduced tubular reabsorption of sodium, similar to thiazide action, but weaker.

Preparations and uses of caffeine and theophylline

Aminophylline. The most generally useful preparation is aminophylline, which is a soluble, irritant salt of theophylline with ethylenediamine (see Asthma, below).

Attempts to make non-irritant, orally reliable preparations of theophylline have resulted in choline theophyllinate and numerous variants. Sustained-release formulations are convenient for asthmatics, but they cannot be assumed to be bio-equivalent, and repeat prescriptions should adhere to the formulation of a particular manufacturer. Suppositories are available. Aminophylline is used in the following conditions:

* Asthma. In severe asthma (given intravenously) when β-adrenoceptor agonists fail to give adequate response; and for chronic asthma (orally) to provide a background bronchodilator effect.
* Neonatal apnoea; caffeine is also effective.

Caffeine is used as an additional ingredient in analgesic tablets; about 60 mg potentiates the effects of NSAIDs; also as an aid in hypotension of autonomic failure (above) and to enhance oral ergotamine absorption in migraine.

Xanthine-containing drinks (see also above)

Coffee, tea and cola drinks in excess can make people tense and anxious. Epidemiological studies indicate either no, or only slight, increased risk (two- to three-fold) of coronary heart disease in heavy (including decaffeinated) coffee

---

[30]The European Union regulations define 'decaffeinated' as coffee (bean) containing 0.3% or less of caffeine (normal content 1–3%).

consumers (more than four cups daily) (see Blood Lipids, below). Slight tolerance to the effects of caffeine (on all systems) occurs. Withdrawal symptoms, attributable to psychological and perhaps mild physical dependence, occur in habitual coffee drinkers (five or more cups/day) 12–16 h after the last cup; they include headache (lasting up to 6 days), irritability and jitteriness; they may occur with transient changes in intake, e.g. high at work, lower at the weekend.

Chronic overdose. Excessive prolonged consumption of caffeine causes anxiety, restlessness, tremors, insomnia, headache, cardiac extrasystoles and confusion. The cause can easily be overlooked if specific enquiry into habits is not made, including children regarding cola drinks. Of coffee drinkers, up to 25% who complain of anxiety may benefit from reduction of caffeine intake. An adult heavy user may be defined as one who takes more than 300 mg caffeine per day, i.e. four cups of 150 mL of brewed coffee, each containing 80 ± 20 mg caffeine per cup or five cups (60 ± 20 mg) of instant coffee. The equivalent for tea would be 10 cups at approximately 30 mg caffeine per cup; and of cola drinks about 2 L. Plainly, caffeine drinks brewed to personal taste of consumer or vendor must have an extremely variable concentration according to source of coffee or tea, amount used, method and duration of brewing. There is also great individual variation in the effect of coffee both among individuals and sometimes in the same individual at different times of life (see Sleep, above).

Decaffeinated coffee contains about 3 mg per cup; cola drinks contain 8–13 mg caffeine per 100 mL; cocoa as a drink, 4 mg per cup; chocolate (solid) 6–20 mg/30 g.

In *young people*, high caffeine intake has been linked to behaviour disorders, and a limit of 125 mg/L has been proposed for cola drinks.

Blood lipids. Drinking five cups of boiled coffee per day increases plasma total cholesterol by up to 10%; this does not occur with coffee made by simple filtration. Cessation of coffee drinking can reduce plasma cholesterol concentration in hypercholesterolaemic men.

Breast-fed infants may become sleepless and irritable if there is high maternal intake. Fetal cardiac arrhythmias have been reported with exceptionally high maternal caffeine intake, e.g. 1.5 L cola drinks per day.

Cannabis

Cannabis is obtained from the annual plant *Cannabis sativa* (hemp),[31] and its varieties *Cannabis indica* and *Cannabis americana*. The preparations that are smoked are called 'marijuana' (also 'grass', 'pot', 'weed') and consist of crushed

leaves and flowers. There is a wide variety of regional names, e.g. 'ganja' (India, Caribbean), 'kif' (Morocco), 'dagga' (Africa). The resin scraped off the plant is known as hashish (hash). The term 'cannabis' is used to include all the above preparations. As most preparations are illegally prepared, it is not surprising that they are impure and of variable potency. The plant grows wild in the Americas,[32] Africa and Asia. It can also be grown successfully in the open in the warmer southern areas of Britain. Some 27% of the adult UK population report having used cannabis in their lifetime.

Pharmacokinetics

Of the scores of chemical compounds that the resin contains, the most important are the oily cannabinoids, including tetrahydrocannabinol (THC), which is the main psychoactive ingredient. Samples of resin vary greatly in the amounts and proportions of these cannabinoids according to their country of origin. As the sample ages, its THC content declines. THC content of samples can vary from 8% to almost zero. Smoke from a cannabis cigarette (the usual mode of use is to inhale and hold the breath to allow maximum absorption) delivers 25–50% of the THC content to the respiratory tract. THC ($t_{1/2}$ 4 days) and other cannabinoids undergo extensive biotransformation in the body, yielding scores of metabolites, several of which are themselves psychoactive. They are extremely lipid-soluble and are stored in body fat from which they are slowly released.[33] Hepatic drug-metabolising enzymes are inhibited acutely but may also be induced by chronic use of crude preparations.

Pharmacodynamics

Cannabinoid CB_1-receptors (expressed by hypothalamic and peripheral neurones, e.g. sensory terminals in the gastro-intestinal tract, and by adipocytes) and CB_2-receptors (expressed only in the periphery by immune cells) together with their endogenous ligands (called 'endocannabinoids') are components of the *endocannabinoid neuromodulatory system*, which has a role in many physiological processes including food intake and energy homeostasis. Cannabinoids act as agonists at CB_1-receptors (mediating addictive effects) and CB_2-receptors. Understanding this system offers scope for developing novel drug therapies (see below).

---

[31]The term derives from cannabis grown for its fibers and used commercially to make, e.g. rope and textiles.

[32]The commonest pollen in the air of San Francisco, California, is said to be that of the cannabis plant, illegally cultivated.
[33]When a chronic user discontinues, cannabinoids remain detectable in the urine for an average of 4 weeks, and it can be as long as 11 weeks before 10 consecutive daily tests are negative (Ellis G M, Mann M A, Judson B A et al 1985 Excretion patterns of cannabinoid metabolites after last use in a group of chronic users. Clinical Pharmacology and Therapeutics 38(5):572–578).

Psychological reactions are very varied, being much influenced by the behaviour of the group. They commence within minutes of starting to smoke and last for 2–3 h. Euphoria is common and is believed to follow stimulation of the limbic system reward pathways causing release of dopamine from the nucleus accumbens (see common mechanism of drugs of dependence Fig. 11.1). There may be giggling or laughter which can seem pointless to an observer. Sensations become more vivid, especially visual, and contrast and intensity of colour can increase, although no change in acuity occurs. Size of objects and distance are distorted. Sense of time can disappear altogether, leaving a sometimes distressing sense of timelessness. Recent memory and selective attention are impaired; the beginning of a sentence may be forgotten before it is finished. The subject is very suggestible and easily distracted. Psychological tests such as mental arithmetic, digit-symbol substitution and pursuit meter tests show impairment. These effects may be accompanied by feelings of deep insight and truth. Memory defect may persist for weeks after abstinence. Once memory is impaired, concentration becomes less effective, because the object of attention is less well remembered. With this may go an insensitivity to danger or the consequences of actions. A striking phenomenon is the intermittent wavelike nature of these effects which affects mood, visual impressions, time sense, spatial sense and other functions.

The desired effects of cannabinoids, as of other psychodysleptics, depend not only on the expectation of the user and the dose, but also on the environmental situation and personality. Genial or revelatory experiences may indeed occur.

Cannabinoids and skilled tasks, e.g. car driving. General performance in both motor and psychological tests deteriorates, more in naïve than in experienced subjects. Effects may be similar to alcohol, but experiments in which the subjects are unaware that they are being tested (and so do not compensate voluntarily) are difficult to do, as with alcohol. In a placebo-controlled trial of airline pilots in a flight simulator, performance was impaired for up to 50 h after the pilots smoked a joint containing THC 20 mg (a relatively low dose by current standards).[34]

Uses

A therapeutic role has been suggested for cannabinoids in a variety of conditions including chronic pain, migraine headaches, muscle spasticity in multiple sclerosis or spinal cord injury, movement disorders, appetite stimulation in patients with AIDS, nausea and vomiting.

THC is currently available as *dronabinol,* a synthetic form and as *nabilone,* a synthetic analogue, and both are approved to alleviate chemotherapy-induced vomiting in patients who have shown inadequate response to conventional antiemetics, and AIDS-related wasting syndrome.

Issues of cannabis and cannabis-based medicines were the subject of a working party report[35] whose main conclusions were:

- Inhibition of cannabinoid action can be used to help obese patients to *lose weight.* The first of a new class of CB_1-receptor antagonists, rimonabant, reduced body-weight and improved cardiovascular risk factors (HDL-cholesterol, triglycerides, insulin resistance) in obese patients over 1 year.[36] It may cause nausea and depression and is contraindicated in pregnancy.
- In *neuropathic pain,* i.e. due to damaged neural tissue, data from well-controlled but limited duration trials suggest that THC is similar to codeine in potency, is safe and is not associated with tolerance or dependence.
- Cannabinoids regulate bone mass, and cannabinoid receptor antagonists may have a role in the treatment of osteoporosis.
- Data on the value of cannabis preparations for multiple sclerosis are not conclusive, although there is some support for a therapeutic effect.

Adverse effects

Acute

The *psychological* effects can be unpleasant, especially in inexperienced subjects. These are: timelessness and the feeling of loss of control of mental processes; feelings of unease, sometimes amounting to anguish and acute panic; 'flashbacks' of previously experienced hallucinations, e.g. on LSD. The effect of an acute dose usually ends in drowsiness and sleep. Increase in appetite is commonly experienced. It has been suggested that acute cannabis use might be associated with acute cardiovascular fatality, but this remains unproven.

Chronic

There is tendency to paranoid thinking. Cognitive defect occurs and persists in relation to the duration of cannabis

---

[34]Yesavage J A, Leirer V O, Denari M, Hollister L E 1985 'Hangover' effects of marijuana intoxication in airline pilots. American Journal of Psychiatry 142:1325–1328.

[35]Working Party Report 2005 Cannabis and Cannabis-Based Medicines: Potential Benefits and Risks to Health. Royal College of Physicians, London.
[36]Van Gaal L F, Rissanen A M, Scheen A J et al 2005 Effects of the cannabinoid-1 receptor blocker rimonabant on weight reduction and cardiovascular risk factors in overweight patients: 1-year experience from the RIO-Europe study. Lancet 365:1389–1397.

use. High or habitual use can be followed by a psychotic state; this is usually reversible, quickly with brief periods of cannabis use, but more slowly after sustained exposures. Evidence indicates that chronic use may precipitate psychosis in vulnerable individuals.[37] Continued heavy use can lead to *tolerance,* and a *withdrawal* syndrome (depression, anxiety, sleep disturbance, tremor and other symptoms). Abandoning cannabis is difficult for many users.

In studies of self-administration by monkeys, spontaneous use did not occur, but, once use was initiated, drug-seeking behaviour developed. Subjects who have become tolerant to LSD or opioids as a result of repeated dosage respond normally to cannabis, but there appears to be cross-tolerance between cannabinoids and alcohol. The term 'amotivational syndrome' signifies an imprecisely characterised state, with features ranging from a feeling of unease and sense of not being fully effective, up to a gross lethargy, with social passivity and deterioration. Yet the reversibility of the state, its association with cannabinoid use, and its recognition by cannabis users make it impossible to ignore. (See Escalation theory, p. 144.)

The smoke produces the usual smoker's cough and delivers much more tar than tobacco cigarettes. In terms of damage to the bronchial epithelium, e.g. squamous metaplasia (a pre-cancerous change), three or four cannabis cigarettes are the equivalent of 20 tobacco cigarettes. Cannabinoids are teratogenic in animals, but effect in humans is unproved, although there is impaired fetal growth with repeated use.

Given the widespread recreational use of cannabis and its potential harmful effects, recent research has the development of strains of the cannabis plant with altered composition with regards to cannabidiol (CBD) and tetrahydrocannabinol (THC). Evidence from both experimental and population-based studies suggests that CBD can protect users from negative effects such as memory impairment, paranoia, psychosis and possibly addiction characterised by use of high THC cannabis products. The skunk strain of cannabis characteristically contains high levels of THC (approximately 15% of total cannabinoids). In the cannabis plant, both CBD and THC are made from a common precursor material cannabigerolic acid (CBGA). Increasing CBD levels in the plant is associated with a corresponding fall in THC levels. The optimum ratio is yet to be determined, but it might be possible to use existing regulatory frameworks to increase availability and access to less harmful cannabis products containing higher ratios of CBD to THC.

[37]Henquet C, Murray R, Linszen D, van Os J 2005 Prospective cohort study of cannabis use, predisposition for psychosis, and psychotic symptoms in young people. British Medical Journal 330:11–14.

Management of adverse reactions to psychodysleptics

Mild and sometimes even severe episodes ('bad trips') can be managed by reassurance including talk, 'talking the patient down' and physical contact, e.g. hand-holding (LSD and mescaline). Sedation of anxious or excited subjects can be effected with diazepam (or haloperidol).

Psychostimulants

Cocaine

Cocaine is found in the leaves of the coca plant *(Erythroxylum coca)*, a bush commonly found growing wild in Peru, Ecuador and Bolivia, and cultivated in many other countries. A widespread and ancient practice among South American peasants is to chew coca leaves with lime to release the alkaloid which gives relief from fatigue and hunger, and from altitude sickness in the Andes, experienced even by natives of the area when journeying; it also induces a pleasant introverted mental state. What may have been (or even still may be) an acceptable feature of these ancient stable societies has now developed into a massive criminal business for the manufacture and export of purified cocaine to developed societies, where its use constitutes an intractable social problem. An estimated 1 million people abused cocaine in the UK in 2009. This increase in use has been fuelled by falling street prices.

Pharmacokinetics and pharmacodynamics. Cocaine hydrochloride, extracted from the coca leaves, is a fine white powder. It is metabolised by plasma esterases; the $t_{1/2}$ is 50 min. It is taken to obtain the immediate characteristic intense euphoria which is often followed in a few minutes by dysphoria. This leads to repeated use (10–45 min) during 'runs' of usually about 12 h. After the 'run' there follows the 'crash' (dysphoria, irritability, hypersomnia), lasting for hours to days. After the 'crash' there may be depression ('cocaine blues') and decreased capacity to experience pleasure (anhedonia) for days to weeks.

Route of administration. Cocaine can be snorted, swallowed, smoked (below) or injected. Intranasal use causes mucosal vasoconstriction, anosmia and eventually necrosis and perforation of the nasal septum. Smoking involves converting the non-volatile cocaine HCl into the volatile 'free base' or 'crack' (by extracting the HCl with alkali).

For use it is vaporised by heat (it pops or cracks) in a special glass 'pipe'; or mixed with tobacco in a cigarette. Inhalation with breath-holding allows pulmonary absorption that is about as rapid as an intravenous injection. It induces an intense euphoric state. The mouth and pharynx become anaesthetised. (See Local anaesthetic action of cocaine, p. 318.) Intravenous use gives the expected rapid effect (kick, flash, rush). Cocaine may be mixed with heroin (as 'speedball').

Mode of action. Cocaine binds to and blocks the dopamine reuptake transporter which plays a key role in controlling entry of dopamine into central nerve terminals after release. Dopamine then accumulates in the synapse and acts on adjacent neurones to produce the characteristic 'high'. The psychotropic effects of cocaine are similar to those of amfetamine (euphoria and excitement) but briefer. Psychological dependence with intense compulsive drug-seeking behaviour is characteristic of even short-term use. Physical dependence is arguably slight or absent. Tachyphylaxis, acute tolerance, occurs.

Overdose is common among users. Up to 22% of heavy users report losing consciousness. The desired euphoria and excitement turn to acute fear, with psychotic symptoms, convulsions, hypertension, haemorrhagic stroke, tachycardia, arrhythmias, hyperthermia. Coronary artery vasospasm (sufficient to present as the acute coronary syndrome with chest pain and myocardial infarction) may occur, and acute left ventricular dysfunction.

Treatment is chosen according to the clinical picture (and the known mode of action), from haloperidol (rather than chlorpromazine) for mental disturbance; diazepam for convulsions; a vasodilator, e.g. a calcium channel blocker, for hypertension; glyceryl trinitrate for myocardial ischaemia (but not a β-blocker which aggravates cocaine-induced coronary vasospasm). Fetal growth is retarded by maternal use, but teratogenicity is uncertain.

> Cocaine-induced coronary artery spasm and myocardial infarction is an increasingly recognised problem and should be suspected in a young person presenting with cardiac chest pain.

Amfetamines

An easily prepared crystalline form of methylamfetamine (known as 'crystal meth' or 'ice') is in widespread illicit use as a psychostimulant. Amfetamine is a racemic compound: the *laevo* form is relatively inactive, but dexamfetamine (the *dextro* isomer) finds use in medicine. Amfetamine will be described, and structurally related drugs only in the ways in which they differ.

Pharmacokinetics. Amfetamine ($t_{1/2}$ 12 h) is readily absorbed by any usual route and is largely eliminated unchanged in the urine. Urinary excretion is pH dependent; being a basic substance, elimination will be greater in an acid urine. As well as oral use, intravenous administration (with the pleasurable 'flash' as with opioids) is employed. *Interactions* are as expected from mode of action, e.g. antagonism of antihypertensives; severe hypertension with MAOIs and β-adrenoceptor blocking drugs.

Mode of action. Amfetamine acts centrally by releasing dopamine stored in nerve endings and peripherally by α- and β-adrenoceptor actions common to indirectly acting sympathomimetics. As with all drugs acting on the CNS, the psychological effects vary with mood, personality and environment, as well as with dose. Subjects become euphoric, and fatigue is postponed. Although physical and mental performance may improve, this cannot be relied on. Subjects may be more confident and show more initiative, and be better satisfied with a more speedy performance that has deteriorated in accuracy. There may be anxiety and a feeling of nervous and physical tension, especially with large doses, and subjects develop tremors and confusion, and feel dizzy. Time seems to pass with greater rapidity. The sympathomimetic effect on the heart, causing palpitations, may intensify discomfort or alarm. Amfetamine increases the peripheral oxygen consumption, and this, together with vasoconstriction and restlessness, leads to hyperthermia in overdose, especially if the subject exercises.

Dependence on amfetamine and similar sympathomimetics is chiefly psychological. There is a withdrawal syndrome, suggesting physical dependence. Tolerance occurs. Severe dependence induces behaviour disorders, hallucinations, even florid psychosis, which can be controlled by haloperidol. Withdrawal is accompanied by lethargy and sleep, desire for food, and sometimes severe depression, which leads to an urge to resume the drug.

Acute poisoning is manifested by excitement and peripheral sympathomimetic effects. Convulsions may occur in acute or chronic overuse; a state resembling hyperactive paranoid schizophrenia with hallucinations develops. Hyperthermia occurs with cardiac arrhythmias, vascular collapse, intracranial haemorrhage and death. Treatment is chlorpromazine with added antihypertensive, e.g. labetalol, if necessary; these provide sedation and β-adrenoceptor blockade (but not a β-blocker alone, see p. 431), rendering unnecessary the optional enhancement of elimination by urinary acidification.

Chronic overdose can cause a psychotic state mimicking schizophrenia. A vasculitis of the cerebral and/or renal vessels can occur, possibly due to release of vasoconstrictor amines from both platelets and nerve endings. Severe hypertension can result from the renal vasculitis.

Structurally related drugs include dexamfetamine, used for narcolepsy and in attention-deficit hyperactivity disorder (ADHD) (see p. 360), methylphenidate (used for ADHD), tenamfetamine (Ecstasy, see p. 157), phentermine, diethylpropion and pemoline.

Khat

The leaves of the khat shrub *(Catha edulis)* contain alkaloids (cathinine, cathine, cathidine) that are structurally like amfetamine and produce similar effects. They are chewed fresh (for maximal alkaloid content). The habit was confined to geographical areas favourable to the shrub (Arabia, East Africa) until modern transportation allowed wider distribution. Use in the UK has been increasingly reported. It has been banned in the USA and Canada. Khat chewers (mostly male) become euphoric, loquacious, excited, hyperactive and even manic. As with some other drug dependencies, subjects may give priority to their drug needs above personal, family, and other social and economic responsibilities. Cultivation takes up serious amounts of scarce arable land and irrigation water.

Volatile substance abuse

Seekers of the 'self-gratifying high' also inhale any volatile substance that may affect the CNS. These include adhesives ('glue sniffing'), lacquer-paint solvents, petrol, nail varnish, any pressurised aerosol, butane liquid gas (the latter especially may 'freeze' the larynx, allowing fatal inhalation of food, drink, gastric contents, or even the liquid itself to flood the lungs). Even solids, e.g. paint scrapings, solid shoe polish, may be volatilised over a fire.

These substances are particularly abused by the young (13–15 years), no doubt largely because they are accessible at home and in ordinary shops, and these children cannot easily buy alcohol or 'street' drugs (although this may be changing as dealers target the youngest).

CNS effects include confusion and hallucinations, ataxia, dysarthria, coma, convulsions, respiratory failure. Liver, kidney, lung and heart damage occur. Sudden cardiac death may be due to sensitisation of the heart to endogenous catecholamines. If the substance is put in a plastic bag from which the user takes deep inhalations, or is sprayed in a confined space, e.g. cupboard, there is particularly high risk.

A 17-year-old boy was offered the use of a plastic bag and a can of hair spray at a beach party. The hair spray was released into the plastic bag and the teenager put his mouth to the open end of the bag and inhaled … he exclaimed, 'God, this stuff hits ya fast!' He got up, ran 100 yards, and died.[38]

Signs of frequent volatile substance abuse include perioral eczema and inflammation of the upper respiratory tract.

---

[38]Bass M 1970 Sudden sniffing death. Journal of the American Medical Association 212:2075.

Guide to further reading

Aubin, H.J., Karila, L., Reynaud, M., 2011. Pharmacotherapy for smoking cessation: present and future. Curr. Pharm. Des. 17, 143–150.

Clark, S., 2005. Personal account: on giving up smoking. Lancet 365, 1855.

Doll, R., 1997. One for the heart. Br. Med. J. 315, 1664–1668.

Edwards, R., 2004. The problem of tobacco smoking. Br. Med. J. 328, 217–219 (and subsequent articles in this series on the 'ABC of Smoking Cessation').

Fergusson, D.M., Poulton, R., Smith, P.F., Boden, J.M., 2006. Cannabis and psychosis. Br. Med. J. 322, 172–176.

Flower, R., 2004. Lifestyle drugs: pharmacology and the social agenda. Trends Pharmacol. Sci. 25, 182–185.

Gerada, C., 2005. Drug misuse: a review of treatments. Clin. Med. (Northfield Il) 5, 69–73.

Gordon, R.J., Lowy, F.D., 2005. Bacterial infections in drug users. N. Engl. J. Med. 353, 1945–1954.

Hartmann-Boyce, J., McRobbie, H., Bullen, C., et al., 2016. Electronic cigarettes for smoking cessation (2016). Cochrane Database Syst. Rev. (9), CD010216. Available at: http://www.cochranelibrary.com/enhanced/doi/10.1002/14651858.CD010216.pub3.

Hser, Y.-I., Liang, D., Lan, Y.-C., et al., 2016. Drug Abuse, HIV, and HCV in Asian Countries. J. Neuroimmune Pharmacol. 11, 383–393.

Jamrozik, K., 2005. Estimate of deaths attributable to passive smoking among UK adults: database analysis. Br. Med. J. 330, 812–815.

Kahan, M., Srivastava, A., Ordean, A., Cirone, S., 2011. Buprenorphine: new treatment of opioid addiction in primary care. Can. Fam. Physician 57, 281–289.

Kosten, T.R., O'Connor, P.G., 2003. Management of drug and alcohol withdrawal. N. Engl. J. Med. 348, 1786–1795.

Lange, R.A., Hillis, L.D., 2001. Cardiovascular complications of cocaine use. N. Engl. J. Med. 345, 351–358.

Malaiyandi, V., Sellers, E.M., Tyndale, R.F., 2005. Implications of CYP2A6 genetic variation for smoking behaviours and nicotine dependence. Clin. Pharmacol. Ther. 77, 145–158.

Minozzi, S., Amato, L., Vecchi, S., et al., 2011. Oral naltrexone maintenance treatment for opioid dependence. Cochrane Database Syst. Rev. (4), CD001333.

Nutt, D., King, L.A., Saulsbury, W., Blakemore, C., 2007. Development of a rational scale to assess the harm of drugs of potential misuse. Lancet 369, 1047–1053.

Ricaurte, G.A., McCann, U.D., 2005. Recognition and management of complications of new recreational drug use. Lancet 365, 2137–2145 (see also p. 2146, the anonymous Personal Account: GHB – sense and sociability).

Rong, C., Lee, Y., Carmona, N.E., et al., 2017. Cannabidiol in medical marijuana: Research vistas and potential opportunities. Pharmacol. Res. 121, 213–218.

Snead, O.C., Gibson, K.M., 2005. g-hydroxybutyric acid. N. Engl. J. Med. 352, 2721–2732.

Schifano, F., Orsolini, L., Papanti, G.D., Corkery, J.M., 2015. Novel psychoactive substances of interest for psychiatry. World Psychiatry 14, 15–26.

Topiwala, A., Allan, C.L., Valkanova, V., et al., 2017. Moderate alcohol consumption as risk factor for adverse brain outcomes and cognitive decline. Longitudinal cohort study. Brit. Med. J. 357, j2353.

Toupal, J.T., Ronan, M.V., Moore, A., Rosenthal, M.D., 2017. Inpatient management of opioid use disorder: A review for hospitalists. J. Hosp. Med. 12, 369–374.

Infection and inflammation

Chapter | **12** |

Chemotherapy of infections

David A. Enoch, Mark Farrington

SYNOPSIS

Infection is a major category of human disease and skilled management of antimicrobial drugs is crucial. The term *chemotherapy* is used for the drug treatment of infections in which the infecting agents (viruses, bacteria, protozoa, fungi and helminths) are destroyed or removed without injuring the host. The use of the term to cover all drug or synthetic drug therapy needlessly removes a distinction which is convenient to the clinician and has the sanction of long usage. By convention the term is also used to include therapy of cancer. This chapter will examine:

- **Classification of antimicrobial drugs.**
- **How antimicrobials act.**
- **Principles of optimal antimicrobial therapy.**
- **Use of antimicrobial drugs: choice; combinations; chemoprophylaxis and pre-emptive suppressive therapy; chemoprophylaxis in surgery.**
- **Special problems with antimicrobial drugs: resistance; superinfection; masking of infections.**
- **Antimicrobial drugs of choice.**

History

Many substances that we now know to possess therapeutic efficacy were first used in the distant past. The Ancient Greeks used male fern, and the Aztecs *Chenopodium*, as intestinal anthelminthics. The Ancient Hindus treated leprosy with Chaulmoogra. For hundreds of years moulds have been applied to wounds, but, despite the introduction of mercury as a treatment for syphilis (16th century), and the use of cinchona bark against malaria (17th century), the history of modern rational chemotherapy did not begin until Ehrlich[1] developed the idea from his observation that aniline dyes selectively stained bacteria in tissue microscopic preparations and could selectively kill them. He invented the word 'chemotherapy' and in 1906 he wrote:

> *In order to use chemotherapy successfully, we must search for substances which have an affinity for the cells of the parasites and a power of killing them greater than the damage such substances cause to the organism itself … This means … we must learn to aim, learn to aim with chemical substances.*

The antimalarials pamaquin and mepacrine were developed from dyes, and in 1935 the first sulfonamide, linked with a dye (Prontosil), was introduced as a result of systematic studies by Domagk.[2] The results obtained with sulfonamides in puerperal sepsis, pneumonia and meningitis were dramatic and caused a revolution in scientific and medical thinking.

In 1928, Fleming[3] accidentally rediscovered the long-known ability of *Penicillium* fungi to suppress the growth of bacterial cultures, but put the finding aside as a curiosity. His Nobel lecture in 1945 was prophetic for our current times:

---

[1]Paul Ehrlich (1854–1915), the German scientist who was the pioneer of chemotherapy and discovered the first cure for syphilis (Salvarsan).
[2]Gerhard Domagk (1895–1964), bacteriologist and pathologist, who made his discovery while working in Germany. Awarded the 1939 Nobel prize for Physiology or Medicine, he had to wait until 1947 to receive the gold medal because of Nazi policy at the time.
[3]Alexander Fleming (1881–1955). He researched for years on antibacterial substances that would not be harmful to humans. His findings on penicillin were made at St Mary's Hospital, London. See http://nobelprize.org/nobel_prizes/medicine/laureates/1945/fleming-lecture.pdf (accessed November 2017).

It is not difficult to make microbes resistant to penicillin in the laboratory by exposing them to concentrations not sufficient to kill them, and the same thing has occasionally happened in the body. The time may come when penicillin can be bought by anyone in the shops. Then there is the danger that the ignorant man may easily underdose himself and by exposing his microbes to non-lethal quantities of the drug, make them resistant.

In 1939, principally as an academic exercise, Florey[4] and Chain[5] undertook an investigation of antibiotics, i.e. substances produced by microorganisms that are antagonistic to the growth or life of other microorganisms.[6] They prepared penicillin and confirmed its remarkable lack of toxicity.[7] When the preparation was administered to a policeman with combined staphylococcal and streptococcal septicaemia, there was dramatic improvement; unfortunately the manufacture of penicillin in the local pathology laboratory could not keep pace with the requirements (it was also extracted from the patient's urine and re-injected); it ran out, and the patient later succumbed to infection.

In recent years, however:

the magic bullets have lost some of their magic. One solution may be to find alternatives to antibiotics when resistance appears, but there is also an urgent need for new antibiotics to be developed. Few pharmaceutical companies are now involved in antibiotic development … The high cost of development, the prolonged safety evaluation, and the probable short duration of field use and the present

tendency for any new compound to induce resistance all militate against major investment in new compounds.[8]

(See the review by Morel and Mossialos[9] on how this perverse economic incentive could be turned around.)

The realisation of this emerging threat is increasing worldwide. In 2013, the Department of Health in England launched a new Five Year Antibiotic Resistance Strategy (2015–2018).[10] It was published as part of a One Health approach, which aimed to address antibiotic resistance in humans, animals, agriculture and the wider environment. Its main objectives were to improve the knowledge and understanding of antibiotic resistance, to conserve and steward the effectiveness of current antibiotics and stimulate the development of new agents, diagnostics and novel therapies. In the strategy and her annual report, published in February 2013, the Chief Medical Officer in England recommended that antibiotic resistance be placed on the national risk register. Seven key priorities were outlined:

1. Optimising prescribing practices (i.e. antimicrobial stewardship)
2. Improving infection prevention and control
3. Raising awareness and changing behaviour
4. Improving the evidence base through research
5. Developing new drugs/vaccines/other diagnostics and treatments
6. Improving evidence base through surveillance
7. Strengthening the UK and international collaboration.

The O'Neill report (chaired by an economist for the Department of Health in England) has subsequently suggested setting up a global antimicrobial resistance innovation fund to boost the number of early research ideas, ensuring that existing drugs are used appropriately, improving the use of diagnostics wherever they can make a difference, attracting and retaining a high-calibre skills base and modernising the surveillance of drug resistance globally.[11] These and other measures are summarized elsewhere.[12]

---

[4]Howard Walter Florey (1898–1969), Professor of Pathology at Oxford University.
[5]Ernest Boris Chain (1906–1979), biochemist. Fleming, Florey and Chain shared the 1945 Nobel prize for Physiology or Medicine.
[6]Strictly, the definition should refer to substances that are antagonistic in dilute solution because it is necessary to exclude various common metabolic products such as alcohols and hydrogen peroxide. The term 'antibiotic' is now commonly used for antimicrobial drugs in general, and it would be pedantic to object to this. Today, many commonly used antibiotics are either fully synthetic or are produced by major chemical modification of naturally produced molecules: hence, 'antimicrobial agent' is perhaps a more accurate term, but 'antibiotic' is the commoner usage.
[7]The importance of this discovery for a nation at war was obvious to these workers, but the time, July 1940, was unpropitious, for invasion was feared. The mood of the time is shown by the decision to ensure that, by the time invaders reached Oxford, the essential records and apparatus for making penicillin would have been deliberately destroyed; the productive strain of *Penicillium* mould was to be secretly preserved by several of the principal workers smearing the spores of the mould into the linings of their ordinary clothes where it could remain dormant but alive for years; any member of the team who escaped (wearing the right clothes) could use it to start the work again (Macfarlane G 1979 Howard Florey, Oxford).

---

[8]Lord Soulsby of Swaffham Prior 2005 Resistance to antimicrobials in humans and animals. British Medical Journal 331:1219.
[9]Morel C M, Mossialos E 2010 Stoking the antibiotic pipeline. British Medical Journal 340:1115–1118.
[10]Department of Health and Department for Environment, Food, and Rural Affairs – UK Five Year Antimicrobial Resistance Strategy 2013 to 2018. Available at: https://www.gov.uk/government/uploads/system/uploads/attachment_data/file/244058/20130902_UK_5_year_AMR_strategy.pdf. Accessed 28th January 2017
[11]O'Neill J. The Review on Antimicrobial Resistance. Available at: https://amr-review.org/sites/default/files/160525_Final%20paper_with%20cover.pdf (accessed 28th January 2017).
[12]Sabtu N, Enoch DA, Brown NM. Antibiotic resistance: what, why, where, when and how? British Mededical Bulletin 2015;116:105–113.

Classification of antimicrobial drugs

Antimicrobial agents may be classified according to the type of organism against which they are active, and in this book we follow the sequence:

1. Antibacterial drugs.
2. Antiviral drugs.
3. Antifungal drugs.
4. Antiprotozoal drugs.
5. Anthelminthic drugs.

A few antimicrobials have useful activity across several of these groups. Metronidazole inhibits obligate anaerobic bacteria as well as some protozoa that rely on anaerobic metabolic pathways (such as *Trichomonas vaginalis*), whilst co-trimoxazole has activity against bacteria, fungi (e.g. *Pneumocystis* spp.) and parasites (e.g. *Isospora* spp.).

Antimicrobial drugs have also been classified broadly into:

- *Bacteriostatic*, i.e. those that act primarily by arresting bacterial multiplication, such as sulfonamides, tetracyclines and chloramphenicol.
- *Bactericidal*, i.e. those which act primarily by killing bacteria, such as penicillins, aminoglycosides and rifampicin.

The classification is in part arbitrary because most bacteriostatic drugs are bactericidal at high concentrations, under certain incubation conditions in vitro, and against some bacteria. However, there is some clinical evidence for efficacy of conventionally bactericidal drugs for infective endocarditis, meningitis and immunosuppressed patients.

Bactericidal drugs act most effectively on rapidly dividing organisms. Thus a bacteriostatic drug, by reducing multiplication, may protect the organism from the killing effect of a bactericidal drug. Such mutual antagonism of antimicrobials may be clinically important, but the matter is complex because of the multiple factors that determine each drug's efficacy at the site of infection. In vitro tests of antibacterial synergy and antagonism may only distantly replicate these conditions.

Probably more important is whether its antimicrobial effect is *concentration*-dependent or *time*-dependent. Examples of the former include the quinolones and aminoglycosides in which the outcome is related to the peak antibiotic concentration achieved at the site of infection in relation to the minimum concentration necessary to inhibit multiplication of the organism (the minimum inhibitory concentration, or MIC). These antimicrobials produce a prolonged inhibitory effect on bacterial multiplication (the post-antibiotic effect, or PAE) which suppresses growth until the next dose is given. In contrast, agents such as the β-lactams and macrolides have more modest PAEs and exhibit

time-dependent killing; their concentrations should be kept above the MIC for a high proportion of the time between each dose (Fig. 12.1).

Fig. 12.1 shows the results of an experiment in which a culture broth initially containing 10^6 bacteria per mL is exposed to various concentrations of two antibiotics, one of which exhibits concentration-dependent and the other time-dependent killing. The 'control' series contains no antibiotic, and the other series contain progressively higher antibiotic concentrations from $0.5 \times$ to $64 \times$ the MIC. Over 6 h incubation, the time-dependent antibiotic exhibits killing, but there is no difference between the $1 \times$ MIC and $64 \times$ MIC. The additional cidal effect of rising concentrations of the antibiotic which has concentration-dependent killing can be clearly seen.

How antimicrobials act – sites of action

It should always be remembered that drugs are seldom the sole instruments of cure but act together with the natural

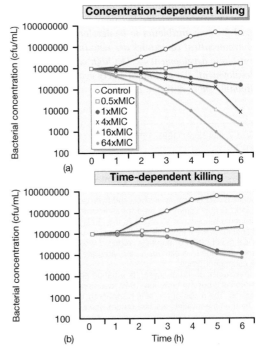

Fig. 12.1 Efficacy of antimicrobials: examples of concentration-dependent and time-dependent killing (see text) (cfu = colony-forming units).

defences of the body. Antimicrobials may act at different sites in the target organism, and these are characteristically structures or metabolic pathways that differ from those in the human host – this allows for 'selective toxicity':

The cell wall. Bacterial multiplication involves breakdown and extension of the cell wall; interference with these processes prevents the organism from resisting osmotic pressures, so that it bursts. Obviously, the drugs are effective principally against growing cells. They include: penicillins, cephalosporins, glycopeptides (e.g. vancomycin), bacitracin and cycloserine.

The cytoplasmic membrane. Drugs that interfere with its structure include: polyenes (nystatin, amphotericin), azoles (e.g. fluconazole, itraconazole), polymyxins (colistin, polymyxin B) and daptomycin.

Protein synthesis. Drugs that interfere at various points with the buildup of peptide chains on microbial ribosomes include: chloramphenicol, macrolides (e.g. erythromycin), fusidic acid, tetracyclines, aminoglycosides, quinupristin/dalfopristin and linezolid.

Nucleic acid metabolism. Drugs may interfere:

- *directly* with microbial DNA or its replication or repair, e.g. quinolones, metronidazole, or with RNA, e.g. rifampicin
- *indirectly* on nucleic acid synthesis, e.g. sulfonamides, trimethoprim.

Principles of antimicrobial chemotherapy

The following principles, many of which apply to drug therapy in general, are a guide to good practice with antimicrobial agents.

Make a diagnosis as precisely as is possible and define the site of infection, the organism(s) responsible and their susceptibility to a range of antimicrobial agents (to give several therapeutic options to cater for different sites of infection and the possibility of allergies or other drug sensitivities in the infected individual). This objective will be more readily achieved if all relevant samples for laboratory culture are taken before treatment is begun. Once antimicrobials have been administered, isolation of the underlying organism by culture may be inhibited, and its place in diagnostic samples may be taken by resistant, colonising bacteria which obscure the true causative pathogen. New diagnostic methods that rely on detecting specific microbial nucleic acids (e.g. the polymerase chain reaction, PCR), lipids or proteins allow detection of the causative pathogen in patients who have already received antimicrobial therapy,

although it is currently less likely simultaneously to determine the antimicrobial susceptibility patterns of these microbes.

It is inconsistent that the assessment of new antibiotics for therapeutic use is very much more rigorously controlled than is the introduction of diagnostic tests that direct their use – Gluud and Gluud propose a harmonised approach to the assessment and regulation of new diagnostic procedures in clinical microbiology.[13]

Remove barriers to cure, e.g. drain abscesses, remove obstruction in the urinary tract and infected intravenous catheters and consider removal of prosthetic devices (e.g. prosthetic joint prostheses).

Decide whether chemotherapy is really necessary. Chronic abscesses or empyemata respond poorly to antibiotics alone and require surgical drainage, although chemotherapeutic cover may be essential if surgery is undertaken in order to avoid dissemination of infection during the operation. Even some acute infections are better managed symptomatically than by antimicrobials; thus the risks of adverse drug reactions for previously healthy individuals might outweigh the modest clinical benefits that follow antibiotic therapy of salmonella gastroenteritis and streptococcal sore throat.

Select the best drug. This involves consideration of the following factors:

- *Specificity:* indiscriminate use of broad-spectrum drugs promotes antimicrobial resistance and encourages opportunistic infections, e.g. with yeasts (see p. 172). At the beginning of treatment, empirical 'best guess' chemotherapy of reasonably broad spectrum must often be given because the susceptibility and identity of the responsible microbe is uncertain. The spectrum **should** be narrowed once these are microbiologically confirmed.
- *Pharmacokinetic factors:* to ensure that the chosen drug is capable of reaching the site of infection in adequate amounts, e.g. by crossing the blood–brain barrier.
- *The patient:* who may previously have exhibited allergy to a group of antimicrobials or whose routes of elimination may be impaired, e.g. by renal disease.

Administer the drug in optimum dose and frequency and by the most appropriate route(s). Inadequate doses may encourage the development of microbial resistance. In general, on grounds of practicability, intermittent dosing is preferred to continuous infusion. There is emerging evidence that glycopeptides may be more effective when given as a continuous infusion, whilst beta-lactams can also be given

---

[13]Gluud C G, Gluud L L 2005 Evidence based diagnostics. British Medical Journal 330:724–726

as extended infusions, particularly in sicker patients. Plasma concentration monitoring can be performed to optimise therapy and reduce adverse drug reactions (e.g. aminoglycosides, glycopeptides).

Antibiotics should also be started as soon as possible in the patient with features of sepsis/severe sepsis (see infection of the blood in Ch. 14).

Continue therapy until apparent cure has been achieved; most acute infections are treated for 5–10 days. There are many exceptions to this, such as typhoid fever, tuberculosis and infective endocarditis, in which relapse is possible long after apparent clinical cure and so the drugs are continued for a longer period determined by comparative or observational trials. Otherwise, prolonged therapy is to be avoided because it increases costs and the risks of adverse drug reactions.

Test for cure. In some infections, microbiological proof of cure is desirable because disappearance of symptoms and signs occurs before the organisms are eradicated. This is generally restricted to especially susceptible hosts, e.g. urinary tract infection in pregnancy. Confirmatory culture must be done, of course, after withdrawal of chemotherapy.

Prophylactic chemotherapy for surgical and dental procedures should be of very limited duration, often only a single large dose being given (see p. 172).

Carriers of pathogenic or resistant organisms should not routinely be treated to remove the organisms, for it may be better to allow natural re-establishment of a normal flora. The potential benefits of clearing carriage must be weighed carefully against the inevitable risks of adverse drug reactions.

Use of antimicrobial drugs

Choice

Identification of the microbe and performing susceptibility tests take time, and therapy at least of the more serious infections must usually be started on the basis of the informed 'best guess' (i.e. 'empirical' therapy). Especially in critically ill patients, choosing initial therapy to which the infecting microbes are susceptible has been shown to improve the outcome – with the worldwide rise in prevalence of multiply resistant bacteria during the past decade, knowledge of local antimicrobial resistance rates is therefore an essential prerequisite. Publication of these rates (and corresponding guidelines for choice of empirical therapy for common infections) is now an important role for clinical diagnostic microbiology laboratories. Such guidelines must be reviewed regularly to keep pace with changing resistance patterns.

When considering 'best guess' therapy, infections may be categorised as those in which:

1. Choice of antimicrobial follows automatically from the clinical diagnosis because the causative organism is always the same, and is virtually always sensitive to the same drug, e.g. meningococcal septicaemia (benzylpenicillin), some haemolytic streptococcal infections, e.g. scarlet fever, erysipelas (benzylpenicillin), typhus (tetracycline), leprosy (dapsone with rifampicin).
2. The infecting organism is identified by the clinical diagnosis, but no safe assumption can be made as to its sensitivity to any one antimicrobial, e.g. tuberculosis.
3. A single infecting organism is not identified by the clinical diagnosis, e.g. in urinary tract infection or abdominal surgical wound infection.

Particularly in the second and third categories, choice of an antimicrobial may be guided by:

Knowledge of the likely pathogens (and their current local susceptibility rates to antimicrobials) in the clinical situation. Thus co-amoxiclav might be a reasonable first choice for lower urinary tract infection (coliform organisms – depending on the prevalence of resistance locally), and benzylpenicillin for meningitis in the adult (meningococcal or pneumococcal).

Rapid diagnostic tests. Rapid detection of markers of infection such as C-reactive protein (CRP) and procalcitonin assays are now available, and evidence is accruing as to how they should best be used. Both CRP and procalcitonin concentrations rise in the serum within a few hours of the commencement of serious bacterial infections, and it appears that clinical decisions on antimicrobial use based on algorithms that include the results of such assays may be more accurate, and may spare some patients from antibiotic exposure.

Use of tests of this type to diagnose involvement of specific pathogens has undergone a revolution with the widespread introduction of affordable, sensitive and specific assays. Increasingly, reliable tests are being introduced which can be used at the patient's bedside ('point of care' (POC) tests). Classically, antimicrobials were selected after direct microscopy of smears of body secretions or tissues – thus flucloxacillin may be indicated when clusters of Gram-positive cocci are found (indicating staphylococci), but glycopeptides would be preferred in those hospitals with a high prevalence of meticillin-resistant *Staphylococcus aureus* (MRSA).

Light microscopy will remain useful in this way for many years to come, but use of PCR to detect DNA sequences specific for individual microbial species or resistance mechanisms greatly speeds up the institution of definitive, reliable therapy. These methods are already widely used for diagnosing meningitis (detecting *Neisseria meningitidis*,

Streptococcus pneumoniae and *Haemophilus influenzae*), tuberculosis (including detection of rifampicin resistance) and most viral infections. Quantitative PCR allows monitoring the response to therapy (e.g. monitoring copy numbers of circulating cytomegalovirus (CMV) DNA in a transplant recipient being treated with ganciclovir). Several rapid non-culture techniques are being assessed for laboratory application (e.g. mass spectroscopy) which allow speciation of bacteria and fungi within a few minutes of their culture in broth or on solid media.

Modification of treatment can be made later if necessary, in the light of conventional culture and susceptibility tests. Treatment otherwise should be changed only after adequate trial, usually 2–3 days, because over-hasty alterations cause confusion and encourage the emergence of resistant organisms.

Route of administration. Parenteral therapy (which may be i.m. or i.v.) is preferred for therapy of serious infections because high therapeutic concentrations are achieved reliably and rapidly. Initial parenteral therapy should be switched to the oral route whenever possible once the patient has improved clinically and as long as a suitable oral antibiotic is available and they are able to absorb it (i.e. not with vomiting, ileus or diarrhoea). Many antibiotics are well absorbed orally, and the long-held assumption that prolonged parenteral therapy is necessary for adequate therapy of serious infections (such as osteomyelitis) is often not supported by the results of clinical trials.

Intravenous therapy was typically restricted to hospital patients in the past. However, continuation parenteral therapy of certain infections in patients in the community is sometimes performed by specially trained nurses (as outpatient parenteral antimicrobial therapy; OPAT). The costs of hospital stays and some risks of health-care-associated infections are avoided, but this type of management is suitable only when the patient's clinical state is stable, oral therapy is not suitable, and the infection is amenable to once-daily administration of a suitable antibiotic (usually one having a prolonged half-life).

Oral therapy of infections is usually cheaper and avoids the risks associated with maintenance of intravenous access; on the other hand, it may expose the gastrointestinal tract to higher local concentrations of antibiotic with consequently greater risks of antibiotic-associated diarrhoea. Some antimicrobial agents are available only for topical use to skin, anterior nares, eye or mouth; in general it is better to avoid antibiotics that are also used for systemic therapy because topical use may be especially likely to select for resistant strains. Topical therapy to the conjunctival sac is used for therapy of infections of the conjunctiva and the anterior chamber of the eye.

Inhalational antibiotics are of proven benefit for pseudomonas colonisation of the lungs in children with cystic fibrosis (twice-daily tobramycin), monthly pentamidine for pneumocystis prophylaxis and zanamivir for patients with oseltamivir-resistant influenza A and B (if commenced within 48 h). In addition, there is probable benefit for colistin in cystic fibrosis and as an adjunct to parenteral antibiotics for Gram-negative pneumonia, for aminoglycosides in bronchiectasis, and for ribavirin for RSV infection in children.

Other routes used for antibiotics on occasion include rectal (as suppositories), intra-ophthalmic, intrathecal (to the CSF), and by direct injection or infusion to infected tissues.

Combinations

Treatment with a single antimicrobial is sufficient for most infections. The indications for use of two or more antimicrobials are:

- to avoid the development of drug resistance, especially in chronic infections where many bacteria are present (hence the chance of a resistant mutant emerging is high), e.g. tuberculosis.
- to broaden the spectrum of antibacterial activity: (1) in a known mixed infection, e.g. peritonitis following gut perforation, or (2) where the infecting organism cannot be predicted but treatment is essential before a diagnosis has been reached, e.g. septicaemia complicating neutropenia or severe community-acquired pneumonia.
- to obtain potentiation (or 'synergy'), i.e. an effect unobtainable with either drug alone, e.g. penicillin plus gentamicin for enterococcal endocarditis.
- to enable reduction of the dose of one component and hence reduce the risks of adverse drug reactions, e.g. flucytosine plus amphotericin B for *Cryptococcus neoformans* meningitis.

Chemoprophylaxis and pre-emptive suppressive therapy

It is sometimes assumed that what a drug can cure it will also prevent, but this is not necessarily so. The basis of effective chemoprophylaxis is the use of a drug in a healthy person to prevent infection by one organism of reliable and predictable susceptibility, e.g. benzylpenicillin against a beta-haemolytic Group A streptococcus. However, the term 'chemoprophylaxis' is commonly extended to include suppression of existing infection.

It is essential to know the organisms causing infection and their local resistance patterns, and the period of time the patient is at risk. A narrow-spectrum antibiotic regimen should be administered only during this period – ideally for a few minutes before until a few hours after the risk period. It is therefore much easier to define chemotherapeutic regimens for short-term exposures (e.g. surgical operations) than it is for longer-term and less well-defined risks. The main categories of chemoprophylaxis may be summarised as follows:

- *True prevention of primary infection*: rheumatic fever,[14] recurrent urinary tract infection.
- *Prevention of opportunistic infections*, e.g. due to commensals getting into the wrong place (coagulase-negative staphylococcal prosthetic joint infection from the patient's skin during the operation, and peritonitis after bowel surgery). Note that these are both high-risk situations of short duration; prolonged administration of drugs before surgery would result in the areas concerned (mouth and bowel) being colonised by drug-resistant organisms with potentially disastrous results (see below). Immunocompromised patients can benefit from longer-term chemoprophylaxis, e.g. of Gram-negative septicaemia complicating neutropenia with an oral quinolone, or of *Pneumocystis carinii* pneumonia with co-trimoxazole.
- *Suppression of existing infection* before it causes overt disease, e.g. tuberculosis, malaria.
- *Prevention of acute exacerbations* of a chronic infection, e.g. bronchitis, cystic fibrosis.
- *Prevention of spread among contacts* (in epidemics and/ or sporadic cases). Spread of influenza A can be partially prevented by oseltamivir; ciprofloxacin may be used when there is a case of meningococcal meningitis in a family.

Long-term prophylaxis of bacterial infection can be achieved often by doses that are inadequate for therapy once the acute infection has been fully treated.

Attempts to use drugs routinely to prevent infection when a wide and unpredictable range of organisms may be involved, e.g. pneumonia in the unconscious patient and urinary tract infection in patients with long-term urinary catheters, have not only failed but have sometimes encouraged infections with less susceptible organisms. Attempts routinely to prevent bacterial infection secondary to virus infections, e.g. in respiratory tract infections and measles, have also not been sufficiently successful to outweigh the disadvantages. In these situations, it is generally better to

be alert for complications and then to treat them promptly and vigorously rather than to try to prevent them.

Chemoprophylaxis in surgery

The principles governing use of antimicrobials in this context are as follows.

Chemoprophylaxis is justified:

- When the risk of infection is high because of large numbers of bacteria at the operative site, e.g. in operations on the large bowel.
- When the risk of infection is low but the consequences of infection would be disastrous, e.g. infection of prosthetic joints or prosthetic heart valves.
- When the risks of infection are low but randomised controlled trials have shown the benefits of prophylaxis to outweigh the risks, e.g. single-dose antistaphylococcal prophylaxis for uncomplicated hernia and breast surgery.

In the UK, controversy followed the publication in 2006 of the updated guidelines of the British Society for Antimicrobial Chemotherapy's working party on the prevention of infective endocarditis (see the Guide to further reading for illustrative articles). The new guidelines advocated a much more restricted policy of administering antimicrobial prophylaxis at the time of medical interventions, including dentistry. This was based on the lack of convincing evidence for the efficacy of this time-honoured practice, with the exception of those patients at highest risk (for example, those with prosthetic heart valves or who had previously suffered episodes of infective endocarditis). This policy was supported by the subsequent publication of evidence-based guidelines from the National Institute for Health and Clinical Excellence (NICE) in England, and similar guidelines have subsequently been promoted in other countries, including the USA.

Antimicrobials should be selected in the light of knowledge of the likely pathogens at the sites of surgery and their locally prevalent antimicrobial susceptibility.

Antimicrobials should be given i.v., i.m. or occasionally rectally at the beginning of anaesthesia and for no more than 48 h. A single preoperative dose, given at the time of induction of anaesthesia, has been shown to give optimal cover for most operations. A glycopeptide is often included in prophylactic regimens when the patient is known to be a carrier of MRSA or its local prevalence is high (ask microbiological advice).

Specific instances are:

1. *Colorectal surgery*: there is a high risk of infection with enterobacteriaceae, *Clostridium* spp., streptococci and

---

[14]Rheumatic fever is caused by a large number of types of Group A streptococci, and immunity is type-specific. Recurrent attacks are commonly due to infection with different strains of these, all of which are sensitive to penicillin and so chemoprophylaxis is effective. Acute glomerulonephritis is also due to Group A streptococci, but only a few types cause it, so that natural immunity is more likely to protect and second attacks are rare. Therefore, chemoprophylaxis is not used.

Bacteroides spp. which inhabit the gut (co-amoxiclav or gentamicin and metronidazole).

2. *Gastroduodenal surgery:* colonisation of the stomach with gut organisms occurs especially when acid secretion is low, e.g. in gastric malignancy, following use of a histamine H_2-receptor antagonist or following previous gastric surgery (co-amoxiclav or gentamicin and metronidazole).

3. *Gynaecological surgery:* because the vagina contains *Bacteroides* spp. and other anaerobes, streptococci and coliforms (co-amoxiclav).

4. *Leg amputation:* because there is a risk of gas gangrene in an ischaemic limb and the mortality is high (benzylpenicillin, or metronidazole for the patient with allergy to penicillin).

5. *Insertion of prostheses – joints, heart valves, vessels:* chemoprophylaxis is justified because infection (*Staphylococcus aureus*, coagulase-negative staphylococci and enterobacteriaceae are commonest) often means that the artificial joint, valve or vessel must be replaced. Single perioperative doses of appropriate antibiotics with plasma elimination half-lives of several hours (e.g. cefotaxime) are adequate, but if short half-life agents are used (e.g. flucloxacillin, +/– gentamicin single dose) several doses should be given during the first 24 h.

6. *General surgery:* clearance of *Staphylococcus aureus* from the anterior nares of carriers with mupirocin is known to reduce the incidence of wound infection by about one-half, and this treatment has recently been shown in one high-quality trial to be effective when targeted only at staphylococcal nasal carriers who were detected by screening nasal swabs with a rapid real-time PCR assay. This strategy is much more potentially attractive than the alternative of treating all patients preoperatively, which has been demonstrated not to reduce infection rates significantly while maximising unnecessary mupirocin exposure.

Problems with antimicrobial drugs

Resistance

Microbial resistance to antimicrobials is a matter of great importance; if sensitive strains are supplanted by resistant ones, then a valuable drug may become useless. Just as 'some are born great, some achieve greatness, and some have greatness thrust upon them',[15] so microorganisms may be naturally ('born') resistant, 'achieve' resistance by mutation or have resistance 'thrust upon them' by transfer of plasmids and other mobile genetic elements.

Resistance may become more prevalent by spread of microorganisms containing resistance genes, and also by dissemination of the resistance genes among different microbial species. Because resistant strains are encouraged (selected) at the population level by use of antimicrobial agents, antibiotics are the only group of therapeutic agents which can alter the actual diseases suffered by other, untreated individuals. About 50% of antimicrobial use is in human medicine – the remainder being given to animals – and 80% of human use occurs in domiciliary practice, out of hospitals.

Problems of antimicrobial resistance have burgeoned during the past few decades in most countries of the world, both in and out of hospital, and fortunately a number of international bodies have been established devoted to the reduction of resistance worldwide: 'Our mission is clear: we must work together to preserve the power of antimicrobials and to return these miracle agents to their rightful position as effective treatments of disease'.[16]

Some resistant microbes are currently mainly restricted to hospital patients or to those who have recently been in hospital, e.g. MRSA, vancomycin-resistant enterococci (VRE). Others more commonly infect patients in the community, e.g. penicillin- and macrolide-resistant *Streptococcus pneumoniae* and multiply resistant *Mycobacterium tuberculosis*. Some (such as enterobacteriaceae that produce 'extended spectrum β-lactamases' (ESBLs)) are commoner in hospital but now also commonly occur in individuals who have never been inpatients. CPE (carbapenemase-producing enterobacteriaceae) are now also emerging in patients with no prior health-care contact (see below).

This is a rapidly changing field, and our technical abilities to detect novel resistance mechanisms and to type resistant strains of microbe have recently improved. As a result, a continuing series of different antimicrobial resistant and virulent microorganisms have been recognised to have emerged recently in Europe and North America. These include: community-acquired, toxin-producing MRSA (primarily affecting previously well young adults and intravenous drug users); multiply resistant *Acinetobacter baumannii* (including strains introduced by transfer of tsunami victims and Gulf War casualties to hospitals in their home countries); and CPE. Carbapenemase-producing enterobacteriaceae are enterobacteriaceae (e.g. *E. coli*, *Klebsiella* spp.) that have acquired a carbapenemase gene, typically by transfer of a plasmid. These plasmids can switch between different species of enterobacteriaceae and are highly transmissible. There are a number of different carbapenemases. The most common ones identified so far include NDM (New Delhi

---

[15]Malvolio in *Twelfth Night*, act 2 scene 5, by William Shakespeare (1564–1616).

[16]Dr Stuart Levy, http://www.tufts.edu/med/apua/.

metallo-beta-lactamase), KPC (Klebsiella pneumoniae carbapenemase), VIM (Verona-integron metallo-beta-lactamase) and OXA-48 (oxacillinase), though this is a rapidly expanding and evolving field. These problems have spawned a new nomenclature for beta-lactamase resistance mechanisms, and for Gram-negative rod resistance in general – 'multidrug-resistant' (MDR) strains are resistant to at least three different antimicrobial drug classes, 'extensively drug-resistant' (XDR) strains are susceptible to only one or two antimicrobial options, while 'pan-drug resistant' (PDR) strains are no longer amenable to antimicrobial treatment.

It is to be hoped that our abilities to treat and prevent such infections will continue to increase in parallel with our abilities to recognise them (laboratory testing methodology also needs to be developed continually because, for example, some of the new beta-lactamases (such as 'AmpC' and OXA-48-producing strains in particular) can be difficult to detect with conventional techniques.

Considerable hope is given by the remarkable reductions in MRSA bacteraemia rates reported from English hospitals in the past 10 years, which have apparently resulted from mandated enforcement of conventional but stringent screening, clearance and infection control measures: there was a 46% fall in the 2 years from July 2008 to September 2010. Hence rising resistance rates are not inevitable.

In well-controlled observational studies, the outcomes of infections with antibiotic-resistant bacteria are generally significantly poorer than those with susceptible strains, and the costs of therapy and associated length of hospital stay are greater.

Mechanisms of resistance act as follows:

- *Naturally resistant strains.* Some bacteria are innately resistant to certain classes of antimicrobial agent, e.g. coliforms and many other Gram-negative bacteria possess outer cell membranes which protect their cell walls from the action of certain penicillins and cephalosporins. Facultatively anaerobic bacteria (such as *Escherichia coli*) lack the ability to reduce the nitro group of metronidazole which therefore remains in an inactive form.
- *Spontaneous mutation* brings about organisms with novel antibiotic resistance mechanisms. If these cells are viable, in the presence of the antimicrobial agent selective multiplication of the resistant strain occurs so that it eventually dominates.
- *Transmission of genes from other organisms* is the commonest and most important mechanism. Genetic material may be transferred, e.g. in the form of *plasmids* which are circular strands of DNA that lie outwith the chromosomes and contain genes capable of controlling various metabolic processes including formation of β-lactamases (that destroy some

penicillins and cephalosporins), and enzymes that inactivate aminoglycosides. Alternatively, genetic transfer may occur through *bacteriophages* (viruses which infect bacteria), particularly in the case of staphylococci.

Resistance is mediated most commonly by the production of enzymes that modify the drug, e.g. aminoglycosides are phosphorylated, β-lactamases hydrolyse penicillins. Other mechanisms include decreasing the passage into or increasing the efflux of drug from the bacterial cell (e.g. meropenem resistance in *Pseudomonas aeruginosa*), modification of the target site so that the antimicrobial binds less effectively (e.g. meticillin resistance in staphylococci), and bypassing of inhibited metabolic pathways (e.g. resistance to trimethoprim in many bacteria). More is becoming known of the complex molecular systems which control expression of antimicrobial resistance, and this knowledge should soon lead to novel compounds that inhibit resistance mechanisms at the genetic and phenotypic levels (see Stix[17] for an example).

Limitation of resistance to antimicrobials may be achieved by 'antibiotic stewardship'. A recent meta-analysis found that antimicrobial stewardship can actually reduce antibiotic use and reduce length of stay without affecting mortality (Davey et al 2017)[18] which includes:

- Avoidance of indiscriminate use by ensuring that the indication for, and the dose and duration of treatment are appropriate; studies of hospital and domiciliary prescribing have shown that up to 35% of antimicrobial courses administered in the UK may be inappropriate – either not indicated at all, or administered for too long. Performing ward rounds in areas of the hospital with high rates of antibiotic use (e.g. intensive care units, acute surgical wards) to assess the justification for treatment of individual patients and to educate other doctors in limiting unnecessary courses of antibiotics has recently become an important role for clinical microbiologists.
- Restricting use of antimicrobial combinations to appropriate circumstances, e.g. tuberculosis.
- The requirement for all antimicrobial prescriptions to have the indication (reason) for the antimicrobial stated, along with its duration, and evidence its review at 48–72 hours (in light of microbiology results). These parameters should be audited regularly

[17]Stix G 2006 An antibiotic resistance fighter. New Scientist April: 80–83.
[18]Davey P, Marwick CA, Scott CL, Charani E, McNeil K, Brown E, Gould IM, Ramsay CR, Michie S. Interventions to improve antibiotic prescribing practices for hospital inpatients. Cochrane Database Syst Rev. 2017 Feb 9;2:CD003543. doi: 10.1002/14651858.CD003543.pub4

and fed back to clinicians in order to improve prescribing practice.

- Constant monitoring of resistance patterns in a hospital or community (changing recommended antibiotics used for empirical treatment when the prevalence of resistance becomes high), and strict infection control in hospitals (e.g. isolation of carriers, hand hygiene practices for ward staff) to prevent the spread of resistant bacteria.
- Restricting drug use, e.g. delaying the emergence of resistance by limiting the use of the newest member of a group of antimicrobials so long as the currently used drugs are effective; restricting use of a drug may become necessary where it promotes the proliferation of resistant strains.
- Avoiding transmission of multiply resistant bacteria among patients and staff in hospital, by health care workers performing careful hand hygiene between each patient contact, and through identification and isolation of carriers.

'The over-riding principle of medicine is "do no harm", yet, in the case of antibiotics, harm is inevitable, for use (even appropriate usage) and selects for resistance, complicating the treatment of future patients.'[19]

Antibiotic policies and guidelines are agreed among clinicians, microbiologists and pharmacists which guide prescribing towards a limited range of agents which provide adequate choice to cover therapy of important infections while limiting confusion and maximising the opportunities for economical purchase in bulk. Analysis of the many trials of 'antibiotic cycling', where first-choice antibiotics for commonly treated infections in a hospital or ward are formally rotated with a periodicity of several months or years, has shown that this strategy does not reduce overall resistance rates or total antibiotic usage. Use of 'delayed prescriptions' in primary health-care management of less serious infections, where a prescription is given to patients for them to take to the pharmacy only if their symptoms fail to improve in 24–48 h, has been shown to reduce antibiotic usage and not impair outcomes in upper and lower respiratory tract infection.

Doctors are encouraged to avoid use of antimicrobial agents whenever possible, and international efforts are being made to educate the general public not to expect an antibiotic prescription for minor ailments such as coughs and colds (see, for example).[20]

Point of care testing of CRP in primary care is also recommended in order to help general practitioners discriminate between viral and bacterial respiratory tract infections[21] and was recommended by the O'Neill report.[22]

Several prospective studies have shown that initial broad-spectrum empirical therapy given to acutely ill patients in hospital can be safely 'rationalised' to narrower-spectrum antimicrobial agents as soon as the results of initial cultures have been obtained (i.e. usually after 48 h).

Evidence is accumulating that resistance rates do not rise inevitably and irreversibly (see page 174). In both hospital and domiciliary practice, reductions in antibiotic usage are often shown to be followed by reductions in the prevalence of microbial resistance, although there can be a 'lag' of months or years. The situation is sometimes complicated by the phenomenon of 'linked multiple resistance' whereby the genes coding resistance mechanisms to several antibiotics are carried on the same genetic elements (e.g. plasmid). In this case, use of any of these antibiotics will select for increased resistance via all the mechanisms carried by the plasmid.

Although clinical microbiology laboratories report microbial susceptibility test results as 'sensitive/susceptible' or 'resistant' to a particular antibiotic, this is not an absolute predictor of clinical response. In a given patient's infection, variables such as absorption of the drug, its penetration to the site of infection, and its activity once there (influenced, for example, by protein binding, pH, concentration of oxygen, metabolic state of the pathogen, intracellular location and concentration of microbes) profoundly alter the likelihood that effective therapy will result.

Superinfection

When any antimicrobial drug is used, there is usually suppression of part of the normal bacterial flora of the patient which is susceptible to the drug. Often, this causes no ill effects, but sometimes a drug-resistant organism, freed from competition, proliferates to an extent which allows an infection to be established. The principal organisms responsible are *Candida albicans* and pseudomonads. But careful clinical assessment of the patient is essential, as the mere presence of such organisms in diagnostic specimens taken from a site in which they may be present as commensals does not necessarily mean they are causing disease.

Antibiotic-associated (or *Clostridium difficile*-associated) colitis is an example of a superinfection. It is caused by

[19]Livermore D M 2006 Minimising antibiotic resistance. Lancet Infectious Diseases 5:450–459.
[20]http://www.biomedcentral.com/1471-2296/10/20 and http://ecdc.europa.eu/en/EAAD/Pages/Home.aspx/.

[21]Little P et al. Effects of internet-based training on antibiotic prescribing rates for acute respiratory-tract infections: a multinational, cluster, randomised, factorial, controlled trial. Lancet 2013; 382 (9899):1175–1182. doi: 10.1016/S0140-6736(13)60994-0.
[22]O'Neill J. The Review on Antimicrobial Resistance. Available at: https://amr-review.org/sites/default/files/160525_Final%20paper_with%20cover.pdf. (accessed 28th January 2017).

alteration of the normal bowel flora, which allows multiplication of *Clostridium difficile* which releases several toxins that damage the mucosa of the bowel and promote excretion of fluid. Almost any antimicrobial agent may initiate this condition, but the drugs most commonly reported today are cephalosporins and quinolones (e.g. ciprofloxacin), though with the reduction in use of these agents in the UK, amoxicillin and co-amoxiclav are increasingly implicated. It takes the form of an acute colitis (pseudomembranous colitis) with diarrhoeal stools containing blood or mucus, abdominal pain, leucocytosis and dehydration. A history of antibiotic use in the previous 3 weeks, even if the drug therapy has been stopped, should alert the physician to the diagnosis, which is confirmed by detection of *C. difficile* toxin in the stools and typical appearances on proctosigmoidoscopy. Recurrence/relapse is common. Mild cases usually respond to discontinuation of the offending antimicrobial, allowing re-establishment of the patient's normal bowel flora or metronidazole. More severe cases merit treatment with oral vancomycin. Some strains have been associated with particularly severe disease and have caused large outbreaks in hospitals – combined therapy with oral vancomycin and parenteral metronidazole plus intensive care support is required for the most serious cases. Intracolonic instillation of vancomycin, intravenous immunoglobulin and surgery (e.g. total colectomy) have also been used. Treatment guidelines are summarised elsewhere.[23] Fidaxomicin (an RNA polymerase inhibitor) has been recently introduced and appears to be as effective as vancomycin for therapy of *C. difficile* infection but may be associated with a reduction in relapse/recurrence rates. Diarrhoea in some cases can be intractable. Instillation of microbiologically screened donor faeces (i.e. faecal transplantation) in an attempt to restore a normal balance of the gut flora – in some cases with surprisingly good response rates of over 80% in therapeutic trials.[24] Several guidelines support its use, though they warn potential risks.

Faecal microbiota transplant for recurrent Clostridium difficile infection. Available at: https://www.nice.org.uk/guidance/ipg485. Accessed November 2017.[25]

C. difficile may be spread among hospitalised patients on the unwashed hands of health-care workers and also survives well (it is a spore-forming organism) in the environment – symptomatic patients should be isolated and the ward cleaned carefully. Hospital outbreaks have responded to combinations of control measures ('care bundles'), especially involving severe restriction of the use of cephalosporin and quinolone antibiotics.

Opportunistic infection arises in patients whose immune systems are compromised or whose phagocytic cellular defences have been reduced by disease (e.g. AIDS, hypogammaglobulinaemia, leukaemia) or drugs (e.g. cytotoxics). Such infections may involve organisms that rarely or never cause clinical disease in normal hosts. Treatment of possible infections in such patients should be prompt, initiated before the results of bacteriological tests are known, and usually involve combinations of bactericidal drugs administered parenterally. Infections of this type include *Pneumocystis carinii* pneumonia, and 'primary' septicaemia in neutropenic patients with gut organisms such as *Escherichia coli* and *Klebsiella* spp. which cross the mucosa of the gut and invade the bloodstream directly. Local defences may also be compromised and allow opportunistic infection with lowly pathogens even in otherwise healthy hosts: the best example is *Staphylococcus epidermidis* infection of intravenous catheters.

Masking of infections

Masking of infections by chemotherapy is an important possibility. For example, a course of penicillin adequate to cure gonorrhoea may prevent simultaneously contracted syphilis from showing primary and secondary stages without effecting a cure, and a serological test for syphilis should therefore be done 3 months after treatment for gonorrhoea.

Drugs of choice

For detailed guidance on the choice of antimicrobial drugs for particular infections, the reader is referred to Chapters 13 and 14, and to a variety of contemporary clinical sources, including textbooks of microbiology and infectious diseases.

In previous editions, we have referred to the current 'Medical Letter on Drugs and Therapeutics' and 'Treatment Guidelines from the Medical Letter' (USA) editions from 2000 to 2010 (current version available online at: http://www.medicalletter.org/downloads/t94-1.pdf), and this is still valuable, although it is of most relevance to North American practice.

[23]Debast SB, Bauer MP, Kuijper EJ, European Society of Clinical M, Infectious D. European Society of Clinical Microbiology and Infectious Diseases: update of the treatment guidance document for Clostridium difficile infection. *Clin Microbiol Infect*. 2014;20 Suppl 2(March):1-26. doi:http://dx.doi.org/10.1111/1469-0691.12418.

[24]Garborg K, Waagsbø B, Stallemo A et al 2010 Results of faecal donor instillation therapy for recurrent *Clostridium difficile*-associated diarrhoea. Scandinavian Journal of Infectious Diseases 42:857–861.

[25]Cammarota G, Ianiro G, Tilg H, et al European FMT Working Group. European consensus conference on faecal microbiota transplantation in clinical practice. Gut. 2017 Apr;66(4):569-580. doi: 10.1136/gutjnl-2016-313017. Epub 2017 Jan 13.

Detailed guidance, intended for use by primary care physicians in England and including evidence-based recommendations on antibiotic choice for particular infections and extensive reference lists, is available via the Public Health England website.[26] We also recommend section 5 of the Electronic British National Formulary (https://www.bnf.org/products/bnf-online/). Tables on drugs for viruses, fungi, protozoa and helminths are provided in Chapter 15.

---

[26]https://www.gov.uk/government/organisations/public-health-england.

Guide to further reading

Ada, G., 2001. Vaccines and vaccination. N. Engl. J. Med. 345, 1042–1053.

Alliance for the Prudent Use of Antibiotics (APUA), The APUA website has a wide range of articles and useful links relating to the control of antimicrobial resistance worldwide. Available at: http://www.tufts.edu/med/apua/. (Accessed November 2017).

Arias, C.A., Murray, B.E., 2009. Antibiotic-resistant bugs in the 21st century – a clinical super-challenge. N. Engl. J. Med. 360, 439–443.

Aymes, S., 2005. Treatment of staphylococcal infection. Prescriptions must be part of a package that includes infection control. Br. Med. J. 330, 976–977.

Bode, L.G., Kluytmans, J.A., Wertheim, H.F., et al., 2010. Preventing surgical-site infections in nasal carriers of Staphylococcus aureus. N. Engl. J. Med. 362, 9–17.

Boudma, L., Luyt, C.E., Tubach, F., et al., 2010. Use of procalcitonin to reduce patients' exposure to antibiotics in intensive care units (PRORATA trial): a multicentre randomized controlled trial. Lancet 375, 463–474.

Broyles, M.R., 2017. Impact of Procalcitonin-Guided Antibiotic Management on Antibiotic Exposure and Outcomes: Real-world Evidence. Open Forum Infect Dis 4 (4), ofx213. doi: 10.1093/ofid/ofx213. eCollection 2017 Fall.

Colebrook, L., Kenny, M., 1939. Treatment with prontosil for puerperal infections. Lancet 2, 1319. (a classic paper).

Connaughton, M., 2008. Commentary: controversies in NICE guidance on infective endocarditis. Available at: http://www.bmj.com/content/336/7647/771.full.pdf. (Accessed November 2017).

Corwin, P., Toop, L., McGeoch, G., et al., 2005. Randomised controlled trial of intravenous antibiotic treatment for cellulitis at home compared with hospital. Br. Med. J. 330, 129–132.

Dancer, S.J., 2004. How antibiotics can make us sick: the less obvious adverse effects of antimicrobial chemotherapy. Lancet Infect. Dis. 4, 611–619.

Deleo, F.R., Otto, M., Kreiswirth, B.N., Chambers, H.F., 2010. Community-acquired meticillin-resistant Staphylococcus aureus. Lancet 375, 1557–1568.

Fletcher, C., 1984. First clinical use of penicillin. Br. Med. J. 289, 1721–1723 (a classic paper).

Gluud, C.G., Gluud, L.L., 2005. Evidence based diagnostics. Br. Med. J. 330, 724–726.

Public Health England. The 'Antimicrobial Resistance' section of the website of the UK Public Health England. Available at: https://www.gov.uk/government/collections/antimicrobial-resistance-amr-information-and-resources. (Accessed November 2017) is a valuable resource of contemporary background information on the prevalence and epidemiology of infectious diseases and antimicrobial resistance in the UK. Also on the PHE website, quarterly-updated reports on MRSA MSSA, E. coli bacteraemia and Clostridium difficile diarrhoea rates in England and Wales can be found at: https://www.gov.uk/government/statistics/mrsa-mssa-and-e-coli-bacteraemia-and-c-difficile-infection-quarterly-epidemiological-commentary. (Accessed November 2017).

Kluytmans, J., Struelens, M., 2009. Meticillin resistant Staphylococcus aureus in the hospital. Br. Med. J. 338, 532–537.

Loudon, I., 1987. Puerperal fever, the streptococcus, and the sulphonamides, 1911–1945. Br. Med. J. 295, 485–490.

Morel, C., Mossailos, E., 2010. Stoking the antibiotic pipeline. Br. Med. J. 340, 1115–1118.

Pitout, J.D., 2010. The latest threat in the war on antimicrobial resistance (NDM beta-lactamases). Lancet Infect. Dis. 10, 578–579.

Pitout, J.D., 2010. Infections with extended-spectrum beta-lactamase-producing Enterobacteriaceae: changing epidemiology and drug treatment choices. Drugs 70, 313–333.

Queenan, A.M., Bush, K., 2007. Carbapenemases: the versatile beta-lactamases. Clin. Microbiol. Rev. 20, 440–458.

Richie, R., Wray, D., Stoken, T., 2008. Prophylaxis against infective endocarditis: summary of NICE guidance. Available online: http://www.bmj.com/content/336/7647/770.full.pdf. (Accessed November 2017).

Ryan, E.T., Wilson, M.E., Kain, K.C., 2002. Illness after international travel. N. Engl. J. Med. 347, 505–516.

Shannon-Lowe, J., Matheson, N.J., Cooke, F.J., Aliyu, S.H., 2010. Prevention and medical management of Clostridium difficile infection. Br. Med. J. 340, 641–646.

Stix, G., 2006. An antibiotic resistance fighter. New Sci. April, 80–83.

Taubert, K.A., Wilson, W., 2017. Is endocarditis prophylaxis for dental procedures necessary? Heart Asia 9 (1), 63–67. doi: 10.1136/heartasia-2016-010810. eCollection 2017.

Chapter | **13** |

Antibacterial drugs

David A. Enoch, Mark Farrington

SYNOPSIS

The range of antibacterial drugs is wide and affords the clinician scope to select with knowledge of microbial susceptibilities and patient factors, e.g. allergy, site of infection, renal disease. Because members of each structural group are usually handled by the body in a similar way and have the same range of adverse effects, antibacterial drugs are here discussed in groups, primarily by their site of antibacterial action, and secondly by molecular structure.

Classification

Inhibition of cell wall synthesis

β-**lactams** the structure of which contains a β-lactam ring. The major subdivisions are:

- *Penicillins,* whose official names usually include, or end in, 'cillin'.
- *Cephalosporins* and *cephamycins,* which are recognised by the inclusion of 'cef' or 'ceph' in their official names. In the UK recently, all these names have been standardised to begin with 'cef'.

Other subcategories of β-lactams include:

- Carbapenems (e.g. meropenem).
- Monobactams (e.g. aztreonam).
- β-lactamase inhibitors (e.g. clavulanic acid).

Other inhibitors of cell-wall synthesis include vancomycin and teicoplanin.

Inhibition of protein synthesis

Aminoglycosides. The names of those that are derived from streptomyces end in 'mycin', e.g. tobramycin. Others include gentamicin (from *Micromonospora purpurea* which is not a fungus, hence the spelling as 'micin') and semi-synthetic drugs, e.g. amikacin.

Tetracyclines, as the name suggests, are four-ringed structures, and their names end in '-cycline'.

Macrolides: e.g. erythromycin. Clindamycin, structurally a lincosamide, has a similar action and overlapping antibacterial activity.

Other drugs that act by inhibiting protein synthesis include quinupristin-dalfopristin, linezolid, chloramphenicol and sodium fusidate.

Inhibition of nucleic acid synthesis

Sulfonamides. Usually their names contain 'sulpha' or 'sulfa'. These drugs and trimethoprim, with which they may be combined, inhibit synthesis of nucleic acid precursors.

Quinolones are structurally related to nalidixic acid; the names of the most recently introduced members of the group end in '-oxacin', e.g. ciprofloxacin. They act by preventing DNA replication.

Azoles all contain an azole ring, and the names end in '-azole', e.g. metronidazole. They act by the production of short-lived intermediates toxic to the DNA of sensitive organisms. Rifampicin inhibits bacterial DNA-dependent RNA polymerase.

Antimicrobials that are restricted to certain specific uses, i.e. tuberculosis, urinary tract infections, are described with the treatment of these conditions in Chapter 14.

Inhibition of cell wall synthesis

β-lactams

Penicillins

Benzylpenicillin (1942) is produced by growing one of the penicillium moulds in deep tanks. In 1957 the penicillin nucleus (6-amino-penicillanic acid) was synthesised and it became possible to add various side-chains and so to make semi-synthetic penicillins with different properties. Penicillins differ widely in antibacterial spectrum. A general account of the penicillins follows and then of the individual drugs insofar as they differ.

Mode of action. Penicillins act by inhibiting the enzymes (penicillin-binding proteins, PBPs) involved in the cross-linking of the peptidoglycan layer of the cell wall, which is weakened, and this leads to osmotic rupture. Penicillins are thus bactericidal and are ineffective against resting organisms which are not making new cell wall. The main defence of bacteria against penicillins is to produce enzymes, β-lactamases, which hydrolyse the β-lactam ring. Other mechanisms that have been described include modifications to PBPs to render them unable to bind β-lactams, reduced permeability of the outer cell membrane of Gram-negative bacteria (porin loss), and up-regulation of efflux pumps in the outer membrane which remove β-lactam molecules. Some particularly resistant bacteria may possess several mechanisms that act in concert. The remarkable safety and high therapeutic index of the penicillins is due to the fact that human cells, while bounded by a cell membrane, lack a cell wall. They exhibit time-dependent bacterial killing (see p. 168).

Pharmacokinetics. Benzylpenicillin is destroyed by gastric acid and is unsuitable for oral use. Others, e.g. phenoxymethylpenicillin, resist acid and are absorbed in the upper small bowel. The plasma $t_{1/2}$ of penicillins is usually <2 h. They are distributed mainly in the body water and enter well into the CSF if the meninges are inflamed. Penicillins are organic acids, and their rapid clearance from plasma is due to secretion into renal tubular fluid by the anion transport mechanism in the kidney. Renal clearance therefore greatly exceeds the glomerular filtration rate (127 mL/min). The excretion of penicillin can be usefully delayed by concurrently giving probenecid, which competes successfully for the transport mechanism. Dosage of penicillins may need to be reduced for patients with severely impaired renal function.

Adverse effects. The main hazard with the penicillins is *allergic reactions*. These include itching, rashes (eczematous or urticarial), fever and angioedema. Rarely (about 1 in 10 000) there is anaphylactic shock, which can be fatal (about 1 in 50 000–100 000 treatment courses). Allergies are least likely when penicillins are given orally and most likely with topical application. Metabolic opening of the β-lactam ring creates a highly reactive penicilloyl group which polymerises and binds with tissue proteins to form the major antigenic determinant. The anaphylactic reaction involves specific IgE antibodies which can be detected in the plasma of susceptible persons.

There is *cross-allergy* between all the various forms of penicillin, probably due in part to their common structure, and in part to the degradation products common to them all. *Partial cross-allergy* exists between penicillins and cephalosporins (1–10%, dependent on the generation of the cephalosporin), which is of particular concern when the reaction to either group of antimicrobials has been angioedema or anaphylactic shock. Carbapenems (meropenem and imipenem-cilastatin) and, especially, the monobactam aztreonam apparently have a lower risk of cross-reactivity. One experimental study estimated the rate of reactivity to meropenem in patients with a previous history of immediate penicillin hypersensitivity reaction as a maximum of 5.2%.

When attempting to predict whether a patient will have an allergic reaction, a reliable history of a previous adverse response to penicillin is valuable. Immediate-type reactions such as urticaria, angioedema and anaphylactic shock can be taken to indicate allergy, but interpretation of maculo-papular rashes is more difficult. Since an alternative drug can usually be found, a penicillin is best avoided if there is suspicion of allergy, although the condition is undoubtedly overdiagnosed and may be transient (see below).

When the history of allergy is not clear-cut and it is necessary to prescribe a penicillin, the presence of IgE antibodies in serum is a useful indicator of reactions mediated by these antibodies, i.e. immediate (type I) reactions. Additionally, an intradermal test for allergy may be performed using standard amounts of a mixture of a major determinant (metabolite) (benzylpenicilloyl polylysine) and minor determinants (such as benzylpenicillin) of the allergic reaction; appearance of a flare and wheal reaction indicates a positive response. The fact that only about 10% of patients with a history of 'penicillin allergy' respond suggests that many who are so labelled are not, or are no longer, allergic to penicillin.

Other adverse effects include diarrhoea due to alteration in normal intestinal flora, which may progress to *Clostridium difficile*-associated diarrhoea. Neutropenia is a risk if penicillins (or other β-lactam antibiotics) are used in high dose and usually for a period of longer than 10 days. Rarely the penicillins cause anaemia, sometimes haemolytic, and thrombocytopenia or interstitial nephritis. Sometimes patients receiving parenteral β-lactams may develop fever with no other signs of an adverse reaction except occasionally for a modestly raised CRP: this should always be considered in the investigation of such patients who seem otherwise well, and cautiously stopping antibiotic therapy usually produces a prompt resolution. Penicillins are presented as their sodium or potassium salts which are inevitably taken in significant amounts for patients with renal or cardiac disease if high dose of antimicrobial is used. Extremely high plasma penicillin concentrations cause convulsions. Co-amoxiclav and flucloxacillin given in high doses for prolonged periods in the elderly may cause hepatic toxicity.

Narrow-spectrum penicillins

Benzylpenicillin

Benzylpenicillin ($t_{1/2}$ 0.5 h) (penicillin G) has to be given with spaced doses that have to be large to maintain a therapeutic concentration, but the large therapeutic ratio of penicillin allows the resulting fluctuations to be tolerable.[1] Benzylpenicillin is eliminated by the kidney, with about 80% being actively secreted by the renal tubule, and this can be blocked by probenecid.

Uses. Benzylpenicillin is highly active against *Streptococcus pneumoniae* and the Lancefield Group A, β-haemolytic streptococcus *(Streptococcus pyogenes)*. Viridans streptococci are usually sensitive unless the patient has recently received penicillin. *Enterococcus faecalis* is less susceptible and, especially for endocarditis, penicillin should be combined with an aminoglycoside, usually gentamicin. This combination is synergistic unless the enterococcus is highly resistant to the aminoglycoside (minimal inhibitory concentration (MIC) of 128 mg/L or above); such strains are becoming more frequent in hospital patients and present major difficulties in therapy. Over 90% of *Staphylococcus aureus* are now resistant in hospital and domiciliary practice. Benzylpenicillin is a drug of choice for infections due to *Neisseria meningitidis* (meningococcal meningitis and septicaemia), *Bacillus anthracis* (anthrax), *Clostridium perfringens* (gas gangrene) and *tetani* (tetanus), *Corynebacterium diphtheriae* (diphtheria), *Treponema pallidum* (syphilis), *Leptospira* spp. (leptospirosis), *Actinomyces israelii* (actinomycosis) and for *Borrelia burgdorferi* (Lyme disease) in children. Penicillin resistance rates in *Neisseria gonorrhoeae* are high in many parts of the world.

Adverse effects are in general uncommon, apart from allergy (above). It is salutary to reflect that the first clinically useful true antibiotic (1942) is still in use and remains among the least toxic.

Preparations and dosage for injection. Benzylpenicillin may be given i.m. or i.v. (by bolus injection or by continuous infusion). For a sensitive infection, benzylpenicillin[2] 600 mg 6-hourly is enough.

For relatively insensitive infections and where sensitive organisms are sequestered within avascular tissue (e.g. infective endocarditis) 7.2 g is given daily i.v. in divided doses. When an infection is controlled, a change may be made to the oral route with phenoxymethylpenicillin (amoxicillin is more reliably absorbed in adults).

Procaine penicillin, given i.m. only, liberates benzylpenicillin over 12–24 h, but it will not give therapeutic blood concentrations for some hours after injection, and peak concentrations are low.

Preparations and dosage for oral use. Phenoxymethylpenicillin (penicillin V) is resistant to gastric acid and so is moderately well absorbed, sometimes erratically in adults. It is less active than benzylpenicillin against *Neisseria gonorrhoeae* and *meningitidis*, and so is unsuitable for use in gonorrhoea and meningococcal meningitis, although satisfactory against *Streptococcus pneumoniae* and *Streptococcus pyogenes*, especially after the acute infection has been controlled by intravenous therapy. The dose is 500 mg 6-hourly.

All oral penicillins are best given on an empty stomach to avoid the absorption delay caused by food.

Antistaphylococcal penicillins

Certain bacteria produce β-lactamases which open the β-lactam ring that is common to all penicillins, thus terminating their antibacterial activity. β-lactamases vary in their activity against different β-lactams, with side-chains attached to the β-lactam ring stearically hindering access of the drug to the enzymes' active sites.

Examples of agents stable to staphylococcal β-lactamases include:

- *Flucloxacillin* ($t_{1/2}$ 1 h) is better absorbed and so gives higher blood concentrations than does cloxacillin. It may cause cholestatic jaundice, particularly when used for more than 2 weeks or given to patients older than 55 years of age.
- *Cloxacillin* ($t_{1/2}$ 0.5 h) has been withdrawn from the market in some countries, including the UK.
- *Methicillin* and *oxacillin*: Their use is now confined to laboratory sensitivity tests. Identification of methicillin-resistant *Staphylococcus aureus* (MRSA) in patients indicates the organisms are resistant to all β-lactam antibiotics and often to other antibacterial drugs.

Broad-spectrum penicillins

The activity of these semi-synthetic penicillins extends to include many Gram-negative bacilli. They do not resist β-lactamases, and their usefulness has reduced markedly in recent years because of the increased prevalence of organisms that produce these enzymes.

---

[1] Is it surprise at the answer that reduces most classes of students to silence when asked the trough:peak ratio for a drug given 6-hourly with a $t_{1/2}$ of 0.5 h? (answer: $2^{12} = 4096$).
[2] 600 mg = 1 000 000 units, 1 mega-unit.

These agents are less active than benzylpenicillin against Gram-positive cocci, but more active than the β-lactamase-resistant penicillins (above). They have useful activity against *Enterococcus faecalis* and many strains of *Haemophilus influenzae*. *Enterobacteriaceae* are unreliably susceptible. Members of this group differ more pharmacologically than antibacterially.

Amoxicillin ($t_{1/2}$ 1 h; previously known as amoxycillin) is a structural analogue of ampicillin (below) and is better absorbed from the gut (especially after food), and for the same dose achieves approximately double the plasma concentration. Diarrhoea is less frequent with amoxicillin than with ampicillin. The oral dose is 250–500 mg 8-hourly; a parenteral form is available but offers no advantage over ampicillin.

Ampicillin ($t_{1/2}$ 1 h) is acid-stable and is moderately well absorbed when swallowed. The oral dose is 250 mg–1 g 6–8-hourly; or i.m. or i.v. 500 mg 4–6-hourly. Approximately one-third of a dose appears unchanged in the urine. The drug is concentrated in the bile.

Co-amoxiclav (Augmentin). *Clavulanic acid* is a β-lactam molecule which has little intrinsic antibacterial activity but binds irreversibly to β-lactamases. Thereby it competitively protects the penicillin against bacterial β-lactamases, acting as a 'suicide' inhibitor. It is formulated in tablets as its potassium salt (equivalent to 125 mg of clavulanic acid) in combination with amoxicillin (250 or 500 mg), as co-amoxiclav, and is a satisfactory oral treatment for infections due to β-lactamase–producing organisms, notably in the respiratory or urogenital tracts. These include many strains of *Staphylococcus aureus*, *Escherichia coli* and an increasing proportion of *Haemophilus influenzae*. It also has useful activity against β-lactamase–producing anaerobes (e.g. *Bacteroides* spp.). The $t_{1/2}$ is 1 h, and the dose one tablet 8-hourly.

Adverse effects. Ampicillin may cause diarrhoea, but the incidence (12%) is less with amoxicillin. Ampicillin and amoxicillin are commonly associated with *Clostridium difficile* diarrhoea, related to the frequency of their use rather than to high innate risk of causing the disease. Ampicillin and its analogues may cause a macular rash resembling measles or rubella, usually unaccompanied by other signs of allergy, and seen in patients with disease of the lymphoid system, notably *infectious mononucleosis* and lymphoid leukaemia. A macular rash should not be taken to imply allergy to other penicillins, which tend to cause a true urticarial reaction. Patients with renal failure and those taking allopurinol for hyperuricaemia also seem more prone to ampicillin rashes. Cholestatic jaundice has been associated with use of co-amoxiclav even up to 6 weeks after cessation of the drug; the clavulanic acid may be responsible.

Mecillinam

Pivmecillinam ($t_{1/2}$ 1 h) is an oral agent active against Gram-negative organisms including many extended-spectrum β-lactamase–producing (ESBL) Enterobacteriaceae, but inactive against *Pseudomonas aeruginosa* and its relatives and Gram-positive organisms. Pivmecillinam is hydrolysed in vivo to the active form mecillinam (which is poorly absorbed by mouth). It has been used to treat urinary tract infection.

Temocillin

Temocillin is a semi-synthetic 6-alpha-methoxy derivative of ticarcillin that is highly stable to most β-lactamases except metallo-carbapenemases (e.g. IMP, NDM, VIM) and OXA-48 like enzymes. It lacks activity against anaerobes, Gram positive bacteria and most Gram-negative non-fermenters such as Pseudomonas aeruginosa and Acinetobacter spp. It does, however, have in vitro activity against ESBL- and AmpC-producing Enterobacteriaceae (Livermore et al. 2006; Rodriguez-Villalobos et al. 2011), KPC-producing E. coli and Klebsiella pneumoniae (Adams-Haduch et al. 2009) and Burkholderia cepacia complex (Bonacorsi et al. 1999).

Clinical studies are limited to non-comparative series. Optimal dosage (≥2 g twice daily) was associated with improved outcome, whilst the presence of AmpC or ESBL did not affect outcome. Two retrospective non-randomised studies of the use of temocillin in cystic fibrosis patients with B. cepacia complex have been published (Kent et al. 2008; Lekkas et al. 2006)

Antipseudomonal penicillins

Carboxypenicillins

These in general have the same antibacterial spectrum as ampicillin (and are susceptible to β-lactamases), but have the additional capacity to destroy *Pseudomonas aeruginosa* and indole-positive *Proteus* spp.

Ticarcillin ($t_{1/2}$ 1 h) is presented in combination with clavulanic acid (as Timentin), so to provide greater activity against β-lactamase – producing organisms. It is given by i.m. or slow i.v. injection or by rapid i.v. infusion.

Ureidopenicillins

These are adapted from the ampicillin molecule, with a side-chain derived from urea. They must be administered parenterally and are eliminated mainly in the urine. Accumulation in patients with poor renal function is less than with other penicillins, as 25% is excreted in the bile. An unusual feature of their kinetics is that, as the dose is increased, the plasma concentration rises disproportionately, i.e. they exhibit *saturation (zero-order) kinetics*.

For pseudomonas septicaemia, a ureidopenicillin plus an aminoglycoside provides a synergistic effect, but the co-administration in the same fluid results in inactivation of the aminoglycoside (as with carboxypenicillins, above).

Piperacillin ($t_{1/2}$ 1 h) is available as a combination with the β-lactamase inhibitor tazobactam (as Tazocin).

Cephalosporins

Cephalosporins were first obtained from a filamentous fungus *Cephalosporium* cultured from the sea near a Sardinian sewage outfall in 1945; their molecular structure is closely related to that of penicillin, and many semi-synthetic forms have been introduced. They now comprise a group of antibiotics having a wide range of activity and low toxicity. The term 'cephalosporins' will be used here in a general sense, although some are strictly cephamycins, e.g. cefoxitin and cefotetan.

Mode of action is that of the β-lactams, i.e. cephalosporins impair bacterial cell wall synthesis and hence are bactericidal. They exhibit time-dependent bacterial killing (see p. 168).

The addition of various side-chains on the cephalosporin molecule confers variety in pharmacokinetic and antibacterial activities. The β-lactam ring can be protected by such structural manoeuvring, which results in compounds with improved activity against Gram-negative organisms, but less anti–Gram-positive activity. The cephalosporins resist attack by some β-lactamases, but resistance is mediated by other means.

Pharmacokinetics. Usually, cephalosporins are excreted unchanged in the urine, but some, including cefotaxime, form a desacetyl metabolite which possesses some antibacterial activity. Many are actively secreted by the renal tubule, a process which can be blocked with probenecid. As a rule, the dose of cephalosporins should be reduced in patients with poor renal function. Cephalosporins in general have a $t_{1/2}$ of 1–4 h, although there are exceptions (e.g. ceftriaxone, $t_{1/2}$ 8 h). Wide distribution in the body allows treatment of infection at most sites, including bone, soft tissue, muscle and (in some cases) CSF. Data on individual cephalosporins appear in Table 13.1.

Table 13.1 The cephalosporins

Drug	$t_{1/2}$ (h)	Excretion in urine (%)	Comment
First generation **Parenteral**			
Cefazolin	2	90	Generally replaced by the newer cephalosporins
Cefradine (also oral)	1	86	
Oral			
Cefaclor	1	86	All very similar. Effective against common respiratory pathogens but (excepting cefaclor) poor activity against *Haemophilus influenzae*. More active against *Escherichia coli* than amoxicillin and trimethoprim. Uncomplicated upper and lower respiratory tract, urinary tract and soft-tissue infections, and follow-on treatment once parenteral drugs have brought infection under control
Cefadroxil	2	88	
Cefalexin	1	88	
Second generation **Parenteral**			
Cefoxitin (a cephamycin) (Cefotetan is similar)	1	90	More resistant to β-lactamases than first-generation drugs; active against *Staphylococcus aureus*, *Streptococcus pyogenes*, *Streptococcus pneumoniae*, *Neisseria* spp., *Haemophilus influenzae* and many Enterobacteriaceae. Cefoxitin also kills *Bacteroides fragilis* in abdominal and pelvic infections. Cefuroxime may be given for community-acquired pneumonia (not when caused by *Mycoplasma pneumoniae*, *Legionella* or *Chlamydia*). The oral form, cefuroxime axetil, is also used for the range of infections listed for the first-generation oral cephalosporins (above)
Cefuroxime (also oral)	1	80	

Table 13.1 The cephalosporins—cont'd

Drug	$t_{1/2}$ (h)	Excretion in urine (%)	Comment
Third generation Parenteral			More effective than second-generation against Gram-negative organisms while retaining activity against Gram-positive bacteria. Cefotaxime and ceftriaxone are used for serious infections such as septicaemia, pneumonia, and for meningitis. Ceftriaxone is also used for gonorrhoea and Lyme disease; also once-per day outpatient i.v. therapy
Cefotaxime	1	60	
Ceftazidime	2	88	
Ceftriaxone	8	56 (44 bile)	
Oral			
Cefixime	4	23 (77 bile)	Active against a range of Gram-positive and Gram-negative organisms including *Staphylococcus aureus* (excepting cefixime), *Streptococcus pyogenes*, *Streptococcus pneumoniae*, *Neisseria* spp., *Haemophilus influenzae* and (excepting cefpodoxime) many Enterobacteriaceae. Used to treat urinary, upper and lower respiratory tract infections
Cefprozil	2	40	
Cefpodoxime proxetil	2	80	Used as a marker in the laboratory for the detection of ESBL
Fourth generation			
Cefpirome	2.3	75	
Cefepime	2	85	
Fifth generation			
Ceftobiprole	3.5	70	Additionally active against MRSA
Ceftaroline	1.6 (2.6 after multiple doses)	88	Additionally active against MRSA
Others			
Ceftolozane-tazobactam	2.5 (2.7 after multiple doses)	95	Additional Gram-negative cover
Ceftazidime avibactam	2	80–90	Additional Gram-negative cover

Classification and uses. The cephalosporins are conventionally categorised by 'generations' sharing broadly similar antibacterial and pharmacokinetic properties; newer agents have rendered this classification less precise but it retains sufficient usefulness to be presented in Table 13.1.

Adverse effects. Cephalosporins are well tolerated. The most usual unwanted effects are allergic reactions of the penicillin type, and gastrointestinal upset. Overall the rate of cephalosporin skin reactions such as urticarial rashes and pruritus lies between 1% and 3%. There is cross-allergy between penicillins and cephalosporins involving 1–10% of patients (depending on generation of cephalosporin); if a patient has had a severe or immediate allergic reaction or if serum or skin testing for penicillin allergy is positive (see p. 182), then a cephalosporin should not be used. Pain may be experienced at the sites of i.v. or i.m. injection. If cephalosporins are continued for more than 2 weeks, reversible thrombocytopenia, haemolytic anaemia, neutropenia, interstitial nephritis or abnormal liver function tests may occur. The broad spectrum of activity of the third-generation cephalosporins may predispose to opportunistic infection with resistant bacteria or *Candida albicans* and to *Clostridium difficile* diarrhoea. In the UK, reduction of broad-spectrum cephalosporin use is one component of the bundle of measures aimed to reduce the incidence of *Clostridium difficile*–associated diarrhoea. Ceftriaxone achieves high concentrations in bile and, as the calcium salt, may precipitate to cause symptoms resembling cholelithiasis (biliary pseudolithiasis).

Ceftobiprole is a parenteral cephalosporin which binds avidly to the mutated penicillin binding protein 2′ responsible for methicillin resistance in staphylococci. It is unusual for cephalosporins in that it has good activity in vitro MRSA and *Enterococcus faecalis* and better activity than ceftriaxone against penicillin-resistant pneumococci. Clinical trials are underway in skin and soft-tissue infection and pneumonia. Ceftaroline has a similar spectrum of activity and range of indications to ceftobiprole. A number of cephalosporins have recently been combined with β-lactam inhibitors. Ceftolozane-tazobactam and ceftazidime-avibactam have extended Gram-negative activity, particularly against *Pseudomonas aeruginosa*.

Other β-lactam antibacterials

Monobactam

Aztreonam ($t_{1/2}$ 2 h) is the first member of this class of β-lactam antibiotic. It is active against Gram-negative organisms including *Pseudomonas aeruginosa*, *Haemophilus influenzae* and *Neisseria meningitidis* and *gonorrhoeae*. Aztreonam is used to treat septicaemia and complicated urinary tract infections, lower urinary tract infections and gonorrhoea.

Adverse effects include reactions at the site of infusion, rashes, gastrointestinal upset, hepatitis, thrombocytopenia and neutropenia. It may be used with caution in penicillin-allergic patients.

Carbapenems

Members of this group have the widest spectrum of all currently available antimicrobials, being bactericidal against most Gram-positive and Gram-negative aerobic and anaerobic pathogenic bacteria. They are resistant to hydrolysis by most β-lactamases, including ESBLs. Only occasional pseudomonas relatives (e.g. *Stenotrophomonas maltophilia*, *Elizabethkingia meningoseptica*) are naturally resistant. Acquired resistance is uncommon but emerging, particularly in Enterobacteriaceae and *Pseudomonas aeruginosa*. This could be due to ESBL with porin loss or, more worryingly, to the emergence of carbapenemases. There are a number of different carbapenemases, and the number of types is increasing. The most common carbapenemases include KPC (*Klebsiella pneumoniae* carbapenemase), NDM (new Delhi metallo-β-lactamase), VIM (Verona integron encoded metallo-β-lactamase) and OXA-48 (oxacillinase). They are often plasmid-borne and readily transmissible; OXA-48 in particular can also be easily missed by standard laboratory methods. All have geographic areas where they are more common, though some patients are infected/colonized with multiple carbapenemases.

Imipenem

Imipenem ($t_{1/2}$ 1 h) is inactivated by metabolism in the kidney to products that are potentially toxic to renal tubules; combining imipenem with cilastatin (as Primaxin), a specific inhibitor of dihydropeptidase – the enzyme responsible for its renal metabolism – prevents both inactivation and toxicity.

Imipenem is used to treat septicaemia, intra-abdominal infection and nosocomial pneumonia. In terms of imipenem, 1–2 g/day is given by i.v. infusion in 3–4 doses.

Adverse effects. It may cause gastrointestinal upset including nausea, blood disorders, allergic reactions, confusion and convulsions.

Meropenem ($t_{1/2}$ 1 h) is similar to imipenem, but is stable to renal dihydropeptidase and can therefore be given without cilastatin. It penetrates into the CSF and is not associated with nausea or convulsions.

Ertapenem ($t_{1/2}$ 4 h) is given as a single daily injection; because of this, it has found a niche indication for parenteral therapy of multiply resistant Gram-negative bacteria out of hospital, such as ESBL-producing coliforms. It is, however, much less active against *Pseudomonas aeruginosa*, *Acinetobacter* and their relatives and *Enterococcus* spp. Adverse events are uncommon, but include diarrhoea (4.8%), infusion vein phlebitis (4.5%) and nausea (2.8%).

Penems

Faropenem ($t_{1/2}$ approximately 1 h) is the first of this group to reach the clinical trial stage. Penems are hybrids of penicillins and cephalosporins, and faropenem is well absorbed by mouth, and is active against a wide range of Gram-positive and Gram-negative pathogens. It is not available in the UK.

Other inhibitors of cell wall synthesis and membrane function

Vancomycin

Vancomycin ($t_{1/2}$ 8 h), a 'glycopeptide', acts on multiplying organisms by inhibiting cell wall formation at a site different from the β-lactam antibacterials. It is bactericidal against most strains of clostridia (including *Clostridium difficile*), almost all strains of *Staphylococcus aureus* (including those that produce β-lactamase and methicillin-resistant strains), coagulase-negative staphylococci, viridans group streptococci and enterococci. Frankly resistant *Staphylococcus aureus* strains have been exceptionally rarely reported, although isolates with raised (but still formally susceptible) vancomycin MICs around 2–3 mg/L have been increasingly recognised and have a somewhat poorer outcome when the drug is used to treat serious, systemic infections such as endocarditis and bacteraemia. Detecting these borderline-susceptible strains reliably in the microbiology laboratory can be technically challenging. Therapeutic drug monitoring is important to keep trough concentrations at the upper end of the acceptable scale.

Vancomycin is poorly absorbed from the gut and is given i.v. for systemic infections, as there is no satisfactory i.m. preparation. It distributes effectively into body tissues and is eliminated by the kidney.

Uses. Oral vancomycin is effective in cases of antibiotic-associated pseudomembranous colitis (caused by *Clostridium difficile*) in a dose of 125–500 mg 6-hourly by mouth. Combined with an aminoglycoside, it may be given i.v. for streptococcal endocarditis in patients who are allergic to benzylpenicillin and for serious infection with methicillin-resistant staphylococci. It is not as effective as flucloxacillin for serious infections caused by methicillin-susceptible *S. aureus*. Dosing is guided by plasma concentration monitoring with the aim of achieving trough concentrations between 15 and 20 mg/L. Trough concentrations of up to 25 mg/L of recent vancomycin formulations have not been associated with significant toxicity, and may give better outcomes for the most severe infections and those with less-susceptible strains. There is actually no strong evidence that monitoring peak and/or trough serum vancomycin concentrations reduces the incidence of nephrotoxicity or ototoxicity. However, achieving adequate serum concentrations clearly correlates with both outcome and avoidance of rises in isolates' vancomycin MICs, so initial doses should be calculated on total body-weight even in obese subjects, and dose adjustments should be based on measured serum concentrations performed at least weekly in subjects with stable renal function (and more often in those with reduced or varying renal function).

Adverse effects. Tinnitus and deafness may occur, but may improve if the drug is stopped. Nephrotoxicity and allergic reactions also occur. Rapid i.v. infusion may cause a maculopapular rash, possibly due to histamine release (the 'red person' syndrome).

Teicoplanin is structurally related to vancomycin and is active against Gram-positive bacteria. The $t_{1/2}$ of 50 h allows once daily i.v. or i.m. administration. It is less likely than vancomycin to cause ototoxicity or nephrotoxicity, but serum monitoring is required to assure adequate serum concentrations for severely ill patients and those with changing renal function. It can be given more rapidly than vancomycin.

Daptomycin ($t_{1/2}$ 9 h) is a recently released lipopeptide antibiotic, naturally produced by the bacterium *Streptomyces roseosporus*, which was first isolated from a soil sample from Mount Ararat in Turkey.[3] It has activity against virtually all Gram-positive bacteria, including penicillin-resistant *Streptococcus pneumoniae* and MRSA, regardless of vancomycin resistance phenotype. It is unable to cross the Gram-negative outer membrane, rendering these bacteria resistant.

Daptomycin demonstrates concentration-dependent bactericidal activity, including moderately so against most enterococci (for which vancomycin is generally bacteriostatic). Initial binding to the Gram-positive cell membrane is followed by a variety of effects including membrane depolarisation (probably via the drug forming an ion channel across the membrane: this seems to be the main cidal mechanism) and reduced lipoteichoic acid and protein synthesis. A few *Clostridium* species appear innately resistant, but resistance has proved difficult to induce in vitro, and reduction in susceptibility during clinical use has rarely been reported to date. The underlying mechanisms of resistance seem to involve a variety of physiological effects including an altered membrane potential. Staphylococci with increased vancomycin MICs are also less susceptible to daptomycin, and resistance to both agents is acquired progressively in a stepwise fashion.

It is administered by single daily intravenous injection, and is over 90% protein bound. Virtually no metabolism occurs, and excretion is predominantly renal, with about 60% of a dose being recoverable unchanged from the urine. The standard dosage is 4 mg/kg per dose, with the frequency of dosing reduced to 48-hourly for patients with creatinine clearances below 30 mL/min. A higher dose of 6 mg/kg/day is licensed for right-sided infective endocarditis. Higher doses (e.g. 10 mg/kg/day) have been used for treating patients with enterococcal bacteraemia/endocarditis; it is not licensed for this indication. CSF penetration is only about 5%, but sufficient concentrations may be achieved to be useful, for example, for penicillin-resistant pneumococcal meningitis.

Adverse drug reactions have been reported at similar rates to vancomycin. Use of a longer dose interval has avoided the problems of skeletal muscle pain and rises in serum creatinine kinase (CK) that were reported when daptomycin was first introduced in the 1980s in a twice-daily regimen. These adverse effects led to an interruption in its development. The effects were fully reversible and probably related to the need to allow recovery time for drug action on the

---

[3]Eisenstein B I, Oleson F B Jr, Baltz R H 2010 Daptomycin: from the mountain to the clinic, with essential help from Francis Tally, MD. Clinical Infectious Diseases 50(Suppl. 1):S10–S15.

myocyte cell membrane, but patients receiving daptomycin should nevertheless be monitored for muscle pain or weakness. Weekly serum CK assays should be performed during prolonged treatment courses; mild elevations are seen in about 7% of patients and are usually insignificant, but occasionally discontinuation of therapy is needed. The eosinophil count should also be monitored, as an eosinophilic pneumonitis has been associated with this drug.

Daptomycin is approved in the UK for treatment of complicated skin and skin structure infections caused by Gram-positive bacteria and right-sided infective endocarditis caused by *Staphylococcus aureus* (mainly seen in i.v. drug users). Wider applications will doubtless appear, and it may prove useful in, for example, endocarditis more generally, osteomyelitis and MRSA infections of orthopaedic hardware. It is usefully employed by outpatient antibiotic therapy clinics because of its single daily dosing and clinical safety. It is not approved for therapy of community-acquired pneumonia because of inferior outcomes which may be related to inhibition by pulmonary surfactant.

Oritavancin, dalbavancin and telavancin are semi-synthetic lipoglycopeptides with high, concentration-dependent bactericidal activity in vitro against most Gram-positive pathogens. Their modes of action probably resemble that of vancomycin, inhibiting the late stages of cell wall peptidoglycan synthesis. The large molecular size of these compounds impairs their diffusion in laboratory agars, creating technical difficulties in some antimicrobial susceptibility tests. The drugs are licensed for clinical use in resistant and difficult Gram-positive infections, initially of skin and the soft tissues. They have been compared to vancomycin and found to be non-inferior. Dalbavancin may be of particular use in outpatient antibiotic therapy clinics since it has a prolonged half-life ($t_{1/2}$ 5–7 days) and re-dosing may be required only weekly, and excretion occurs via both urine and faeces.

Cycloserine is used for drug-resistant tuberculosis (see p. 212).

Inhibition of protein synthesis

Aminoglycosides

In the purposeful search that followed the demonstration of the clinical efficacy of penicillin, streptomycin was obtained from *Streptomyces griseus* in 1944, cultured from a heavily manured field, and also from a chicken's throat. Aminoglycosides resemble each other in their mode of action and pharmacokinetic, therapeutic and toxic properties.

Mode of action. The aminoglycosides act inside the cell by binding to the ribosomes in such a way that incorrect amino acid sequences are entered into peptide chains. Aminoglycosides are bactericidal and exhibit concentration-dependent bacterial killing (see p. 168).

Pharmacokinetics. Aminoglycosides are water-soluble and do not readily cross cell membranes. Poor absorption from the intestine necessitates their administration i.v. or i.m. for systemic use, and they distribute mainly to the extracellular fluid; transfer to the cerebrospinal fluid is poor even when the meninges are inflamed. Their $t_{1/2}$ is 2–5 h.

Aminoglycosides are eliminated unchanged mainly by glomerular filtration, and attain high concentrations in the urine. Significant accumulation occurs in the renal cortex. Plasma concentration should be measured regularly (and frequently in renally impaired patients). With prolonged therapy, e.g. endocarditis (gentamicin), monitoring must be meticulous.

Current practice is to administer aminoglycosides as a single daily dose. Algorithms are available to guide such dosing according to patients' weight and renal function, and in this case only trough concentrations need to be assayed. Lean body-weight should be used because aminoglycosides distribute poorly in adipose tissue. Single daily dose therapy is probably less ototoxic and nephrotoxic than divided-dose regimens, and appears to be as effective. The immediate high plasma concentrations that result from single daily dosing are advantageous, e.g. for acutely ill septicaemic patients, as aminoglycosides exhibit concentration-dependent killing (see p. 168). Twice- or thrice-daily dosing regimens are used for endocarditis; post-dose levels are required in addition to pre-dose levels.

Antibacterial activity. Aminoglycosides are in general active against staphylococci and aerobic Gram-negative organisms including almost all the Enterobacteriaceae and many pseudomonads. Bacterial resistance to aminoglycosides is an increasing but patchily distributed problem, notably by acquisition of plasmids (see p. 174) which carry genes coding for the formation of drug-destroying enzymes. Gentamicin resistance is rare in community-acquired pathogens in many hospitals in the UK.

Uses include:

- *Gram-negative bacillary infection*, particularly septicaemia, renal, pelvic and abdominal sepsis. Gentamicin remains the drug of choice, but tobramycin may be preferred for *Pseudomonas aeruginosa*. Amikacin has the widest antibacterial spectrum of the aminoglycosides but is best reserved for infection caused by gentamicin-resistant organisms. If local resistance rates are low, an aminoglycoside may be included in the initial best-guess regimen for treatment of serious septicaemia. A potentially less toxic antibiotic may be substituted when culture results are known

(48–72 h), and toxicity is very rare after such a short course.

- *Bacterial endocarditis.* An aminoglycoside, usually gentamicin, usually comprises part of the antimicrobial combination for enterococcal or streptococcal infection of the heart valves.
- *Other infections*: tuberculosis, tularaemia, plague, brucellosis.
- *Topical uses.* Neomycin and framycetin, too toxic for systemic use, are effective for topical treatment of infections of the conjunctiva or external ear. Tobramycin is given by inhalation for therapy of infective exacerbations of cystic fibrosis: sufficient systemic absorption may occur to recommend assay of serum concentrations in such patients.

Adverse effects. Aminoglycoside toxicity is a risk when the dose administered is high or of long duration, and the risk is higher if renal clearance is inefficient (because of disease or age), other potentially nephrotoxic drugs are co-administered (e.g. loop diuretics, amphotericin B) or the patient is dehydrated. It may take the following forms:

- *Ototoxicity.* Both vestibular (especially with gentamicin and streptomycin) and auditory (amikacin, neomycin) damage may occur, causing hearing loss, vertigo, nystagmus and tinnitus which may be permanent (see above). Tinnitus may give warning of auditory nerve damage. Early signs of vestibular toxicity include motion-related headache, dizziness or nausea. Serious ototoxicity can occur with topical application, including ear drops. At least five mutations in the mitochondrial gene encoding 12 S rRNA have been found that predispose patients to irreversible aminoglycoside hearing loss, and the possibility of screening individuals before commencing therapy is being investigated. Anti–free radical agents such as salicylate may reduce aminoglycoside toxicity. Audiology should be performed at the start of and during therapy, particularly if it is prolonged.
- *Nephrotoxicity.* Dose-related changes, which are usually reversible, occur in renal tubular cells, where aminoglycosides accumulate. Low blood pressure, loop diuretics and advanced age are recognised as added risk factors.
- *Neuromuscular blockade.* Aminoglycosides may impair neuromuscular transmission and aggravate (or reveal) myasthenia gravis, or cause a transient myasthenic syndrome in patients whose neuromuscular transmission is normal.
- *Other reactions* include rashes and haematological abnormalities, including marrow depression, haemolytic anaemia and bleeding due to antagonism of factor V.
- For gentamicin and tobramycin, ototoxicity and nephrotoxicity are increased if peak concentrations exceed 12–14 mg/L consistently, or troughs exceed 2 mg/L. For amikacin the corresponding concentrations are 32–34 mg/L and 10 mg/L.

Individual aminoglycosides

Gentamicin is active against aerobic Gram-negative bacilli including *Escherichia coli*, *Enterobacter*, *Klebsiella*, *Proteus* and *Pseudomonas*. In streptococcal and enterococcal endocarditis, gentamicin is combined with benzylpenicillin or amoxicillin (true synergy is seen provided the enterococcus is not highly resistant to gentamicin).

Dose is 3–7 mg/kg body-weight per day (the highest dose for more serious infections) either as a single dose or in three equally divided doses. The rationale behind single-dose administration is to achieve high peak plasma concentrations (10–14 mg/L, which correlate with therapeutic efficacy) and more time at lower trough concentrations (16 h at <1 mg/L, which are associated with reduced risk of toxicity). Therapy should rarely exceed 7 days. Patients with cystic fibrosis eliminate gentamicin rapidly and require higher doses. Gentamicin applied to the eye gives effective corneal and aqueous humour concentrations.

Tobramycin is similar to gentamicin; it is more active against most strains of *Pseudomonas aeruginosa* and may be less nephrotoxic.

Amikacin is mainly of value because it is more resistant to aminoglycoside-inactivating bacterial enzymes than gentamicin. It is finding new application in the initial management of multiply resistant Gram-negative sepsis, especially in areas with high rates of ESBL-producing coliforms. Peak plasma concentrations should be kept between 20–30 mg/L and trough concentrations below 10 mg/L.

Netilmicin is active against some strains of bacteria that resist gentamicin and tobramycin; it may be less ototoxic and nephrotoxic.

Neomycin and *framycetin* are principally used topically for skin, eye and ear infections. Enough absorption can occur from both oral and topical use to cause eighth cranial nerve damage, especially if there is renal impairment.

Streptomycin, superseded as a first-line choice for tuberculosis, may be used to kill resistant strains of the organism.

Spectinomycin is active against Gram-negative organisms, but its clinical use is confined to gonorrhoea in patients allergic to penicillin, or to infection with gonococci that are β-lactam drug resistant, although resistance to it is reported.

Tetracyclines and glycylcyclines

Tetracyclines have a broad range of antimicrobial activity, and differences among the individual members have traditionally been small, but new tetracyclines and tetracycline derivatives are now being developed with even wider spectra of activity that include some bacteria with acquired resistance to other classes of antibiotic.

Mode of action. Tetracyclines interfere with protein synthesis by binding to bacterial ribosomes, and their selective action is due to higher uptake by bacterial than by human cells. They are bacteriostatic.

Pharmacokinetics. Most tetracyclines are only partially absorbed from the alimentary tract, enough remaining in the intestine to alter the flora and cause diarrhoea. They are distributed throughout the body and cross the placenta. Tetracyclines in general are excreted mainly unchanged in the urine and should be avoided when renal function is severely impaired, although doxycycline and minocycline are eliminated by non-renal routes and are preferred for patients with impaired renal function.

Uses. Tetracyclines are active against nearly all Gram-positive and Gram-negative pathogenic bacteria, but increasing bacterial resistance and low innate activity limit the clinical use of most members of the class. Although 4-quinolone usage has replaced them especially in the developed world, they remain drugs of first choice for infection with chlamydiae (psittacosis, trachoma, pelvic inflammatory disease, lymphogranuloma venereum), mycoplasma (pneumonia), rickettsiae (Q fever, typhus), *Bartonella* spp., and borreliae (Lyme disease, relapsing fever) (for use in acne, see p. 283). Doxycycline is used in therapeutic and prophylactic regimens for malaria (see p. 236) and is active against amoebae and a variety of other protozoa. Their most common other uses are as second-line therapy of minor skin and soft-tissue infections especially in β-lactam–allergic patients; surprisingly, many MRSA strains currently remain susceptible to tetracyclines in the UK.

An unexpected use for a tetracycline is in the treatment of chronic hyponatraemia due to the syndrome of inappropriate antidiuretic hormone secretion (SIADH) when water restriction has failed. Demeclocycline produces a state of unresponsiveness to ADH, probably by inhibiting the formation and action of cyclic AMP in the renal tubule. It is effective and convenient to use in SIADH because this action is both dose-dependent and reversible.

Adverse reactions. Heartburn, nausea and vomiting due to gastric irritation are common, and attempts to reduce this with milk or antacids impair absorption of tetracyclines (see below). Diarrhoea and opportunistic infection may supervene. Disorders of epithelial surfaces, perhaps due partly to vitamin B complex deficiency and partly to mild opportunistic infection with yeasts and moulds, lead to sore mouth and throat, black hairy tongue, dysphagia and perianal soreness. Vitamin B preparations may prevent or arrest alimentary tract symptoms.

Due to their chelating properties with calcium phosphate, tetracyclines are selectively taken up in the teeth and growing bones of the fetus and of children. This causes hypoplasia of dental enamel with pitting, cusp malformation, yellow or brown pigmentation and increased susceptibility to caries. After the 14th week of pregnancy and in the first few months of life, even short courses can be damaging. Prolonged tetracycline therapy can also stain the fingernails at all ages.

The effects on the bones after they are formed in the fetus are of less clinical importance because pigmentation has no cosmetic disadvantage and a short exposure to tetracycline is unlikely significantly to delay growth.

Inhibition of protein synthesis in man causes blood urea to rise (the anti-anabolic effect); the increased nitrogen load can be clinically important in renal failure and in the elderly.

Tetracyclines induce photosensitisation and other rashes. Liver and pancreatic damage can occur, especially in pregnancy and with renal disease, when the drugs have been given i.v. Rarely tetracyclines cause benign intracranial hypertension (not always benign, because permanent visual damage may occur: signs and symptoms of raised intracranial pressure present, also known as 'pseudotumour cerebri'), dizziness and other neurological reactions. These may develop after tetracyclines have been taken for 2 weeks or 1 year, and the visual function of any patient taking tetracyclines who develops headaches or visual disturbance should be assessed carefully and their fundi examined.

Interactions. Dairy products reduce absorption to a degree, but antacids and iron preparations do so much more, by chelation to calcium, aluminium and iron.

Individual tetracyclines

Tetracycline is eliminated by the kidney and in the bile ($t_{1/2}$ 6 h). Because of incomplete absorption from the gut, i.v. doses need be less than one-half of the oral dose to be similarly effective. The dose is 250–500 mg 6-hourly by mouth.

Doxycycline is well absorbed from the gut, even after food. It is excreted in the bile, in the faeces which it re-enters by diffusing across the small intestinal wall and, to some extent, in the urine ($t_{1/2}$ 16 h). These non-renal mechanisms compensate effectively when renal function is impaired and no reduction of dose is necessary; 200 mg is given on the first day, then 100–200 mg/day.

Minocycline differs from other tetracyclines in that its antibacterial spectrum includes *Neisseria meningitidis* and it has been used for meningococcal prophylaxis. It is well absorbed from the gut, even after a meal, partly metabolised in the liver and partly excreted in the bile and urine ($t_{1/2}$ 15 h). Dose reduction is not necessary when renal function is impaired; 200 mg initially is followed by 100 mg 12-hourly. Minocycline, but not other tetracyclines, may cause a reversible vestibular disturbance with dizziness, tinnitus and impaired balance, especially in women.

Other tetracyclines include demeclocycline (see above), lymecycline and oxytetracycline.

Tigecycline ($t_{1/2}$ 42 h) is the first of the glycylcyclines to be licensed. These are close relatives of the tetracyclines; tigecycline shares the same molecular structure as minocycline with the addition of a 9-glycylamide group as a side chain on the tetracycline ring. The molecule binds to the 30 S bacterial ribosomal subunit, blocking entry of amino-acyl tRNA molecules to the A site and preventing amino acid chain elongation. Probably because of stearic hindrance from the 9-glycylamide structure and avid ribosomal binding, tigecycline is unaffected by the two commonest tetracycline resistance mechanisms – ribosomal alteration and efflux pumps. Consequently the compound displays useful bacteriostatic activity against a wide range of pathogens including streptococci and staphylococci (including vancomycin-resistant enterococci (VRE) and MRSA), Gram-negative bacilli (including *Legionella* spp. and *Acinetobacter baumannii*, although not *Proteus* spp. or *Pseudomonas* spp. and their relatives) and anaerobes.

It is licensed for skin and soft-tissue infection, complicated intra-abdominal infections and community-acquired pneumonia, in which trial outcomes have shown equivalent efficacy to carbapenems and other similar agents. Resistance has emerged during treatment of a variety of serious infections. A somewhat higher mortality rate than comparator agents (4% vs. 3%) has been reported by post-marketing surveillance during treatment of a range of serious infections: this observation requires scientific investigation before tigecycline's use is re-evaluated, but caution is warranted.

It is only available for parenteral use and is administered as a 100-mg first dose followed by 50 mg twice daily. Distribution is widespread throughout the body, although little crosses the blood–brain barrier and concentrations achieved in the urine are below the tigecycline MIC of many pathogens. Limited metabolism occurs, with about 60% of a dose eliminated via the gut and bile and 33% in the urine (only 22% as unchanged tigecycline). No dosage adjustment is required in renal failure or dialysis, and a dose reduction is required only in severe hepatic failure. A similar range and rate of side-effects to the tetracyclines has been reported.

Macrolides and lincosamides

Erythromycin

Erythromycin ($t_{1/2}$ 2–4 h) binds to bacterial ribosomes and interferes with protein synthesis; it is bacteriostatic and exhibits time-dependent killing (see p. 168). It is effective against Gram-positive organisms because these accumulate the drug more efficiently, and its antibacterial spectrum is similar to that of penicillin. It also has some activity against some Gram-negative bacteria such as *Legionella* spp., *Campylobacter* spp. and *Bordetella pertussis*.

Absorption after oral administration is best with erythromycin estolate, even if there is food in the stomach. Hydrolysis of the estolate in the body releases the active erythromycin which diffuses readily into most tissues; the $t_{1/2}$ is dose-dependent, and elimination is almost exclusively in the bile and faeces.

Uses. Erythromycin is the drug of choice for:

- *Mycoplasma pneumoniae* in children, although in adults a tetracycline may be preferred.
- *Legionella* spp., with or without rifampicin, although some authorities prefer a quinolone.
- Diphtheria (including carriers), pertussis and for some chlamydial infections.

In gastroenteritis caused by *Campylobacter jejuni*, erythromycin is effective in eliminating the organism from the faeces, although it does not reduce the duration of the symptoms unless given very early in the illness.

Erythromycin is an effective alternative choice for penicillin-allergic patients infected with *Staphylococcus aureus, Streptococcus pyogenes, Streptococcus pneumoniae* or *Treponema pallidum*.

Acne; see page 283.

Dose is 250 mg 6-hourly or twice this in serious infection and four times for legionnaires' disease.

Adverse reactions. Erythromycin is remarkably non-toxic, but the estolate can cause cholestatic hepatitis. This is probably an allergy, and recovery is usual, but the estolate should not be given to a patient with liver disease. Other allergies are rare. Gastrointestinal disturbances occur frequently (up to 28%), particularly diarrhoea and nausea, but opportunistic infection is uncommon.

Interactions. Erythromycin and the other macrolides are enzyme inhibitors and interfere with the cytochrome P450 metabolic inactivation of some drugs, e.g. warfarin, cyclosporin, tacrolimus, digoxin, carbamazepine, theophylline, disopyramide, increasing their effects. Reduced inactivation of terfenadine may lead to serious cardiac arrhythmias, and of ergot alkaloids may cause ergotism. Increased serum erythromycin concentrations are seen with co-administration of azole antifungal agents, some calcium channel blockers and anti-HIV protease inhibitors (ritonavir, saquinavir). Combination of erythromycin with strong inhibitors of P450 enzymes has been associated with an increased risk of sudden cardiac death (azole antifungal agents, diltiazem, verapamil and troleandomycin).

Clarithromycin acts like erythromycin and has a similar spectrum of antibacterial activity, i.e. mainly against Gram-positive organisms, although it is usefully more active against *Haemophilus influenzae*. The usual dose is 250–500 mg 12-hourly. It is rapidly and completely absorbed from the gastrointestinal tract, 60% of a dose is inactivated by metabolism which is saturable (note that the $t_{1/2}$ increases with dose: 3 h after 250 mg, 9 h after 1200 mg) and the remainder is eliminated in the urine. Clarithromycin is used for respiratory tract infections including atypical pneumonias and soft-tissue infections. It is concentrated intracellularly, achieving concentrations which allow effective therapy in combination for non-tuberculous mycobacterial infections such as *Mycobacterium avium-intracellulare*. Gastrointestinal tract adverse effects are uncommon (7%). Interactions: see erythromycin (above).

Azithromycin has additional activity against a number of important Gram-negative organisms including *Haemophilus influenzae* and *Neisseria gonorrhoeae*, and also *Chlamydiae*, but is a little less effective than erythromycin against Gram-positive organisms.

Azithromycin achieves high concentrations in tissues relative to those in plasma. It remains largely unmetabolised and is excreted in the bile and faeces ($t_{1/2}$ 50 h). Azithromycin is used to treat respiratory tract and soft-tissue infections and sexually transmitted diseases, especially genital *Chlamydia* infections, and is effective for travellers' diarrhoea, especially when combined with loperamide. It has been used in patients with cystic fibrosis who are colonised with *Pseudomonas aeruginosa*: azithromycin may have synergistic activity with other anti-pseudomonal agents, and its modest anti-inflammatory effects may also reduce the intensity of symptoms. Gastrointestinal effects (9%) are less than with erythromycin, but diarrhoea, nausea, dyspepsia and abdominal pain occur. In view of its high hepatic excretion, use in patients with liver disease should be avoided. Interactions: see erythromycin (above).

Telithromycin ($t_{1/2}$ 10 h) is the first of the ketolides, semi-synthetic relatives of the macrolides which bind to the 50 S bacterial ribosomal subunit, preventing translation and ribosome assembly. Its molecular differences from erythromycin make it more acid stable and less susceptible to bacterial export pumps, while increasing its ribosomal binding. Its spectrum of activity includes most erythromycin-resistant strains of *Streptococcus pneumoniae*, but it is not active against erythromycin-resistant staphylococci, including most health-care–associated MRSA.

It is licensed for once-daily oral therapy of upper and lower respiratory tract infections, and good efficacy has been demonstrated with relatively short courses (e.g. 5 days). Bioavailability is approximately 57% and is unaffected by food intake. It is generally well tolerated, although it causes diarrhoea more commonly than the newer macrolides and some patients experience transient visual disturbance (blurred or double vision). Rare cases of serious hepatotoxicity have been reported, although dose adjustment is not required in hepatic failure. Some authorities recommend halving the daily dose with severe renal failure, and it is a potent inhibitor of cytochrome P450 liver enzymes, resulting in interactions with, for example, itraconazole, rifampicin, midazolam and atorvastatin.

Clindamycin, structurally a lincosamide rather than a macrolide, binds to bacterial ribosomes to inhibit protein synthesis. Its antibacterial spectrum is similar to that of erythromycin (with which there is partial cross-resistance – so-called 'inducible MLS resistance') and flucloxacillin. It also has activity against some anaerobes; inducible resistance is variable in prevalence in common pathogens in different parts of the world, with the result that clindamycin can be a useful second-line agent for oral treatment of some difficult infections (e.g. MRSA osteomyelitis) as long as susceptibility testing is correctly performed. Clindamycin is well absorbed from the gut and distributes to most body tissues including bone. The drug is metabolised by the liver, and enterohepatic cycling occurs with bile concentrations 2–5 times those of plasma ($t_{1/2}$ 3 h). Significant excretion of metabolites occurs via the gut.

Clindamycin is used for staphylococcal bone and joint infections, dental infections and serious intra-abdominal sepsis (in the last, it is usually combined with an agent active against Gram-negative pathogens such as gentamicin). Because of its ability to inhibit production of bacterial protein toxins, it is the antibiotic of choice for serious invasive *Streptococcus pyogenes* infections (although surgical resection of affected tissue plays a prime role), and it is also an alternative to linezolid for treatment of Panton-Valentine leukocidin-producing strains of *Staphylococcus aureus* (see p. 219). It is a second choice in combination for some *Toxoplasma* infections (see p. 244). Topical preparations are used for therapy of severe acne and non-sexually transmitted infection of the genital tract in women.

The most serious **adverse effect** is antibiotic-associated (pseudomembranous) colitis (see p. 175); clindamycin should be stopped if any diarrhoea occurs.

Other inhibitors of protein synthesis

Chloramphenicol

Chloramphenicol has a broad spectrum of activity and is primarily bacteriostatic, but may be bactericidal against *Haemophilus influenzae*, *Neisseria meningitidis* and *Streptococcus pneumoniae*.

Pharmacokinetics. Chloramphenicol succinate is hydrolysed to active chloramphenicol, and there is much individual variation in the capacity to perform this reaction. Chloramphenicol is inactivated by conjugation with glucuronic acid in the liver ($t_{1/2}$ 5 h in adults). In the neonate, the process of glucuronidation is slow, and plasma concentrations are extremely variable, especially in premature neonates in whom monitoring of plasma concentration is essential. Chloramphenicol penetrates well into all tissues, including the CSF and brain, even in the absence of meningeal inflammation.

Uses. Chloramphenicol's role in meningitis and brain abscess has largely been superseded, but it is a second-line agent for these indications. Chloramphenicol may be used for salmonella infections (typhoid fever, salmonella septicaemia), but ciprofloxacin is now preferred. Topical administration is effective for bacterial conjunctivitis.

Adverse effects. Systemic use of chloramphenicol is dominated by the fact that it can cause rare (between 1 : 18 000 and 1 : 100 000 courses) though serious bone marrow damage which may be a dose-dependent, reversible depression of erythrocyte, platelet and leucocyte formation that occurs early in treatment (type A adverse drug reaction), or an idiosyncratic (probably genetically determined), non–dose-related, and usually fatal aplastic anaemia which may develop during, or even weeks after, prolonged treatment, and sometimes on re-exposure to the drug (type B adverse reaction). This has also occurred, very rarely, with eye drops. Marrow depression may be detected at an early and recoverable stage by frequent checking of the full blood count.

The 'grey baby' syndrome occurs in neonates as circulatory collapse in which the skin develops a cyanotic grey colour. It is caused by failure of the liver to conjugate, and of the kidney to excrete the drug.

Sodium fusidate

Sodium fusidate is a steroid antimicrobial which is used almost exclusively against staphylococci. Because staphylococci may rapidly become resistant via a one-step genetic mutation, the drug should be combined with another antistaphylococcal drug, e.g. flucloxacillin. Sodium fusidate is readily absorbed from the gut and distributes widely in body tissues including bone. It is metabolised and very little is excreted unchanged in the urine; the $t_{1/2}$ is 5 h.

Uses. Sodium fusidate is a valuable drug for treating severe staphylococcal infections, including osteomyelitis, and is available as i.v. and oral preparations. In an ointment or gel, sodium fusidate is used topically for staphylococcal skin infection. Another gel preparation is used for topical application to the eye: this contains such a high fusidic acid concentration that it possesses useful activity against most bacteria that cause conjunctivitis.

Adverse effects. It is well tolerated, but mild gastrointestinal upset is frequent. Jaundice may develop, particularly with high doses given intravenously, and liver function should be monitored.

Resistance to antimicrobials: linezolid, quinupristin-dalfopristin and fosfomycin

Linezolid and quinupristin-dalfopristin (Synercid) were developed in response to the emergence of multiply resistant Gram-positive pathogens during the 1990s. Both have clinically useful activity against MRSA (including vancomycin-intermediate and -resistant strains), vancomycin-resistant enterococci and penicillin-resistant *Streptococcus pneumoniae*. They are currently reserved for treatment of infections caused by such bacteria and for use in patients who are allergic to more established antibiotics. Difficult decisions are being faced about how such novel but expensive antimicrobial agents should be used:

> *No antibiotic should be used recklessly, however difficult it appears to be to select for resistance in vitro. On the other hand, the attitude that 'All new antibiotics should be locked away' risks stifling innovation whilst denying life-saving treatments … Debates on the use of new anti-Gram-positive agents are sure to intensify … and it is vital that they take place on a basis of science not knee-jerk restrictions or over-zealous marketing.[4]*

These agents are inactive against most Gram-negative bacteria.

Linezolid, a synthetic oxazolidinone, is the first member of the first totally new class of antibacterial agents to be released to the market for 20 years, the first new agent approved for therapy of MRSA for over 40 years, and the first oral antibiotic active against VRE. It binds to domain

---

[4]Livermore D M 2000 Quinupristin/dalfopristin and linezolid: where, when, which and whether to use? Journal of Antimicrobial Chemotherapy 46:347–350.

V of the 23 S component of the 50 S ribosomal subunit and inhibits formation of the initiation complex between transfer-RNA, messenger RNA and the ribosomal subunits. It is bacteriostatic against most Gram-positive bacteria, but is bactericidal against pneumococci.

Resistance has been reported so far in enterococcus and *Staphylococcus aureus* isolates from immunocompromised patients and others with chronic infections who had been treated with linezolid for long periods; a handful of examples from other species have also been found. Linezolid-resistant isolates possess modified 23 S ribosomal RNA genes, and the level of resistance correlates with the number of gene copies the organisms carry. Most Gram-negative bacteria are resistant by virtue of possessing membrane efflux pumps. Many obligate anaerobes are susceptible.

It is eliminated via both renal and hepatic routes ($t_{1/2}$ 6 h) with 30–55% excreted in the urine as the active drug. Oral and parenteral formulations are available, and the usual dose is 600 mg 12-hourly by both routes; absorption after oral administration is rapid, little affected by food, and approaches 100%. Dose modification in hepatic or renal impairment is not necessary. Distribution includes to the CSF, eye and respiratory tract, although variability in concentrations achieved is seen with systemic sepsis, cystic fibrosis and burn injuries and also in neonates, and it is noteworthy that linezolid resistance has developed during treatment of patients with low serum concentrations.

Linezolid is licensed in the UK for skin, soft-tissue and respiratory tract infections, and it is usually restricted on grounds of cost to those caused by multiply resistant pathogens. The oral formulation has proven useful for follow-on therapy of severe and chronic infections caused by bacteria resistant to other agents, e.g. MRSA osteomyelitis, although its drug cost is high for both oral and parenteral preparations.

Adverse effects include nausea, vomiting and headache, with much the same frequency as with penicillin and macrolide therapy. Reversible optic and irreversible peripheral neuropathy have been reported and, importantly, marrow suppression may occur, especially where there is pre-existing renal disease or patients are also receiving other drugs that may have adverse effects on marrow or platelet function, so full blood counts and neurological assessments should be performed regularly. Patients should not generally receive linezolid for longer than 4 weeks unless available alternatives carry disadvantages; this is frequently the case, for example, during treatment of multiply resistant pathogens such as MRSA, where comparative studies have generally shown equivalent efficacy and similar rates of adverse events. Linezolid is active against multi-drug and extensively drug-resistant *Mycobacterium tuberculosis*, non-tuberculous mycobacteria and *Nocardia* spp. and seems effective therapeutically, although course lengths have been limited by high rates of myelosuppression and neuropathy. Potentiation of the pressor activity of monoamine oxidase inhibitors and other interactions with adrenergic, serotonergic and dopaminergic drugs may occur, and it may also interact with foods of high tyramine content such as aged meats, cheese, beer and wine. Tedizolid is a second-generation oxazolidinone derivative that is 4-to-16-fold more potent against staphylococci and enterococci compared to linezolid. The recommended dosage for treatment is 200 mg once daily for a total duration of 6 days, either orally (with or without food) or through an intravenous injection (if the patient is older than 18 years of age). It is licensed for the treatment of skin and soft-tissue infections. Guidance suggests that monitoring of platelets and white blood cells is not required.

Quinupristin-dalfopristin is a 30%:70% combination of two streptogramin molecules: the dalfopristin component binds first to the 50 S bacterial ribosome, inducing a conformational change which allows the additional binding of quinupristin. The combination results in inhibition of both aminoacyl-tRNA attachment and the peptidyl transferase elongation step of protein synthesis, resulting in premature release of polypeptide chains from the ribosome. The summative effect is bactericidal. Acquired resistance is currently rare, but a variety of possible mechanisms of resistance have been reported including methylation of the 23 S RNA molecule (also involved in erythromycin resistance), enzymatic hydrolysis and phosphorylation and efflux pumps. Most strains of *Enterococcus faecalis* are naturally resistant, but *E. faecium* is susceptible, as are the respiratory pathogens *Legionella pneumophila*, *Moraxella catarrhalis* and *Mycoplasma pneumoniae*. Other Gram-negative bacteria have impermeable membranes and hence are resistant. The $t_{1/2}$ is 1.5 h. Quinupristin-dalfopristin is available for administration only by i.v. injection; the usual dose is 7.5 mg/kg every 8 h.

It is licensed in the UK for *Enterococcus faecium* infections, skin and soft-tissue infections, and hospital-acquired pneumonia, but recently supplies have become difficult to obtain.

Injection to peripheral veins frequently causes phlebitis, so a central line is required. Arthralgia and myalgia are seen in about 10% of patients. No dosage reduction is recommended in renal impairment, but the dose should be reduced in moderate hepatic impairment and it should generally be avoided if the impairment is severe.

Fosfomycin, a phosphonic acid derivative, was originally extracted from a *Streptomyces* sp. bacterium in 1969, but is now fully synthetic. Oral preparations have been used in a number of countries for over 20 years mainly for urinary tract infection, and a disodium derivative is available for intravenous and intramuscular use.

Fosfomycin is bactericidal against many Gram-positive and Gram-negative bacteria via inhibition of uridine diphosphate-GlcNAc enol-pyruvyltransferase (MurA). It enters bacterial and mammalian cells via an active transport system. Susceptible bacteria include most Enterobacteriaceae, *Staphylococcus aureus* and *epidermidis*, *Streptococcus pneumoniae* and *Enterococcus faecalis*. In some cases, synergy has been demonstrated with β-lactam antibiotics. Predictably resistant species include *Acinetobacter* spp., *Listeria monocytogenes* and anaerobes, while few *Pseudomonas aeruginosa* or *Enterococcus faecium* are inhibited. Fosfomycin has a small molecular size and relatively long $t_{1/2}$ (5.7 h) and so penetrates most tissues, including the CSF and eye. Few data are available on drug interactions, although reported adverse events are uncommon, mainly including mild gastrointestinal disturbance (5–6%) and rashes (4%), and pain and inflammation at the infusion and injection site of the parenteral preparation (3%). Caution is advised when fosfomycin is used in patients with cardiac insufficiency, hypertension, hyperaldosteronism, hypernatraemia or pulmonary oedema. A high sodium load associated with the use of fosfomycin may result in decreased levels of potassium in serum or plasma.

Most published experience is with single 3-g oral doses for lower urinary tract infection, where fosfomycin activity persists in the urine for 48 h and is as effective as 3–5-day courses of conventional agents: it is one convenient choice for ESBL-producing Enterobacteriaceae. A 3-g alternate day regimen for 5 days (i.e. on days 1, 3 and 5) may be used for complicated urinary tract infection. Prolonged and successful use is reported for a wide variety of serious infections where treatment had been complicated by bacterial resistance and host allergy to other agents, including infections with penicillin-resistant pneumococci, MRSA, ESBL and CPE Enterobacteriaceae and vancomycin-resistant *E. faecalis*. Resistance can emerge during therapy of the individual, mediated by conjugation of glutathione to the antibiotic molecule by bacterial metalloglutathione transferase, but surveys in countries where the drug has been used for two decades have shown a consistently low (3%) primary resistance rate in urinary tract pathogens, and there is no cross-resistance to other antimicrobial classes.

Inhibition of nucleic acid synthesis

Sulfonamides and sulfonamide combinations

Sulfonamides now have their place in medicine mainly in combination with trimethoprim. Because of the risks of adverse drug reactions associated with their use, this is generally restricted to specific indications where other therapeutic agents have clearly inferior efficacy. Many sulfonamide compounds have recently been withdrawn from the market. Their individual names are standardised in the UK to begin with 'sulfa-'.

The enzyme dihydrofolic acid (DHF) synthase converts *p*-aminobenzoic acid (PABA) to DHF, which is subsequently converted to tetrahydric folic acid (THF), purines and DNA. The sulfonamides are structurally similar to PABA, successfully compete with it for DHF synthase, and thus ultimately impair DNA formation. Most bacteria do not use preformed folate, but humans derive DHF from dietary folate which protects their cells from the metabolic effect of sulfonamides. Trimethoprim acts at the subsequent step by inhibiting DHF reductase, which converts DHF to THF. The drug is relatively safe because bacterial DHF reductase is much more sensitive to trimethoprim than is the human form of the enzyme. Both sulfonamides and trimethoprim are bacteriostatic.

Pharmacokinetics. Sulfonamides for systemic use are absorbed rapidly from the gut. The principal metabolic path is acetylation, and the capacity to acetylate is genetically determined in a bimodal form, i.e. there are slow and fast acetylators (see Pharmacogenetics), but the differences are of limited practical importance in therapy. The kidney is the principal route of excretion of drug and acetylate.

Systemic use

Sulfonamide-trimethoprim combination. *Co-trimoxazole* (sulfamethoxazole plus trimethoprim); the optimum synergistic in vitro effect against most susceptible bacteria is achieved with a 5:1 ratio of sulfamethoxazole to trimethoprim, although concentrations achieved in the tissues vary considerably. Each drug is well absorbed from the gut, has a $t_{1/2}$ of 10 h and is 80% excreted by the kidney; consequently, the dose of co-trimoxazole should be reduced when renal function is impaired.

Trimethoprim on its own is now used in many conditions for which the combination was originally recommended, and it may cause fewer adverse reactions (see below). The combination is, however, retained for the following:

* Prevention and treatment of pneumonia due to *Pneumocystis carinii* infection in immunosuppressed patients (for therapy, high doses of 120 mg/kg/day in 2–4 divided doses are used and therapeutic drug monitoring is essential).
* Prevention and treatment of toxoplasmosis, and treatment of nocardiasis, *Elizabethkingia meningoseptica* and *Stenotrophomonas maltophilia* infection (90–120 mg/kg/day dosing).

Sulfadiazine ($t_{1/2}$ 10 h), sulfametopyrazine ($t_{1/2}$ 38 h) and sulfadimidine (sulfamethazine) ($t_{1/2}$ approximately 6 h, dose dependent) are available in some countries for urinary tract infections, meningococcal meningitis and other indications, but resistance rates are high.

Silver sulfadiazine is used topically for prophylaxis and treatment of infected burns, leg ulcers and pressure sores because of its wide antibacterial spectrum (which includes pseudomonads).

Miscellaneous

Sulfasalazine (salicylazosulfapyridine) is used in inflammatory bowel disease (see p. 575); in effect the sulfapyridine component acts as a carrier to release the active 5-aminosalicylic acid in the colon (see also rheumatoid arthritis, p. 261).

Adverse effects of sulfonamides include malaise, diarrhoea and rarely cyanosis (due to methaemoglobinaemia). These may all be transient and are not necessarily indications for stopping the drug. Crystalluria may rarely occur.

Allergic reactions include: rash, fever, hepatitis, agranulocytosis, purpura, aplastic anaemia, peripheral neuritis and polyarteritis nodosa. Rarely, severe skin reactions including erythema multiforme bullosa (Stevens-Johnson syndrome) and toxic epidermal necrolysis (Lyell's syndrome) occur.

Haemolysis may occur in glucose-6-phosphate dehydrogenase–deficient subjects. Patients with AIDS have a high rate of allergic systemic reactions (fever, rash) to co-trimoxazole used for treatment of *Pneumocystis carinii* pneumonia.

Trimethoprim

Trimethoprim ($t_{1/2}$ 10 h) has emerged as a useful broad-spectrum antimicrobial on its own, active against many Gram-positive and Gram-negative aerobic organisms excepting the enterococci and *Pseudomonas aeruginosa*; the emergence of resistant organisms is becoming a problem, especially for treatment of urinary tract infection. The drug is rapidly and completely absorbed from the gastrointestinal tract and is largely excreted unchanged in the urine. Trimethoprim is effective as sole therapy in treating urinary and respiratory tract infections and for low-dose prophylaxis of urinary tract infections.

Adverse effects are fewer than with co-trimoxazole and include: skin rash, anorexia, nausea, vomiting, abdominal pain and diarrhoea. Trimethoprim should not be given to pregnant women, premature infants or infants during the first few weeks of life. Although trimethoprim is excreted in breast milk, it is not necessarily contraindicated for short-term therapy during lactation.

Nitrofurantoin

Nitrofurantoin is a useful agent for the treatment of urinary tract infection. It only attains low concentrations in renal tissue and the bloodstream so should not be used if pyelonephritis or bacteraemia is suspected. Treatment may fail if used for ascending infection. Furthermore, if a patient has a reduced glomerular filtration rate, urinary concentrations may be inadequate for nitrofurantoin. eGFR frequently declines with age, on average by between 6 and 9 mL/min/1.73 m² per decade. Around one-half of women older than 75 years and men older than 85 years of age will have an eGFR less than 60 mL/min/1.73 m². Long-term and/or repeated courses of nitrofurantoin are associated with severe pulmonary fibrosis, which can be fatal. Nitrofurantoin is poorly tolerated by some patients, but the modified release form has fewer unwanted effects. A review and meta-analysis suggested a clinical cure rate almost equivalent to comparators but with a 5-day rather than 3-day course.[5]

Toxicity was mainly gastrointestinal effects and no pulmonary adverse events were reported, though this may be a reflection of short follow-up periods.[5] There are no specific studies of nitrofurantoin in urinary infection caused by ESBL-producing organisms, but urinary tract infections that are susceptible to nitrofurantoin have a similar response rate irrespective of ESBL production if the patient has an adequate GFR.

Quinolones

(4-quinolones, fluoroquinolones)

The first widely used quinolone, nalidixic acid, was discovered serendipitously as a by-product of chloroquine synthesis. It is effective for urinary tract infections because it is concentrated in the urine, but it has little systemic activity. Fluorination of the quinolone structure was subsequently found to produce compounds that were up to 60 times more active than nalidixic acid and killed a wider range of organisms. These newer '4-quinolones' act principally by inhibiting bacterial (but not human) DNA gyrase (topoisomerase II and IV), thus preventing the supercoiling of DNA, a process that is necessary for compacting chromosomes in the bacterial cell; they are bactericidal and exhibit concentration-dependent bacterial killing (see p. 168). In general quinolones are extremely active against Gram-negative organisms, and most have useful activity against *Pseudomonas aeruginosa*, mycobacteria and *Legionella pneumophila*. Most are less active against Gram-positive organisms (resistance commonly emerges) and anaerobes. Resistance typically arises via mutation of the target enzymes, and these are coded on mobile plasmids; efflux pumps may also contribute. Quinolone resistance rates of a wide range of Gram-negative bacteria have risen alarmingly worldwide

[5]Huttner A, Verhaegh E M, Harbarth S, Muller A E, Theuretzbacher U, Mouton J W. 2015. Nitrofurantoin revisited: a systematic review and meta-analysis of controlled trials. Journal of Antimicrobial Chemotherapy 70:2456–2464. Available from: PM:26066581.

during the past 15 years, and clinical cross-resistance across all members of the group is common. Resistance is particularly a problem in *Pseudomonas aeruginosa* (where quinolones are the only oral agent with activity against them), ESBL and carbapenemase-producing Enterobacteriaceae and N. *gonorrhoeae.*

Pharmacokinetics. Quinolones are well absorbed from the gut, and widely distributed in tissue. Mechanisms of inactivation (hepatic metabolism, renal and biliary excretion) are detailed below for individual members. There is substantial excretion and re-absorption via the colonic mucosa, and patients with renal failure or intestinal malfunction, e.g. ileus, are prone to accumulate quinolones.

Uses vary between individual drugs (see below).

Adverse effects include gastrointestinal upset and allergic reactions (rash, pruritus, arthralgia, photosensitivity and anaphylaxis). High rates of quinolone usage in hospitals have been associated with outbreaks of diarrhoea caused by *Clostridium difficile*, so reduced use is one component of the bundles of recommended control measures (see p. 175). CNS effects may develop with dizziness, headache and confusion. Convulsions have occurred during treatment (avoid or use with caution where there is a history of epilepsy or concurrent use of NSAIDs, which potentiate this effect). Reversible arthropathy has developed in weight-bearing joints in immature animals exposed to quinolones. Quinolones should be used only for serious infections and then with caution in children and adolescents; however, ciprofloxacin is licensed for treatment of *Pseudomonas aeruginosa* lung infection in children older than 5 years of age with cystic fibrosis. Rupture of tendons, notably the Achilles, has occurred, more commonly in the elderly and those taking corticosteroids concurrently. Levofloxacin and ofloxacin are less likely than ciprofloxacin to cause corneal precipitates during topical therapy to the eye and are preferred for this as much as for their enhanced anti–Gram-positive activity.

Some are potent liver enzyme inhibitors and impair the metabolic inactivation of other drugs including warfarin, theophylline and sulphonylureas, increasing their effect. Magnesium- and aluminium-containing antacids impair absorption of quinolones from the gastrointestinal tract, probably through forming a chelate complex; ferrous sulphate and sucralfate also reduce absorption.

Individual members of the group include the following:

Ciprofloxacin ($t_{1/2}$ 3 h) is effective against a range of bacteria but particularly the Gram-negative organisms (see above). Chlamydia and mycoplasma are susceptible. Ciprofloxacin is indicated for use in infections of the urinary, gastrointestinal and respiratory tracts, skin and soft-tissue infections, gonorrhoea and septicaemia. It has proven especially useful for oral therapy of chronic Gram-negative infections such as osteomyelitis, and for acute exacerbations of *Pseudomonas*

infection in cystic fibrosis. It has been used for the prophylaxis and therapy of anthrax, including cases resulting from bioterrorism. The dose is 250–750 mg 12-hourly by mouth, 400 mg 12-hourly i.v. but halved when the glomerular filtration rate is <20 mL/min. Ciprofloxacin impairs metabolism of theophylline and of warfarin, both of which should be monitored carefully when co-administered.

Norfloxacin ($t_{1/2}$ 3 h) is used for acute or chronic recurrent urinary tract infections.

Ofloxacin ($t_{1/2}$ 4 h) has modestly greater Gram-positive, but less Gram-negative activity than ciprofloxacin. It is used for urinary and respiratory tract infections, gonorrhoea, and topically for eye infection.

Nalidixic acid ($t_{1/2}$ 6 h) is now used principally for the prevention of urinary tract infection. It may cause haemolysis in glucose-6-phosphate dehydrogenase–deficient subjects.

Others. *Levofloxacin* ($t_{1/2}$ 7 h) has greater activity against *Streptococcus pneumoniae* than ciprofloxacin and is used for respiratory and urinary tract infection. *Moxifloxacin* ($t_{1/2}$ 9–12 h) has strong anti–Gram-positive activity and is also effective against many anaerobes, but it is only weakly active against *Pseudomonas*. It is recommended as a second-line agent for upper and lower respiratory tract infections including those caused by 'atypical' pathogens, penicillin-resistant *Streptococcus pneumoniae* and mycobacteria. QT prolongation occurs, and moxifloxacin is contraindicated in patients with cardiac failure or rhythm disorders. It has balanced renal and hepatic excretion, so dose modification in renal failure is not necessary.

Azoles

This group includes:

- Metronidazole and tinidazole (antibacterial and antiprotozoal), which are described here.
- Fluconazole, itraconazole, clotrimazole, econazole, ketoconazole, isoconazole and miconazole, which are described under Antifungal drugs (p. 232).
- Albendazole, mebendazole and thiabendazole, which are described under Anthelminthic drugs (p. 244).

Metronidazole

In obligate anaerobic microorganisms (but not in aerobes), metronidazole is converted into an active form by reduction of its nitro group: this binds to DNA and prevents nucleic acid formation; it is bacteriostatic.

Pharmacokinetics. Metronidazole is well absorbed after oral or rectal administration and distributed widely. It is eliminated in the urine, partly unchanged and partly as metabolites. The $t_{1/2}$ is 8 h.

Uses. Metronidazole's clinical indications are:

- treatment of sepsis to which anaerobic organisms, e.g. *Bacteroides* spp. and anaerobic cocci, are contributing, including post-surgical infection, intra-abdominal infection and septicaemia, osteomyelitis and abscesses of brain or lung.
- antibiotic-associated pseudomembraneous colitis (caused by *Clostridium difficile*).
- trichomoniasis of the urogenital tract in both sexes.
- amoebiasis *(Entamoeba histolytica)*, including both intestinal and extra-intestinal infection.
- Giardiasis *(Giardia lamblia)*.
- acute ulcerative gingivitis and dental infections (*Fusobacterium* spp. and other oral anaerobic flora).
- anaerobic vaginosis (*Gardnerella vaginalis* and vaginal anaerobes).

Dose. Established anaerobic infection is treated with metronidazole by mouth 400 mg 8-hourly; by rectum 1 g 8-hourly for 3 days followed by 1 g 12-hourly; or by i.v. infusion 500 mg 8-hourly. A topical gel preparation is useful for reducing the odour associated with anaerobic infection of fungating tumours.

Adverse effects include nausea, vomiting, diarrhoea, furred tongue and an unpleasant metallic taste in the mouth; also headache, dizziness and ataxia. Rashes, urticaria and angioedema occur. Peripheral neuropathy occurs if treatment is prolonged, and epileptiform seizures if the dose is high. Large doses of metronidazole are carcinogenic in rodents, and the drug is mutagenic in bacteria; long-term studies have failed to discover oncogenic effects in humans.

A disulfiram-like effect (see p. 150) occurs with alcohol because metronidazole inhibits alcohol and aldehyde dehydrogenase; patients should be warned appropriately.

Tinidazole is similar to metronidazole in use and adverse effects, but has a longer $t_{1/2}$ (13 h). It is excreted mainly unchanged in the urine. The longer duration of action of tinidazole may be an advantage, e.g. in giardiasis, trichomoniasis and acute ulcerative gingivitis, in which tinidazole 2 g by mouth in a single dose is as effective as a course of metronidazole.

Minor antimicrobials

These are included because they are effective topically without serious risk of allergy, while toxicity or chemical instability limits or precludes their systemic use.

Mupirocin is primarily active by inhibition of tRNA synthetase in Gram-positive organisms, including those commonly associated with skin infections. It is available as an ointment for use, e.g. in folliculitis and impetigo, and to eradicate *Staphylococcus aureus* site, e.g. in carriers of resistant staphylococci and to clear nasal carriage before surgery (see p. 173). It is also effective at reducing rates of staphylococcal peritonitis in patients receiving chronic ambulatory peritoneal dialysis, and for this indication it needs only to be applied to the nares for a few days per month. Re-colonisation after eradication of carriage occurs quite swiftly, with 5–30% being positive around 4 days after treatment, and 85–100% after 1 month.

Moderate resistance (by mutation of the of tRNA synthetase enzyme) is quite common in staphylococci in hospitals that have extensive mupirocin usage. Such strains may fail to be eradicated from the nares, but their numbers are usually significantly reduced so that therapeutic aims may still be achieved (i.e. reduction of the numbers of staphylococci entering the patient's wound perioperatively, hence a reduction in postoperative wound infection rates). However, high-level resistance (MIC of 512 mg/L or above) is transferable by a plasmid and leads to failure rates of around 75%. Mupirocin is rapidly hydrolysed in the tissues.

Retapamulin, a tricyclic pleuromutilin derived from the edible mushroom *Clitopilus scyphoides*, binds to a site on the 50 S bacterial ribosomal subunit and is active against streptococci and staphylococci, including MRSA, anaerobes, but almost no Gram-negative bacteria. For treatment of infected eczema and similar conditions, it is applied in a thin layer to the skin twice daily and covered with a sterile bandage or gauze dressing if desired. Systemic absorption is very low, and the most commonly reported adverse reaction is allergy at the application site.

Polypeptide (polymyxin) antibiotics

Colistin (polymyxin E; $t_{1/2}$ 6 h) is a polypeptide effective against most Gram-negative organisms. It is sometimes used orally for bowel decontamination, by inhalation via a saline nebuliser in patients with cystic fibrosis who are infected with *Pseudomonas aeruginosa*, and is applied to skin, including external ear infections. It can also be used systemically for severe infections with multiply resistant Gram-negative pathogens such as pseudomonads and *Acinetobacter* when no alternative agents are available and can be given intrathecally as well. Having received marketing approval in the 1950s, the polymyxins were not subjected to the drug development procedures and regulatory scrutiny needed for modern drugs. Thus, information to guide their clinical use has been scarce. Inhalational use is also being assessed for adjunctive therapy of Gram-negative ventilator-associated pneumonia (usually in combination with intravenous colistin therapy). Adverse effects of systemic administration include nephrotoxicity, neurological symptoms and neuromuscular blockade; renal function should be monitored daily and the dose reduced to 12–18-hourly in patients with creatinine clearance <10–20 mL/min. Recently published case series of parenteral use have reported few problems of serious toxicity even in patients who received prolonged courses of therapy.

Polymyxin B is also active against Gram-negative organisms, particularly *Pseudomonas aeruginosa*. Its principal use now is topical application for skin, eye and external ear infections.

Gramicidin is used in various topical applications as eye and ear drops, combined with neomycin and framycetin.

Guide to further reading

Cunha, B.A., 2006. New uses for older antibiotics: nitrofurantoin, amikacin, colistin, polymyxin B, doxycycline, and minocycline revisited. Med. Clin. North Am. 90, 1089–1107.

Drawz, S.M., Bonomo, R.A., 2010. Three decades of beta-lactamase inhibitors. Clin. Microbiol. Rev. 23, 160–201.

Falagas, M.E., Kastoris, A.C., Kapaskelis, A.M., et al., 2010. Fosfomycin for the treatment of multidrug-resistant, including extended-spectrum beta-lactamase producing, enterobacteriaceae infections: a systematic review. Lancet Infect. Dis. 10, 43–50.

Sánchez García, M., De la Torre, M.A., Morales, G., et al., 2010. Clinical outbreak of linezolid-resistant *Staphylococcus aureus* in an intensive care unit. J. Am. Med. Assoc. 303, 2260–2264.

Gaynes, R.P., 2010. Preserving the effectiveness of antibiotics. J. Am. Med. Assoc. 303, 2293–2294.

Holgate, S., 1988. Penicillin allergy: how to diagnose and when to treat. Br. Med. J. 296, 1213.

Howden, B.P., Davies, J.K., Johnson, P.D., et al., 2010. Reduced vancomycin susceptibility in *Staphylococcus aureus*, including vancomycin-intermediate and heterogeneous vancomycin-intermediate strains: resistance mechanism, laboratory detection and clinical implications. Clin. Microbiol. Rev. 23, 99–139.

Huttner, A., Verhaegh, E.M., Harbarth, S., et al., 2015. Nitrofurantoin revisited: a systematic review and meta-analysis of controlled trials. J. Antimicrob. Chemother. 70, 2456–2464. Available from: PM:26066581.

Kelkar, P.S., Li, J.T.C., 2001. Cephalosporin allergy. N. Engl. J. Med. 345, 804–809.

McLean-Tooke, A., Aldridge, C., Stroud, C., et al., 2011. Practical management of antibiotic allergy in adults. J. Clin. Pathol. 64, 192–199. Available at: http://jcp.bmj.com/content/early/2010/12/20/jcp.2010.077289.full.pdf. (Accessed May 2017).

Romano, A., Viola, M., Guéant-Rodriguez, R.M., et al., 2007. Tolerability of meropenem in patients with IgE-mediated hypersensitivity to penicillins. Ann. Intern. Med. 146, 266–269.

Rybak, M., Lomaestro, B., Rotschafer, J.C., et al., 2009. Therapeutic monitoring of vancomycin in adult patients: a consensus review of the American Society of Health-System Pharmacists, the Infectious Diseases Society of America, and the Society of Infectious Diseases Pharmacists. Am. J. Health Syst. Pharm. 66, 82–98. Available at: http://www.ajhp.org/cgi/reprint/66/1/82. (Accessed May 2017).

Torres, M.J., Blanca, M., 2010. The complex clinical picture of beta-lactam hypersensitivity: penicillins, cephalosporins, monobactams, carbapenems, and clavams. Med. Clin. North Am. 94, 805–820.

Van Rijen, M., Bonten, M., Wenzel, R., Kluytmans, J., 2010. Mupirocin ointment for preventing *Staphylococcus aureus* infections in nasal carriers. Cochrane Database Syst. Rev. (4), cd006216, 2008.

Williams, D.N., 2016. Antimicrobial resistance: are we at the dawn of the post-antibiotic era? J. R. Coll. Physicians Edinb. 46, 150–156.

Chapter | 14

Chemotherapy of bacterial infections

David A. Enoch, Mark Farrington, Surender K. Sharma

SYNOPSIS

We live in a world heavily populated by microorganisms of astonishing diversity. This chapter considers the bacteria that cause disease in individual body systems, the drugs that combat them, and how they are best used. The chapter discusses infection of:

- Blood.
- Paranasal sinuses and ears.
- Throat.
- Bronchi, lungs and pleura.
- Endocardium.
- Meninges.
- Intestines.
- Urinary tract.
- Genital tract.
- Bones and joints.
- Eye.

It also discusses mycobacteria that infect many sites.

Infection of the blood

Bacteraemia is defined as the presence of bacteria in the bloodstream. Bacteraemia with clinical features of sepsis is defined as **septicaemia**. Septicaemia is a medical emergency that moves clinically from sepsis (systemic inflammatory response syndrome, 'SIRS') via organ dysfunction ('severe sepsis') to septic shock as the associated mortality rates progress from 16% to 46%. In a shocked patient (i.e. with low blood pressure that does not promptly respond to circulatory volume enhancement), survival rates fall by over 7% for each hour of delay in commencing effective antibiotics. Urgent support of the circulation and other organs is necessary for survival. Rapid assessment by senior medical staff and early involvement of infection specialists have also been associated with an improved outcome and lowest antibiotic costs during treatment.

Usually, the infecting organism(s) is not known at the time of presentation and treatment must be instituted on the basis of a 'best guess' (i.e. 'empirical therapy'). The clinical circumstances and knowledge of local resistance patterns may provide clues. Examples of suitable choices are given in the list below; patients who have been in hospital for some time before presenting with septicaemia need antibiotic regimens that provide more reliable cover for multiply resistant pathogens, and examples of these are given in square brackets:

- Septicaemia accompanied by a spreading rash that does not blanch with pressure should be assumed to be meningococcal, and the patient must be referred to hospital urgently (after an immediate parenteral dose of benzylpenicillin): ceftriaxone.
- Community-acquired pneumonia: co-amoxiclav + clarithromycin.
- When septicaemia follows gastrointestinal or genital tract surgery, *Escherichia coli* (or other enterobacteriaceae), anaerobic bacteria, (e.g. *Bacteroides* spp.), streptococci or enterococci are likely pathogens: piperacillin-tazobactam or gentamicin plus benzylpenicillin plus metronidazole [meropenem if prior extended spectrum beta-lactamases, ESBL, plus vancomycin if prior MRSA, methicillin-resistant *Staphylococcus aureus*].
- Septicaemia related to urinary tract infection usually involves *Escherichia coli* (or other Gram-negative bacteria), enterococci: gentamicin + co-amoxiclav or

piperacillin-tazobactam alone [meropenem if prior ESBL].

- Neonatal septicaemia is usually due to Lancefield Group B streptococcus or enterobacteriaceae: benzylpenicillin plus gentamicin [vancomycin + ceftazidime].
- Staphylococcal septicaemia may be suspected where there is an abscess, e.g. of bone or lung, or with acute infective endocarditis or infection of intravenous catheters: high-dose flucloxacillin [vancomycin if prior MRSA]. Uncomplicated *Staphylococcus aureus* bacteraemia should be treated for ≥14 days to reduce the risk of metastatic infection: patients with prolonged bacteraemia or who fail to settle promptly should be considered for treatment as for staphylococcal endocarditis.
- Severe cellulitis, bites and necrotising fasciitis accompanied by septicaemia should be treated with optimal cover for Lancefield Group A streptococcus, anaerobes and coliforms: piperacillin-tazobactam + clindamycin [meropenem + clindamycin].
- Septicaemia in patients rendered neutropenic by cytotoxic drugs frequently involves coliforms and *Pseudomonas* spp. translocating to the circulation directly from the bowel, while coagulase-negative staphylococci also commonly arise from central venous catheter infection: piperacillin-tazobactam (+/− gentamicin). Vancomycin could be added if line infection is clinically suspected.

    Staphylococcal toxic shock syndrome occurs in circumstances that include healthy women using vaginal tampons, in abortion or childbirth, and occasionally with skin and soft-tissue infection and after packing of body cavities, such as the nose. Flucloxacillin is used, and elimination of the source by removal of the tampon and drainage of abscesses is also important.

Patients with features of sepsis should be given their antimicrobials IV initially, and their combination with optimal circulatory and respiratory support and glycaemic control.

Patients who have had a splenectomy or have hyposplenism are at risk of fulminant septicaemia especially from capsulate bacteria, e.g. *Streptococcus pneumoniae, Neisseria meningitidis*. The risk is greatest in the first 2 years after splenectomy (but is lifelong), in children, and in those with splenectomy for haematological malignancy. Patients must be immunised against appropriate pathogens and receive continuous low-dose oral prophylaxis with phenoxymethylpenicillin (penicillin V), or erythromycin in those allergic to penicillin. Refer to a reliable source, e.g. British National Formulary, for the most recent advice, including about vaccination.

Infection of paranasal sinuses and ears

Sinusitis

As oedema of the mucous membrane hinders the drainage of pus, a logical first step is to open the obstructed passage with a sympathomimetic vasoconstrictor, e.g. ephedrine nasal drops. Antibiotic therapy produces limited additional clinical benefit, but the common infecting organism(s) – *Streptococcus pneumoniae, Haemophilus influenzae, Streptococcus pyogenes, Moraxella catarrhalis* – usually respond to oral amoxicillin (with or without clavulanic acid) or doxycycline. It is necessary to treat around 15 patients with antibiotic to cure one patient faster than the natural resolution rate.

In chronic sinusitis, correction of the anatomical abnormalities (polypi, nasal septum deviation) is often important, and diverse organisms, many of them normal inhabitants of the upper respiratory tract, may be cultured, e.g. anaerobic streptococci, *Bacteroides* spp. Judgement is required as to whether any particular organism is acting as a pathogen. Choice of antibiotic should be guided by culture and sensitivity testing; therapy may need to be prolonged. Fungi can also infect sinuses. Whilst allergic rhinitis is the most common manifestation, invasive fungal sinusitis (e.g. due to *Aspergillus* spp. and mucoraceous moulds) should be suspected in immunosuppressed patients (e.g. with haematological malignancy or poorly controlled diabetes mellitus).

Otitis media

Mild cases are normally viral and often resolve spontaneously, needing only analgesia and observation. A bulging, inflamed eardrum indicates bacterial otitis media usually due to *Streptococcus pneumoniae, Haemophilus influenzae, Moraxella catarrhalis, Streptococcus pyogenes* (Group A) or *Staphylococcus aureus*. Amoxicillin or co-amoxiclav is satisfactory, but the clinical benefit of antibiotic therapy is small in controlled trials, and good outcomes with reduced use of antibiotics have been demonstrated if patients are given a prescription which they only fill if they worsen or fail to improve after 48 h (sometimes known as a 'WASP' – a 'wait-and-see' prescription). Children younger than 2 years of age with bilateral otitis and those with acute aural discharge (otorrhoea) benefit most from antibiotic treatment. Chemotherapy has not removed the need for myringotomy when pain is very severe, and also for later cases, as sterilised pus may not be completely absorbed and may leave adhesions that impair hearing. Chronic infection presents a similar problem to that of chronic sinus infection, above. Pneumococcal vaccination is modestly effective at reducing recurrences in children who are prone to them.

Otitis externa

Otitis externa is an inflammatory reaction of the meatal skin. Many cases recover after thorough cleansing of the external ear canal by suction. If infection is present, topical agents are typically appropriate such as aluminium acetate or antibacterial agents with activity against organisms such as *S. aureus* and Gram-negative bacteria (e.g. enterobacteriaceae and *P. aeruginosa*). These include neomycin or gentamicin. Solutions containing a topical corticosteroid may also be useful if eczema is present.

Systemic antibiotics are required if there is spreading cellulitis, if the patient is systemically unwell or if invasive otitis externa is suspected (e.g. pain, tenderness of the tissue around the ear, discharging pus from the ear). Invasive otitis externa typically occurs in elderly or diabetic patients. Imaging and surgery may be required for this condition. Flucloxacillin (to cover *S. aureus*) and ciprofloxacin (to cover *P. aeruginosa*) may be required.

Infection of the throat

Pharyngitis is usually viral, but the more serious cases may be due to *Streptococcus pyogenes* (Group A) (always sensitive to benzylpenicillin), which cannot be differentiated clinically from virus infection with any certainty. Prevention of complications is more important than relief of the symptoms, which seldom last long, and corticosteroids are much more effective than antibiotics at shortening the period of pain. There is no general agreement as to whether chemotherapy should be employed in mild sporadic sore throat, and expert reviews reflect this diversity of opinion.[1-3]

The disease usually subsides in a few days, septic complications are uncommon and rheumatic fever rarely follows. It is reasonable to withhold penicillin unless streptococci are cultured or the patient develops a high fever; some primary care physicians take a throat swab and give the patient a WASP for penicillin which is only filled if streptococci are isolated. Severe sporadic or epidemic sore throat is likely to be streptococcal, and the risk of these complications is limited by phenoxymethylpenicillin by mouth (clarithromycin or an oral cephalosporin in the penicillin-allergic),

given, ideally, for 10 days, although compliance is poor once the symptoms have subsided, and 5 days should be the minimum objective. Azithromycin (500 mg daily p.o.) for 3 days is effective as long as the streptococci are susceptible, with improved compliance, and 5-day courses of oral cephalosporins are as effective as 10 days of penicillin. Do not use amoxicillin if the circumstances suggest pharyngitis due to infectious mononucleosis, as the patient is very likely to develop a rash (see p. 181). In a closed community, chemoprophylaxis of unaffected people to stop an epidemic may be considered, for instance with oral phenoxymethylpenicillin 125 mg 12-hourly.

In scarlet fever and erysipelas, the infection is invariably streptococcal (Group A), and benzylpenicillin should be used even in mild cases, to prevent rheumatic fever and nephritis.

Chemoprophylaxis

Chemoprophylaxis of streptococcal (Group A) infection with phenoxymethylpenicillin is necessary for patients who have had one attack of rheumatic fever. Continue for at least 5 years or until 20 years of age, whichever is the longer period (although some hold that it should continue for life). Chemoprophylaxis should be continued for life after a second attack of rheumatic fever. A single attack of acute nephritis is not an indication for chemoprophylaxis. Ideally, chemoprophylaxis should continue throughout the year but, if the patient is unwilling to submit to this, cover at least the colder months (see also footnote p. 172).

Adverse effects are uncommon. Patients taking penicillin prophylaxis are liable to have penicillin-resistant viridans type streptococci in the mouth, so that during even minor dentistry, e.g. scaling, there is a risk of bacteraemia and thus of infective endocarditis with a penicillin-resistant organism in those with any residual rheumatic heart lesion. Patients taking penicillins are also liable to be carrying resistant staphylococci and pneumococci.

Other causes of pharyngitis

Vincent's infection (microbiologically complex, including anaerobes, spirochaetes) responds readily to benzylpenicillin; a single i.m. dose of 600 mg is often enough except in a mouth needing dental treatment, when relapse may follow. Metronidazole 200 mg 8-hourly by mouth for 3 days is also effective.

Diphtheria (*Corynebacterium diphtheriae*). Antitoxin 10 000–100 000 units i.v. in two divided doses 0.5–2 h apart is given to neutralise toxin already formed. The dose varies according to the severity of the disease. Erythromycin or benzylpenicillin is also used, to prevent the production of more toxins.

[1]Cooper R J, Hoffman J R, Bartlett J G et al 2001 Principles of appropriate antibiotic use for acute pharyngitis in adults: background. Annals of Internal Medicine 134:506.
[2]Del Mar C B, Glasziou P, Spinks A B 2008 Antibiotics for sore throat (Cochrane review). Available at: http://www2.cochrane.org/reviews/en/ab000023.html (accessed November 2011).
[3]Thomas M, Del Mar C, Glasziou P 2000 How effective are treatments other than antibiotics for acute sore throat? British Journal of General Practice 50:817.

Whooping cough *(Bordetella pertussis)*. Chemotherapy is needed in unvaccinated children whose defences are compromised, have damaged lungs or are younger than 3 years of age. Erythromycin is usually recommended at the catarrhal stage and should be continued for 14 days (also as prophylaxis in cases of special need). It may curtail an attack if given early enough (before paroxysms have begun, and certainly within 21 days of exposure to a known case) but is not dramatically effective; it also reduces infectivity to others. A corticosteroid, salbutamol and physiotherapy may be helpful for relief of symptoms, but reliable evidence of efficacy is lacking.

Lemierre's disease refers to infectious thrombophlebitis of the internal jugular vein. It typically develops as a complication of a bacterial sore throat infection in young, otherwise healthy adults. The thrombophlebitis may lead to further systemic complications such as bacteraemia or septic emboli. Lemierre's disease occurs most often when a bacterial (typically *Fusobacterium necrophorum*) throat infection progresses to the formation of a peritonsillar abscess. Spread of infection to the nearby internal jugular vein provides a gateway for the spread of bacteria through the bloodstream. The inflammation surrounding the vein and compression of the vein may lead to blood clot formation.

Infection of the bronchi, lungs and pleura

Bronchitis

Most cases of acute bronchitis are viral; where bacteria are responsible, the usual pathogens are *Streptococcus pneumoniae* and/or *Haemophilus influenzae*. It is questionable whether there is a role for antimicrobials in uncomplicated acute bronchitis, but amoxicillin, a tetracycline or trimethoprim is appropriate if treatment is considered necessary. Whether newer antimicrobials, e.g. moxifloxacin, confer significant outcome advantages to justify their expense and side effects is debatable.

In chronic bronchitis, suppressive chemotherapy with amoxicillin or trimethoprim may be considered during the colder months (in temperate, colder regions), for patients with symptoms of pulmonary insufficiency, recurrent acute exacerbations or permanently purulent sputum.

For intermittent therapy, the patient is given a supply of the drug and told to take it in full dose at the first sign of a 'chest' cold, e.g. purulent sputum, and to stop the drug after 3 days if there is rapid improvement. Otherwise, the patient should continue the drug until recovery takes place.

If the exacerbation lasts for more than 10 days, there is a need for clinical reassessment.

Pneumonias

The clinical setting is a useful guide to the causal organism and hence to the 'best guess' early choice of antimicrobial. It is not possible reliably to differentiate between pneumonias caused by 'typical' and 'atypical' pathogens on clinical grounds alone, and most experts advise initial cover for both types of pathogen in seriously ill patients. However, there is no strong evidence that adding 'atypical' cover to empirical parenteral treatment with a β-lactam antibiotic improves the outcome.[4]

Published guidelines often recommend hospital admission and parenteral and broader-spectrum therapy for the most severely affected patients as assessed by the 'CURB-65' score (one point is scored for each of *C*onfusion, elevated serum *U*rea, *R*espiratory rate >30 breaths per minute, low *B*lood pressure, and age of *65* years or older). A score of ≥3 is associated with increased mortality, and patients require IV therapy. Delay of 4 hours or more in commencing effective antibiotics in the most seriously ill patients is associated with increased mortality.

Pneumonia in previously healthy people (community acquired)

Disease that is segmental or lobar in its distribution is usually due to *Streptococcus pneumoniae* (pneumococcus). *Haemophilus influenzae* is a rare cause in this group, although it more often leads to exacerbations of chronic bronchitis. Benzylpenicillin i.v. or amoxicillin or clarithromycin p.o. are the treatments of choice if pneumococcal pneumonia is very likely; use clarithromycin, doxycycline or moxifloxacin in a penicillin-allergic patient. Seriously ill patients should receive benzylpenicillin (to cover the pneumococcus) plus ciprofloxacin (to cover *Haemophilus* and 'atypical' pathogens), and co-amoxiclav plus clarithromycin is an alternative that may have a lower propensity to promote *Clostridium difficile* diarrhoea. Where penicillin-resistant pneumococci are common, i.v. ceftriaxone is a reasonable 'best guess' choice pending confirmation of susceptibilities from the laboratory, with vancomycin as an alternative. A wide variety of new antibiotics is under investigation for use in penicillin-resistant pneumococcal infections, including cephalosporins, e.g. ceftobiprole; penicillin relatives, 'respiratory' quinolones (e.g. moxifloxacin and levofloxacin); lipoglycopeptides, e.g. dalbavancin; and ketolides, e.g. cethromycin.

---

[4]https://www.nice.org.uk/guidance/cg191/evidence/full-guideline-pdf-193389085.

Pneumonia following influenza is often caused by *Staphylococcus aureus*, and 'best guess' therapy usually involves adding flucloxacillin to the benzylpenicillin-containing regimens above. When staphylococcal pneumonia is proven, rifampicin p.o. plus flucloxacillin i.v. should be used in combination. Staphylococcal pneumonia that involves strains producing Panton-Valentine leucocidin toxin is frequently necrotising in nature, and linezolid or clindamycin have been shown to reduce toxin production at the ribosomal level so are recommended for inclusion when this condition is suspected.

'Atypical' cases of pneumonia may be caused by *Mycoplasma pneumoniae* or more rarely *Chlamydia pneumoniae* or *psittaci* (psittacosis/ornithosis), *Legionella pneumophila* or *Coxiella burnetii* (Q fever), and doxycycline or clarithromycin should be given by mouth. Treatment of ornithosis should continue for 10 days after the fever has settled, and that of mycoplasma pneumonia and Q fever for 3 weeks to prevent relapse.

At an early stage (i.e. at 24–48 h), once there is clinical improvement, i.v. administration should change to oral.

Pneumonia acquired in hospital

Pneumonia is usually defined as being nosocomial (Greek: *nosokomeian*, hospital) if it presents after at least 48 h in hospital. It occurs primarily among patients admitted with medical problems or recovering from abdominal or thoracic surgery and those who are on mechanical ventilators. The common pathogens are *Staphylococcus aureus*, Enterobacteriaceae, *Streptococcus pneumoniae*, *Pseudomonas aeruginosa* and *Haemophilus influenzae*, and anaerobes after aspiration. Mild cases can be given co-amoxiclav unless they are known to be colonised with resistant bacteria, but for severe cases it is reasonable to initiate therapy with piperacillin-tazobactam (plus vancomycin if the local prevalence of MRSA is high) pending the results of sputum culture and susceptibility tests. Vancomycin or teicoplanin are equally effective for MRSA pneumonia as linezolid, and have an overall lower rate of adverse reactions.

Pneumonia in people with chronic lung disease

Normal commensals of the upper respiratory tract proliferate in damaged lungs especially following virus infections, pulmonary congestion or pulmonary infarction. Antibiotics should not be given to patients who do not demonstrate two or more of increased dyspnoea, sputum volume and sputum purulence. Mixed infection is common, and as *Haemophilus influenzae* and *Streptococcus pneumoniae* are often the pathogens, amoxicillin or trimethoprim is a reasonable choice in domiciliary practice; if response is inadequate, co-amoxiclav or a quinolone should be substituted, but

there is no evidence that they are superior first line to the older choices.

Klebsiella pneumoniae is a rare cause of lung infection (Friedlander's pneumonia), particularly if cavitating, in the alcoholic and debilitated elderly. Piperacillin-tazobactam, possibly plus an aminoglycoside, is recommended, though cephalosporins, quinolones and carbapenems also have activity.

Moraxella catarrhalis, a commensal of the oropharynx, may be a pathogen in patients with chronic bronchitis; because many strains produce β-lactamase, co-amoxiclav, a tetracycline or clarithromycin is used.

Pneumonia in immunocompromised patients

Pneumonia is common, e.g. in acquired immune deficiency syndrome (AIDS) or in those who are receiving immunosuppressive drugs.

Common pathogenic bacteria may be responsible *(Staphylococcus aureus, Streptococcus pneumoniae)*, but often organisms of lower natural virulence (Enterobacteriaceae, viruses, fungi) are causal and necessitate strenuous efforts to identify the microbe including, if feasible, bronchial washings or lung biopsy.

- Until the pathogen is known, the patient should receive broad-spectrum antimicrobial treatment, such as piperacillin-tazobactam or an aminoglycoside plus ceftazidime.
- Aerobic Gram-negative bacilli, e.g. Enterobacteriaceae, *Klebsiella* spp., are pathogens in one-half of the cases, especially in neutropenic patients, and respond to piperacillin-tazobactam or ceftazidime. These and *Pseudomonas aeruginosa* may respond better with addition of an aminoglycoside.

  Pneumocystis carinii is an important respiratory pathogen in patients with deficient cell-mediated immunity; treat with co-trimoxazole 120 mg/kg daily by mouth or i.v. in two to four divided doses for 14 days, as modified by serum assay, or with pentamidine (see p. 244).

Legionnaires' disease

Legionella pneumophila responds to erythromycin 4 g/day i.v. in divided doses, or clarithromycin, with the addition of rifampicin in more severe infections. Ciprofloxacin is probably a little more effective, although at the expense of a higher risk of adverse reactions.

Pneumonia due to anaerobic microorganisms

Pneumonia often follows aspiration of material from the oropharynx, or accompanies other lung pathology such as pulmonary infarction or bronchogenic carcinoma. In addition to conventional microbial causes, pathogens include anaerobic and aerobic streptococci, *Bacteroides* spp. and *Fusobacterium* spp. Co-amoxiclav or piperacillin-tazobactam may be needed for several weeks to prevent relapse.

Pulmonary abscess: treat the identified organism, and employ aspiration or formal surgical drainage if necessary.

Empyema: aspiration or drainage is essential, followed by antibiotic treatment of the isolated organism.

Endocarditis

When there is suspicion, at least three sets of blood cultures should be taken from different sites and at different times. The time frame of this depends on how 'sick/septic' the patient is: blood cultures should be taken over a few hours if the patient is septic and at risk of acute endocarditis (with antibiotics commenced immediately after the final set), whereas they can be taken over a period of several days if the patient is stable. Antimicrobial treatment should be adjusted later in the light of the results. Delay in treating only exposes the patient to the risk of grave cardiac damage or systemic embolism. Streptococci, enterococci and staphylococci are causal in 80% of cases, with viridans group streptococci having recently been overtaken by *Staphylococcus aureus* as the most common pathogens. In intravenous drug users, *Staphylococcus aureus* is particularly likely, although the potential list of pathogens is extensive in this group. Culture-negative endocarditis (in 8–10% of cases in contemporary practice) is usually due to previous antimicrobial therapy or to special culture requirements of the microbe; it is best regarded as being due to streptococci and treated accordingly.

Endocarditis on prosthetic valves presenting in the first few months after the operation usually involves *Staphylococcus aureus*, coagulase-negative staphylococci or occasionally Gram-negative rods. The infecting flora then becomes progressively more characteristic of native valve infections as time progresses.

Principles for treatment

- Use high doses of bactericidal drugs because the organisms are difficult to access in avascular vegetations on valves.
- Give drugs parenterally and preferably by i.v. bolus injection to achieve the necessary high peak concentration to penetrate the vegetations.
- Examine the infusion site daily and change it regularly to prevent opportunistic infection, which is usually with coagulase-negative staphylococci or fungi. A central venous catheter or peripherally inserted central catheter is optimal.

- Continue therapy, usually for 2–6 weeks, and, in the case of infected prosthetic valves, 6 weeks. Prolonged courses may also be indicated for patients infected with enterococci or other strains with penicillin minimum inhibitory concentrations (MICs) above 0.5 mg/L, whose presenting symptoms have been present for over 6 weeks, for those with large vegetations, and those whose clinical symptoms and signs are slow to settle after treatment has started. Highly susceptible streptococcal endocarditis (penicillin MIC of 0.1 mg/L or below) can be treated successfully with 2-week courses.
- Valve replacement may be needed at any time during and after antibiotic therapy if cardiovascular function deteriorates or the infection proves impossible to control.
- Adjust the dose according to the sensitivity of the infecting organism – use the MIC test (see p. 168).

Dose regimens

The following regimens are commonly recommended (the reader is referred to the British Society for Antimicrobial Chemotherapy treatment guidelines 2012):

1. Initial ('best guess') treatment should comprise benzylpenicillin (7.2 g i.v. daily in six divided doses), plus gentamicin (1 mg/kg body-weight 8-hourly – synergy allows this dose of gentamicin and minimises risk of adverse effects). Regular serum gentamicin assay is vital: trough concentrations should be below 1 mg/L and peak concentrations 3–5 mg/L; if *Staphylococcus aureus* is suspected, high-dose flucloxacillin plus rifampicin should be used. Patients allergic to penicillin and those with intracardiac prostheses or suspected MRSA infection should receive vancomycin plus rifampicin plus gentamicin. Patients presenting acutely (suggesting infection with *Staphylococcus aureus*) should receive flucloxacillin (8–12 g/day in four to six divided doses) plus gentamicin.

2. When an organism is identified and its sensitivity determined:
   - *Viridans group streptococci*: the susceptibility of the organism determines the antimicrobial(s) and its duration of use, ranging from benzylpenicillin plus gentamicin for 2 weeks, to vancomycin plus gentamicin for 6 weeks. Patients with uncomplicated endocarditis caused by very sensitive strains may be managed as outpatients; ceftriaxone 2 g/day for 4 weeks may be suitable for these patients.
   - *Enterococcus faecalis* (Group D): amoxicillin 2 g 4-hourly or benzylpenicillin 2.4 g 4-hourly plus

gentamicin 1 mg/kg 8–12-hourly i.v. for 4–6 weeks. The prolonged gentamicin administration carries a significant risk of adverse drug reactions, but is essential to assure eradication of the infection. Streptococci from endocarditis are checked for high-level gentamicin resistance (MIC above 128 mg/L) because cidal synergy is not seen with β-lactams in such strains. Alternative regimens for such infections include amoxicillin plus streptomycin (if not similarly high-level resistant) or high-dose amoxicillin alone.

- *Staphylococcus aureus*: flucloxacillin 2 g 4–6-hourly i.v. for at least 4 weeks. In the presence of intracardiac prostheses, flucloxacillin is combined with rifampicin orally (or fusidic acid) for at least the first 2 weeks, and MRSA may be treated with vancomycin plus rifampicin plus fusidic acid (or gentamicin) for 4–6 weeks.
- *Staphylococcus epidermidis* infecting native heart valves is managed as for *Staphylococcus aureus* if the organism is sensitive.
- *Coxiella* or *Chlamydia*: give doxycycline 100 mg once daily orally, plus ciprofloxacin 500 mg 8-hourly for at least 3 years. Valve replacement is advised in many cases.
- *Fungal endocarditis*: amphotericin B plus flucytosine has been used, although experience is growing with the echinocandins, and specialist advice should be sought. Valve replacement is usually essential.
- *Culture-negative endocarditis*: benzylpenicillin plus gentamicin i.v. are given for 4–6 weeks.

Prophylaxis

Transient bacteraemia is provoked by dental procedures that induce gum bleeding, surgical incision of the skin, instrumentation of the urinary tract and parturition. However, even seemingly innocent activities such as brushing the teeth result in bacteraemia and are lifelong risks, whereas medical interventions are usually single. Adding this to the fact that even single antibiotic doses carry inevitable risks and the evidence base for their efficacy is lacking, expert working parties have re-evaluated the traditional wisdom of advocating prophylactic antibiotics for many procedures in patients with acquired or congenital heart defects.

Meningitis

Speed of initiating treatment and accurate bacteriological diagnosis are the major factors determining the fate of the patient, especially with invasive meningococcal disease where fulminant meningococcal septicaemia still carries a 20–50% mortality rate (and supporting the circulation in the intensive care unit is as important a determinant of outcome as the rapid commencement of antibiotic therapy). With suspected meningococcal disease, unless the patient has a history of penicillin anaphylaxis, benzylpenicillin should be started by the general practitioner before transfer to hospital; the benefit of rapid treatment outweighs the reduced chance of identifying the causative organism. Molecular diagnostic methods such as the polymerase chain reaction (PCR) for bacterial DNA in CSF or blood enable rapid diagnosis, even when the causative organisms have been destroyed by antibiotics.

Drugs must be given i.v. in high dose. The regimens below provide the recommended therapy, with alternatives for patients allergic to first choices, and septic shock requires appropriate management (see p. 198). Intrathecal therapy is now considered unnecessary (except for neurosurgical infections in association with indwelling CSF drains and shunts) and can be dangerous, e.g. encephalopathy with penicillin.

Initial therapy

Initial therapy should be sufficient to kill all pathogens, which are likely to be:

All ages older than 5 years

For *Neisseria meningitidis* and *Streptococcus pneumoniae*, give benzylpenicillin 2.4 g 4-hourly. Some prefer ceftriaxone 2 g i.v. 12-hourly in all cases pending the results of susceptibility tests, and this may be generally preferred depending upon the local prevalence of penicillin resistance. In such cases, in those 50 years of age and older, pregnant or immunocompromised patients it is prudent to add amoxicillin (2 g i.v. 4-hourly) initially to cover the possibility of listeria involvement as cephalosporins have no activity against *Listeria monocytogenes*. Optimal therapy for known or suspected penicillin-resistant pneumococcal meningitis comprises ceftriaxone 2 g i.v. 12-hourly plus vancomycin 15 mg/kg i.v. 12-hourly plus rifampicin 300 mg i.v. 12-hourly.

Children younger than 5 years

Neisseria meningitidis is now commonest. *Haemophilus influenzae*, formerly a frequent pathogen, is rarely isolated following immunisation programmes. *Streptococcus pneumoniae* is also less common than in older patients. Give a cephalosporin, e.g. ceftriaxone.

Neonates

For *Escherichia coli*, give cefotaxime or ceftazidime perhaps with gentamicin. For Group B streptococci, give benzylpenicillin plus gentamicin. Consult a specialist text for details of doses. Add amoxicillin if *Listeria monocytogenes* is suspected.

Dexamethasone given i.v. (0.15 mg/kg 6-hourly for 4 days) and early appears to reduce long-term neurological sequelae, especially sensorineural deafness, in infants and children. In adults there is evidence to support dexamethasone therapy in pneumococcal meningitis, but outcome is not affected in meningitis caused by other pathogens.

β-lactam anaphylaxis

Chloramphenicol with vancomycin remains a good alternative for 'blind' therapy in patients giving a history of β-lactam anaphylaxis. Co-trimoxazole is required to cover for listeria in patients with risk factors (mentioned above).

Subsequent therapy

Necessarily, i.v. administration should continue until the patient can take drugs by mouth, but whether or when continuation therapy should be oral or i.v. is a matter of debate. Antimicrobials (except aminoglycosides) enter well into the CSF when the meninges are inflamed; relapse may be due to restoration of the blood–CSF barrier as inflammation reduces. The following are recommended (adult doses).

Neisseria meningitidis. Give benzylpenicillin 2.4 g 4-hourly or ceftriaxone 2 g i.v. 12-hourly for a minimum of 5 days.

Streptococcus pneumoniae. Give ceftriaxone 2 g i.v. 12-hourly or benzylpenicillin 2.4 g 4-hourly (if the organism is penicillin-sensitive), and continue for 10 days after the patient has become afebrile.

Haemophilus influenzae. Give ceftriaxone 2 g i.v. 12-hourly or chloramphenicol 100 mg/kg daily for 10 days after the temperature has settled. Subdural empyema, often presenting as persistent fever, is relatively common after meningitis due to *Haemophilus influenzae* and may require surgical drainage.

Listeria monocytogenes. Give amoxicillin 2 g i.v. 6-hourly for 21 days plus gentamicin 5 mg/kg for the first week. Co-trimoxozole 15 mg/kg i.v. 6–8-hourly is required in penicillin allergy.

Chemoprophylaxis

The three common pathogens (below) are spread by respiratory secretions. Asymptomatic nasopharyngeal carriers seldom develop meningitis but may transmit the pathogens to close personal contacts. Rifampicin by mouth is effective at reducing carriage rates.

Meningococcal meningitis often occurs in epidemics in closed communities, but also in isolated cases. Patients and close personal contacts should receive a single dose of ciprofloxacin (500 mg by mouth) or ceftriaxone (250 mg i.m. or i.v.); the latter is of particular value for pregnant women.

Haemophilus influenzae type b has similar infectivity to that of the meningococcus; give rifampicin 600 mg by mouth daily for 4 days to unimmunised contacts.

Pneumococcal meningitis tends to occur in isolated cases, and contacts do not need chemoprophylaxis.

Infection of the intestines

(For Helicobacter pylori, see p. 567)

Both wit and truth are contained in the aphorism that 'travel broadens the mind but opens the bowels'. Antimicrobial therapy should be reserved for specific conditions with identified pathogens where benefit has been shown; acute diarrhoea can be caused by bacterial toxins in food, dietary indiscretions, anxiety and by drugs as well as by infection. Even if diarrhoea is infective, it may be due to viruses; or, if bacterial, antimicrobial agents may not reduce the duration of symptoms and may aggravate the condition by permitting opportunistic infection and encouraging *Clostridium difficile*–associated diarrhoea. Maintaining water and electrolyte balance either orally or by i.v. infusion with a glucose–electrolyte solution, and administration of an antimotility drug (except in small children, and those with bloody, dysenteric stools, and in *Clostridium difficile* infection), are the mainstays of therapy in such cases (see Oral rehydration therapy, p. 571). Some specific intestinal infections do benefit from chemotherapy:

Campylobacter **spp.** Clarithromycin, azithromycin or ciprofloxacin by mouth eliminates the organism from the stools but is only clinically effective if commenced within the first 24–48 h of the illness and if the patient is severely affected. Ciprofloxacin resistance has become common in parts of the world (e.g. Thailand).

Shigella **spp.** Mild disease requires no specific antimicrobial therapy, but toxic shigellosis with high fever should be treated with i.v. ceftriaxone or ciprofloxacin/azithromycin by mouth for 5 days.

Salmonella **spp.** Give an antimicrobial for severe salmonella gastroenteritis, or for bacteraemia or salmonella enteritis in an immunocompromised patient. The choice lies between ciprofloxacin, azithromycin or a parenteral cephalosporin (i.e. ceftriaxone): ciprofloxacin resistance is rising in incidence in salmonella (including in *S. typhi*), especially in the Indian subcontinent.

Typhoid fever is a generalised infection and requires treatment with 14 days of i.v. ceftriaxone, oral or i.v. ciprofloxacin, or oral azithromycin. Chloramphenicol, amoxicillin or co-trimoxazole are less effective alternatives. Initial parenteral therapy can be switched to oral once the patient has improved and susceptibility of the causative pathogen determined. A longer period of treatment may be required for those who develop complications such as osteomyelitis or abscess.

A carrier state develops in a few individuals who have no symptoms of disease but who can infect others.[5] Organisms reside in the biliary or urinary tracts. Ciprofloxacin in high dose by mouth for 3–6 months may be successful for what can be a very difficult problem, requiring investigation for urinary tract abnormalities or even cholecystectomy.

Escherichia coli is a normal inhabitant of the bowel, but some enterotoxigenic strains are pathogenic and are frequently a cause of travellers' diarrhoea. A quinolone, e.g. ciprofloxacin, azithromycin or the non-absorbable rifampicin-relative rifaximin are alternatives (see Travellers' diarrhoea, p. 571). Prophylactic use of an antimicrobial is not usual but, should it be deemed necessary, a quinolone or rifaximin is effective.

Verotoxic *Escherichia coli* (VTEC; O157) may cause severe bloody diarrhoea and systemic effects such as the haemolytic uraemic syndrome (HUS); antibiotic therapy has been shown in some trials to worsen the prognosis. In general, avoid using an antibiotic for bloody diarrhoea unless VTEC has been excluded bacteriologically.

Vibrio cholerae. Death in cholera is due to electrolyte and fluid loss in the stools, and this may exceed 1 L/h. Prompt replacement and maintenance of water and electrolyte balance with i.v. and oral electrolyte solutions is vital. A single dose of doxycycline, given early, significantly reduces the amount and duration of diarrhoea and eliminates the organism from the faeces (thus lessening the contamination of the environment). Ciprofloxacin or a macrolide (clarithromycin or azithromycin) are alternatives for resistant organisms. Oral zinc acetate supplements have been shown modestly to reduce the volume and duration of cholera diarrhoea in combination with antibiotics, probably by improving gut mucosal integrity and function in malnourished patients. Carriers may be treated by doxycycline by mouth in high dose for 3 days.

Selective decontamination of the gut may reduce the risk of nosocomial infection from gut organisms (including fungi) in patients who are immunocompromised or receiving intensive care (notably mechanical ventilation). The commonest regimen involves combinations of topical non-absorbable (colistin, nystatin and amphotericin B) and i.v. (cefotaxime) antimicrobials to reduce the number of Gram-negative bacilli and yeasts while maintaining a normal anaerobic flora. Alternatives include using the topical agents alone, or administering oral ciprofloxacin. Selective decontamination should be used with great care in hospitals with a high incidence of multiply resistant bacteria or *Clostridium difficile* diarrhoea.

Peritonitis is usually a mixed infection, and antimicrobial choice must take account of coliforms and anaerobes, although the need to include cover for the other major component of the bowel flora, streptococci and enterococci, is less certain. Co-amoxiclav with gentamicin or piperacillin-tazobactam alone, or a combination of gentamicin, benzylpenicillin plus metronidazole, or meropenem alone (if prior ESBL isolated) is usually appropriate, and can be stopped after the patient is clinically improved and their inflammatory markers (e.g. C-reactive protein) have normalised. Short courses of antibiotics (5–7 days) are associated with a good outcome for intestinal perforations that are surgically corrected within 1 or 2 days. Surgical drainage of peritoneal collections and abscesses may need to be repeated.

Chemoprophylaxis in surgery. See p. 172.

Antibiotic-associated colitis and *Clostridium difficile* diarrhoea. See p. 175.

Traveller's diarrhoea. See p. 571.

Infection of the urinary tract

(Excluding sexually transmitted infections)

Common pathogens include *Escherichia coli* (commonest in all patient groups), *Proteus* spp., *Klebsiella* spp., other Enterobacteriaceae, *Pseudomonas aeruginosa*, *Enterococcus* spp. and *Staphylococcus saprophyticus*.

Patients with abnormal urinary tracts, e.g. renal stones, prostatic hypertrophy, indwelling urinary catheters, are likely to be infected with a more varied and antimicrobial-resistant microbial flora. Identification of the causative organism and of its sensitivity to drugs is important because of the range of organisms and the prevalence of resistant strains.

For infection of the lower urinary tract a low dose may be effective, as many antimicrobials are concentrated in the urine. Infections of the substance of the kidney require the doses needed for any systemic infection. A large urine volume

---

[5]The most famous carrier was Mary Mallon ('Typhoid Mary') who worked as a cook in New York City, USA, using various assumed names and moving through several different households. She caused at least 10 outbreaks with 51 cases of typhoid fever and three deaths. To protect the public, she was kept in detention for 23 years.

(over 1.5 L/day) and frequent micturition hasten elimination of infection.

Drug treatment of urinary tract infection falls into several categories:

Lower urinary tract infection (cystitis)

This is most commonly seen in young women with normal urinary tracts. Antibiotic treatment shortens the duration of symptoms but may cause adverse reactions, and 20–30% are free from symptoms at 5–7 days even without antibiotics. Initial treatment with nitrofurantoin or trimethoprim is usually satisfactory (Durojaiye & Healey 2015). Co-amoxiclav, cephalexin or ciprofloxacin are other options but are associated with increased risks of *C. difficile* so are generally used as second-line therapy (cephalexin is typically reserved for pregnant women). Current resistance rates of 20–50% among common pathogens for trimethoprim and amoxicillin threaten their value for empirical therapy in many parts of the world. Therapy should normally last for 3 days and may need to be altered once the results of bacterial sensitivity are known.

Upper urinary tract infection

Acute pyelonephritis may be accompanied by septicaemia and is usually marked by fever and loin pain. In such patients it is advisable to start with co-amoxiclav with gentamicin i.v. or alternatively piperacillin-tazobactam (meropenem if prior ESBL) i.v. If oral therapy is considered suitable, co-amoxiclav (14 days) or ciprofloxacin (7 days) is recommended. This is an infection of the kidney substance and so needs adequate blood as well as urine concentrations, although a switch to an oral agent (guided by the results of susceptibility testing) to complete the course is recommended after the patient has clinically improved.

Upper or lower tract infection with extended-spectrum β-lactamase (ESBL) enterobacteriaceae strains has become more common in some locales, even in patients with no prior hospital contact (see p. 191). Such bacteria are usually resistant also to ciprofloxacin, parenteral cephalosporins and gentamicin. Parenteral meropenem, ertapenem or amikacin, or oral pivmecillinam, nitrofurantoin or fosfomycin may be effective.

Recurrent urinary tract infection

Attacks following rapidly with the same organism may be relapses and indicate a failure to eliminate the original infection. Attacks with a longer interval between them and produced by differing bacterial types may be regarded as due to reinfection, most often by ascending infection from the perineal skin. Repeated short courses of antimicrobials

should overcome most recurrent infections but, if these fail, 7–14 days of high-dose treatment may be given, following which continuous low-dose prophylaxis may be needed with trimethoprim, nitrofurantoin or an oral cephalosporin. Daily ingestion of cranberry juice may reduce the frequency of relapse in women, perhaps by sugars within the juice interfering with adhesion of bacteria to the urinary epithelium. Vesicoureteric reflux (passage of bladder urine back up the ureter to the kidney) accounts for about one-third of urinary tract infections in children, and causes progressive renal damage. Long-term oral antibiotic prophylaxis in such patients is modestly effective at reducing symptomatic infections.

Asymptomatic infection ('asymptomatic bacteriuria')

This may be found by routine urine testing of pregnant women or patients with known structural abnormalities of the urinary tract. Such infection may explain micturition frequency or incontinence in the elderly. Appropriate antimicrobial therapy should be given, chosen on the basis of susceptibility tests, and normally for 7–10 days. Amoxicillin or a cephalosporin is preferred in pregnancy, although nitrofurantoin may be used if imminent delivery is not likely (see below).

Prostatitis

The commonest pathogens here are Gram-negative aerobic bacilli, although chlamydia may also be involved. A quinolone such as ciprofloxacin is commonly used, although trimethoprim, doxycycline or erythromycin are also effective. Being lipid soluble, these drugs penetrate the prostate in adequate concentration; they may usefully be combined. Response to a single, short course is often good, but recurrence is common and patients can be regarded as cured only if they have been symptom-free without resort to antimicrobials for 1 year. Four weeks of oral therapy is often given for recurrent attacks. Treatment of prostatitis with ESBL or carbapenemase-producing enterobacteriaceae is problematic due to the poor penetration of β-lactams and aminoglycosides into the prostate. Evidence is emerging that fosfomycin may be a suitable agent for this indication.

Chemoprophylaxis

Chemoprophylaxis is sometimes undertaken in patients liable to recurrent attacks or acute exacerbations of ineradicable infection. It may prevent progressive renal damage in children who are found to have asymptomatic bacteriuria on routine screening. Nitrofurantoin (50–100 mg/day) or trimethoprim (100 mg/day) is satisfactory. The drugs are best given as a single oral dose at night.

Tuberculosis of the genitourinary tract is treated on the principles described for pulmonary infection (see p. 211).

Special drugs for urinary tract infections

General antimicrobials used for urinary tract infections are described elsewhere. A few agents find use solely for infection of the urinary tract:

Nitrofurantoin, a synthetic antimicrobial, is active against the majority of urinary pathogens except pseudomonads and *Proteus* spp., and has increased in importance recently because it has retained activity against a useful proportion of urinary tract coliforms that have acquired resistance to trimethoprim, oral β-lactams and quinolones. It is well absorbed from the gastrointestinal tract and is concentrated in the urine ($t_{1/2}$; 1 h), but plasma concentrations are too low to treat infection of kidney tissue. Excretion is reduced when there is renal insufficiency, rendering the drug both more toxic and less effective. Adverse effects include nausea and vomiting (much reduced with the macrocrystalline preparation) and diarrhoea. Peripheral neuropathy occurs, especially in patients with significant renal impairment, in whom the drug is contraindicated. Allergic reactions include rashes, generalised urticaria and pulmonary infiltration with lung consolidation or pleural effusion. Nitrofurantoin is safe in pregnancy, except near to term (because it may cause neonatal haemolysis), and it must be avoided in patients with glucose-6-phosphate dehydrogenase deficiency (see p. 103).

Nalidixic acid. See p. 195.

Pivmecillinam 400 mg p.o. initially, then 200–400 mg p.o. three or four times daily. Evidence for its use in treating ESBL-producing enterobacteriaceae is limited. Some authors suggest levels may be increased by the addition of clavulanate (found in co-amoxiclav).

Fosfomycin trometamol 3 g p.o. in a single dose is suitable for simple cystitis. 3 g p.o. (on alternate days; day 1; day 3 and day 5) may be suitable for complicated UTI. Daily oral therapy may be required if treating prostatitis.

Genital tract infections

A general account of orthodox literature is given below, but treatment is increasingly the prerogative of specialists, who, as is so often the case, get the best results. Interested readers are referred to specialist texts. Sexually transmitted infections are commonly multiple. Tracing and screening of contacts plays a vital part in controlling spread and reducing re-infection. Recommended treatment regimens vary to some extent among countries, and this is in response to differences in antimicrobial susceptibility of the relevant pathogens and availability of antimicrobial agents.

Gonorrhoea

The problems of β-lactam and quinolone resistance in *Neisseria gonorrhoeae* infection are increasing (ciprofloxacin resistance rates rose from 2.1% in 2000 to 39% in 2015. Resistance to azithromycin was 10% in 2015. In 2015, the world's first documented case of treatment failure to dual ceftriaxone and azithromycin therapy was reported in England. Effective treatment requires exposure of the organism briefly to a high concentration of the drug. Single-dose regimens are practicable and improve compliance. The following schedules are effective:

Uncomplicated anogenital infections. Current first-line treatment for gonorrhoea involves dual therapy with ceftri-axone (500 mg i.m.) and azithromycin (1 g p.o.), but treatment effectiveness is threatened by antimicrobial resistance.

Pharyngeal gonorrhoea responds less reliably, and i.m. ceftriaxone is recommended.

Coexistent infection. *Chlamydia trachomatis* is frequently present with *Neisseria gonorrhoeae*; tetracycline by mouth for 7 days or a single oral dose of azithromycin 1 g or ofloxacin 400 mg will treat the chlamydial urethritis.

Non-gonococcal urethritis

The vast majority of cases of urethritis with pus in which gonococci cannot be identified are due to sexually transmitted organisms, usually *Chlamydia trachomatis* (the most common bacterial sexually transmitted infection worldwide) and sometimes *Ureaplasma urealyticum*. Tetra-cycline for 1 week, or single-dose azithromycin by mouth are effective.

Pelvic inflammatory disease

Several pathogens are usually involved, including *Chlamydia trachomatis, Neisseria gonorrhoeae* and *Mycoplasma hominis,* and there may be superinfection with bowel and other urogenital tract bacteria. A combination of antimicrobials is usually required, e.g. ceftriaxone plus doxycycline plus metronidazole i.v. for severe, acute infection where chlamydia involvement is likely, or co-amoxiclav alone for post-partum chorioamnionitis.

Syphilis

Primary and secondary syphilis are effectively treated by a single dose of 2.4 million units (MU) benzathine penicillin i.m. Doxycycline or erythromycin orally for 2 weeks may be used for penicillin-allergic patients, and a single oral dose of 2 g azithromycin appears to have equivalent efficacy. *Treponema pallidum* is invariably sensitive to penicillin, but macrolide resistance has rarely been reported worldwide except in infections in men who have sex with men.

Tertiary syphilis responds to doxycycline for 28 days or to 3 weekly doses of 2.4 MU benzathine penicillin i.m. *Neurosyphilis* requires higher serum concentrations for cure and should be treated with procaine penicillin 2.4 megaunits i.m. once daily for 17 days with oral probenecid 500 mg four times a day.

Congenital syphilis in the newborn should be treated with benzylpenicillin for 10 days at least. Some advocate that a pregnant woman with syphilis should be treated as for primary syphilis in each pregnancy, in order to avoid all danger to children. Therapy is best given between the third and sixth month, as there may be a risk of abortion if it is given earlier.

Results of treatment of syphilis with penicillin are excellent. Follow-up of all cases is essential, for 5 years if possible.

The Jarisch–Herxheimer reaction is probably caused by cytokine (mainly tumour necrosis factor) release following massive destruction of spirochaetes. Presenting as pyrexia, it is common during the few hours after the first penicillin injection; other features include tachycardia, headache, myalgia and malaise, which last for up to 1 day. It cannot be avoided by giving graduated doses of penicillin. Prednisolone may prevent it and should probably be given if a reaction is specially to be feared, e.g. in a patient with syphilitic aortitis.

Chancroid

The causal agent, *Haemophilus ducreyi*, normally responds to erythromycin for 7 days or a single dose of ceftriaxone or azithromycin.

Granuloma inguinale

Calymmatobacterium granulomatis infection responds to co-trimoxazole or doxycycline for 2 weeks or a single dose of azithromycin weekly for 4 weeks.

Bacterial vaginosis (bacterial vaginitis, anaerobic vaginosis)

Bacterial vaginosis is a common form of vaginal discharge in which neither *Trichomonas vaginalis* nor *Candida albicans* can be isolated and inflammatory cells are not present: it is diagnosed from the characteristic Gram stain appearances of a vaginal swab. The condition is associated with overgrowth of several normal commensals of the vagina including *Gardnerella vaginalis*, Gram-negative curved bacilli and anaerobic organisms, the latter being responsible for the characteristic fishy odour of the vaginal discharge. The condition responds well to a single dose of metronidazole 2 g or 400 mg thrice daily for 1 week by mouth, with 7 days of topical clindamycin cream offering an alternative.

Candida vaginitis. See p. 231.

Trichomonas vaginitis. See p. 244.

Infection of bones and joints

Causative bacteria of **osteomyelitis** may arrive via the bloodstream or be implanted directly (through a compound fracture, chronic local infection of local tissue, or surgical operation). *Staphylococcus aureus* is the commonest isolate in all patient groups, and *Salmonella* species in the tropics. Chronic osteomyelitis of the lower limbs (especially when underlying chronic skin infection in the elderly) frequently involves obligate anaerobes (such as *Bacteroides* spp.) and enterobacteriaceae.

Strenuous efforts should be made to obtain bone for culture because superficial and sinus cultures are poorly predictive of the underlying flora, and prolonged therapy is required for chronic osteomyelitis (usually 6–8 weeks, sometimes longer). Surgical removal of dead bone improves the outcome of chronic osteomyelitis.

Definitive therapy is guided by the results of culture, but commonly used regimens include co-amoxiclav (community-acquired cases in adults), flucloxacillin with or without fusidic acid (for *Staphylococcus aureus*), ceftriaxone or co-amoxiclav (in children), and ciprofloxacin (for enterobacteriaceae). Short courses of therapy (3–6 weeks) may suffice for acute osteomyelitis, but vertebral body osteomyelitis requires at least 8 weeks of treatment.

Septic arthritis is a medical emergency if good joint function is to be retained. *Staphylococcus aureus* is the commonest pathogen, but a very wide range of bacteria may be involved including streptococci, enterobacteriaceae and *Neisseria* spp. Aspiration of the joint allows specific microbiological diagnosis, differentiation from non-infectious causes such as crystal synovitis, and has therapeutic benefit, e.g. for the hip joint, where formal drainage is recommended. Initial therapy is as for chronic osteomyelitis, and continuation guided by culture results for 4–6 weeks is usually required. Switching to oral therapy is often possible with satisfactory progress.

Infection of prosthetic joints may also involve a range of bacteria, but is most commonly staphylococcal (*S. aureus* and coagulase-negative staphylococci). Debridement of the prosthesis and culture of adjacent bone biopsy samples fulfils both therapeutic and diagnostic needs, and prolonged antibiotic therapy guided by culture is successful (with retention of the prosthesis in situ) in 60% of cases or more as long as it is commenced within a few weeks of first presentation of the infection and the prosthesis is stable.

Eye infections

Superficial infections, caused by a variety of organisms, are treated by chloramphenicol, fusidic acid, framycetin, gentamicin, ciprofloxacin, levofloxacin, ofloxacin or neomycin in drops or ointments. Ciprofloxacin, ofloxacin, levofloxacin, gentamicin or tobramycin is used for *Pseudomonas aeruginosa*, and fusidic acid principally for *Staphylococcus aureus*. Preparations often contain hydrocortisone or prednisolone, but the steroid masks the progress of the infection; should it be applied with an antimicrobial to which the organism is resistant (bacterium or virus), it may aggravate the disease by suppressing protective inflammation. Local chemoprophylaxis without corticosteroid is used to prevent secondary bacterial infection in viral conjunctivitis. A variety of antibiotics may be given by direct injection to the chambers of the eye for treatment of bacterial endophthalmitis.

Chlamydial conjunctivitis. In the developed world, the genital (D–K) serotypes of the organism are responsible, and the reservoir and transmission is maintained by sexual contact. Endemic trachoma in developing countries is usually caused by serotypes A, B and C. In either case, oral tetracycline is effective. Pregnant or lactating women may receive systemic erythromycin. Neonatal ophthalmia responds to systemic erythromycin and topical tetracycline.

Herpes keratitis. See p. 225.

Fungal keratitis. Keratitis due to *Fusarium* spp., *Aspergillus* spp. and other moulds may occur, particularly in patients with contact lenses and prior antibiotic use. Treatment is typically with systemic voriconazole and topical therapy (natamycin +/– topical amphotericin B or voriconazole).

Mycobacterial infections

Pulmonary tuberculosis

Nearly one-third of the world's population is infected with *Mycobacterium tuberculosis*, and it is the second leading cause of death due to an identified pathogen, after HIV infection. Drug therapy has transformed tuberculosis from a disabling and often fatal disease into one in which almost 100% cure is obtainable, although the recent emergence of multiply drug-resistant tuberculosis (MDR-TB) and extensively drug-resistant tuberculosis (XDR-TB) strains and their interaction with HIV infection has disturbed this optimistic view. Chemotherapy was formerly protracted, but a better understanding of the mode of action of antituberculosis drugs and of effective immune reconstitution in HIV infection has allowed the development of shorter-course regimens.

Principles of antituberculosis therapy

- Kill a large number of actively multiplying bacilli: *isoniazid* achieves this.
- Treat persisters, i.e. semi-dormant bacilli that metabolise slowly or intermittently: *rifampicin* and *pyrazinamide* are the most efficacious.
- Prevent the emergence of drug resistance by multiple therapy to suppress single-drug–resistant mutants that may exist de novo or emerge during therapy: *isoniazid* and *rifampicin* are best.
- Combined formulations are used to ensure that poor compliance does not result in monotherapy with consequent drug resistance.

Most contemporary regimens employ an initial *intensive* phase with rifampicin, isoniazid, pyrazinamide and ethambutol, to reduce the bacterial load as rapidly as possible (usually for 2 months), followed by a *continuation* phase with rifampicin and isoniazid given for at least 4 months (Fig. 14.1) based on sensitivity data.

All short-course regimens include isoniazid, pyrazinamide, rifampicin and ethambutol. After extensive clinical trials, the following have been found satisfactory:

1. An *unsupervised* regimen of daily dosing comprising isoniazid and rifampicin for 6 months, plus pyrazinamide and ethambutol for the first 2 months.
2. A *supervised* (directly observed therapy, DOT) regimen for patients who cannot be relied upon to comply with treatment, comprising thrice-weekly dosing with isoniazid and rifampicin for 6 months, plus pyrazinamide and ethambutol for the first 2 months (isoniazid and pyrazinamide are given in higher dose than in the unsupervised regimen). Daily DOT is more effective than thrice-weekly dosing. With both of the above regimens, ethambutol by mouth or streptomycin i.m. should be added for the first 2 months if there is a likelihood of drug-resistant organisms, or if the patient is severely ill with extensive active lesions. Ethambutol should not be administered in small children as they are unable to report visual side-effects.

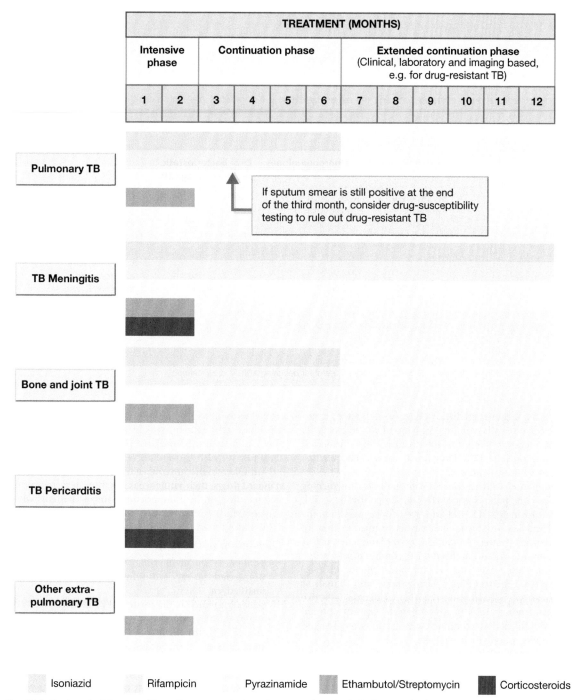

Fig. 14.1 Treatment of drug-sensitive pulmonary and extrapulmonary tuberculosis. Daily supervised treatment is preferred. Intermittent, thrice-weekly treatment administered under direct observation equally effective. Monitor adverse effects (hepatic functions, serum uric acid) periodically.

Table 14.1 General principles for MDR-TB and XDR-TB drug regimen according to drug-susceptibility testing

- Include at least five drugs
- Include any first-line drug to which *Mycobacterium tuberculosis* is susceptible
- Include an injectable for a prolonged period
- Include a quinolone
- Consider regional drug resistance data and the patient's treatment history while planning a drug regimen

First-line oral agents	Second-line drugs			Drugs with uncertain efficacy[e]
	Injectable agents	**Fluoroquinolones**	**Oral bacteriostatic second-line agents**	
Pyrazinamide	Streptomycin[b]	Ofloxacin	Cycloserine/terizidone	Clofazimine
Ethambutol	Kanamycin[c]	Levofloxacin	Ethionamide/	Thioacetazone
Rifabutin[a]	Amikacin[c]	Moxifloxacin	prothionamide[d]	High-dose isoniazid
	Capreomycin		PAS[d]	Linezolid
				Amoxicillin-clavulanate
				Clarithromycin/
				azithromycin
				Imipenem/cilastin

MDR-TB, multiply drug-resistant tuberculosis; XDR-TB, extensively drug-resistant tuberculosis.
[a]High degree of cross-resistance common between rifampicin and rifabutin
[b]First-line drug
[c]Cross-resistance common
[d]Gastrointestinal adverse effects and hypothyroidism common with both
[e]Not recommended for routine use in MDR-TB, but may be useful for designing XDR-TB drug regimen

All of the regimens are highly effective, with relapse rates of 1–2% in those who continue for 6 months; even if patients default after, say, 4 months, tuberculosis can be expected to recur in only 10–15%. Drug resistance seldom develops with any of these regimens.

Compliance is often a concern with multiple drug therapy given for long periods, especially in the developing world, and (surprisingly) DOT did improve relapse rates in many trials. Fixed-dose combination therapy is assumed to improve compliance; however, bio-availability of rifampicin remains a matter of concern in fixed-dose combinations; some commonly used fixed-dose combinations include Rifater (rifampicin, isoniazid plus pyrazinamide), and Rifinah or Rimactazid (rifampicin plus isoniazid). In all cases, effective control of tuberculosis in a population requires optimal therapy of index cases combined with careful screening and case finding among their contacts.

Special problems

Drug resistant organisms. Initial drug resistance occurs in about 4% of isolates in the UK, usually to isoniazid. Patients with multiply drug-resistant tuberculosis (defined as resistant to rifampicin and isoniazid at least) should be treated with three or four drugs to which the organisms are sensitive, and treatment should extend for 12–24 months after cultures become negative (Table 14.1 and Fig. 14.2). Treatment of such cases requires expert management.

Non-tuberculous mycobacteria are often resistant to standard drugs; their virulence is low, but they can produce serious infection in immunocompromised patients which may respond, e.g. to macrolide (clarithromycin), ethambutol or rifabutin, often in combination.

Chemoprophylaxis may be either:

- *primary*, i.e. the giving of antituberculous drugs to uninfected but exposed individuals, which is seldom justified, or
- *secondary*, which is the treatment of infected but symptom-free individuals, e.g. those known to be in contact with the disease and who develop a positive tuberculin reaction. Secondary chemoprophylaxis may be justified in children younger than 3 years of age because they have a high risk of disseminated disease; isoniazid alone for 6–9 months may be used, as there is little risk of resistant organisms emerging because the organism load is low. Shorter treatment regimens with an alternative drug (rifampicin for 4 months or 3 months) or drug combinations

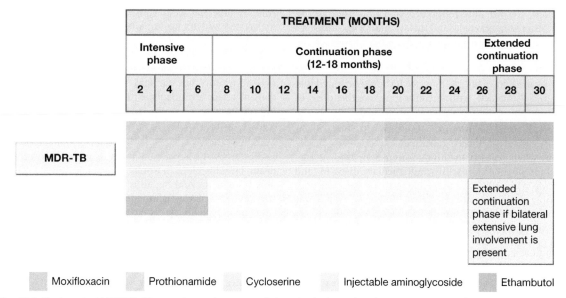

TREATMENT (MONTHS)														
Intensive phase			Continuation phase (12-18 months)									Extended continuation phase		
2	4	6	8	10	12	14	16	18	20	22	24	26	28	30

MDR-TB

Extended continuation phase if bilateral extensive lung involvement is present

Moxifloxacin   Prothionamide   Cycloserine   Injectable aminoglycoside   Ethambutol

Fig. 14.2 Treatment of MDR-TB. The number and category of drugs in the intensive phase may vary according to country's national programme. Monitor adverse effects (neuropsychiatric, renal, hepatic and thyroid functions) periodically. In patients with MDR-TB who have not been previously treated with second-line drugs and in whom resistance to fluoroquinolones and second-line injectables has been excluded or is considered unlikely, a shorter MDR-TB regimen of 9–12 months may be used instead of the conventional longer duration regimen. MDR-TB, multiply drug-resistant tuberculosis.

(rifampicin plus isoniazid for 3 months) have better adherence rates. Combined use of rifampicin and pyrazinamide for 2 months in HIV-negative contacts is not recommended as it produces severe drug-induced hepatitis.

Pregnancy. Drug treatment should never be interrupted or postponed during pregnancy. On the general principle of limiting exposure of the fetus, the standard four-drug, 6-month course (no. 1 above) is best. Exclude streptomycin from any regimen (danger of fetal eighth cranial nerve damage).

Treatment of MDR-TB is not contraindicated during pregnancy. While treating MDR-TB, risks and benefits should be discussed with the mother. Treatment should be started in the second trimester or earlier if the disease is severe; to avoid teratogenic effects, drugs should not be administered in the first trimester. Injectables should be avoided. Capreomycin is the injectable of choice in an unavoidable situation but carries the risk of ototoxicity. Ethionamide should be avoided as it aggravates nausea and vomiting and also has teratogenic effects.

Extrapulmonary tuberculosis. The principles of treatment, i.e. multiple therapy and prolonged follow-up, are the same as for pulmonary tuberculosis (see Fig. 14.1). Many chronic tuberculosis lesions may be relatively inaccessible to drugs

as a result of avascularity, so treatment frequently has to be prolonged and dosage high, especially if damaged tissue cannot be removed by surgery, e.g. tuberculosis of bones.

Meningeal tuberculosis It is essential to use isoniazid and pyrazinamide, which penetrate well into the CSF. Rifampicin and streptomycin enter inflamed meninges well, but non-inflamed meninges less so, whereas ethambutol has poor penetration. An effective regimen is isoniazid, rifampicin, pyrazinamide and streptomycin. Treatment is required for 12 months in total. Surgery may be required if there is evidence of raised intracranial pressure.

Bone and joint tuberculosis. Six-month drug regimens containing rifampicin are effective (see Fig. 14.1). Surgery is indicated when chemotherapy fails with evidence of ongoing infection and for relief of cord compression with persistent or recurrent neurological deficits or instability of the spine.

Lymph node tuberculosis. In drug-susceptible lymph node tuberculosis, a 6-month regimen is adequate. The course remains even if the node has been surgically removed. Affected lymph nodes may enlarge while the patient is on treatment or after the end of treatment without any evidence of mycobacterial relapse (immune reconstitution inflammatory syndrome [IRIS]). Cold abscesses of lymph nodes require needle drainage.

Adrenal steroid and tuberculosis. Corticosteroids are administered in adrenal gland involvement with Addison's disease, in meningeal and pericardial tuberculosis (see Fig. 14.1). Prednisolone or dexamethasone are typically commenced at a high dose at the start of anti-TB therapy and then weaned down after 4–8 weeks. It should be noted that rifampicin interacts with prednisolone, so the dose of prednisolone should be increased accordingly.

Tuberculosis in the immunocompromised. Such patients require special measures because they may be infected more readily when exposed; their infections usually involve large numbers of tubercle bacilli (multibacillary disease), and patients with AIDS are more likely to be infected with multiply antibiotic-resistant strains. While treating patients co-infected with HIV and tuberculosis, antituberculosis treatment (ATT) is started first and antiretroviral treatment (ART) is started subsequently. ART-naïve HIV/AIDS patients should be started on ART between 2 weeks and 2 months after anti-TB drugs, depending on CD4 cell counts. Patients already on ART require some modification in treatment; efavirenz should be used in place of nevirapine. Rifabutin should be preferred over rifampicin while using protease inhibitors (less interaction issues). Patients while on ART and ATT may develop IRIS (within 3 months of treatment). In this paradoxical reaction, patients initially show some improvement and subsequently reveal either aggravation of existing lesions or appearance of fresh lesions. Development of IRIS does not require stopping of ART, and usually non-steroidal anti-inflammatory drugs (NSAIDs) are sufficient. Drug-resistant TB should be ruled out. Usually at least four drugs are started, and patients are isolated until bacteriological results have been obtained and they have shown clinical improvement. If infections are proved to involve antibiotic-susceptible mycobacteria, therapy can continue with a conventional 6-month regimen with careful follow-up. Particular problems may occur with multiple drug interactions during antituberculous treatment of patients receiving antiretroviral therapy.

Antituberculosis drugs

Isoniazid

Isoniazid (INH, isonicotinic acid hydrazide) is selectively effective against *Mycobacterium tuberculosis* because it prevents the synthesis of components that are unique to mycobacterial cell walls. Hence it is bactericidal against actively multiplying bacilli (whether within macrophages or at extracellular sites) but is bacteriostatic against non-dividing bacilli; it has little or no activity against other bacteria. Isoniazid is well absorbed from the alimentary tract and is distributed throughout the body water, including CSF. It should always be given in cases where there is special risk of meningitis (miliary tuberculosis and primary infection). Isoniazid is inactivated by conjugation with an acetyl group, and the rate of the reaction is bimodally distributed. The $t_{1/2}$ is 1 h in fast and 4 h in slow acetylators; fast acetylators achieve less than one-half the steady-state plasma concentration of slow acetylators, but standard oral doses (300 mg/day) on daily regimens give adequate tuberculocidal concentrations in both groups.

Adverse effects. Isoniazid is in general well tolerated. The most severe adverse effect is liver damage, ranging from a moderate rise in hepatic enzymes to severe hepatitis and death. Liver histology in isoniazid hepatitis is indistinguishable from acute viral hepatitis. It is probably caused by a chemically reactive metabolite(s), e.g. acetylhydrazine. Most cases are in patients older than 35 years of age, and develop within the first 8 weeks of therapy; liver function should be monitored monthly during this period at least. High-dose isoniazid (16–20 mg/kg/day) may be useful in DR-TB.

Isoniazid is a structural analogue of pyridoxine and accelerates its excretion, the principal result of which is peripheral neuropathy with numbness and tingling of the feet, motor involvement being less common. Neuropathy is more frequent in slow acetylators, malnourished people, pregnant and breast-feeding women, the elderly and those with HIV infection, liver disease, diabetes mellitus and alcoholism, chronic renal failure, malnutrition. Patients should therefore receive pyridoxine 10 mg/day by mouth, which prevents neuropathy and does not interfere with the therapeutic effect. Other adverse effects include mental disturbances, incoordination, optic neuritis and convulsions.

Isoniazid inhibits the metabolism of phenytoin, carbamazepine and ethosuximide, increasing their effect. Blood levels of these drugs should be monitored (therapeutic drug monitoring).

Rifampicin

Rifampicin has bactericidal activity against the tubercle bacillus, comparable to that of isoniazid. It is also used in leprosy.

It acts by inhibiting RNA synthesis, bacteria being sensitive to this effect at much lower concentrations than mammalian cells; it is particularly effective against mycobacteria that lie semi-dormant within cells. Rifampicin has a wide range of antimicrobial activity. Other uses include leprosy, severe legionnaires' disease (with erythromycin or ciprofloxacin), the chemoprophylaxis of meningococcal meningitis (though ciprofloxacin is now recommended), and severe staphylococcal infection (with flucloxacillin or vancomycin).

Rifampicin is well absorbed from the gastrointestinal tract and penetrates most tissues. Entry into the CSF when meninges are inflamed is sufficient to maintain therapeutic concentrations at normal oral doses, but transfer is reduced as inflammation subsides in 1–2 months.

Enterohepatic recycling takes place, and eventually about 60% of a single dose is eliminated in the faeces; urinary excretion of unchanged drug also occurs. The $t_{1/2}$ is 4 h after initial doses, but shortens on repeated dosing because rifampicin is a very effective enzyme inducer and increases its own metabolism (as well as that of several other drugs; see below).

Adverse reactions. Rifampicin rarely causes any serious toxicity. Adverse reactions include flushing and itching with or without a rash, and thrombocytopenia. Rises in plasma levels of bilirubin and hepatic enzymes may occur when treatment starts, but are often transient and are not necessarily an indication for stopping the drug; fatal hepatitis, however, has occurred. Hepatic function should be checked before starting treatment and at least for the first few months of therapy. Intermittent dosing, i.e. less than twice weekly, either as part of a regimen or through poor compliance, promotes an influenza-like syndrome (malaise, headache and fever, shortness of breath and wheezing), acute haemolytic anaemia and thrombocytopenia, and acute renal failure sometimes with haemolysis. These may have an immunological basis. Red discoloration of urine, tears and sputum is a useful indication that the patient is taking the drug. Rifampicin also causes an orange discoloration of soft contact lenses.

Interactions. Rifampicin is a powerful enzyme inducer and speeds the metabolism of numerous drugs, including warfarin, steroids (including contraceptives), narcotic analgesics, oral antidiabetic agents, phenytoin, triazole antifungal agents and dapsone. Appropriate increase in dosage, and alternative methods of contraception, are required to compensate for increased drug metabolism (see also paracetamol overdose, p. 254).

Rifabutin ($t_{1/2}$ 36 h) has similar activity and adverse reactions, and is used for prophylaxis of *Mycobacterium avium* infection in patients with AIDS, and for treatment of tuberculous and non-tuberculous mycobacterial infection in combination with other drugs. All rifamycins have high levels of cross-resistance. It is preferred over rifampicin when protease inhibitors are used for treating HIV-TB co-infection. Rifabutin and saquinavir should not be used together. Rifabutin and protease inhibitors are costlier drugs; dose reduction of rifabutin is required, as most protease inhibitors are inhibitors of CYP3A4 isoenzyme and significantly reduce clearance of rifabutin. The dose of rifabutin should be increased from 300 mg/day to 450–600 mg/day when it is co-administered with efavirenz. Adverse effects include gastrointestinal intolerance, bone marrow suppression, hepatotoxicity, uveitis and skin discoloration with normal serum bilirubin (pseudojaundice).

Rifaximin is a semi-synthetic rifamycin that is not absorbed from the gastrointestinal tract (less than 0.4%). Because of the very high faecal concentrations achieved after a 400-mg oral dose (about 8000 µg/g faeces), it has broad activity against the common bacterial causes of travellers' diarrhoea and has proved as effective as an oral quinolone or azithromycin (see p. 571), and adverse effects are rare. Efficacy of rifaximin treatment in acute hepatic encephalopathy is well documented. Its protective effect against breakthrough episodes of hepatic encephalopathy along with lactulose on a long-term basis is being evaluated, as rifaximin has a low risk of inducing bacterial resistance.

Pyrazinamide

Pyrazinamide is a derivative of nicotinamide and is included in first-choice combination regimens because of its particular ability to kill intracellular persisters, i.e. mycobacteria that are dividing or semi-dormant, often within cells. Its action is dependent on the activity of intrabacterial pyrazinamidase, which converts pyrazinamide to the active pyrazinoic acid; this enzyme is most effective in an acidic environment such as the interior of cells. In drug-sensitive tuberculosis, it should not be administered beyond 2 months. It is inactive against *Mycobacterium bovis*. Pyrazinamide is well absorbed from the gastrointestinal tract and metabolised in the liver, with very little unchanged drug appearing in the urine ($t_{1/2}$ 9 h). CSF concentrations are almost identical to those in the blood. Pyrazinamide is safe to use in pregnancy.

Adverse effects include hyperuricaemia and arthralgia, which is relatively frequent with daily but less so with intermittent dosing and, unlike gout, affects both large and small joints. Pyrazinoic acid, the principal metabolite of pyrazinamide, inhibits renal tubular secretion of urate. Symptomatic treatment with a non-steroidal anti-inflammatory drug is usually sufficient, and it is rarely necessary to discontinue pyrazinamide because of arthralgia. Incidence of hepatitis which occurred with high doses has decreased with modern short-course schedules, but still requires close clinical and laboratory monitoring. Sideroblastic anaemia and urticaria also occur.

Ethambutol

Ethambutol, being bacteriostatic, is used in conjunction with other antituberculous drugs to delay or prevent the emergence of resistant bacilli. It is well absorbed from the gastrointestinal tract, and effective concentrations occur in most body tissues including the lung; in tuberculous meningitis, sufficient amounts may reach the CSF to inhibit mycobacterial growth, but insignificant amounts enter the CSF if the meninges are not inflamed. Excretion is mainly by the kidney, by tubular secretion as well as by glomerular filtration ($t_{1/2}$ 4 h); the dose should be reduced when renal function is impaired.

Adverse effects. In recommended oral doses (15 mg/kg/day), with dose adjustment for reduced renal function, ethambutol is relatively non-toxic. The main problem is rare *optic neuritis* (unilateral or bilateral) causing loss of visual acuity, central scotomata, occasionally also peripheral vision loss and red–green colour blindness. The changes reverse if treatment is stopped promptly; if not, the patient may go blind. It is prudent to note any history of eye disease and to get baseline tests of vision, including colour vision, before starting treatment with ethambutol. The drug should not be given to a patient with reduced vision who may not notice further deterioration. Patients should be told to read small print in newspapers regularly (with each eye separately) and, if there is any deterioration, to stop the drug immediately and seek advice. Patients who cannot understand and comply (especially children) should be given alternative therapy if possible. The need for repeated specialist ophthalmological monitoring is controversial. Peripheral neuritis occurs but is rare.

Antituberculosis drug-induced hepatitis

Among the first-line antituberculosis drugs, rifampicin, isoniazid and pyrazinamide are potentially hepatotoxic drugs. Additionally, rifampicin can cause asymptomatic jaundice without evidence of hepatitis. Rifampicin rarely causes hepatitis when administered alone, and rifampicin and isoniazid are ~ 3 times less toxic in the absence of pyrazinamide. It is essential to rule out acute viral hepatitis by performing markers for viral hepatitis before diagnosing antituberculosis drug-induced hepatitis in developing nations. Drug-induced hepatitis can be life-threatening if drugs are continued despite its occurrence. All hepatotoxic drugs should be immediately stopped until complete biochemical recovery occurs. In the interim period, ethambutol, streptomycin and one of the fluoroquinolones should be administered. The best approach to reintroducing antituberculosis drugs is still debatable. The approach could be sequential or simultaneous. Some advocate reintroduction of all three drugs one by one as it allows identification of the culprit drug, while others prefer to use rifampicin first followed by isoniazid and if the patient tolerates both drugs avoid pyrazinamide.

Streptomycin

See p. 186.

Thiacetazone

Thiacetazone is tuberculostatic and is used with isoniazid to inhibit the emergence of resistance to the latter drug. It is absorbed from the gastrointestinal tract, partly metabolised and partly excreted in the urine ($t_{1/2}$ 13 h). Usual adult dose is 150 mg/day. It is not used in HIV-TB co-infection because of severe cutaneous reactions; Asian patients may have higher incidence of Stevens–Johnson syndrome.

Adverse reactions include gastrointestinal symptoms, conjunctivitis and vertigo. More serious effects are erythema multiforme, haemolytic anaemia, agranulocytosis, cerebral oedema and hepatitis.

Second-line antituberculosis drugs

Kanamycin and amikacin

Both kanamycin ($t_{1/2}$ 2–4 h) and amikacin ($t_{1/2}$ 2–4 h) are bactericidal drugs of the aminoglycoside class, valuable in patients with resistance to streptomycin. Cross-resistance between kanamycin and amikacin is usual. The optimal dose of amikacin is 15 mg/kg body-weight, usually 0.75–1 g/day i.m. Adverse effects are similar to streptomycin.

Capreomycin

Capreomycin ($t_{1/2}$ 4–6 h) is a bactericidal aminoglycoside derived from *Streptomyces capreolus*. There is no cross-resistance with other aminoglycosides. The usual dose is 20 mg/kg/day up to 1 g in a single dose daily i.m. for 40–120 days; the dose is then reduced to 2–3 times weekly as the risk of adverse effects increases sharply. Adverse effects are similar to streptomycin. Hypokalaemia, hypocalcaemia and hypomagnesaemia have been reported. Rarely, hepatitis and general cutaneous reactions may occur.

Thioamides

Ethionamide and prothionamide. Ethionamide ($t_{1/2}$ 2–3 h) and prothionamide ($t_{1/2}$ 2–3 h) are bactericidal drugs. Their chemical structure resembles thioacetazone, and there is frequent partial cross-resistance. The maximum optimum dose is 15–20 mg/kg/day up to 1 g/day, and the usual dose is 750 mg/day in patients weighing 50 kg or more (or can be split in two doses: 500 mg in the morning and 250 mg in the evening) and 500 mg/day in patients weighing <50 kg. These drugs are more acceptable when administered with orange juice or milk. Adverse reactions include gastrointestinal side-effects, depression, hallucinations, hepatitis, hypothyroidism and peripheral neuropathy. The drugs should be avoided during pregnancy.

Cycloserine and terizidone

Cycloserine ($t_{1/2}$ 10 h) is bacteriostatic at the usual dosage, and terizidone is a combination of two molecules of cycloserine. The maximum daily dose is 15–20 mg/kg; the usual dose of cycloserine and terizidone is 500–750 mg/day (250 mg in the morning and 500 mg 12 hours later). Main adverse effects are related to the central nervous system (less with terizidone) and include headache, tremors, insomnia, depression, convulsions, altered behaviour and suicidal tendencies. Addition of pyridoxine (50 mg/250 mg of cycloserine and terizidone is recommended) decreases these adverse effects.

Fluoroquinolones

Ciprofloxacin ($t_{1/2}$ 3–5 h) is no longer recommended to treat drug-susceptible or drug-resistant tuberculosis. The most potent available fluoroquinolones, in descending order, include: moxifloxacin ($t_{1/2}$ 9–10 h) (400 mg/day) or gatifloxacin ($t_{1/2}$ 8 h) (400 mg/day) > levofloxacin ($t_{1/2}$ 6–8 h) (750 mg/day) > ofloxacin ($t_{1/2}$ biphasic: 4–5 h and 20–25 h [accounts for <5%]) (800 mg/day). Though moxifloxacin and gatifloxacin have equal potency, the latter is not favoured in those with diabetes mellitus because of the risk of hyperglycaemia, hypoglycaemia and new-onset diabetes mellitus. Later-generation fluoroquinolones have some efficacy against ofloxacin-resistant strains and are recommended for the treatment of XDR-TB. Close monitoring is required as safety data on long-term use are limited. Prolonged QT interval occurs with moxifloxacin. Side effects of fluoroquinolones have been described previously.

Para-aminosalicylic acid (PAS)

Usual dose of para-aminosalicylic acid (PAS) ($t_{1/2}$ 1 h) is 8–12 g/day in divided doses. Commonly observed adverse effects include gastrointestinal upset, hepatic dysfunction and hypothyroidism; it should be administered cautiously in patients with cardiac and renal insufficiency because of the sodium load.

Bedaquiline. Bedaquiline is a novel oral diarylquinoline anti-mycobacterial agent with a unique mechanism of action: the specific and selective inhibition of mycobacterial ATP synthase, essential for energy generation in *M. tuberculosis*. Bedaquiline was granted accelerated approval in 2012, based on Phase IIb data.[6] Bedaquiline may be added to a WHO-recommended regimen in adult patients with MDR-TB when an effective treatment regimen containing four second-line drugs in addition to pyrazinamide according to WHO recommendations cannot be designed and when there is

documented evidence of resistance to any fluoroquinolones in addition to MDR-TB (WHO, 2013).[7] The most commonly reported adverse events in the bedaquiline arm were nausea, arthralgia, headache and vomiting. Additional adverse events were dizziness, increased transaminases, myalgia, diarrhoea and QT prolongation on ECG. Main safety concerns included QT prolongation, cardiac events, and deaths (10 deaths in the bedaquiline arm versus two in the placebo arm).

Delamanid. Delamanid is a novel nitro-dihydro-imidazo-oxazole derivative that specifically inhibits mycolic acid biosynthesis. The antibacterial activity is specific for mycobacteria. It is described as a pro-drug that undergoes reductive metabolism by *M. tuberculosis* to produce an active free radical. Delamanid resistance has occurred during treatment, and therefore it must be administered along with other drugs predicted to be effective. Mycobacterial resistance to delamanid may develop due to a mutation in one of the five coenzyme F420 genes necessary for the activation of delamanid.

It is authorised by the European Commission for the treatment of adults with pulmonary MDR-TB on the basis of Phase IIb trial data under the provisions for orphan medicinal products. Delamanid, as part of an appropriate combination regimen, can increase the proportion of patients achieving sputum culture conversion at 2 months in adult patients with pulmonary MDR-TB in whom standard MDR-TB regimens cannot otherwise be composed for reasons of resistance or tolerability. The main safety concern of delamanid is QT interval prolongation. Further evidence is needed to assess safety and efficacy.

Clofazimine. Discussed below.

Linezolid. Usual adult dose is 600 mg twice a day for 4–6 weeks, and subsequently the dose is reduced to 600 mg/day to reduce the adverse effects. See also p. 191.

Clarithromycin 500 mg twice a day. See also p. 190.

Leprosy

Effective treatment of leprosy is complex and requires much experience to obtain the best results. Problems of resistant leprosy now require that multiple drug therapy be used and involve:

- For *paucibacillary disease*: dapsone and rifampicin for 6 months.
- For *multibacillary disease*: dapsone, rifampicin and clofazimine for 2 years. Follow-up for 4–8 years may be necessary.

[6]Diacon AH, Pym A, Grobusch MP, et al.; TMC207-C208 Study Group (2014) Multidrug-resistant tuberculosis and culture conversion with bedaquiline. New Engl and Journal of Medicine 371:723–732.

[7]World Health Organization (2013) The use of bedaquiline in the treatment of multidrug-resistant tuberculosis: interim policy guidance. Geneva: WHO.

Dapsone is a bacteriostatic sulphone (related to sulphonamides, acting by the same mechanism; see p. 193). It has long been the standard drug for all forms of leprosy. Irregular and inadequate duration of treatment with a single drug has allowed the emergence of primary and secondary resistance to become a major problem. Dapsone is also used to treat dermatitis herpetiformis and *Pneumocystis carinii* pneumonia (with trimethoprim), and (with pyrimethamine) for malaria prophylaxis. The $t_{1/2}$ is 27 h. Adverse effects range from gastrointestinal symptoms to agranulocytosis, haemolytic anaemia and generalised allergic reactions that include exfoliative dermatitis.

Rifampicin (see above) is bactericidal, and is safe and effective when given once monthly. This long interval renders feasible the directly observed administration of rifampicin which the above regimens require.

Clofazimine has leprostatic and anti-inflammatory effects (preventing erythema nodosum leprosum). It causes gastrointestinal symptoms. Reddish discoloration of the skin and other cutaneous lesions also occur and may persist for months after the drug has been stopped. The $t_{1/2}$ is 70 days.

Other antileprotics include ethionamide and prothionamide. Thalidomide (see p. 261), despite its notorious past, still finds a use with corticosteroid in the control of allergic lepromatous reactions.

Other non-tuberculous mycobacteria

Mycobacterium abscessus is an increasingly recognised cause of infection due to the rise in immunocompromised patients. Treatment typically comprises an induction phase of 2–8 weeks (with amikacin and imipenem being the favoured option for induction; alternatives include cefoxitin or tigecycline). Options for the maintenance phase include clarithromycin, linezolid, moxifloxacin or clofazimine.

Mycobacterium avium complex (MAC) is intrinsically resistant to many antibiotics and antituberculosis drugs but is fairly susceptible to macrolides, rifamycins, ethambutol, clofazimine, fluoroquinolones (e.g. ciprofloxacin, levofloxacin, moxifloxacin) and aminoglycosides.

In general, MAC infection is treated with 2 or 3 antimicrobials for at least 12 months.

Other bacterial infections

Burns. Infection may be reduced by application of silver sulfadiazine cream, although evidence for clinical benefit is weak. Substantial absorption can occur from any raw surface, and use of aminoglycoside preparations, e.g. neomycin, can cause ototoxicity. Use of systemic antibiotics for days 4 to 14 in patients with large burns has been shown to reduce mortality by nearly 50% at the expense of a significant rise in the prevalence of antibiotic resistance.

Gas gangrene. The skin between the waist and the knees is normally contaminated with anaerobic faecal organisms. However assiduous the skin preparation for orthopaedic operations or thigh amputations, this will not kill or remove all the spores. Surgery performed for vascular insufficiency where tissue oxygenation may be poor is likely to be followed by infection. Gas gangrene (*Clostridium perfringens*) may occur; prophylaxis with benzylpenicillin or metronidazole is used.

Cellulitis (inflammation of the skin) is most commonly a β-haemolytic streptococcal infection, although *Staphylococcus aureus* may also be implicated, and a wide range of bacteria including obligate anaerobes may be involved in cases associated with arterial insufficiency (e.g. lower limb infections in diabetes mellitus). Mild streptococcal/staphylococcal cases will usually respond to flucloxacillin, although more clinically severe infections may require the addition of high-dose parenteral benzylpenicillin or clindamycin. Occasionally the infection may progress to a rapidly spreading infection of the tissues, with necrosis of the overlying skin (so-called 'necrotising fasciitis'); to halt its spread requires urgent surgical resection of all non-viable tissues, and addition of clindamycin to the antibiotic regimen is recommended. Clindamycin exerts its beneficial effects by inhibiting production of streptococcal toxins at the ribosomal level. Care must be used when giving clindamycin due to the risks of *C. difficile* infection.

Wounds. Systemic antibiotic therapy is necessary at least for several days in dirty wounds, and in penetrating wounds of body cavities. Flucloxacillin is probably best, but in the case of penetrating abdominal wounds metronidazole should be added and consideration given to adding an agent active against aerobic Gram-negative bacteria, e.g. gentamicin (see also Tetanus). In some hospitalised patients, vancomycin or another glycopeptide might be prudent to cover the possibility of MRSA involvement.

Bites from humans and other mammals are common and involve the inoculation of the rich bacterial flora of the mouth to the deep tissues. Secondary infection is frequent (up to 80% of cat bites become infected) and may involve *Pasteurella multocida* which can cause rapidly spreading cellulitis and is resistant to flucloxacillin and erythromycin. Appropriate management beyond direct care of the wound includes prevention of tetanus, wound infection and transmission of viruses such as hepatitis B and C, and HIV and rabies in endemic areas. Antibiotic prophylaxis reduces wound infection risks in bites of the hand and those made by humans or cats, and co-amoxiclav is considered the best choice; doxycycline and metronidazole would be suitable for penicillin-allergic patients. *Pasteurella* spp. are typically resistant to macrolides.

Abscesses and infections in serous cavities are treated according to the antimicrobial sensitivity of the organism concerned, but require high doses because of poor penetration. Aspiration or surgical drainage of such collections of pus shortens the period of illness, and antibiotic therapy may on occasion be avoided for smaller abscesses after drainage.

Acne (see Ch. 17) is in part caused and exacerbated by infection with *Propionibacterium acnes*. Erythromycin and tetracyclines (such as doxycycline or minocycline) produce modest benefit when combined with topical therapy with benzoyl peroxide.

Health care–associated infections (HCAIs) comprising ventilator-associated pneumonia, surgical wound infection, intravenous catheter-associated bacteraemia, meningitis following neurosurgery and infection of prosthetic devices such as joint replacements and heart valves may involve conventional pathogens such as *Staphylococcus aureus* and Lancefield Group A β-haemolytic streptococcus, but a number of antibiotic-resistant pathogens are also commonly involved. These isolates can pose difficult therapeutic problems, especially because the infections often present in patients with multiple pre-existing pathologies, including liver and renal impairment. The causative bacteria include MRSA and multiply resistant coagulase-negative staphylococci, ESBL and carbapenemase-producing enterobacteriaceae (see p. 207), and a number of normally weakly pathogenic Gram-negative bacteria such as *Stenotrophomonas maltophilia* and *Acinetobacter* spp. These bacteria can be resistant to all conventional antimicrobial agents, and discussion with a microbiologist or infectious diseases physician is recommended before treatment is attempted. A number of unusual combinations of antibiotics have been recommended, and previously outdated agents have been resurrected for treatment of infections with these pathogens: for example, colistin, fosfomycin and chloramphenicol.

Actinomycosis. The anaerobe *Actinomyces israelii* is sensitive to several drugs, but not to metronidazole, and drug access

> **Community-acquired MRSA (CA-MRSA)** has caused large outbreaks of infection in North American cities, and clusters in other parts of the world. Many reported strains produce a toxin, the Panton–Valentine leucocidin, and affected patients may suffer recurrent cutaneous abscesses and necrotizing fasciitis and pneumonia. Recommended treatment regimens include antibiotics active at the ribosome to reduce toxin production – especially linezolid and clindamycin – and topical mupirocin and fucidin, although these strains are often more susceptible to non–β-lactam antibiotics than traditional health care–associated MRSA.

is poor because of granulomatous fibrosis. High doses of benzylpenicillin or amoxicillin are given for weeks or months; the infections are often mixed with other anaerobic bacteria, so metronidazole is often given in addition to ensure activity against all components of the mixture. Co-amoxiclav may be a convenient alternative. Surgery is likely to be needed.

Leptospirosis. To be maximally effective against *Leptospira*, start chemotherapy within 4 days of the onset of symptoms. Benzylpenicillin is recommended for severe disease, and ceftriaxone is an alternative; a Herxheimer reaction may be induced (see syphilis). Doxycycline and amoxicillin are alternatives for milder illnesses. General supportive management is important, including attention to fluid balance and observation for signs of hepatic, renal or cardiac failure.

Lyme disease. Keeping the skin covered and use of insect repellents are probably effective to prevent tick bites; tick removal shortly after attachment (within 24 h) should prevent infection. A single dose of doxycycline 200 mg within 72 h of a recognised tick bite is 87% effective as prophylaxis, but should be used only in high-risk areas (expert advice should be sought). In most manifestations of the established disease, *Borrelia burgdorferi* responds to amoxicillin or doxycycline orally for up to 21 days, but invasion of the central nervous system calls for large doses of ceftriaxonee i.v. for 14 days.

Guide to further reading

Algorithm for the early management of suspected bacterial meningitis and meningococcal septicaemia in immunocompetent adults. Available at: http://www.meningitis.org/health-professionals (Accessed June 2017).

Bhan, M.K., Bahl, R., Bhatnagar, S., 2005. Typhoid and paratyphoid fever. Lancet 366, 749–762.

Bharti, A.R., Nally, J.E., Ricaldi, J.N., et al., 2003. Leptospirosis: a zoonotic disease of global importance. Lancet Infect. Dis. 3, 757–771.

British Association of Sexual Health and HIV, 2017. United Kingdom National Guidelines. Available at: https://www.bashh.org/guidelines (Accessed June 2017).

Gould, F.K., Denning, D.W., Elliott, T.S., et al., 2012. Guidelines for the diagnosis and antibiotic treatment of endocarditis in adults: a report of the Working Party of the British Society for Antimicrobial Chemotherapy. Antimicrob. Chemother. 67, 269–289.

Mathews, C.J., Weston, V.C., Jones, A., et al., 2010. Bacterial septic arthritis in adults. Lancet 375, 846–855.

Matthews, P.C., Berendt, A.R., McNally, M.A., et al., 2009. Diagnosis and management of prosthetic joint infection. Br. Med. J. 338, 1378–1383.

NICE, 2016. Pneumonia in adults: diagnosis and management. Clinical guideline [CG191] 2014. NICE: London. Available at: https://www.nice.org.uk/guidance/cg191 (Accessed June 2017).

NICE, 2016. Prophylaxis against infective endocarditis: antimicrobial prophylaxis against infective endocarditis in adults and children undergoing interventional procedures. Clinical guideline [CG64] 2016. NICE: London. Available at: https://www.nice.org.uk/guidance/cg64 (Accessed June 2017).

Scottish Intercollegiate Guidelines Network, 2012. Management of suspected bacterial urinary tract infection in adults: a national clinical guideline. Available at: http://www.sign.ac.uk/assets/sign88.pdf (Accessed June 2017).

Spiro, D.M., Tay, K.Y., Arnold, D.H., et al., 2006. Wait-and-see prescription for the treatment of acute otitis media: a randomized controlled trial. J. Am. Med. Assoc. 296, 1235–1241.

Surviving Sepsis Campaign. Available at: http://www.survivingsepsis.org/ (Accessed June 2017).

World Health Organization, 2017. World Health Organization guidelines for treatment of drug-susceptible tuberculosis and patient care (2017 update). World Health Organization, Geneva. Available at: http://www.who.int/tb/publications/2017/dstb_guidance_2017/en/ (Accessed June 2017).

Chapter | 15 |

Viral, fungal, protozoal and helminthic infections

Sani Aliyu

SYNOPSIS

- Viruses present a more difficult problem of chemotherapy than do higher organisms, e.g. bacteria, for they are intracellular parasites that use the metabolism of host cells.[1] Highly selective toxicity is, therefore, harder to achieve. In the past 20 years, identification of the molecular differences between viral and human metabolism has led to the development of many effective antiviral agents; four were available in 1990, now there are over 40.

- Fungal infections range from inconvenient skin conditions to life-threatening systemic diseases; the latter have become more frequent as opportunistic infections in patients immunocompromised by drugs or AIDS, or in those receiving intensive medical and surgical interventions in intensive care units.

- Protozoal infections. Malaria is the major transmissible parasitic disease in the world. Drug resistance is an increasing problem and differs with geographical location, and species of plasmodium.

- Helminthic infestations cause considerable morbidity. The drugs that are effective against these organisms are summarised.

---

[1]'The large-scale screening for natural compounds able to kill bacteria in vitro, which was the basis for the boom of antibiotics in the 1950s, was not successful for antivirals ... The driving force for the boom of antivirals in this period has been the pressure to contain the HIV pandemic, combined with the increased understanding of the molecular mechanisms ... which has allowed the identification of new targets for therapeutic intervention.' (Rappuoli R 2004 From Pasteur to genomics: progress and challenges in infectious diseases. Nature Medicine 10:1177–1185.)

Viral infections

Antiviral agents are most active when viruses are replicating. The earlier that treatment is given, therefore, the better the result. Apart from primary infection, viral illness is often the consequence of reactivation of latent virus in the body. Patients whose immune systems are compromised may suffer particularly severe illness. Viruses are capable of developing resistance to antimicrobial drugs, with similar implications for the individual patient, for the community and for drug development. An overview of drugs that have proved effective against viral diseases appears in Table 15.1.

Herpes simplex and varicella zoster

Aciclovir

Aciclovir ($t_{1/2}$ 3 h) is a nucleoside analogue that is selectively phosphorylated by virus-specific thymidine kinase. Phosphorylated aciclovir inhibits viral replication by acting as a substrate for viral DNA polymerase, thus accounting for its high therapeutic index. It is effective against susceptible herpes viruses if started early in the course of infection, but it does not eradicate persistent infection because viral DNA is integrated in the host genome. About 20% is absorbed from the gut, but this is sufficient for oral systemic treatment of some infections. It distributes widely in the body; the concentration in CSF is approximately half that of plasma, and the brain concentration may be even lower. These differences are taken into account in dosing for viral encephalitis (for which aciclovir must be given i.v.). Dose adjustment is required for patients with impaired renal function, as the drug is predominantly excreted in the urine. For oral and

Table 15.1 Drugs of choice for virus infections

Organism	Drug of choice	Alternative
Varicella zoster		
chickenpox	Aciclovir	Valaciclovir or famciclovir
zoster	Aciclovir or famciclovir	Valaciclovir
Herpes simplex		
keratitis	Aciclovir (topical)	
labial	Aciclovir (topical and/or oral)	Valaciclovir or famciclovir
genital	Aciclovir (topical and/or oral)	Valaciclovir
	Famciclovir (oral)	Penciclovir
encephalitis	Aciclovir	
disseminated	Aciclovir	Foscarnet
Human immunodeficiency virus (HIV)	Lamivudine/emtricitabine	Abacavir
	Tenofovir	Didanoside
	Zidovudine	Stavudine
	Lopinavir/ritonavir	Saquinavir
	Atazanavir	Darunavir
	Fosamprenavir	Tipranavir
	Efavirenz	Nevirapine
	Etravirine	Dolutegravir
	Raltegravir	
	Enfuvirtide	
	Maraviroc	
Hepatitis B	Pegylated interferon α-2a and interferon 2b, lamivudine	Adefovir, tenofovir, entecavir, telbivudine
Hepatitis C	Pegylated interferon α-2a or interferon 2b plus ribavirin	
Hepatitis D	Interferon-α	Pegylated interferon α-2a and interferon 2b
Influenza A	Zanamivir, oseltamivir	Amantadine
Cytomegalovirus (CMV)	Valganciclovir, ganciclovir	Foscarnet, cidofovir
Respiratory syncytial virus	Ribavirin	Palivizumab
Papillomavirus (genital warts)	Imiquimod	
Molluscum contagiosum	Imiquimod	Cidofovir

topical use, the drug is given five times daily. It can be given twice daily orally for suppressive therapy.

Indications. The indications for aciclovir include:

Herpes simplex virus:
- Skin infections, including initial and recurrent labial and genital herpes, most effective when new lesions are forming; skin and mucous membrane infections (as tablets or oral suspension).
- Ocular keratitis (topical treatment with ophthalmic ointment is standard, oral treatment is also effective).
- Prophylaxis and treatment in the immunocompromised (oral, as tablets or suspension).
- Encephalitis and disseminated disease (i.v.).
- Aciclovir-resistant herpes simplex virus has been reported in patients with AIDS but remains rare in

immunocompetent patients. Foscarnet (p. 230) and cidofovir (p. 230) have been used in these cases.

Varicella zoster virus:

- Chickenpox, particularly in the immunocompromised (i.v.) or in the immunocompetent with pneumonitis or hepatitis (i.v.).
- Shingles in immunocompetent persons (as tablets or suspension, and best started within 48 h of the appearance of the rash). Immunocompromised persons will often have more severe symptoms and require i.v. administration.

Adverse reactions. These are remarkably few. The ophthalmic ointment causes a mild transient stinging sensation and a diffuse superficial punctate keratopathy which clears when the drug is stopped. Oral or i.v. use may cause gastrointestinal symptoms, headache and neuropsychiatric reactions. Extravasation following i.v. administration causes severe local inflammation. Crystal-induced acute renal failure is an important complication of i.v. therapy that can be avoided by ensuring good hydration during treatment.

Valaciclovir. This is a prodrug (ester) of aciclovir, i.e. after oral administration the parent aciclovir is released. It has an improved bio-availability (about 60%) due to the addition of an ester side chain, thus allowing for a less frequent, 8-hourly, dosing. It is used for treating herpes zoster infections and herpes simplex infections of the skin and mucous membranes.

Famciclovir ($t_{1/2}$ 2 h) is a prodrug of penciclovir, which is similar to aciclovir; it is used for herpes zoster and genital herpes simplex infections, and a single dose is effective at reducing the time to healing of labial herpes simplex. It need be given only 8-hourly. Penciclovir is also available as a cream for treatment of labial herpes simplex.

Idoxuridine. The first widely available antiviral drug; it is variably effective topically for ocular and cutaneous herpes simplex, with few adverse reactions. It has been superseded by aciclovir.

Human immunodeficiency virus (HIV)

According to UNAIDS data, 36.7 million people worldwide were living with human immunodeficiency virus (HIV) in 2015, with about 2 million new infections and 1 million deaths yearly; only 17 million people were accessing treatment in 2015.

General comments

- The aims of antiretroviral therapy are to delay disease progression and prolong survival by suppressing the replication of the virus. Optimal suppression also prevents the emergence of drug resistance and reduces the risk of onward transmission to sexual partners and the unborn children of HIV-infected mothers. Virological failure may be defined as primary where there is inability to reduce plasma HIV viral load to fewer than 50 copies per microlitre despite 6 months of antiretroviral therapy, or secondary if there is failure to maintain viral load suppression at less than 50 copies per microlitre.
- No current antiviral agents or combinations eliminate HIV infection, but the most effective combinations (so-called 'highly active antiretroviral therapy', HAART) produce profound suppression of viral replication in many patients and allow useful reconstitution of the immune system, measured by a fall in the plasma viral load and an increase in the numbers of cytotoxic T cells (CD4 count). Rates of opportunistic infections such as *Pneumocystis carinii* pneumonia and cytomegalovirus (CMV) retinitis are reduced when CD4 counts are restored, and life expectancy is markedly increased.
- Combination therapy reduces the risk of emergence of resistance to antiretroviral drugs, which is increasing in incidence, even in patients newly diagnosed with HIV. Mutations in the viral genome either prevent binding of the drug to the active site of the protease or reverse transcriptase enzymes, or lead to removal of the drug from the reverse transcriptase active site. The potential for rapid development of resistance is immense because untreated HIV replicates rapidly (50% of circulating virus is replaced daily), the spontaneous mutation rate is high, the genome is small, the virus will develop single mutations at every codon every day, and for many antiretroviral agents a single mutation will render the virus fully resistant.
- The decision to begin antiretroviral therapy used to be based primarily on the CD4 cell count, but current recommendations now require antiretroviral therapy to be commenced as soon as possible after diagnosis. Early initiation of antiretroviral therapy is particularly important for patients with advanced HIV infection (CD4 cell count below 200 cells per microlitre or a low CD4 percentage (e.g. <14%), those with an AIDS diagnosis (e.g. Kaposi sarcoma), hepatitis B and HIV co-infection where treatment is indicated, and in conditions where achieving a suppressed viral load is desired in order to prevent transmission (e.g. in pregnancy).
- There are currently more than 30 approved antiretroviral agents in six classes, plus various fixed drug combinations (Table 15.2).

Table 15.2 Classification and mechanism of antiretrovirals

Classification		Mechanism of action	Examples
Reverse transcriptase inhibitors	Nucleoside and nucleotide analogue reverse transcriptase inhibitors (NRTIs)	Nucleoside analogues are incorporated into growing viral DNA chain, leading to chain termination	Zidovudine Lamivudine Emtricitabine Abacavir Tenofovir disoproxil Stavudine Didanoside
	Non-nucleoside reverse transcriptase inhibitors (NNRTIs)	Bind to a hydrophobic pocket near the active site of the reverse transcriptase enzyme, inhibiting DNA synthesis	Efavirenz Nevirapine Etravirine
Entry inhibitors	Entry blockers	Bind to CCR5 receptors on the surface of some CD4 cells, blocking entry of HIV virion	Maraviroc
	Fusion inhibitors	Bind to gp41, an HIV surface protein, interfering with fusion and T cell entry	Enfuvirtide
Protease inhibitors		Inhibit protease enzyme, required for cleavage of viral proteins and assembly	Amprenavir Atazanavir Darunavir Fosamprenavir Indinavir Lopinavir Nelfinavir Ritonavir Saquinavir Tipranavir
Integrase inhibitors		Block integrase, essential for insertion of viral DNA into host DNA	Raltegravir Dolutegravir

- Current HAART regimens use a combination of drugs that act at different phases of the viral life cycle. The most frequently used combinations employ a backbone of two nucleoside analogue reverse transcriptase inhibitors (NRTIs) plus either a non-nucleoside reverse transcriptase inhibitor (NNRTI), a ritonavir-boosted protease inhibitor (rPI) or an integrase strand transfer inhibitor. The choice for the individual patient is best made after reference to contemporary, expert advice (see the websites listed in the Guide to further reading).
- Alternative combinations are used if these variables deteriorate or unwanted drug effects occur. Antiretroviral resistance testing, both genetic (by searching viral RNA for sequences coding for resistance) and phenotypic (by testing antiretroviral agents against the patient's virus in cell culture), also guide the choice of drug regimen, especially after virological failure.

- Pregnancy and breast feeding pose special problems. The objectives of therapy are to minimise drug toxicity to the fetus while reducing the maternal viral load and the catastrophic results of HIV transmission to the neonate. Prevention of maternal–fetal and maternal–infant spread is the most cost-effective way of using antiretroviral drugs in less developed countries. Maternal–fetal transmission rates are related to maternal viral load, with rates of 0.1% reported when maternal viral load is less than 50 copies per microlitre while on HAART. Where resources permit, access to safe alternatives to breast feeding should be provided to infected mothers.
- Combination antiretroviral therapy, especially the thymidine nucleoside analogue reverse transcriptase inhibitors zidovudine and stavudine, causes redistribution of body fat in some patients – the 'lipodystrophy syndrome'. Protease inhibitors can disturb lipid and glucose metabolism to a degree that

warrants a change to drugs with limited effects on lipid metabolism, e.g. ritonavir-boosted atazanavir, and the introduction of lipid-lowering agents.

- Impaired cell-mediated immunity leaves the host prey to opportunistic infections including: candidiasis, coccidioidomycosis, cryptosporidiosis, CMV disease, herpes simplex, histoplasmosis, *Pneumocystis carinii* pneumonia, toxoplasmosis and tuberculosis (often with multiply resistant organisms). Treatment of these conditions is referred to elsewhere in this text.[2]

- Improvement in immune function as a result of antiretroviral treatment may provoke an inflammatory reaction against residual opportunistic organisms (immune reconstitution inflammatory syndrome, IRIS). Although infrequent, this may present with development of new infections or worsening opportunistic infections, e.g. tuberculosis and cryptococcal disease.

- Antiretroviral drugs may also be used in combination to reduce the risk of infection with HIV from injuries, e.g. from HIV-contaminated needles and following sexual exposure to a high-risk partner (post-exposure prophylaxis or PEP). The drugs may also be given on a regular continuous basis to people engaged in high-risk sexual activity (pre-exposure prophylaxis or PrEP). The decision to offer PrEP or PEP, and the optimal combination of drugs used, is a matter for experts; for PEP to be effective, administration must begin within a few hours of exposure and continue for 28 days.

- Some drugs described here have found additional indications, or are used only for therapy of non-HIV infections, e.g. adefovir for chronic hepatitis B infection.

Nucleoside and nucleotide reverse transcriptase inhibitors

The HIV replicates by converting its single-stranded RNA into double-stranded DNA, which is incorporated into host DNA; this crucial conversion, the reverse of the normal cellular transcription of nucleic acids, is accomplished by the enzyme *reverse transcriptase*. Nucleoside reverse transcriptase inhibitors (NRTIs) have a high affinity for the *reverse transcriptase* enzyme and are integrated by it into the viral DNA chain, causing premature chain termination. While all NRTIs require activation by host enzymes to triphosphates prior to incorporation into the DNA chain, tenofovir (as the only nucleotide analogue) is unique in requiring only two phosphorylations for activation.

---

[2]For a comprehensive review, see http://aidsinfo.nih.gov/guidelines.

Zidovudine (AZT, Retrovir)

Zidovudine, a thymidine analogue, is the first antiretroviral licensed for the treatment of HIV-1. Resistance develops rapidly when used as monotherapy through the sequential accumulation of thymidine analogue mutations (TAMs) at codon 41, 67, 70, 215 and 219; conversely, point mutations at codon 184 selected by lamivudine and emtricitabine therapy enhance susceptibility to zidovudine (and stavudine) by delaying the emergence of TAMs.

Pharmacokinetics. Zidovudine is well absorbed from the gastrointestinal tract (it is available as capsules and syrup) and is rapidly cleared from the plasma ($t_{1/2}$ 1 h); concentrations in cerebrospinal fluid (CSF) are approximately one-half of those in plasma. Zidovudine is also available i.v. for patients temporarily unable to take oral medications, for neonates and for intrapartum use. The drug is inactivated mainly by glucuronidation in the liver, but 20% is excreted unchanged by the kidney. Zidovudine competitively inhibits the intracellular phosphorylation of stavudine, therefore use in combination with stavudine should be avoided.

Uses. Zidovudine is indicated for the treatment of HIV infection as part of a combination regimen. It is an established choice for the prevention of maternal–fetal transmission, both as part of a combination regimen antenatally in the mother and as monotherapy in the newborn. The enhanced CNS penetration of zidovudine makes it an important option for the treatment of HIV-associated neurocognitive disease (HAND). The drug is available as part of a fixed drug combination with lamivudine (as Combivir), and with abacavir and lamivudine (as Trizivir). This drug is less frequently used nowadays due to the availability of less toxic regimens.

Adverse reactions early in treatment may include anorexia, nausea, vomiting, headache, dizziness, malaise and myalgia, but tolerance develops to these and usually the dose does not need to be altered. More serious are anaemia and neutropenia, which develop more commonly when the dose is high, with advanced disease, and in combination with ganciclovir, interferon-α and other marrow suppressive agents. A toxic myopathy (not easily distinguishable from HIV-associated myopathy) may develop with long-term use. Rarely, a syndrome of hepatic necrosis with lactic acidosis may occur with zidovudine (and with other reverse transcriptase inhibitors).

Didanosine

Didanosine (ddI) is a thymidine analogue with similar activity to zidovudine. It has a short plasma $t_{1/2}$ (1 h) but a much longer intracellular duration than zidovudine, and thus prolonged antiretroviral activity. Didanosine is rapidly but incompletely absorbed from the gastrointestinal tract (30–40%) and is widely distributed in body water; 30–65%

is recovered unchanged in the urine. Drug absorption is affected by food, and therefore it has to be taken on an empty stomach or at least 2 h after a meal. Didanosine may cause pancreatitis, lactic acidosis, hepatomegaly with steatosis and peripheral neuropathy. Other adverse effects include hyperuricaemia and diarrhoea, any of which may give reason to reduce the dose or discontinue the drug. Retinal changes and optic neuritis have also been reported. The combination of stavudine and didanosine is associated with a high risk of toxicity and should be avoided. Dose adjustment of didanosine is required when used in combination with tenofovir and in patients with renal insufficiency. Similar to zidovudine, didanoside is rarely used nowadays due to its high toxicity profile.

Lamivudine and emtricitabine

Lamivudine (3TC) is a reverse transcriptase inhibitor with a relatively long intracellular $t_{1/2}$ (14 h; plasma $t_{1/2}$ 6 h). Lamivudine is the most common nucleoside analogue used in HAART regimens due to its excellent tolerance profile. A nucleoside backbone of lamivudine with zidovudine (Combivir), abacavir (Kivexa) or emtricitabine and tenofovir (Truvada) as fixed drug combinations, appears to reduce viral load effectively and to be well tolerated. The drug is well absorbed from the gastrointestinal tract (86%) and excreted mainly by the kidney with minimal metabolism; dose modification is necessary in renal impairment.

Lamivudine was the first nucleoside analogue to be licensed for therapy of chronic hepatitis B infection, for which it should be used in combination with tenofovir (as part of a HAART regimen) in HIV co-infected patients. Emergence of resistant mutants of hepatitis B is troublesome (due to mutations of the viral reverse transcriptase/DNA polymerase), occurring in up to about 30% of patients after 1 year and 70% after 5 years of therapy.

The most common unwanted effects include headache and gastrointestinal upset. Lactic acidosis and severe hepatomegaly with steatosis, including fatal cases, have been reported. A higher dose of lamivudine is required for the treatment of HIV than for hepatitis B infection; patients with co-infection should receive doses appropriate for treatment of HIV.

Emtricitabine

Emtricitabine has a similar structure, tolerability, efficacy and resistance profile. It should not be used in combination with lamivudine, as it contains the same active constituent.

Abacavir

Abacavir ($t_{1/2}$ 2 h) has high therapeutic efficacy; it is usually well tolerated, but adverse effects include hypersensitivity reactions especially during the first 6 weeks of therapy,

affecting about 8% of patients; the drug must be stopped immediately and avoided in future if hypersensitivity is suspected. The presence of the HLA-B*5701 allele predicts increased risk of hypersensitivity reaction in the Caucasian population; patients should be tested for the presence of this allele prior to starting therapy.

Tenofovir

Tenofovir ($t_{1/2}$ 17 h), administered orally as the prodrug tenofovir disoproxil fumarate (TDF), is also effective against hepatitis B virus. Some 80% is excreted renally, and dose adjustment is recommended in patients with a creatinine clearance of less than 50 mL/min. Monitor closely for signs of new onset or acute renal impairment, electrolyte and renal tubular disturbance (Fanconi syndrome); avoid concomitant nephrotoxic drugs while on tenofovir.

Severe acute exacerbation of hepatitis has been described following cessation of therapy for hepatitis B infection. There are now two formulations of tenofovir; the standard TDF and tenofovir alafenamide (TAF). Unlike TDF, TAF undergoes intracellular phosphorylation to tenofovir diphosphate, thus allowing for higher intracellular levels of the active drug with a much lower oral dose and thence less renal and bone toxicity when compared to TDF.

Stavudine

Stavudine (d4T) inhibits reverse transcriptase by competing with the natural substrate deoxythymidine triphosphate, and additionally is incorporated into viral DNA, causing termination of chain elongation ($t_{1/2}$ 1.5 h). Troublesome lipoatrophy has limited its use by most authorities outside the developing world. Hepatic toxicity and pancreatitis are reported, and a dose-related peripheral neuropathy may occur, all probably related to mitochondrial toxicity. Stavudine is more frequently associated with lactic acidosis than other nucleoside analogues.

Adefovir

Adefovir dipivoxil is a nucleoside analogue used for chronic hepatitis B infection, including against lamivudine-resistant strains. It is administered as the oral prodrug (plasma $t_{1/2}$ 8 h, intracellular $t_{1/2}$ of active metabolite 17 h). Adverse effects are uncommon, but include headache, abdominal pain and diarrhoea. Resistance emerges over time (30% after 5 years), but much less commonly than with lamivudine therapy, possibly due to the flexibility of the adefovir molecule, which allows it to conform to mutated binding sites. Dose adjustment is required for patients with renal impairment. Adefovir should not be co-prescribed with tenofovir. The recommended adefovir dose for hepatitis B therapy will not suppress HIV infection; HIV status should therefore be confirmed prior to commencing adefovir for hepatitis B infection, as unrecognised co-infection may lead to the emergence of HIV resistance.

Protease inhibitors

In its process of replication, HIV produces precursor proteins, which are subsequently cleaved by the protease enzyme into component parts and reassembled into virus particles; protease inhibitors disrupt this essential process.

Protease inhibitors reduce viral RNA concentration ('viral load'), increase the CD4 count and improve survival when used in combination with other agents. They are metabolised extensively by isoenzymes of the cytochrome P450 system, notably by CYP 3A4, and most protease inhibitors inhibit these enzymes. They have a plasma $t_{1/2}$ of 2–4 h, except for fosamprenavir (8 h) and atazanavir (7 h with food). The drugs have broadly similar therapeutic effects. Members of the group include:

- amprenavir, atazanavir, fosamprenavir (a prodrug of amprenavir), lopinavir, ritonavir, saquinavir, tipranavir, indinavir and darunavir.

Adverse effects include gastrointestinal disturbance, headache, dizziness, sleep disturbance, raised liver enzymes, neutropenia, pancreatitis and rashes. Unique side-effects include asymptomatic reversible unconjugated hyper-bilirubinaemia with atazanavir and nephrolithiasis with indinavir.

Interactions. Involvement with the cytochrome P450 system provides scope for numerous drug–drug interactions. Agents that induce P450 enzymes, e.g. rifampicin, St John's wort, accelerate their metabolism, reducing plasma concentration and therapeutic efficacy; enzyme inhibitors, e.g. ketoconazole, cimetidine, raise their plasma concentration with risk of toxicity.

The powerful inhibiting effect of ritonavir on CYP 3A4 and CYP 2D6 is harnessed usefully by its combination in low (subtherapeutic) dose with other protease inhibitors; the result is to decrease the metabolism and increase the therapeutic efficacy of the concurrently administered protease inhibitors (called ritonavir 'boosting' or 'potentiation'), i.e. a *beneficial* drug–drug interaction. Ritonavir boosting is particularly advantageous in patients infected with low-level resistant virus where the high drug levels help improve efficacy, but this may be at the detriment of increased gastrointestinal side-effects and metabolic disturbances. Ritonavir boosting is now a recommended treatment standard for all protease inhibitor–containing regimens. Cobicistat is another CYP3A4 inhibitor with similar pharmacokinetic boosting as ritonavir but with fewer GI side effects. It is available as a single pill on its own or as a combination regime with either darunavir, atazanavir or a single-tablet triple regime with an integrase strand inhibitor (elvitegravir), emtricitabine and tenofovir (Stribild®).

Non-nucleoside reverse transcriptase inhibitors

This group is structurally different from the reverse transcriptase inhibitors; members are active against the subtype HIV-1 but not HIV-2, a subtype encountered mainly in West Africa. Non-nucleoside reverse transcriptase inhibitors are metabolised by CYP 450 enzymes and hence the potential for significant drug–drug interactions. The drugs have considerably longer half-lives when compared to nucleoside reverse transcriptase inhibitors.

Efavirenz is taken once per day ($t_{1/2}$ 52 h). Rash is relatively common during the first 2 weeks of therapy, but resolution usually occurs within a further 2 weeks; the drug should be stopped if the rash is severe or if there is blistering, desquamation, mucosal involvement or fever. Neurological adverse reactions occur in about 50% of patients, usually insomnia, depression and abnormal dreams; this may be reduced by taking the drug before retiring at night; gastrointestinal side-effects and occasional hepatitis and pancreatitis have also been reported. Efavirenz is teratogenic, so should be avoided in pregnancy. Resistance is associated with mutations at codon 103 and 181, which also confers cross-resistance to nevirapine.

Nevirapine is used in combination with at least two other antiretroviral drugs. It is commonly prescribed in the developing world and is relatively safe in pregnancy. It penetrates the CSF well, and undergoes hepatic metabolism ($t_{1/2}$ 28 h); it induces its own metabolism, and the dose should be increased gradually. Nevirapine is initially commenced as a once-daily regimen, with a 2-week lead-in period to twice daily if tolerated. Rash (including Stevens–Johnson syndrome) is seen in up to 20% of patients and, occasionally, fatal hepatitis. The risk of an adverse drug event is closely related to the CD4 count; nevirapine is contraindicated in females with CD4 counts above 250 per microlitre and males with CD4 counts above 400 per microlitre.

Etravirine ($t_{1/2}$ 41 h) is administered twice daily after meals; rash is the commonest adverse effect, generally appearing within the first 6 weeks of therapy, and peripheral neuropathy. Etravirine has activity against NNRTI-resistant HIV strains and should be used in combination with other antiretroviral agents. Due to potentially significant drug interactions, etravirine should not be co-administered with other NNRTIs, unboosted protease inhibitors and ritonavir-boosted tipranavir, fosamprenavir and atazanavir.

Rilpivirine ($t_{1/2}$ 50 h) is administered once daily. The drug bio-availability is improved with low gastric pH and therefore needs to be taken with food. It should not be taken with CYP3A enzyme inducers or other agents that increase gastric pH. Rilpivirine is available either as a single pill or in combination with emtricitabine and tenofovir as Eviplera®.

It should not be used in patients with a baseline HIV viral load >100 000 copies/mL.

Entry inhibitors

Enfuvirtide is the first antiretroviral agent to target the host cell attachment/entry stage in the HIV replication cycle; the linear 36–amino acid synthetic peptide inhibits fusion of the cellular and viral membranes. It is given by subcutaneous injection ($t_{1/2}$ 4 h). The drug seems most effective when combined with several antiretroviral agents to which the virus is susceptible and is licensed for use in treatment-experienced patients with extensive drug resistance. Enfuvirtide does not inhibit cytochrome P450 enzymes and therefore has limited drug interactions.

Adverse effects are usually limited to mild injection-site reactions, although hypersensitivity, peripheral neuropathy and other adverse reactions are reported rarely. HIV isolates with decreased susceptibility have been recovered from enfuvirtide-treated patients; these exhibit mutations in the gp41 outer envelope glycoprotein of the virus (which plays a key role in infection of CD4 cells by fusing the HIV envelope with the host cell membrane).

Maraviroc is an entry inhibitor that specifically targets and blocks the chemokine co-receptor CCR5, which is used by HIV for fusion and cell entry. Maraviroc has no activity against HIV virions that preferentially bind to another surface chemokine co-receptor (CXCR4), found in about 60% of antiretroviral experienced patients. Hence a 'Trofile assay' is required to determine if a susceptible (CCR5 tropic) strain is present as the dominant quasispecies in a patient prior to commencing maraviroc therapy. It is recommended as part of a combination regimen in treatment-experienced patients with multiply drug-resistant strains.

Integrase inhibitors

Raltegravir ($t_{1/2}$ 41 h) targets the HIV integrase enzyme, which is essential in integrating viral genetic material into the DNA of the host target cell. It is generally well tolerated and metabolised by glucuronidation. It has a low genetic barrier to resistance (arising from mutations in the integrase gene) and should be used with caution in patients at increased risk of myopathy or rhabdomyolysis.

Dolutegravir ($t_{1/2}$ 13–14 h) has a similar mechanism of action and side-effect profile to raltegravir. Due to its more potent activity and higher barrier to resistance when compared to raltegravir, dolutegravir is frequently used as part of a regimen in treatment-experienced patients facing virological failure. Dolutegravir can be taken with or without food but should not be co-administered with

magnesium-aluminium antacids, iron and calcium preparations nor with drugs that induce CYP3A4.

Fixed-dose combinations of antiretroviral drugs are convenient, help to lessen pill burden and may improve compliance, but the components of the combination may differ in their dependence on metabolic inactivation or renal excretion; particular attention to these is necessary when use in patients with renal or hepatic impairment is proposed.

Fixed-dose combination antiretrovirals	
Combivir	zidovudine and lamivudine
Kivexa (Europe), Epzicom (USA)	abacavir and lamivudine
Truvada	tenofovir (TDF) and emtricitabine
Trizivir	zidovudine and lamivudine and abacavir
Atripla	Tenofovir (TDF) and emtricitabine and efavirenz
Kaletra	lopinavir and ritonavir
Eviplera	tenofovir (TDF) and emtricitabine and rilpivirine
Evotaz	atazanavir and cobicistat
Rezolsta (Prezcobix in the USA)	darunavir and cobicistat
Stribild	tenofovir (TDF) and emtricitabine and elvitegravir and cobicistat
Genvoya	tenofovir alafenamide (TAF) and emtricitabine and elvitegravir and cobicistat
Descovy	tenofovir alafenamide (TAF) and emtricitabine
Odefsey	tenofovir alafenamide (TAF) and emtricitabine and rilpivirine

Influenza A

Neuraminidase inhibitors are highlighted by the emergence of avian influenza viruses with the potential for mutation to cause pandemic spread in the human population, although their clinical effectiveness is not high. The two antiviral drugs oseltamivir and zanamivir were widely used for the public health control of the 2009 influenza A (H1N1) pandemic.

Amantadine

Amantadine is effective only against influenza A; it acts by interfering with the uncoating and release of viral genome into the host cell. It is well absorbed from the gastrointestinal tract and is eliminated in the urine ($t_{1/2}$ 3 h). Following the emergence of the 2009 influenza A (H1N1) virus as the predominant circulating strain, resistance to amantadine is now almost universal; for this reason, amantidine is no longer recommended for the treatment of influenza.

Adverse reactions include dizziness, nervousness, light-headedness and insomnia. Drowsiness, hallucinations, delirium and coma may occur in patients with impaired renal function. Convulsions may be induced, and amantadine should be avoided in epileptic patients.

Amantadine for Parkinson's disease: see p. 384.

Zanamivir (Relenza)

Zanamivir is a viral neuraminidase inhibitor that blocks both entry of influenza A and B viruses to target cells and the release of their progeny. It is administered as a dry powder twice daily in a 5-day course by a special inhaler. The limited bio-availability (2%) of zanamivir has made it the preferred antiviral in pregnancy. The duration of symptoms is reduced from about 6 to 5 days, with a smaller reduction in the meantime taken to return to normal activities. In high-risk groups, the reduction in duration of symptoms is a little greater, and fewer patients need antibiotics. It is also effective for prophylaxis given as a once-daily inhalation.

The UK National Institute for Health and Clinical Excellence (NICE) recommends that zanamivir be reserved for:

- at-risk patients (those with chronic respiratory or cardiovascular disease, immunosuppression or diabetes mellitus, or older than 65 years of age).
- when virological surveillance in the community indicates that influenza virus is circulating.
- only those presenting within 48 h of the onset of influenza-like symptoms.

Zanamivir retains activity against amantadine-resistant and some oseltamivir-resistant strains.

Unwanted effects are uncommon, but bronchospasm may be precipitated in asthmatics, and gastrointestinal disturbance and rash are occasionally seen.

Oseltamivir (Tamiflu)

Oseltamivir is an oral prodrug of a viral neuraminidase inhibitor. It reduces the severity and duration of symptoms caused by influenza A or B in adults and children if commenced within 36 h of the onset of symptoms. More specifically, the risk of respiratory complications such as secondary pneumonia, antibiotic use and hospital admission are reduced. It is effective for post-exposure prophylaxis, where it should be started within 48 h of contact with the index case and continued daily for 10 days, a usage that might be appropriate for health-care workers and those especially likely to suffer serious complications from pre-existing illness. Prophylaxis may be given for 2 weeks after influenza immunisation while protective antibodies are being produced.

Oseltamivir is one option for treatment and prophylaxis of avian H5N1 and 2009 influenza A (H1N1) virus. In the event of a pandemic, treatment for 5 days and prophylactic use for up to 6 weeks (or until 48 h after last exposure) are suggested.

Unwanted effects are uncommon; some people experience gastrointestinal symptoms that are reduced by taking the drug with food.

Resistance to oseltamivir emerged in late 2007 among seasonal influenza A H1N1 viruses as a result of a spontaneous mutation at position 274 (His274Tyr) in the neuraminidase enzyme. So far, this mutation appears to be confined mostly to seasonal influenza A H1N1 strains, with the majority of 2009 influenza A (H1N1) viruses still susceptible to oseltamivir; the mutation also does not appear to confer resistance to zanamivir.

Peramivir is an experimental neuraminidase inhibitor formulated for intravenous use and currently undergoing phase III trials. The drug was granted temporary emergency use authorisation by the US Food and Drug Administration (FDA) during the 2009 influenza A (H1N1) pandemic for hospitalised patients with severe suspected or confirmed influenza A (H1N1) infection where oseltamivir or zanamivir therapy had failed or the inhalational or oral routes were considered unreliable.

Cytomegalovirus

Ganciclovir

Ganciclovir resembles aciclovir in its mode of action, but is much more toxic. An acyclic analogue of guanosine, the drug is converted to a triphosphate form which competitively inhibits virion DNA polymerase, leading to chain termination. It is given i.v. and is eliminated in the urine, mainly unchanged ($t_{1/2}$ 4 h). Ganciclovir is active against several types of virus, but toxicity limits its i.v. use to life- and sight-threatening CMV infection in immunocompromised patients, including CMV retinitis, pneumonitis, colitis and disseminated disease.

Valganciclovir is an oral prodrug of ganciclovir that provides systemic concentrations almost as high as those following i.v. therapy. It is used for treatment of CMV retinitis (acute treatment of peripheral retinal lesions and maintenance suppressive therapy) in patients with AIDS, and to prevent CMV disease in patients receiving immunosuppressive therapy following organ transplantation (especially liver transplants). A combined approach of ganciclovir-releasing intraocular implant plus oral valganciclovir is sometimes considered in patients with immediate sight-threatening CMV retinitis.

Ganciclovir-resistant CMV isolates have been reported, and require treatment with foscarnet or cidofovir.

Adverse reactions include neutropenia and thrombocytopenia, which are usually but not always reversible. Concomitant use of potential marrow-depressant drugs, e.g. co-trimoxazole, amphotericin B, azathioprine, zidovudine, should be avoided, and co-administration of granulocyte colony-stimulating factor may ameliorate the myelosuppressive effects. Other reactions are fever, rash, gastrointestinal symptoms, confusion and seizure (the last especially when imipenem is co-administered).

Foscarnet

Foscarnet finds use i.v. for CMV retinitis in patients with HIV infection when ganciclovir is contraindicated, and for aciclovir-resistant herpes simplex virus infection (see p. 221). It is generally less well tolerated than ganciclovir; adverse effects include renal toxicity (usually reversible), nausea and vomiting, neurological reactions and marrow suppression. Hypocalcaemia is seen especially when foscarnet is given with pentamidine, e.g. during treatment of multiple infections in patients with AIDS. Renal toxicity can be minimised with good hydration and dose modification. Foscarnet causes a contact dermatitis which can lead to unpleasant genital ulcerations due to high urine drug concentrations; this is potentially preventable with good urinary hygiene.

Cidofovir

Cidofovir is given by i.v. infusion (usually every 1–2 weeks) for CMV retinitis in patients with AIDS when other drugs are unsuitable or resistance is a problem. It has also been used i.v. and topically to produce resolution of molluscum contagiosum skin lesions in immunosuppressed patients, and it may be effective in other poxvirus infections. Nephrotoxicity is common with i.v. use, but is reduced by hydration with i.v. fluids before each dose and co-administration with probenecid. Other unwanted effects include bone marrow suppression, nausea and vomiting, and iritis and uveitis, and cause about 25% of patients to discontinue therapy.

Fomivirsen

Fomivirsen, an antisense oligonucleotide, is available in some countries as an intravitreal injection for CMV retinitis in HIV-infected patients who cannot tolerate or who have failed treatment with other drugs.

Respiratory syncytial virus (RSV)

Ribavirin is a synthetic nucleoside used for RSV bronchiolitis in infants and children, inhaled by a special ventilator. As therapeutic efficacy for this indication is controversial, it is usually reserved for the most severe cases and those with coexisting illnesses, such as immunosuppression. Systemic absorption by the inhalational route is negligible.

Ribavirin is effective by mouth ($t_{1/2}$ 45 h) for reducing mortality from Lassa fever and hantavirus infection (possibly also other viral haemorrhagic fevers and West Nile virus) and, when combined with interferon α-2b or peg-interferon, for chronic hepatitis C infection (see below). It does not cross the blood–brain barrier, so is unlikely to be effective in viral encephalitides. Systemic ribavirin is an important teratogen, and it may cause cardiac, gastrointestinal and neurological adverse effects. It may also cause haemolytic anaemia, for which close monitoring is required.

Palivizumab is a humanised monoclonal antibody directed against the F glycoprotein on the surface of RSV. It is given by monthly i.m. injection in the winter and early spring to infants and children younger than 2 years of age at high risk of RSV infection. Transient fever and local injection site reactions are seen, and rarely, gastrointestinal disturbance, rash, leucopenia or disturbed liver function occur. Anaphylaxis has occurred rarely (1 in 10 000).

Drugs that modulate the host immune system

Interferons. Virus infection stimulates the production of protective glycoproteins (interferons) which act:

- *directly* on uninfected cells to induce enzymes that degrade viral RNA
- *indirectly* by stimulating the immune system
- to modify cell regulatory mechanisms and inhibit neoplastic growth.

Interferons are classified as α, β or γ according to their antigenic and physical properties. α-Interferons (subclassified -2a, -2b and -N1) are effective against conditions that include hairy cell leukaemia, chronic myelogenous leukaemia, recurrent or metastatic renal cell carcinoma, Kaposi's sarcoma in patients with AIDS (an effect that may be due partly to its activity against HIV) and condylomata acuminata (genital warts).

Interferon α-2a and -2b also improve the manifestations of viral hepatitis, but responses differ according to the infecting agent. In about one-third of patients with chronic hepatitis B, therapy with interferon α-2b leads to loss of circulating 'e' antigen, a return to normal liver enzyme levels, histological improvement in liver architecture, and a lowered rate of progression of liver disease. It is contraindicated in patients with decompensated liver disease.

Pegylated (bound to polyethylene glycol) interferon α-2a is more effective than standard interferon α and is now the standard of care for patients with chronic hepatitis C infection. Over 50% of patients with hepatitis C respond to the combination of pegylated interferon plus ribavirin, and 30–40% to peg-interferon alone. Successful treatment results in the serum concentration of viral RNA becoming undetectable by polymerase chain reaction (PCR). Hepatitis D (δ agent co-infection with hepatitis B) requires a much larger dose of interferon to obtain a response, and relapse may yet occur when the drug is withdrawn. Interferon α-2b may be effective in West Nile virus encephalitis.

See also p. 588 for lamivudine and adefovir, use in chronic hepatitis B infection.

Adverse reactions are common and include an influenza-like syndrome (naturally produced interferon may be responsible for symptoms in natural influenza infection), fatigue and depression, which respond to lowering the dose but tend to improve after the first week. Other effects are anorexia (sufficient to induce weight loss), alopecia, convulsions, hypotension, hypertension, cardiac arrhythmias and bone marrow depression (which may respond to granulocyte colony-stimulating factors and erythropoietin). Interferons inhibit the metabolism of theophylline, increasing its effect, and autoimmune diseases such as thyroiditis may be induced or exacerbated.

Imiquimod is used topically for genital warts (caused by papillomaviruses). Treatment for 2–3 months results in gradual clearance of warts in about 50% of patients, and recurrence is less common than after physical removal, e.g. with liquid nitrogen.

Inosine pranobex is reported to stimulate the host immune response to virus infection and has been used for mucocutaneous herpes simplex, genital warts and subacute sclerosing panencephalitis. It is administered by mouth and metabolised to uric acid, so should be used with caution in patients with hyperuricaemia or gout.

Fungal infections

Widespread use of immunosuppressive chemotherapy and the emergence of AIDS have contributed to a rise in the incidence of opportunistic infection ranging from comparatively trivial cutaneous infections to systemic diseases that demand prolonged treatment with potentially toxic agents.

Superficial mycoses

Dermatophyte infections (ringworm, tinea)

Longstanding remedies such as Compound Benzoic Acid Ointment (Whitfield's ointment) are still acceptable for mild infections, but a topical imidazole (clotrimazole, econazole, miconazole, sulconazole), which is also effective against candida, is now usually preferred. Tioconazole is effective topically for nail infections. When multiple areas are affected, especially if the scalp or nails are included, and when topical therapy fails, oral itraconazole or terbinafine are used.

Candida infections

Cutaneous infection is generally treated with topical amphotericin, clotrimazole, econazole, miconazole or nystatin. Local hygiene is also important. An underlying explanation should be sought when a patient fails to respond to these measures, e.g. diabetes, the use of a broad-spectrum antibiotic or of immunosuppressive drugs.

Candidiasis of the alimentary tract mucosa responds to amphotericin, fluconazole, ketoconazole, miconazole or nystatin as lozenges (to suck, for oral infection), gel (held in the mouth before swallowing), suspension or tablets.

Vaginal candidiasis is treated by clotrimazole, econazole, isoconazole, ketoconazole, miconazole or nystatin as pessaries or vaginal tablets or cream inserted once or twice a day with cream or ointment on surrounding skin. Failure may be due to a concurrent intestinal infection causing re-infection, and nystatin tablets may be given by mouth 8-hourly with the local treatment. Alternatively, oral fluconazole may be used, now available without prescription ('over the counter') in the UK. The male sexual partner may use a similar antifungal ointment for his benefit and for the patient's (to prevent re-infection).

Fluconazole is often given orally or i.v. to heavily immunocompromised patients, e.g. during periods of profound granulocytopenia, and to severely ill patients on intensive care units to reduce the incidence of systemic candidiasis. *Candida albicans* is rarely (1% of clinical isolates) resistant to fluconazole, but other *Candida* species may be, more commonly in hospitals where prophylactic fluconazole use is extensive.

Isolation of candida from the bloodstream or intravenous catheter tips of patients with predisposing factors for systemic candidasis, e.g. prolonged intravenous access, neutropenia, is associated with a significant risk of serious sequelae, e.g. retinal or renal deposits, and should be treated with an effective antifungal for at least 3 weeks; fluconazole, amphotericin or any of the echinocandins will be appropriate.

Systemic mycoses

The principal treatment options are summarised in Table 15.3.

Classification of antifungal agents

- Drugs that disrupt the fungal cell membrane:
  - *polyenes,* e.g. amphotericin
  - *azoles:* imidazoles, e.g. ketoconazole, triazoles, e.g. fluconazole
  - *allylamine:* terbinafine.
- Drugs that disrupt the fungal cell wall:
  - *echinocandins,* e.g. caspofungin, anidulafungin, micafungin.
- Drugs that inhibit mitosis: griseofulvin.
- Drugs that inhibit DNA synthesis: flucytosine.

Pneumocystosis, caused by *Pneumocystis jirovecii,* is an important cause of potentially fatal pneumonia in the immunosuppressed, especially HIV-positive patients. It is treated with high-dose co-trimoxazole at 120 mg/kg daily in two to four divided doses for 21 days by mouth or i.v. infusion; monitoring of plasma concentrations is recommended. Patients with more severe illness should also receive corticosteroid. Although co-trimoxazole resistance is rare, patients who fail to respond or are intolerant may benefit from pentamidine or primaquine plus clindamycin. Other options include atovaquone for mild disease. Co-trimoxazole, dapsone (with pyrimethamine if toxoplasma prophylaxis is indicated) or atovaquone by mouth, or intermittent inhaled pentamidine, are used for primary and secondary prophylaxis in patients with AIDS.

Drugs that disrupt the fungal cell membrane

Polyenes

These act by binding tightly to sterols present in cell membranes. The resulting deformity of the membrane allows leakage of intracellular ions and enzymes, causing cell death.

Table 15.3 Drugs of choice for some fungal infections

Infection	Drug of first choice	Alternative
Aspergillosis	Amphotericin or voriconazole	Caspofungin, itraconazole, posaconazole
Blastomycosis[a]	Itraconazole or amphotericin	Fluconazole
Candidiasis		
mucosal	Fluconazole or amphotericin	Caspofungin, voriconazole or fluconazole
systemic	Fluconazole or amphotericin ± flucytosine	Caspofungin, micafungin, anidulafungin, voriconazole
Coccidioidomycosis[a]	Fluconazole, amphotericin or itraconazole	
Cryptococcosis	Amphotericin + flucytosine (followed by fluconazole)	Fluconazole
Fusariosis	Voriconazole	Amphotericin
Histoplasmosis	Itraconazole or amphotericin	Fluconazole
chronic suppression[b]	Itraconazole	Amphotericin
Mucormycosis	Amphotericin	Posaconazole
Paracoccidioidomycosis	Itraconazole or amphotericin	Ketoconazole[c]
Pseudallescheriasis	Voriconazole, ketoconazole or itraconazole	
Sporotrichosis		
cutaneous	Itraconazole	Potassium iodide
deep	Amphotericin	Itraconazole or fluconazole
Tinea pedis	Terbinafine cream or topical azole (miconazole, clotrimazole, econazole)	Fluconazole

[a]Patients with severe illness, meningitis, AIDS or some other causes of immunosuppression should receive amphotericin.
[b]For patients with AIDS.
[c]Continue treatment for 6–12 months.
This table was drawn substantially from The Medical Letter on Drugs and Therapeutics (2005, USA). The authors are grateful to the Chairman of the Editorial Board for permission to publish the material.

Those polyenes that have useful antifungal activity bind selectively to ergosterol, the most important sterol in fungal (but not mammalian) cell walls.

Amphotericin (amphotericin B)

Amphotericin is absorbed negligibly from the gut and must be given by i.v. infusion for systemic infection; about 10% remains in the blood, and the fate of the remainder is not known but is probably bound to tissues. The $t_{1/2}$ is 15 days and, after stopping treatment, drug persists in the body for several weeks.

Amphotericin is at present the drug of choice for most systemic fungal infections (but see Table 15.3). The diagnosis of systemic infection should, whenever possible, be firmly established; tissue biopsy and culture may be necessary, and methods using the PCR to detect aspergillus DNA may revolutionise management of invasive infection.

A conventional course of treatment for filamentous fungal infection lasts 6–12 weeks, during which at least 2 g amphotericin is given (usually 0.7–1 mg/kg daily, and up to 10 mg/kg daily of lipid-associated formulations for the most severe, invasive infections), but lower total and daily doses (e.g. 0.6 mg/kg daily) are used for candida infections, with correspondingly better tolerance. Antifungal drugs may be combined with immune-stimulating agents, e.g. granulocyte colony-stimulating factor, and clinical response in neutropenic episodes is closely related to return of normal neutrophil counts.

Lipid-associated formulations of amphotericin offer the prospect of reduced risk of toxicity while retaining therapeutic efficacy. In an aqueous medium, a lipid with hydrophilic and hydrophobic properties will form vesicles (liposomes) comprising an outer lipid bilayer surrounding an aqueous centre. The AmBisome formulation incorporates amphotericin in a lipid bilayer (55–75 nm diameter) from which the drug is released. Other lipid-associated complexes include Abelcet ('amphotericin B lipid complex') and Amphocil ('amphotericin B colloidal dispersion'). Lipid-associated formulations may be more effective for some indications because higher doses (3 mg/kg daily) may be given rapidly and safely. They are the first choice when renal function is impaired. Treatment often begins with the conventional formulation in those with normal kidneys, resorting to lipid-associated formulations if the patient's renal function deteriorates.

Adverse reactions. Gradual escalation of the dose limits toxic effects, which may be deemed justifiable in life-threatening infection if conventional amphotericin is used. A strategy of continuous i.v. infusion appears to combine therapeutic efficacy with tolerability. Renal impairment is invariable, although reduced by adequate hydration; nephrotoxicity is reversible, at least in its early stages. Hypokalaemia and hypomagnesaemia (due to distal renal tubular acidosis) may necessitate replacement therapy. Other adverse effects include anorexia; nausea; vomiting; malaise; abdominal, muscle and joint pains; loss of weight; anaemia; and fever. Aspirin, an antihistamine (H_1-receptor) or an antiemetic may alleviate symptoms. Severe febrile reactions are mitigated by hydrocortisone 25–50 mg before each infusion. Lipid-formulated preparations are associated with adverse reactions much less often, but fever, chills, nausea, vomiting, nephrotoxicity, electrolyte disturbance and occasional nephrotoxicity and hepatotoxicity are reported.

Nystatin

(named after New York State Health Laboratory)

Nystatin is too toxic for systemic use. It is not absorbed from the alimentary canal and is used to prevent or treat superficial candidiasis of the mouth, oesophagus or intestinal tract (as suspension, tablets or pastilles), for vaginal candidiasis (pessaries) and cutaneous infection (cream, ointment or powder).

Azoles

The antibacterial, antiprotozoal and anthelminthic members of this group are described in the appropriate sections. Antifungal azoles comprise the following:

- *Imidazoles* (ketoconazole, miconazole, fenticonazole, clotrimazole, isoconazole, tioconazole) interfere with fungal oxidative enzymes to cause lethal accumulation of *hydrogen peroxide;* they also reduce the formation of *ergosterol,* an important constituent of the fungal cell wall which thus becomes permeable to intracellular constituents. Lack of selectivity in these actions results in important adverse effects.
- *Triazoles* (fluconazole, itraconazole, voriconazole, posaconazole) damage the fungal cell membrane by inhibiting *lanosterol 14-α-demethylase,* an enzyme crucial to ergosterol synthesis, resulting in accumulation of toxic sterol precursors. Triazoles have greater selectivity against fungi, better penetration of the CNS, resistance to degradation and cause less endocrine disturbance than do the imidazoles.

Ketoconazole

Ketoconazole is well absorbed from the gut (poorly where there is gastric hypoacidity; see below); it is widely distributed in tissues, but concentrations in CSF and urine are low; its action is terminated by metabolism by cytochrome P450 3A ($t_{1/2}$ 8 h). For systemic mycoses, ketoconazole (see Table 15.3) has been superseded by fluconazole and itraconazole on the grounds of improved pharmacokinetics, tolerability and efficacy. Impairment of steroid synthesis by ketoconazole has been put to other uses, e.g. inhibition of testosterone synthesis lessens bone pain in patients with advanced androgen-dependent prostatic cancer.

Adverse reactions include nausea, giddiness, headache, pruritus and photophobia. Impairment of testosterone synthesis may cause gynaecomastia and decreased libido in men. Of particular concern is impairment of liver function, ranging from a transient increase in levels of hepatic transaminases and alkaline phosphatase to severe injury and death.

Interactions. Drugs that lower gastric acidity, e.g. antacids, histamine H_2-receptor antagonists, impair the absorption of ketoconazole from the gastrointestinal tract. Like all imidazoles, ketoconazole binds strongly to several cytochrome P450 isoenzymes, inhibiting their action and thereby increasing effects of oral anticoagulants, phenytoin and ciclosporin, and increasing the risk of cardiac arrhythmias with terfenadine. A disulfiram-like reaction occurs with alcohol. Concurrent use of rifampicin, by enzyme induction of CYP 3A, markedly reduces the plasma concentration of ketoconazole.

Other imidazoles. Miconazole is an alternative. Clotrimazole is widely used as an effective topical agent for dermatophyte, yeast and other fungal infections (intertrigo, athlete's foot, ringworm, pityriasis versicolor, fungal nappy rash). Econazole and sulconazole are similar. Tioconazole is used for fungal nail infections, and isoconazole and fenticonazole for vaginal candidiasis.

Fluconazole

Fluconazole is absorbed from the gastrointestinal tract and is excreted largely unchanged by the kidney ($t_{1/2}$ 30 h). It is effective by mouth for oropharyngeal and oesophageal candidiasis, and i.v. for systemic candidiasis and cryptococcosis (including cryptococcal meningitis; it penetrates the CSF well). It is used prophylactically in a variety of conditions predisposing to systemic candida infections, including at times of profound neutropenia after bone marrow transplantation, and in patients in intensive care units who have intravenous lines in situ, are receiving antibiotic therapy and have undergone bowel surgery. It may cause gastrointestinal discomfort, headaches, reversible alopecia, increased levels of liver enzymes and allergic rash, but is generally well tolerated. Animal studies demonstrate embryotoxicity, and there have been reports of multiple congenital abnormalities in women treated with long-term high-dose fluconazole, therefore fluconazole should be avoided in pregnant women. High doses increase the effects of phenytoin, ciclosporin, zidovudine and warfarin.

Itraconazole

Itraconazole is available for oral (suspension and capsule) and i.v. administration ($t_{1/2}$ 25 h, increasing to 40 h with continuous treatment). The intravenous preparation is not available in many countries. Absorption from the gut is about 55%, but variable. It is improved by ingestion with food, but decreased by fatty meals and therapies that reduce gastric acidity. Plasma concentrations should be monitored during prolonged use for critical indications. The oral suspension formulation has significantly improved bio-availability compared to the capsule formulation and is much less affected by gastric hypoacidity. Itraconazole is heavily protein bound, and virtually none is found within the CSF. It is almost completely oxidised in the liver (by CYP 3A) and excreted in the bile; little unchanged drug enters the urine.

Itraconazole is used for a variety of superficial mycoses, as a prophylactic agent for aspergillosis and candidiasis in the immunocompromised, and i.v. for treatment of histoplasmosis. It is licensed in the UK as a second-line agent for *Candida*, *Aspergillus* and *Cryptococcus* infections, and it may be convenient as 'follow-on' therapy after systemic aspergillosis has been brought under control by an amphotericin preparation. It appears to be an effective adjunct treatment for allergic bronchopulmonary aspergillosis.

Adverse effects are uncommon, but include transient hepatitis and hypokalaemia. Prolonged use may lead to cardiac failure, especially in those with pre-existing cardiac disease. Co-administration of a calcium channel blocker adds to the risk. Cyclodextrin (used as a vehicle for the i.v. formulation) accumulates and causes sodium overload in renally impaired patients, but the oral formulation avoids this problem.

Interactions. Enzyme induction of CYP 3A, e.g. by rifampicin, reduces the plasma concentration of itraconazole. Additionally, its affinity for several P450 isoforms, notably CYP 3A4, causes it to inhibit the oxidation of a number of drugs, including phenytoin, warfarin, ciclosporin, tacrolimus, midazolam, triazolam, cisapride and terfenadine (see above), increasing their intensity and/or duration of effect.

Voriconazole

Voriconazole ($t_{1/2}$ 7 h) is more active in vitro than itraconazole against *Aspergillus* because of more avid binding of the sterol synthetic enzymes of filamentous fungi; it also appears to have synergistic activity against *Aspergillus* in combination with amphotericin. It is as active as the other triazoles against yeasts and is more reliably and rapidly absorbed than itraconazole by mouth, but cross-resistance between these agents is usual. It is more effective than conventional amphotericin in invasive aspergillosis, and probably equivalent to lipid-associated formulations. Oral absorption is not significantly reduced by gastric hypoacidity. CSF and brain tissue concentrations are at least 50% of those in the plasma, and are sufficient for effective therapy of fungal infections of the eye and CNS.

Adverse effects. Administration i.v. gives rise rapidly to transient visual disturbance in 30% of patients (blurring, alerted visual perception such as reversal of light and dark, visual hallucinations and photophobia). These often resolve after the first week of therapy, and almost all of those affected are able to continue with the course of treatment.

Accumulation of the cyclodextrin vehicle (see above) may cause sodium retention in renally impaired patients with i.v. use. Patients with hepatic cirrhosis should receive a standard loading, but only one-half of the daily maintenance dose. Transiently raised liver enzyme levels are seen in up to 20% of patients, but serious liver impairment is rare. Rashes and photosensitivity appear to be more common than with the other triazoles.

Extensive metabolism of voriconazole by the cytochrome P450 system (predominantly CYP 2C19) may lead to unwanted interaction with patients receiving rifampicin, ciclosporin or tacrolimus.

Posaconazole

Posaconazole ($t_{1/2}$ 20 h) is structurally related to itraconazole and has similar in vitro antifungal activity to voriconazole. It is fungistatic against *Candida* spp. but fungicidal against *Aspergillus* spp., and is also active against a range of other filamentous fungi. It provides effective prophylaxis against invasive fungal infection in leukaemia and bone marrow transplant patients. The oral bio-availability is high (90%), especially when taken with a fatty meal. More than 75% of the dose is excreted in the faeces.

Adverse effects are uncommon, but include gastrointestinal disturbance, dizziness and fatigue, neutropenia (7% of patients) and transient disturbance of liver function. Dose adjustment is not required for renal or hepatic impairment.

Allylamine

Terbinafine

Terbinafine interferes with ergosterol biosynthesis, and thereby with the formation of the fungal cell membrane. It is absorbed from the gastrointestinal tract and undergoes extensive metabolism in the liver ($t_{1/2}$ 14 h). Terbinafine is used topically for dermatophyte infections of the skin and orally for infections of hair and nails where the site, e.g. hair, severity or extent of the infection renders topical use inappropriate (see pp. 280–281). Treatment may need to continue for several weeks. Terbinafine may cause nausea, diarrhoea, dyspepsia, abdominal pain, headaches and cutaneous reactions.

Drugs that disrupt the fungal cell wall

Echinocandins

The echinocandins are large lipopeptide molecules that inhibit synthesis of β-(1,3)-d-glucan, a vital component of the cell walls of many fungi (excepting *Cryptococcus*

neoformans, against which they have no useful activity). In vitro and in vivo, the echinocandins are rapidly fungicidal against most *Candida* spp. and fungistatic against *Aspergillus* spp. Echinocandins have no activity against emerging pathogens such as *Fusarium* sp., *Scedosporium* sp. and zygomycetes. They are available as i.v. preparations only.

Caspofungin ($t_{1/2}$ 10 h) is the first member of this group. It is licensed for i.v. treatment of invasive candidiasis, suspected fungal infections in febrile neutropenic patients, and *Aspergillus* infections in patients who have not responded to amphotericin or itraconazole. Caspofungin retains activity against most triazole- and polyene-resistant yeasts, and is also active against *Pneumocystis jiroveci*. It is widely distributed through body tissues and highly protein bound. It penetrates the CSF poorly, but clinical responses in fungal CNS infection have been reported.

Caspofungin is generally well tolerated, but headache, fever, raised liver function tests and hypokalaemia occur. Patients with significant liver impairment should receive a reduced dose. Patients might experience histamine-induced reactions when the drug is infused too rapidly.

Micafungin has similar activity to caspofungin and is licensed for the treatment of invasive candida infections (oesophagitis, peritonitis and candidaemia) and for prophylaxis of *Candida* spp. and *Aspergillus* infection in patients undergoing haemopoetic stem cell transplantation. It is highly protein bound and, unlike caspofungin and anidulafungin, does not require a loading dose. Micafungin was found to induce the development of liver tumours in rats after treatment for 3 months and longer; close monitoring of patients for liver damage is advised.

Anidulafungin is a semi-synthetic echinocandin derived from *Aspergillus nidulans*. It has a much longer elimination $t_{1/2}$ than the other echinocandins (27 h) and is not metabolised by the liver, but undergoes slow chemical degradation to inactive metabolites. It has no significant drug–drug interactions, with no dose adjustment required in renal or hepatic impairment. Anidulafungin is approved for the treatment of invasive candidiasis in adult non-neutropenic patients.

Other antifungal drugs

Griseofulvin

Griseofulvin prevents fungal growth by binding to microtubular proteins and inhibiting mitosis. The therapeutic efficacy of griseofulvin depends on its capacity to bind to keratin as it is being formed in the cells of the nail bed, hair follicles and skin, for dermatophytes specifically infect keratinous tissues. Griseofulvin does not kill fungus already established; it merely prevents infection of new keratin so that the duration of treatment is governed by the time that it takes for infected keratin to be shed. On average, hair and skin infection should be treated for 4–6 weeks, although toenails may need 1 year or more. Treatment must continue for a few weeks after both visual and microscopic evidence has disappeared. Fat in a meal enhances absorption of griseofulvin; it is metabolised in the liver and induces hepatic enzymes ($t_{1/2}$ 15 h).

Griseofulvin is effective against all superficial ringworm (dermatophyte) infections, but ineffective against pityriasis versicolor, superficial candidiasis and all systemic mycoses.

Adverse reactions include gastrointestinal upset, rashes, photosensitivity, headache and various CNS disturbances.

Flucytosine

Flucytosine (5-fluorocytosine) is metabolised in the fungal cell to 5-fluorouracil, which inhibits nucleic acid synthesis. It is well absorbed from the gut, penetrates effectively into tissues, and almost all is excreted unchanged in the urine ($t_{1/2}$ 4 h). The dose should be reduced for patients with impaired renal function, and the plasma concentration monitored. The drug is well tolerated when renal function is normal. *Candida albicans* rapidly becomes resistant to flucytosine, which ought not to be used alone; it may be combined with amphotericin (see Table 15.3), but this increases the risk of adverse effects (leucopenia, thrombocytopenia, enterocolitis) and it is reserved for serious infections where the risk:benefit balance is favourable, e.g. *Cryptococcus neoformans* meningitis.

Protozoal infections

Malaria

About one-half of the world's population is exposed to malaria, with an estimated 250 million cases and 1 million deaths annually, mainly in sub-Saharan African children (where a child dies from malaria on average every 30 seconds). In terms of socioeconomic impact, malaria is the most important of the transmissible parasitic diseases.

Quinine as cinchona bark was introduced into Europe from South America in 1631 (by Agostino Salumbrino, a Jesuit priest and trained apothecary, who sent a small quantity of bark to Rome where much of the terrain was swampy and fevers were common – hence the term 'Jesuit's bark'). It was used for all fevers, among them malaria, the occurrence of which was associated with damp places with bad air (*'mal aria'*).

Life cycle of the malaria parasite and sites of drug action

The incubation period of malaria is 10–35 days. The principal features of the life cycle (Fig. 15.1) of the malaria parasite must be known in order to understand its therapy.

Female anopheles mosquitoes require a blood meal for egg production, and in the process of feeding they inject salivary fluid containing *sporozoites* into humans. As no drugs are effective against sporozoites, infection with the malaria parasite cannot be prevented.

Hepatic cycle

(site 1 in Fig. 15.1)

Sporozoites enter liver cells where they develop into schizonts, which form large numbers of merozoites which, after 5–16 days, but sometimes after months or years, are released into the circulation. *Plasmodium falciparum* differs in that it has no persistent hepatic cycle.

Primaquine, proguanil and tetracyclines (*tissue schizontocides*) act at this site and are used for:

- *Radical cure*, i.e. an attack on persisting hepatic forms (*hypnozoites*, i.e. sleeping) once the parasite has been cleared from the blood; this is most effectively accomplished with primaquine; proguanil is only weakly effective.
- *Preventing the initial hepatic cycle*. This is also called *causal prophylaxis*. Primaquine was long regarded as too toxic for prolonged use, but evidence now suggests it may be used safely, and it is inexpensive; proguanil is weakly effective. Doxycycline may be used short term.

Vaccine development against both falciparum and vivax malaria concentrates mostly on surface antigens (e.g. circumsporozoite protein) involved in the pre-erythrocytic stages, before invasion of liver cells (stage 1).

Erythrocyte cycle

(site 2 in Fig. 15.1)

Merozoites enter red cells, where they develop into schizonts, which form more merozoites that are released when the cells burst, giving rise to the features of the clinical attack. The merozoites re-enter red cells, and the cycle is repeated.

Chloroquine, quinine, mefloquine, halofantrine, proguanil, pyrimethamine and tetracyclines (blood schizontocides) kill these asexual forms. Drugs that act at this stage in the cycle of the parasite may be used for:

- *Treatment* of acute attacks of malaria.
- *Prevention* of attacks by early destruction of the erythrocytic forms. This is called *suppressive prophylaxis* as it does not cure the hepatic cycle (above).

Sexual forms

(site 3 in Fig. 15.1)

Some merozoites differentiate into male and female gametocytes in the erythrocytes and can develop further

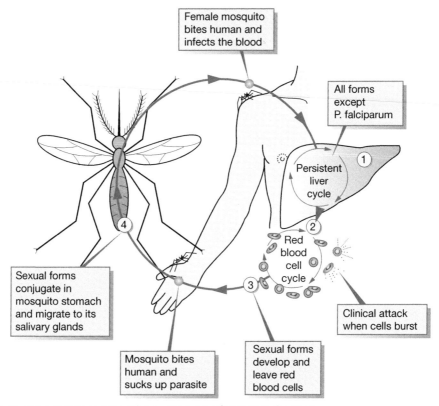

Fig. 15.1 Life cycle of the malaria parasite. (The numbers are referred to in the text.)

only if they are ingested by a mosquito, where they form *sporozoites* (site 4 in Fig. 15.1) and complete the transmission cycle.

Quinine, mefloquine, chloroquine, artesunate, artemether and primaquine (gametocytocides) act on sexual forms and prevent transmission of the infection because the patient becomes non-infective and the parasite fails to develop in the mosquito (site 4).

In summary, drugs may be selected for:

- treatment of clinical attacks
- prevention of clinical attacks
- radical cure.

Drugs used for malaria, and their principal actions, are classified in Table 15.4.

Drug-resistant malaria

Drug-resistant parasites constitute a persistent problem. *Plasmodium falciparum* is now resistant to chloroquine and sulfadoxine-pyrimethamine in many parts of the world. Areas of high risk for resistant parasites include sub-Saharan Africa, Latin America, Oceania (Papua New Guinea, Solomon Islands, Vanuatu) and some parts of Southeast Asia. Mefloquine resistance is rare outside Southeast Asia. There are concerns with emerging artesunate resistance in western Cambodia due to monotherapy. Chloroquine-resistant *Plasmodium vivax* is also reported. Hyperparasitaemia and inappropriate or low dosing of antimalarials are important drivers of resistance.

Resistance can be reduced by combining antimalarials with different mechanisms of action, usually in the form of artemisinin-based combination therapies (ACTs). ACTs are often more effective than single-agent therapy or non–artemisinin-based combinations and are now recommended by the World Health Organization (WHO) for the treatment of *Plasmodium falciparum* malaria globally.

Any physician who is unfamiliar with the resistance pattern in the locality from which patients have come, or to which they are going, is well advised to check the current position. Because prevalence and resistance rates are so variable, advice on therapy and prophylaxis in this section is given for general guidance only, and readers are referred to specialist sources for up-to-date information.

Table 15.4 Antimalarial drugs and their sites of action

Drug	Biological activity	
	Blood schizontocide	Tissue schizontocide
4-Aminoquinolone chloroquine	++	0
Arylaminoakohols quinine	++	0
mefloquine	++	0
Phenanthrene methanol halofantrine	++	0
lumefantrine	++	0
Antimetabolites proguanil	+	+
pyrimethamine	+	0
sulfadoxine	+	0
dapsone	+	0
Antibiotics tetracycline	+	+
doxycycline	+	+
minocycline	+	+
8-Aminoquinolone primaquine	0	+
Sesquiterpenes artesunate	+	0
artemether	+	0

Chemotherapy of an acute attack of malaria[3]

Successful management demands attention to the following points of principle:

- Whenever possible, the diagnosis should be confirmed before treatment by examination of blood smears; this is not often possible in the developing world, where clinically diagnosed illnesses may receive unnecessary courses of antimalarials, thus increasing the risk of plasmodial resistance.
- When the infecting organism is not known or infection is mixed, treatment should begin as for *Plasmodium falciparum* (below).
- Drugs used to treat *Plasmodium falciparum* malaria must always be selected with regard to the prevalence of local patterns of drug resistance.

- Patients not at risk of re-infection should be re-examined several weeks after treatment for signs of recrudescence, which may result from inadequate chemotherapy or survival of persistent hepatic forms.

Falciparum ('malignant') malaria

Falciparum malaria in the non-immune is a medical emergency, and malaria of unknown infecting species should be treated as though it were falciparum. The regimen depends on the condition of the patient; the doses quoted are for adults. Chloroquine resistance is now widespread; therefore this drug should not be used for the treatment of falciparum malaria.

If the patient can swallow and there are no serious complications such as impairment of consciousness, treatment options are as follows:

- A quinine salt:[4] 600 mg 8-hourly by mouth for 5–7 days, followed by doxycycline 200 mg daily for at least

---

[3]Treatment regimens vary in detail; those quoted here accord with the recommendations in the *British National Formulary* 2010 and national UK specialist guidelines; the BNF is a good source of contact numbers, addresses and websites to obtain expert advice on therapy and prophylaxis of malaria.

[4]Acceptable as quinine hydrochloride, dihydrochloride or sulfate, but not quinine bisulfate, which contains less quinine.

7 days. This additional therapy is necessary, as quinine alone tends to be associated with a higher rate of relapse. Clindamycin (450 mg four times daily for 7 days) may be given as an alternative follow-on therapy instead of doxycycline, and is particularly suitable for pregnant women. If the parasite is likely to be sensitive, Fansidar (pyrimethamine plus sulfadoxine) 3 tablets as a single dose is an alternative.

- Malarone (atovaquone and proguanil hydrochloride): 4 tablets once daily for 3 days.
- Riamet (artemether plus lumefantrine): if weight >35 kg, 4 tablets initially, followed by five further doses of 4 tablets given at 8, 24, 36, 48 and 60 h.
- Mefloquine is also effective, but resistance has been reported in several regions, including Southeast Asia. It is not necessary to use follow-on therapy after Riamet, mefloquine or Malarone.

Seriously ill patients should be treated with:

- A quinine salt:[4] 20 mg/kg as a loading dose[5] (maximum 1.4 g) infused i.v. over 4 h, followed 8 h later by a maintenance infusion of 10 mg/kg (maximum 700 mg) infused over 4 h, repeated every 8 h[6] until the patient can swallow tablets to complete the 7-day course. Patients at increased risk of arrhythmias and the elderly should have ECG monitoring while on the infusion.
- Doxycycline or clindamycin should be given subsequently, as above (mefloquine is an alternative, but this must begin at least 12 h after parenteral quinine has ceased).
- Intravenous artesunate showed a clear benefit when compared to quinine in patients with severe falciparum malaria.[7] A large randomised trial showed a 34% reduction in mortality with intravenous artesunate when compared to quinine; the number needed to treat to prevent one death was 13.[8] Intravenous artesunate is not licensed in the European Union, but should be considered on a 'named patient' basis for severe cases not responsive to quinine or if quinine resistance is suspected, or there is a high parasite count (>20%). Intravenous artesunate should be accompanied by a 7-day course of doxycycline.

Treatment in pregnancy should always be based on expert advice.

Non-falciparum ('benign') malarias

These are usually due to *Plasmodium vivax* or less commonly to *Plasmodium ovale* or *Plasmodium malariae*.

The drug of choice is *chloroquine*, which should be given by mouth as follows:

- Initial dose: 620 mg (base),[9] then 310 mg as a single dose 6–8 h later.
- Second day: 310 mg as a single dose.
- Third day: 310 mg as a single dose.

The total dose of chloroquine base over 3 days should be approximately 25 mg/kg base. This is sufficient for *Plasmodium malariae* infection, but for *Plasmodium vivax* and *Plasmodium ovale* eradication of the hepatic parasites is necessary to prevent relapse, by giving:

- Primaquine, 15 mg/day for 14 days started after the chloroquine course has been completed. *Plasmodium vivax* infections require 30 mg/day for 14 days. Primaquine can lead to haemolysis in patients with G6PD deficiency (if mild G6PD deficiency, lower dosing of 45 mg once-weekly for 8 weeks may suffice without undue risk of haemolysis).

Chemoprophylaxis of malaria

Geographically variable plasmodial drug resistance has become a major factor. The WHO gives advice in its annually revised booklet *Vaccination Certificate Requirements and Health Advice for International Travel*, and national bodies publish recommendations, e.g. British National Formulary, that apply particularly to their own residents.

General principles

- Chemoprophylaxis aims to prevent deaths from falciparum malaria, but only ever gives relative protection; travellers should guard against bites by using mosquito nets and repellents, and wearing

---

[5]The loading dose should not be given if the patient has received quinine, quinidine or mefloquine in the previous 24 h; see also warnings about halofantrine (below).
[6]Reduced to 5–7 mg/kg of quinine salt if the infusion lasts for more than 48 h.
[7]A Cochrane Review of six clinical trials showed a significantly reduced risk of death, reduced parasite clearance time and hypoglycaemia when artesunate was compared with quinine for the treatment of severe malaria. Jones K L, Donegan S, Lalloo D G 2007 Artesunate versus quinine for treating severe malaria. Cochrane Database Systematic Review Oct 17;(4):CD005967.
[8]Dondorp A, Nosten F, Stepniewska K, et al 2005 Artesunate versus quinine for treatment of severe falciparum malaria: a randomised trial. Lancet 366:717–725.

[9]The active component of many drugs, whether acid or base, is relatively insoluble and may present a problem in formulation. This is overcome by adding an acid to a base or vice versa; the weight of the salt differs according to the acid or base component, i.e. chloroquine base 150 mg = chloroquine sulfate 200 mg = chloroquine phosphate 250 mg (approximately). Where there may be variation, therefore, the amount of drug prescribed is expressed as the weight of the active component, in the case of chloroquine, the base.

well-covering clothing especially during high-risk times of day (after dusk).

- Mefloquine, doxycycline and atovaquone-proguanil (Malarone) are the most commonly advised prophylactic regimens, and are particularly recommended for areas of chloroquine-resistant falciparum malaria. Chloroquine, alone or in combination with proguanil, may be considered in areas of the world where the risk of acquiring chloroquine-resistant falciparum malaria is low, although there is considerable concern regarding the protective efficacy of this regimen. Due to widespread *P. falciparum* resistance to proguanil, single-agent prophylaxis with this agent is rarely appropriate for most regions of the world.
- Effective chemoprophylaxis requires that there be a plasmodicidal concentration of drug in the blood when the first infected mosquito bites, and that it be sustained safely for long periods.
- The progressive rise in plasma concentration to *steady state* (after $t_{1/2} \times 5$), sometimes attained only after weeks (consider mefloquine $t_{1/2}$ 21 days, chloroquine $t_{1/2}$ 50 days), allows unwanted effects (which can impair compliance or be unsafe) to be delayed, in some instances until after a subject has entered a malarial area. Thus, it is advised that prophylaxis begin long enough before travel to reveal acute intolerance and to impress on the subject the importance of compliance (to relate drug-taking to a specific daily or weekly event).
- Prompt achievement of efficacy and safety, i.e. *plasmodicidal concentrations*, by one (or two) doses is plainly important for travellers who cannot wait on dosage schedules to deliver both only when steady-state blood concentrations are attained; the schedules must reflect this need.
- Prophylaxis should continue for at least 4 weeks after leaving an endemic area to kill parasites that are acquired about the time of departure, are still incubating in the liver and will develop into the erythrocyte phase. Malarone, however, only needs to be taken for a week after return. The traveller should be aware that any illness occurring within 1 year, and especially within 3 months, of return, may be malaria.
- Chloroquine and proguanil may be used for periods of up to 5 years, and mefloquine for up to 1–2 years; expert advice should be taken by long-term travellers, especially those going to areas for which other prophylactic drugs are recommended.
- *Naturally acquired immunity* offers the most reliable protection for people living permanently in endemic areas (below). Repeated attacks of malaria confer partial immunity, and the disease often becomes no more than an occasional inconvenience. Vaccines to confer active immunity are under development.

- A short course of prophylaxis (4–6 weeks) may be considered for pregnant women and young children returning to their permanent homes in malarious areas after a prolonged period of stay in a non-endemic area, pending suitable arrangements for health care.
- As a rule, the *partially immune* should not take a prophylactic. The reasoning is that immunity is sustained by the red cell cycle, loss of which through prophylaxis diminishes their resistance and leaves them highly vulnerable to the disease. There are, however, exceptions to this general advice, and the partially immune may or should use a prophylactic:
    - if it is virtually certain that they will never abandon its use
    - if they go to another malarial area where the strains of parasite may differ
    - during the last few months of pregnancy in areas where *Plasmodium falciparum* is prevalent (to avert the risk of miscarriage).

Examples of standard prophylactic regimens

- Chloroquine: 300 mg (base) once weekly (start 1 week before travel).
- Proguanil: 200 mg once daily (start 1 week before travel).
- Chloroquine plus proguanil in the above doses.
- Malarone: 1 tablet daily (start 1–2 days before travel).
- Mefloquine: 250 mg once weekly (start 1 week, preferably 2–3 weeks, before travel).
- Doxycycline: 100 mg once daily (start 1–2 days before travel).

For 'last minute' travellers. The standard regimens normally provide immediate protection, but it will be sensible to avoid mefloquine (if an alternative antimalarial is available) in the last minute traveller with no history of previous mefloquine exposure or who is intolerant of the drug. Current UK national guidelines do not recommend giving a loading dose of prophylactic antimalarials for the purpose of rapidly achieving steady-state plasma concentration.

Drug interactions. Where subjects are already taking other drugs, e.g. antiepileptics and cardiovascular drugs, it is desirable to start prophylaxis as much as 2–3 weeks in advance to establish safety.

Antimalarial drugs and pregnancy

Women living in endemic areas in which *Plasmodium falciparum* remains sensitive to chloroquine should take chloroquine prophylactically throughout pregnancy. Proguanil (an 'antifol', see below) may be taken for prophylaxis provided it is accompanied by folic acid 5 mg/day. Chloroquine may be used in full dose to treat chloroquine-sensitive infections. Quinine is the only widely available drug that is acceptable as suitable for treating chloroquine-resistant infections during pregnancy. Mefloquine is teratogenic in animals, and a woman should avoid pregnancy while taking it, and for 3 months afterwards (although evidence is accruing that it may be safe for use in chloroquine-resistant areas). Doxycycline is contraindicated throughout pregnancy, and Malarone (proguanil plus atovaquone) should be avoided unless there is no suitable alternative.

Individual antimalarial drugs

Chloroquine

Chloroquine ($t_{1/2}$ 50 days) is concentrated within parasitised red cells and forms complexes with plasmodial DNA. It is active against the blood forms and also the gametocytes (formed in the mosquito) of *Plasmodium vivax*, *Plasmodium ovale* and *Plasmodium malariae*; it is ineffective against many strains of *Plasmodium falciparum* and also its immature gametocytes. Chloroquine is readily absorbed from the gastrointestinal tract and is concentrated several-fold in various tissues, e.g. erythrocytes, liver, spleen, heart, kidney, cornea and retina; the long $t_{1/2}$ reflects slow release from these sites. A priming dose is used in order to achieve adequate free plasma concentration (see acute attack, above). Chloroquine is partly inactivated by metabolism, and the remainder is excreted unchanged in the urine.

Adverse effects are infrequent at doses normally used for malaria prophylaxis and treatment, but are more common with the higher or prolonged doses given for resistant malaria or for rheumatoid arthritis or lupus erythematosus (see p. 260).

Corneal deposits of chloroquine may be asymptomatic or may cause halos around lights or photophobia. These are not a threat to vision and reverse when the drug is stopped. Retinal toxicity is more serious, and may be irreversible. In the early stage, it takes the form of visual field defects; late retinopathy classically gives the picture of macular pigmentation surrounded by a ring of pigment (the 'bull's-eye' macula). The functional defect can take the form of scotomas, photophobia, defective colour vision and decreased visual acuity resulting, in the extreme case, in blindness.

Other reactions include pruritus, which may be intolerable and is common in Africans, headaches, gastrointestinal disturbance, precipitation of acute intermittent porphyria in susceptible individuals, mental disturbances and interference with cardiac rhythm, the latter especially if the drug is given i.v. in high dose (it has a quinidine-like action). Long-term use is associated with reversible bleaching of the hair and pigmentation of the hard palate.

Acute overdose may be rapidly fatal without treatment, and indeed has even been described as a means of suicide.[10] Pulmonary oedema is followed by convulsions, cardiac arrhythmias and coma; as little as 50 mg/kg can be fatal. These effects are principally due to the profound negative inotropic action of chloroquine. Diazepam was found fortuitously to protect the heart, and adrenaline/epinephrine reduces intraventricular conduction time; this combination of drugs, given by separate i.v. infusions, improves survival.

Halofantrine

Halofantrine ($t_{1/2}$ 2.5 days) is active against the erythrocytic forms of all four *Plasmodium* species, especially *Plasmodium falciparum* and *Plasmodium vivax*, and at the schizont stage. Its mechanism of action is not fully understood. Absorption of halofantrine from the gastrointestinal tract is variable, incomplete and substantially increased (6–10-fold) by taking the drug with food (see below). It is converted to an active metabolite, and no unchanged drug is recovered in the urine. Due to cardiotoxicity concerns, halofantrine is not included in any of the WHO-approved artemisinin combination therapy (ACT) options for treatment of uncomplicated *Plasmodium falciparum* malaria. It is no longer recommended for the treatment of drug-resistant *Plasmodium vivax* malaria and should also not be used for prophylaxis.

Lumefantrine

Lumefantrine ($t_{1/2}$ 3 days) has a similar structure and mechanism of action to halofantrine. It is only available as a fixed drug combination with artemether (Riamet or Co-artem). It has variable bio-availability; absorption is substantially increased by fatty meals, with plasma levels peaking about 10 h after oral intake. Unlike halofantrine, there are no cardiotoxicity concerns and it is well tolerated.

Mefloquine

Mefloquine ($t_{1/2}$ 21 days) is similar in several respects to quinine, although it does not intercalate with plasmodial DNA. It is used for malaria chemoprophylaxis, and occasionally to treat uncomplicated *Plasmodium falciparum* (both chloroquine-sensitive and chloroquine-resistant) and chloroquine-resistant *Plasmodium vivax* malaria. Mefloquine is rapidly absorbed from the gastrointestinal tract, and its action is terminated by metabolism. When used for prophylaxis, 250 mg (base)/week should be taken, commencing 1–3 weeks before entering and continued for 4 weeks after leaving a malarious area. It should not be given to patients with hepatic or renal impairment.

Adverse effects include nausea, dizziness, disturbance of balance, vomiting, abdominal pain, diarrhoea and loss of

---

[10]Report 1993 Chloroquine poisoning. Lancet 307:49.

appetite. More rarely, hallucinations, seizures and psychoses occur. Mefloquine should be avoided in patients taking β-adrenoceptor and calcium channel antagonists, because it causes sinus bradycardia; quinine can potentiate these and other dose-related effects of mefloquine.

Neuropsychiatric events, including seizures and psychoses, occur after high-dose therapy in about 1 in 10 000 of those using the drug for prophylaxis. Less severe reactions including headache, dizziness, depression and insomnia have been reported, but there is uncertainty as to whether these can be ascribed to mefloquine. The drug should not be used in travellers with a history of neuropsychiatric disease including convulsions and depression, and in those whose activities require fine coordination or spatial performance, e.g. airline flight-deck crews.

Primaquine

Primaquine ($t_{1/2}$ 6 h) acts at several stages in the development of the plasmodial parasite, possibly by interfering with its mitochondrial function. Its unique effect is to eliminate the hepatic forms of *Plasmodium vivax* and *Plasmodium ovale* after standard chloroquine therapy, but only when the risk of re-infection is absent or slight. Primaquine also has weak activity against blood forms of the parasite. Due to its antigametocidal effect, single-dose primaquine is now recommended at the end of an ACT course of therapy for falciparum malaria in areas where malaria elimination is a priority. Primaquine is well absorbed from the gastrointestinal tract, is only moderately concentrated in the tissues, and is rapidly metabolised.

Adverse effects include anorexia, nausea, abdominal cramps, methaemoglobinaemia, granulocytopenia and haemolytic anaemia, especially in patients with genetic deficiency of erythrocyte glucose-6-phosphate dehydrogenase (G6PD). Subjects should be tested for G6PD and, in those who are mildly deficient, the risk of haemolytic anaemia is greatly reduced by giving primaquine in reduced dose. Primaquine is not recommended during pregnancy, severe G6PD deficiency and conditions that predispose to granulocytopenia, e.g. rheumatoid arthritis and systemic lupus erythematosus.

Proguanil (chloroguanide)

Proguanil ($t_{1/2}$ 17 h) inhibits dihydrofolate reductase, which converts folic to folinic acid, deficiency of which inhibits plasmodial cell division. Plasmodia, like most bacteria but unlike humans, cannot make use of preformed folic acid. Pyrimethamine and trimethoprim, which share this mode of action, are collectively known as the 'antifols'. Their plasmodicidal action is markedly enhanced by combination with sulfonamides or sulfones because there is inhibition of sequential steps in folate synthesis. It is used alone (usually with chloroquine) for malaria prophylaxis, and is also available with atovaquone (as Malarone: proguanil hydrochloride 100 mg plus atovaquone 250 mg) for prophylaxis and treatment.

Proguanil is moderately well absorbed from the gut and is excreted in the urine either unchanged or as an active metabolite. Being little stored in the tissues, proguanil must be used daily when given for prophylaxis. It is rarely recommended alone (as a single agent) for prophylaxis.

Adverse effects. In prophylactic doses, proguanil is well tolerated. Mouth ulcers and stomatitis have been reported. The drug should be avoided or used in reduced dose for patients with impaired renal function.

Pyrimethamine

Pyrimethamine ($t_{1/2}$ 4 days) inhibits plasmodial dihydrofolate reductase, for which it has a high affinity. It is well absorbed from the gastrointestinal tract and is extensively metabolised. It is seldom used alone (see below). Pregnant women should receive supplementary folic acid when taking pyrimethamine.

Adverse effects reported include anorexia, abdominal cramps, vomiting, ataxia, tremor, seizures and megaloblastic anaemia.

Pyrimethamine with sulfadoxine

Pyrimethamine acts synergistically with sulfadoxine (as Fansidar) to inhibit folic acid metabolism (see 'antifols', above); sulfadoxine is excreted in the urine. In the past, this combination was used with quinine to treat acute attacks of malaria caused by susceptible strains of *Plasmodium falciparum*; the widespread emergence of pyrimethamine-sulfadoxine–resistant falciparum and vivax malaria has led to changes in the use of this drug. An ACT regimen of artesunate and pyrimethamine-sulfadoxine is now available as separate scored tablets for the treatment of uncomplicated falciparum malaria in Africa, but should not be used in areas of multiple-drug resistance, such as Southeast Asia. Pyrimethamine-sulfadoxine, either as a single agent or combined with artesunate, is no longer considered an appropriate choice for the treatment of *Plasmodium vivax* malaria.

Adverse effects. Any sulphonamide-induced allergic reactions can be severe, e.g. erythema multiforme, Stevens–Johnson syndrome and toxic epidermal necrolysis. Because of its 'antifol' action, the combination should not be used by pregnant women unless they take a folate supplement.

Pyrimethamine with dapsone

This fixed drug combination (Maloprim or Deltaprim) of 12.5 mg pyrimethamine and 100 mg of dapsone was used for many years as prophylaxis against *Plasmodium falciparum* malaria. Due to toxicity concerns (agranulocytosis) and increasing resistance to pyrimethamine, this regimen is no longer recommended for prophylaxis, although it continues to be available in parts of Africa, in particular Zimbabwe and neighbouring countries.

Quinine

Quinine ($t_{1/2}$ 9 h; 18 h in severe malaria) is obtained from the bark of the South American cinchona tree. It binds to plasmodial DNA to prevent protein synthesis, but its exact mode of action remains uncertain. It is used to treat *Plasmodium falciparum* malaria in areas of multiple-drug resistance. Apart from its antiplasmodial effect, quinine is used for myotonia and muscle cramps because it prolongs the muscle refractory period. Quinine is included in dilute concentration in tonics and aperitifs for its desired bitter taste.

Quinine is well absorbed from the gastrointestinal tract and is almost completely metabolised in the liver.

Adverse effects include tinnitus, diminished auditory acuity, headache, blurred vision, nausea and diarrhoea (common to quinine, quinidine, salicylates and called 'cinchonism'). Idiosyncratic reactions include pruritus, urticaria and rashes. Hypoglycaemia may be significant when quinine is given by i.v. infusion, and supplementary glucose may be required.

When large amounts are taken, e.g. (unreliably) to induce abortion or in attempted suicide, ocular disturbances, notably constriction of the visual fields, may occur and even complete blindness, the onset of which may be very sudden. Vomiting, abdominal pain and diarrhoea result from local irritation of the gastrointestinal tract. Quinidine-like effects include hypotension, disturbance of atrioventricular conduction and cardiac arrest. Activated charcoal should be given. Supportive measures are employed thereafter, as no specific therapy has proven benefit.

Quinidine, the dextrorotatory isomer of quinine, has antimalarial activity, but is used mainly as a cardiac antiarrhythmic (see p. 453).

Artesunate and artemether Artesunate and artemether are soluble derivatives of artemisinin, which is isolated from the leaves of the Chinese herb qinghaao (Artemisia annua). Both drug formulations are available for oral, intramuscular and i.v. administration. Artemether is lipid soluble whereas artesunate is water soluble and hence also available as an i.v. formulation. They are rapidly effective against the blood forms of the plasmodia including multi-resistant strains and in severe infections. They are well tolerated but should be used with caution in patients with chronic cardiac disease as they prolong the PR and QTc interval in some experimental animals. Intramuscular preparations are widely used in the developing world as pre-referral treatment for patients with severe falciparum malaria who are unable to reach the nearest health facility safely in good time. Intravenous aretesunate

is now the preferred antimalarial for severe falciparum malaria in the developed world. Artemisinins are not appropriate for prophylaxis (because of their short $t_{1/2}$) and should never be used as monotherapy for unconplicated falciparum malaria.

Artemisinin-based combination therapies (ACTs)

Riamet, a combination of artemether 20 mg and lumefantrine 120 mg, is licensed for acute uncomplicated falciparum malaria. Lumefantrine has the advantage of not being available as a single agent (unlike other ACTs), and hence less likely to generate resistance as a result of selection pressure due to inappropriate monotherapy. Riamet is highly effective, with cure rates exceeding 96%, even in areas with drug-resistant falciparum malaria. It is the first fixed dose ACT to satisfy stringent international quality and efficacy criteria and is now widely used as the standard of care for the treatment of uncomplicated falciparum malaria. The drug is given as a complex 6-dose regimen over a 60-hour period. Adverse effects are uncommon, but irreversible hearing loss is reported.

Other WHO-approved ACTs include:

- Artesunate plus mefloquine.
- Artesunate plus amodiaquine.
- Artesunate plus sulfadoxine-pyrimethamine.
- Dihydroartemisinin plus piperaquine.

Although the combination of artesunate and mefloquine shows similar efficacy to Riamet, there are concerns with tolerability of mefloquine, particularly among African children. ACTs containing amodiaquine and pyrimethamine-sulfadoxine should be avoided in areas where resistance to these agents exceeds 20%, e.g. parts of Southeast Asia.

Amoebiasis

Infection occurs when mature cysts are ingested and pass into the colon, where they divide into trophozoites; these forms either enter the tissues or form cysts. Amoebiasis occurs in two forms, both of which need treatment:

- *Bowel lumen amoebiasis* is asymptomatic, and trophozoites (non-infective) and cysts (infective) are passed into the faeces. Treatment is directed at eradicating cysts with a luminal amoebicide; *diloxanide furoate* is the drug of choice; *iodoquinol* or *paromomycin* are alternatives.
- *Tissue-invading amoebiasis* gives rise to dysentery, hepatic amoebiasis and liver abscess. A systemically active drug (tissue amoebicide) effective against trophozoites must be used, e.g. *metronidazole, tinidazole, ornidazole*. Parenteral forms of these are

Table 15.5 Drugs for some protozoal infections

Infection	Drug and comment
Giardiasis	Metronidazole, tinidazole or mepacrine
Leishmaniasis	
visceral	Sodium stibogluconate or meglumine antimoniate; resistant cases may benefit from combining antimonials with paromomycin, miltefosine or amphotericin (including AmBisome). Pentamidine is rarely used now due to toxicity concerns
cutaneous	Mild lesions heal spontaneously, fluconazole; antimonials or paromomycin may be injected intralesionally
Toxoplasmosis	Most infections are self-limiting in the immunologically normal patient. Pyrimethamine with sulfadiazine for chorioretinitis, and active toxoplasmosis in immunodeficient patients; folinic acid is used to counteract the inevitable megaloblastic anaemia. Alternatives include pyrimethamine with clindamycin or azithromycin or atovaquone. Spiramycin for primary toxoplasmosis in pregnant women. Expert advice is essential
Trichomoniasis	Metronidazole or tinidazole is effective
Trypanosomiasis	
African (sleeping sickness)	Suramin or pentamidine is effective during the early stages but not for the later neurological manifestations for which melarsoprol should be used. Eflornithine is effective for both early and late stages. Expert advice is recommended
American (Chagas' disease)	Prolonged (1–3 months) treatment with benznidazole or nifurtimox may be effective

available for patients too ill to take drugs by mouth. In severe cases of amoebic dysentery with suspected or confirmed peritonitis, broad-spectrum antibiotics should be administered and surgical intervention considered.

Treatment with tissue amoebicides should always be followed by a course of a luminal amoebicide to eradicate the source of the infection.

Dehydroemetine (from ipecacuanha), less toxic than the parent emetine, is claimed by some authorities to be the most effective tissue amoebicide. It is reserved for the treatment of metronidazole-resistant amoebiasis and in dangerously ill patients, but these are more likely to be vulnerable to its cardiotoxic effects. When dehydroemetine is used to treat amoebic liver abscess, chloroquine should also be given.

The drug treatment of other protozoal infections is summarised in Table 15.5.

Notes on drugs for protozoal infections

Atovaquone is a quinone; it may cause gastrointestinal and mild neurological side-effects, and rare hepatotoxicity and blood dyscrasias.

Benznidazole is a nitroimidazole that may occasionally cause peripheral neuritis but is generally well tolerated, including by infants.

Dehydroemetine inhibits protein synthesis; it may cause pain at the site of injection, weakness and muscular pain, hypotension, precordial pain and cardiac arrhythmias.

Diloxanide furoate may cause troublesome flatulence, and pruritus and urticaria may occur.

Eflornithine inhibits protozoal DNA synthesis; it may cause anaemia, leucopenia and thrombocytopenia, and seizures.

Iodoquinol may cause abdominal cramps, nausea and diarrhoea. Skin eruptions, pruritus ani and thyroid gland enlargement have been attributed to its iodine content. The recognition of severe neurotoxicity with the related drug, clioquinol, in Japan in the 1960s must give cause for caution in its use.

Meglumine antimonate is a pentavalent antimony compound, similar to sodium stibogluconate (below).

Melarsoprol, a trivalent organic arsenical, acts through its high affinity for sulphydryl groups of enzymes. Adverse effects include encephalopathy, myocardial damage, proteinuria and hypertension.

Mepacrine (quinacrine) was formerly used as an antimalarial but is now an alternative to metronidazole or tinidazole for giardiasis. It may cause gastrointestinal upset, occasional acute toxic psychosis, hepatitis and aplastic anaemia.

Nifurtimox is a nitrofuran derivative. Adverse effects include anorexia, nausea, vomiting, gastric pain, insomnia, headache, vertigo, excitability, myalgia, arthralgia and convulsions. Peripheral neuropathy may necessitate stopping treatment.

Paromomycin, an aminoglycoside, is not absorbed from the gut; it is similar to neomycin.

Pentamidine is a synthetic aromatic amidine; it must be administered parenterally or by inhalation as it is absorbed unreliably from the gastrointestinal tract; it does not enter the CSF. Given systemically it frequently causes nephrotoxicity, which is reversible; acute hypotension and syncope are common especially after rapid i.v. injection. Pancreatic damage may cause hypoglycaemia due to insulin release.

Sodium stibogluconate (Pentostam) is an organic pentavalent antimony compound; it may cause anorexia, vomiting, coughing and substernal pain. Used in mucocutaneous leishmaniasis, it may lead to severe inflammation around pharyngeal or tracheal lesions which may require control with corticosteroid. *Meglumine antimoniate* is similar.

Suramin forms stable complexes with plasma protein and is detectable in urine for up to 3 months after the last injection; it does not cross the blood–brain barrier. It may cause tiredness, anorexia, malaise, polyuria, thirst, and tenderness of the palms and soles.

Miltefosine is a phosphocholine analogue that was originally developed as an oral antineoplastic. It is the only effective oral treatment for cutaneous and visceral leishmaniasis. The main adverse effects are vomiting, diarrhoea and raised transaminases. The drug is teratogenic in animals, and therefore should be avoided in pregnancy and used with caution in women of reproductive age.

Helminthic infections

Helminths have complex life cycles, special knowledge of which is required by those who treat infections. Table 15.6 will suffice here. Drug resistance has not so far proved to be a clinical problem, though it has occurred in animals on continuous chemoprophylaxis.

Drugs for helminthic infections

Albendazole is similar to mebendazole (below).

Diethylcarbamazine kills both microfilariae and adult worms. Fever, headache, anorexia, malaise, urticaria, vomiting and asthmatic attacks following the first dose are due to products of destruction of the parasite, and reactions are minimised by slow increase in dosage over the first 3 days.

Ivermectin may cause immediate reactions due to the death of the microfilaria (see diethylcarbamazine). It can be effective in a single dose, but is best repeated at intervals of 6–12 months.

Levamisole paralyses the musculature of sensitive nematodes which, unable to maintain their anchorage, are expelled by normal peristalsis. It is well tolerated, but may cause abdominal pain, nausea, vomiting, headache and dizziness.

Mebendazole blocks glucose uptake by nematodes. Mild gastrointestinal discomfort may be caused, and it should not be used in pregnancy or in children younger than 2 years of age.

Metriphonate is an organophosphorus anticholinesterase compound that was originally used as an insecticide. Adverse effects include abdominal pain, nausea, vomiting, diarrhoea, headache and vertigo.

Niclosamide blocks glucose uptake by intestinal tapeworms. It may cause some mild gastrointestinal symptoms.

Piperazine may cause hypersensitivity reactions, neurological symptoms (including 'worm wobble') and may precipitate epilepsy.

Praziquantel paralyses both adult worms and larvae. It is metabolised extensively. Praziquantel may cause nausea, headache, dizziness and drowsiness; it cures with a single dose (or divided doses in 1 day).

Pyrantel depolarises neuromuscular junctions of susceptible nematodes, which are expelled in the faeces. It cures with a single dose. It may induce gastrointestinal disturbance, headache, dizziness, drowsiness and insomnia.

Tiabendazole inhibits cellular enzymes of susceptible helminths. Gastrointestinal, neurological and hypersensitivity reactions, liver damage and crystalluria may be induced.

Table 15.6 Drugs for helminthic infections		
Infection	Drug	Comment
Cestodes (tapeworms) Beef tapeworm *Taenia saginata*	Niclosamide or praziquantel	Praziquantel cures with single dose
Pork tapeworm *Taenia solium*	Niclosamide or praziquantel	Praziquantel cures with single dose
Cysticercosis *Taenia solium*	Albendazole or praziquantel	Treat in hospital as dying and disintegrating cysts may cause cerebral oedema
Fish tapeworm *Diphyllobothrium latum*	Niclosamide or praziquantel	

Continued

Table 15.6 Drugs for helminthic infections—cont'd

Infection	Drug	Comment
Hydatid disease *Echinococcus granulosus*	Albendazole	Surgery for operable cyst disease
Nematodes (intestinal)		
Ascariasis *Ascaris lumbricoides*	Levamisole, mebendazole, pyrantel pamoate, piperazine or albendazole	
Hookworm *Ancylostoma duodenale*	Mebendazole, albendazole or pyrantel pamoate	Anaemic patients require iron or blood transfusion
Necator americanus	Albendazole	
Strongyloidiasis *Strongyloides stercoralis*	Thiabendazole or ivermectin	Alternatively, albendazole is better tolerated
Threadworm (pinworm) *Enterobius vermicularis*	Pyrantel pamoate, mebendazole, albendazole or piperazine salts	
Whipworm *Trichuris trichiuria*	Mebendazole or albendazole	
Nematodes (tissue)		
Cutaneous larva migrans *Ancylostoma braziliense; Ancylostoma caninum*	Thiabendazole (topical for single tracks); ivermectin, albendazole or oral thiabendazole (for multiple tracks)	Calamine lotion for symptom relief
Guinea worm *Dracunculus medinensis*	Metronidazole, mebendazole	Rapid symptom relief
Trichinellosis *Trichinella spiralis*	Mebendazole	Prednisolone may be needed to suppress allergic and inflammatory symptoms
Visceral larva migrans *Toxocara canis; Toxocara cati*	Diethylcarbamazine, albendazole or mebendazole	Progressive escalation of dose lessens allergic reactions to dying larvae; prednisolone suppresses inflammatory response in ophthalmic disease
Lymphatic filariasis *Wuchereria bancrofti; Brugia malayi; Brugia timori*	Diethylcarbamazine	Destruction of microfilia may cause an immunological reaction (see below)
Onchocerciasis (river blindness) *Onchocerca volvulus*	Ivermectin	Cures with single dose. Suppressive treatment; a single annual dose prevents significant complications
Schistosomiasis (intestinal)		
Schistosoma mansoni; Schistosoma japonicum	Praziquantel	Oxamniquine only for *Schistosoma mansoni*
Schistosomiasis (urinary)		
Schistosoma haematobium	Praziquantel	Metriphonate only for *Schistosoma haematobium*
Flukes (intestinal, lung, liver)	Praziquantel	Alternatives: niclosamide for intestinal fluke, bithionol for lung fluke

Guide to further reading

American Centers for Disease Control and Prevention (CDC-P). Their website includes a comprehensive travel section that contains high-quality and up-to-date information about prophylaxis, avoidance, diagnosis and treatment of infectious diseases of travel. Available at: http://www.cdc.gov/travel (Accessed May 2017).

Beigel, J.H., Farrar, J., Han, A.M., et al., of the Writing Committee of WHO Consultation on Human Influenza A/H5, 2005. Avian influenza A (H5N1) infection in humans. N. Engl. J. Med. 353, 1374–1385.

Bethony, J., Brooker, S., Albonico, M., et al., 2006. Soil-transmitted helminth infections: ascariasis, trichuriasis, and hookworm. Lancet 367, 1521–1532.

Bouchaud, O., Imbert, P., Touze, J.E., et al., 2009. Fatal cardiotoxicity related to halofantrine: a review based on a worldwide safety data base. Malar. J. 8, 289.

British HIV Association, The Association provides a wealth of information on best practice management of HIV infection and opportunistic infections. Available at: http://www.bhiva.org/ClinicalGuidelines.aspx (Accessed May 2017).

Bruce-Chwatt, L.J., 1988. Three hundred and fifty years of the Peruvian fever bark. BMJ 296, 1486–1487.

Chiodini, P., Hill, D., Lalloo, D., et al., 2007. Guidelines for Malaria Prevention in Travellers to the United Kingdom. Health Protection Agency, London. January 2007.

Edwards, G., Biagini, G.A., 2006. Resisting resistance: dealing with the irrepressible problem of malaria. Br. J. Clin. Pharmacol. 61, 690–693.

Esté, J.A., Telenti, A., 2007. HIV entry inhibitors. Lancet 370, 81–88.

European Group for Blood and Bone Marrow Transplantation. Their website has an Infectious Diseases Working Party section containing recent evidence-based recommendations for managing fungal and viral infections. See European Conference on Infection in Leukaemia (ECIL-3) Working Party Guidelines. Available at: http://www.ebmt.org (Accessed May 2017).

Fit for Travel. Another useful contemporary source is 'Fit for Travel', the NHS public access website providing travel health information for people travelling abroad from the UK. Available at: http://www.fitfortravel.scot.nhs.uk/ (Accessed May 2017).

Franco-Paredes, C., Santos-Preciado, J.I., 2006. Problem pathogens: prevention of malaria in travellers. Lancet Infect. Dis. 6, 139–149.

Geisbert, T.W., Jahrling, P.B., 2004. Exotic emerging viral diseases: progress and challenges. Nat. Med. 10 (Suppl. review), S110–S121.

Greenwood, B.M., Bojang, K., Whitty, C.J., Targett, G.A., 2005. Malaria. Lancet 365, 1487–1498.

Gryseels, B., Polman, K., Clerinx, J., Kestens, L., 2006. Human schistosomiasis. Lancet 368, 1106–1118.

Health Protection Agency [now part of Public Health England]. The Agency website has detailed information and links to common travel associated infections. Available at: www.hpa.org.uk (Accessed November 2011).

Jefferson, T., Demicheli, V., Rivetti, D., et al., 2006. Antivirals for influenza in healthy adults: systematic review. Lancet 367, 303–313.

Lalloo, D.G., Shingadia, D., Pasvol, G., et al., 2007. UK malaria treatment guidelines. J. Infect. 54, 111–121.

Lever, A.M.L., Aliyu, S.H., 2009. HIV and AIDS. Medicine 37, 313–390.

McManus, D.P., Zhang, W., Li, J., Bartley, P.B., 2003. Echinococcosis. Lancet 362, 1295–1304.

Merson, M.H., 2006. The HIV-AIDS pandemic at 25 – the global response. N. Engl. J. Med. 354, 2414–2417.

Montoya, J.G., Liesenfeld, O., 2004. Toxoplasmosis. Lancet 363, 1965–1976.

Murray, H.W., Berman, J.D., Davies, C.R., Saravia, N.G., 2005. Advances in leishmaniasis. Lancet 366, 1561–1577.

Patterson, T.F., 2005. Advances and challenges in management of invasive mycoses. Lancet 366, 1013–1025.

Sepkowitz, K.A., 2006. One disease, two epidemics – AIDS at 25. N. Engl. J. Med. 354, 2411–2414.

Snow, R.W., Marsh, K., 2010. Malaria in Africa: progress and prospects in the decade since the Abuja Declaration. Lancet 376, 137–139.

University of Liverpool interactive charts on antiretroviral drug interactions, information about advances in therapeutic drug monitoring and other resources. Available at: http://www.hiv-druginteractions.org (Accessed May 2017).

US Department of Health and Human Services guidelines on use of antiretroviral agents in adults and adolescents, and children, which are updated several times per year. Available at: http://www.aidsinfo.nih.gov (Accessed May 2017).

World Health Organization, data on HIV infection. Available at: http://www.who.int/topics/hiv_infections/en (Accessed May 2017).

WHO. Guidelines for the treatment of malaria, third edition. World Health Organisation, Geneva, April 2015.

Chapter | 16 |

Drugs for inflammation and joint disease

Clare Thornton, Justin C. Mason

SYNOPSIS

A vast burden of human disease involves the process of inflammation and the engagement of an immune response, often entirely appropriately as in the case of defence against infection. By contrast, a number of organ-specific and multi-system rheumatic diseases are characterised by a primary abnormality within the immune response, requiring treatments that modify or suppress it. This chapter reviews the process of inflammation, drugs in current use and those in development that act to modify it, and the management of certain common inflammatory diseases. The chapter covers the following areas:

- **Acute inflammation.**
- **Adaptive immune system.**
- **Glucocorticoids.**
- **NSAIDs/aspirin/paracetamol.**
- **Immunomodulatory drugs.**
- **Biologics.**
- **Management of common rheumatic diseases.**

Introduction

The immune system is a complex of interrelated genetic, molecular and cellular components that provides defence against invading microorganisms and aberrant native cells and repairs tissues once the pathogen is eradicated. The central process by which these are achieved is inflammation: the sequence of events by which a pathogen is detected, cells of the immune system are recruited, the pathogen is eliminated and resulting tissue damage repaired.

Inflammation is appropriate as a response to physical damage, microbial infection or malignancy. A number of illnesses result from abnormal activation or prolongation of the immune response. These include allergy (hay fever, asthma), autoimmunity (rheumatoid arthritis (RA), systemic lupus erythematosus (SLE)), and allograft rejection.

Anti-inflammatory drugs, by acting on and modifying the response of the innate immune system to a challenge, are useful in many settings to damp down an over-exuberant or pathologically prolonged inflammatory response. Immunomodulatory agents, which act on components of the adaptive immune response, are important for the treatment of complex autoimmune diseases and in preventing allograft rejection. Many drugs used in the treatment of these diseases have complex mechanisms of action, working on multiple arms of the immune response, and in some cases the principal way in which they exert their effects is not clear. Partly this is due to the complexity of the immune system itself; many components have overlapping functions, leading to redundancy, and many have several apparently unrelated actions.

Research over the last few decades has vastly improved our appreciation of the complexity of the immune system and of the pathogenesis of many autoimmune diseases. Although there does not appear to be one single factor that leads inexorably to the development or perpetuation of any inflammatory disease, certain mediators that play central roles in specific diseases have been identified. The advent of monoclonal antibodies, fusion proteins and other new drug development technology has allowed the manufacture of a rapidly expanding group of new agents ('biologicals') that target specific components of the immune response thought to be driving particular diseases. These drugs have dramatically changed treatment paradigms, and hopefully will lead to significant improvements in the future outlook for patients suffering rheumatic disease.

Inflammation

The process of acute inflammation is initiated when resident tissue leucocytes (macrophages or mast cells) detect a challenge, for example pathogenic bacteria, or monosodium urate crystals in the case of gout. This sets off a cascade of intracellular signalling that results in activation of the cell, release of soluble cytokines such as tumour necrosis factor-α (TNFα), interleukin-1 (IL-1) and interleukin-6 (IL-6) and other mediators such as histamine and prostaglandins. IL-1, IL-6 and TNFα stimulate endothelial cells at the site of injury to express cellular adhesion molecules, which attract and bind circulating leucocytes, principally neutrophils, and induce them to leave the circulation and migrate into the affected area. They also have systemic effects such as the development of fever and the production of acute phase proteins including C-reactive protein (CRP).

Neutrophils, along with macrophages, phagocytose the injurious stimulus and destroy it. Neutrophils and macrophages may also cause damage to the surrounding host tissue through the release of digesting enzymes such as matrix metalloproteinases and collagenases. The inflammatory process therefore needs to be halted rapidly once the invading organism has been cleared. This occurs partly because neutrophils have a very short lifespan and die quickly once they have left the circulation, and partly through the release of anti-inflammatory mediators.

Several drugs in current use act on the various stages of this inflammatory process. Antagonists of TNFα, IL-1 and IL-6 are available (see Biologic agents, p. 262). Colchicine, used in the treatment of gout, interferes with neutrophil chemotaxis, thus inhibiting their recruitment to the site of inflammation.

Many leucocytes, including mast cells and macrophages, as well as endothelial cells, synthesise pro-inflammatory eicosanoids and platelet-activating factor (PAF) (Fig. 16.1). These are 20-carbon unsaturated fatty acids derived from phospholipid substrates in the plasma membrane by the enzymes phospholipase A_2, cyclo-oxygenase (COX) and lipo-oxygenase (which are induced by IL-1). The prostaglandins, thromboxanes and leukotrienes have diverse pro-inflammatory roles. Leukotrienes promote the activation and accumulation of leucocytes at sites of inflammation. Prostaglandins induce vasodilatation of the microcirculation and are important in pain signalling from locally inflamed tissue. Platelet-activating factor and thromboxane A_2 affect the coagulation and fibrinolytic cascades. Non-steroidal anti-inflammatory drugs (NSAIDs), including aspirin, inhibit COX and hence prostaglandin and thromboxane synthesis. Glucocorticoids act by inducing the synthesis of lipocortin-1, a polypeptide that inhibits phospholipase A_2, and thereby

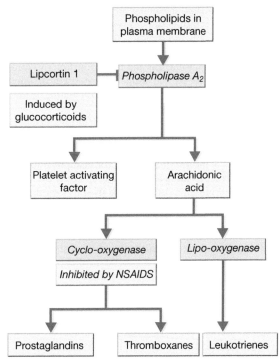

Fig. 16.1 Synthesis of eicosanoids and platelet-activating factor, and drugs acting on this pathway. The enzymes phospholipase A_2, cyclo-oxygenase and lipo-oxygenase are involved in the synthesis of prostaglandins, thromboxanes, leukotrienes and platelet-activating factor, all of which are derived from phospholipid substrates in plasma membranes. Glucocorticoids induce lipocortin 1, which inhibits phospholipase A_2. NSAIDs inhibit cyclo-oxygenases 1 and 2, preventing formation of prostaglandins and thromboxanes.

exert a broad anti-inflammatory effect. The leukotriene receptor antagonists montelukast and zafirlukast cause bronchodilatation and are used to treat asthma.

The adaptive immune response

The adaptive immune response, although integrated into the process of inflammation, becomes active at later stages. Its key properties are (1) specificity: each B and T lymphocyte recognises a single specific peptide sequence; and (2) memory: when an invading pathogen has been recognised once, a small number of specific cells remain dormant within the lymph tissue for many years. If that pathogen is detected again, a very rapid response is mounted to eradicate it before the development of clinical symptoms.

An adaptive immune response is initiated when a helper T cell recognises a peptide antigen presented on the surface of an antigen-presenting cell (APC) and is activated (Fig. 16.2). The activated helper T cell is then able to activate other types of T cells and B cells. This results in the proliferation of adaptive cellular effectors, the generation and release of antibodies by plasma cells and the production of a range of cytokines by the participating leucocytes. On occasion, amplification loops may become self-perpetuating, leading to chronic autoimmune disease.

Many immunomodulatory drugs, such as the calcineurin inhibitors, seek to break these loops by inhibiting lymphocyte proliferation. Other newer approaches target specific components of the immune system. For example, rituximab binds CD20, a cell surface molecule found only on B lymphocytes and not memory cells. It is used to treat diseases in which pathogenic autoantibody production is prominent, such as rheumatoid arthritis and SLE. Abatacept blocks co-stimulatory signals, which are required when a helper T cell is activated, by recognising bound antigen presented by an APC. This is a central process in the pathogenesis of rheumatoid arthritis, and abatacept is licensed to treat this.

Pharmacological manipulation of inflammatory mediators

Glucocorticoids

Glucocorticoids (GCs) are among the most widely prescribed anti-inflammatory drugs, due to their profound efficacy, long history of use and familiarity. Besides their anti-inflammatory actions, they exert effects on carbohydrate, protein and lipid metabolism, some of which contribute to their substantial adverse effect profile.

GCs are used in acute and chronic settings to treat inflammatory conditions ranging from asthma and allergy, to prevention of allograft rejection, to rheumatoid arthritis and systemic vasculitis. Because of their rapid onset of action (less than 24 h) and potency, they remain the preferred acute treatment for severe inflammatory disease in a wide variety of settings despite their adverse effects. In chronic disease, the aim now is to minimise cumulative exposure

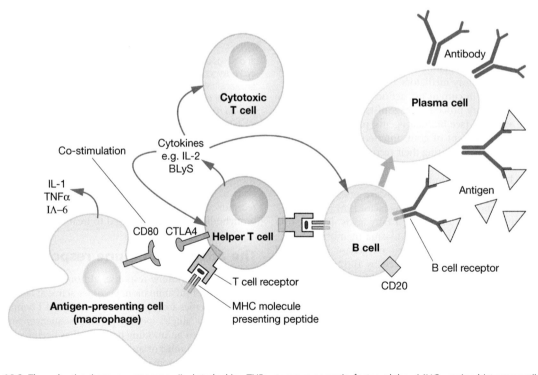

Fig. 16.2 The adaptive immune response. IL, interleukin; TNFa, tumour necrosis factor alpha; MHC, major histocompatibility complex; BLyS, B-lymphocyte stimulating factor. Helper T cells are activated through interaction with antigen presenting cells, leading to cytokine release and activation of cytotoxic T cells and B cells. B cells bind specific antigens, and mature into plasma cells.

by using other immunomodulatory 'steroid-sparing' drugs, and proactively to manage potential long-term side-effects such as osteoporosis.

Mode of action

GCs, being lipophilic, diffuse across the cell membrane and bind the cytosolic glucocorticoid receptor (GR) (Fig. 16.3). Receptor polymorphisms influence the strength of the receptor interaction, and represent one source of variation in sensitivity to exogenous steroids. Once bound, the GC-GR complex translocates to the nucleus where it acts in at least two ways to alter gene transcription:

1. The GC-GR complex binds to the glucocorticoid response element within target gene promoters, increasing transcription of various anti-inflammatory genes. These include I-κB, which inhibits the activation of nuclear factor (NF)-κB, and the cytokines IL-4, IL-10, IL-13 and transforming growth factor (TGF)β, which have immunosuppressive and anti-inflammatory activity.

2. The GC-GR complex interferes with the binding of the transcription factors activating protein (AP)-1 and NF-κB to their response elements. This action decreases the transcription of a range of pro-inflammatory mediators. These include IL-1β and TNFα; IL-2, which stimulates T-cell proliferation; a range of chemokines and cellular adhesion molecules; metalloproteinases; COX-2; and inducible nitric oxide synthase.

3. GCs increase synthesis of the polypeptide lipocortin-1, which inhibits phospholipase A_2 and thereby the synthesis of prostaglandins, thromboxane A_2 and PAF (see Fig. 16.1).

At the cellular level, GCs reduce the numbers of circulating lymphocytes, eosinophils and monocytes. This is maximal 4–6 hours after administration and is achieved by a combination of apoptosis induction and inhibition of proliferation. Chronic administration of GC is associated with a neutrophilia caused by release of neutrophils from the bone marrow and reduced adherence to vascular walls.

In inflammatory disease, the choice of GC preparation will reflect the site and the extent of inflamed tissue, e.g. oral or parenteral for systemic disease, inhaled in asthma, topical in cutaneous, ocular, oral or rectal disease. Different corticosteroid preparations, their pharmacokinetics, modes of delivery and adverse effects are discussed elsewhere, except for the management of steroid-induced osteoporosis, which is found in the section on management of rheumatoid arthritis at the end of this chapter.

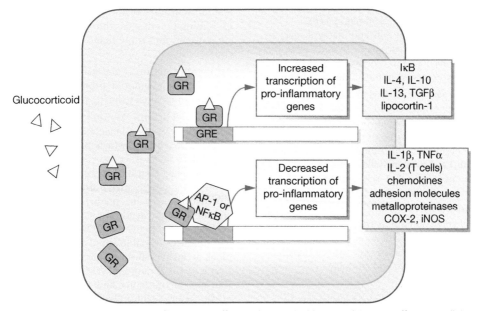

Fig. 16.3 Mechanisms of glucocorticoid anti-inflammatory effects. Glucocorticoids exert pleiotropic effects on cellular metabolism. They increase transcription of a number of genes encoding anti-inflammatory proteins and decrease transcription of pro-inflammatory genes. AP-1, activating protein-1; COX, cyclo-oxygenase; GR, glucocorticoid receptor; GRE, glucocorticoid response element; IL, interleukin; iNOS, inducible nitric oxide synthase; NF, nuclear factor; TGF, transforming growth factor.

Non-steroidal anti-inflammatory drugs (NSAIDs)

NSAIDs are an extremely widely prescribed group of drugs that are mainly used for their analgesic effects. They possess a single common mode of action: inhibition of cyclo-oxygenase, thereby reducing prostaglandin synthesis. This is also the mode of action of paracetamol (acetaminophen) and aspirin.

Recently concern has arisen over the effect of traditional NSAIDs and COX-2 inhibitors on the cardiovascular system, with analysis of the VIGOR[1] study showing that rofecoxib in particular increases the risk of myocardial infarction (rofecoxib has since been withdrawn from use). While they retain an important role in the treatment of acute gout, inflammatory arthritis, ankylosing spondylitis and dysmenorrhea, long-term prescription should only be undertaken following a full discussion with the patient regarding the balance of risks and benefits.

Mode of action

NSAIDs inhibit cyclo-oxygenase (COX), which catalyses the synthesis of prostaglandins and thromboxane from arachidonic acid (see Fig. 16.1). There are two isoforms of COX:

- COX-1 is *constitutively*[2] expressed in most cell types.
- COX-2 is *induced* when inflammatory cells (fibroblasts, endothelial cells and macrophages) are activated by cytokines such as IL-1β and TNFα. It is also often upregulated in cancer cells, and is constitutively expressed in the kidney and brain.

Both isoforms generate prostaglandins during an inflammatory response, while COX-1 activity is required for prostaglandin synthesis for tissue homeostasis. Thus, many NSAID adverse effects are due to reductions in beneficial prostaglandin production, for example in the gastric mucosa (PGI_2 and PGE_2) and renal medulla. Recognition of this led to the development of COX-2–selective drugs.

NSAIDs can be categorised according to their COX specificity as:

- COX-2–*selective* compounds (coxibs), which inhibit COX-2 with at least five times greater potency than COX-1. The group includes celecoxib, etoricoxib, lumiracoxib, meloxicam and etodolac.

- *Non–COX-2–selective* compounds, which comprise all other NSAIDs. These drugs inhibit COX-1 as well as COX-2.

Pharmacokinetics

NSAIDs are absorbed almost completely from the gastrointestinal tract, tend not to undergo first-pass elimination (see p. 89), are highly protein bound and have small volumes of distribution. Their $t_{1/2}$ values in plasma tend to group into short (1–5 h) or long (10–60 h). Differences in $t_{1/2}$ are not necessarily reflected proportionately in duration of effect, as peak and trough drug concentrations at their intended site of action following steady-state dosing are much less than those in plasma. The vast majority of NSAIDs are weak organic acids and localise preferentially in the synovial tissue of inflamed joints (see pH partition hypothesis, p. 82).

Uses

Analgesia. All NSAIDs are analgesics and are particularly effective for disorders with an inflammatory component, as the analgesic action is due to COX inhibition, both in the brain and at the site of inflammation. The non-selective and COX-2-selective agents have generally comparable analgesic efficacies.

Anti-inflammatory action. The majority of NSAIDs are anti-inflammatory because they inhibit COX in the periphery. COX inhibition in most chronic inflammatory conditions, while useful for symptomatic relief, does not modify the course of disease.

Antipyretic action. Paracetamol and all other NSAIDs reduce cytokine-induced prostaglandin synthesis in the hypothalamus, thus reducing fever.

Antiplatelet action. Aspirin irreversibly acetylates a serine residue in COX-1. In platelets, the main result is inhibition of thromboxane A_2 (which promotes platelet adhesion, coagulation and vasoconstriction) production for the life of the platelet (7 days). This is the basis for the use of aspirin to prevent and treat arterial thromboses secondary to atherosclerosis and other predisposing illnesses such as the antiphospholipid syndrome.

Other non-selective NSAIDs bind reversibly to COX-1 and produce a variable antiplatelet action. Ibuprofen may block access of aspirin to the active site on platelets and interfere with its cardioprotective effect when taken regularly (but not intermittently, and aspirin taken 2 h before ibuprofen may avoid the problem). Other NSAIDs do not appear to have this interaction.

It has been suggested that inhibition of COX-2 reduces synthesis of endothelial PGI_2 (prostacyclin – which acts to prevent platelet aggregation and causes vasodilatation), while

---

[1]Bombardier C, Laine L, Reicin A et al 2000 Comparison of upper gastrointestinal toxicity of rofecoxib and naproxen in patients with rheumatoid arthritis. VIGOR study group. New England Journal of Medicine 343:1520–1528.
[2]Continuously produced, rather than depending on the presence of an inducer.

allowing the continued production of COX-1–derived thromboxane A_2. In theory, this could alter the balance within the vasculature in favour of thromboxane A_2 and increase the risk of cardiovascular events, although the relative contributions of COX-1 and COX-2 in endothelial prostacyclin synthesis remain to be determined.

Colorectal cancer. Long-term administration of an NSAID reduces the incidence of colonic cancer by approximately 50%. This appears to be related to the inhibition of COX-2, which is up-regulated in colon tumours.

Adverse effects

Gastrointestinal. Dyspepsia is one of the commonest side-effects of NSAIDs. The propensity to gastrointestinal (GI) ulceration may result in occult or overt blood loss. Use of NSAIDs is associated with an approximately four-fold increased incidence of severe GI haemorrhage, and such complications account for between 700 and 2000 deaths in the UK each year. In addition, ulceration and stricture of the small intestine can result in anaemia, diarrhoea and malabsorption, similar to Crohn's disease. The risk of NSAID-induced GI haemorrhage is associated with high doses and prolonged use; age older than 65 years; previous history of peptic ulceration; concomitant use of glucocorticoids, anticoagulants or other NSAIDs; heavy smoking and alcohol use; and the presence of *Helicobacter pylori* infection.

NSAID-associated GI disease appears to result from the inhibition of COX-1–mediated production of cytoprotective mucosal prostaglandins, especially PGI_2 and PGE_2, which inhibit acid secretion in the stomach, promote mucus production and enhance mucosal perfusion. Several large randomised controlled trials have investigated the incidence of GI adverse effects in traditional NSAIDs compared with coxibs. The VIGOR (rofecoxib versus naproxen), CLASS[3] (celecoxib versus ibuprofen and diclofenac) and TARGET[4] (lumiracoxib versus ibuprofen and naproxen) studies all indicate that coxib use leads to an approximately 50% reduction of upper GI adverse events.

The GI toxicity of traditional NSAIDs may be reduced by co-prescription of a proton pump inhibitor, e.g. omeprazole, an H_2-receptor blocker, e.g. ranitidine, or the prostaglandin analogue misoprostol. Proton pump inhibitors are more effective than the other classes of gastroprotective agent and should be considered in all patients with at least one of the above risk factors. In fact, it is now recommended by the UK National Institute for Health and Clinical Effectiveness (NICE) that all patients older than 45 years prescribed an NSAID, whether COX-2 selective or not, also receive a proton pump inhibitor.

Cardiovascular. The VIGOR and APPROVE[5] trials reported increased thrombotic cardiovascular events in patients treated with rofecoxib, leading to concerns about a class effect of the coxibs. It was suggested that COX-2 selectivity resulted in an imbalance between prostacyclin and thromboxane production, an effect which would not be seen with traditional NSAIDs, which inhibited the synthesis of both equally. Subsequent data from the prospective MEDAL[6] and TARGET trials have not supported a class effect based on COX-2 selectivity. These studies suggest that treatment with either a coxib or an NSAID results in a small increase in cardiovascular risk. The risk is dose-related, and rofecoxib, particularly at doses exceeding 50 mg/day, confers the highest cardiovascular risk in the majority of studies. A recent study of more than 1 million patients quantified cardiovascular risk as a composite of coronary death, non-fatal myocardial infarction and fatal and non-fatal stroke, and reported that diclofenac and rofecoxib were associated with the highest cardiovascular risk, while naproxen and perhaps celecoxib at doses ≤200 mg/day were the least likely to cause a cardiovascular event.[7] NICE guidelines recommend that patients with pro-thrombotic risk, coronary artery or cerebrovascular disease should not be prescribed NSAIDs or a coxib. For other patients, treatment decisions should be made on an individual patient basis taking into account both cardiovascular and GI risk factors. The medication should be prescribed for the shortest possible time and regularly reviewed.

Renal. NSAIDs decrease renal perfusion in individuals with congestive cardiac failure, chronic renal disease and cirrhosis with ascites: states in which renal perfusion is dependent upon prostaglandin-mediated vasodilatation. NSAIDs may also promote sodium and water retention, causing oedema and hypertension in some individuals. Papillary necrosis and interstitial nephritis are rare complications, often in the context of chronic and excessive NSAID use.

[3]Silverstein F E, Faich G, Goldstein J L et al 2000 Gastrointestinal toxicity with celecoxib vs nonsteroidal anti-inflammatory drugs for osteoarthritis and rheumatoid arthritis: the CLASS study: a randomized controlled trial. Celecoxib Long-term Arthritis Safety Study. Journal of the American Medical Association 284:1247–1255.
[4]Farkouh M E, Kirshner H, Harrington R A et al 2004 Comparison of lumiracoxib with naproxen and ibuprofen in the Therapeutic Arthritis Research and Gastrointestinal Event Trial (TARGET), cardiovascular outcomes: randomised controlled trial. Lancet 364:675–684.

[5]Bresalier R S, Sandler R S, Quan H et al 2005 Cardiovascular events associated with rofecoxib in a colorectal adenoma chemoprevention trial. New England Journal of Medicine 352:1092–1102.
[6]Cannon C P, Curtis S P, FitzGerald G A et al 2006 Cardiovascular outcomes with etoricoxib and diclofenac in patients with osteoarthritis and rheumatoid arthritis in the Multinational Etoricoxib and Diclofenac Arthritis Long-term (MEDAL) programme: a randomised comparison. Lancet 368:1771–1781.
[7]Fosbøl E L, Folke F, Jacobsen S et al 2010 Cause-specific cardiovascular risk associated with nonsteroidal antiinflammatory drugs among healthy individuals. Circulation, Cardiovascular Quality and Outcomes 3:395–405.

Worsening of asthma. NSAID intolerance in asthmatics probably reflects diversion of arachidonic acid metabolism towards excessive products of the lipo-oxygenase pathway. It is not immune-mediated but clinically may resemble hypersensitivity, with manifestations including vasomotor rhinitis, urticaria, bronchoconstriction, flushing, hypotension and shock.

Other unwanted effects include headache, confusion, photosensitivity, erythema multiforme, toxic epidermal necrolysis, deranged liver function, cytopenias, haemolytic anaemia and inhibition of ovulation.

Principal interactions

NSAID interactions include:

- Angiotensin-converting enzyme (ACE) inhibitors and angiotensin II receptor blockers: there is a risk of renal impairment and hyperkalaemia.
- Quinolone antimicrobials: convulsions may occur if NSAIDs are co-administered.
- Anticoagulant (warfarin) and antiplatelet agents (dypiridamole, clopidogrel): there is an increased risk of GI bleeding with NSAIDs.
- Antihypertensives: their effect is lessened due to sodium retention by inhibition of renal prostaglandin formation.
- Ciclosporin and tacrolimus: their nephrotoxic effect is exacerbated by NSAIDs.
- Cytotoxics: renal tubular excretion of methotrexate is reduced by competition with NSAIDs, with risk of methotrexate toxicity (low-dose methotrexate given weekly avoids this hazard).
- Diuretics: NSAIDs cause sodium retention and reduce diuretic efficacy, and there is a risk of hyperkalaemia with potassium-sparing diuretics.
- Lithium: NSAIDs delay the excretion of lithium by the kidney and may cause lithium toxicity.

Paracetamol (acetaminophen)

Mode of action and uses. Paracetamol is an effective treatment for mild-moderate pain and for relieving fever. It does not affect platelet function or disrupt the GI mucosal barrier. Paracetamol has analgesic efficacy equivalent to aspirin, but in therapeutic doses it has only weak anti-inflammatory effects, a functional separation that reflects its differential inhibition of enzymes responsible for prostaglandin synthesis.[8] For this reason, some would not class paracetamol as an NSAID.

Pharmacokinetics. Paracetamol ($t_{1/2}$ 2 h) is well absorbed from the GI tract. It is inactivated in the liver, principally by conjugation as glucuronide and sulphate. Minor metabolites of paracetamol are also formed, of which one oxidation product, N-acetyl-p-benzoquinone imine (NAPQI), is highly reactive chemically. This substance is normally rendered harmless by conjugation with glutathione. The supply of hepatic glutathione is limited, and if the amount of NAPQI formed is greater than the amount of glutathione available, the excess metabolite oxidises thiol (SH-) groups on key enzymes, causing cell death. This is the mechanism of hepatic necrosis in paracetamol overdose.

Dose. The oral dose is 0.5–1 g every 4–6 h; maximum daily dose 4 g.

Adverse effects. Paracetamol is usually well tolerated. Allergic reactions and rash sometimes occur. Maximal, long-term, daily dosing may predispose to chronic renal disease.

Acute overdose. Severe hepatocellular damage and renal tubular necrosis can result from taking 150 mg/kg body-weight (about 10 or 20 tablets) in one dose.[9] Patients at particular risk include:

- Those whose enzymes are induced as a result of taking drugs or alcohol; their liver and kidneys form more NAPQI.
- Those who are malnourished (chronic alcohol abuse, eating disorders, HIV infection) to the extent that the liver and kidneys are depleted of glutathione to conjugate with NAPQI.

Clinical signs of hepatic damage (jaundice, abdominal pain, hepatic tenderness) and increased liver enzymes do not become apparent for 24–48 h after the overdose. Hepatic failure may ensue 2–7 days later; and is best monitored using prothrombin time.

The plasma concentration of paracetamol is of predictive value; if it lies above a semi-logarithmic graph joining points between 200 mg/L (1.32 mmol/L) at 4 h after ingestion to 50 mg/L (0.33 mmol/L) at 12 h, then serious hepatic damage is likely (plasma concentrations measured earlier than 4 h are unreliable because of incomplete absorption). Patients who are malnourished are regarded as being at risk at 50% of these plasma concentrations.

The general principles for limiting drug absorption apply if the patient is seen within 4 h. Activated charcoal by mouth

---

[8]Aronoff D M, Oates J A, Boutaud O et al 2006 New insights into the mechanism of action of acetaminophen: its clinical pharmacological characteristics reflect inhibition of the two prostaglandin H_2 synthases. Clinical Pharmacology and Therapeutics 79:9–19.

[9]A 73-year-old woman was taking paracetamol for pain relief but added a paracetamol-containing proprietary preparation for cold relief, in effect nearly doubling the dose. She died of paracetamol poisoning. Her husband said that his wife 'knew that too much paracetamol was dangerous but she did not realise there was paracetamol in [the proprietary preparation]' which she bought at a supermarket that did not have a dispensary counter where she could have received advice. Report 2011 British Medical Journal 342:971.

is effective and should be considered if paracetamol in excess of 150 mg/kg body-weight or 12 g, whichever is the smaller, is thought to have been ingested within the previous hour. The decision to use activated charcoal must take into account its capacity to bind the oral antidote methionine.

Specific therapy involves replenishing stores of liver glutathione, which conjugates NAPQI and so diminishes the amount available to do harm. Glutathione itself cannot be used as it penetrates cells poorly, but N-acetylcysteine (NAC) and methionine are effective as they are precursors for the synthesis of glutathione. NAC is administered intravenously – an advantage if the patient is vomiting. The regimen is: 150 mg/kg in 200 mL 5% dextrose over 15 min; then 50 mg/kg in 500 mL 5% dextrose over 4 h; then 100 mg/kg in 1000 mL 5% dextrose over 16 h. While it is most effective if administered within 8 h of the overdose, evidence shows that continuing treatment for up to 72 h still provides benefit. Methionine alone may be used to initiate treatment when facilities for infusing NAC are not immediately available. The earlier such therapy is instituted the better, and it should be started if:

- a patient is estimated to have taken more than 150 mg/kg body-weight, without waiting for the measurement of the plasma concentration
- plasma concentration indicates the likelihood of liver damage (above), or
- there is uncertainty about the amount taken, or its timing.

Aspirin (acetylsalicylic acid)

In the 18th century, the Reverend Edmund Stone wrote about the value of an extract of bark from the willow tree (of the family *Salix*) for alleviating pain and fever. The active ingredient was salicin, which is metabolised to salicylic acid in vivo. Sodium salicylate manufactured from salicin proved highly successful in the treatment of rheumatic fever and gout, but it was a gastric irritant. In 1897, Felix Hoffman, a chemist at the Bayer Company, whose father developed abdominal pain with sodium salicylate, succeeded in producing acetylsalicylic acid in a form that was chemically stable. The new preparation proved acceptable to his father and paved the way for the production of aspirin.

Mode of action. The anti-inflammatory, analgesic and antipyretic actions of aspirin are those of NSAIDs in general (see above). The following additional actions are relevant:

- An antiplatelet effect due to permanent inactivation, by acetylation, of COX-1 in platelets, preventing synthesis of thromboxane A_2. Platelets cannot regenerate the enzyme, and the resumption of thromboxane A_2 production is dependent on the entry of new platelets into the circulation (platelet

lifespan is 7 days). Thus a continuous antiplatelet effect is achieved with low doses.
- Respiratory stimulation is a characteristic of aspirin intoxication and occurs both directly by stimulation of the respiratory centre and indirectly through increased carbon dioxide production.
- Although aspirin in high dose reduces renal tubular reabsorption of uric acid so increasing its elimination, other treatments for hyperuricaemia are preferred. Indeed aspirin should be avoided in gout, as low doses inhibit uric acid secretion and on balance its effects on uric acid elimination are adverse.

Uses. The main use of aspirin is as an antiplatelet agent to prevent arterial thrombotic events due to atherosclerosis. It has largely been overtaken by NSAIDs and paracetamol as an analgesic. In high doses, it is used to treat inflammation in Kawasaki disease, in combination with intravenous immunoglobulin, but in other inflammatory illnesses it has now been superseded by other, more effective agents with fewer side-effects.

Pharmacokinetics. Aspirin ($t_{1/2}$ 15 min) is well absorbed from the stomach and upper GI tract. Hydrolysis removes the acetyl group, and the resulting salicylate ion is inactivated largely by conjugation with glycine. At low doses, this reaction proceeds by first-order kinetics with a $t_{1/2}$ of about 4 h, but at high doses and in overdose the process becomes saturated, i.e. kinetics become zero order, and most of the drug in the body is present as the salicylate. The challenge in overdose is to remove salicylate.

Dose. Doses of 75–150 mg/day are used to prevent thrombotic vascular occlusion; 300 mg as immediate treatment for myocardial infarction; 300–900 mg every 4–6 h for analgesia.

Adverse effects. Gastrointestinal effects are those of NSAIDs in general. Effects particularly associated with aspirin are:

- *Salicylism* (the symptoms of an excessive dose): tinnitus and hearing difficulty, dizziness, headache and confusion.
- *Allergy.* Aspirin is a common cause of allergic or pseudoallergic symptoms and signs. Patients exhibit severe rhinitis, urticaria, angioedema, asthma or shock. Those who already suffer from recurrent urticaria, nasal polyps or asthma are more susceptible.
- *Reye's syndrome.* Epidemiological evidence relates aspirin use to the development of the rare Reye's syndrome (encephalopathy, liver injury) in children recovering from febrile viral infections. Consequently, aspirin should not be given to children younger than 15 years of age.

Acute overdose. A moderate overdose (plasma salicylate 500–750 mg/L) will cause nausea, vomiting, epigastric discomfort, tinnitus, deafness, sweating, pyrexia, restlessness, tachypnoea and hypokalaemia. A large overdose (plasma salicylate concentration above 750 mg/L) may result in pulmonary oedema, convulsions and coma, with severe dehydration and ketosis. Bleeding is unusual, despite the antiplatelet effect of aspirin.

Adults who have taken a single large quantity usually develop a respiratory alkalosis. Metabolic acidosis suggests severe poisoning, but a mixed picture is commonly seen. In children younger than 4 years of age, severe metabolic acidosis is more likely than respiratory alkalosis, especially if the drug has been ingested over many hours (e.g. mistaken for sweets).

Serial measurements of plasma salicylate are necessary to monitor the course of the overdose, for the concentration may rise in the early hours after ingestion. The general management of overdose applies, but the following are relevant for salicylate overdose:

- *Activated charcoal* 50 g by mouth prevents salicylate absorption from the GI tract. Gastric lavage or the use of an emetic is no longer recommended.
- *Correction of dehydration,* using dextrose 5% i.v. is often indicated.
- *Acid–base disturbance.* Alkalosis or mixed alkalosis/acidosis need no specific treatment. Metabolic acidosis is treated with sodium bicarbonate, which alkalinises the urine and accelerates the removal of salicylate in the urine.
- *Haemodialysis* may be necessary if renal failure develops or the plasma salicylate concentration exceeds 900 mg/L.

Colchicine

Colchicine is derived from the autumn crocus (*Colchicum autumnale*). Its anti-inflammatory properties have long been recognised: Alexander of Tralles recommended colchicum for gout in the 6th century AD. Nowadays, in addition to relieving inflammation in acute gout attacks, it is used to treat other inflammatory disorders including Behçet's syndrome and the hereditary fever syndrome familial Mediterranean fever. The precise way in which colchicine reduces inflammation is not completely understood but relates to its effects on neutrophils (which play a prominent role in the pathology of these conditions). It inhibits the assembly of microtubules, thus interfering with mitotic spindle formation and arresting cell division as well as inhibiting cell migration.

The most common adverse effect of colchicine is diarrhoea, due to its effects on rapidly proliferating GI epithelial cells.

If this is ignored, severe neutropenia may follow, and it is therefore a sign to stop the drug and restart at a lower dose. Agranulocytosis and aplastic anaemia may complicate chronic use.

Immunomodulatory drugs

Immunomodulatory drugs are used both to control symptoms and to retard or arrest the progression of chronic inflammatory diseases. They act to inhibit inflammation in a variety of ways, and reduce the proliferation and activation of lymphocytes.

The terminology surrounding immunomodulatory drugs has evolved separately in different specialties, although the underlying management principles are similar. Rheumatologists use the term 'disease-modifying anti-rheumatic drugs' (DMARDs) to describe those agents that reduce inflammatory disease activity and prevent radiologically determined disease progression in illnesses such as rheumatoid or psoriatic arthritis. Treatment regimens for systemic vasculitis or severe organ involvement in the connective tissue diseases make use of terminology drawn from oncology, with 'remission induction' followed by 'maintenance' phases. Many of these drugs are described as 'steroid-sparing' as their concomitant use with glucocorticoids substantially reduces the total cumulative dose of steroid required for disease suppression. Many can be used in combination: with steroids, with each other or with biologic agents. This is discussed in the section on specific disease management at the end of the chapter.

The choice and combination of immunomodulatory agent in an individual patient depends on the following considerations:

- Severity of disease: this determines the risk:benefit ratio. For example, cerebral or renal lupus is more hazardous than rash or arthritis, and therefore a more potent but potentially more toxic drug regimen is justified.
- Adverse-effect profile: both the probability and severity of potential adverse effects need to be considered.
- Evidence base: this, disappointingly, is often patchy but where it exists affords greater confidence for the prescribing physician.
- Age: the risk of future malignancy is less significant in elderly patients.
- Co-morbidity: drugs causing hypertension or adverse lipid profiles may be avoided in patients with high cardiovascular risk.
- Pregnancy/breast feeding: an absolute contraindication for many immunomodulatory drugs.

- Importance of future fertility: cyclophosphamide is likely to decrease fertility; leflunomide requires a long washout period prior to pregnancy.

Most conventional immunomodulatory agents act by inhibiting activation or reducing proliferation of lymphocytes. Many have more than one mechanism of action, and often the precise way in which they exert their effects is unknown. Moreover, their antiproliferative and cytotoxic effects are in most cases not specific to the immune system but will affect any rapidly dividing cell population. This is one of the major causes of toxicity. Fig. 16.4 presents an overview of these drugs and the known mechanisms of action that are relevant to the following discussion.

Methotrexate, azathioprine, mycophenolate mofetil and leflunomide are antimetabolites, interfering with the *de novo* synthesis of purines and pyrimidines, on which proliferating (but not resting) lymphocytes depend. Methotrexate is thought to have additional anti-inflammatory effects. The calcineurin antagonists (ciclosporin and tacrolimus) and

sirolimus selectively inhibit T-cell activation and proliferation, by inhibiting cytokine expression and cytokine-driven proliferation, respectively. Cyclophosphamide is an alkylating agent that is cytotoxic in dividing cells and, in an autoimmune response, is particularly toxic to rapidly proliferating lymphocytes. Intravenous immunoglobulin has immunomodulatory effects through interference with Fcγ receptor signalling, among other mechanisms. The precise mechanisms of action of sulfasalazine, hydroxychloroquine, thalidomide, dapsone and gold are less clear, but they have been shown to influence the expression of a range of pro-inflammatory cytokines.

Immunomodulatory drugs have well recognised and occasionally very serious toxic side-effects, but these only occur in a proportion of patients and/or are reversible on cessation of drug. They also often have less impact on quality of life than the inevitable effects of chronic high-dose glucocorticoid.

The complexity of prescribing and monitoring of toxicity with most immunomodulatory drugs demands collaboration between specialists, general practitioners and a well-informed

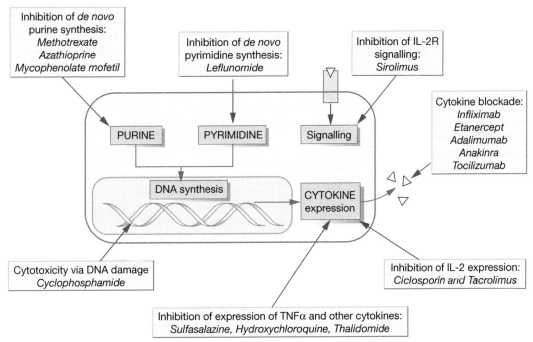

Fig. 16.4 Overview of action of immunomodulatory drugs. Many conventional immunomodulatory drugs used in rheumatology practice are anti-metabolites, inhibiting *de novo* synthesis of purines or pyrimidines; pathways upon which activated lymphocytes are particularly dependent. The mechanisms of action of sulfasalazine, hydroxychloroquine and thalidomide appear to involve inhibition of expression of pro-inflammatory cytokines. The calcineurin inhibitors and sirolimus interfere with either the expression of IL-2 or signalling downstream of the IL-2 receptor; these effects target activated T cells. Cyclophosphamide is a cytotoxic agent that indiscriminately targets proliferating cells. Several biological agents block specific pro-inflammatory cytokines. Agents in current use include those targeting TNFα, IL-1 and IL-6.

patient. All should only be initiated under specialist supervision, and all call for close monitoring, for example of bone marrow, liver, kidney or other organs, as known toxicity dictates. Live vaccines in general should not be given to immunosuppressed patients as there is a risk of disseminated infection.

Methotrexate

Methotrexate was first developed as an anticancer drug 50 years ago. Studies in the 1980s demonstrated its efficacy in rheumatoid arthritis, and it is now the principal DMARD used in this disease. It is also used to treat many other chronic inflammatory illnesses, particularly psoriatic arthritis, and in the maintenance phase of therapy for systemic vasculitis.

Mechanism of action. As a folate analogue, methotrexate inhibits folate-dependent enzymes involved in purine biosynthesis, thus reducing lymphocyte proliferation, and this was originally thought to be its principal mechanism of action (and is likely to be the source of many of its toxic effects). In recent years, however, it has become clear that methotrexate has a number of other anti-inflammatory effects, and inhibition of 5-aminoimidazole-4-carboxamide ribonucleotide (AICAR) transformylase, another folate-dependent enzyme, is now thought to be the likely pathway responsible for its efficacy in chronic inflammatory conditions.[10] This results in a rise in intracellular levels of AICAR, which then inhibits adenosine deaminase and prevents the degradation of adenosine. Increased plasma concentrations of adenosine are thought to mediate many anti-inflammatory effects such as decreased TNFα and IFNγ production.

Prescription. Methotrexate is usually prescribed orally, starting at 7.5–10 mg once weekly and increasing as bone marrow and liver function allows, up to 25 mg. Parenteral administration is also possible, but is principally used in paediatric practice. Folic acid is usually prescribed (variably 5 mg weekly, three times weekly or on all days apart from on the methotrexate dosing day), in order to mitigate the adverse effects. This appears to have little effect on the blockade of *de novo* purine synthesis, unlike folinic acid (tetrahydrofolic acid).

Adverse effects. The most serious adverse effects of methotrexate are bone marrow toxicity, hepatic toxicity and pneumonitis; regular (at least monthly) monitoring of full blood count and liver function testing are recommended, and a baseline chest X-ray is performed prior to first prescription. Methotrexate is also embryotoxic (see below). Mouth ulcers and nausea occur commonly but may be improved by co-prescription of folic acid.

Interactions. Methotrexate used with trimethoprim, co-trimoxazole or sulphonamides creates a risk of megaloblastic anaemia and pancytopenia due to the additive antifolate effect. Folinic acid rescue may be effective should this occur.

Contraindications. Methotrexate should not be prescribed to patients with moderate to severe renal impairment, liver disease or an active infection. Because of its teratogenicity, it must not be prescribed for women who are or may become pregnant or who are breast feeding. Both men and women should be counselled to use effective contraception while taking methotrexate and for 6 months afterwards.

Azathioprine

Azathioprine is another antimetabolite which acts by inhibiting purine biosynthesis, thus preferentially acting on proliferating lymphocytes. Besides its use to prevent rejection in organ transplant recipients, it has a well-established role as a disease-modifying or steroid-sparing agent in the maintenance phase of treatment of chronic inflammatory diseases, such as SLE, ANCA-associated and large vessel vasculitis, and interstitial lung disease.

Mechanism of action. Azathioprine undergoes reduction in the presence of glutathione to 6-mercaptopurine and then to 6-thioguanine. This forms a false purine nucleotide that is then incorporated into DNA, thus inhibiting DNA replication and cell proliferation. It may also trigger apoptosis. These actions result in a reduction in circulating B and T lymphocytes, reduced IL-2 secretion and reduced IgM and IgG synthesis.

Azathioprine and 6-mercaptopurine are metabolised predominantly by methylation and oxidation in the liver and/or erythrocytes, via thiopurine methyltransferase (TPMT).

Prescription. Azathioprine is taken orally, starting at 25–50 mg and rising over the course of several weeks to a daily dose of 1.5–2.5 mg/kg. Polymorphisms in the gene encoding TPMT are associated with variable catabolism and hence toxicity, and in most centres erythrocyte TPMT activity is assessed prior to its prescription, to guide use, dose and escalation.

Adverse effects. The major serious reactions are bone marrow suppression resulting in leucopenia, anaemia and thrombocytopenia; hepatotoxicity; increased susceptibility to infection; and in the long term an increased risk of neoplasia. As with methotrexate, regular monitoring of full blood count and liver function is mandatory. Other side-effects include nausea, alopecia and, rarely, allergy.

Interactions. Xanthine oxidase, the enzyme inhibited by allopurinol and febuxostat to therapeutic effect in the

---

[10]Chan E S, Cronstein B N 2010 Methotrexate – how does it really work? Nature Reviews Rheumatology 6:175–178.

management of gout, is involved in the catabolism of aza-thioprine. Concomitant use of xanthine oxidase inhibitors and azathioprine may result in profound myelosuppression and should be avoided. If the combination is unavoidable, azathioprine must be decreased to 25–33% of the usual dose. Sulfasalazine and NSAIDs inhibit TPMT and thereby the metabolism of azathioprine, also increasing the risk of myelotoxicity. Lastly, co-prescription of angiotensin-converting enzyme inhibitors and azathioprine increases the risk of myelosuppression; the mechanism is incompletely understood but has assumed greater importance with the recent appreciation that patients with SLE and other chronic inflammatory disorders have an increased risk of cardiovascular disease and are thus more likely to be prescribed both.

Contraindications. Experience with azathioprine in pregnant women with renal transplants indicates that it is relatively safe, probably because the fetus cannot metabolise 6-mercaptopurine. Although a teratogenic metabolite is present in breast milk, its concentration is low and no evidence for harm exists; nevertheless, breast feeding while taking azathioprine is best regarded as unsafe.

Mycophenolate mofetil

Mycophenolate mofetil (MMF) is also an antimetabolite that inhibits purine synthesis. It is licensed for the prophylaxis of acute rejection following organ transplantation and is also used (unlicensed in the UK) as a treatment for SLE nephritis, other connective tissue diseases with severe major organ involvement and systemic vasculitis.

Mechanism of action. MMF is metabolised to mycophenolic acid, which inhibits inosine monophosphate dehydrogenase, an enzyme in the guanine nucleotide synthesis pathway used by lymphocytes. As other cells have salvage pathways, MMF selectively inhibits lymphocyte proliferation.

Adverse effects. These are similar to azathioprine and include GI disturbances (diarrhoea is particularly common), myelosuppression, hepatotoxicity, electrolyte disturbances, adverse lipid profile, increased risk of malignancy and pancreatitis. MMF is teratogenic and thus is contraindicated during pregnancy.

Leflunomide

The active metabolite of leflunomide (A77 1726) inhibits dihydro-orotate dehydrogenase, a mitochondrial enzyme required for the synthesis of pyrimidines.[11] It arrests the proliferation of activated lymphocytes and is licensed for the treatment of rheumatoid arthritis and psoriatic arthritis.

Adverse effects. Diarrhoea is commonest; other GI disturbances, hepatitis, leucopenia, alopecia, hypertension and allergy also occur. In the event of a serious adverse event, the elimination of leflunomide can be accelerated by colestyramine (8 g three times daily).

Contraindications. Leflunomide is contraindicated in liver disease, severe hypoproteinaemia, immunodeficiency, pregnancy, breast feeding or if there is a possibility of future pregnancy. A gap of at least 2 years is recommended between cessation of leflunomide treatment and conception.

Calcineurin inhibitors

The calcineurin inhibitors ciclosporin and tacrolimus inhibit cytokine-driven activation and proliferation of activated T cells by interfering with synthesis of IL-2. Both bind cytosol receptors called 'immunophilins' (ciclophilin and FKBP-12, respectively) and form complexes that inhibit IL-2 production via the calcineurin pathway. They are used orally to prevent rejection after solid organ transplantation and in chronic inflammatory disorders including cutaneous psoriasis, Behçet's syndrome, systemic vasculitis and, occasionally, rheumatoid arthritis. However, other preparations are also becoming accepted: topical tacrolimus is used in cutaneous SLE and severe atopic dermatitis.

Adverse effects. The use of ciclosporin has in recent years been curtailed a little by the substantial incidence of hypertension and nephrotoxicity associated with long-term use, and the development of more effective, less toxic competitors. Both ciclospoin and tacrolimus can cause myelosuppression and hepatotoxicity, and regular blood monitoring is required; GI problems are also common, particularly diarrhoea with tacrolimus.

Sirolimus

Sirolimus (rapamycin) is a macrolide antibiotic, structurally very similar to tacrolimus, that is licensed for use in preventing rejection after solid organ transplantation, and is occasionally used (unlicensed) to treat autoimmune inflammatory disorders such as SLE and Behçet's syndrome. Sirolimus-coated stents are also commonly used in percutaneous coronary artery intervention, as the presence of sirolimus reduces neo-intimal proliferation. It acts by binding FKBP-12, like tacrolimus, but the complex in this case has no effect on the calcineurin pathway and instead binds to and inhibits activation of mTOR (mammalian target of rapamycin), an important signalling kinase. This in turn suppresses cytokine-driven T-cell and B-cell proliferation and antibody production. Adverse effects are similar to those of tacrolimus.

---

[11]Anonymous 2000 Leflunomide for rheumatoid arthritis. Drug and Therapeutics Bulletin 38:52–54.

Cyclophosphamide

Cyclophosphamide, an alkylating cytotoxic agent, damages DNA by forming cross-links which trigger apoptosis in dividing cells. In autoimmunity, it is particularly toxic to rapidly proliferating lymphocytes and has also been used as a cancer chemotherapy drug. It is used to induce remission in severe inflammatory conditions with life-threatening organ involvement such as SLE nephritis, ANCA-associated vasculitis causing nephritis or pulmonary haemorrhage, or rapidly progressive interstitial lung disease.

Prescription and adverse effects. In rheumatological practice, cyclophosphamide is most commonly given as an intravenous pulse, repeated at 3–4 week intervals, for six pulses. Oral cyclophosphamide is less frequently used due to the larger cumulative dose and thus increased risk of long-term toxicities. A serious consequence is haemorrhagic cystitis, due to the action of acrolein (a drug metabolite) on the urinary tract epithelium. This is minimised by intravenous pre-hydration and oral administration of 2-mercaptoethane sulphonate (mesna), which reacts with and inactivates acrolein. Other adverse effects are highly significant and include bone marrow toxicity and consequent increased risk of opportunistic infection, infertility, teratogenicity, severe nausea and increased incidence of malignancy, especially of the bladder. In male patients, sperm may be stored prior to cyclophosphamide treatment.

Hydroxychloroquine

Hydroxychloroquine, an antimalarial drug, is used commonly for mild manifestations of SLE and other connective tissue diseases, particularly rashes and arthralgia, at doses of 200–400 mg daily. In rheumatoid arthritis, it is used as an adjunct to other disease-modifying agents.

Mechanism of action. It is not well understood how hydroxychloroquine exerts its disease-modifying effects. In vitro studies suggest that chloroquine and hydroxychloroquine can reduce the production of pro-inflammatory cytokines including TNFα and IL-1β, and both are known to be concentrated in lysosomes, inhibiting the metabolism of deoxyribonucleotides.

Adverse effects. Hydroxychloroquine is normally very well tolerated and has a low incidence of side-effects. GI disturbances, rashes, and, rarely, blood dyscrasias may occur. Retinal toxicity may rarely occur with long-term use; measurement of visual acuity initially and at annual intervals is recommended.[12]

Contraindications. Hydroxychloroquine should be used with caution in hepatic or renal impairment, in neurological disorders, in glucose 6-phosphate dehydrogenase deficiency and in porphyria. The manufacturer's instructions advise against use in pregnancy and breast feeding, but data on over 250 pregnancies in women with connective tissue disease who were taking hydroxychloroquine provide evidence that the treatment is safe in pregnancy, and probably also during breast feeding.[13]

Sulfasalazine

Sulfasalazine (SSZ) is a conjugate of mesalazine (5-amino-salicylic acid, 5-ASA) coupled to sulfapyridine. It is used to treat rheumatoid arthritis, either alone or in combination with methotrexate, and peripheral joint involvement in the spondyloarthropathies, including ankylosing spondylitis and reactive arthritis.

Mechanism of action. SSZ is cleaved by bacterial azoreductases in the colon to release 5-ASA and sulfapyridine (Fig. 16.5). 5-ASA is retained mostly in the colon and excreted, but 30% of intact SSZ and all sulfapyridine are absorbed. Anti-inflammatory effects of mesalazine, both in the colonic epithelial cell and in peripheral blood mononuclear cells, include inhibition of cyclo-oxygenase and lipo-oxygenase, scavenging of free radicals, and inhibition of the production of pro-inflammatory cytokines and immunoglobulins. In the treatment of inflammatory bowel disease, preparations containing 5-ASA alone have efficacy comparable to that of SSZ, but with fewer side-effects. In contrast, the sulfapyridine component appears to be the active moiety in rheumatoid arthritis. SSZ has been shown to reduce rheumatoid factor titres, inhibit IL-2–induced T-cell proliferation and inhibit macrophage IL-1 and IL-12 production, but the relative importance of these effects on its anti-inflammatory activity remains unclear.

Adverse effects. Sulfasalazine is associated with a number of adverse effects including cytopenias and hepatitis, which appear to be caused by the sulfapyridine moiety. A lupus-like syndrome may occur; the risk of this is higher in rheumatoid patients who are antinuclear antibody-positive.

Intravenous immunoglobulin

Intravenous immunoglobulin (IvIg) was first used in 1952 to treat primary immune deficiencies. It is composed of pooled IgG extracted from the plasma of 3000–10 000 blood donors, and contains the entire repertoire of naturally

---

[12]Fielder A, Graham E, Jones S et al 1998 Royal College of Ophthalmologists guidelines: ocular toxicity and hydroxychloroquine. Eye 12:907–909.

[13]Costedoat-Chalumeau N, Amoura Z, du Huong L T et al 2005 Safety of hydroxychloroquine in pregnant patients with connective tissue diseases. Review of the literature. Autoimmunity Reviews 4:111–115.

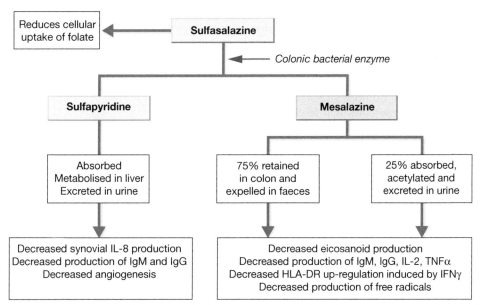

Fig. 16.5 Metabolism and activity of sulfasalazine. Sulfasalazine is reduced to sulfapyridine and mesalazine in the colon by bacterial azoreductases. The two components have distinct anti-inflammatory activities.

occurring antibodies. Besides its uses as a treatment for primary immune deficiencies and hypogammaglobulinaemia, it has immunomodulatory properties, making it an effective therapy for a number of autoimmune conditions. However, it has also been used in scenarios where there is no evidence of efficacy and little theoretical basis to suggest benefit. As there is a national shortage, the UK NHS has recently introduced guidelines to restrict its use only to those conditions in which there is a known benefit.[14]

Diseases in which IvIg is known to be of benefit include: Kawasaki disease, immune thrombocytopenic purpura (ITP), dermatomyositis, Guillain–Barré syndrome and chronic inflammatory demyelinating polyneuropathy. There are many others in which it may be used as part of a range of treatments.

Mechanism of action. The immunomodulatory mechanism of action of IvIg is thought primarily to be through the Fc region of the IgG molecule. Binding to Fc receptors and altering Fc receptor signalling in macrophages, other phagocytes and B cells has been shown to be an important effect in ITP and other autoimmune cytopenias. In dermatomyositis and Kawasaki disease, modulation of complement cascade activation is important. IvIg binds C3b and C4b, thus inhibiting formation of the membrane attack complex. Other functions of IvIg such as suppression of

autoantibodies and of cytokines and chemokines have also been demonstrated.

Adverse effects. These include infusion reactions during or shortly after treatment, acute renal failure and rarely thrombosis, hyperproteinaemia and disseminated intravascular coagulation. As IvIg contains trace amounts of IgA, IgA-deficient patients may develop a hypersensitivity reaction following repeated infusions, which may progress to anaphylaxis.

Thalidomide

Thalidomide is rightly notorious for its teratogenic effects. In recent years it has re-emerged as a treatment for certain inflammatory dermatoses, including discoid lupus erythematosus, Behçet's disease, erythema nodosum leprosum, and graft-versus-host disease. The mechanism of action of its anti-inflammatory effects is not fully understood, but it has been shown to inhibit anti-TNFα production and also has anti-angiogenic properties. Apart from the known teratogenicity, the use of thalidomide is limited by cumulative peripheral nerve damage, and nerve conduction studies should be monitored annually.

Dapsone

Dapsone, traditionally used to treat mycobacterial (principally leprosy) and occasionally protozoal infections, also has

---

[14]www.ivig.nhs.uk (accessed November 2011)

anti-inflammatory properties. It can be used to treat discoid lupus and other inflammatory dermatological disorders characterised by neutrophil infiltration. Although it is clear that its antimicrobial activity stems from inhibition of folate synthesis, this does not appear to be the mechanism of its anti-inflammatory effects. These are less well understood, but may involve impairing neutrophil chemotaxis and stabilisation of neutrophil lysosomes, thus inhibiting the respiratory burst. Common adverse effects include rashes, haemolysis and liver dysfunction; it may also rarely cause blood dyscrasias and methaemoglobinaemia. It should be avoided in patients suffering from glucose 6-phosphate dehydrogenase deficiency (see p. 103).

Biologic agents

The biggest change in treatment of inflammatory disease over the last 10 years has been the development of mono-clonal antibodies and fusion proteins that target a specific component of the inflammatory response. This allows selective modification of the abnormal immune response underlying many chronic inflammatory diseases, resulting in greater efficacy and potentially fewer side-effects than conventional 'dirtier' immunosuppressants. The first drugs of this sort to enter widespread clinical use were TNFα antagonists, which now have an established role in the treatment of rheumatoid arthritis, juvenile idiopathic arthritis, ankylosing spondylitis, psoriasis and Crohn's disease.

In recent years there has been a dramatic increase in the variety of different biological drugs, and their indications. Their major drawbacks, shared by all, are an increased susceptibility to infection, and price, which in the UK at least severely curtails their use. A brief overview only is given here.

Anti-TNFα therapies

TNFα, a pro-inflammatory cytokine, is produced predomi-nantly by macrophages and in smaller amounts by CD4 + Th1 lymphocytes. It plays an important role in macrophage activation and the eradication of intracellular bacterial and fungal infections. TNFα is also a key mediator of the inflam-matory response seen in chronic granulomatous conditions such as rheumatoid arthritis and Crohn's disease. TNFα blockade by biological agents has proved highly effective for many chronic inflammatory diseases, and there are now several different agents selectively targeting TNFα available, with more in development.

Infliximab is a chimeric monoclonal IgG1 antibody (Fig. 16.6). In rheumatoid arthritis, it is administered by intra-venous infusion at 3 mg/kg, repeated 2 and 6 weeks after

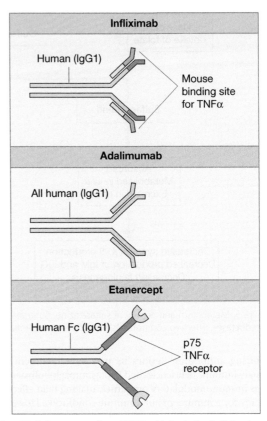

Fig. 16.6 Structure of anti-TNFα biologicals. Infliximab and adalimumab are monoclonal antibodies. Etanercept is a fusion molecule composed of two p75 TNFα receptors coupled to a human immunoglobulin Fc component.

the initial infusion and then at 8-week intervals. In ankylosing spondylitis, psoriasis and Crohn's disease, it is used at doses of 5 mg/kg. Methotrexate is co-prescribed to limit the development of neutralising antibodies.

Adalimumab is a fully human monoclonal IgG1 antibody (see Fig. 16.6). The recommended dose is 40 mg by sub-cutaneous injection fortnightly, in combination with methotrexate. It is licensed for use in rheumatoid arthritis, ankylosing spondylitis and psoriatic arthritis.

Etanercept is a fusion protein consisting of two human p75 TNFα receptors coupled to an Fc component of human IgG1 (see Fig. 16.6). It is licensed for weekly subcutaneous injection in adult patients with rheumatoid arthritis (50 mg), for children older than 4 years of age with polyarticular juvenile idiopathic arthritis (400 µg/ kg; maximum dose 50 mg), psoriasis and ankylosing spondylitis.

Table 16.1 New drugs for inflammation and joint disease

1. mAb – Cytokine modulator	Anti IL-12 and IL-23
Principal example	Ustekinumab (Stelara)
Licensed indication(s)	Psoriasis, psoriatic arthritis, Crohn's disease
Comment	Licensed for TNFi-refractory PsA and Crohn's and for psoriasis. Works well for psoriasis, but only a subset of PsA patients respond.
2. mAb – Cytokine modulator	Anti IL-17a
Principal example	Secukinumab (Cosentyx)
Licensed indication(s)	Ankylosing spondylitis, psoriatic arthritis
Comment	Will be used for patients who have not responded to TNF blockade in these conditions
3. Phosphodiesterase-4 inhibitor	
Principal example	Apremilast (Otezla)
Licensed indication(s)	Psoriasis, psoriatic arthritis
Comment	Oral treatment used alongside conventional DMARDs, before biologics are prescribed (NICE approved for psoriasis but not PsA)
4. Janus kinase inhibitor	
Principal example	Tofacitinib
Licensed indication(s)	Rheumatoid arthritis
Comment	Oral agent, likely to be used alongside conventional DMARDs, before biologic drugs (NICE technology appraisal awaited)
Biosimilars	New versions of biologic drugs made as patents for original molecules expire
Principal examples	Benepali (etanercept) Remsima, inflectra (infliximab)
Licensed indication(s)	As for TNFi

The mechanism of action of etanercept differs from that of the monoclonal IgG antibodies in that it:

- does not fix complement and therefore does not cause lysis of cells that express TNFα on their surface
- binds trimeric (active) TNFα only, in contrast with infliximab, which binds both monomeric (inactive) and trimeric (active) TNFα
- also binds lymphotoxin (TNFβ).

There are two further anti-TNFα antibodies that have recently entered clinical practice in the UK. **Golimumab** is a fully human monoclonal antibody to TNFα which is taken monthly; and **certolizumab pegol** is a pegylated humanised Fab fragment directed against TNFα.

Finally, a new development in anti-TNF therapies is the availability of biosimilar molecules, as the originators come off patent. Benepali (biosimilar etanercept) and remsima (biosimilar infliximab) are increasingly used in the UK (Table 16.1).

Adverse effects

The major risk with anti-TNF therapy is increased susceptibility to infection, particularly with intracellular pathogens

such as *Mycobacteria tuberculosis* (M.Tb). In the case of M.Tb, this may be reactivation of latent disease, but there is also a risk of new infection with M.Tb, other mycobacteria or intracellular pathogens such as histoplasmosis, coccidiomycosis or nocardiosis. Guidelines for assessing risk and for managing infection with *Mycobacterium tuberculosis* in the context of anti-TNFα agents are available.[15] Chemoprophylaxis must be started prior to treatment in patients with latent infection.

Antinuclear antibodies develop twice as commonly in rheumatoid arthritis patients taking anti-TNFα agents. The risk of developing anti–double-stranded DNA antibodies is also increased, but the clinical significance of these autoantibodies is unclear in the majority of cases. Anti-TNFα–induced lupus is a rare complication.

Infusion reactions may occur with infliximab administration, e.g. fever, pruritus, urticaria, chest pain, hypotension and dyspnoea. These usually resolve if the infusion rate is

[15]British Thoracic Society Standards of Care Committee 2005 BTS recommendations for assessing risk and for managing *Mycobacterium tuberculosis* infection and disease in patients due to start anti-TNF-α treatment. Thorax 60:800–805.

slowed or suspended temporarily and then restarted at a slower rate.

Symptoms and/or radiological evidence of demyelination may be exacerbated, as may severe cardiac failure.

TNFα blockade presents a theoretical risk of increasing the incidence of malignancy. In patients with rheumatoid arthritis, current data do not suggest an overall augmented tumour risk, but the chance of developing lymphoma may be increased.

B-cell depletion

Rituximab[16] is a chimeric monoclonal IgG1 antibody specific for CD20, which is expressed on B cells but not plasma cells. Initially used for B-cell lymphomas, it is now prescribed for a variety of autoimmune disorders, including rheumatoid arthritis and SLE, in which autoantibody production is a significant disease-causing mechanism. Targeting CD20 removes the pathogenic antibody-producing cells, leaving the memory plasma cells needed to mount a response to infection intact. It is administered by intravenous infusion in doses of 1 g 2 weeks apart. The B-cell count is then monitored to check for depletion. Patients can be re-treated if their B-cell count recovers and the disease recurs. The major adverse effects are increased susceptibility to infection, and infusion reactions.

Belimumab is a monoclonal antibody that blocks B-lymphocyte stimulator (BLyS), preventing the proliferation of B cells. It recently received FDA approval as a treatment for SLE.

Inhibition of T-cell activation

Abatacept[16] is a fusion protein formed from the extracellular domain of human CTLA4 (cytotoxic T lymphocyte antigen-4) linked to the Fc portion of human IgG1. Normally, CTLA4 on the T-cell membrane binds CD80 and CD86 on antigen presenting cells to provide the co-stimulation signal required for full T-cell activation when it recognises a Class II MHC-antigen complex. Abatacept competes with T-cell-bound CTLA4 and binds CD80 or CD86 itself, thus preventing co-stimulation, and this leads to a reduction in T-cell proliferation and cytokine production. It has been shown to be effective in reducing rheumatoid arthritis activity and is given as an intravenous infusion.

Other biologic anticytokine agents

Interleukin-1 (IL-1) is a pro-inflammatory cytokine with a central role in the activation of an inflammatory response.

Anakinra is recombinant IL-1Ra, an endogenous antagonist of the IL-1 receptor. Clinical trials in rheumatoid arthritis, SLE and psoriasis have had disappointing results, but anakinra is dramatically effective in treating rare hereditary fever syndromes characterised by excess IL-1 signalling. These include cryopyrin-associated periodic syndromes (CAPS) such as Muckle–Wells syndrome, and hyper-IgD syndrome. Anakinra is also effective in treating systemic onset juvenile inflammatory arthritis and adult-onset Still's disease, and may be effective in severe gout.

Interleukin-6 (IL-6) is another pro-inflammatory cytokine that is of critical importance to the mounting of an immune response, and is the most abundant cytokine found in the synovium of rheumatoid arthritis patients. **Tocilizumab** is a monoclonal antibody that binds IL-6 receptors and inhibits their intracellular signalling. It has been shown to be effective in controlling disease activity in rheumatoid arthritis,[17] and is licensed for use in this condition in the UK. It is given by intravenous infusion on a monthly basis.

For psoriatic arthritis, psoriasis and ankylosing spondylitis, two further mAb have become available in the last couple of years. Ustekinumab (stelara) targets IL-12 and IL-23, and is licensed and approved by NICE to treat psoriasis and psoriatic arthritis (see Table 16.1). Secukinumab (cosentyx) targets IL-17 and is used to treat both psoriatic arthritis and ankylosing spondylitis (see Table 16.1).

Other strategies

Two further agents have reached clinical practice in the last 2 years, through drug discovery programmes. Apremilast (otezla) inhibits phosphodiesterase-4, and is licensed to treat psoriatic arthritis (see Table 16.1). Tofacitinib (xeljanz) is an inhibitor of the intracellular signalling pathway JAK-STAT, and is effective in treating rheumatoid arthritis (see Table 16.1). These two agents have the advantage of being oral preparations, and could potentially in future be used alongside DMARDs, before progressing to biologic agents.

Management of diseases affecting the joints

Osteoarthritis

Osteoarthritis (OA) is the most common form of arthritis, with radiographic evidence of knee OA in up to 15% of people older than 55 years of age. It reflects a dynamic bone and cartilage response to joint trauma and ageing. OA is a

---

[16]BMJ Group 2008 Rituximab and abatacept for rheumatoid arthritis. Drug and Therapeutics Bulletin 46:57–61.

[17][No authors listed] 2010 Tocilizumab for rheumatoid arthritis. Drug and Therapeutics Bulletin 48(1):9–12.

common cause of disability, particularly in the elderly, and is the major indication for joint replacement.

The aims of management of OA are to control pain, reduce progression of joint damage and minimise disability. The major strategies employed are non-pharmacological; there are no disease-modifying drugs in clinical use. Patient education in pain management is important to minimise the adverse effects of analgesics. NSAIDs have been shown to be marginally more effective but are associated with more adverse effects than paracetamol.[18] Regular paracetamol or co-dydramol should therefore be tried before introducing an NSAID. Other options include topical NSAID gel, which may provide a modest improvement in symptoms at least in the short term. For patients with large-joint OA, occasional intra-articular injection of corticosteroid and local anaesthetic can provide some respite for up to 6 weeks.

Gout

- Gout is a recurrent acute inflammatory arthritis caused by monosodium urate (MSU) crystals within synovial joints, affecting 1.4% of the UK population. Hyperuricaemia is due to over-production or under-excretion of uric acid. Both mechanisms may operate in the same patient, but reduced renal clearance is the main cause of hyperuricaemia in most cases. Drugs may influence these processes as follows:
  - Over-production of uric acid occurs if there is excessive cell destruction releasing nucleic acids. This may occur when myeloproliferative and lymphoproliferative disorders are first treated.
  - Under-excretion of uric acid is caused by thiazide and loop diuretics, low-dose aspirin (see earlier), ethambutol, pyrazinamide, nicotinic acid, ciclosporin and alcohol (which increases uric acid synthesis and also causes a rise in serum lactic acid that inhibits tubular secretion of uric acid). Conversely, a small number of drugs have a mild uricosuric effect and increase renal clearance of urate. Losartan and fenofibrate are examples of this.

Patients with gout but no visible tophi have a uric acid pool that is two to three times normal. This exceeds the amount that can be carried in solution in extracellular fluid, so MSU crystals precipitate and form deposits in tissues, including the joints and occasionally in subcutaneous tissues (tophi). These crystals then trigger acute attacks of inflammatory arthritis.

The priority in an acute attack is to relieve the intense pain by reducing the inflammatory response. NSAIDs are most commonly prescribed, but if contraindicated, colchicine (EULAR[19] guidelines suggest 0.5 mg three times daily) is an alternative. A short course of oral prednisolone or intra-articular corticosteroid is also effective, although the severity of joint pain may preclude intra-articular injection during an acute attack.

Management of chronic gout should include a review of modifiable risk factors for hyperuricaemia, including obesity, hypertension, excessive alcohol consumption, high dietary intake of purines (red meat, game, seafood, legumes) and drugs (see above). If these measures are insufficient, plasma uric acid levels may be reduced by inhibiting the formation of uric acid (allopurinol, febuxostat), or increasing renal excretion (sulfinpyrazone, probenecid or benzbromarone). In treatment-resistant cases, 'biologic' therapy with recombinant uricase, which metabolises urate further, can be considered. Rapid lowering of plasma uric acid by any means can precipitate an acute flare, probably by causing the dissolution of crystal deposits. Colchicine prescribed concomitantly for up to 6 months or an NSAID for 6 weeks protect against this.

Allopurinol inhibits xanthine oxidase, the enzyme that converts xanthine and hypoxanthine to uric acid. Patients taking allopurinol excrete less uric acid and more xanthine and hypoxanthine in the urine. It is readily absorbed from the GI tract, metabolised in the liver to oxypurinol, which is also a xanthine oxidase inhibitor, and excreted unchanged by the kidney. Allopurinol is indicated in recurrent gout and during treatment of myeloproliferative disorders where cell destruction creates a high uric acid load. It prevents the hyperuricaemia due to diuretics and may be combined with a uricosuric agent.

Adverse effects of allopurinol include precipitation of an acute gout attack and the allopurinol hypersensitivity syndrome (AHS) which is rare but can be severe. Features include hepatitis, desquamating erythematous rash, eosinophilia and worsening renal function. For this reason, allopurinol should not be commenced unless the diagnosis is certain, and attacks of gout are frequent despite lifestyle changes. It also interferes with the metabolism of azathioprine, and co-prescription may cause severe myelosuppression.

Febuxostat is a newly licensed non-purine selective xanthine oxidase inhibitor. Although it is at least as effective, if not more, than allopurinol at lowering serum urate levels, its safety in patients who are allergic to allopurinol has not been fully established. Diarrhoea, liver function disturbance

---

[18]Pincus T, Koch G G, Sokka T et al 2001 A randomized, double-blind, crossover clinical trial of diclofenac plus misoprostol versus acetaminophen in patients with osteoarthritis of the hip or knee. Arthritis and Rheumatism 44:1587–1598.

[19]European League Against Rheumatism.

and other GI symptoms are the commonest adverse effects. Febuxostat also interferes with azathioprine metabolism.

Sulfinpyrazone competitively inhibits the active transport of organic anions across the kidney tubule, both from the plasma to the tubular fluid and vice versa. The effect is dose-dependent: at low dose sulfinpyrazone prevents secretion of uric acid into tubular fluid, and at high dose, and more powerfully, it prevents reabsorption, increasing its excretion in the urine. A net beneficial uricosuric action is obtained with an initial dose of 100–200 mg/day by mouth with food, increasing over 2–3 weeks to 600 mg/day, which should be continued until the plasma uric acid level is normal. The dose may then be reduced for maintenance, to as little as 200 mg daily. During initial therapy, ensure that fluid intake is at least 2 L/day to prevent uric acid crystalluria. Other adverse effects are mainly gastrointestinal; sulfinpyrazone is contraindicated in peptic ulcer.

Rasburicase is a recombinant uricase which converts urate into allantoin, a more soluble metabolite which is readily excreted renally. It rapidly and profoundly lowers serum uric acid concentration and is licensed for use in tumour lysis syndrome. It has also been used in small numbers of patients with gout, but antibody development limits its effectiveness with repeated infusions, as would be needed to treat chronic tophaceous gout. A pegylated uricase (pegloticase),[20] which has a longer $t_{1/2}$ and is less immunogenic, has shown promise in recent trials.

Rheumatoid arthritis

Rheumatoid arthritis (RA) is a chronic symmetrical polyarthritis affecting approximately 1% of the UK population. The principal pathology is inflammation within synovial joints, causing pain, swelling and stiffness and progressing to erosion and eventually joint destruction. RA is a systemic autoimmune inflammatory disorder and may cause extra-articular manifestations affecting blood vessels, bone marrow, GI tract, skin, lungs and eyes. Further sources of morbidity reflect the interaction of the disease process with adverse effects of medication and include osteoporosis, GI haemorrhage and accelerated atherosclerosis. Mortality in patients with RA is increased up to three-fold compared with the general population; most of the excess is due to cardiovascular disease.

The initial management of a patient presenting with new inflammatory polyarthritis consists of reducing systemic inflammation, joint pain and stiffness while the diagnosis is confirmed.[21] This may be achieved by short-term glucocorticoids such as Depo-Medrone 120 mg i.m., combined with analgesia and an NSAID (e.g. diclofenac 50 mg three times daily).

Once a diagnosis of RA is made, a DMARD should be initiated. As these reduce the progression of joint damage, it is imperative to start treatment in early disease; it is not acceptable to attempt to treat patients with early RA solely symptomatically. Methotrexate is the most common first-line DMARD. Careful education and counselling of the patient is important to ensure regular monitoring (of bone marrow, liver and lung function) and early detection of adverse effects. Folic acid 5 mg (up to 6 days weekly) is co-prescribed to reduce side-effects such as mouth ulcers.

Hydroxychloroquine is often used as an adjunct DMARD with methotrexate, and combination therapy of methotrexate, sulfasalazine and hydroxychloroquine can have added benefits beyond that of the individual drugs. Where methotrexate is contraindicated, ineffective or toxic, sulfasalazine alone, leflunomide or gold are alternatives. At any point in the disease course, glucocorticoids can be used as an adjunct to control flares, administered orally, intra-articularly or intra-muscularly.

If adequate disease control is not achieved after use of two DMARDs, UK guidelines recommend starting anti-TNFα agents: infliximab, etanercept or adalimumab. If this is not effective, current practice involves switching to an alternative anti-TNFα agent with a different mechanism of action, or to the anti-CD20 mAb, rituximab. In 2010, tocilizumab (anti IL-6R) and abatacept (T-cell co-stimulation blockade) were approved for those patients who have not responded to other biologics. Many other biologic agents targeting cytokine expression, immune cell subtypes and intracellular signalling are currently in development.

It is particularly important to address cardiovascular risk reduction in patients with RA, given the increased risk of cardiovascular disease associated with chronic inflammation. Aggressive management of RA with DMARDs may reduce cardiovascular disease incidence at the same time as controlling inflammation. Moreover, atorvastatin has been reported to improve disease activity scores in RA.[22]

Protection against osteoporosis is particularly important for patients who receive long-term glucocorticoids; even doses less than prednisolone 7.5 mg daily increase fracture risk. The UK guideline[23] for the prevention and treatment

---

[20]Sundy J S, Baraf H S, Becker M A et al 2008 Efficacy and safety of intravenous (IV) pegloticase (PGL) in subjects with treatment failure gout (TFG): phase 3 results from GOUT1 and GOUT2 [Abstract]. Arthritis and Rheumatism 58(Suppl.):S400.

[21]Kennedy T, McCabe C, Struthers G et al 2005 BSR guidelines on standards of care for persons with rheumatoid arthritis. Rheumatology (Oxford) 44:553–556.

[22]McCarey D W, McInnes I B, Madhok R et al 2004 Trial of atorvastatin in rheumatoid arthritis (TARA): double-blind, randomised placebo-controlled trial. Lancet 363:2015–2021.

[23]Bone and Tooth Society, National Osteoporosis Society and Royal College of Physicians. Glucocorticoid-induced osteoporosis – guidelines for prevention and treatment. 2002. Available at: http://www.rcplondon.ac.uk/pubs/books/glucocorticoid/.

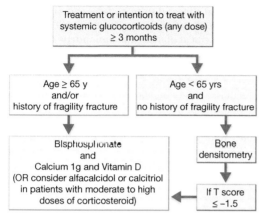

Treatment or intention to treat with
systemic glucocorticoids (any dose)
≥ 3 months

Age ≥ 65 y
and/or
history of fragility fracture

Age < 65 yrs
and
no history of fragility fracture

Bisphosphonate
and
Calcium 1g and Vitamin D
(OR consider alfacalcidol or calcitriol
in patients with moderate to high
doses of corticosteroid)

Bone
densitometry

If T score
≤ −1.5

Fig. 16.7 Prevention and treatment of glucocorticoid-induced osteoporosis. UK guidelines for osteoprotection in patients treated with glucocorticoids.

of glucocorticoid-induced osteoporosis is summarised in Fig. 16.7. Bone loss is most rapid in the first few months of treatment, therefore protection must be considered at the onset of treatment, whenever the intention is to continue for more than 3 months, at any dose. Strategies include minimising the dose of corticosteroid, concomitant prescription of vitamin D 800 IU and calcium 1 g daily and advice on smoking cessation, alcohol intake, nutrition and exercise. Bisphosphonates should be prescribed for all patients older than 65 years of age, or those with a history of a fragility fracture. Other patients should undergo bone densitometry and should be prescribed a bisphosphonate if the T score is −1.5 or less[24] at either lumbar spine or hip.

Patients with RA have a five-fold increased risk of GI haemorrhage compared with the general population, mainly due to NSAID use, alone or in combination with corticosteroids. Any patient with RA taking regular NSAIDs should also be prescribed a proton pump inhibitor or other gastroprotective agent.

Psoriatic arthritis

Cutaneous psoriasis affects 2% of the population, of whom 10% develop psoriatic arthritis (PsA), an inflammatory arthritis that can lead to erosions and joint destruction. The objectives of management are to relieve symptoms and prevent joint damage.

As with RA, symptomatic management strategies include use of NSAIDs and intra-articular corticosteroids. The evidence base for the use DMARDs in PsA is generally poor, but methotrexate is most commonly used. Sulfasalazine and leflunomide can be tried if methotrexate is ineffective or contraindicated. Anti-TNFα therapy is effective in psoriatic arthritis and in severe cutaneous psoriasis,[25] in contrast to the anti–T-cell biologic agents efalizumab and alefacept which, although effective for skin disease, have not been shown in trials to have dramatic benefits in PsA.

Ankylosing spondylitis

Ankylosing spondylitis (AS) is an inflammatory disorder of the spine and sacroiliac joints, sometimes associated with peripheral arthritis, anterior uveitis and aortitis, that affects 0.1% of the population. The traditional objectives in its management were to relieve pain and stiffness and maintain mobility through a combination of regular NSAIDs and physiotherapy. No DMARDs have shown efficacy in treating spinal disease, although sulfasalazine is effective for peripheral arthritis. Management of AS has been revolutionised by the discovery that anti-TNFα therapy can dramatically improve spinal disease activity.[26] Evidence from serial magnetic resonance imaging indicates that bone oedema regresses following TNFα blockade.

Systemic lupus erythematosus

Systemic lupus erythematosus (SLE) is a chronic multi-organ autoimmune condition affecting primarily young women, that may have life-threatening manifestations. Management depends on the degree and severity of organ involvement, which may range from mild rashes and arthralgia to pancytopenia or renal and cerebral vasculitis.

Mild lupus may be treated with hydroxychloroquine and lifestyle advice, such as avoidance of sun exposure or extreme stress, but many require a more potent immunomodulator, such as azathioprine or mycophenolate mofetil (MMF). Flares may be controlled by pulses of glucocorticoid i.v. or i.m. or a progressively reduced oral course, although some patients require long-term low-dose GC. Topical or intra-articular steroids are used if appropriate. Severe manifestations such as lupus nephritis are traditionally managed with i.v. pulses of methylprednisolone and cyclophosphamide. MMF is now increasingly used, in light of the risk of infertility

[24]The T score is the number of standard deviations above or below the mean bone mineral density of a 25-year-old (sex-matched) individual. A T score below −2.5 indicates osteoporosis.

[25]Kyle S, Chandler D, Griffiths C E M et al 2005 Guideline for anti-TNF-alpha therapy in psoriatic arthritis. Rheumatology (Oxford) 44:390–397.
[26]Keat A, Barkham N, Bhalla A et al 2005 BSR guidelines for prescribing TNF-α blockers in adults with ankylosing spondylitis. Report of a working party of the British Society for Rheumatology. Rheumatology (Oxford) 44:939–947.

associated with cyclophosphamide. B-cell depletion with rituximab may also be effective.

Co-morbidities result from both the disease and its treatment; in addition to excess cardiovascular mortality, there is a risk long term of developing other autoimmune diseases or malignancy as well as osteoporosis or opportunistic infection. Patients with SLE should be screened for antiphospholipid antibodies, and antiplatelet therapy should be considered in those who are positive.

Polymyalgia rheumatica and giant cell arteritis

These are chronic inflammatory conditions that occur mainly in patients older than 60 years of age and present with proximal pain and stiffness, fever and night sweats or headache. The most feared complication is sudden visual loss due to involvement of the ophthalmic artery. They respond exquisitely to corticosteroids. If giant cell arteritis is suspected or diagnosed, high-dose prednisolone (0.5–1 mg/kg daily) is used. Polymyalgia rheumatica responds to lower doses, e.g. prednisolone 15 mg daily. Other immunomodulators such as azathioprine or methotrexate do not have proven efficacy but are sometimes used in patients whose disease requires unacceptably high doses of glucocorticoid for suppression. As treatment is normally required for at least 2 years, osteoprotection and gastroprotection must be used.

Guide to further reading

Barnes, P.J., 2006. Corticosteroids: the drugs to beat. Eur. J. Pharmacol. 533, 2–14.

Baschant, U., Tuckermann, J., 2010. The role of the glucocorticoid receptor in inflammation and immunity. J. Steroid Biochem. Mol. Biol. 120, 69–75.

Braun, J., 2016. New targets in psoriatic arthritis. Rheumatology (Oxford) 55 (Suppl. 2), ii30–ii37.

Cohen, S., Fleischmann, R., 2010. Kinase inhibitors: a new approach to rheumatoid arthritis treatment. Curr. Opin. Rheumatol. 22, 330–335.

D'Cruz, D., Khamashta, M., Hughes, G., 2007. Systemic lupus erythematosus. Lancet 369, 587–596.

Dasgupta, B., Borg, F.A., Hassan, N., et al., 2010. BSR and BHPR guidelines for the management of giant cell arteritis. Rheumatology 49, 1594–1597.

Dasgupta, B., Borg, F.A., Hassan, N., et al., 2010. BSR and BHPR guidelines for the management of polymyalgia rheumatica. Rheumatology 49, 186–190.

Elwood, P.C., Gallagher, A.M., Duthie, G.G., et al., 2009. Aspirin, salicylates, and cancer. Lancet 373, 1301–1309.

Fearon, D., 2003. Innate immunity. In: Warrell, D.A. (Ed.), Oxford Textbook of Medicine, forth ed. Oxford University Press, Oxford. (Chapter 5.5).

Gabay, C., Lamacchia, C., Palmer, G., 2010. IL-1 pathways in inflammation and human diseases. Nat. Rev. Rheumatol. 6, 232–241.

McMichael, A., 2003. Principles of immunology. In: Warrell, D.A., Cox, T.M., Firth, J.D., Benz, E.J. (Eds.), Oxford Textbook of Medicine, forth ed. Oxford University Press, Oxford. (Chapter. 5.1).

National Institute for Health and Clinical Excellence. Osteoarthritis: the care and management of osteoarthritis in adults. NICE Guidance CG59. Available at: http://guidance.nice.org.uk/CG59 (accessed November 2011).

National Institute for Health and Clinical Excellence. Rheumatoid arthritis: the management of rheumatoid arthritis in adults. NICE Guidance CG79. Available at: http://guidance.nice.org.uk/CG79 (accessed November 2011).

Østensen, M., Förger, F., 2009. Management of RA medications in pregnant patients. Nat. Rev. Rheumatol. 5, 382–390.

Østensen, M., Motta, M., 2007. Therapy insight: the use of anti-rheumatic drugs during nursing. Nat. Clin. Pract. Rheumatol. 3, 490–496.

Richette, P., Doherty, M., Pascual, E., et al., 2016 updated EULAR evidence-based recommendations for the management of gout Annals of the Rheumatic Diseases Published Online First: 25 July 2016. doi: 10.1136/annrheumdis-2016-209707.

Šenolt, L., Vencovský, J., Pavelka, K., et al., 2009. Prospective new biological therapies for rheumatoid arthritis. Autoimmun. Rev. 9, 102–107.

Shepard, H.M., Phillips, G.L., Thanos, C., et al., 2017. Developments in therapy with monoclonal antibodies and related proteins. Clin Med (Lond) 17 (3), 220–232.

Sieper, J., 2016. New treatment targets for axial spondyloarthritis. Rheumatology (Oxford) 55 (Suppl. 2), ii38–ii42.

Terkeltaub, R., 2010. Update on gout: new therapeutic strategies and options. Nat. Rev. Rheumatol. 6, 30–38.

Chapter 17

Drugs and the skin

Thomas K. K. Ha

SYNOPSIS

This account is confined to therapy directed primarily at the skin and covers the following topics:

- **Dermal pharmacokinetics.**
  - **Vehicles for presenting drugs to the skin.**
- **Selected topical preparations.**
  - **Emollients and barrier preparations**
  - **Topical analgesics**
  - **Antipruritics**
  - **Analgesics**
  - **Adrenal corticosteroids**
  - **Sunscreens**
  - **Drug-specific rashes.**
- **Approaches to some skin disorders.**
  - **Psoriasis**
  - **Acne**
  - **Urticaria**
  - **Atopic dermatitis.**

Dermal pharmacokinetics

Human skin is a highly efficient self-repairing barrier that permits terrestrial life by regulating heat and water loss while preventing the ingress of noxious chemicals and microorganisms. A drug applied to the skin may diffuse from the stratum corneum into the epidermis and then into the dermis, to enter the capillary microcirculation and thus the systemic circulation (Fig. 17.1). The features of components of the skin in relation to drug therapy, whether for local or systemic effect, are worthy of examination.

The principal barrier to penetration resides in the multiple-layered lipid-rich stratum corneum. The passage of a drug through this layer is influenced by its:

- *Physicochemical features:* lipophilic drugs can utilise the *intra*cellular route because they readily cross cell walls, whereas hydrophilic drugs principally take the *inter*cellular route, diffusing in fluid-filled spaces between cells.
- *Molecular size:* most therapeutic agents suitable for topical delivery measure 100–500 Da.

Drugs are presented in vehicles (bases[1]), designed to vary in the extent to which they increase hydration of the stratum corneum; e.g. oil-in-water creams promote hydration (see below). Increasing the water content of the stratum corneum via occlusion or hydration generally increases the penetration of both lipophilic and hydrophilic materials. This may be due to an increased fluid content of the lipid bilayers. The stratum corneum and stratum granulosum layers become more similar with hydration and occlusion, thus lowering the partition coefficient of the molecule passing through the interface. Some vehicles also contain substances intended to enhance penetration by reducing the barrier properties of the stratum corneum, e.g. fatty acids, terpenes, surfactants. Encapsulation of drugs into vesicular liposomes may enhance drug delivery to specific compartments of the skin, e.g. hair follicles.

Absorption through normal skin varies with site. From the sole of the foot and the palm of the hand, it is relatively low; it increases progressively on the forearm, trunk, head and neck; and on the scrotum and vulva, absorption is very high. Where the skin is damaged by inflammation, burn or exfoliation, barrier function is reduced and absorption is further increased.

---

[1]The chief ingredient of a mixture.

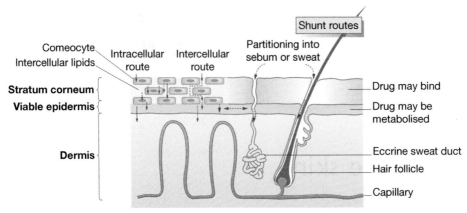

Fig. 17.1 Principal pathways operating during topical drug delivery.

If an occlusive dressing (impermeable plastic membrane) is used, absorption increases by as much as 10-fold (plastic pants for babies are occlusive, and some ointments are partially occlusive). Systemic toxicity can result from use of occlusive dressing over large areas.

Transdermal delivery systems are now used to administer drugs via the skin for systemic effect; the advantages and disadvantages of this route are discussed on p. 91.

Vehicles for presenting drugs to the skin

Dermatological formulations tend to be classified by their physical properties. The formulations below are described in order of decreasing water content. All water-based formulations must contain preservatives, e.g. chlorocresol, but these rarely cause allergic contact dermatitis.

Liquid formulations

Water or a solvent is the most important component. The preparation can be a soak, a bath or a paint. Wet dressings are generally used to cleanse, cool and relieve pruritus in acutely inflamed lesions, especially where there is much exudation, e.g. atopic eczema. The frequent reapplication and the cooling effect of evaporation of the water reduce the inflammatory response by inducing superficial vasoconstriction (an effect enhanced when alcohol is present in the formulation). Sodium chloride solution 0.9%, stringent substances, e.g. aluminium acetate lotion, or potassium permanganate soaks or compresses of approximately 0.01–0.05% can be used. The use of *lotions* (wet dressings) over very large areas can reduce body temperature dangerously in the old or the very ill.

Two-phase or multiple liquid shake lotions, e.g. calamine lotion, are essentially a convenient way of applying a powder to the skin with additional cooling due to evaporation of the water. They are contraindicated when there is much exudate, because crusts form. Lotions, after evaporation, sometimes produce excessive drying of the skin, but this can be reduced if oils are included, as in oily calamine lotion.

Creams

These are emulsions of either oil in water (washable; cosmetic 'vanishing' creams) or water in oil. The water content allows the cream to rub in well. A cooling effect (cold creams) is obtained with both groups as the water evaporates.

Oil-in-water creams, e.g. aqueous cream (see emulsifying ointment, below), mix with serous discharges and are especially useful as vehicles for water-soluble drugs. They may contain a wetting (surface tension–reducing) agent (cetomacrogol). Various other ingredients, e.g. calamine, zinc, may be added to it.

Water-in-oil creams, e.g. oily cream, zinc cream, behave like oils in that they do not mix with serous discharges, but their chief advantage over ointments (below) is that the water content makes them easier to spread and they give a better cosmetic effect. They act as lubricants and emollients, and can be used on hairy parts. Water-in-oil creams can be used as vehicles for lipid-soluble substances.

Creams, being less occlusive and effective at hydrating the stratum corneum, are not as effective for drug delivery as ointments.

Ointments

Ointments are greasy and thicker than creams. Some are both lipophilic and hydrophilic, i.e. by occlusion they promote dermal hydration, but are also water miscible. Other ointment bases are composed largely of lipid; by preventing water loss, they have a hydrating effect on skin and are used in chronic dry conditions. Ointments contain fewer preservatives and are less likely to sensitise. There are two main kinds:

Water-soluble ointments include mixtures of macrogols and polyethylene glycols; their consistency can be varied readily. They are easily washed off and are used in burn dressings, as lubricants and as vehicles that readily allow passage of drugs into the skin, e.g. hydrocortisone.

Emulsifying ointment is made from emulsifying wax (cetostearyl alcohol and sodium lauryl sulphate) and paraffins. Aqueous cream is an oil-in-water emulsion of emulsifying ointment.

Non-emulsifying ointments do not mix with water. They adhere to the skin to prevent evaporation and heat loss, i.e. they can be considered a form of occlusive dressing (with increased systemic absorption of active ingredients); skin maceration may occur. Non-emulsifying ointments are helpful in chronic dry and scaly conditions, such as atopic eczema, and as vehicles; they are not appropriate where there is significant exudation. They are difficult to remove except with oil or detergents and are messy and inconvenient, especially on hairy skin. Paraffin ointment contains beeswax, paraffins and cetostearyl alcohol.

Collodions and gels

Collodions are preparations of a thickening agent, e.g. cellulose nitrate (pyroxylin) dissolved in an organic solvent. The solvent evaporates rapidly and the resultant flexible film is used to hold a medicament, e.g. salicylic acid, in contact with the skin. They are irritant and inflammable, and are used to treat only small areas of skin.

Gels or *jellies* are semi-solid colloidal solutions or suspensions used as lubricants and as vehicles for drugs. They are sometimes useful for treating the scalp.

Pastes

Pastes, e.g. zinc compound paste, are stiff, semi-occlusive ointments containing insoluble powders. They are very adhesive and are valuable for treating highly circumscribed lesions while preventing spread of active ingredients on to surrounding skin. Their powder content enables them to absorb a moderate amount of discharge. They can be used as vehicles, e.g. coal tar paste, which is zinc compound paste with 7.5% coal tar. Lassar's paste is used as a vehicle for dithranol in the treatment of well-circumscibed plaque psoriasis.

Solid preparations

Solid preparations such as dusting powders, e.g. zinc starch and talc,[2] may cool by increasing the effective surface area of the skin, and they reduce friction between skin surfaces by their lubricating action. Although usefully absorbent, they cause crusting if applied to exudative lesions. They may be used alone or as specialised vehicles for, e.g., fungicides.

Emollients and barrier preparations

Emollients hydrate the skin and soothe and smooth dry scaly conditions. They need to be applied frequently, as their effects are short lived. There is a variety of preparations, but aqueous cream, in addition to its use as a vehicle (above), is effective when used as a soap substitute. Various other ingredients may be added to emollients, e.g. menthol, camphor or phenol for its mild antipruritic effect, and zinc and titanium dioxide as astringents.[3]

Barrier preparations. Many different kinds have been devised for use in medicine, in industry and in the home to reduce dermatitis. They rely on water-repellent substances, e.g. silicones (dimethicone cream), and on soaps, as well as on substances that form an impermeable deposit (titanium, zinc, calamine). The barrier preparations are useful in protecting skin from discharges and secretions (colostomies, nappy rash) but are ineffective when used under industrial working conditions. Indeed, the irritant properties of some barrier creams can enhance the percutaneous penetration of noxious substances. A simple after-work emollient is more effective.

Silicone sprays and *occlusives*, e.g. hydrocolloid dressings, may be effective in preventing and treating pressure sores. Masking creams (camouflaging preparations) for obscuring unpleasant blemishes from view are greatly valued by patients.[4] They may consist of titanium oxide in an ointment base with colouring appropriate to the site and the patient.

Topical analgesics

Counterirritants and rubefacients are irritants that stimulate nerve endings in intact skin to relieve pain in skin (e.g. post-herpetic), viscera or muscle supplied by the same nerve root. All produce inflammation of the skin, which becomes flushed – hence the term 'rubefacients'. The best

---

[2]Talc is magnesium silicate. It must not be used for dusting surgical gloves as it causes granulomas if it gets into mounds or body cavities.
[3]Astringents are weak protein precipitants, e.g. tannins, salts of aluminium and zinc.
[4]In the UK, the Red Cross offers a free cosmetic camouflage service through hospital dermatology departments.

counterirritants are physical agents, especially heat. Many compounds have been used for this purpose, and suitable preparations contain salicylates, nicotinates, menthol, camphor and capsaicin. Specific transient receptor potential (TRP) cation channels involved in sensory perception in skin can be stimulated by these drugs. The moderate heat receptor TRPV1 is sensitive to capsaicin as well as moderate heat (42–52 °C), whereas TRPM8 is stimulated specifically by temperatures below 26 °C and by menthol.

Topical non-steroidal anti-inflammatory drugs (NSAIDs) can be used to relieve musculoskeletal pain.

Local anaesthetics. Lidocaine and prilocaine are available as gels, ointments and sprays to provide reversible block of conduction along cutaneous nerves. Benzocaine and amethocaine (tetracaine) carry a high risk of sensitisation.

Volatile aerosol sprays, beloved by sports people, produce analgesia by cooling and by placebo effect.

Antipruritics

Mechanisms of itch are both peripheral and central. Itch (at least histamine-induced itch) is not a minor or low-intensity form of pain. Cutaneous histamine injection stimulates a specific group of C fibres with very low conduction speeds and large fields, distinct from those that signal pain. Second-order neurones then ascend via the spinothalamic tract to the thalamus. In the central nervous system, endogenous opioid peptides are released (the opioid antagonist naloxone can relieve some cases of intractable itch). Itch signalling appears to be under tonic inhibition by pain. If pain after histamine injection is reduced by opioid then itch results and, if pain is ablated by lidocaine, itch sensation increases. Prolonged inflammation in the skin may lead to peripheral and central sensitisation, thus leading non-itchy stimuli to be reinterpreted as itch.

Liberation of histamine and other autacoids in the skin also contributes and may be responsible for much of the itch of urticarial allergic reactions. Histamine release by bile salts may explain some, but not all, of the itch of obstructive jaundice. It is likely that other chemical mediators, e.g. serotonin, progesterone metabolites, endogenous opioids and prostaglandins, are involved.

Generalised pruritus

In the absence of a primary dermatosis, it is important to search for an underlying cause, e.g. iron deficiency, liver or renal failure and lymphoma, but there remain patients in whom the cause either cannot be removed or is not known. Antihistamines (H₁-receptor), especially chlorphenamine and hydroxyzine orally, are used for their sedative or anxiolytic effect (except in urticaria); they should not be applied topically over a prolonged period because of risk of allergy. In severe pruritus, a sedative antidepressant may also help.

The itching of obstructive jaundice might be relieved by the anion exchange resin colestyramine, an endoscopically placed nasobiliary drain or phototherapy with ultraviolet B light. Naltrexone offers short-term relief of the pruritus associated with haemodialysis.

Localised pruritus

Scratching or rubbing seems to give relief by converting the intolerable persistent itch into a more bearable pain. A vicious cycle can be set up in which itching provokes scratching, and scratching leads to infected skin lesions that itch, as in prurigo nodularis. Covering the lesion or enclosing it in a medicated bandage so as to prevent any further scratching or rubbing may help. Multiple intralesional triamcinolone injections and thalidomide may be used in recalcitrant cases of prurigo nodularis.

Topical corticosteroid preparations are used to treat the underlying inflammatory cause of pruritus, e.g. in eczema. A cooling application such as 0.5–2% menthol in aqueous cream is temporarily antipruritic.

Calamine and *astringents* (aluminium acetate, tannic acid) may help. Local anaesthetics do not offer any long-term solution and, as they are liable to sensitise the skin, they are best avoided. Topical doxepin can be helpful in localised pruritus, but extensive use induces sedation and may cause allergic contact dermatitis.

Pruritus ani is managed by attention to any underlying disease, e.g. haemorrhoids, parasites and hygiene. Emollients, e.g. washing with aqueous cream and a weak corticosteroid with antiseptic/anticandida application, may be used briefly to settle any acute eczema or superinfection. Some cases are a form of neurodermatitis, and an antihistamine with anti-anxiolytic properties, e.g. hydroxyzine, or a low-dose sedative antidepressant, e.g. doxepin, and mirtazapine, may be helpful. Secondary contact sensitivity, e.g. to local anaesthetics, must be considered.

Adrenocortical steroids

Actions. Adrenal steroids possess a range of actions, of which the following are relevant to topical use:

- Inflammation is suppressed, particularly when there is an allergic factor, and immune responses are reduced.
- Antimitotic activity suppresses proliferation of keratinocytes, fibroblasts and lymphocytes (useful in psoriasis, but also causes skin thinning).
- Vasoconstriction reduces ingress of inflammatory cells and humoral factors to the inflamed area; this action

Table 17.1 Fingertip unit dosimetry for topical corticosteroids (distance from the tip of the adult index finger to the first crease)

Age	Face/neck	Arm/hand	Leg/foot	Trunk (front)	Trunk (back, including buttocks)
3–6 months	1	1	1.5	1	1.5
1–2 years	1.5	1.5	2	2	3
3–5 years	1.5	2	3	3	3.5
6–10 years	2	2.5	4.5	3.5	5
Adult	2.5	Arm: 3 Hand: 1	Leg: 6 Foot: 2	7	7

(blanching effect on human skin) has been used to measure the potency of individual topical corticosteroids (see below).

Penetration into the skin is governed by the factors outlined at the beginning of the chapter. The vehicle should be appropriate to the condition being treated: an ointment for dry, scaly conditions; a water-based cream for weeping eczema.

Uses. Adrenal corticosteroids should be considered a symptomatic and sometimes curative, but not preventive, treatment. Ideally a potent steroid (see below) should be given only as a short course and reduced as soon as the response allows. Corticosteroids are most useful for eczematous disorders (atopic, discoid, contact), whereas dilute corticosteroids are especially useful for flexural psoriasis (where other therapies are highly irritant). Adrenal corticosteroids of highest potency are reserved for recalcitrant dermatoses, e.g. lichen simplex, lichen planus, nodular prurigo and discoid lupus erythematosus.

Topical corticosteroids should be applied sparingly. The 'fingertip unit'[5] is a useful guide in educating patients (Table 17.1). The difficulties and dangers of systemic adrenal steroid therapy are sufficient to restrict such use to serious conditions (such as pemphigus and generalised exfoliative dermatitis) not responsive to other forms of therapy.

Guidelines for the use of topical corticosteroids:
- Use for symptom relief and not prophylactically.
- Choose the appropriate therapeutic potency (Table 17.2), e.g. mild for the face. In cases likely to be resistant, use a very potent preparation, e.g. for 3 weeks, to gain control, after which change to a less potent preparation.

- Choose the appropriate vehicle, e.g. a water-based cream for weeping eczema, an ointment for dry, scaly conditions.
- Prescribe in small but adequate amounts so that serious overuse is unlikely to occur without the doctor knowing, e.g. weekly quantity by group (see Table 17.2): very potent, 15 g; potent, 30 g; other, 50 g.
- Occlusive dressing should be used only briefly. Note that babies' plastic pants are an occlusive dressing as well as being a social amenity.
- If it's wet, dry it; if it's dry, wet it. The traditional advice contains enough truth to be worth repeating.
- One or two applications per day are all that is usually necessary.

Choice. Topical corticosteroids are classified according to both drug and potency, i.e. therapeutic efficacy in relation to weight (see Table 17.2). Their potency is determined by the amount of vasoconstriction a topical corticosteroid produces (McKenzie skin-blanching test[6]) and the degree to which it inhibits inflammation. Choice of preparation relates both to the disease and the site of intended use. High-potency preparations are commonly needed for lichen planus and discoid lupus erythematosus; weaker preparations (hydrocortisone 0.5–2.5%) are usually adequate for eczema, for use on the face and in childhood.

When a skin disorder requiring a corticosteroid is already infected, a preparation containing an antimicrobial is added, e.g. fusidic acid or clotrimazole. When the infection has been eliminated, the corticosteroid may be continued alone.

---

[5]The distance from the tip of the index finger to the first skin crease.

[6]McKenzie A W, Stoughton R B 1962 Method for comparing percutaneous absorption of steroids. Archives of Dermatology 86:608–610.

Table 17.2 Topical corticosteroid formulations conventionally ranked according to therapeutic potency

Potency	Formulations
Very potent	Clobetasol (0.05%); also formulations of diflucortolone (0.3%), halcinonide
Potent	Beclometasone (0.025%); also formulations of betamethasone, budesonide, desoximetasone, diflucortolone (0.1%), fluclorolone, fluocinolone (0.025%), fluocinonide, fluticasone, hydrocortisone butyrate, mometasone (once daily), triamcinolone
Moderately potent	Clobetasone (0.05%); also formulations of alclometasone, clobetasone, desoximetasone, fluocinolone (0.00625%), fluocortolone, fluandrenolone
Mildly potent	Hydrocortisone (0.1–1.0%); also formulations of alclomethasone, fluocinolone (0.0025%), methylprednisolone

Important note: the ranking is based on agent and its concentration; the same drug appears in more than one rank.

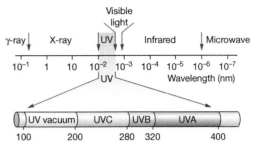

Fig. 17.2 The ultraviolet component of the electromagnetic spectrum.

reduce the risk of systemic toxicity. Suppression of the hypothalamic–pituitary axis occurs readily with overuse of the very potent agents, and when 20% of the body is under an occlusive dressing with mildly potent agents.

Other complications of occlusive dressings include infections (bacterial, candidal) and even heat stroke when large areas are occluded. Antifungal cream containing hydrocortisone and used for vaginal candidiasis may contaminate the urine and misleadingly suggest Cushing's syndrome.[7]

Applications to the eyelids may get into the eye and cause glaucoma.

Rebound exacerbation of the disease can occur after abrupt cessation of therapy. This can lead the patient to reapply the steroid and so create a vicious cycle.

Allergy. Corticosteroids, particularly hydrocortisone and budesonide or other ingredients in the formulation, may cause allergic contact dermatitis. The possibility of this should be considered when expected benefit fails to occur, e.g. varicose eczema.

Intralesional injections are used occasionally to provide high local concentrations without systemic effects in chronic dermatoses, e.g. hypertrophic lichen planus and discoid lupus erythematosus.

Adverse effects. Used with restraint, topical corticosteroids are effective and safe. Adverse effects are more likely with formulations ranked therapeutically as very potent or potent in Table 17.2.

Short-term use. Infection may spread.

Long-term use. Skin atrophy can occur within 4 weeks and may or may not be fully reversible. It reflects loss of connective tissue, which also causes striae (irreversible) and generally occurs at sites where dermal penetration is high (face, groins, axillae).

Other effects include: local hirsutism; perioral dermatitis (especially in young women), which responds to steroid withdrawal and may be mitigated by tetracycline by mouth for 4–6 weeks; depigmentation (local); monomorphous acne (local). Potent corticosteroids should not be used on the face unless this is unavoidable. Systemic absorption can lead to all the adverse effects of systemic corticosteroid use. Fluticasone propionate and mometasone furoate are rapidly metabolised following cutaneous absorption, which may

Sunscreens (sunburn and photosensitivity)

Ultraviolet (UV) solar radiation (Fig. 17.2) is defined as:

- UVA (320–400 nm), which damages collagen, contributes to skin cancer and drug photosensitivity.
- UVB (280–320 nm), which is 1000 times more active than UVA, acutely causes sunburn and chronically skin cancer and skin ageing.
- UVC (200–280 nm), which is prevented, at present, from reaching the earth at sea level by the stratospheric ozone layer, although it can cause skin injury at high altitude.

[7]Kelly C J G, Ogilvie A, Evans J R et al 2001 Raised cortisol excretion rate in urine and contamination by topical steroids. British Medical Journal 322:594.

Protection of the skin

Protection from UV radiation is effected by:

Absorbent sunscreens. These organic chemicals absorb UVB and UVA at the surface of the skin (generally more effective for UVB).

UVB protection is provided by aminobenzoic acid and aminobenzoates (padimate-O), cinnamates, salicylates, camphors.

UVA protection is provided by benzophenones (mexenone, oxybenzone), dibenzoylmethanes.

Reflectant sunscreens. Opaque inorganic minerals such as titanium dioxide, zinc oxide and calamine act as a physical barrier to UVB and UVA (especially zinc oxide); they are cosmetically unattractive, but the newer micronised preparations are more acceptable. Because they are able to protect against visible light, they are especially useful in photosensitivity disorders, e.g. porphyria.

The performance of a sunscreen is expressed as the sun protective factor (SPF), which refers to UVB (UVA is more troublesome to measure, and the protection is indicated by a star rating system, with four stars providing the greatest). An SPF of 10 means that the dose of UVB required to cause erythema must be 10 times greater on protected than on unprotected skin. The SPF should be interpreted only as a rough guide; consumer use is more haphazard, and less liberal amounts are applied to the skin in practice. The benefits of using active agents including vitamins, antioxidants, osmolytes and DNA repair enzymes in sunscreens and cosmetics to counteract the inherent photochemical processes that can induce DNA damage in skin cells is unproven.

Sunscreens should protect against both UVB and UVA. Absorbent and reflectant components are combined in some preparations. The washability of the preparation (including removal by sweat and swimming) is also relevant to efficacy and frequency of application; some penetrate the stratum corneum (padimate-O) and are more persistent than others.

Uses. Sunscreens are no substitute for light-impermeable clothing and sun avoidance (especially during peak hours of UV light). Daily application of sunscreen appears to protect more against UV-induced skin changes than intermittent use of the product. Methodical use has been demonstrated to reduce the incidence of cutaneous squamous cell carcinoma. Sunscreens are especially beneficial in protecting those who are photosensitive due to drugs (below) or disease, i.e. for photodermatoses such as photosensitivity dermatitis, polymorphic light eruption, cutaneous porphyrias and lupus erythematosus.

Treatment of mild sunburn is usually with a lotion such as oily calamine lotion. Severe cases are helped by topical corticosteroids. NSAIDs, e.g. indometacin, can help if given early, by preventing the formation of prostaglandins.

Drug photosensitivity

Drug photosensitivity means that an adverse effect occurs as a result of drug plus light, usually UVA; sometimes even the amount of UV radiation from fluorescent light tubes is sufficient.

Systemically taken drugs that can induce photosensitivity are many, the most common being the following:[8]

- Antimitotics: dacarbazine, vinblastine, taxanes, methotrexate.
- Antimicrobials: demeclocycline, doxycycline, nalidixic acid, sulfonamides.
- Antipsychotics: chlorpromazine, prochlorperazine.
- Cardiac arrhythmic: amiodarone.
- Diuretics: furosemide, chlorothiazide, hydrochlorothiazide.
- Fibric acid derivatives, e.g. fenofibrate.
- Hypoglycaemics: tolbutamide.
- NSAIDs: piroxicam.
- Psoralens (see below).
- Antifungals: voriconazole (extreme phototoxicity and heightened risk of squamous cell carcinoma and melanoma).

Topically applied substances that can produce photosensitivity include:

- Para-aminobenzoic acid and its esters (used as sunscreens).
- Coal tar derivatives.
- Psoralens from juices of various plants, e.g. bergamot oil.
- 6-Methylcoumarin (used in perfumes, shaving lotions, sunscreens).

There are two forms of photosensitivity:

Phototoxicity, like drug toxicity, is a normal effect of too high a dose of UV light in a subject who has been exposed to the drug. The reaction is like severe sunburn. The threshold returns to normal when the drug is withdrawn. Some drugs, notably NSAIDs, induce a 'pseudoporphyria', clinically resembling porphyria cutanea tarda and presenting with skin fragility, blisters and milia on sun-exposed areas, notably the backs of the hands.

Photoallergy, like drug allergy, is a cell-mediated immunological effect that occurs only in some people, and which may be severe with a small dose. Photoallergy due to drugs is the result of a photochemical reaction caused by UVA in which the drug combines with tissue protein to form an antigen. Reactions may persist for years after the drug is withdrawn; they are usually eczematous.

---

[8]Data from The Medical Letter 1995;37:35.

Systemic protection, as opposed to application of drug to exposed areas, should be considered when the topical measures fail.

Antimalarials such as hydroxychloroquine may be effective for short periods in polymorphic light eruption and in cutaneous lupus erythematosus.

Psoralens (obtained from citrus fruits and other plants), e.g. methoxsalen, are used to induce photochemical reactions in the skin. After topical or systemic administration of the psoralen and subsequent exposure to UVA, there is an erythematous reaction that goes deeper than ordinary sunburn and may reach its maximum only after 48 h (sunburn maximum is 12–24 h). Melanocytes are activated and pigmentation occurs over the following week. This action is used to repigment areas of disfiguring depigmentation, e.g. vitiligo in black-skinned persons.

In the presence of UVA, the psoralen interacts with DNA, forms thymine dimers and inhibits DNA synthesis. Psoralen plus UVA (PUVA) treatment is used chiefly in severe psoriasis (a disease characterised by increased epidermal proliferation) and cutaneous T-cell lymphoma.

Severe *adverse reactions* can occur with psoralens and UV radiation, including sunburn, increased risk of skin cancer (due to mutagenicity inherent in their action), cancer of the male genitalia, cataracts and accelerated skin ageing; the treatment is used only by specialists.

Chronic exposure to sunlight induces wrinkling and yellowing due to the changes in the dermal connective tissue. Topical retinoids are used widely in an attempt to reverse some of these tissue changes. Public pursuit of novel tanning strategies, including the unregulated subcutaneous self-administration of synthetic analogues of alpha–melanocyte-stimulating hormone (alpha-MSH), has been reported. Medical practitioners should be aware that these agents can complicate the clinical presentation of patients with changing moles and suspected melanoma.

Miscellaneous compounds

Keratolytics are used to destroy unwanted tissue, including warts and corns. Great care is obviously necessary to avoid ulceration. They include trichloroacetic acid, salicylic acid and many others. Resorcinol and sulphur are mild keratolytics used in acne. Salicylic acid may enhance the efficacy of a topical steroid in hyperkeratotic disorders.

Tars are mildly antiseptic, antipruritic and inhibit keratinisation in an ill-understood way. They are safe in low concentrations and are used in psoriasis. Photosensitivity occurs, and tar–UVB regimens are highly effective therapies for extensive psoriasis. There are very many preparations, which usually contain other substances, e.g. coal tar and salicylic acid ointment.

Ichthammol is a sulphurous, tarry, distillation product of fossilised fish (obtained in the Austrian Tyrol); it has a weaker effect than coal tar.

Zinc oxide provides mild astringent, barrier and occlusive actions. Calamine is basic zinc carbonate that owes its pink colour to added ferric oxide. It has a mild astringent action, and is used as a dusting powder and in shake and oily lotions.

Urea is used topically to assist skin hydration, e.g. in ichthyosis.

Insect repellents, e.g. against mosquitoes, ticks, fleas, such as DEET (diethyl toluamide), dimethyl phthalate. These are applied to the skin and repel insects principally by vaporisation. They must be applied to all exposed skin, and sometimes also to clothes, if their objective is to be achieved (some damage plastic fabrics and spectacle frames). Their duration of effect is limited by the rate at which they vaporise (dependent on skin and ambient temperature), by washing off (sweat, rain, immersion) and by mechanical factors causing rubbing (physical activity). They can cause allergic and toxic effects, especially with prolonged use.

Benzyl benzoate may be used on clothes; it resists one or two washings.

Cutaneous drug reactions

Drugs applied locally or taken systemically often cause rashes. These take many different forms, and the same drug may produce different rashes in different people. Types of drug rash include:

- Exanthems.
- Acute generalised exanthematous pustulosis.
- Fixed drug rash.
- Stevens–Johnson syndrome/erythema multiforme/ toxic epidermal necrolysis.
- Hypersensitivity reaction including DRESS (drug rash with eosinophilia and systemic symptoms), e.g. hepatitis. The pathogenesis of DRESS is likely to be multifactorial. The factors include deficient detoxification of a drug metabolite in patients who are genetically susceptible, drug interactions, and direct effects of drug-specific T cells. Recent reports of co-infection with human herpesvirus (HHV)-6 or HHV-7 and a transient hypogammaglobulinaemia may prove important in anticonvulsant hypersensitivity.

Some of the mechanisms involved in drug-induced cutaneous reactions are described in Box 17.1.

Although drugs may change, the clinical problems remain depressingly the same: a patient develops a rash; he or she

Box 17.1 **Mechanisms of cutaneous drug reactions**

Immunological mechanisms

- IgE dependent
- Cytotoxic
- Immune complex mediated
- Cell mediated

Non-immunological mechanisms

- Overdosage
- Cumulative toxicity
- Delayed toxicity
- Drug–drug–food interactions
- Exacerbation of disease

Idiosyncratic

- Drug rash with eosinophilia and systemic symptoms (DRESS)
- Toxic epidermal necrolysis/Stevens–Johnson syndrome
- Drug reactions in setting of HIV
- Drug-induced lupus

is taking many different tablets; which, if any, of these caused the eruption, and what should be done about it? It is no answer simply to stop all drugs, although the fact that this can often be done casts some doubt on the patient's need for them in the first place. All too often, potentially valuable drugs are excluded from further use on totally inadequate grounds. Clearly some guidelines are useful, but no simple set of rules exists that can cover this complex subject:[9]

1. *Can other skin diseases be excluded, and are the skin changes compatible with a drug cause?* Clinical features that indicate a drug cause include the type of primary lesion (blisters, pustules), distribution of lesions (acral lesions in erythema multiforme), mucosal involvement and evidence of systemic involvement (fever, lymphadenopathy, visceral involvement).
2. *Which drug is most likely to be responsible?* Document all of the drugs the patient has been exposed to and the date of introduction of each drug. Determine the interval between commencement date and the date of the skin eruption. Chronology is important, with most reactions occurring about 10–12 days after starting a new drug or within 2–3 days in previously exposed patients. A search of standard literature sources of adverse reactions, including the

pharmaceutical company data, can be helpful in identifying suspect drugs.
3. *Are any further tests worthwhile?* Excluding infectious causes of skin eruptions is important, e.g. viral exanthems, mycoplasma. A skin biopsy in cases of non-specific dermatitis is helpful, as a predominance of eosinophils would support a drug precipitant.
4. *Is any treatment needed?* Supporting the ill patient and stopping the causative drug is crucial.

Drug-specific rashes

Despite great variability, some hints at drug-specific or characteristic rashes from drugs taken systemically can be discerned; some examples are as follows:

- *Acne and pustular:* corticosteroids, androgens, ciclosporin, penicillins.
- *Allergic vasculitis:* sulfonamides, NSAIDs, thiazides, chlorpropamide, phenytoin, penicillin, retinoids.
- *Anaphylaxis:* X-ray contrast media, penicillins, angiotensin-converting enzyme (ACE) inhibitors.
- *Bullous pemphigoid:* furosemide (and other sulfonamide-related drugs), ACE inhibitors, penicillamine, penicillin, PUVA therapy.
- *Eczema:* penicillins, phenothiazines.
- *Exanthematic/maculopapular* reactions are the most frequent; unlike a viral exanthem, the eruption typically starts on the trunk; the face is relatively spared. Causes include antimicrobials, especially ampicillin, sulfonamides and derivatives (sulfonylureas, furosemide and thiazide diuretics).
- *Morbilliform* (measles-like) eruptions typically recur on rechallenge.
- *Erythema multiforme:* NSAIDs, sulfonamides, barbiturates, phenytoin, paclitaxel.
- *Erythema nodosum:* dermatitis and sulfonamides, oral contraceptives, prazosin.
- *Exfoliative erythroderma:* gold, phenytoin, carbamazepine, allopurinol, penicillins, neuroleptics, isoniazid.
- *Fixed eruptions* are eruptions that recur at the same site, often circumoral, with each administration of the drug: phenolphthalein (laxative self-medication), sulfonamides, quinine (in tonic water), tetracycline, barbiturates, naproxen, nifedipine.
- *Hair loss:* cytotoxic anticancer drugs, acitretin, oral contraceptives, heparin, androgenic steroids (women), sodium valproate, gold.
- *Hypertrichosis:* corticosteroids, ciclosporin, doxasosin, minoxidil.
- *Lichenoid eruption:* β-adrenoceptor blockers, chloroquine, thiazides, furosemide, captopril, gold, phenothiazines.

[9]Hardie R A, Savin J A 1979 Drug-induced skin diseases. British Medical Journal 1:935 (to whom we are grateful for the quotation and classification).

- *Lupus erythematosus:* hydralazine, isoniazid, procainamide, phenytoin, oral contraceptives, sulfazaline.
- *Purpura:* thiazides, sulfonamides, sulfonylureas, phenylbutazone, quinine. Aspirin induces a capillaritis (pigmented purpuric dermatitis).
- *Photosensitivity:* see above.
- *Pemphigus:* penicillamine, captopril, piroxicam, penicillin, rifampicin.
- *Pruritus* unassociated with rash: oral contraceptives, phenothiazines, rifampicin (cholestatic reaction).
- *Pigmentation:* oral contraceptives (chloasma in photosensitive distribution), phenothiazines, heavy metals, amiodarone, chloroquine (pigmentation of nails and palate, depigmentation of the hair), minocycline.
- *Psoriasis* may be aggravated by β-blockers, lithium and antimalarials.
- *Scleroderma-like:* bleomycin, sodium valproate, tryptophan contaminants (eosinophilia–myalgia syndrome).
- *Serum sickness:* immunoglobulins and other immunomodulatory blood products.
- *Stevens–Johnson syndrome and toxic epidermal necrolysis* (TENS): e.g. anticonvulsants, sulfonamides, aminopenicillins, NSAIDs, allopurinol, chlormezanone, corticosteroids.
- *Urticaria and angioedema:* penicillins, ACE inhibitors, gold, NSAIDs, e.g. aspirin, codeine.
- Patients with the acquired immunodeficiency syndrome (AIDS) have an increased risk of adverse reactions, which are often severe. Recovery after withdrawal of the causative drug generally begins within a few days, but lichenoid reactions may not improve for weeks.

Diagnosis

The patient's drug history may give clues. Reactions are commoner during early therapy (days) than after the drug has been given for months. Diagnosis by purposeful read-ministration of the drug (challenge) is not recommended, especially in patients suffering a generalised effect or with mucosal involvement, as it may precipitate toxic epidermal necrolysis.

Patch and photopatch tests are useful in contact dermatitis, as they reproduce the causative process, but should be performed only by those with special experience. Fixed drug eruptions can sometimes be reproduced by patch testing with the drug over the previously affected site.

Intradermal tests introduce all the problems of allergy to drugs, e.g. metabolism, combination with protein, fatal anaphylaxis.

Treatment

Treatment involves supportive care and removal of the causative drug. Use cooling applications and antipruritics; use a histamine H_1-receptor blocker systemically for acute urticaria. The use of adrenal corticosteroids is controversial. It may be useful for severe exanthems if the incriminated drug is crucial for other concurrent disease, and is useful for internal organ disease involvement in DRESS. The use of human-derived immunoglobulin infusions is increasingly advocated in the treatment of toxic epidermal necrolysis.

Safety monitoring

Several drugs commonly used in dermatology should be monitored regularly for (principally systemic) adverse effects. These include:

- *Aciclovir* (plasma creatinine).
- *Azathioprine* (blood count and liver function).
- *Colchicine* (blood count, plasma creatinine).
- *Ciclosporin* (plasma creatinine).
- *Dapsone* (liver function, blood count including reticulocytes).
- *Methotrexate* (blood count, liver function).
- *PUVA* (liver function, antinuclear antibodies).
- *Aromatic retinoids* (liver function, plasma lipids).

The patient and doctor must always remain vigilant about drug–drug and drug–food interactions that may result in toxicity, e.g. methotrexate/trimethoprim, ciclosporin/grapefruit juice.

Individual disorders

Table 17.3 is not intended to give the complete treatment of even the commoner skin conditions but merely to indicate a reasonable approach. Secondary infections of ordinarily uninfected lesions may require added topical or systemic antimicrobials. Analgesics, sedatives or tranquilisers may be needed in painful or uncomfortable conditions, or where the disease is intensified by emotion or anxiety.

Psoriasis

In psoriasis there is increased epidermal undifferentiated cell proliferation and inflammation of the epidermis and dermis. The consequence of increased numbers of immature horn cells containing abnormal keratin is that an abnormal stratum corneum is formed. Drugs are used to:

- dissolve keratin (keratolysis)
- inhibit cell division.

An emollient such as aqueous cream will reduce the inflammation. The proliferated cells may be eliminated by a *dithranol* (antimitotic) preparation applied accurately to the lesions (but not on the face or scalp) for 1 h and then removed, as it is irritant to normal skin and stains skin, blond hair and fabrics. A suitable regimen may begin with 0.1% dithranol, increasing to 1%. Dithranol is available in cream bases or in Lassar's paste (the preparations are not interchangeable). It is used daily until the lesions have disappeared and may produce prolonged remissions of psoriasis.

Table 17.3 Summary of treatment for selected skin disorders

Condition	Treatment	Remarks
Androgenic alopecia	Topical 2% or 5% minoxidil is worth trying. Finasteride can stop hair loss and increase hair density in 50% of men	The response occurs in 4–12 months; hair loss resumes when therapy is stopped
Alopecia areata	Potent topical or intralesional corticosteroids may be useful in the short term	Although distressing, the condition is often self-limiting. A few individuals have responded to PUVA or contact sensitisation induced by diphencyprone
Dermatitis herpetiformis	Dapsone is typically effective in 24 h, or sulfapyridine. Long-term gluten-free diet	Methaemoglobinaemia may complicate dapsone therapy
Hirsutism in women	Combined oestrogen–progestogen contraceptive pill: cyproterone plus ethinylestradiol (Dianette). Spironolactone, cimetidine have been used	Local cosmetic approaches: epilation by wax or electrolysis; depilation (chemical), e.g. thioglycollic acid, barium sulfide. The result of laser epilation is transient and may paradoxically induce excess hair growth in certain individuals
Hyperhidrosis	Astringents reduce sweat production, especially aluminium chloride hexahydrate. Antimuscarinics, e.g. glycopyrrolate (topical or systemic), may help and may be used with iontophoresis. Botulinum toxin can be used to provide temporary remission (3–4 months) and is most useful for the axilla. Sympathectomy is used occasionally but may be complicated by compensatory hyperhidrosis	The characteristic smell is produced by bacterial action, so cosmetic deodorants contain antibacterials rather than substances that reduce sweatimpetigo
Impetigo	Topical antibiotics, e.g. mupirocin, fusidic acid	In severe cases (resistant organisms) systemic macrolide, cephalosporin antibiotics
Intertrigo	Cleansing lotions, powders to cleanse, lubricate and reduce friction. A dilute corticosteroid with anticandidal cream is often helpful	No evidence that new azoles are superior to nystatin
Larva migrans	Cryotherapy. Albendazole (single dose) or topical thiabendazole	
Lichen planus	Antipruritics (menthol); potent topical corticosteroid	PUVA or retinoids in severe cases
Lichen simplex (neurodermatitis)	Antipruritics (menthol); topical corticosteroid; sedating antihistamines	Occluding the lesion so as to prevent scratch–itch cycle to patient. Focused cognitive behaviour therapy may be helpful

Continued

Table 17.3 Summary of treatment for selected skin disorders—cont'd

Condition	Treatment	Remarks
Lupus erythematosus	Photoprotection (including against UVA) is essential. Potent adrenal corticosteroid topically or intralesionally. Hydroxychloroquine or mepacrine. Monitor for retinal toxicity when treatment is long term. Other agents include acetretin and auranofin	
Malignancies	Actinic keratoses and Bowen's disease can be treated with topical 5-fluorouracil (skin irritation is to be expected) or cryotherapy. Imiquimod is a possible topical alternative. Extensive lesions may respond to photodynamic therapy: the skin is sensitised using a topical haematoporphyrin derivative, e.g. aminolaevulinic acid, and irradiated with a visible light or laser source. Cutaneous T-cell lymphoma in its early stages is best treated conservatively; PUVA will often clear lesions for several months or years; alternatives include topical nitrogen mustard, e.g. carmustine, radiotherapy and the retinoid bexarotene	
Nappy rash	Prevention: rid re-usable nappies of soaps, detergents and ammonia by rinsing. Change frequently, and use an emollient cream, e.g. aqueous cream, to protect skin. Costly disposable nappies are useful but must also be changed regularly. Cure: zinc cream or calamine lotion plus above measures	
Onychomycosis	Confirm dermatophyte infection with microscopy and culture. Terbinafine, 2 pulses of itraconazole or 6–9 months of once-weekly fluconazole is used for fingernail onychomycosis. For toenail disease, terbinafine is used for 12–16 weeks; 3–4 pulses of itraconazole or fluconazole once per week for 9–15 months can be used	The newer oral antifungals have not been approved for use in children. Surgical removal of infected nail maybe required and reinfection is common
Pediculosis (lice)	Permethrin, phenothrin, carbaryl or malathion (anticholinesterases, with safety depending on more rapid metabolism in humans than in insects, and on low absorption)	Usually two applications 7 days apart to kill lice from eggs that survive the first dose. Physical measures including regular combing and keeping hair short are important
Pemphigus and pemphigoid	Milder cases can be treated with topical corticosteroids and tetracyclines. Systemic steroids and immunosuppressants (azathioprine, mycophenylate) are useful for severe disease. Plasmapheresis, IVIg and rituximab may also be useful for resistant cases	
Pityriasis rosea	Antipruritics and emollients as appropriate; UVB phototherapy	The disease is self-limiting

Table 17.3 Summary of treatment for selected skin disorders—cont'd

Condition	Treatment	Remarks
Pyoderma gangrenosum	Topical therapies may include corticosteroids, tacrolimus. Systemic corticosteroids are usually effective. Immunosuppressives, e.g. ciclosporin, may be used for steroid-sparing effect. Some patients respond to dapsone, minocycline or clofazamine	
Rosacea	Topical metronidazole and systemic tetracycline. Retinoids are useful for severe cases	Control pustulation in order to prevent secondary scarring and rhinophyma
Scabies (Sarcoptes scabiei)	Permethrin dermal cream. Alternatives include benzyl benzoate or ivermectin (single dose), especially for outbreaks in closed communities. Crotamiton or calamine for residual itch. Topical corticosteroid to settle persistent hypersensitivity	Apply to all members of the household, immediate family or partner. Change underclothes and bedclothes after application
Seborrhoeic dermatitis: dandruff (Pityriasis capitis)	A proprietary shampoo with pyrithione, selenium sulfide or coal tar; ketoconazole shampoo in more severe cases. Occasionally a corticosteroid lotion may be necessary	
Tinea capitis	In children, griseofulvin for 6–8 weeks is effective and safe. Terbinafine for 4 weeks is effective against Trichophyton spp. Microsporum will respond to 6 weeks' therapy with terbinafine	Antifungal shampoos can reduce active shedding in patients treated with oral antifungals
Tinea pedis	Most cases will respond to tolnaftate or undecenoic acid creams. Allylamine (terbinafine) creams are possibly more effective than azoles in resistant cases	
Venous leg ulcers	Limb compression is the mainstay of therapy. Other agents including pentoxifylline and skin grafts are useful adjuncts to compression therapy	
Viral warts	All treatments are destructive and should be applied with precision. Salicylic acid in collodion daily. Many other caustic (keratolytic) preparations exist, e.g. salicylic and lactic acid paint or gel. For plantar warts, formaldehyde or glutaraldehyde; for plantar or anogenital warts, podophyllin (antimitotic). Follow the manufacturer's instructions meticulously. If one topical therapy fails, it is worth trying a different type. Topical imiquimod is an alternative for genital warts; it is irritant. Careful cryotherapy (liquid nitrogen)	Warts often disappear spontaneously. Cryotherapy can cause ulceration, damage the nail matrix and leave permanent scars

Tar (antimitotic) preparations are used in a similar way, are less irritating to normal skin and are commonly used for psoriasis of the scalp.[10]

Topical adrenal corticosteroids act principally by reducing inflammation. Application, especially under occlusive dressings, can be very effective at suppressing the disease, but increased doses (concentrations) become necessary, and rebound, which may be severe, follows withdrawal. For this reason, potent corticosteroids should never be used except for lesions on the scalp, palms and soles. Corticosteroids of mild potency may be used for flexural psoriasis where other drugs are too irritating.

Systemic corticosteroid administration should be avoided, for high doses are needed to suppress the disease, which is liable to recur in a more unstable form when treatment is withdrawn, as it must be if complications of long-term steroid therapy are to be avoided.

Calcipotriol and tacalcitol are analogues of calcitriol, the most active natural form of vitamin D. They inhibit cell proliferation and encourage cell differentiation. Although they have less effect on calcium metabolism than does calcitriol, excessive use (more than 100 g/week) can raise the plasma calcium concentration.

Vitamin A (retinols) plays a role in epithelial function, and the retinoic acid derivative *acitretin* (orally) inhibits psoriatic hyperkeratosis over 4–6 weeks. Acitretin should be used in courses (6–9 months) with intervals (3–4 months). It is teratogenic, like the other vitamin A derivatives. It is not recommended for use in women of childbearing potential because the drug is stored in the liver and in fat, and active metabolites are released many months after cessation of therapy.

UVB light is effective in guttate psoriasis and potentiates the effects of topical agents such as calcipotriol (act by reducing cell division), antimitotic agents like tar (Goeckerman's regimen) and dithranol (Ingram's regimen). Oral psoralen followed by UVA light (PUVA) may be used to clear severe cases of psoriasis, with remissions of more than 1 year being achievable. Long-term PUVA therapy is associated with an increased risk of cutaneous squamous cell carcinoma and melanoma development (especially in those given maintenance treatment).

Ciclosporin, the systemic calcineurin inhibitor (see p. 558), has been instrumental in shifting the focus of psoriasis research from keratinocyte abnormalities to immune perturbations. It has a rapid onset of action and is useful in achieving remissions in all forms of psoriasis. Monitoring of blood pressure and renal function is mandatory. Severe adverse effects, including renal toxicity, preclude its being used as long-term suppressive therapy.

Since the introduction of ciclosporin for psoriasis, much research has focused on new ways of disrupting T lymphocytes and the cytokines involved in the induction and maintenance of psoriasis. These drugs target specific cellular events, e.g. induction of T-lymphocytic apoptosis, inhibition of tumour necrosis factor. The exact role of these promising therapies is still evolving.

Folic acid antagonists, e.g. methotrexate, can also suppress epidermal activity and inhibit T and B lymphocytes, and are especially useful when psoriasis is severe and remits rapidly with other treatments. Methotrexate is particularly of use if there is associated disabling arthritis. Platelet count and renal and liver function must be monitored regularly. When 1.5 g of the total dose has been taken, liver biopsy should be considered, especially in those with predisposing hepatic steatosis.

The last decade has witnessed a significant advance in the management of refractory moderate-to-severe psoriasis with the introduction of biological therapies to clinical practice. These drugs target specific cellular events, e.g. induction of T-lymphocytic apoptosis, inhibition of tumour necrosis factor. Three classes of biological therapies have been used: T-cell inhibitors, tumour necrosis factor (TNF)-α inhibitors and interleukin (IL-12 and IL-23) inhibitors. The first of these to be introduced, the T-cell inhibitor efalizumab, was withdrawn because of a rare association with progressive multifocal leukoencephalopathy (PML). In contrast, anti-TNF treatments are now firmly established, offering a high level of efficacy and a good safety record. Ustekinumab, by targeting the p40 subunit common to interleukins 12 and 23, offers a viable alternative to anti-TNFs in the treatment of moderate-to-severe psoriasis. The identification of PML as a serious but statistically rare risk associated with efalizumab demonstrates the strengths and weaknesses of the current drug approval and pharmacovigilance processes for fully measuring the safety of a drug. Patients and clinicians need to be aware of the relative completeness and limitations of existing safety data of a drug when selecting a treatment.

It is plain from this brief outline that treatment of psoriasis requires considerable judgement, and choice will depend on the patient's sex, age and the severity of the condition. Topical therapies such as calcipotriol, tar or dithranol-containing compounds should be the mainstay of limited mild psoriasis. Topical corticosteroids can be used for psoriasis inversus under close supervision, as overuse can lead to cutaneous atrophy. Phototherapy is useful for widespread psoriasis where compliance with topical

---

[10]But are not without risk. A 46-year-old man whose psoriasis was treated with topical corticosteroids, UV light and tar was seen in the hospital courtyard bursting into flames. A small ring of fire began several centimetres above the sternal notch and encircled his neck. The patient promptly put out the fire. He admitted to lighting a cigarette just before the fire, the path of which corresponded to the distribution of the tar on his body (Fader D J, Metzman M S 1994 Smoking, tar, and psoriasis: a dangerous combination. New England Journal of Medicine 330:1541).

treatments is difficult. Resistant disease is best managed by the specialist who may utilise a rotation of treatments, including retinoids, methotrexate, ciclosporin, UVB plus dithranol and PUVA plus acitretin, to reduce the unwanted effects of any single therapy. Fumaric acid compounds, hydroxyurea and specific biological agents are useful for severe cases.

Acne

Acne vulgaris results from disordered function of the pilosebaceous follicle whereby abnormal keratin and sebum (the production of which is androgen driven) form debris that plugs the mouth of the follicle. *Propionibacterium acnes* colonises the debris. Bacterial action releases inflammatory fatty acids from the sebum, resulting in inflammation. Acne is a chronic disorder and if uncontrolled can lead to irreversible scarring.

The following measures are used progressively and selectively as the disease becomes more severe; they may need to be applied for up to 3–6 months:

- *Mild keratolytic* (exfoliating, peeling) formulations unblock pilosebaceous ducts, e.g. benzoyl peroxide, sulphur, salicylic acid, azelaic acid.
- *Systemic or topical antimicrobial therapy* (tetracycline, erythromycin, lymecycline) is used over months (expect 30% improvement after 3 months). Bacterial resistance is not a problem; benefit is due to suppression of bacterial lipolysis of sebum, which generates inflammatory fatty acids. (Avoid minocycline because of adverse effects, including raised intracranial pressure and drug-induced lupus.)
- *Vitamin A (retinoic acid) derivatives* reduce sebum production and keratinisation. Vitamin A is a teratogen. *Tretinoin* (Retin-A) is applied topically (but not in combination with other keratolytics). Tretinoin should be avoided in sunny weather and in pregnancy. Benefit is seen in about 10 weeks. *Adapalene*, a synthetic retinoid, may be better tolerated as it is less irritant. *Isotretinoin* (Roaccutane) orally is highly effective (a single course of treatment to a cumulative dose of 100 mg/kg is curative in 94% of patients), but is known to be a *serious teratogen;* its use should generally be confined to the more severe cystic and conglobate cases, where other measures have failed. Fasting blood lipids should be measured before and during therapy (levels of cholesterol and triglycerides may rise). Women of childbearing potential should be fully informed of this risk, pregnancy-tested before commencement and use contraception for 4 weeks before, during and for 4

weeks after cessation.[11] Other adverse effects are described, including mood change and severe depression.
- *Hormone therapy.* The objective is to reduce androgen production or effect by using (1) oestrogen, to suppress hypothalamic–pituitary gonadotrophin production, or (2) an antiandrogen (cyproterone). An oestrogen alone as initial therapy to get the acne under control or, in women, the cyclical use of an oral contraceptive containing 50 µg of oestrogen diminishes sebum secretion by 40%. A combination of ethinylestradiol and cyproterone (Dianette) orally is also effective in women (it has a contraceptive effect, which is desirable as the cyproterone may feminise a male fetus).

Urticaria

Acute urticaria (named after its similarity to the sting of a nettle, *Urtica*) and *angioedema* usually respond well to H_1-receptor antihistamines, although severe cases are relieved more quickly with use of adrenaline/epinephrine (adrenaline injection 1 mg/mL:0.1–0.3 mL s.c.). A systemic corticosteroid may be needed in severe cases, e.g. urticarial vasculitis.

In some individuals, urticarial weals are provoked by physical stimuli, e.g. friction (dermographism), heat or cold. Exercise may induce weals, particularly on the upper trunk (cholinergic urticaria). Physical urticarias are particularly challenging to treat.

Chronic urticaria usually responds to an H_1-receptor antihistamine with low sedating properties, e.g. cetirizine or loratidine. Terfenadine is also effective, but may cause dangerous cardiac arrhythmias if the recommended dose is exceeded or if it is administered with drugs (or grapefruit juice) that inhibit its metabolism. But lack of sleep increases the intensity of itch (similar to pain), and a sedating antihistamine may be useful at night. H_2-receptor antihistamines may be added for particularly resistant cases. In some patients with antibodies against the Fc receptor on mast cells, immunosuppressive therapies (e.g. ciclosporin, methotrexate or intravenous immunoglobulin) may be required.

---

[11]The risk of birth defect in a child of a woman who has taken isotretinoin when pregnant is estimated at 25%. Thousands of abortions have been performed in such women in the USA. It is probable that hundreds of damaged children have been born. There can be no doubt that there has been irresponsible prescribing of this drug, e.g. in less severe cases. The fact that a drug with such a grave effect is still permitted to be available is attributed to its high efficacy. In Europe, women of childbearing age must comply with a pregnancy prevention programme and be monitored monthly while on a course of isotretinoin. In the USA, patients and their doctors and pharmacists are required by the US Food and Drug Administration (FDA) to register with the mandatory iPLEDGE distribution programme in order to receive this medication.

Omalizumab is a humanised monoclonal antibody that binds to circulating IgE. This prevents IgE binding to high-affinity receptors (FcεRI) on the surface of mast cells and basophils, thus reducing receptor expression and the release of inflammatory mediators. Currently licensed as add-on therapy for patients with severe, persistent allergic asthma via subcutaneous injection, omalizumab has been reported to be highly effective in treating severe chronic spontaneous urticaria in teenagers and adults.

Omalizumab has also been reported to demonstrate efficacy in the treatment of inducible or physical urticaria, such as solar urticaria or cold urticaria, which does not respond well to antihistamines.[12]

Hereditary angioedema, with deficiency of C_1-esterase inhibitor (a complement inhibitor), may not respond to antihistamines or corticosteroid but only to fresh frozen plasma or, preferably, C_1-inhibitor concentrate. Delay in initiating the treatment may lead to death from laryngeal oedema (try adrenaline/epinephrine i.m. in severe cases). Icatibant is a selective and specific antagonist of bradykinin B_2 receptors. It has been approved in Europe for the symptomatic treatment of acute attacks of hereditary angioedema (HAE) in adults (with C_1-esterase–inhibitor deficiency). For long-term prophylaxis, an androgen (stanozolol, danazol) can be effective. Hereditary angioedema does not manifest as simple urticaria.

Atopic dermatitis

Atopic dermatitis is a chronic condition, and treatment must be individualised and centred around preventive measures. Successful management includes the elimination of precipitating and exacerbating factors, and maintaining the skin barrier function by use of topical or systemic agents.

Immunological triggers of atopic dermatitis vary and can include aeroallergens, detergents (including soaps), irritants, climate and microorganisms. Identification and modification of these factors is useful.

Antiseptic-containing soap substitutes are useful in reducing pro-inflammatory *Staphylococcus aureus* colonies.

In *acute* weeping dermatitis, lotions, wet dressing or soaks (sodium chloride, potassium permanganate) are used.

In *subacute* and *chronic* disease, skin care with occlusive emollients helps to offset the xerosis (dryness) that creates microfissures in the skin and disturbs its normal barrier function. Topical corticosteroids form the cornerstone of pharmacological therapy. In general, the lowest-potency topical steroid should be used initially and higher-potency agents

considered only if these fail, the aim being to switch to intermittent steroid use protocols once the disease has been controlled. Higher-potency agents are usually inappropriate for young children and highly permeable areas. Very potent steroids should not be used for longer than 2 consecutive weeks to minimise the likelihood of unwanted effects.

The calcineurin inhibitors, tacrolimus and pimecrolimus, are effective topically. Local irritation may result, but they do not cause skin atrophy and so are especially useful on the face. Long-term safety data are still lacking, and the US Food and Drug Administration cautions against long-term use in children on the grounds of cutaneous carcinogenesis.

Sedating H_1-receptor antihistamines with anxiolytic properties may assist with sleep and nocturnal itch. A 2-week course of systemic corticosteroid is useful, especially in cases of acute allergic contact dermatitis. Long-term oral immunosuppression with ciclosporin, mycophenylate or azathioprine should be undertaken only in specialist centres. Although there is minimal objective improvement in atopic dermatitis with UVB phototherapy, patients have consistently reported subjective improvement in itch.

Dupilumab is an innovative first-in-class biologic agent for moderate-to-severe atopic dermatitis. A fully human monoclonal antibody directed against the shared IL-4 receptor alpha subunit, dupilumab blocks signalling from both IL-4 and IL-13, which are key cytokines that are required for the initiation and maintenance of the Th2 (Type 2 helper T-cell) immune response, which is believed to be a critical pathway in allergic inflammation.[13]

Skin infections

Superficial bacterial infections, e.g. impetigo, eczema, are commonly staphylococcal or streptococcal. They are treated with a topical antimicrobial for less than 2 weeks, applied twice daily after removal of crusts that prevent access of the drug, e.g. with a povidone–iodine preparation. Very extensive cases need systemic treatment.

Topical *sodium fusidate* and *mupirocin* are preferred (as they are not used ordinarily for systemic infections and therefore development of drug-resistant strains is less likely to have any serious consequences). Framycetin and polymyxins are also used. Absorption of neomycin from all topical preparations can cause serious injury to the eighth cranial nerve. It is also a contact sensitiser.

When prolonged treatment is required, topical antiseptics (e.g. chlorhexidine) are preferred and bacterial resistance is less of a problem.

[12]Goldstein S, Gabriel S, Kianifard F, Ortiz B, Skoner DP, 2017, Clinical features of adolescents with chronic idiopathic or spontaneous urticaria: Review of omalizumab clinical trials. Annals of Allergy Asthma and Immunology 118:500–504.

[13]Blakely K, Gooderham M, Papp K 2016 Dupilumab, A Monoclonal Antibody for Atopic Dermatitis: A Review of Current Literature. Skin Therapy Letter 2016;21:1–5.

Combination of an antimicrobial drug with a corticosteroid (to suppress inflammation) can be useful for secondarily infected eczema.

The *disadvantages* of antimicrobials are contact allergy and developments of resistant organisms (which may cause systemic, as well as local, infection). Failure to respond may be due to the development of a contact allergy (which may be masked by corticosteroid).

Infected leg ulcers generally do not benefit from long-term antimicrobials, although topical metronidazole is useful when the ulcer is malodorous due to colonisation with Gram-negative organisms. An antiseptic (plus a protective dressing with compression) is preferred if antimicrobial therapy is needed.

Nasal carriers of staphylococci may be cured (often temporarily) by topical mupirocin or neomycin plus chlorhexidine.

Deep bacterial infections, e.g. boils, generally do not require antimicrobial therapy, but if they do it should be systemic. Cellulitis requires systemic chemotherapy initially with benzylpenicillin and flucloxacillin.

Infected burns are treated with a variety of antimicrobials, including silver sulfadiazine and mupirocin.

Fungal infections. Superficial dermatophyte or *Candida* infections purely involving the skin can be treated with a topical imidazole, e.g. clotrimazole, miconazole. Pityriasis versicolor, a yeast infection, primarily involves the trunk in young adults. It responds to topical antifungals or selenium sulfide preparations; severe infection may require systemic itraconazole. It tends to recur, and regular treatments are frequently necessary. Invasion of hair or nails by a dermatophyte or a deep mycosis requires systemic therapy; terbinafine is the most effective drug. Terbinafine and griseofulvin are ineffective against yeasts, for which itraconazole is an alternative. Itraconazole can be used in weekly pulses each month for 3–4 months; it is less effective against dermatophytes than terbinafine.

Viral infections. Topical antivirals, e.g. aciclovir, penetrate the stratum corneum poorly. Aciclovir is used systemically for severe infections, e.g. eczema herpeticum.

Parasitic infection. Topical parasiticides (see Table 17.3 for details).

Disinfection and cleansing of the skin. Numerous substances are used according to circumstances:

- For skin preparation prior to injection: ethanol or isopropyl alcohol.
- For disinfection: chlorhexidine salts, cationic surfactant (cetrimide), soft soap, povidone–iodine (iodine complexed with polyvinylpyrrolidone), phenol derivatives (hexachlorophene, triclosan) and hydrogen peroxide.

Guide to further reading

Bystryn, J.C., Rudolph, J., 2005. Pemphigus. Lancet 366, 61–73.

Currie, B.J., McCarthy, J.S., 2010. Permethrin and ivermectin for scabies. N. Engl. J. Med. 362, 717–725.

Hwang, S.T., Janik, J.E., Jaffe, E.S., Wilson, W.H., 2008. Mycosis fungoides and Sézary syndrome. Lancet 371, 945–957.

James, W.D., 2005. Acne. N. Engl. J. Med. 352, 1463–1472.

Kaplan, K.P., 2002. Chronic urticaria and angioedema. N. Engl. J. Med. 346, 175–179.

Kullavanijaya, P., Lim, H.W., 2005. Photoprotection. J. Am. Acad. Dermatol. 52, 937–958.

Madan, V., Lear, J.T., Szeimies, R.M., 2010. Non-melanoma skin cancer. Lancet 375, 673–685.

Naldi, L., Rebora, A., 2009. Clinical practice. Seborrheic dermatitis. N. Engl. J. Med. 360, 387–396.

Nestle, F.O., Kaplan, D.H., Barker, J., 2009. Psoriasis. N. Engl. J. Med. 361, 496–509.

Powell, F.C., 2005. Rosacea. N. Engl. J. Med. 352, 793–803.

Rosenfield, R.L., 2005. Hirsutism. N. Engl. J. Med. 353, 2578–2588.

Schwartz, R.A., 2004. Superficial fungal infections. Lancet 364, 1173–1182.

Smith, C.H., Barker, J.N.W.N., 2006. Psoriasis and its management. Br. Med. J. 333, 380–384.

Stern, R.S., 2004. Treatment of photoaging. N. Engl. J. Med. 350, 1526–1534.

Thompson, J.F., Scolyer, R., Kefford, R., 2005. Cutaneous melanoma. Lancet 365, 687–701.

Williams, H.C., 2005. Atopic dermatitis. N. Engl. J. Med. 352, 2314–2324.

Yosipovitch, G., Greaves, M., Schmelz, M., 2003. Itch. Lancet 361, 690–694.

Section | 4 |

Nervous system

Chapter | 18 |

Pain and analgesics

Michael C. Lee, Mark Abrahams

Pain and analgesics

'The work which you are accomplishing is immensely important for the good of humanity, as you seek the ever more effective control of physical pain and of the oppression of mind and spirit that physical pain so often brings with it.'

[Pope John Paul II (26 July 1987). Pope John Paul II. Letter handed to John Bonica on the occasion of the Fifth World Congress on Pain. In: Benedetti C, Chapman CR, Giron G eds. Opioid Analgesia: Recent advances in Systemic Administration (Advances in Pain Research and Therapy, vol. 14). New York, NY: Raven Press, 1990.]

Definition of pain

The International Association for the Study of Pain defines pain as 'an unpleasant sensory and emotional experience associated with actual or potential tissue damage, or described in terms of such damage'. This implies that the degree of pain experienced by the patient may be unrelated to the extent of underlying tissue damage and that emotional or spiritual distress can add to the patient's experience of pain (Fig. 18.1).

This chapter focuses on the use of drugs for pain relief and illustrates the use of many analgesics that may be encountered in clinical practice. However, clinicians should

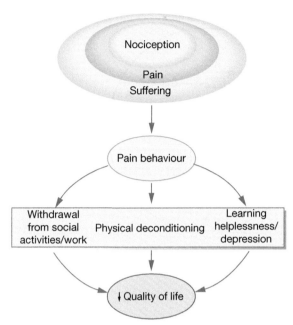

Fig. 18.1 A model of pain perception. *(Modified with permission from Carr D B, Loese J L, Morris D (eds) 2005 Narrative, pain, and suffering. The challenge of narrative to pain. Progress in Pain Research and Management series, vol. 34. IASP Press, Seattle.)*

recognise that the experience of pain is influenced by physical, emotional and psychological factors. While drug therapy is an expedient (and familiar) form of treatment, successful management of pain requires a more holistic approach that addresses all the components of pain.[1]

Nociception

Pain alerts us to ongoing or potential tissue damage, and the ability to sense pain is vital to our survival. The physiological process by which pain is perceived is known as *nociception*. While the neurobiology of nociception is complex, its appreciation provides a useful framework for understanding the way analgesics work (Fig. 18.2).

Our nervous system is alerted to actual or potential tissue injury by the activation of the peripheral terminals of highly specialised primary sensory neurons called *nociceptors*. Nociceptors have unmyelinated (C-fibre) or thinly myelinated (Aδ-fibre) axons. Their cell bodies lie in the dorsal root ganglia of the spinal cord or in the trigeminal ganglia. Different nociceptors encode discrete intensities and modalities of pain, depending upon their expression of ion-channel receptors. These receptors are *transducers*. They convert noxious stimuli into action potentials. Some of these transducers have been identified, including those that respond to heat (>46 °C), cold (<10 °C) and direct chemical irritants such as capsaicin.

Action potentials that result from the transduction of noxious stimuli are conducted along the axon of the sensory neuron into the spinal cord. Conduction of the action potentials in sensory neurons depends on voltage-gated sodium channels, including two that are predominately expressed in nociceptors: $Na_v1.7$ and $Na_v1.8$.

The central terminal of the nociceptor makes synaptic contact with *dorsal horn neurons* within the spinal cord. Glutamate, an amino acid, is the main excitatory neurotransmitter released at these synapses. Its release can be inhibited by ligands that act to activate receptors found on the central terminal of the nociceptors (pre-synaptic inhibition). These include the opioids, cannabinoids, gamma-amino butyric acid (GABA) receptor ligands and the anticonvulsants, gabapentin and pregabalin. Opioids and GABA also influence the action of glutamate on the dorsal horn neurons. They act on post-synaptic receptors to open potassium or chloride channels. This results in hyperpolarisation of the neuron, which inhibits its activity.

Other neurotransmitters may also be released by the central terminal of the nociceptors. For example, substance P is released during high-intensity and repetitive noxious stimulation. It mediates slow excitatory post-synaptic potentials and results in a localised depolarisation that facilitates the activation of N-methyl-D-aspartate (NMDA) receptors by glutamate. The end result is a progressive increase in the output from dorsal horn neurons. This amplified output is thought to be responsible for the escalation of pain when the skin is repeatedly stimulated by noxious heat; a phenomenon known as *wind-up*.

Nociceptive output from the spinal cord is further modulated by descending inhibitory neurons that originate from supra-spinal sites such as the periaqueductal gray or the rostral ventromedial medulla and terminate on nociceptive neurons in the spinal cord as well as on spinal inhibitory inter-neurons that store and release opioids. Stimulation of these brain regions, either electrically or chemically

---

[1]'Another event at Elsterhorst had a marked effect on me. The Germans dumped a young Soviet prisoner in my ward late one night. The ward was full, so I put him in my room as he was moribund and screaming and I did not want to wake the ward. I examined him. He had obvious gross bilateral cavitation and a severe pleural rub. I thought the latter was the cause of the pain and the screaming. I had no morphia, just aspirin, which had no effect. I felt desperate. I knew very little Russian then and there was no one in the ward who did. I finally instinctively sat down on the bed and took him in my arms, and the screaming stopped almost at once. He died peacefully in my arms a few hours later. It was not the pleurisy that caused the screaming but loneliness. It was a wonderful education about the care of the dying. I was ashamed of my misdiagnosis and kept the story secret.' Cochrane AL (with M Blythe). London: BMJ (Memoir Club), 1989, p 82.

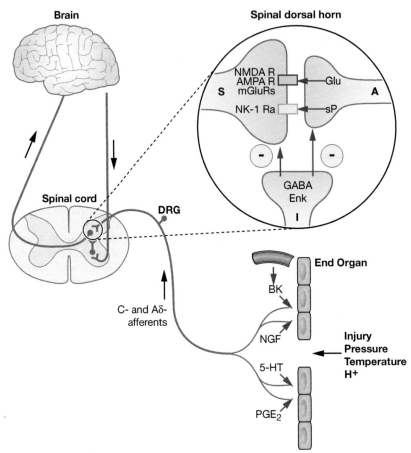

Fig. 18.2 Schematic representation of nociceptive pathways. Noxious stimuli such as protons (H+), temperature (temp) etc. applied to end organs activate nociceptors. Injury leads to the release of prostaglandins such as prostaglandin E_2 (PGE_2), serotonin (5-HT), nerve growth factor (NGF) etc. from damaged cells, bradykinin (BK) from blood vessels and substance P (sP) from nociceptors. These agents either activate nociceptors directly or sensitise them to subsequent stimuli by parallel activation of intracellular kinases by G-protein–coupled receptors and tyrosine kinase receptors. Primary nociceptive afferents (C-fibres, Aδ-fibres) of dorsal root ganglion (DRG) neurons synapse on second-order neurons (S) in the spinal dorsal horn (magnified in inset). Here, glutamate (Glu) and sP released from primary afferent terminals (A) activate glutamate receptors (NMDA R, AMPA R, mGluRs) and neurokinin-1 (NK-1) receptors, respectively, located post-synaptically on spinal neurons. These synapses are negatively modulated by spinal inhibitory interneurons (I), which employ enkephalins (Enk) or gamma-amino-butyric acid (GABA) as neurotransmitters. Spinal neurons convey nociceptive information to the brain and brainstem. Activation of descending noradrenergic and/or serotonergic systems, which originate in the brain and brainstem, leads to the activation of spinal inhibitory interneurons (I), thereby resulting in antinociception.

(e.g. opioids), produces analgesia in humans. Transmission through these inhibitory pathways is facilitated by monoamine neurotransmitters such as norepinephrine and serotonin.

Finally, dorsal horn neurons send projections to supraspinal areas in the brainstem, hypothalamus and thalamus and then, through relay neurons, to the cortex where the sensation of pain is perceived. The mechanism by which the cortex produces the conscious appreciation of pain is the focus of much research.

Classification of clinical pain

Rational pharmacological treatment of clinical pain depends on a number of factors, including the underlying cause and duration of pain, the patient's general medical condition and prognosis. Clinically, pain is generally conveniently classified as either acute or chronic, based on duration of pain. Where possible, pain should be further classified based on mechanism or initiating disease, for example neuropathic pain or cancer-related.

Acute pain, such as that experienced after trauma or surgery, typically resolves with healing of the injured tissue and can usually be effectively managed with the appropriate use of pharmacotherapy. Poorly controlled post-surgical pain is associated with the development of complications such as pneumonia, myocardial ischaemia, paralytic ileus and thromboembolism, as well as an increased risk of the patient developing chronic pain. In this setting, effective analgesia not only reduces patient anxiety and provides subjective comfort but also helps to blunt autonomic and somatic reflex responses. Effective analgesia can promote early mobilisation and increased appetite, and this, in turn, can improve postoperative outcome. Moreover, research suggests that analgesia given before surgical incision may reduce subsequent postoperative pain. Clinicians have attempted to exploit the concept of pre-emptive analgesia with varying success.

Chronic pain is commonly defined as pain that persists beyond the period expected for healing or pain that is associated with progressive, non-malignant disease. Chronic pain may be due to the persistent stimulation of nociceptors in areas of ongoing tissue damage (e.g. from an inflammatory process in rheumatoid arthritis). However, in many instances, chronic pain can persist long after the healing of damaged tissue. In some patients, chronic pain presents without any identified ongoing tissue damage or antecedent injury.

Neuropathic pain is a form of chronic pain resulting from damage to the somatosensory nervous system. Neuropathic pain can be due to damage to the sensory afferents, such as patients with diabetic or AIDS polyneuropathy, post-herpetic neuralgia or lumbar radiculopathy, or due to the central somatosensory pathway, such as patients with spinal cord injury, multiple sclerosis or stroke. The mechanisms of neuropathic pain remain the subject of much research.

Cancer-related pain refers to pain that is the result of primary tumour growth, metastatic disease or the toxic effects of chemotherapy and radiation, such as neuropathies due to neurotoxic antineoplastic drugs.

Evaluation of pain

The optimal pharmacological management of the patient's pain will depend on the type and cause of pain, as well as the psychological and physical condition of the patient. A comprehensive evaluation of the pain is, therefore, essential

if we are to treat the patient successfully and safely. Underlying or treatable pathology must be excluded unless an obvious cause of pain is apparent (e.g. after recent surgery or trauma).

Once disease pathology is excluded or optimally managed, additional tests are usually unhelpful. The illusory sense of progress such tests provide for both physician and patient may perpetuate maladaptive behaviour and impede the return to more normal function.

The evaluation of persistent pain should include pain location, quality, severity, duration, course, timing (including frequency of remissions and degree of fluctuation), exacerbating and relieving factors, and co-morbidities associated with the pain (with emphasis on psychological issues, depression and anxiety). The efficacy and adverse effects of currently or previously used drugs and other treatments should also be determined.

If appropriate, the patient should be asked whether litigation is ongoing or whether financial compensation for injury will be sought. A personal or family history of chronic pain can often give insight into the current problem. The patient's level of function should be assessed in detail, focusing on family relationships (including sexual), social network and employment or vocation. The interviewer should elicit how the patient's pain affects the activities of normal living.

It is also important to determine what the pain means to the patient. In some patients, reporting pain may be more socially acceptable than reporting feelings of depression or anxiety. Pain and suffering should also be distinguished. In cancer patients in particular, suffering may be due as much to loss of function and fear of impending death as to pain. The patient's expression of pain represents more than the pathology intrinsic to the disease.

Thorough physical examination is essential and can often help to identify underlying causes and to evaluate, further, the degree of functional impairment. A basic neurological (sensory) examination of the affected region may identify features associated with neuropathic pain including:

- *Allodynia* – pain due to a stimulus which does not normally provoke pain, e.g. light touch on the skin
- *Hyperalgesia* – an increased response to a stimulus which is normally painful
- *Paraesthesia* – abnormal or loss of normal sensation, e.g. 'pins and needles'
- *Dyaesthesia* – a painful paraesthesia, e.g. burning foot pain in diabetic neuropathy.

Pharmacotherapy

An *analgesic* is defined as a drug that relieves pain. Analgesics are classified as *opioids* and *non-opioids* (e.g. NSAIDs).

Co-analgesics or adjuvants are drugs that have a primary indication other than pain but are analgesic in some conditions. For example, anti-depressants and anticonvulsants also act to reduce nociceptive transmission in neuropathic pain.

The efficacy and effectiveness of any given analgesic varies widely between individuals. Analgesics also have a relatively narrow therapeutic window, and drug dosages may be limited by the onset of adverse effects. For these reasons, an analgesic should be titrated for an individual patient until an acceptable balance is achieved between subjective pain relief and adverse drug effects.

Non-opioid analgesics

NSAIDS (non-steroidal anti-inflammatory drugs)

Mechanism of analgesia

Endothelial damage produces an inflammatory response in tissues. Damaged cells release intracellular contents, such as adenosine triphosphate, hydrogen and potassium ions. Inflammatory cells recruited to the site of damage produce cytokines, chemokines and growth factors. A profound change to the chemical environment of the peripheral terminal of nociceptors occurs. Some chemical factors act directly on the nociceptor terminal to activate it and produce pain, and others sensitise the terminal so that it becomes hypersensitive to subsequent stimuli. This process is known as 'peripheral sensitisation'.

Prostanoid is a major sensitiser that is produced at the site of tissue injury. NSAIDs act by inhibiting cyclooxygenase, an enzyme involved in the production of prostanoid, as well as other prostaglandins. This enzyme has a number of isoforms, the most studied being cyclooxgenase-1 (COX-1) and cyclooxygenase-2 (COX-2). Their actions are inhibited by NSAIDs. Increased COX-2 production is induced by tissue injury and accounts for the efficacy of COX-2–specific inhibitor drugs (COXIBs). The inhibitory effect of NSAIDs on the production of other prostaglandins is responsible for the common side-effects of these drugs. Among other functions, the prostaglandins produced by cyclooxygenase act to protect the gastric mucosa, maintain normal blood flow in the kidney and preserve normal platelet function. Inhibition of prostaglandin production, therefore, can cause gastric irritation, damage to the kidney and an increased risk of bleeding.

Clinical use

NSAIDs are among the most commonly prescribed analgesics and, unless contraindicated, are effective and appropriate analgesics for use in acute inflammatory pain. There is much evidence to suggest that NSAIDs are effective in cancer-related pain. The benefit of NSAIDs in chronic non–cancer-related pain is less certain, with efficacy only proven in chronic inflammatory musculoskeletal pain, mainly from studies in rheumatoid arthritis. NSAIDs are generally ineffective in neuropathic pain conditions, and a careful risk–benefit assessment should be made prior to use in view of the side-effects associated with long-term use.

Choice of NSAID and route of administration

There is little difference in the clinical benefit conferred by any particular NSAID. However, NSAIDs differ in their pharmacokinetic properties and side-effects. This should be taken into account when choosing a non-steroidal agent for long-term use. For example, the oxicams (e.g. piroxicam, tenoxicam) are metabolised slowly and have a high degree of enteropathic circulation. These NSAIDs have long elimination half-lives (but also higher incidences of gastrointestinal and renal side-effects).

NSAIDs should be given orally when possible. The same dose of NSAID is equally effective whether the dose is injected or taken orally. Topical application of NSAIDs for musculoskeletal pain is an exception as it is effective and is associated with a lower incidence of side-effects.

Adverse effects

All NSAIDs are associated with dose-dependent adverse effects. In particular, there is a risk of gastrointestinal bleed, renal toxicity and a possibility of cardiac-related complications. The morbidity related to gastrointestinal adverse effects is considerable (~5 per 1000 patients per year of treatment), and catastrophic bleeding can occur without any preceding warning symptoms. For this reason, it is recommended that, when used in the longer term NSAIDs should be prescribed along with an appropriate gastroprotective agent.

COX-2–specific NSAIDs provide analgesia with a reduced risk of gastrointestinal bleed (but have a similar risk of renal toxicity). Trials have shown a slightly increased risk of cardiac complications in at-risk patients. Subsequent trials, however, have indicated that increased cardiac risk may also be associated with the use of non-selective NSAIDs. Current guidelines suggest that all cyclooxygenase-inhibiting drugs should be used with caution, at the lowest effective dose and for the shortest possible time, in patients with known cardiovascular or cerebrovascular disease.

Acetaminophen (Paracetamol)

The major advantage of acetaminophen over NSAIDs is its relative lack of adverse effects; this justifies its use as a first-line analgesic. It can be used on its own, or synergistically with non-steroidal drugs or opioids. Acetaminophen is also an antipyretic with very weak anti-inflammatory properties. There is increasing evidence that its analgesic effect is central and results from the activation of descending serotonergic pain-inhibiting pathways, but its primary site of action may still be inhibition of prostaglandin synthesis (via COX-3 inhibition). Its major drawback is the liver toxicity seen in acute overdose due to the accumulation in the liver of benzoquinones. Recent reviews suggest that long-term use of paracetamol (especially at higher doses) may also be associated with a small increased risk of adverse events including myocardial infarction, gastrointestinal bleeds and renal impairment.

Nefopam (3,4,5,6-tetrahydro-5-methyl-I-I-phenyl-1H-2.5-benoxazocine hydrochloride)

Nefopam is chemically distinct and pharmacologically unrelated to any presently known analgesic. It has been used in Europe for intravenous and oral administration since 1976. It is a racemic mixture of its two enantiomers. Although its mechanism of action remains largely unknown, Nefopam is thought to increase the inhibiting tone of serotonergic and norepinephrinergic descending pathways by inhibiting the synaptic uptake of dopamine, norepinephrine and serotonin. Compared to NSAIDs and opioids, nefopam has the advantage of minimally affecting platelet aggregation and having no central nervous system (CNS) depressive effect. However, there have been rare fatal overdoses with the oral form of the drug, characterised by convulsions and arrhythmia. Its sympathomimetic action renders it contraindicated in patients with limited coronary reserve, prostatitis and glaucoma. Minor side-effects (nausea, dizziness and sweating) are observed in 15–30% of treated patients. Nefopam has been abused primarily for its psycho-stimulant effects, which are probably linked to its dopamine-reuptake inhibition properties.

Opioid analgesics

Opium (the dried juice of the seed head of the opium poppy) was used in prehistoric times. Modern medical practice still benefits from the use of its alkaloids, employing them as analgesics, tranquillisers, antitussives and in the treatment of diarrhoea.

The principal active ingredient in crude opium was isolated in 1806 by Friedrich Sertürner, who tested pure morphine on himself and three young men. He observed that the drug caused cerebral depression and relieved toothache, and named it after Morpheus, the Greek god of dreams. Opium contains many alkaloids, but the only important opiates (drugs derived from opium) are morphine (10%) and codeine. Papaverine is occasionally used as a vasodilator.

'Opioid' is a generic term for natural or synthetic substances that bind to specific opioid receptors in the CNS, producing an agonist action.

Mechanism of action of opioids

Opioids produce their effects by activating specific G-protein–coupled receptors in the brain, spinal cord and peripheral nervous system. There are three major classes of opioid receptor – δ-opioid (OP1,DOR), κ-opioid (OP2,KOR) and μ-opioid (OP3,MOR) – that correspond respectively to their endogenous ligands: enkephalin, dynorphin and β-endorphin. Although studies suggest the existence of subtypes of all three major opioid receptor classes, the evidence is controversial and the sub-classification is of little practical value except, perhaps, to explain the change in adverse-effect profile sometimes seen during opioid rotation in long-term opioid use or cancer-related pain.

Agonist activity at opioid receptors acts to open potassium channels and prevent the opening of voltage-gated calcium channels. This reduces neuronal excitability and inhibits the release of pain neurotransmitters.

Classification of opioid drugs

Opioids have been traditionally classified as *strong, intermediate*, and *weak*, according to their perceived analgesic properties and propensity for addiction. This classification can be misleading, as it implies that weak opioids such as codeine are less effective but safe. Codeine may be less potent than morphine but can cause respiratory depression if given in sufficient quantities. Codeine-like drugs are also frequently abused. Opioids may also be classified according to their structure. As described later, the properties of opioids may be predicted on the basis of activity on opioid and other receptor systems. The functional classification is probably of most clinical use (Table 18.1).

Opioid pharmacodynamics

Opioids act to reduce the intensity and unpleasantness of pain. The common adverse effects are due to their action on different opioid receptors. They include sedation, euphoria, dysphoria, respiratory depression, constipation, pruritus, and nausea and vomiting. It is important to note, however, that many of these effects tend to diminish with time as tolerance to the opioid develops. Constipation and dry mouth (leading

293

Table 18.1 Classification of opioids

Traditional

Strong	Intermediate	Weak
Morphine Diamorphine Fentanyl	Partial agonists Mixed agonist-antagonist	Codeine

Structural

Morphinans	Phenylperidines	Diphenylprophylamines	Esters
Morphine Codeine	Meperidine Fentanyl	Methadone Dextropropoxyphene	Remifentanil

Functional

Pure agonists	Partial agonists	Mixed action	Antagonists
Morphine Codeine	Buprenorphine	Pentazocine Nalbupine Butorphanol	Naxolone

to increased risk of dental caries), however, are more resistant to the development of tolerance and remain problems with long-term use. Impairment of hypothalamic function also occurs with long-term opioid use and may result in loss of libido, impotence and infertility.

Adverse effects associated with the use of opioids in acute pain (and occasionally in chronic non-malignant pain) can often be managed simply by reducing the opioid dose or switching to a different opioid. In palliative medicine, adverse effects related to long-term opioid use are often treated pro-actively. Laxatives are used for the treatment of constipation. Excessive sedation can be treated by methylphenidate or dextroamphetamine. Rotating to another opioid, or using more frequent but smaller doses of opioids may also help.

Systemic effects of opioid analgesics

Central nervous system

Opioids reduce the intensity and unpleasantness of pain. Patients taking opioid analgesics often report less distress, even when they can still perceive pain. Sedative effects occur frequently, particularly in the early stages of treatment, but often resolve. Sedation can remain a problem, especially at higher doses, and is a common cause of drug discontinuation in the chronic pain population. The sensitivity of the respiratory centre to hypercarbia and hypoxaemia is reduced by opioids. Hypoventilation, due to a reduction in respiratory rate and tidal volume, ensues. Cough is inhibited by a central action. Prolonged apnea and respiratory obstruction can occur during sleep. These effects are more pronounced when the respiratory drive is impaired by disease, for example in chronic obstructive pulmonary disease, obstructive sleep apnea and raised intracranial pressure.

In clinical practice, opioid-related respiratory depression is more common in patients being treated for acute pain than in patients established on long-term opioids. Respiratory depression in the acute pain patient is caused by an increase in opioid concentrations in the blood. This may be due to the use of an inappropriately large dose that fails to account for differences in patient physiology (e.g. the hypovolaemic trauma patient or the elderly patient) or because the patient is unable to excrete the drug efficiently (e.g. the patient with renal impairment). Respiratory depression is unusual in patients established on long-term opioids due to the development of tolerance. However, sudden changes to the patient's physiological state (e.g. the development of acute renal failure) may produce increases in blood opioid concentration and precipitate toxic effects.

Nausea and vomiting are common in patients receiving opioids for acute pain relief. The mechanism of action is thought to be the activation of opioid receptors within the chemoreceptor trigger zone within the medulla, although opioid effects on the gastrointestinal tract and vestibular function probably play a role. Anti-emetics are often pre-scribed for the prophylaxis or treatment of nausea.

Miosis occurs due to an excitatory effect on the parasym-pathetic nerve innervating the pupil. Pin-point pupils are characteristic of acute poisoning; at therapeutic doses the pupils are merely smaller than normal.

Cardiovascular system

Opioids cause peripheral vasodilatation and impair sympathetic vascular reflexes. Hypotension may occur on rising from the supine position, but this is seldom troublesome in the reasonably fit patient and is rare with long-term use. Intravenous administration of opioids to patients who are hypovolaemic or have poor cardiac reserve can result in marked hypotension. However, intravenous morphine titrated carefully may benefit patients with acute myocardial infarct and left ventricular failure as morphine reduces sympathetic drive (from pain and anxiety) and preload (by venodilatation), thereby reducing the work of the heart.

Gastrointestinal tract

Opioids cause a tonic increase of smooth muscle tone along the gastrointestinal tract. Reduced peristalsis (propulsion) and delayed gastric emptying results in constipation. Delay in the passage of the intestinal contents results in greater absorption of water and increased viscosity of faeces, and this contributes to constipation (this effect is useful in the treatment of diarrhoea). Opioid-induced constipation commonly occurs in palliative care and can be managed by increasing the fibre content of the diet to >10 g/day (unless bowel obstruction exists) and prescribing a stool softener (e.g. docusate sodium 100 mg b.i.d. or t.i.d.), usually along with a stimulant laxative (e.g. senna or bisacodyl). Stimulant laxatives should be started at a low dose (e.g. Senna 15 mg o.d.) but can be increased if necessary. Persisting constipation can be managed with an osmotic laxative (e.g. magnesium citrate) given q 2–3 days or with lactulose given daily (e.g. 15 mL b.i.d.). If opioid-induced constipation does not respond to conventional laxative therapy, prescription of methylnaltrexone may be indicated. Methylnaltrexone is a quaternary mu-opioid receptor antagonist and hence does not cross the blood–brain barrier to reverse the central analgesic effects of opiates. It is administered subcutaneously, usually once every other day under specialist supervision.

Pressure within the biliary tree due to spasm of the sphincter of Oddi is increased after opioid administration. Colicky pain due to morphine administration can occur in some patients. This can be both diagnosed and relieved by titrating a small dose of the opioid antagonist, naloxone. It is a commonly held belief that meperidine (pethidine) produces less spasm in the sphincter of Oddi than other opioids due to its atropine-like effects and, therefore, should be the opioid of choice for treatment of biliary tree and pancreatic pain. At higher equianalgesic doses, however, its effect on the sphincter is similar to other opioids, and meperidine confers no advantage.

Urogenital tract

The increased contraction of the ureters is probably clinically unimportant. Increased tone in the detrusor muscle and contraction of the external sphincter, together with inhibition of the voiding reflexes may cause urinary retention.

Others

Opioid administration is often associated with cutaneous vasodilation that results in the flushing of the face, neck and thorax. This may, in part, be due to histamine release. Pruritus is common with epidural or intrathecal administration of opioids and appears to be mediated by opioid receptor activation, as it is reversed by naloxone.

Opioid pharmacokinetics

Bioavailability varies among opioids after oral administration but is generally poor. Methadone is an exception (80%) (Table 18.2).

Most opioids have a large volume of distribution, and many have similar elimination half-lives. Notable exceptions with short half-lives are alfentanil and remifentanil. Methadone has a low clearance and a large volume of distribution. This results in its very prolonged half-life ($t_{1/2}$). There is a risk of delayed toxicity associated with the use of methadone, as steady-state plasma levels are not approached until 4–5 half-lives have passed. Controlled-release opioids typically require days to approach steady-state plasma levels.

Table 18.2 Approximate oral bioavailability of opioids

Opioid	Approximate oral bioavailability %
Hydromorphone	20
Morphine	30
Diamorphine	30
Meperidine	30
Codeine	60
Oxycodone	60
Levorphanol	70
Tramadol	80
Methadone	80

Duration of analgesia usually correlates with $t_{1/2}$ unless the parent drug has active metabolites (morphine) or if the drug has a high affinity for opioid receptors (buprenorphine). One must also consider inter-individual variation in the pharmacodynamic response to opioids. For example, opioid sensitivity is increased in the neonate and in the elderly. This variability and the narrow therapeutic index of opioids make it imperative that the dose of opioid should be titrated and its effects monitored for each patient. For opioid-naïve patients with acute pain, frequent monitoring of pain relief, sedation, respiratory rate and blood pressure is necessary to guide dosage adjustment.

Route of administration

The oral route is preferred as it is simple, non-invasive and relatively affordable. It requires little in the form of direct medical supervision or complex delivery equipment. However, the slower onset of action renders this route less convenient for use in acute pain. The oral route is also unsuitable when patients suffer from emesis, dysphagia, gastrointestinal obstruction or malabsorption or in acute trauma where the patient may have delayed gastric emptying.

If parenteral administration is necessary, the intravenous route is preferable to intramuscular injection for repeated boluses because it is less painful. Also, intramuscular or subcutaneous routes of administration should not be used if the patient is peripherally vasoconstricted (e.g. in the acute trauma patient), as the establishment of normal peripheral blood flow, as the patient is resuscitated, may result in a sudden redistribution of the drug to the central circulation. Continuous intravenous or subcutaneous infusion should be considered if repeated parenteral doses produce a prominent bolus effect (i.e. toxicity) at peak levels early in the dosing interval or breakthrough pain at trough levels. Patient-controlled analgesia (PCA) systems (in which the patient can trigger additional drug delivery) can be added to an infusion to provide supplementary doses. These systems are safe for both home and hospitalised patients but are contraindicated for sedated and confused patients.

Epidural and intrathecal administration of opioids requires special expertise. The dorsal horn of the spinal cord is rich in opioid receptors, and equivalent analgesia can be provided using a lower dose of opioid, resulting in fewer systemic side-effects. However, rostral spread of the drug can result in delayed toxicity (e.g. respiratory depression) during acute administration, and the cost of infusion systems, staffing and monitoring must also be taken into account. The use of intraventricular morphine appears to be beneficial in treating recalcitrant pain due to head and neck malignancies and tumours (e.g. superior sulcus tumours, breast carcinoma) that affect the brachial plexus.

Pharmacology of individual opioids

Opioid agonist drugs

Morphine

Morphine remains the most widely used opioid analgesic for the treatment of severe pain. It is the gold standard against which other opioids are compared. It is commonly given intramuscularly, intravenously or orally; however, it can also be administered per rectum and into the epidural space or cerebrospinal fluid. Unlike most opioids, it is relatively water soluble. Metabolism is by hepatic conjugation, and its half-life is about 2–4 h. The duration of useful analgesia provided by morphine is about 3–6 h but varies greatly with different drug preparations and routes of administration.

Morphine 6-glucuronide (M6G), one of its major metabolites, is an agonist at the μ receptor and also at the distinct M6G receptor. It is more potent than morphine. As it is excreted in the urine, it accumulates if renal function is impaired. With repeated use of morphine, morphine 6-glucuronide is responsible for a significant amount of pharmacological activity.

Diamorphine

Diamorphine (3,6 diacetyl morphine), or heroin, is a semi-synthetic drug that was first made from morphine at St Mary's Hospital, London, in 1874. In almost every country, except the UK, the manufacture of diamorphine, even for use in medicine, is now illegal.

Diamorphine has no direct activity at the μ receptor. It is rapidly converted within minutes to morphine and 6-monoacetylmorphine, a metabolite of both drugs. The effects of diamorphine are principally due to the actions of morphine and 6-monoacetylmorphine on the μ- and, to a lesser extent, the κ-receptors.

Diamorphine given parenterally has a $t_{1/2}$ of 3 min. When given orally, it is subject to complete pre-systemic or first-pass metabolism, and only morphine ($t_{1/2}$ 3 h) and other metabolites reach the systemic circulation. Thus oral diamorphine is essentially a prodrug. It is likely that there are no significant differences in the pharmacodynamics of diamorphine when compared to morphine when used for acute pain, despite the common belief that diamorphine is associated with more euphoria and less nausea and vomiting. Its greater potency (greater efficacy in relation to weight and, therefore, requiring a smaller volume) and lipid-solubility makes diamorphine suitable for delivery by subcutaneous infusion through a syringe driver when continuous pain control is required in palliative care that can no longer be achieved by the enteral route (oral, buccal, rectal).

Codeine

Codeine is obtained naturally or by methylation of morphine. It has a low affinity for opioid receptors, and most of its analgesic effects result from its metabolism (about 10%) to morphine. The polymorphic CYP2D6 enzyme is responsible for this transformation, and it is absent in some individuals (e.g. 7% of the Caucasian population), suggesting that these patients will derive little benefit from codeine.

Codeine alone is a relatively poor analgesic but can be effective for mild to moderate pain, especially when combined with paracetamol. It can also be useful for the short-term symptomatic control of persistent cough or mild diarrhoea. Prolonged use is often associated with chronic constipation, especially at higher doses (more than 30 mg q.i.d.).

Dihydrocodeine

Dihydrocodeine (DF118) is a low-efficacy opioid with an analgesic potency similar to that of codeine. It is used to relieve moderate acute and chronic pain on its own or as a compound tablet (co-dydramol; dihydrocodeine 10 mg plus paracetamol 500 mg). Although active metabolites (dihydromorphine and dihydromorphine-6-O-glucuronide) account for some of its pharmacological effects, dihydrocodeine itself has analgesic activity and may be a more reliable analgesic when compared to codeine.

Oxycodone

Oxycodone is a semi-synthetic opioid that has been in clinical use since 1917. Its potency is approximately twice that of morphine. Oxycodone is currently used as a controlled-release preparation for cancer and chronic non-malignant pain. The immediate-release solution and tablets are available for acute or breakthrough pain. Parental oxycodone is an alternative when opioids cannot be given orally. Both oxycodone and morphine provide effective analgesia in acute and chronic pain. However, oxycodone may have a more favourable pharmacokinetic profile. Its oral bioavailability, at about 80%, is significantly higher. This results in reduced inter-individual variation in plasma concentrations after oral administration. It has a similar adverse-effect profile to morphine with a slightly reduced incidence of psychotropic effects.

A fixed-dose oral formulation (Targinact) of oxycodone combined with naloxone has been shown to be effective in patients who derive benefit from opioid therapy, but where use of the opioid is limited because of intractable constipation. Naxolone provides competitive antagonism of the opioid-receptor–mediated effects of oxycodone in the gut, thus reducing constipation. Since the bioavailability of naloxone after oral administration is less than 3%, systemic effects from the antagonist drug are unlikely. The recommended maximum daily dose of Targinact is 80 mg oxycodone hydrochloride and 40 mg naloxone hydrochloride.

Hydromorphone

Hydromorphone is a semi-synthetic opioid used primarily for the treatment of cancer-related pain. It can be administered intravenously, orally, and rectally. Hydromorphone is five times as potent as morphine when given by the oral route and eight to nine times as potent when given intravenously, with a similar duration of action. The liver is its principle site of metabolism. In contrast to morphine, the 6-glucuronide metabolite is not produced in any significant amount, the main metabolite being hydromorphone-3-glucuronide. Some metabolites are active, but they are present in such small amounts that they are unlikely to have a significant effect except perhaps in renal failure.

Methadone

Methadone is a synthetic opioid used commonly as a maintenance drug in opioid addicts and increasingly used in cancer and chronic non-malignant pain. It is rapidly absorbed after oral administration and is extensively metabolised to products that are excreted in the urine. The principal feature of methadone is its long duration of action, due to high protein binding and slow liver metabolism. The elimination $t_{1/2}$ of methadone is 20–45 h, making it suitable for use in long-term therapy but less useful for acute pain. Steady-state concentration is only reached after several days with regular administration, and dosages must be carefully titrated.

When used in cancer-related pain or chronic non-malignant pain, an opioid of short $t_{1/2}$ should be provided for breakthrough pain, rather than an extra dose of methadone. The long duration of action also favours its use for the treatment of opioid withdrawal.

Fentanyl

Fentanyl is one of the first short-acting opioids developed for use in anaesthesia. It is approximately 100 times more potent than morphine but undergoes hepatic metabolism to produce inactive metabolites. At low doses, it has a short duration of action due to redistribution of the drug. However, its terminal $t_{1/2}$ is relatively long (1.5–6 h) and, at higher doses, when tissue sites are saturated, its duration of action is much higher. The long $t_{1/2}$ and high lipid solubility makes fentanyl ideal for use as a transdermal patch. These preparations are used commonly in cancer-related pain and chronic non-malignant pain.

Oral transmucosal fentanyl citrate offers a unique way of treating breakthrough and incident pain. The transmucosal route offers rapid onset of action in 5–15 min, with peak plasma concentrations at 22 min. Absorption takes place at the buccal and sublingual mucosa, first-pass effect is avoided, and overall bioavailability is 50%.

Alfentanil

Alfentanil is less potent and has a shorter $t_{1/2}$ than fentanyl. However, despite its lower lipid solubility, it has a more rapid onset of action. This is because a greater proportion of the unbound drug is unionised and able to diffuse freely across the blood–brain barrier. However, like fentanyl, it accumulates with prolonged infusion and the plasma $t_{1/2}$ increases with the duration of infusion.

Remifentanil

Remifentanil is a μ opioid receptor agonist with an analgesic potency similar to fentanyl and a speed of onset similar to alfentanil. It is broken down by blood and tissue esterases and has a short and predictable $t_{1/2}$ (approximately 5 min) which is not affected by renal or hepatic function or plasma cholinesterase deficiency.

Its main metabolite is a carboxylic acid derivative which is excreted by the kidneys. Although this accumulates in renal failure, significant pharmacological effects are unlikely as its potency relative to remifentanil is only 0.1–0.3%.

Remifentanil is unique in that its plasma $t_{1/2}$ remains constant even after prolonged infusion. This property favours its use during anaesthesia, when a rapid wake-up time is desirable (e.g. after neurosurgery).

Papaveretum

Papaveretum is a mixture of opium alkaloids, the principle constituents being morphine (50%), codeine, papaverine and noscapine. Noscapine may be teratogenic and is no longer a component of commercially available papaveretum in UK.

Partial agonist opioid analgesics

Buprenorphine

Buprenorphine is a partial agonist at the μ-receptor. The partial agonist activity, however, is thought to occur at a higher dose than would be normally used therapeutically and is, therefore, rarely clinically significant. It is 30 times more potent than morphine, and its receptor affinity (tenacity of binding) is high. This means that it dissociates from the receptor very slowly. Thus, its peak effect may occur up to

3 h after administration, and its duration of action as long as 10 h. In theory, a partial agonist has less potential for respiratory depression and abuse. However, respiratory depression can occur with buprenorphine overdose and, because of the drug's affinity with the μ-receptor, may only be partially reversed by naloxone. A respiratory stimulant (doxapram) may be needed in overdose or, occasionally, mechanical ventilation.

Because of extensive first-pass metabolism when swallowed, buprenorphine is normally given by the buccal (sublingual) route or by i.m. or slow i.v. injection. It is a useful analgesic in acute pain because administration by injection can be avoided (for children, or for patients with a bleeding disorder or needle phobia). Its low incidence of drug dependency has led to its increased use in withdrawing opioid addicts and in chronic non-malignant pain. Its prolonged $t_{1/2}$ and high lipid solubility makes it suitable for use as a transdermal patch preparation.

Meptazinol

Meptazinol is a high-efficacy partial agonist opioid with central cholinergic activity that is thought to add to its analgesic effect. It is used to relieve acute or chronic pain of moderate intensity. It is thought to have a low incidence of confusion and a low potential for abuse. Its poor oral bioavailability and partial agonist activity makes it less useful in severe pain.

Mixed agonist-antagonist opioid analgesics

Drugs in this class include pentazocine, butorphanol and nalbuphine. They act as partial agonists at the κ receptor and weak antagonists at the μ receptor. Consequently, they may cause withdrawal symptoms in patients dependent on other opioids. As analgesics, mixed agonist-antagonist opioids are not as efficacious as pure μ agonists. Compared to morphine, they produce less dependence (but this definitely occurs), more psychotomimetic effects (κ receptor) and less sedation and respiratory depression (naloxone can reverse the respiratory depression in overdose). They are given to relieve moderate to severe pain, but dysphoric adverse effects often limit their usefulness.

Pentazocine is one-sixth as potent as morphine, nalbuphine is slightly less potent than morphine and butorphanol is five to nine times as potent. Adverse effects include nausea, vomiting, dizziness, sweating, hypertension, palpitations, tachycardia and CNS disturbances such as euphoria, dysphoria and psychotomimesis (mimicking the symptoms of psychosis, e.g. delusions and/or delirium). Pentazocine has effects on the cardiovascular system, raising systolic blood pressure and pulmonary artery pressure, and should be avoided in myocardial infarction.

Opioids with action on other systems

Meperidine

Meperidine (Pethidine) was discovered in 1939 during a search for atropine-like compounds. Its use as a treatment for asthma was abandoned when its opioid agonist properties were appreciated.

Meperidine is primarily a μ-receptor agonist. Despite its structural dissimilarity to morphine, meperidine shares many similar properties, including antagonism by naloxone. It is extensively metabolised in the liver, and the parent drug and metabolites are excreted in the urine. Normeperidine is a pharmacologically active metabolite. It can cause central excitation and, eventually, convulsions, if it accumulates after prolonged intravenous administration or in renal impairment.

Meperidine has atropine-like effects, including dry mouth and blurred vision (cycloplegia and sometimes mydriasis, though usually miosis). It can produce euphoria and is associated with a high incidence of dependence. Its use as an analgesia in obstetric practice was based on early clinical research which showed that, unlike morphine, meperidine did not appear to delay labour. However, the doses of meperidine used in these early studies were low, and it is now established that meperidine confers no added advantage over other opioids at higher equianalgesic doses.

Meperidine is eight to ten times less potent than morphine and has poor and variable oral absorption, with a short duration of action in the range of 2–3 h. For all these reasons, it is recommended that meperidine should be avoided if alternatives are available.[2]

Tramadol

Tramadol is presented as a mixture of two stereoisomers. It is a centrally acting analgesic with relatively weak μ-opioid receptor activity. However, it also inhibits neuronal reuptake of norepinephrine and enhances serotonin release, and this is thought to account for some of its analgesic action.

It is rapidly absorbed from the gastrointestinal tract; 20% of an oral dose undergoes first-pass metabolism, and less than 30% of a dose is excreted unchanged in the urine. Production of the O-desmethyltramadol metabolite is dependent on the cytochrome CYP2D6 enzyme. This metabolite is an active μ agonist with a greater receptor affinity than tramadol. Tramadol is approximately as effective as meperidine for postoperative pain.

Tramadol is less likely to depress respiration and has a lower incidence of constipation compared to opioids, but has a high incidence of nausea and dizziness. It can cause seizures (rare) and should be used with caution in susceptible patients.

Tapentadol

Tapentadol is currently approved for clinical use in the USA, Australia and the UK. Like tramadol, tapentadol is also a centrally acting analgesic with μ-opioid receptor activity. Unlike tramadol, tapentadol is an open-chain molecule, and this structure confers three main pharmacological differences. First, tapentadol has no active metabolites. Second, the μ-opioid receptor agonist activity of tapentadol is several-fold greater than tramadol. Finally, tapentadol is selective for norepinephrine reuptake inhibition. Clinical trials report tapentadol has fewer gastrointestinal adverse events when compared with an equi-analgesic dose of opioid (for example, oxycodone). To date, there are currently no published clinical trials demonstrating the superiority of tapentadol over tramadol.

Opioid antagonists

Naloxone

Naloxone is a competitive antagonist at μ-, δ-, κ- and σ-opioid receptors and acts to reverse the effects of most opioid analgesics. It acts within minutes when given intravenously and slightly less rapidly when given intramuscularly. However, the duration of antagonism (approximately 20 min) is usually shorter than that of opioid-induced respiratory depression. Close monitoring of the patient and repeated doses of naloxone may therefore be necessary.

A common starting dosage in an opioid-naïve patient with acute opioid overdosage is 0.4 mg i.v. every 2–3 min until effect. For patients receiving long-term opioid therapy, it should be used only to reverse respiratory depression and must be administered more cautiously to avoid precipitating withdrawal or severe pain. A reasonable starting dose is 0.04 mg (dilute a 0.4-mg ampoule in 10 mL saline) i.v. every 2–3 min until the respiratory rate improves.

Choice of opioid analgesic

An opioid may be preferred because of favourable experience, lower cost (methadone is least expensive), availability, route of administration or duration of action. Opioids with a

---

[2]WHO Expert Committee on the Selection and Use of Essential Medicines. The selection and use of essential medicines: report of the WHO Expert Committee, 2003 (including the 13th model list of essential medicines). Geneva, World Health Organization, 2003)..

Table 18.3 Relative potency of opioids

Drug	Oral:parenteral potency ratio*	Parenteral potency relative to morphine**
Morphine	1:6	1.0
Codeine	2:3	0.1
Hydromorphone	1:5	6.0
Meperidine	1:4	0.15
Oxycodone	1:2	1.0
Methadone	1:2	1.0

*Oral-parenteral ratio: for example, morphine is six times more potent parenterally than orally.
**Parenteral potency relative to morphine: for example, hydromorphone is six times more potent than an equal dose of morphine when given parenterally.
Mitchell JP: General Care of the Patient, in Manual of Medical Therapeutics, 26th ed by Claiborne D and Ridner M (eds). Little, Brown and Co. 1989. p 5.

Table 18.4 Opioid oral analgesic equivalents

Analgesic	Single dose	Equianalgesic dose Oral morphine
Codeine	60 mg	5 mg
Dihydrocodeine	60 mg	8 mg
Tramadol	50 mg	10 mg
Meptazinol	200 mg	8 mg
Buprenorphine sublingual	200 µg	10 mg
Hydromorphone	1.3 mg	10 mg
Methadone	1 mg	10 mg
Oxycodone	5 mg	10 mg

short $t_{1/2}$ (morphine and diamorphine) should be used as first-line agents for acute pain but may be replaced with longer-acting drugs if pain persists.

Knowledge of equianalgesic doses of opioids is essential when changing drugs or routes of administration (Tables 18.3 and 18.4). Cross-tolerance between drugs is incomplete, so when one drug is substituted for another, the equianalgesic dose should be reduced by 50%. The only exception is methadone, which should be reduced by 75–90%. Opioid rotation is commonly used in palliative care when life expectancy is limited as a means of reducing side-effects and limiting the development of tolerance.

The prolonged use of opioids for chronic non-malignant pain is currently under scrutiny. Poor prescribing practices in the USA in the last decade have led to an alarming increase in deaths from overdose and misuse. Clinical trial data are unavailable for outcomes beyond 3 months of use, and there are concerns that comfort afforded by opioid analgesia therapy does not translate to improvements in physical or emotion functioning and is associated with increased morbidity related to drug-induced side-effects. Adverse effects, including abnormalities in endocrine and immune function, increased risk in cardiovascular events and, surprisingly, a risk of gastrointestinal bleeding similar to that of non-selective NSAID drugs, are dose-related, and there appears to be a significant increase in drug-related side-effects beyond morphine equivalent doses of 120 mg/day. Hence, we recommend that chronic opioid use should only be pre-scribed by clinicians working within a multidisciplinary setting where access to non-pharmacological approaches to pain is available. Expertise for tapering opioid therapy, or indeed any analgesic, should be available if the long-term drug proves ineffective, unsuitable or is no longer required for pain management.

Tolerance, dependence and addiction

Although the use of strong opioid analgesics in cancer-related pain is well-established, physicians are often reluctant to prescribe opioids in acute, and especially in chronic, non-malignant pain. Patients (and their families, friends and employers) are, likewise, wary about the long-term use of opioids. The reasons for this reluctance may stem from previous experiences of the genuine problems associated with long-term opioid use in patients or, more often, due to the perception of opioids as dangerous and addictive drugs. Patients and physicians also frequently confuse toler-ance and dependence with drug addiction.

Tolerance indicates the need to increase the dose of a drug with time to achieve the same analgesic effect. It is due to physiological adaptation to the drug. In practice, tolerance can be managed by increasing the dose of the opioid drug over time. However, tolerance to the adverse effects of opioids (e.g. constipation) is often less-predictable, and the development of side-effects may prevent further escalation of the drug.

It is important to distinguish a gradual reduction in efficacy of an analgesic that is due to the development of tolerance, from the onset of pain due to progression of the underlying disease process or new pathology. In addition, there are animal data suggesting that opioids can paradoxically increase pain when administered at high doses and for prolonged periods of time. The phenomenon is termed 'opioid-induced hyperalgesia'. The few case reports of patients with opioid-induced hyperalgesia described high doses of opioids (more than 180 mg morphine equivalent per day), with worse pain on dose escalation, which improves with gradual reduction in opioid therapy.

Dependence is the physical manifestation of tolerance, and its effects are observed soon after abrupt withdrawal of a long-term opioid. The severity of withdrawal symptoms varies depending on the patient, the drug and the length of treatment, and includes symptoms such as coryza, tremor, sweating, abdominal cramps, myalgia, vomiting and diarrhoea. Acute withdrawal can usually be avoided by reducing the drug dose gradually at the end of treatment by about 50% every 2 days (but may require a slower rate of withdrawal in some long-term patients). Patients on long-term opioid therapy should not be given mixed agonist/antagonist drugs, as they can precipitate withdrawal.

Addiction is a behavioural problem characterised by drug-seeking activity in the individual in order to experience its psychotropic effects. This drug-seeking behaviour may persist despite the knowledge that continued use of the drug will result in considerable physical, emotional, social or economic harm. The incidence of iatrogenic addiction in patients taking opioid medications for acute post-surgical or traumatic pain is negligible, and the risk is also extremely low in patients prescribed opioids for cancer-related pain. However, in patients taking opioids for chronic non-malignant pain, the prevalence of past or present opioid use disorder is thought to be approximately 8–12%. While the risk of *de novo* addiction remains low in well-managed patients, the decision to prescribe should be taken with caution, especially in at-risk patients (e.g. in patients with history of mental illness or prior history of drug or alcohol misuse).

Pain management in opioid addicts

Drug addicts can suffer from pain. Physicians, particularly in hospitals, are often guilty of withholding or under-prescribing opioids for drug-addicted patients in acute pain. This stems from unfounded fears of 'worsening' the addiction, distrust of the patient's motives or misguided attempts to 'cure' the patient of his addiction.

Before treating opioid addicts with acute pain, physicians should attempt to establish the patient's daily opioid intake prior to hospital admission. The patient should then be maintained with an equivalent daily dose of opioid medication throughout his or her admission. Physicians should be aware that the strength of street drugs is highly variable. The addicted patient may also have an acute medical condition that alters opioid pharmacokinetics unpredictably. It is safer, therefore, to first prescribe an appropriate dose of an opioid with a short duration of action on an 'as-required' basis, in order to assess opioid requirements, before conversion to longer-acting opioids for maintenance.

The opioid-addicted patient with acute pain will require appropriate analgesia in addition to the calculated maintenance dose. Non-opioid analgesics are useful adjuncts but should not be used as a substitute for opioid analgesia. The use of opioid agonist-antagonist compounds in known or suspected active opioid addicts is absolutely contraindicated, as these drugs may precipitate withdrawal.

Co-analgesics

Co-analgesics (adjuvant analgesics) are important for the treatment of cancer-related and chronic non-malignant pain. These agents provide an 'opioid-sparing' effect and are effective for the treatment of neuropathic pain associated with many cancers. In chronic non-malignant pain, co-analgesics are frequently used as 'first-line' drugs and form the mainstay of treatment for chronic neuropathic pain. As co-analgesics are generally used in other medical conditions (e.g. as anticonvulsants or antidepressants), their basic pharmacology will be covered in the relevant chapters elsewhere. This chapter highlights the use of co-analgesics in the context of pain management.

Multipurpose adjuvant analgesics

Corticosteroids

Corticosteroids are amongst the most widely used adjuvant analgesics in palliative care. They improve quality of life in cancer patients by virtue of their analgesic effects and other beneficial effects on appetite, nausea, mood and malaise. Corticosteroids may also reduce oedema around metastases or damaged nerve plexuses. Patients with advanced cancer who experience pain and other symptoms often respond favourably to a relatively small dose of corticosteroid (e.g. dexamethasone 1–2 mg twice daily).

Neuroleptics

Methotrimeprazine has proven very useful in bedridden patients with advanced cancer who experience pain associated with anxiety, restlessness or nausea. In this setting, the

301

sedative, anxiolytic and antiemetic effects of this drug can be useful, and side-effects, such as orthostatic hypotension, are less clinically significant. Treatment can be started at 6–25 mg/day in three divided doses at mealtimes and increased until optimum effect. Alternatively, as a sedative, a single nighttime dose of 10–25 mg can be given.

Benzodiazepines

Benzodiazepines have limited analgesic effects but are often used as a short-term treatment for painful muscle spasm. Their use, however, must be balanced by the potential for side-effects, including sedation and confusion. With the important exception of clonazepam, which is widely accepted for use in the management of neuropathic pain, these drugs are generally prescribed only if another indication exists, such as anxiety or insomnia.

Adjuvant analgesics used in neuropathic pain

Antidepressants

At present, the evidence for analgesic efficacy is greatest for the tertiary amine tricyclic drugs, such as amitriptyline, doxepin and imipramine. The secondary amine tricyclic antidepressants (such as desipramine and nortriptyline) have fewer side-effects and are preferred when there are serious concerns about sedation, anticholinergic effects or cardiovascular toxicity. Dual-reuptake inhibitors (venlafaxine, duloxetine) may be beneficial for patients who obtain relief from tricyclics but find the adverse effects a problem. Duloxetine is currently licensed for the treatment of pain from diabetic neuropathy and fibromyalgia and has been shown to be effective in clinical trials. There is little evidence, however, to suggest that duloxetine is more efficacious compared to tricyclic antidepressant drugs for the treatment of neuropathic pain.

The dose of duloxetine required to treat pain is 60–120 mg, which also has clinically relevant antidepressant effects. This is in contrast to other antidepressant drugs used in neuropathic pain, where the analgesic effect of the drugs occurs at a smaller dose and within a shorter time from onset (1–2 weeks) than any antidepressant effect. The drugs should be started at a low dose to minimise initial side-effects (e.g. amitriptyline 10 mg o.d. in the elderly and 10–25 mg o.d. in younger patients). Education of the patient is essential. They should be informed that the analgesic effect of the antidepressant medication can take days or weeks to develop and that the drug must be taken on a regular basis for effect. It is common for patients to report taking the medication intermittently as a supplement to simple analgesics 'when the pain is bad'. Patient compliance is often improved when physicians emphasise that the drugs are being prescribed for their analgesic effects and not for their antidepressant properties.

Abrupt withdrawal of the antidepressant drugs should be avoided, as it can cause a variety of unpleasant symptoms thought to be related to rebound cholinergic activity. These include vivid dreams, restlessness and gastrointestinal hyperactivity. These symptoms can be minimised if the drug dose is reduced gradually at intervals of 5–10 days.

Anticonvulsants

In 1853, Alfred Trousseau, then director of the medical clinic at Hotel-Dieu in Paris, suggested that painful paroxysms seen in trigeminal neuralgia were due to discharges in the trigeminal system that were similar to the neuronal discharges seen in epilepsy. Trousseau's hypothesis was tested by Bergouigan, who successfully used phenytoin to treat trigeminal neuralgia. Carbamazepine was studied in the same condition during a placebo-controlled double-blind design that was among the first of its kind in pain medicine. Since then, anticonvulsants have been extensively used in a wide variety of neuropathic pain syndromes, particularly those associated with 'lancinating' or 'shooting' pain. Animal studies have shown that peripheral nerve fibres in persistent pain syndromes have altered expression of certain ion channels, particularly novel sodium channels, and N-type calcium channels.

Carbamazepine, phenytoin and sodium valproate have been used for many years to treat neuropathic pain. However, carbamazepine remains the only anticonvulsant licensed within the UK for the treatment of trigeminal neuralgia. All anticonvulsants produce side-effects such as dizziness and drowsiness. Carbamazepine, in particular, may suppress bone marrow function and cause hyponatraemia. Its use requires regular blood monitoring.

Gabapentin and pregabalin are newer anticonvulsant agents that show good efficacy in clinical trials of neuropathic pain. These drugs bind to the $\alpha_2\delta$-1 subunit of voltage-dependent calcium channels and may work by preventing the formation of excitatory synapses within the CNS. Gabapentin is generally better tolerated than the older anticonvulsants and has a license in the UK for the treatment of neuropathic pain. It is not metabolised by the liver and has few clinically significant drug interactions. It should be started at a dose of 300 mg at night (100 mg in the elderly) and titrated upwards as tolerated or to a dose of 600–1200 mg t.i.d. A saturable gut transport mechanism limits bioavailability at high oral doses (but also protects against overdosage). Pregabalin shares a similar mode of action to gabapentin, but has the advantage of more linear pharmacokinetics and can be given as a twice-daily preparation (normal maintenance dose up to 300 mg b.i.d.).

Local anaesthetics

Local anaesthetic agents are specifically developed to provide local and regional anaesthesia. The use of systemic local anaesthetics in neuropathic pain was first suggested in the 1950s and was popularised by subsequent studies that showed effectiveness in the treatment of painful diabetic neuropathy. Parenteral administration is, however, impractical for long-term treatment. Lidocaine infusions are mostly used to identify the subgroup of patients with neuropathic pain who respond to sodium channel blockade. Patients who respond favourably to lidocaine infusion may proceed to a trial of its oral analogue, mexiletine or other sodium channel–blocking drugs.

A topical lidocaine patch preparation, consisting of an adhesive dressing infused with a preparation containing 5% lidocaine may be useful for the treatment of post-herpetic neuralgia and other peripheral neuropathic pain conditions. Lidocaine 5% transdermal patches show reasonable efficacy in clinical trials with minimal systemic absorption of the local anaesthetic agent. Their ease of use and lack of side-effects may encourage use for the treatment of post-herpetic neuralgia and other neuropathic pain disorders.

Capsaicin

Capsaicin (derived from chili peppers) activates specific vanilloid receptors found in C-nociceptors. Initial topical application causes a transient burning sensation. With repeated applications, however, desensitisation of the nociceptors occurs. This is the basis for its use in chronic pain conditions.

Clinical trials using topically applied 0.025–0.075% capsaicin cream (applied four times daily) show good results for pain due to diabetic neuropathy and post-herpetic neuralgia. However, repeated applications for several weeks are required, and compliance is often poor.

A topical patch preparation containing 8% capsaicin is now available for use in peripheral neuropathic pain conditions. This preparation has been shown to provide longer-lasting pain relief (~3 months) with a single 30–60-minute application. However, application of the patch requires preparation of the skin beforehand with local anaesthetic.

Clonidine

Clonidine has agonist activity at α_2 and imidazoline receptors and is an effective analgesic when given intravenously or via the epidural or intrathecal routes. Oral preparations also exist and are well-absorbed, with 75–95% bioavailability. Its greater potency, when given centrally means that analgesic efficacy can be obtained with smaller doses and a reduced incidence of side-effects. Clonidine has been shown to augment the analgesic potency of epidural local anaesthetic agents and opioids and has proven efficacy in chronic pain disorders, including cancer pain. The major side-effects are sedation and hypotension. The latter is caused primarily by central sympatholysis and may be compounded by concomitant bradycardia. Chronic administration leads to a risk of rebound hypertension if withdrawn suddenly.

Cannabinoids

Delta-9-tetrahydrocannabinol (THC) is the only constituent of cannabis with clinically significant analgesic properties. THC is a partial agonist at the cannabinoid-1 receptor (CB-1r), which mediates its analgesic effects. However, the CB-1r is widely expressed throughout the CNS (including the brain), which accounts for the psychotropic effects of THC. Clinical trials continue to suggest that THC is useful for the treatment of refractory chronic pain, particularly in multiple sclerosis, cancer or HIV. Additionally, the cannabinoid is an anti-emetic and stimulates the appetite.

THC and related cannabinoids are formulated for the oral and oro-mucosal routes. The oral preparations are pure and synthetically derived. The oro-mucosal preparation (Sativex®) is plant-derived and composed of THC and cannabidiol (CBD) in equal proportions. Cannabidiol does not possess analgesic properties but may attenuate the psychoactivity of THC via an anxiolytic effect. Sativex® is currently licensed in Canada for the symptomatic relief of neuropathic pain in multiple sclerosis and pain from cancer.

The oral bioavailability of THC is poor and varies highly between individuals. Peak plasma concentration improves with fasting and occurs 2–4 h after drug ingestion. The oro-mucosal route avoids the hepatic first-pass effect and consequently has a quicker onset and greater bioavailability. Consequently, patients may themselves adjust the dose of Sativex® until pain relief is achieved with tolerable side-effects.

Ziconotide

Ziconotide (previously called SNX-111) is the synthetic form of the hydrophilic conopeptide ω-MVIIA, which is found in the venom of the Pacific fish-hunting snail, C magus. Notably, ziconotide is the only truly novel analgesic that has emerged from decades of pharmaceutical research and development.

Ziconotide binds reversibly and tightly to a subset of voltage-sensitive calcium channels (N-type channels). These N-type channels are found in the dorsal horn of the spinal cord and localised to the pre-synaptic central terminals of primary afferent neurons. The binding of ziconotide inhibits these channels, which reduces nociceptive transmission at the spinal level. However, N-type calcium channels are found throughout the CNS and account for the adverse effects of ziconotide. Common adverse effects are dizziness, nausea, confusion and headache. More severe, but rare, side-effects are hallucinations, thoughts of suicide and new or worsening depression. Consequently, the drug is contraindicated in patients with a history of psychosis, schizophrenia, clinical depression and bipolar disorder.

Ziconotide is only administered intrathecally to minimise side-effects. The optimal dose is achieved by slow titration over weeks as an infusion via an intrathecal pump. The method of delivery is complex, costly and invasive. Consequently, ziconotide is only approved for the management of severe chronic pain in patients for whom intrathecal therapy is warranted and who have been shown to be intolerant of, or refractory to, other treatment, such as systemic analgesics, adjunctive therapies or IT morphine. Drug tolerance does not occur, and there are minimal withdrawal effects after prolonged infusion.

Ketamine

Ketamine is a non-competitive NMDA antagonist that acts at the phencyclidine (PCP) binding site in the NMDA receptor. Controlled studies show good analgesic efficacy in peripheral and central neuropathic pain, fibromyalgia and chronic ischaemic pain. The drug can be given using various routes of administration, but trials most frequently report the use of intravenous boluses of 0.1–0.45 mg/kg, followed in some studies by infusions of around 5–7 μg/kg/min. Oral bioavailability is poor and impaired by poor taste, but the drug is now available as a more tolerably flavoured oral ketamine solution. Use of the drug is often associated with adverse effects, including unpleasant dreams, hallucinations and visual and auditory disturbances, and long-term use has been associated with bladder and renal complications. Ketamine may have a synergistic effect when combined with opioids.

Adjuvants used for bone pain

Bisphosphonates

Bisphosphonates (previously known as diphosphonates) are analogues of inorganic pyrophosphate that inhibit osteoclast activity and, consequently, reduce bone resorption in a variety of illnesses. This effect, presumably, underlines the putative analgesic efficacy of these compounds in bone pain. Currently the evidence for analgesic effects is best for pamidronate. Potential differences in the analgesia produced by the various drugs in this class require additional study, and neither dose-dependent effects nor long-term risks or benefits in cancer patients are established. The use of any bisphosphonate requires monitoring of serum calcium, phosphate, magnesium and potassium.

Pharmacotherapy of acute migraine headaches

Migraine is a neurological disorder characterised by episodic attacks of moderate–severe throbbing headache with a number of associated symptoms that include nausea, vomiting, photophobia and phonophobia (a persistent, abnormal and unwarranted fear of sound). In around one-third of patients with migraine, the headache can be accompanied by focal neurological symptoms (aura). In Europe and the USA, about 18% of women and 6% of men suffered at least one migraine attack in the past year. Migraine has been ranked among the world's most disabling medical illnesses. Its socio-economic impact is substantial, with an estimated annual cost of $17 billion for treatment alone.

The pathophysiology of migraine is complex, but a likely causative factor is the release of vasoactive peptides from the sensory nerve terminals that innervate meningeal blood vessels. This causes dilatation of the arteries in the meninges, perivascular inflammation and amplification of the nociceptive afferent nerve supply. Sensory input from dural and cerebrovascular sensory fibres are amplified and perceived as pain (allodynia). Activation of the sympathetic nervous system is the likely cause of autonomic symptoms such as nausea and vomiting. Sensory symptoms (aura) are produced by a transient, spreading disturbance in cortical function. Migraine possesses features of inflammatory and functional pain, as well as objective neurologic dysfunction. Diagnosis is based on the headache's characteristics and associated symptoms.[3]

Management of migraine

Migraine is best thought of, and managed as, a chronic pain syndrome. Non-pharmacological management of migraine involves helping patients to identify and avoid triggering factors such as stress, foods containing vasoactive amines (e.g. chocolate, cheese), bright lights, loud noises, hormonal changes and hypoglycaemia. Other behavioural and psychological interventions used for prevention include relaxation training, thermal biofeedback combined with relaxation training, electromyography biofeedback and cognitive behavioural therapy.

Pharmacotherapy of migraine is either abortive or preventive.

[3]International Headache Society, 2004. International classification of headache disorders. Cephalalgia 24 (Suppl. 1), 1–160. Iovino, M., Feifel, U., Young, C.L., Wolters, J.M., Wallenstein, G., 2004.

Abortive treatment of migraine

Drugs used to abort an acute attack of migraine are either non-specific (analgesics) or specific (triptans and ergots).

Simple analgesics such as acetylsalicylic acid (900 mg) or acetaminophen (1000 mg), with or without the addition of caffeine, can often be effective for mild to moderate headaches. The addition of domperidone (10 mg p.o.), prochlorperazine (50 mg p.o.) or metoclopramide (10 mg p.o.) may help reduce nausea, and may have an abortive effect, even in the absence of nausea. NSAIDs, such as naproxen (500–1000 mg p.o. or p.r. with an antiemetic), ibuprofen (400–800 mg p.o.), or tolfenamic acid (200 mg p.o.) can also be very useful, when tolerated. All tend to be most effective when given early during the headache.

With frequent use, these medications tend to increase headache frequency and may cause a state of refractory daily or near-daily headache; so-called 'analgesic-associated chronic daily headache (CDH)'. Codeine-containing compound analgesics are notorious, and their use requires careful monitoring for worsening symptoms. Patients who require regular analgesics may be more easily treated with standard preventatives.

When simple measures fail, or more aggressive treatment is required, more specific drugs are required.

Selective 5-HT$_1$ agonists (triptans)

Triptans are serotonin (5-hydroxytryptamine or 5-HT) antagonists with high affinity for 5-HT$_{1B}$ or 5-HT$_{1D}$ receptors. Action at the 5-HT$_{1B}$ receptors on blood vessels produces cranial vasoconstriction. Action at pre-synaptic 5-HT$_{1D}$ receptors inhibits the release of vasoactive peptides and nociceptive neurotransmitters. Recent comparative randomised trials of triptans show efficacy rates similar to that of simple analgesics and NSAIDs. In patients without cardiovascular contraindications, triptans are safe, effective and appropriate first-line treatments for patients who have a moderate to severe headache and in patients in whom simple or combination analgesics have failed to provide adequate relief. Triptan therapy is most effective when used early when the headache is mild, but it is uncertain if they are best used after resolution of the aura, and the optimal timing is probably patient-dependent.

The choice of triptan also depends upon patient preference, as well as the character, duration and severity of the headache, convenience and cost. Non-oral administration may be beneficial in cases when the headache intensifies rapidly or severe nausea and emesis are early features of the headache. Sumatriptan and zolmitriptan are available intranasally, and sumatriptan can be given subcutaneously.

The onset of action of most triptans is 20–60 min (10 min for sumatriptan). If necessary, patients can take another dose after 2 or 4 h. If the appropriate dose of triptan is ineffective or has unacceptable side-effects, consider a switch to an alternative triptan formulation. The drugs can be used in combination with other simple analgesics, NSAIDs and antiemetics. There is a risk of developing serotonin syndrome if given in combination with other serotonin-reuptake inhibitor drugs (e.g. SSRI or MAOI antidepressants). While the risk of causing birth defects is probably low, triptans should not be used routinely during pregnancy.

Minor adverse effects such as flushing and neck or chest tightness are very common. In most cases, this is not caused by coronary vasoconstriction. However, there are reported cases of serious cardiovascular events, and triptans should be avoided in patients who have, or are at high risk of developing, coronary heart disease and those with cerebral or peripheral vascular disease.

Frequent use of triptans is also associated with the development of analgesic-associated chronic daily headache and, in general, the use of the drugs should be limited to an average of 2 days per week.

Sumatriptan

Sumatriptan (Imigran, Imitrex) is rapidly absorbed after oral administration and undergoes extensive (84%) pre-systemic metabolism. Its elimination $t_{1/2}$ is 2.5 h. The oral dose is 25–50 mg and should not exceed 200 mg in a 24-hour period. The oral route may be avoided by giving sumatriptan 5–20 mg intranasally (disagreeable taste). This can be repeated once after 2 h, but no more than 40 mg should be given in 24 h. When a rapid response is required, sumatriptan 6 mg can be given subcutaneously (bioavailability by the subcutaneous route is 96%), with an onset of action of 10–15 min. This can be repeated once in a 24-hour period.

Sumatriptan is generally well tolerated. As well as the commonly reported symptoms of neck and chest tightness, sumatriptan is also associated with malaise, fatigue, dizziness, vertigo and sedation. Nausea and vomiting may follow oral or s.c. administration.

Other triptans include zolmitriptan, naratriptan, rizatriptan, almotriptan, frovatriptan and eletriptan. All have similar safety profiles but varying duration of action. The therapeutic response and adverse effects of different triptans is often idiosyncratic, and several drugs may have to be tried before one is found that offers relief with minimal adverse events.

Ergotamine

Although ergotamine is a useful anti-migraine compound, it is not considered a first-line drug for migraine because of its adverse effects and, in the UK, is no longer recommended by the National Institute for Health and Care

Excellence (NICE). Ergots have much greater receptor affinity at serotonergic ($5\text{-}HT_{1A}$, $5\text{-}HT_2$), adrenergic and dopaminergic receptors compared to triptans. Peripheral vasoconstriction that results from ergotamine administration can persist for as long as 24 h, and repeated doses lead to cumulative effects long outlasting the migraine attack. It may precipitate angina pectoris, probably by increasing cardiac pre- and after-load. Ergotamine should never be used for prophylaxis of migraine.

Preventive treatment for migraine

For patients who are unable to achieve adequate pain relief with the use of the standard analgesic medications and triptans, the use of medications to reduce the frequency and intensity of migraine attacks may be appropriate. Other indications for preventative medications includes troublesome adverse events from standard drug therapies, acute drug overuse, very frequent headaches (more than two per week), special circumstances such as hemiplegic migraine or attacks with a risk of permanent neurological injury.

Medications that are used for migraine prophylaxis include β-adrenergic blockers, non-steroidal anti-inflammatory drugs and antineuropathic medications such as the antidepressants, calcium-channel antagonists and anticonvulsants. Drugs with the best documented effectiveness are β-adrenergic blockers, and the anticonvulsant drugs, sodium valproate and topiramate, but they have variable efficacy, and on average, with longer-term use, they reduce migraine frequency by 50% in only about 40–45% of patients. In addition, adherence is often poor in long-term use due to adverse effects.

Choice of migraine prophylactic agent is based on effectiveness, adverse events and coexistent and co-morbid conditions. Women of childbearing potential should be educated about the risk of drugs in pregnancy and encouraged to consider contraception. Because of the risk of adverse effects, especially drowsiness, on commencing treatment, all the migraine prophylactic drugs should be started at a low dose and increased slowly until therapeutic effects develop or the maximum dose is reached. A full therapeutic trial may take 2–6 months. Patients should try to avoid overusing drugs for acute attacks during the trial period. If headaches are well-controlled, treatment can be tapered down and may be discontinued if the patient remains symptom-free.

Beta-adrenergic Blockers

Comparison trials demonstrate similar efficacy to other preventative strategies such as valproic acid and topiramate, but perhaps with improved tolerability. Unwanted effects include sedation, dizziness, blurred vision and fatigue, and the drugs are contraindicated in asthma, heart block and peripheral vascular disease. Propranolol (maintenance dose 40–240 mg/day p.o. in divided doses) inhibits triptan metabolism, potentially increasing the risk of side-effects, and concurrent use of triptans should be avoided or used with caution.

Valproic acid

The anticonvulsant GABAergic drug, valproic acid, has been used for migraine prevention since the 1980s. Treatment is usually started at 250 mg p.o. at night and titrated upwards to effect, with an optimal dose around 500–600 mg in divided doses. There is little evidence that higher doses (up to 1500 mg daily) provide greater efficacy. Common adverse effects include sedation, dizziness and weight gain. There is a rare risk of serious reactions, including liver and pancreatic failure. Valproic acid is teratogenic and should be avoided in women of childbearing age.

Topiramate

Topiramate is an anticonvulsant with a number of different actions that includes enhanced GABA activity, voltage-gated Na^+ and Ca^{2+} channel inhibition, reduced activity of glutamate at AMPA/kainite post-synaptic receptors and inhibition of the pre-synaptic release of calcitonin gene-related protein (CGRP). The net result is a reduction in excitatory transmission and an increase in inhibitory neurotransmission.

In clinical trials, topiramate has been shown to reduce the frequency of migraine attacks. The drug should be started at 25 mg p.o. at night and increased gradually as tolerated. Trials demonstrated optimal effect at a dose of 100 mg daily, with little effect at 50 mg, and an increased incidence of side-effects at higher doses. Positive effects were usually seen within the first month of treatment and continued with longer-term use.

Adverse effects include paraesthesia, fatigue and dizziness. Unlike many of the antineuropathic medications, topiramate is not associated with weight gain. Topiramate is associated with a risk of fetal abnormalities and can impair the effectiveness of hormonal contraceptives, and women of childbearing potential must be advised and offered suitable contraception.

Other drugs used in migraine prevention

There have been numerous trials of alternative medications for use in migraine prophylaxis, overall with limited evidence of success, and possible new targets for the treatment and prevention of migraine continue to generate much interest in pharmaceutical trials. Riboflavin (Vitamin B$_2$) at high dose (400 mg p.o. daily) has been shown to reduce the frequency of migraine attacks. Botulinum Toxin A (Botox), given as a series of injections to the face and scalp musculature, has been shown to reduce the frequency of headache days and, although the effect is modest, has been approved by the US Food and Drug Administration and, in 2012, by NICE in the UK, for treatment of migraine headache unresponsive to other prophylactic medications.

Guide to further reading

Dowell, D., Haegerich, T.M., Chou, R., 2016. CDC guideline for prescribing opioids for chronic pain— United States. JAMA 315, 1624–1645.

Diener, H., Charles, A., Goadsby, P.J., Holle, D., 2015. New therapeutic approaches for the prevention and treatment of migraine. Lancet Neurol. 14, 1010–1022.

Lee, M.C., Tracey, I., 2013. Imaging pain: a potent means for investigating pain mechanisms in patients. Br. J. Anaesth. 111, 64–72.

Portenoy, R.K., 2011. Treatment of cancer pain. Lancet 377, 2236–2247.

Turk, D.C., Wilson, H.D., Cahana, A., 2011. Treatment of chronic non-cancer pain. Lancet 377, 2226–2235.

Woolf, C.J., 2007. Nociceptors – noxious stimulus detectors. Neuron 55, 353–364.

Wu, C.L., Raja, S.N., 2011. Treatment of acute post-operative pain. Lancet 377, 2226–2235.

Chapter 19

Anaesthesia and neuromuscular block

Jerry P. Nolan

SYNOPSIS

The administration of general anaesthetics and neuromuscular blocking drugs is generally confined to trained specialists. Nevertheless, non-specialists are involved in perioperative care and will benefit from an understanding of how these drugs act. Doctors from a variety of specialties use local anaesthetics, and the pharmacology of these drugs is discussed in detail:

- **General anaesthesia.**
- **Pharmacology of anaesthetics.**
- **Inhalation anaesthetics.**
- **Intravenous anaesthetics.**
- **Muscle relaxants: neuromuscular blocking drugs.**
- **Local anaesthetics.**
- **Obstetric analgesia and anaesthesia.**
- **Anaesthesia in patients already taking drugs.**
- **Anaesthesia in the diseased, the elderly and children; sedation in intensive therapy units.**

General anaesthesia

Until the mid-19th century, such surgery as was possible had to be undertaken at tremendous speed. Surgeons did their best for terrified patients by using alcohol, opium, cannabis, hemlock or hyoscine.[1] With the introduction of general anaesthesia, surgeons could operate for the first time with careful deliberation. The problem of inducing quick, safe and easily reversible unconsciousness for any desired length of time in humans began to be solved only in the 1840s when the long-known substances nitrous oxide, ether and chloroform were introduced in rapid succession.

The details surrounding the first use of surgical anaesthesia were submerged in bitter disputes on priority following an attempt to anaesthetise a patient with ether. The key events around this time were:

- 1842 – W.E. Clarke of Rochester, New York, administered ether for a dental extraction; however, the event was not made widely known at the time.
- 1844 – Horace Wells, a dentist in Hartford, Connecticut, introduced nitrous oxide to produce anaesthesia during dental extraction.
- 1846 – On 16 October William Morton, a Boston dentist, successfully demonstrated the anaesthetic properties of ether.
- 1846 – On 21 December Robert Liston performed the first surgical operation in England under ether anaesthesia.[2]
- 1847 – James Y. Simpson, professor of midwifery at the University of Edinburgh, introduced chloroform for the relief of labour pain.

The next important developments in anaesthesia were in the 20th century, when the appearance of new drugs, both

---

[1] A Japanese pioneer in about 1800 wished to test the anaesthetic efficacy of a herbal mixture including solanaceous plants (hyoscine-type alkaloids). His elderly mother volunteered as subject as she was anyway expected to die soon. But the pioneer administered it to his wife for, 'as all three agreed, he could find another wife, but could never get another mother' (Journal of the American Medical Association 1966;197:10).

[2] Frederick Churchill, a butler from Harley Street, had his leg amputated at University College Hospital, London. After removing the leg in 28 s, a skill necessary to compensate for the previous lack of anaesthetics, Robert Liston turned to the watching students, and said, 'This Yankee dodge, gentlemen, beats mesmerism hollow'. That night he anaesthetised his house surgeon in the presence of two women (Merrington W R 1976 University College Hospital and its Medical School: A History. Heinemann, London).

as primary general anaesthetics and as adjuvants (muscle relaxants), new apparatus and clinical expertise in rendering prolonged anaesthesia safe enabled surgeons to increase their range. No longer was the duration and type of surgery determined by patients' capacity to endure pain.

Phases of general anaesthesia

Balanced surgical anaesthesia (*hypnosis, analgesia* and *muscle relaxation*) with a single drug would require high doses that would cause adverse effects such as slow and unpleasant recovery, and depression of cardiovascular and respiratory function. In modern practice, different drugs are used to attain each objective so that adverse effects are minimised.

The perioperative period may be divided into three phases, and several factors determine the choice of drugs given in each of these. In brief:

Before surgery, an assessment is made of:

- the patient's physical and psychological condition
- any concurrent illness
- the relevance of any existing drug therapy.

All of these may influence the choice of anaesthetic technique and anaesthetic drugs.

During surgery, drugs will be required to provide:

- unconsciousness
- analgesia
- muscular relaxation when necessary
- control of blood pressure, heart rate and respiration.

After surgery, drugs will play a part in:

- reversal of neuromuscular block (if required)
- relief of pain, and nausea and vomiting
- other aspects of postoperative care, including intensive or high-dependency care.

Patients are often already taking drugs affecting the central nervous and cardiovascular systems, and there is considerable potential for interaction with anaesthetic drugs.

The techniques for giving anaesthetic drugs and the control of ventilation and oxygenation are of great importance, but are outside the scope of this book.

Before surgery (premedication)

The principal aims are to provide:

Anxiolysis and amnesia. A patient who is going to have a surgical operation is naturally apprehensive; this anxiety is reduced by reassurance and a clear explanation of what to expect. Very anxious patients will secrete a lot of adrenaline/epinephrine from the suprarenal medulla, and this may make them more liable to cardiac arrhythmias with some

anaesthetics. In the past, sedative premedication was given to virtually all patients undergoing surgery. This practice has changed dramatically because of the increasing proportion of operations undertaken as 'day cases' (in the UK 80% of elective surgical procedures are undertaken as day cases) and the recognition that sedative premedication prolongs recovery. Sedative premedication is now prescribed very rarely and is reserved for those who are particularly anxious. Benzodiazepines, such as temazepam (10–20 mg for an adult), provide anxiolysis and amnesia for the immediate presurgical period.

Analgesia is indicated if the patient is in pain before surgery, or the analgesia can be given pre-emptively to prevent postoperative pain. Severe preoperative pain is treated with a parenteral opioid such as morphine. Non-steroidal anti-inflammatory drugs (NSAIDs) and paracetamol are commonly given orally before operation to prevent postoperative pain after minor surgery. For moderate or major surgery, these drugs are supplemented with an opioid towards the end of the procedure.

Timing. Premedication is given about 1 hour before surgery.

Gastric contents. Pulmonary aspiration of gastric contents can cause severe pneumonitis. Patients at risk of aspiration are those with full stomachs, in the third trimester of pregnancy or with an incompetent gastro-oesophageal sphincter. A single dose of an antacid, e.g. sodium citrate, may be given before a general anaesthetic to neutralise gastric acid in high-risk patients. Alternatively or additionally, a histamine H_2-receptor blocker, e.g. ranitidine, or proton pump inhibitor, e.g. omeprazole, will reduce gastric secretion volume as well as acidity. Metoclopramide usefully hastens gastric emptying, increases the tone of the lower oesophageal sphincter and is an antiemetic.

During surgery. The aim is to induce *unconsciousness, analgesia* and *muscle relaxation* – the anaesthetic triad. Total muscular relaxation (paralysis) is required for some surgical procedures, e.g. intra-abdominal surgery, but most surgery can be undertaken without neuromuscular blockade. A typical general anaesthetic consists of:

Induction

1. Usually intravenous: pre-oxygenation is followed by a small dose of an opioid, e.g. fentanyl or alfentanil to provide analgesia and sedation, followed by propofol or, less commonly, thiopental, etomidate or ketamine to induce anaesthesia. Airway patency is maintained with a supraglottic airway device (e.g. laryngeal mask airway (LMA) or i-gel), a tracheal tube or, for very short procedures, an oral airway and facemask. Insertion of a tracheal tube usually requires paralysis with a neuromuscular blocker and is undertaken if

there is a risk of pulmonary aspiration from regurgitated gastric contents or from blood.

2. Inhalational induction, usually with sevoflurane, is undertaken less commonly. It is used in children, particularly if intravenous access is difficult.

Maintenance

1. Most commonly with oxygen and air (occasionally nitrous oxide is used instead of air), plus a volatile agent, e.g. sevoflurane, desflurane or isoflurane. Additional doses of a neuromuscular blocker or opioid are given as required.
2. Many anaesthetists now prefer to use a continuous intravenous infusion of propofol to maintain anaesthesia. This technique of *total intravenous anaesthesia* provides a quality of recovery that is better than after inhalational anaesthesia. The propofol infusion is often combined with an infusion of remifentanil, an ultra-short-acting opioid.

When appropriate, peripheral nerve block with a local anaesthetic, or neural axis block, e.g. spinal or epidural, provides intraoperative analgesia and muscle relaxation. These local anaesthetic techniques provide excellent post-operative analgesia.

After surgery

The anaesthetist ensures that the effects of neuromuscular blocking drugs and opioid-induced respiratory depression have either worn off or have been adequately reversed by an antagonist; the patient is not left alone until conscious, with protective reflexes restored, and with a stable circulation.

Relief of pain after surgery can be achieved with several techniques. An *epidural infusion* of a mixture of local anaesthetic and opioid provides excellent pain relief after major surgery such as laparotomy. *Parenteral morphine,* given intermittently by a nurse or a patient-controlled system, will also relieve moderate or severe pain but has the attendant risk of nausea, vomiting, sedation and respiratory depression. Patient-controlled fentanyl is often preferred to morphine because it has faster onset of action and is less likely than morphine to cause nausea. The addition of regular paracetamol and an NSAID, given orally or parenterally (the rectal route is used much less commonly now), will provide additional pain relief and reduce the requirement for morphine.

Postoperative nausea and vomiting (PONV) is common after laparotomy and major gynaecological surgery, e.g. abdominal hysterectomy. The use of propofol, particularly when given to maintain anaesthesia, has reduced the incidence of PONV. Antiemetics, such as ondansetron, cyclizine, and metoclopramide may be helpful. Dexamethasone also reduces the incidence of PONV. Many anaesthetists use a combination of two (ondansetron and dexamethasone is a common choice) or three of these drugs, a strategy which has been shown to be particularly effective.

Some special techniques

Dissociative anaesthesia is a state of profound analgesia and anterograde amnesia with minimal hypnosis during which the eyes may remain open; it can be produced by ketamine (see p. 314). It is particularly useful where modern equipment is lacking or where access to the patient is limited, e.g. in prehospital or military settings.

Sedation and amnesia without analgesia is provided by intravenous midazolam or, less commonly nowadays, by diazepam. These drugs can be used alone for procedures causing mild discomfort, e.g. endoscopy, and with a local anaesthetic where more pain is expected, e.g. removal of impacted wisdom teeth. Benzodiazepines produce anterograde, but not retrograde, amnesia. By definition, the sedated patient remains responsive and cooperative. (For a general account of benzodiazepines and the competitive antagonist flumazenil, see Ch. 20.)

Benzodiazepines can cause respiratory depression and apnoea, especially in the elderly and in patients with respiratory insufficiency. The combination of an opioid and a benzodiazepine is particularly dangerous. Benzodiazepines depress laryngeal reflexes and place the patient at risk of inhalation of oral secretions or dental debris. A continuous infusion of low-dose propofol provides very effective sedation that can be rapidly titrated to produce the desired effect. Use of propofol in this way should be undertaken only by those with advanced airway skills, such as anaesthetists and some emergency physicians.

Entonox, a 50:50 mixture of nitrous oxide and oxygen, is breathed by the patient using a demand valve. It is particularly useful in the prehospital environment and for brief procedures, such as splinting limbs.

Methoxyflurane, a volatile anaesthetic, which is no longer used for general anaesthesia, is available in a handheld inhaler enabling self-administration for relief of acute pain, particularly in the prehospital environment.

Pharmacology of anaesthetics

All successful general anaesthetics are given intravenously or by inhalation because these routes enable closest control over blood concentrations and thus of effect on the brain.

Mode of action

General anaesthetics act on the brain, primarily on the midbrain reticular activating system, and the spinal cord. Many anaesthetics are lipid soluble, and there is good correlation between this and anaesthetic effectiveness (the Overton–Meyer hypothesis); the more lipid-soluble tend to be the more potent anaesthetics, but such a correlation is not invariable. Some anaesthetic agents are not lipid soluble and many lipid-soluble substances are not anaesthetics.

Until recently it was thought that the principal site of action of general anaesthetics was relatively non-specific action in the neuronal lipid bilayer membrane. The current view is that anaesthetic agents interact with proteins to alter the activity of specific neuronal ion channels, particularly the fast neurotransmitter receptors such as nicotinic acetylcholine, γ-aminobutyric acid (GABA) and glutamate receptors. The suppression of motor responses to painful stimuli by anaesthetics is mediated mainly by the spinal cord, whereas hypnosis and amnesia are mediated within the brain.

Comparison of the efficacy of inhalational anaesthetics is made by measuring the minimum alveolar concentration (MAC) in oxygen required to prevent movement in response to a standard surgical skin incision in 50% of subjects. The MAC of the volatile agent is reduced by the co-administration of nitrous oxide.

Inhalation anaesthetics

The preferred inhalation anaesthetics are those that are minimally irritant and non-flammable, and comprise nitrous oxide and the fluorinated hydrocarbons, e.g. sevoflurane.

Pharmacokinetics (volatile liquids, gases)

The depth of anaesthesia is correlated with the tension (partial pressure) of anaesthetic drug in brain tissue. This is driven by the development of a series of tension gradients from the high partial pressure delivered to the alveoli and decreasing through the blood to the brain and other tissues. The gradients are dependent on the blood/gas and tissue/gas solubility coefficients, as well as on alveolar ventilation and organ blood flow.

An anaesthetic that has *high* solubility in blood, i.e. a high blood/gas partition coefficient, will provide a slow induction and adjustment of the depth of anaesthesia. Here, the blood acts as a reservoir (store) for the drug so that it does not enter the brain readily until the blood reservoir is filled. A rapid induction can be obtained by increasing the concentration of drug inhaled initially and by hyperventilating the patient.

Anaesthetics with *low* solubility in blood, i.e. a low blood/gas partition coefficient (nitrous oxide, desflurane, sevoflurane), provide rapid induction of anaesthesia because the blood reservoir is small and anaesthetic is available to pass into the brain sooner.

During induction of anaesthesia, the blood is taking up anaesthetic selectively and rapidly, and the resulting loss of volume in the alveoli leads to a flow of anaesthetic into the lungs that is independent of respiratory activity. When the anaesthetic is discontinued, the reverse occurs and it moves from the blood into the alveoli. In the case of nitrous oxide, this can account for as much as 10% of the expired volume and so can significantly lower the alveolar oxygen concentration. Mild hypoxia occurs and lasts for as long as 10 min. Oxygen is given to these patients during the last few minutes of anaesthesia and the early post-anaesthetic period. This phenomenon, *diffusion hypoxia*, occurs with all gaseous anaesthetics, but is most prominent with gases that are relatively insoluble in blood, for they will diffuse out most rapidly when the drug is no longer inhaled, i.e. just as induction is faster, so is elimination. Nitrous oxide is especially powerful in this respect because it is used at concentrations of up to 70%.

Nitrous oxide

Nitrous oxide (1844) is a gas with a slightly sweetish smell that is neither flammable nor explosive. It produces light anaesthesia without demonstrably depressing the respiratory or vasomotor centre provided that normal oxygen tension is maintained.

Advantages. Nitrous oxide reduces the requirement for other more potent and intrinsically more toxic anaesthetics. It has a strong analgesic action; inhalation of 50% nitrous oxide in oxygen (Entonox) may have similar effects to standard doses of morphine. Induction is rapid and not unpleasant, although transient excitement may occur, as with all anaesthetics. Recovery time rarely exceeds 4 min, even after prolonged administration.

Disadvantages. Nitrous oxide is expensive to buy and to transport. It must be used in conjunction with more potent anaesthetics to produce full surgical anaesthesia.

Uses. Nitrous oxide is still used occasionally to maintain surgical anaesthesia in combination with other anaesthetic agents, e.g. sevoflurane or propofol, and, if required, muscle relaxants. Entonox provides analgesia for obstetric practice and for emergency treatment of injuries.

Dosage and administration. For the maintenance of anaesthesia, nitrous oxide must always be mixed with at least 30% oxygen. For analgesia, a concentration of 50% nitrous oxide with 50% oxygen usually suffices.

Contraindications. Any closed, distensible, air-filled space expands during administration of nitrous oxide, which moves into it from the blood. It is therefore contraindicated in patients with: demonstrable collections of air in the pleural, pericardial or peritoneal spaces; intestinal obstruction; arterial air embolism; decompression sickness; severe chronic obstructive airway disease; emphysema. Nitrous oxide will cause pressure changes in closed, non-compliant spaces such as the middle ear, nasal sinuses and the eye.

Precautions. Continued administration of oxygen may be necessary during recovery, especially in elderly patients (see diffusion hypoxia, above).

Adverse effects. The incidence of nausea and vomiting increases with the duration of anaesthesia. Exposure to nitrous oxide for more than 4 h can cause megaloblastic changes in the bone marrow. Because prolonged and repeated exposure of staff, as well as of patients, may be associated with bone marrow depression and teratogenic risk, scavenging systems are used to minimise ambient concentrations in operating theatres.

Halogenated anaesthetics

Halothane was the first halogenated agent to be used widely, but in the developed world it has been largely superseded by isoflurane, sevoflurane and desflurane. A description of isoflurane is provided, and of the others in so far as they differ. The MAC in oxygen of some volatile anaesthetics is:

Isoflurane 1.2%
Enflurane 1.7%
Sevoflurane 2.0%
Desflurane 6.0%
Halothane 0.74%.

Isoflurane

Isoflurane is a volatile colourless liquid that is not flammable at normal anaesthetic concentrations. It is relatively insoluble and has a lower blood/gas coefficient than halothane or enflurane, which enables rapid adjustment of the depth of anaesthesia. It has a pungent odour and can cause bronchial irritation, making inhalational induction unpleasant. Isoflurane is minimally metabolised (0.2%), and none of the breakdown products has been related to anaesthetic toxicity.

Respiratory effects. Isoflurane causes respiratory depression and diminishes the ventilatory response to carbon dioxide. Although it irritates the upper airway, it is a bronchodilator.

Cardiovascular effects. Anaesthetic concentrations of isoflurane, i.e. 1–1.5 MAC, cause only slight impairment of myocardial contractility. Isoflurane causes peripheral vasodilation and reduces blood pressure. It does not sensitise the heart to catecholamines. In low concentrations (<1 MAC), cerebral blood flow, intracranial pressure and cerebral autoregulation are maintained. Isoflurane is a potent coronary vasodilator and in the presence of a coronary artery stenosis it may cause redistribution of blood away from an area of inadequate perfusion to one of normal perfusion. This phenomenon of 'coronary steal' may cause regional myocardial ischaemia.

Other effects. Isoflurane relaxes voluntary muscles and potentiates the effects of non-depolarising muscle relaxants. Isoflurane depresses cortical EEG activity and does not induce abnormal electrical activity or convulsions.

Sevoflurane

Sevoflurane is less chemically stable than the other volatile anaesthetics in current use. About 2.5% is metabolised in the body and it is degraded by contact with carbon dioxide absorbents, such as soda lime. The reaction with soda lime causes the formation of a vinyl ether (compound A), which may be nephrotoxic. Sevoflurane is less soluble than isoflurane and is very pleasant to breathe, which makes it an excellent choice for inhalational induction of anaesthesia, particularly in children. The respiratory and cardiovascular effects of sevoflurane are very similar to isoflurane, but sevoflurane does not cause 'coronary steal'. In many hospitals, sevoflurane has displaced isoflurane as the most commonly used volatile anaesthetic.

Desflurane

Desflurane has the lowest blood/gas partition coefficient of any inhaled anaesthetic agent and thus gives particularly rapid onset and offset of effect. As it undergoes negligible metabolism (0.03%), any release of free inorganic fluoride is minimised; this characteristic favours its use for prolonged anaesthesia. Desflurane is extremely volatile and cannot be administered with conventional vaporisers. It has a very pungent odour and causes airway irritation that limits its rate of induction of anaesthesia. Despite this limitation, its very rapid recovery characteristics, even after very prolonged anaesthesia, make it an increasingly popular choice for major surgery.

Halothane

Halothane has the highest blood/gas partition coefficient of the volatile anaesthetic agents, and recovery from halothane anaesthesia is comparatively slow. It is pleasant to breathe.

Halothane reduces cardiac output more than any of the other volatile anaesthetics. It sensitises the heart to the arrhythmic effects of catecholamines and hypercapnia; arrhythmias are common, in particular atrioventricular dissociation, nodal rhythm and ventricular extrasystoles. Halothane can trigger malignant hyperthermia in those who are genetically predisposed (see p. 322).

About 20% of halothane is metabolised and it induces hepatic enzymes, including those of anaesthetists and operating theatre staff. Hepatic damage occurs in a small proportion of exposed patients. Typically fever develops 2–3 days after anaesthesia, accompanied by anorexia, nausea and vomiting. In more severe cases, this is followed by transient jaundice or, very rarely, fatal hepatic necrosis. Severe hepatitis is a complication of repeatedly administered halothane anaesthesia (incidence of 1 in 50 000) and follows immune sensitisation to an oxidative metabolite of halothane in susceptible individuals. This serious complication, along with the other disadvantages of halothane and the popularity of sevoflurane for inhalational induction, has almost eliminated its use in the developed world. It remains in common use in other parts of the world because it is comparatively inexpensive.

Oxygen in anaesthesia

Supplemental oxygen is always used with inhalational anaesthetics to prevent hypoxia, even when air is used as the carrier gas. The concentration of oxygen in inspired anaesthetic gases is usually at least 30%, but oxygen should not be used for prolonged periods at a greater concentration than is necessary to prevent hypoxaemia. After prolonged administration, concentrations greater than 80% have a toxic effect on the lungs, which presents initially as a mild substernal irritation, progressing to pulmonary exudation and atelectasis. Use of unnecessarily high concentrations of oxygen in incubators causes retrolental fibroplasia and permanent blindness in premature infants.

Intravenous anaesthetics

Intravenous anaesthetics should be given only by those fully trained in their use and who are experienced with a full range of techniques of managing the airway, including tracheal intubation.

Pharmacokinetics

Intravenous anaesthetics enable an extremely rapid induction because the blood concentration can be raised quickly, establishing a steep concentration gradient and expediting diffusion into the brain. The rate of transfer depends on the lipid solubility and arterial concentration of the unbound, non-ionised fraction of the drug. After a single induction dose of an intravenous anaesthetic, recovery occurs quite rapidly as the drug is redistributed around the body and the plasma concentration reduces. Recovery from a single dose of intravenous anaesthetic is thus dependent on redistribution rather than rate of metabolic breakdown. With the exception of propofol, repeated doses or infusions of intravenous anaesthetics will cause considerable accumulation and prolong recovery. Attempts to use thiopental as the sole anaesthetic in war casualties led to it being described as an ideal form of euthanasia.[3]

It is common practice to induce anaesthesia intravenously and then to use a volatile anaesthetic for maintenance. When administration of a volatile anaesthetic is stopped, it is eliminated quickly through the lungs and the patient regains consciousness. The recovery from propofol is rapid, even after repeated doses or an infusion, and it is now by far the most popular intravenous anaesthetic.

Propofol

Induction of anaesthesia with 1.5–2.5 mg/kg occurs within 30 s and is smooth and pleasant with a low incidence of excitatory movements. Some preparations of propofol cause pain on injection, but adding lidocaine 20 mg to the induction dose eliminates this. The recovery from propofol is rapid, and the incidence of nausea and vomiting is extremely low, particularly when propofol is used as the sole anaesthetic. Recovery from a continuous infusion of propofol is relatively rapid, as the plasma concentration decreases by both redistribution and metabolic clearance (predominantly as the glucuronide). Special syringe pumps incorporating pharmacokinetic algorithms enable the anaesthetist to select a target plasma or effect-site propofol concentration (e.g. 4 µg/mL for induction of anaesthesia) once details of the patient's age and weight have been entered. This technique of target-controlled infusion (TCI) provides a convenient method for giving a continuous infusion of propofol.

Central nervous system. Propofol causes dose-dependent cortical depression and is an anticonvulsant. It depresses laryngeal reflexes more than barbiturates, which is an advantage when inserting a supraglottic airway.

Cardiovascular system. Propofol reduces vascular tone, which lowers systemic vascular resistance and central venous pressure. The heart rate remains unchanged, and the result is a fall in blood pressure to about 70–80% of

---

[3]Halford J J 1943 A critique of intravenous anaesthesia in war surgery. Anesthesiology 4:67.

the pre-induction level and a small reduction in cardiac output.

Respiratory system. Unless it is undertaken very slowly, induction with propofol causes transient apnoea. On resumption of respiration, there is a reduction in tidal volume and an increase in rate.

Thiopental

Thiopental is a very short-acting barbiturate[4] that induces anaesthesia smoothly, within one arm-to-brain circulation time. The typical induction dose is 3–5 mg/kg. Rapid distribution (initial $t_{1/2}$ 4 min) allows swift recovery after a single dose. The terminal $t_{1/2}$ of thiopental is 11 h, and repeated doses or continuous infusion lead to significant accumulation in fat and very prolonged recovery. Thiopental is metabolised in the liver. The incidence of nausea and vomiting after thiopental is slightly higher than that after propofol. The pH of thiopental is 11, and extravasation causes considerable local damage. Accidental intra-arterial injection will also cause serious injury distal to the injection site. In recent years, use of thiopental as an anaesthetic induction drug has been largely confined to obstetric practice because it is thought not to affect the fetus as much as propofol. However, as today's anaesthetists become progressively less familiar with thiopental, even in obstetric practice, propofol is becoming the preferred anaesthetic induction drug.

Central nervous system. Thiopental has no analgesic activity and may be antanalgesic. It is a potent anticonvulsant. Cerebral metabolic rate for oxygen consumption ($CMRO_2$) is reduced, causing cerebral vasoconstriction, reduction in cerebral blood flow and intracranial pressure.

Cardiovascular system. Thiopental reduces vascular tone, causing hypotension and a slight compensatory increase in heart rate. Antihypertensives or diuretics may augment the hypotensive effect.

Respiratory system. Thiopental reduces respiratory rate and tidal volume.

Methohexitone

Methohexitone is a barbiturate similar to thiopental, but its terminal $t_{1/2}$ is considerably shorter. Since the introduction of propofol, its use is confined almost entirely to inducing anaesthesia for electroconvulsive therapy (ECT). Propofol

shortens seizure duration and may reduce the efficacy of ECT; despite this, supply problems with methohexitone have made propofol a common choice for ECT.

Etomidate

Etomidate is a carboxylated imidazole. It causes pain on injection, and excitatory muscle movements are common on induction of anaesthesia. There is a 20–50% incidence of nausea and vomiting associated with its use. Etomidate causes adrenocortical suppression by inhibiting 11β- and 17β-hydroxylase, and for this reason is not used for prolonged infusion. Even after a single dose of etomidate, adrenocortical suppression can last for as long as 72 h and in septic patients is associated with an increased incidence of organ failure. Despite all of these disadvantages, it is still used occasionally, particularly for emergency anaesthesia, because it causes less cardiovascular depression and hypotension than thiopental or propofol. It should not be used in patients with sepsis.

Ketamine

Ketamine is a phencyclidine (hallucinogen) derivative and an antagonist of the NMDA receptor.[5] In anaesthetic doses, it produces a trancelike state known as *dissociative anaesthesia* (sedation, amnesia, dissociation, analgesia).

Advantages. Anaesthesia persists for up to 15 min after a single intravenous injection and is characterised by profound analgesia. Ketamine may be used as the sole analgesic for diagnostic and minor surgical interventions. In contrast to most other anaesthetic drugs, ketamine usually causes tachycardia and increases blood pressure and cardiac output, making it an increasingly popular choice for inducing anaesthesia in shocked patients. Because pharyngeal and laryngeal reflexes are only slightly impaired, the airway may be less at risk than with other general anaesthetic techniques. It is a potent bronchodilator and is sometimes used to treat severe bronchospasm in asthmatics requiring mechanical ventilation.

Disadvantages. Ketamine produces no muscular relaxation. It increases intracranial and intraocular pressure. Hallucinations with delirium can occur during recovery (the emergence reaction) but are minimised if ketamine is used solely as an induction drug and followed by a conventional inhalational anaesthetic. Their incidence is reduced by giving a benzodiazepine both as a premedication and after the procedure.

Uses. Subanaesthetic doses of ketamine can be used to provide analgesia for painful procedures of short duration such as the dressing of burns, radiotherapeutic procedures, marrow sampling and minor orthopaedic procedures.

---

[4]Johan Adolf Bayer discovered malonylurea (the parent compound of barbiturates) on 4 December 1863. That same day he visited a tavern patronised by artillery officers, and it transpired that 4 December was also the feast day of Saint Barbara, the patron saint of artillery officers, so he named the new compound 'barbituric acid' (Cozanitis D A 2004 One hundred years of barbiturates and their saint. Journal of the Royal Society of Medicine 97:594–598).

[5]N-methyl-D-aspartate.

Ketamine can be used for induction of anaesthesia before giving inhalational anaesthetics or for both induction and maintenance of anaesthesia for short-lasting diagnostic and surgical interventions that do not require skeletal muscle relaxation. It is of particular value for children requiring frequent, repeated anaesthetics. It is increasingly popular for inducing anaesthesia in critically ill patients.

Dosage and administration.

Induction. A dose of 2 mg/kg i.v. over a period of 60 s produces surgical anaesthesia within 1–2 min, lasting for 5–10 min; alternatively 5–10 mg/kg by deep intramuscular injection produces surgical anaesthesia within 3–5 min, lasting for up to 25 min.

Maintenance. Serial doses of 50% of the original intravenous dose or 25% of the intramuscular dose are given to prevent movement in response to surgical stimuli. Tonic and clonic movements resembling seizures occur in some patients but do not indicate a light plane of anaesthesia or a need for additional doses of the anaesthetic.

Recovery of consciousness is gradual. Emergence reactions (above) are lessened by benzodiazepine premedication and by avoiding unnecessary disturbance of the patient during recovery.

Contraindications include: moderate to severe hypertension, cerebral trauma (although this is controversial and many clinicians would use ketamine in such patients), intracerebral mass or haemorrhage, or other causes of raised intracranial pressure; eye injury and increased intraocular pressure; psychiatric disorders such as a schizophrenia and acute psychoses.

Use in pregnancy. Ketamine is contraindicated in pregnancy before term, as it has oxytocic activity. It is also contraindicated in patients with eclampsia or pre-eclampsia. It may be used for assisted vaginal delivery by an experienced anaesthetist. Ketamine is better suited for use during caesarean section; it causes less fetal and neonatal depression than other anaesthetics.

Muscle relaxants

Neuromuscular blocking drugs

A lot of surgery, especially of the abdomen, requires that voluntary muscle tone and reflex contraction be inhibited. This could be attained by deep general anaesthesia (but with risk of cardiovascular depression, respiratory complications and slow recovery) or by regional nerve blockade (which may be difficult to do or contraindicated, e.g. if there is a haemostatic defect).

Selective relaxation of voluntary muscle with neuromuscular blocking drugs enables surgery under light general anaesthesia with analgesia; it also facilitates tracheal intubation, quick induction and quick recovery. However, mechanical ventilation and technical skill are required. Neuromuscular blocking drugs should be given only after induction of anaesthesia.

Neuromuscular blocking drugs first attracted scientific notice because of their use as arrow poisons by the natives of South America, who used the most famous of all, curare, for killing food animals[6] as well as enemies. In 1811 Sir Benjamin Brodie smeared 'woorara paste' on wounds of guinea pigs and noted that death could be delayed by inflating the lungs through a tube introduced into the trachea. Though he did not continue until complete recovery, he did suggest that the drug might be of use in tetanus.

Despite attempts to use curare for a variety of diseases including epilepsy, chorea and rabies, the lack of pure and accurately standardised preparations, as well as the absence of convenient techniques of mechanical ventilation if overdose occurred, prevented it from gaining any firm place in medical practice until 1942, when these difficulties were removed.

Drugs acting at the myoneural junction produce complete paralysis of all voluntary muscle so that movement is impossible and mechanical ventilation is needed. It is plainly important that a paralysed patient should be unconscious during surgery.[7]

Using modern anaesthetic techniques and monitoring, awareness while paralysed for a surgical procedure is

---

[6]Curare was obtained from several sources but most commonly from the vine *Chondrodendron tomentosum*. The explorers Humboldt and Bonpland in South America (1799–1804) reported that an extract of its bark was concentrated as a tarlike mass and used to coat arrows. The potency was designated 'one tree' if a monkey, struck by a coated arrow, could make only one leap before dying. A more dilute ('three tree') form was used to paralyse animals so that they could be captured alive – an early example of a dose–response relationship.
[7]The introduction of tubocurarine into surgery made it desirable to decide once and for all whether the drug altered consciousness. Doubts were resolved in a single experiment: A normal subject was slowly paralysed (curarised) after arranging a detailed and complicated system of communication. Twelve minutes after beginning the slow infusion of curare, the subject, having artificial respiration, could move only his head. He indicated that the experience was not unpleasant, that he was mentally clear and did not want an endotracheal tube inserted. After 22 min, communication was possible only by slight movement of the left eyebrow, and after 35 min paralysis was complete and direct communication lost. An airway was inserted. The subject's eyelids were then lifted for him, and the resulting inhibition of alpha rhythm of the electroencephalogram suggested that vision and consciousness were normal. After recovery, aided by neostigmine, the subject reported that he had been mentally 'clear as a bell' throughout, and confirmed this by recalling what he had heard and seen. The insertion of the tracheal tube had caused only minor discomfort, perhaps because of the prevention of reflex muscle spasm. During artificial respiration, he had 'felt that [he] would give anything to be able to take one deep breath' despite adequate oxygenation (Smith S M et al 1947 Anesthesiology 8:1). *Note*: a randomised controlled trial is not required for this kind of investigation.

extremely rare. In the UK, general anaesthesia using volatile agents should always be monitored with agent analysers, which measure and display the end-tidal concentration of volatile agent. Increasing use of depth of anaesthesia monitors (e.g. bispectral index (BIS), which is based on the processed electroencephalogram) should further reduce the incidence of awareness. In the past, misguided concerns about the effect of volatile anaesthetics on the newborn led many anaesthetists to use little, if any, volatile agent when giving general anaesthesia for caesarean section. Under these conditions, some mothers were conscious and experienced pain while paralysed. Despite its extreme rarity nowadays,[8] fear of awareness under anaesthesia is still a leading cause of anxiety in patients awaiting surgery.

Mechanisms

When an impulse passes down a motor nerve to voluntary muscle, it causes release of acetylcholine from the nerve endings into the synaptic cleft. This activates receptors on the membrane of the motor endplate, a specialised area on the muscle fibre, opening ion channels for momentary passage of sodium, which depolarises the endplate and initiates muscle contraction.

Neuromuscular blocking drugs used in clinical practice interfere with this process. Natural substances that prevent the release of acetylcholine at nerve endings exist, e.g. *Clostridium botulinum* toxin and some venoms.

There are two principal mechanisms by which drugs used clinically interfere with neuromuscular transmission:

1. *By competition* with acetylcholine (atracurium, cisatracurium, mivacurium, pancuronium, rocuronium, vecuronium). These drugs are competitive antagonists of acetylcholine. They do not cause depolarisation themselves but protect the endplate from depolarisation by acetylcholine. The result is a flaccid paralysis. Reversal of this type of neuromuscular block can be achieved with anticholinesterase drugs, such as neostigmine, which prevent the destruction by cholinesterase of acetylcholine released at nerve endings, enable the concentration to build up and so reduce the competitive effect of a blocking agent. Rocuronium and vecuronium can also be reversed with the modified γ-cyclodextrin, sugammadex (see below).
2. *By depolarisation* of the motor endplate (suxamethonium). Such agonist drugs activate the acetylcholine receptor on the motor endplate; at their

first application, voluntary muscle contracts, but as they are not destroyed immediately, like acetylcholine, the depolarisation persists. It might be expected that this prolonged depolarisation would cause muscles to remain contracted, but this is not so (except in chickens).

Competitive antagonists

Atracurium is unique in that it is altered spontaneously in the body to an inactive form ($t_{1/2}$ 30 min) by a passive chemical process (Hofmann elimination). The duration of action (15–35 min) is thus uninfluenced by the state of the circulation, the liver or the kidneys, a significant advantage in patients with hepatic or renal disease and in the aged. It has very little direct effect on the cardiovascular system, but at doses of greater than 0.5–0.6 mg/kg histamine release may cause hypotension and bronchospasm.

Cisatracurium is a stereoisomer of atracurium; it is less prone to cause histamine release.

Vecuronium is a synthetic steroid derivative that produces full neuromuscular blockade about 3 min after a dose of 0.1 mg/kg, lasting for 30 min. It has no cardiovascular side-effects and does not cause histamine release.

Rocuronium is another steroid derivative that has the advantage of a rapid onset of action, such that 1.0 mg/kg allows tracheal intubation to be achieved after 60 s. It has negligible cardiovascular effects and a similar duration of action to vecuronium.

Mivacurium belongs to the same chemical family as atracurium and is the only non-depolarising neuromuscular blocker that is metabolised by plasma cholinesterase. It is comparatively short acting (10–15 min), depending on the initial dose. Mivacurium can cause some hypotension because of histamine release.

Pancuronium was the first steroid-derived neuromuscular blocker in clinical use. It is longer acting than vecuronium and causes a slight tachycardia.

Tubocurarine is now obsolete and no longer available in the UK. It is a potent antagonist at autonomic ganglia and causes significant hypotension.

Antagonism of competitive neuromuscular block

Neostigmine

The action of competitive acetylcholine blockers is antagonised by anticholinesterase drugs, which enable accumulation of acetylcholine. Neostigmine (see also p. 396) is given intravenously, mixed with glycopyrronium to prevent

---

[8] In a recent UK national audit, the incidence of accidence awareness during general anaesthesia was approximately 1 in 20,000 anaesthetics (Pandit JJ, Andrade J, Bogod DG et al. 2014 The 5th National Audit Project (NAP5) on accidental awareness during general anaesthesia: summary of main findings and risk factors. Anaesthesia 69:1089–101).

bradycardia caused by the parasympathetic autonomic effects of the neostigmine. It acts in 4 min, and its effects last for about 30 min. Too much neostigmine can cause neuromuscular block by depolarisation, which will cause confusion unless there have been some signs of recovery before neostigmine is given. Progress should be monitored with a neuromuscular monitor.

Sugammadex

Sugammadex comprises a ringlike structure of low molecular weight sugars and became available in the UK in 2008. This γ-cyclodextrin was designed specifically to encapsulate rocuronium: the negatively charged hydrophilic outer core attracts the positively charged rocuronium and pulls the drug into its lipophilic core. The result is an inactive water-soluble complex that is excreted by the kidneys. A full neuromuscular block from rocuronium can be reversed with sugammadex in less than 3 min. Neostigmine can be used only when the block from rocuronium has started to recover spontaneously (perhaps 30 min after initial injection), and it has many unwanted effects that are not a feature of sugammadex. Vecuronium can also be reversed by sugammadex.

Depolarising neuromuscular blocker

Suxamethonium (succinylcholine)

Paralysis is preceded by muscle fasciculation, and this may be the cause of the muscle pain experienced commonly after its use. The pain may last for 1–3 days and can be minimised by preceding the suxamethonium with a small dose of a competitive blocking agent.

Suxamethonium is the neuromuscular blocker with the most rapid onset and the shortest duration of action (although the onset of rocuronium is almost as fast and with sugammadex the recovery is faster than that of suxamethonium). Tracheal intubation is possible in less than 60 s, and total paralysis lasts for up to 4 min with 50% recovery in about 10 min ($t_{1/2}$ for effect). It is indicated for rapid sequence induction of anaesthesia in patients who are at risk of aspiration – the ability to secure the airway rapidly with a tracheal tube is of the utmost importance. If intubation proves impossible, recovery from suxamethonium and resumption of spontaneous respiration are relatively rapid. Unfortunately, if it is impossible to ventilate the paralysed patient's lungs, recovery may not be rapid enough to prevent the onset of hypoxaemia.

Suxamethonium is destroyed by *plasma pseudocholinesterase* and so its persistence in the body is increased by neostigmine, which inactivates that enzyme, and in patients with hepatic disease or severe malnutrition whose plasma enzyme concentrations are lower than normal. Approximately 1 in 3000 of the European population have hereditary defects in amount or kind of enzyme, and cannot destroy the drug as rapidly as normal individuals.[9] Paralysis can then last for hours, and the individual requires ventilatory support and sedation until recovery occurs spontaneously.

Repeated injections of suxamethonium can cause bradycardia, extrasystoles and even ventricular arrest. These are probably due to activation of cholinoceptors in the heart and are prevented by atropine. It can be used in Caesarean section as it does not cross the placenta readily. Suxamethonium depolarisation causes a release of potassium from muscle, which in normal patients will increase the plasma potassium by 0.5 mmol/L. This is a problem only if the patient's plasma potassium concentration was already high, for example in acute renal failure. In patients with spinal cord injuries and those with major burns, suxamethonium may cause a grossly exaggerated release of potassium from muscle, sufficient to cause cardiac arrest.

Uses of neuromuscular blocking drugs

Only those who are competent in tracheal intubation and ventilation of the patient's lungs should use these drugs. The drugs are used:

- to provide muscular relaxation during surgery, to enable intubation in the emergency department, and occasionally to assist mechanical ventilation in intensive therapy units
- during electroconvulsive therapy to prevent injury to the patient from excessive muscular contraction.

Other muscle relaxants

Drugs that reduce spasm of the voluntary muscles without impairing voluntary movement can be useful in spastic states, low back syndrome and rheumatism with muscle spasm.

Baclofen is structurally related to γ-aminobutyric acid (GABA), an inhibitory central nervous system (CNS) transmitter; it inhibits reflex activity mainly in the spinal cord. Baclofen reduces spasticity and flexor spasms, but, as it has no action on voluntary muscle power, function is commonly not improved. Ambulant patients may need their leg spasticity to provide support, and reduction of spasticity may expose the weakness of the limb. It benefits some cases of trigeminal neuralgia. Baclofen is given orally ($t_{1/2}$ 3 h).

Dantrolene acts directly on muscle and prevents the release of calcium from sarcoplasm stores (see malignant hyperthermia, p. 322).

---

[9]There are wide inter-ethnic differences. When cases are discovered, the family should be investigated for low plasma cholinesterase activity and affected individuals warned.

Anaphylaxis

Anaphylaxis can have either immunological or non-immunological causes. Immunological anaphylaxis is caused by interaction of antigens with immunoglobulin (Ig) E antibodies or less commonly IgG antibodies, or by immune complex/complement-mediated reactions. Non-immunological anaphylaxis is caused by massive mast cell or basophil degranulation in the absence of immunoglobulins. Intravenous anaesthetics and muscle relaxants can cause immunological or non-immunological anaphylaxis; which can be fatal. Muscle relaxants are responsible for 70% of anaphylactic reactions during anaesthesia, and suxamethonium accounts for almost one-half of these.

Local anaesthetics

Cocaine had been suggested as a local anaesthetic for clinical use when Sigmund Freud investigated the alkaloid in Vienna in 1884 with Carl Koller. The latter had long been interested in the problem of local anaesthesia in the eye, for general anaesthesia has disadvantages in ophthalmology. Observing that numbness of the mouth occurred after taking cocaine orally, Koller realised that this was a local anaesthetic effect. He tried cocaine on animals' eyes and introduced it into clinical ophthalmological practice, while Freud was on holiday. The use of cocaine spread rapidly, and it was soon being used to block nerve trunks. Chemists then began to search for less toxic substitutes, with the result that procaine was introduced in 1905.

Desired properties

Innumerable compounds have local anaesthetic properties, but few are suitable for clinical use. Useful substances must be water soluble, sterilisable by heat, have a rapid onset of effect, a duration of action appropriate to the operation to be performed, be non-toxic, both locally and when absorbed into the circulation, and leave no local after-effects.

Mode of action

Local anaesthetics prevent the initiation and propagation of the nerve impulse (action potential). By reducing the passage of sodium through voltage-gated sodium ion channels, they raise the threshold of excitability; in consequence, conduction is blocked at afferent nerve endings, and by sensory and motor nerve fibres. The fibres in nerve trunks are affected in order of size, the smallest (autonomic, sensory) first, probably because they have a proportionately greater surface area, and then the larger (motor) fibres. Paradoxically the effect in the CNS is stimulation (see below).

Pharmacokinetics

The distribution rate of a single dose of a local anaesthetic is determined by diffusion into tissues with concentrations approximately in relation to blood flow (plasma $t_{1/2}$ of only a few minutes). By injection or infiltration, local anaesthetics are usually effective within 5 min and have a useful duration of effect of 1–1.5 h, which in some cases may be doubled by adding a vasoconstrictor (below).

Most local anaesthetics are used in the form of the acid salts, as these are both soluble and stable. The acid salt (usually the hydrochloride) dissociates in the tissues to liberate the free base, which is biologically active. This dissociation is delayed in abnormally acid, e.g. inflamed, tissues, but the risk of spreading infection makes local anaesthesia undesirable in infected areas.

Absorption from mucous membranes on topical application varies according to the compound. Those that are well absorbed are used as surface anaesthetics (cocaine, lidocaine, prilocaine). Absorption of topically applied local anaesthetic can be extremely rapid and give plasma concentrations comparable to those obtained by injection. This has led to deaths from overdosage, especially via the urethra.

For topical effect on intact skin for needling procedures, a eutectic[10] mixture of bases of prilocaine or lidocaine is used (EMLA – *e*utectic *m*ixture of *l*ocal *a*naesthetics). Absorption is very slow, and a cream is applied under an occlusive dressing for at least 1 h. Tetracaine gel 4% (Ametop) is more effective than EMLA cream and enables pain-free venepuncture 30 min after application.

Ester compounds (cocaine, procaine, tetracaine, benzocaine) are hydrolysed by liver and plasma esterases, and their effects may be prolonged where there is a genetic enzyme deficiency.

Amide compounds (lidocaine, prilocaine, bupivacaine, levobupivacaine, ropivacaine) are dealkylated in the liver. Impaired liver function, whether caused by primary cellular insufficiency or low liver blood flow as in cardiac failure, may both delay elimination and cause higher peak plasma concentrations of both types of local anaesthetic. This is likely to be important only with large or repeated doses or infusions.

Prolongation of action by vasoconstrictors

The effect of a local anaesthetic is terminated by its removal from the site of application. Anything that delays its absorption into the circulation will prolong its local action and can reduce its systemic toxicity when large doses are used. Most local anaesthetics, with the exception of cocaine, cause vascular dilation. The addition of a vasoconstrictor such as adrenaline/epinephrine reduces local blood flow, slows the rate of absorption of the local anaesthetic, and prolongs its effect; the duration of action of lidocaine is doubled from 1 h to 2 h. Normally, the final concentration of adrenaline/epinephrine should be 1 in 200 000, although dentists use up to 1 in 80 000.

Do not use a vasoconstrictor for nerve block of an extremity (finger, toe, nose, penis). For obvious anatomical reasons, the whole blood supply may be cut off by intense vasoconstriction so that the organ may be damaged or even lost. Enough adrenaline/epinephrine can be absorbed to affect the heart and circulation, and reduce the plasma potassium concentration.

This can be dangerous in cardiovascular disease, and with co-administered tricyclic antidepressants and potassium-losing diuretics. An alternative vasoconstrictor is *felypressin* (synthetic vasopressin), which, in the concentrations used, does not affect the heart rate or blood pressure and may be preferable in patients with cardiovascular disease.

Other effects

Local anaesthetics also have the following clinically important effects in varying degree:

- Excitation of parts of the CNS, which may manifest as anxiety, restlessness, tremors, euphoria, agitation and even convulsions, which are followed by depression.
- Quinidine-like actions on the heart.

Uses

Local anaesthesia is generally used when loss of consciousness is neither necessary nor desirable, and to provide postoperative analgesia after major surgery. It can be used for major surgery, often with sedation. It is invaluable when the operator must also be the anaesthetist, which is often the case in some parts of the developing world.

Local anaesthetics may be used in several ways to provide the following:

- Surface anaesthesia, as solution, jelly, cream or lozenge.
- Infiltration anaesthesia, to block the sensory nerve endings and small cutaneous nerves.
- Regional anaesthesia.

Regional anaesthesia

Regional anaesthesia requires considerable knowledge of anatomy and attention to detail for both success and safety.

Nerve block means the anaesthetising of a region, small or large, by injecting the drug around, not into, the appropriate nerves, usually either a peripheral nerve or a plexus. The routine use of ultrasound guidance has increased significantly the success rate of peripheral nerve or plexus blocks. Nerve block provides its own muscular relaxation as motor fibres are blocked as well as sensory fibres, although with care differential block, affecting sensory more than motor fibres, can be achieved. There are various specialised forms: brachial plexus, paravertebral, femoral nerve block. Sympathetic nerve blocks may be used in vascular disease to induce vasodilation.

Intravenous. A double cuff is applied to the arm, inflated above arterial pressure after elevating the limb to drain the venous system, and the veins filled with local anaesthetic, e.g. 0.5–1% lidocaine without adrenaline/epinephrine. The arm is anaesthetised in 6–8 min, and the effect lasts for up to 40 min if the cuff remains inflated. The cuff must not be deflated for at least 20 min. The technique is useful in providing anaesthesia for the treatment of injuries speedily and conveniently, and many patients can leave hospital soon after the procedure. The technique must be meticulously conducted, for sudden release of the full dose of local anaesthetic accidentally into the general circulation may cause severe toxicity and even cardiac arrest. Bupivacaine is no longer used for intravenous regional anaesthesia as cardiac arrest caused by it is particularly resistant to treatment.

Extradural (epidural) anaesthesia is used in the thoracic, lumbar and sacral (caudal) regions. Lumbar epidurals are used widely in obstetrics, and low thoracic epidurals provide excellent analgesia after laparotomy. The drug is injected into the *extradural space* where it acts on the nerve roots. This technique is less likely to cause hypotension than spinal anaesthesia. Continuous analgesia is achieved if a local anaesthetic, often mixed with an opioid, is infused through an epidural catheter.

Subarachnoid (intrathecal) block (spinal anaesthesia). The drug is injected *into the cerebrospinal fluid (CSF)*, and by using a solution of appropriate specific gravity and tilting the patient, it can be kept at an appropriate level. Sympathetic nerve blockade causes hypotension. Headache due to CSF leakage is virtually eliminated by using very narrow atraumatic 'pencil point' needles.

Serious local neurological complications, e.g. infection and nerve injury, are extremely rare.

Opioid analgesics are used intrathecally and extradurally. They diffuse into the spinal cord and act on its opioid receptors (see p. 293); they are highly effective in skilled hands for post-surgical and intractable pain. Respiratory depression may occur. The effect begins in 20 min and lasts for up to 12 h.

Diamorphine or other more lipid-soluble opioids, such as fentanyl, may be used.

Adverse reactions

Excessive absorption causes paraesthesiae (face and tongue), anxiety, tremors and even convulsions. The latter are very dangerous, are followed by respiratory depression and may require diazepam or thiopental for control. Cardiovascular collapse and respiratory failure occur with higher plasma concentrations of the local anaesthetic; the cause is direct myocardial depression compounded by hypoxia associated with convulsions. Cardiopulmonary resuscitation must be started immediately. Intravenous lipid may improve resuscitation success after cardiac arrest caused by local anaesthetics.

Anaphylaxis is very rare with *amide* local anaesthetics, and some of those reported have been due to preservatives. Most reported reactions to amide local anaesthetics are due to co-administration of adrenaline/epinephrine, intravascular injection or psychological effects (vasovagal episodes). Reactions with *ester* local anaesthetics are more common.

Individual local anaesthetics

See Table 19.1.

Amides

Lidocaine is a first choice drug for surface use as well as for injection, combining efficacy with comparative lack of toxicity; the $t_{1/2}$ is 1.5 h. It is also useful in cardiac

Table 19.1 Licensed doses for three widely used amide local anaesthetics

	Solution	Dose by volume	Duration of effect (adult)
Lidocaine			1.5 h
Infiltration	0.25–0.5% + adrenaline/epinephrine	up to 60 mL	
Nerve block (peripheral)	1% + adrenaline/epinephrine 2% + adrenaline/epinephrine	up to 50 mL up to 25 mL	
Surface anaesthesia	2% 4%	up to 20 mL up to 5 mL	
Bupivacaine			3–4 h
Infiltration	0.25%	up to 60 mL	
Nerve block (peripheral)	0.25% 0.5%	up to 60 mL up to 30 mL	
Prilocaine			1.5–3 h
Infiltration	0.5%	up to 80 mL	
Nerve block (peripheral)	1% 2% 3% + felypressin (dental use)	up to 40 mL up to 20 mL up to 20 mL	

Notes:
1. Time to peak effect is about 5 min, except bupivacaine (see text).
2. Maximum doses of local anaesthetic plus vasoconstrictor are toxic in absence of the vasoconstrictor, and so substantially less should be used. All doses are only approximate; larger amounts may be safe, but deaths have occurred with smaller amounts, so that the minimum dose that will suffice should be used.
3. Maximum dose of adrenaline/epinephrine is 500 µg (see below).
4. Concentrations of solutions and dose of drug: errors of calculation occur, with sometimes fatal results. 1% means 1 g in 100 mL = 1000 mg in 100 mL = 10 mg/mL; 2% = 20 mg/mL; and so on. It is traditional to express adrenaline/epinephrine concentrations as 1 in 200 000, or 1 in 80 000, or 1 in 1000. 1 in 1000 means 1000 mg (1 g) in 1000 mL = 1 mg/mL. 1 in 200 000 means 1000 mg (1 g) in 200 000 mL = 5 µg/mL. Thus the maximum dose of adrenaline/epinephrine, 500 µg (see above), is contained in 100 mL of 1 in 200 000 solution.

arrhythmias, although it has been largely replaced by amiodarone for this purpose.

Prilocaine is used similarly to lidocaine ($t_{1/2}$ 1.5 h), but it is slightly less toxic. It used to be the preferred drug for intravenous regional anaesthesia, but it is no longer available as a preservative-free solution and most clinicians now use lidocaine instead. Crystals of prilocaine and lidocaine base, when mixed, dissolve in one another to form a eutectic emulsion that penetrates skin and is used for dermal anaesthesia (EMLA; see p. 318), e.g. before venepuncture in children.

Bupivacaine is long acting ($t_{1/2}$ 3 h) (see Table 19.1) and is used for peripheral nerve blocks, and for epidural and spinal anaesthesia. Although onset of effect is comparable to that of lidocaine, peak effect occurs later (30 min).

Levobupivacaine is the S-enantiomer of racemic bupivacaine. The relative therapeutic ratio (levobupivacaine:racemic bupivacaine) for CNS toxicity is 1.03, indicating that levobupivacaine is marginally less toxic.

Ropivacaine may provide better separation of motor and sensory nerve blockade; effective sensory blockade can be achieved without causing motor weakness (although this claim is controversial). The rate of onset of ropivacaine is similar to that of bupivacaine, but its absolute potency and duration of effect are slightly lower. The indications for ropivacaine are similar to those of bupivacaine.

Esters

Cocaine (alkaloid) is used medicinally solely as a surface anaesthetic (for abuse toxicity, see p. 161) usually as a 4% solution, because adverse effects are both common and dangerous when it is injected. Even as a surface anaesthetic, sufficient absorption may take place to cause serious adverse effects, and cases continue to be reported; only specialists should use it, and the dose must be checked and restricted.

Cocaine prevents the uptake of catecholamines (adrenaline/epinephrine, noradrenaline/norepinephrine) into sympathetic nerve endings, thus increasing their concentration at receptor sites, so that cocaine has a built-in vasoconstrictor action, which is why it retains a (declining) place as a surface anaesthetic for surgery involving mucous membranes, e.g. nose. Other local anaesthetics do not have this action; indeed, most are vasodilators, and added adrenaline/epinephrine is not so efficient.

Obstetric analgesia and anaesthesia

Although this soon ceased to be considered immoral on religious grounds, it has been a technically controversial topic since 1853 when it was announced that Queen Victoria had inhaled chloroform during the birth of her eighth child. *The Lancet* recorded 'intense astonishment … throughout the profession' at this use of chloroform, 'an agent which has unquestionably caused instantaneous death in a considerable number of cases'. But the Queen (perhaps ignorant of these risks) took a different view, writing in her private journal of 'that blessed chloroform' and adding that 'the effect was soothing, quieting and delightful beyond measure'.[10]

The ideal drug must relieve labour pain without making the patient confused or uncooperative. It must not interfere with uterine activity nor must it influence the fetus, e.g. to cause respiratory depression by a direct action, by prolonging labour or by reducing uterine blood supply. It should also be suitable for use by a midwife without supervision.

Pethidine has been used widely in obstetric practice; however, its popularity is diminishing because it is not a very potent μ agonist and has an active metabolite (norpethidine) which can make the neonate sleepy with changes in neuro-behaviour for up to 72 h post-partum. Pethidine remained popular for many years because of familiarity, safety (weak μ agonist) and the fact that it could be prescribed by midwives without a doctor's prescription. Diamorphine provides more effective analgesia for labour pain; it has fewer unpleasant effects than pethidine, and because the metabolites are non-sedative the babies feed better. Many delivery units now have patient group directives so that midwives can prescribe and administer diamorphine to mothers in labour without a doctor's prescription.

Nitrous oxide and oxygen (50% of each: Entonox) may be administered for each contraction from a machine the patient works herself or supervised by a midwife (about 10 good breaths are needed for maximal analgesia).

Epidural local anaesthesia provides the most effective pain relief, but the technique should be undertaken only after adequate training. In the UK, only anaesthetists insert epidural catheters.

Spinal anaesthesia is now used much more commonly than epidural anaesthesia for caesarean section. The vast majority of caesarean sections are now undertaken with regional rather than general anaesthesia.

---

[10]The chloroform was administered by John Snow (1813–1858) who invented the ether inhaler and first applied science to anaesthesia. This was the same John Snow who in 1854 traced the source of an outbreak of cholera to sewage contamination of a well in Soho in London by mapping the emergence of new cases in the area. It convinced the local council sufficiently to disable the well pump by removing its handle. More generally, Snow's analysis helped to demonstrate that cholera was a specific, water-borne disease and not a 'miasma' in the air; it turned out to be a founding event in the new science epidemiology.

General anaesthesia during labour presents special problems. Gastric regurgitation and aspiration are a particular risk (see p. 309). The safety of the fetus must be considered; all anaesthetics and analgesics in general use cross the placenta in varying amounts and, apart from respiratory depression, produce no important effects except that high doses interfere with uterine contraction and may be followed by uterine haemorrhage. Neuromuscular blocking drugs can be used safely.

Anaesthesia in patients already taking medication

Anaesthetists are in an unenviable position. They are expected to provide safe service to patients in any condition, taking any drugs. Sometimes there is opportunity to modify drug therapy before surgery, but often there is not. Anaesthetists require a particularly detailed drug history from the patient.

Drugs that affect anaesthesia

Adrenal steroids. Chronic corticosteroid therapy with the equivalent of prednisolone 5 mg daily for 1 month or more suppresses the hypothalamic–pituitary–adrenal (HPA) system. Without corticosteroid supplementation perioperatively, the patient may fail to respond appropriately to the stress of surgery and become hypotensive (see Ch. 35).

Antibiotics. Aminoglycosides, e.g. neomycin, gentamicin, potentiate neuromuscular blocking drugs.

Anticholinesterases can potentiate suxamethonium.

Antiepilepsy drugs. Continued medication is essential to avoid status epilepticus. Drugs must be given parenterally (e.g. phenytoin, sodium valproate) or rectally (e.g. carbamazepine) until the patient can absorb enterally.

Antihypertensives of all kinds; hypotension may complicate anaesthesia. Angiotensin-converting enzyme inhibitors and angiotensin-II receptor antagonists should be withheld on the morning of surgery, but other anti-hypertensive medication, especially β-adrenoceptor blockers, should be continued. Hypertensive patients are particularly liable to excessive increase in blood pressure and heart rate during intubation, which can be dangerous if there is ischaemic heart disease. After surgery, parenteral therapy may be needed for a time.

β-Adrenoceptor blocking drugs can prevent the homeostatic sympathetic cardiac response to cardiac depressant anaesthetics and to blood loss.

Diuretics. Hypokalaemia, if present, will potentiate neuromuscular blocking agents and perhaps general anaesthetics.

Oral contraceptives containing oestrogen, and postmenopausal hormone replacement therapy predispose to thromboembolism.

Psychotropic drugs. Neuroleptics potentiate or synergise with opioids, hypnotics and general anaesthetics.

Antidepressants. Monoamine oxidase inhibitors can cause hypertension when combined with certain amines, e.g. pethidine, or indirectly acting sympathomimetics, e.g. ephedrine. Tricyclics potentiate catecholamines and some other adrenergic drugs.

Anaesthesia in the diseased, and in particular patient groups

The normal response to anaesthesia may be greatly modified by disease. Some of the more important aspects include:

Respiratory disease and smoking predispose the patient to postoperative pulmonary complications, principally infective. The site of operation, e.g. upper abdomen, chest, and the severity of pain influence the impairment to ventilation and coughing.

Cardiac disease. The aim is to avoid the circulatory stress (with increased cardiac work, which can compromise the myocardial oxygen supply) caused by hypertension and tachycardia. Intravenous drugs are normally given slowly to reduce the risk of overdosage and hypotension.

Patients with fixed cardiac output, e.g. with aortic stenosis or constrictive pericarditis, are at special risk from reduced cardiac output with drugs that depress the myocardium and vasomotor centre, for they cannot compensate. Induction with propofol or thiopental is particularly liable to cause hypotension in these patients. Hypoxia is obviously harmful. Skilled technique rather than choice of drugs on pharmacological grounds is the important factor.

Hepatic or renal disease is generally liable to increase drug effects and should be taken into account when selecting drugs and their doses.

Malignant hyperthermia (MH) is a rare pharmacogenetic syndrome with an incidence of between 1 in 15 000 and 1 in 150 000 in North America, exhibiting autosomal dominant inheritance with variable penetrance. The condition occurs during or immediately after anaesthesia and may be precipitated by potent inhalation agents (halothane, isoflurane, sevoflurane) or suxamethonium. The patient may have experienced an uncomplicated general anaesthetic previously. The mechanism involves an abnormally increased release of calcium from the sarcoplasmic reticulum, often caused by an inherited mutation in the gene for the ryanodine receptor, which resides in the sarcoplasmic reticulum membrane. High calcium concentrations stimulate muscle contraction, rhabdomyolysis and a hypermetabolic state. MH is a life-threatening medical emergency. Oxygen consumption increases by up to three times the normal value, and body temperature may increase as fast as 1°C every 5 min, reaching as high as 43°C. Rigidity of voluntary muscles may not be evident at the outset or in mild cases.

Dantrolene 1 mg/kg i.v. is given immediately. Further doses are given at 10-min intervals until the patient responds, to a cumulative maximum dose of 10 mg/kg. Dantrolene ($t_{1/2}$ 9 h) probably acts by preventing the release of calcium from the sarcoplasm store that ordinarily follows depolarisation of the muscle membrane.

Non-specific treatment is needed for the hyperthermia (cooling, oxygen), and insulin and dextrose are given for hyperkalaemia caused by potassium release from contracted muscle. Hyperkalaemia and acidosis may trigger severe cardiac arrhythmias.

Once the immediate crisis has resolved, the patient and all immediate relatives should undergo investigation for MH. This involves a muscle biopsy, which is tested for sensitivity to triggering agents.

Anaesthesia in MH-susceptible patients is achieved safely with total intravenous anaesthesia using propofol and opioids. Dantrolene for intravenous use must be available immediately in every location where general anaesthesia is given. The relation of MH syndrome with neuroleptic malignant syndrome (for which dantrolene may be used as adjunctive treatment, see p. 343) is uncertain.

Muscle diseases. Patients with myasthenia gravis are very sensitive to (intolerant of) competitive, but not to depolarising, neuromuscular blocking drugs.

Those with myotonic dystrophy may recover less rapidly than normal from central respiratory depression and neuromuscular block; they may fail to relax with suxamethonium.

Sickle cell disease. Hypoxia and dehydration can precipitate a crisis.

Atypical (deficient) pseudocholinesterase. There is delay in the metabolism of suxamethonium and mivacurium. The duration of neuromuscular block depends on the level of pseudocholinesterase activity.

Raised intracranial pressure will be made worse by high expired concentration inhalation agents, by hypoxia or hypercapnia, and in response to intubation if anaesthesia is inadequate. Without support from a mechanical ventilator, excessive doses of opioids will cause hypercapnia and increase intracranial pressure.

The elderly (see p. 108) are liable to become confused by cerebral depressants, especially by hyoscine. Atropine also crosses the blood–brain barrier and can cause confusion in the elderly; glycopyrronium is preferable. In general, elderly patients require smaller doses of all drugs than the young. The elderly tolerate hypotension poorly; they are prone to cerebral and coronary ischaemia.

Children (see p. 105). The problems with children are more technical, physiological and psychological than pharmacological.

Sedation in critical care units is used to reduce patient anxiety and improve tolerance to tracheal tubes and mechanical ventilation. Whenever possible, patients are sedated only to a level that enables them to open their eyes to verbal command; over-sedation is harmful. Commonly used drugs include propofol and midazolam, and opioids such as fentanyl, alfentanil, morphine or remifentanil, and the centrally acting α_2 agonists clonidine and dexmedetomidine.

Neuromuscular blockers are required only rarely to assist mechanical ventilation. If pain is treated properly and patient-triggered modes of ventilation are used, many patients in the critical care unit will not require sedation. Reassurance from sympathetic nursing staff is extremely important and far more effective than drugs.

Diabetes mellitus. See page 619.

Thyroid disease. See page 630.

Porphyria. See page 117.

Guide to further reading

Chau, P.L., 2010. New insights into the molecular mechanisms of general anaesthetics. Br. J. Pharmacol. 161, 288–307.

Columb, M.O., Cegielski, D., Haley, D., 2017. Local anaesthetic agents. Anaesth. Intensive Care Med. 18, 150–154.

Farooq, K., Hunter, J.M., 2017. Neuromuscular blocking and reversal agents. Anaesth. Intensive Care Med. 18, 279–284.

Medlock, R.M., Pandit, J.J., 2015. Intravenous anaesthetic agents. Anaesth. Intensive Care Med. 17, 155–162.

Scarth, E., Smith, S. (Eds.), 2016. Drugs in Anaesthesia and Intensive Care, fifth ed. Oxford University Press, Oxford.

Sneyd, J.R., Rigby-Jones, A.E., 2010. New drugs and technologies, intravenous anaesthesia is on the move (again). Br. J. Anaesth. 105, 246–254.

Chapter 20

Psychotropic drugs

David Nutt, Simon Davies, Blanca M. Bolea-Alamanac

SYNOPSIS

Psychiatric disorders are some of the most common illnesses. Advances in drug treatment have revolutionised the practice of psychiatry over the past seven decades. This chapter considers pharmacological treatments in the following areas:

Drugs for:

- Depression (antidepressants).[1]
- Psychosis (antipsychotics 'neuroleptics').
- Bipolar disorder (mood stabilisers).
- Anxiety and sleep disorders.
- Dementia.
- Attention deficit/hyperactivity disorder.

Diagnostic issues

Older classifications of psychiatric disorder divided diseases into 'psychoses' and 'neuroses'. The term 'psychosis' is still widely used to describe a severe mental illness with some combination of hallucinations, delusions, extreme abnormalities of behaviour including marked overactivity, retardation and catatonia, usually with lack of insight. Psychotic disorders include schizophrenia, severe depression and mania.

Psychosis may also be due to illicit substances or organic conditions. Clinical features of schizophrenia are subdivided into 'positive symptoms', which include hallucinations, delusions and thought disorder, and 'negative symptoms' such as apathy, flattening of affect and poverty of speech.

Disorders formerly grouped under 'neuroses' include anxiety disorders (e.g. panic disorder, generalised anxiety disorder, obsessive–compulsive disorder, phobias and post-traumatic stress disorder), eating disorders (e.g. anorexia nervosa and bulimia nervosa), depression (provided there are no 'psychotic' symptoms) and sleep disorders.

Also falling within the scope of modern psychiatric diagnostic systems are organic mental disorders (e.g. dementia in Alzheimer's disease), disorders due to substance misuse (e.g. alcohol and opiate dependence; see Ch. 11), personality disorders, disorders of childhood and adolescence (e.g. attention deficit/hyperactivity disorder, Tourette's syndrome), and mental retardation (learning disabilities).

Drug therapy in relation to psychological treatment

No account of drug treatment strategies for psychiatric illness is complete without considering psychological therapies. Psychotherapies range widely, from simple counselling (supportive psychotherapy) through psychoanalysis to newer techniques such as cognitive behavioural therapy.

As a general rule, *psychotic illnesses* (e.g. schizophrenia, mania and depressive psychosis) require drugs as first-line treatment, with psychotherapy being adjunctive, for instance in promoting drug compliance, improving family relationships and helping individuals cope with distressing symptoms. By contrast, for *depression* and *anxiety disorders*, such as panic disorder and obsessive–compulsive disorder, forms of psychotherapy are available that provide

---

[1]A new system of terminology for psychotropic drugs, known as 'Neuroscience-based nomenclature' (NbN), is currently in the process of being introduced. Once fully implemented, terms such as 'drugs for depression' and 'drugs for psychosis' will be preferred to the traditional terms 'antidepressants' and 'antipsychotics'. See the NbN website and the paper by Zohar J, Stahl S, Moller H J, et al 2015 A review of the current nomenclature for psychotropic agents and an introduction to the Neuroscience-based Nomenclature, European Neuropsychopharmacology 25:2318–2325. However, for the present edition we have continued to use the traditional terminology.

alternative first-line treatment to medication. The choice between drugs and psychotherapy depends on treatment availability, previous history of response, patient preference and the ability of the patient to work appropriately with the chosen therapy. In many cases, there is scope and sometimes advantage to the use of drugs and psychotherapy in combination.

Taking depression as an example, an extensive evidence base exists for the efficacy of several forms of *psychotherapy*. These include cognitive therapy (which normalises depressive thinking), interpersonal therapy (which focuses on relationships and roles), brief dynamic psychotherapy (a time-limited version of psychoanalysis) and cognitive analytical therapy (a structured time-limited therapy that combines the best points of cognitive therapy and traditional analysis).

All doctors who prescribe drugs engage in a 'therapeutic relationship' with their patients. A depressed person whose doctor is empathic, supportive and appears to believe in the efficacy of the drug prescribed is more likely to take the medication and to adopt a hopeful mindset than if the doctor seemed aloof and ambivalent about the value of psychotropic drugs. Remembering that placebo response rates of 30–40% are common in double-blind trials of antidepressants, we should never underestimate the importance of our relationship with the patient in enhancing the pharmacological efficacy of the drugs we use.

Antidepressant drugs

Antidepressants can be broadly divided into five main categories (Table 20.1), *selective serotonin reuptake inhibitors* (SSRIs), serotonin-noradrenaline reuptake inhibitors (SNRIs), tricyclics (TCAs, named after their three-ringed structure), *monoamine oxidase inhibitors* (MAOIs) and a variety of *novel compounds*, some of which are related to TCAs or SSRIs. Clinicians who wish to have a working knowledge of antidepressants would be advised to be familiar with the use of at least one drug from each of the five main categories tabulated. A more thorough knowledge-base would demand awareness of the distinct characteristics of the subgroups of

Table 20.1 Classification of antidepressants

Selective serotonin reuptake inhibitors	Serotonin noradrenaline reuptake inhibitors*	Tricyclics	Monoamine oxidase inhibitors
Fluoxetine	Venlafaxine	Dosulepin	Phenelzine
Paroxetine	Duloxetine	Amitriptyline	Isocarboxazid
Sertraline		Lofepramine	Tranylcypromine
Citalopram[a]		Clomipramine	Moclobemide (RIMA)
Escitalopram[a]		Imipramine	
Fluvoxamine		Trimipramine	
		Doxepin	
		Nortriptyline	
		Protriptyline	
		Desipramine	

Novel compounds

Mainly Noradrenergic	Mixed	Mainly Serotonergic
Reboxetine (NaRI)	Mirtazapine (NaSSa)[b]	Trazodone[b]
Bupropion (NDRI)		Vortioxetine (multimodal)
	Others	
	Agomelatine[c]	

*Other SNRIs not available in the UK include desvenlafaxine, milnacipran and levomilnacipran.
RIMA, reversible inhibitor of monoamine oxidase; NaRI, noradrenaline/norepinephrine reuptake inhibitor; NDRI, noradrenaline/dopamine reuptake inhibitor; NaSSA, noradrenaline/norepinephrine and specific serotonergic antidepressant.
[a]Escitalopram is the active S-enantiomer of citalopram.
[b]Trazodone and mirtazapine have been classed as 'receptor-blocking' antidepressants based on their antagonism of serotonin receptors and presynaptic α$_2$-adrenoceptors
[c]Agomelatine is a melatonin receptor agonist and serotonin receptor blocker.

novel compounds (e.g. mirtazapine, reboxetine, bupropion, vortioxetine and agomelatine) and differences between individual SSRIs, SNRIs and TCAs and between the original MAOIs and the reversible inhibitor of monoamine oxidase (RIMA), moclobemide. As antidepressants are largely similar in their therapeutic efficacy, awareness of profiles of unwanted effects is of particular importance.

An alternative categorisation is based solely on mechanism of action (Fig. 20.1). The majority of antidepressants, including SSRIs, SNRIs, and most TCAs are *reuptake inhibitors*. Some, e.g. trazodone and mirtazapine, are *receptor blockers*, whereas MAOIs including RIMAs are *enzyme inhibitors*.

The first TCAs (imipramine and amitriptyline) and MAOIs appeared between 1957 and 1961 (see Fig. 20.1). The MAOIs were developed from antituberculous agents that unexpectedly improved mood. Imipramine was a chlorpromazine derivative that showed antidepressant rather than antipsychotic properties. Over the next 25 years, the TCA class enlarged to more than 10 agents with heterogeneous pharmacological profiles, and further modifications of the original three-ringed structure gave rise to the pharmacologically distinct agent trazodone.

In the 1980s, an entirely new class of antidepressant arrived with the SSRIs. The first was zimelidine, but unfortunately this was withdrawn due to associations with Guillain–Barré syndrome. Next came fluvoxamine, followed by fluoxetine (Prozac®). Within 10 years, the SSRI class accounted for one-half of antidepressant prescriptions in the UK. Further developments in the evolution of antidepressants have been the arrival of the SNRIs (e.g. venlafaxine and duloxetine) and of novel compounds, including reboxetine (a noradrenaline reuptake blocker), agomelatine (a melatonin receptor agonist), and most recently, vortioxetine (a multimodal agent) and a reversible MAOI, moclobemide.

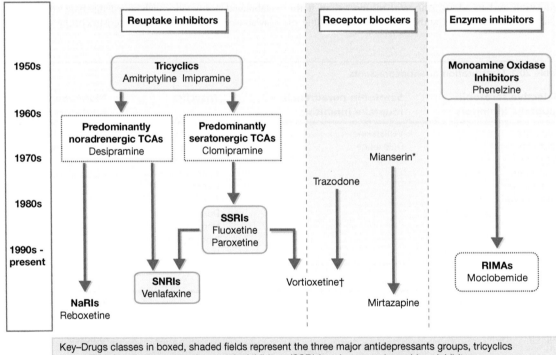

Key–Drugs classes in boxed, shaded fields represent the three major antidepressants groups, tricyclics (TCAs), selective serotonin reuptake inhibitors (SSRIs) and monoamine oxidase inhibitors.
Novel compounds are left unboxed.
NaRI–noradrenaline reuptake inhibitor
SNRI–serotonin, and noradrenaline reuptake inhibitor
RIMA–reversible inhibitor of monoamine oxidase
*–Mianserin is rarely used due to associations with aplastic anaemia
†–Vortioxetine is both a reuptake inhibitor and receptor blocker, as well as acting as an agonist at other 5HT receptors

Fig. 20.1 Flowchart of the evolution of antidepressant drugs, and classification by mechanism of action.

Mechanism of action

The *monoamine hypothesis* proposes that, in depression, there is deficiency of the neurotransmitters *noradrenaline/norepinephrine* and *serotonin* in the brain which can be restored by antidepressants. Drugs that alleviate depression also enhance monoamine availability and release (Fig. 20.2), increasing activity at postsynaptic receptors. It is relevant that (older) antihypertensive agents, e.g. reserpine, which reduced the availability of noradrenaline/norepinephrine, caused depression.

SSRIs act, as their name indicates, predominantly by preventing serotonin reuptake by blocking the cell-surface serotonin transporter; with little effect on noradrenaline/norepinephrine reuptake. *Tricyclic antidepressants* and *reboxetine* inhibit noradrenaline/norepinephrine reuptake, but tricyclic effects on serotonin reuptake vary widely; nortriptyline has little effect on serotonin reuptake, whereas clomipramine is about five times more potent at blocking serotonin than

noradrenaline/norepinephrine reuptake. *SNRIs* are capable of inhibiting reuptake of both transmitters, in most cases being more potent at blocking serotonin reuptake compared with noradrenaline. For example, venlafaxine requires a dose of at least 150 mg/day for noradrenaline/norepinephrine uptake blockade to be exerted.

Mirtazapine also achieves an increase in noradrenergic and serotonergic neurotransmission, but through antagonism of presynaptic α_2 autoreceptors (receptors that mediate negative feedback for transmitter release, i.e. an autoinhibitory feedback system) and to antagonism of α_2 heteroreceptors. Additionally, it selectively blocks certain serotonin receptors ($5HT_2$ and $5HT_3$) while increasing transmission at the $5HT_{1A}$ receptor. Other novel antidepressants include *trazodone*, which alongside weak serotonin reuptake inhibition blocks several types of serotonin receptor (including the $5HT_{2A}$ and $5HT_{2C}$ receptors) as well as α-adrenoceptors and histaminergic receptors and acts as a partial agonist at the $5HT_{1A}$ receptor, and *agomelatine* which acts both as an agonist of

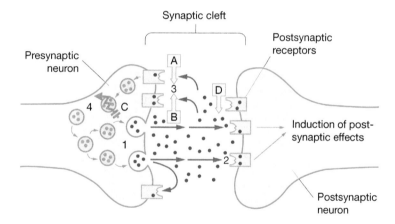

Synaptic cleft

Postsynaptic receptors

Presynaptic neuron

Induction of post-synaptic effects

Postsynaptic neuron

Physiological processes at the synapse:
1. When an electrical signal reaches the presynaptic terminal, presynaptic amine vesicles fuse with the neuronal membrane and release their contents into the synaptic cleft.
2. Amines in the synaptic cleft bind to postsynaptic receptors to produce a postsynaptic response.
3. Amines may be removed from the synaptic cleft by reuptake into the presynaptic neuron.
4. The monoamine oxidase enzyme breaks down presynaptic amines.

Effects of antidepressants:
A. Tricyclics prevent presynaptic reuptake of the amines noradrenaline and serotonin
B. SSRIs predominantly block reuptake of serotonin.
C. MAOIs reduce the activity of monoamine oxidase in breaking down presynaptic amines (leaving more available for release into the presynaptic cleft).
D. Some antidepressants (e.g. agomelatine) block postsynaptic receptors directly.

Fig. 20.2 Mechanism of action of antidepressant drugs at the synapse.

melatonin receptors and a blocker of the serotonin $5HT_{2C}$ receptor, the combined effects of these actions leading to a rise in frontal cortex dopamine availability.

Bupropion (amfebutamone) inhibits reuptake of both dopamine and noradrenaline/norepinephrine. It was originally developed and used as a treatment for depression and is licensed for this indication in most of the world (though for historic reasons not in the UK) but is frequently used to assist smoking cessation (see p. 335). It is also prescribed in attention deficit hyperactivity disorder (see p. 360). The most recent addition to the antidepressant group is vortioxetine. This 'multimodal antidepressant' is both a reuptake inhibitor through its ability to block serotonin reuptake, a blocker of several serotonin receptors particularly the $5HT_3$ one and an agonist of the $5HT_{1A}$ receptor. It has a positive impact on cognitive deficits associated with depression.

MAOIs increase the availability of noradrenaline/ norepinephrine and serotonin by preventing their destruction by the monoamine oxidase type A enzyme in the presynaptic terminal (see Ch. 21, Table 21.3). The older MAOIs, phenelzine, tranylcypromine and isocarboxazid, bind irreversibly to monamine oxidase by forming strong (covalent) bonds. The enzyme is thus rendered permanently ineffective such that amine metabolising activity can be restored only by production of fresh enzyme, which takes weeks. These MAOIs are thus called 'hit and run' drugs as their effects greatly outlast their detectable presence in the blood. Moclobemide, however, as a reversible inhibitor of monoamine oxidase (RIMA) inhibits the enzyme competitively, meaning that its effects can be overcome much more rapidly.

But how do changes in monoamine transmitter levels produce an eventual elevation of mood? Raised neurotransmitter concentrations produce immediate alterations in postsynaptic receptor activation, leading to changes in second-messenger (intracellular) systems and to gradual modifications in cellular protein expression. Most antidepressants increase a cyclic AMP response element binding (CREB) protein, which in turn is involved in regulating the transcription of genes that influence survival of other proteins, including brain-derived neurotrophic factor (BDNF), which exerts effects on neuronal growth.

Although the monoamine hypothesis of depression is conceptually straightforward, it is in reality an oversimplification of a complicated picture. Other systems that are implicated in the aetiology of depression (and which provide potential targets for drug therapy) include the hypothalamic–pituitary–thyroid (HPT) axis and the hypothalamic–pituitary–adrenal (HPA) axis. The finding that 50% of depressed patients have raised plasma cortisol concentrations constitutes evidence that depression may be associated with increased HPA drive.

Pharmacokinetics

The antidepressants listed in Table 20.1 are generally well absorbed after oral administration. Steady-state plasma concentrations of TCAs and SSRIs show great individual variation but correlate with therapeutic effect. Where there is a failure of response, measurement of plasma concentration can be useful, as the failure may be attributable to low plasma levels due to ultra-rapid metabolism (though it is often not available). Antidepressants in general are metabolised principally by hepatic cytochrome P450 enzymes. Of the many isoenzymes identified, the most important in antidepressant metabolism are CYP P450 2D6 (Table 20.2A) and CYP 3A4 (Table 20.2B). Other important P450 enzymes are CYP 1A2 (inhibited by the SSRI fluvoxamine, induced by cigarette smoking; substrates include caffeine and the atypical antipsychotics clozapine, olanzapine and asenapine) and the CYP 2C group (including CYP 2C19 which is inhibited by fluvoxamine and fluoxetine, involved in breakdown of escitalopram and moclobemide). Sometimes several CYP enzymes are capable of mediating the same metabolic step. For example, at least five isoenzymes, including CYP 2D6, 3A4 and 2C9, can mediate the desmethylation of the SSRI sertraline to its major metabolite.

Several of these drugs produce active metabolites that prolong their action (e.g. fluoxetine is metabolised to norfluoxetine, $t_{1/2}$ 200 h). The metabolic products of certain TCAs are antidepressants in their own right, e.g. nortriptyline (from amitriptyline), and imipramine (from clomipramine). Half-lives ($t_{1/2}$) of SSRIs lie from 15 h (fluvoxamine) to 72 h (fluoxetine – and longer for the active metabolite), while SNRIs have shorter $t_{1/2}$ (5 h for venlafaxine and 14 h for duloxetine).

Around 7% of the Caucasian population have very limited CYP 2D6 enzyme activity. Such 'poor metabolisers' may find standard doses of TCAs intolerable, and it is often worth prescribing them at a very low dose. If the drug is then tolerated, plasma concentration assay may confirm the suspicion that the patient is a poor metaboliser. There is also a genetic polymorphism influencing CYP 2C19 activity which has a clinically important effect on metabolism of escitalopram.

Therapeutic efficacy

Provided antidepressant drugs are prescribed at an adequate dose and taken regularly, 60–70% of patients with depression should respond within 4 weeks. Conventional meta-analyses have shown little evidence that any particular drug or class of antidepressant is more efficacious than others, but there are some possible exceptions to this general statement:

Table 20.2A Psychotropic (and selected other) drugs known to be CYP 2D6 substrates, inhibitors and inducers

CYP 2D6 inhibitors

Antidepressants	Other drugs
Paroxetine	Cimetidine
Fluoxetine	Quinidine
Bupropion	Terbinafine
Duloxetine	
Sertraline (weak)	

CYP 2D6 substrates

Antidepressants	Antipsychotics	Miscellaneous
All SSRIs	Chlorpromazine	Atomoxetine
Venlafaxine	Haloperidol	Codeine
Duloxetine	Perphenazine	Dexfenfluramine
Many tricyclics:	Risperidone	Dextromethorphan
e.g. imipramine,		
amitriptyline,		
clomipramine,		
nortriptyline		
Reboxetine	Zuclopenthixol	Dihydrocodeine
		Donepezil
		Hydrocodone
		Tramadol
		MDMA (ecstasy)
		Some β-blockers:
		propranolol
		metoprolol, timolol
		bufaralol, carvidelol

A *substrate* is a substance that is acted upon and changed by an enzyme. Where two substrates of the same enzyme are prescribed together, they will compete, and, if present in sufficient quantities, the metabolism of one or other, or both, drugs may also be inhibited, resulting in increased plasma concentration and possibly in enhanced therapeutic or adverse effects. An enzyme *inducer* accelerates the metabolism of co-prescribed drugs that are substrates of the same enzyme, reducing their effects. An enzyme *inhibitor* retards metabolism of co-prescribed drugs, increasing their effects.

- Venlafaxine, in high dose (>150 mg/day) and escitalopram may have greater efficacy than other antidepressants.
- Amitriptyline appears to be slightly more effective than other TCAs and also SSRIs for severe depression, but this advantage is compromised by its poor tolerability (due to muscarinic, histamine and noradrenaline α_1-receptor blockade) and lack of safety in overdose relative to more modern agents.

- The older MAOIs (e.g. phenelzine) may be more effective than other classes in 'atypical' depression, a form of depressive illness where mood reactivity is preserved, lack of energy may be extreme and biological features are the opposite of the normal syndrome, i.e. excess sleep and appetite with weight gain.

Selection

An antidepressant should be selected to match individual patients' requirements, such as the need or otherwise for a sedative effect, or the avoidance of antimuscarinic effects (especially in the elderly). In the absence of special factors, the choice rests on the weight of evidence of efficacy, the tolerability, the safety in overdose and the likelihood of an effective dose being reached. SSRIs, SNRIs and certain other newer drugs (e.g. mirtazapine, and in some centres bupropion), are highlighted as best meeting these needs.

Mode of use

Antidepressants usually require 3–4 weeks for the full therapeutic effect to be achieved. When a minimal response is seen, an antidepressant can usefully be extended to 6 weeks to see whether further benefit is achieved. By contrast, patients may experience unwanted effects, especially 'jitteriness' or 'activation' symptoms such as increased anxiety and irritability,[2] soon after starting treatment (they should be warned about this possibility), but such symptoms usually diminish with time. Some drugs have the advantage that they can be started at a dose which would be considered adequate for the therapeutic effect (e.g. most SSRIs), but in contrast many others need to be started at a low and generally tolerable starting dose and increased gradually to the therapeutic dose. For example, the tricyclic imipramine should be started at 25–50 mg/day, with gradual increments to a recognised 'minimum therapeutic' dose, around 125 mg/day. Low starting doses are particularly important for elderly patients. Only when the drug has reached the minimum therapeutic dose and been taken for at least 4 weeks can response or non-response be adequately established. However, some patients do achieve response or remission at 'subtherapeutic' doses, for reasons of drug kinetics and limited capacity to metabolise, the self-limiting nature of depression, or by a placebo effect (reinforced by the experience of side-effects, suggesting that the drug must be having some action).

---

[2]Sinclair L I, Christmas D M, Hood S D et al 2009 Antidepressant-induced jitteriness/anxiety syndrome: systematic review. British Journal of Psychiatry 194:483–490.

Table 20.2B Psychotropic (and selected other) drugs known to be CYP 3A4 substrates, inhibitors and inducers

CYP 3A4 inhibitors

Antidepressants	Other drugs
Fluoxetine	Cimetidine
	Clarithromycin
	Erythromycin
	Fluconazole
	Ketoconazole (grapefruit juice)
	Verapamil
	HIV antivirals (e.g. indinavir, ritonavir)

CYP 3A4 substrates

Antidepressants[a]	Anxiolytics, hypnotics and antipsychotics	Miscellaneous
Some SSRIs (fluoxetine, escitalopram/citalopram, sertraline)	Alprazolam	Buprenorphine
Some tricyclics (e.g. amitriptyline, imipramine, nortriptyline)	Buspirone	Carbamazepine
Mirtazapine	Diazepam	Cortisol
Trazodone	Midazolam	Dexamethasone
	Triazolam	Methadone
	Zopiclone	Testosterone
	Aripiprazole	Most calcium channel blockers (e.g. amlodipine, diltiazem, nifedipine, verapamil)
	Haloperidol	Amiodarone
	Lurasidone	Omeprazole
	Quetiapine	Some lipid-lowering drugs (e.g. atorvastatin, simvastatin)
	Zuclopenthixol	

CYP 3A4 inducers

St John's wort
Carbamazapine
Modafinil
Phenytoin
Phenobarbital
Rifampin
HIV antivirals (efavirenz, nevirapine)

A *substrate* is a substance that is acted upon and changed by an enzyme. Where two substrates of the same enzyme are prescribed together, they will compete, and, if present in sufficient quantities, the metabolism of one or other, or both, drugs may also be inhibited, resulting in increased plasma concentration and possibly in enhanced therapeutic or adverse effects. An enzyme *inducer* accelerates the metabolism of co-prescribed drugs that are substrates of the same enzyme, reducing their effects. An enzyme *inhibitor* retards metabolism of co-prescribed drugs, increasing their effects.
[a]Many drugs, including SSRIs and other antidepressants are metabolized by multiple CYP enzymes.

For SSRIs, dose titration is often unnecessary as the minimum therapeutic dose can usually be tolerated as a starting dose. Divided doses are not usually required, and administration is by a single morning or evening dose. Evidence suggests that patients commencing treatment on SSRIs are more likely to reach an effective dose than those starting on TCAs. Of the novel compounds, trazodone usually requires titration to a minimum therapeutic dose of at least 200 mg/day. Response to the SNRIs (venlafaxine and duloxetine), and novel compounds such as mirtazapine and agomelatine may occur at the starting dose, but some dose titration is commonly required. Venlafaxine is licensed for treatment-resistant depression by gradual titration from 75 to 375 mg/day. There is some need for dose titration when using MAOIs. Unlike other drug classes, reduction to a lower maintenance dose is recommended after a response is achieved if unwanted effects are problematical.

Changing and stopping antidepressants

When an antidepressant fails through lack of efficacy despite an adequate trial or due to unacceptable adverse effects, a change to a drug of a different class is generally advisable. For a patient who has not responded to an SSRI, it is logical to switch to either an SNRI (venlafaxine or duloxetine) or one of the novel compounds. Among these, mirtazapine and bupropion are generally considered to be the preferred options. Each of these four drugs should offer a greater increase in synaptic noradrenaline/norepinephrine than the ineffective SSRI. Agomelatine, trazodone, vortioxetine, reboxetine, tricyclics and RIMAs/MAOIs remain as further options for switching. Evidence also suggests that patients failing on one SSRI may respond to a different drug within the class, an approach that is particularly useful where other antidepressant classes have been unsuccessful previously, are contraindicated, or have characteristics that the patient or doctor feels are undesirable. Awareness of biological differences between drugs within a class may also be helpful when patients cannot tolerate other drug classes. For instance, among SSRIs, paroxetine has the most affinity for the serotonin transporter and fluoxetine the least. When changing between antidepressant doses, a conservative approach would be to reduce the first antidepressant progressively over 2 or more weeks before starting the new drug. The gradual reduction is particularly important with paroxetine and venlafaxine, which are known to cause 'discontinuation syndromes' if stopped abruptly, and less important with fluoxetine due to its long $t_{1/2}$ active metabolite which offers 'built-in' protection against withdrawal problems. A more proactive approach would involve 'cross-tapering' the second antidepressant – i.e. starting it while the first antidepressant is being reduced and gradually titrating the dose up. However, an important exception concerns changes to or from MAOIs, which must be handled with great caution due to the dangers of interactions between antidepressants (see below). Therefore MAOIs cannot safely be introduced within 2 weeks of stopping most antidepressants (3 weeks for imipramine and clomipramine; combination of the latter with tranylcypromine is particularly dangerous), and not until 5 weeks after stopping fluoxetine, due to its long $t_{1/2}$ active metabolite. Similarly, other antidepressants should not be introduced until 2–3 weeks have elapsed from discontinuation of MAOI (as these are irreversible inhibitors; see p. 328). No washout period is required when using the reversible MAOI, moclobemide.

When a patient achieves remission, the antidepressant should be continued for at least 9 months at the dose that returned mood to normal. Premature dose reduction or withdrawal is associated with increased risk of relapse. In cases where three or more depressive episodes have occurred, evidence suggests that long-term continuation of an anti-depressant offers protection, as otherwise further relapse is very likely in the next 3 years.

When ceasing use of an antidepressant, the dose should be reduced gradually to avoid discontinuation syndromes (symptoms include anxiety, agitation, nausea and mood swings). Discontinuation of paroxetine and venlafaxine (which have relatively short $t_{1/2}$ and do not have an active metabolite) are associated additionally with dizziness, electric shock–like sensations and paraesthesia.

Augmentation

Augmentation, the addition of a second drug to an existing antidepressant, can be used when two or more standard antidepressants have successively failed to alleviate depressive symptoms despite treatment at an adequate dose for an adequate time. Some of the augmentations discussed may even be used earlier than this if there is an indication or justification for the augmenting drug specific to the individual patient.

One strategy which has come to prominence is to augment (or combine) an SSRI or SNRI antidepressant with the novel antidepressant *mirtazapine*. The initial justification for this combination stems from mirtazapine's unorthodox mechanism of action – the idea being that the presynaptic adjustments effected by mirtazapine could act additively or even synergistically with the monoamine reuptake inhibition of SSRIs and SNRIs. A second justification is more practical – mirtazapine is known to improve the quality of sleep and serotonin reuptake inhibitors may initially disrupt this, thus mirtazapine can be added both to boost the antidepressant effect and to address an unresolved problem with sleep. An evidence base does exist both for mirtazapine–venlafaxine and mirtazapine–fluoxetine co-prescription in depression, with both combinations reported as providing significantly higher remission rates than fluoxetine alone. Ease of initiation of these combinations, along with the evidence of enhanced effectiveness, means that these are currently the most commonly used augmentation strategies for treatment of depression in psychiatry inpatients in the UK. A further logical alternative to augmenting an SSRI with mirtazapine is to augment with bupropion, since this combination is thought to provide reuptake inhibition of all three monoamine transmitters – i.e. serotonin, noradrenaline and dopamine.

Another important augmentation strategy employs the mood stabiliser *lithium carbonate*. Controlled trials suggest that up to 50% of patients who have not responded to standard antidepressants can respond after lithium augmentation, but the evidence is stronger for augmenting tricyclics than for augmenting SSRIs. Addition of lithium requires careful titration of the plasma concentration up to the therapeutic range, with periodic checks thereafter and monitoring for toxicity (see p. 344).

More recently, augmentation of SSRIs with some drugs primarily used for psychosis (antipsychotics) has been effective in clinical trials. Quetiapine and aripiprazole are most commonly used, but adequate evidence exists also for *olanzapine* and *risperidone*. Antipsychotics also have important potential for side-effects, which must be taken into account before their introduction (see p. 339).

Tri-iodothyronine (T3) also aids antidepressant action, and most evidence points to added benefit with TCAs. When co-prescribing TCAs with thyroid hormone derivatives, be aware that the combination of lofepramine with the *levo* isomer of thyroxine is contraindicated. The amino acid L-*tryptophan* and the β-adrenoceptor blocker *pindolol* may also be used to augment. Tryptophan increases 5-hydroxytryptamine (5HT) production, and pindolol may act by blocking negative feedback of 5HT on to $5HT_{1A}$-autoreceptors.

Other indications

Some antidepressants may benefit most forms of *anxiety disorder*, including panic disorder, generalised anxiety disorder, post-traumatic stress disorder, obsessive–compulsive disorder and social phobia (see p. 347). SSRIs are recognised as a first-line drug treatment for all five of these anxiety disorders, while venlafaxine also has a good evidence base in all of them.

Fluoxetine is effective in milder cases of the eating disorder *bulimia nervosa*, in higher doses (60 mg/day) than are required for depression. This effect is independent of that on depression (which may coexist) and may therefore involve a different mode of action. Antidepressants appear to be ineffective in anorexia nervosa. Antidepressants also have a role in pain control. The SNRI drug *duloxetine* is licensed for diabetic neuropathy, while considerable trial evidence exists for use of imipramine and amitriptyline for the control of chronic pain.

Adverse effects

As most antidepressants have similar therapeutic efficacy, the decision regarding which drug to select often rests on adverse-effect profiles and potential to cause toxicity.

Selective serotonin reuptake inhibitors

SSRIs have a range of unwanted effects including nausea, anorexia, dizziness, gastrointestinal disturbance including increased risk of gastrointestinal bleeding, agitation, akathisia (motor restlessness) and anorgasmia (failure to experience an orgasm). They lack direct sedative effect, an advantage over older drugs in patients who need to drive motor vehicles or need to work or study. SSRIs can disrupt the pattern of sleep with increased awakenings, transient reduction in the amount of rapid eye movement (REM) and increased REM latency, but eventually sleep improves due to improved mood. SSRIs lack the side-effects of postural hypotension, antimuscarinic and antihistaminergic effects seen with TCAs. In contrast to both TCAs and mirtazapine, some SSRIs may induce weight loss through their anorectic effects, at least in the short term, although paroxetine appears to be associated more robustly with weight gain. SSRIs are relatively safe in overdose. In recent years an association of citalopram at higher doses has emerged, with QTc prolongation and risk of arrhythmias leading some jurisdictions to advise limiting the dose to 40 mg/day and 20 mg/day in the elderly. Similar advice has been given for escitalopram, but evidence of risk appears to be less robust.

Serotonin syndrome is a rare but dangerous complication of using antidepressants that inhibit serotonin reuptake including SSRIs, SNRIs and vortioxetine. It features restlessness, tremor, shivering and myoclonus, possibly leading to hyperpyrexia, convulsions and delirium. The risk is increased by co-administration with drugs that enhance serotonin transmission, especially MAOIs, the antimigraine triptan drugs and St John's wort. The combination of fluoxetine or paroxetine with tramadol can also cause serotonin syndrome. These SSRIs inhibit the metabolism of tramadol to its active metabolite (which is responsible for the pain relief), leaving a buildup of unmetabolised tramadol which has sufficient serotonergic activity itself to interact with the SSRIs and enhance the risk of serotonin syndrome.

SNRIs

Venlafaxine produces unwanted effects that resemble those of SSRIs with a higher incidence of nausea. Sustained hypertension (due to blockade of noradrenaline/norepinephrine reuptake) is a problem in a small proportion of patients at high dose, and blood pressure should be monitored when more than 200 mg/day is taken. Venlafaxine appears to have some association with cardiac arrhythmias, but whether this is to a degree that is clinically significant is unclear.

Duloxetine may cause early nausea, which tends to subside quickly. Other unwanted effects are somnolence, dizziness and constipation.

Novel compounds

Mirtazapine has benefits in rarely being associated with sexual dysfunction and in improving sleep independent of mood, but it may cause unwanted sedation and weight gain.

Trazodone is an option for depressed patients where sedation is required. It also has the advantages of lacking antimuscarinic effects and of being relatively safe in overdose. Males should be warned of the possibility of priapism (painful penile erections), attributable to the drug's blockade of α_1-adrenoceptors.

Agomelatine is given at night when it appears to resynchronise circadian rhythms, and therefore promotes improved sleep. Like mirtazapine it is rarely associated with sexual dysfunction, but its use necessitates early liver function tests.

Bupropion may be associated with insomnia, nausea and headache. This drug should generally be avoided in patients with a history of epilepsy.

Vortioxetine side-effects are similar to those of SSRIs and include sexual dysfunction. Withdrawal effects are uncommon.

Tricyclic antidepressants

The commonest unwanted effects are those of antimuscarinic action, i.e. dry mouth, constipation, blurred vision and difficulty with accommodation, raised intraocular pressure (glaucoma may be precipitated) and bladder neck obstruction (may lead to urinary retention in older males).

Patients may also experience postural hypotension (through inhibition of α-adrenoceptors), which is often a limiting factor in the elderly; interference with sexual function; weight gain (through blockade of histamine H_1 receptors); prolongation of the QTc interval of the ECG, which predisposes to cardiac arrhythmias especially in overdose (use after myocardial infarction is contraindicated).

Some TCAs (especially trimipramine and amitriptyline) are heavily sedating through a combination of antihistaminergic and α_1-adrenergic–blocking actions, and this presents special problems to those whose lives involve driving vehicles or performing skilled tasks. In selected patients, sedation may be beneficial, e.g. a severely depressed person who has a disrupted sleep pattern or marked agitation.

There is great heterogeneity in adverse-effect profiles among TCAs. Imipramine and lofepramine cause relatively little sedation, and lofepramine is associated with milder antimuscarinic effects (but is contraindicated in patients with severe liver disease).

Overdose. Depression is a risk factor for both parasuicide and completed suicide, and TCAs are commonly taken by those who deliberately self-harm. *Dosulepin* and *amitriptyline* are particularly toxic in overdose. Lofepramine is at least 15 times less likely to cause death from overdose; clomipramine and imipramine occupy intermediate positions.

Clinical features of overdose reflect the pharmacology of TCAs. Antimuscarinic effects result in warm, dry skin from vasodilatation and inhibition of sweating, blurred vision from paralysis of accommodation, papillary dilatation and urinary retention.

Consciousness is commonly dulled, and respiration depression and hypothermia may develop. Neurological signs including hyperreflexia, myoclonus, divergent strabismus and extensor plantar responses may accompany lesser degrees of impaired consciousness and provide scope for diagnostic confusion, e.g. with structural brain damage. Convulsions occur in a proportion of patients. Hallucinations and delirium occur during recovery of consciousness, often accompanied by a characteristic plucking at bedclothes.

Sinus tachycardia (due to vagal blockade) is a common feature, but abnormalities of cardiac conduction accompany moderate to severe intoxication and may proceed to dangerous tachyarrhythmias or bradyarrhythmias. Hypotension may result from a combination of cardiac arrhythmia, reduced myocardial contractility and dilatation of venous capacitance vessels.

Supportive treatment suffices for the majority of cases. Activated charcoal by mouth is indicated to prevent further absorption from the alimentary tract and may be given to the conscious patient in the home prior to transfer to hospital. Convulsions are less likely if unnecessary stimuli are avoided, but severe or frequent seizures often precede cardiac arrhythmias and arrest, and their suppression with diazepam is important. Cardiac arrhythmias do not need intervention if cardiac output and tissue perfusion are adequate. Correction of hypoxia with oxygen, and acidosis by intravenous infusion of sodium bicarbonate are reasonable first measures and usually suffice.

Reboxetine is not structurally related to tricyclic agents but like lofepramine and nortriptyline acts predominantly by noradrenergic reuptake inhibition. Pseudo-antimuscarinic effects, particularly urinary hesitancy and dry mouth, trouble a minority of patients. Postural hypotension may occur, as may impotence in males. It is relatively safe in overdose.

Monoamine oxidase inhibitors

Adverse effects include postural hypotension (especially in the elderly) and dizziness. Less common are headache, irritability, apathy, insomnia, fatigue, ataxia, gastrointestinal disturbances including dry mouth and constipation, sexual dysfunction (especially anorgasmia), blurred vision, difficult micturition, sweating, peripheral oedema, tremulousness, restlessness and hyperthermia. Appetite may increase inappropriately, causing weight gain.

Interactions

Antidepressant use offers considerable scope for adverse interaction with other drugs, and it is prudent always to check specific sources for unwanted outcomes whenever a new drug is added or removed to a prescription list that includes an antidepressant.

Pharmacodynamic interactions

- Most antidepressants (including SSRIs, SNRIs and tricylics) may cause central nervous system (CNS) toxicity if co-prescribed with the dopaminergic drugs entacapone and selegiline (for Parkinson's disease). SSRIs and SNRIs increase the risk of the serotonin syndrome when combined with drugs that enhance serotonin transmission, e.g. the antimigraine triptan drugs which are $5HT_1$-receptor antagonists, and the antiobesity drug sibutramine.

- Most antidepressants lower the convulsion threshold, complicate the drug control of epilepsy and lengthen seizure time in electroconvulsive therapy (ECT). The situation is made more complex by the capacity of carbamazepine to induce the metabolism of antidepressants and of certain antidepressants to inhibit carbamazepine metabolism (see below).

- SSRIs are known to interfere with platelet aggregation and may increase the risk of gastrointestinal bleeding, especially in those with existing risk factors.

- Trazodone and many tricyclics cause sedation, and therefore co-prescription with other sedative agents such as opioid analgesics, H_1-receptor antihistamines, anxiolytics, hypnotics and alcohol may lead to excessive drowsiness and daytime somnolence.

- The majority of tricyclics have undesirable cardiovascular effects, in particular prolongation of the QTc interval, as does the SSRI citalopram at higher doses. Numerous other drugs also prolong the QTc interval, e.g. amiodarone, disopyramide, procainamide, propafenone, quinidine, terfenadine, and psychotropic agents such as pimozide. Their use in combination with antidepressants that prolong QTc enhances the risk of ventricular arrhythmias.

- Tricyclics potentiate the effects of catecholamines and other sympathomimetics, but not those of β_2-receptor agonists used in asthma. Even the small amounts of adrenaline/epinephrine or noradrenaline/norepinephrine in dental local anaesthetics may produce a serious rise in blood pressure.

Pharmacokinetic interactions

Metabolism by cytochrome P450 enzymes provides ample opportunity for interaction of antidepressants with other drugs by inhibition of, competition for, or induction of enzymes. Tables 20.2A and 20.2B indicate examples of mechanisms by which interaction that may occur when relevant drugs are added to, altered in dose or discontinued from regimens that include antidepressants.

Enzyme inhibition. In depression with psychotic features, antidepressants are commonly prescribed with antipsychotics, and there is potential for enhanced drug effects with paroxetine plus aripiprazole (CYP 2D6), fluoxetine plus quetiapine (3A4), and fluvoxamine plus olanzapine (1A2). Tranquillisation with zuclopenthixol acetate (see p. 341) of an agitated patient who is also taking fluoxetine or paroxetine can result in toxic plasma concentrations with excessive sedation and respiratory depression due to inhibition of zuclopenthixol metabolism by CYP 2D6 and CYP 3A4. P450 enzyme inhibition by fluoxetine or paroxetine may also augment effects of alcohol, tramadol (danger of serotonin syndrome), methadone, terfenadine (danger of cardiac arrhythmia), -caine anaesthetics and theophylline.

Enzyme-inducing drugs, e.g. carbamazepine, several other antiepilepsy drugs (oxcarbazepine, phenytoin) and certain antiviral agents accelerate the metabolism of antidepressants by inducing specific CYP enzymes, most commonly CYP 3A4. This will reduce their therapeutic efficacy and require adjustment of dose. Epilepsy is a particularly common co-morbid illness in patients who have both psychiatric illness and learning disabilities, and the combination of an anticonvulsant and an antidepressant or major psychotropic drug is to be anticipated.

Monoamine oxidase inhibitors

Hypertensive reactions. Patients taking MAOIs are vulnerable to highly dangerous hypertensive reactions. Firstly, as MAOIs increase catecholamine stores in adrenergic and dopaminergic nerve endings, the action of sympathomimetics that act indirectly by releasing stored noradrenaline/norepinephrine is augmented. Secondly, patients taking an MAOI are deprived of the protection of the MAO enzyme present in large quantities in the gut wall and liver. Thus orally administered sympathomimetics that would normally be inactivated by MAO are absorbed intact. (Note that enhanced effects are not as great as might be expected from adrenaline/epinephrine, noradrenaline/norepinephrine and isoprenaline, which are chiefly destroyed by another enzyme, catechol-O-methyltransferase, in the blood and liver.)

Symptoms include severe, sudden throbbing headache with slow palpitation, flushing, visual disturbance, nausea, vomiting and severe hypertension. If headache occurs without hypertension, it may be due to histamine release. The hypertension is due both to vasoconstriction from activation of α-adrenoceptors and to increased cardiac output consequent on activation of cardiac β-adrenoceptors. The mechanism is thus similar to that of the episodic hypertension in a patient with phaeochromocytoma.

The rational and effective treatment is an α-adrenoceptor blocker (phentolamine 5 mg i.v.), with a β-blocker later added in case of excessive tachycardia.

Patient education. It is essential to warn patients taking MAOIs of possible sources of the hypertensive reaction.

Many simple remedies sold direct to the public, e.g. for nasal congestion, coughs and colds, contain sympathomimetics (ephedrine, phenylpropanolamine).

Foods likely to produce hypertensive effects in patients taking MAOIs include:
- Cheese, especially if well matured.
- Red wines (especially Chianti) and some white wines; some beers (non- or low-alcohol varieties contain variable but generally low amounts of tyramine).
- Yeast extracts (Marmite, Oxo, Bovril).
- Some pickled herrings.
- Broad bean pods (contain dopa, a precursor of adrenaline/epinephrine).
- Over-ripe bananas, avocados, figs.
- Game.
- Stale foods.
- Fermented bean curds including soy sauce.
- Fermented sausage, e.g. salami, shrimp paste.
- Flavoured textured vegetable protein (Vegemite).

This list may be incomplete, and any partially decomposed food may cause a reaction. Milk and yoghurt appear safe.

Foods to avoid are those that contain sympathomimetics, most commonly *tyramine*, which acts by releasing noradrenaline/norepinephrine from nerve vesicles. Degradation of the protein, casein, by resident bacteria in well-matured cheese can produce tyramine from the amino acid tyrosine (hence the general term 'cheese reaction' to describe provocation of a hypertensive crisis).

Stale foods present a particular danger, as any food subjected to autolysis or microbial decomposition during preparation or storage may contain pressor amines resulting from decarboxylation of amino acids.

The newer drug moclobemide offers the dual advantages of selective MAO-A inhibition; in theory, this should avoid the 'cheese' reaction by sparing the intestinal MAO, which is mainly MAO-B, and of being a competitive, reversible inhibitor. Whereas the irreversible inhibitors inactivate the MAO enzyme and can therefore continue to cause dangerous interactions in the 2–3 weeks after withdrawal, until more enzyme can be synthesised, the reversible nature of MAO inhibition means it is incomplete except during peak plasma concentrations. As the inhibition is competitive, tyramine can then displace the inhibitor from the active site of the MAO enzyme. Consequently, there are fewer dietary restrictions for patients using moclobemide, although hypertensive reactions have been reported.

MAOI interactions with other drugs. The mechanisms of many of the following interactions are obscure, and some are probably due to inhibition of drug-metabolising enzymes other than MAO enzyme, as MAOIs are not entirely selective in their action. Effects last for up to 2–3 weeks after discontinuing the MAOI.

Antidepressants. Combination with tricyclic antidepressants has the potential to precipitate a hypertensive crisis complicated by CNS excitation with hyperreflexia, rigidity and hyperpyrexia.

MAOI-SSRI or MAOI-SNRI combinations may provoke the life-threatening 'serotonin syndrome' (see above). Strict rules apply regarding washout periods when switching between MAOIs and other drugs (see above, Changing and stopping antidepressants, p. 331). Very occasionally, MAOIs are prescribed with other antidepressants, but as many combinations are highly dangerous, such practice should be reserved for specialists only and then as a last resort.

Narcotic analgesics. With co-prescribed pethidine, respiratory depression, restlessness, even coma, and hypotension or hypertension may result (probably due to inhibition of its hepatic demethylation). Interaction with other opioids occurs but is milder.

Other drugs that cause minor interactions with MAOIs include antiepileptics (convulsion threshold lowered), dopaminergic drugs, e.g. selegiline (MAO-B inhibitor) may cause dyskinesias, antihypertensives and antidiabetes drugs (metformin and sulphonylureas potentiated). Concomitant use with bupropion, sibutramine (weight reduction) and $5HT_1$-agonists (migraine) should be avoided. Because of the use of numerous drugs during and around surgery, an MAOI is best withdrawn 2 weeks before, if practicable.

Overdose with MAOIs can cause hypomania, coma and hypotension or hypertension. General measures are used as appropriate with minimal administration of drugs: chlorpromazine for restlessness and excitement; phentolamine for hypertension; no vasopressor drugs for hypotension, because of risk of hypertension (use posture and plasma volume expansion).

St John's wort

The herbal remedy St John's wort *(Hypericum perforatum)* has found favour in some patients with mild to moderate depression. The active ingredients in the hypericum extract have yet to be identified, and their mode of action is unclear. Several of the known mechanisms of action of existing antidepressants are postulated, including inhibition of monoamine reuptake and the MAO enzyme, as well as a stimulation of GABA receptors. Much of the original research into the efficacy of St John's wort was performed in Germany, where its use is well established. Several direct comparisons with tricyclic antidepressants have shown equivalent rates of response, but the interpretation of these studies is complicated by the fact that many failed to use standardised ratings for depressive symptoms, patients tended to receive TCAs below the minimum therapeutic dose, and patients sometimes received St John's wort in doses above the maximum recommended in commercially available preparations. Use of St John's wort is further complicated by the lack of standardisation of the ingredients. A large multi-centre trial found only limited evidence of benefit for St John's wort over placebo in significant major depression.[3]

Despite these reservations, there is certainly a small proportion of patients who, when presented with all the available facts, express a strong desire to take only St John's wort, perhaps from a preference for herbally derived compounds over conventional medicine. For patients with mild depression, it seems reasonable on existing evidence to accede to this preference rather than impair the therapeutic alliance and risk prescribing a conventional antidepressant that will not be taken.

Adverse effects. Those who wish to take St John's wort should be made aware that it may cause dry mouth, dizziness, sedation, gastrointestinal disturbance and confusion. Importantly also, it induces hepatic P450 enzymes (CYP 1A2 and CYP 3A4) with the result that the plasma concentration and therapeutic efficacy of warfarin, oral contraceptives, some anticonvulsants, antipsychotics and HIV protease/reverse transcriptase inhibitors are reduced. Concomitant use of tryptophan and St John's wort may cause serotonergic effects including nausea and agitation.

Electroconvulsive therapy

ECT involves the passage of a small electrical charge across the brain by electrodes applied to the frontotemporal aspects of the scalp with the aim of inducing a tonic–clonic seizure. Reference to it is made here principally to indicate its place in therapy.

ECT requires the patient to be under a general anaesthetic, so it carries the small risks associated with general anaesthesia in minor surgical operations. It may cause memory problems,

although these are generally transient. For these reasons, as well as the relative ease of use of antidepressant drugs, ECT is usually reserved for psychiatric illness where pharmacological treatments have been unsuccessful or where the potential for rapid improvement characteristic of ECT treatment is important. This may arise where patients are in acute danger from their mental state, for instance the severely depressed patient who has stopped eating or drinking, or those with florid psychotic symptoms. Modern-day ECT is a safe and effective alternative to antidepressant treatment and remains a first-line option in clinical circumstances where a rapid response is desired, when it can be life saving.

Repetitive Transcranial Magnetic Stimulation (rTMS) is a non-invasive technique in which alternating magnetic fields emanating from a coil device are used to generate small electric currents directed at specific cortical areas, most commonly the left dorsolateral prefrontal cortex. Since the first device was approved for use in depression in the USA in 2008, the technique has gained acceptance in many countries as an alternative approach to depression resistant to drug treatment, and is supported by a growing evidence base of randomized controlled trials.

Ketamine

Ketamine was originally used as a 'field anaesthetic'. This term refers to its utility in the military context, which was primarily due to its dissociative anaesthetic properties. Ketamine and related compounds which moderate the glutamate system through antagonism of the NMDA receptor have been the subject of a number of recent trials in the treatment of depression, and the evidence underpinning ketamine specifically has been endorsed by a Cochrane Review. Initial trials used ketamine administered by the intravenous route, but more recently ketamine inhaled intranasally has been reported to be effective. At higher doses, ketamine may produce delusions and hallucinations, for which it has attracted attention as a drug of abuse. However, under careful supervision there may be a role for lower-dose ketamine in treatment-resistant depression.

Antipsychotics

Classification

Originally tested as an antihistamine, *chlorpromazine* serendipitously emerged as an effective treatment for psychotic illness in the 1950s. Chlorpromazine-like drugs were originally termed 'neuroleptics' or 'major tranquillisers', but the preferred usage now is drugs for psychosis or 'antipsychotics'.

---

[3]Shelton R C, Keller M B, Gelenberg A et al 2001 Effectiveness of St John's wort in major depression. A randomised control trial. Journal of the American Medical Association 285:1978–1986.

Classification is by chemical structure, e.g. phenothiazines, butyrophenones. Within the large phenothiazine group, compounds are divided into three types on the basis of the side-chain, as this tends to predict adverse-effect profiles (Table 20.3). The continuing search for greater efficacy and better tolerability led researchers and clinicians to reinvestigate *clozapine,* a drug that was originally licensed in the 1960s but subsequently withdrawn because of toxic haematological effects. Clozapine appeared to offer greater effectiveness in treatment-resistant schizophrenia, to have efficacy against 'negative' in addition to 'positive' psychiatric symptoms (Table 20.4), and to be less likely to cause extrapyramidal motor symptoms. It regained its licence in the early 1990s with strict requirements on dose titration and haematological monitoring. The renewed interest in clozapine and its unusual efficacy and tolerability stimulated researchers to examine other 'atypical' antipsychotic drugs.

Thus the most important distinction in modern-day classification of antipsychotic drugs is between the *classical* (typical) agents, such as chlorpromazine, haloperidol and zuclopenthixol, and the so-called *atypical* antipsychotics, which include clozapine and now risperidone, olanzapine, quetiapine, amisulpride, aripiprazole, lurasidone, asenapine and others. These latter are 'atypical' in their mode of action, their relative lack of extrapyramidal motor symptoms and their adverse-effect profiles which differ markedly from the classical agents. Categorisation of atypical agents by their chemical structure is of limited value clinically as they are very heterogeneous. Similarly classification through a shared affinity for a particular receptor system has not been possible; as discussed below, the atypical antipsychotics are very heterogeneous in their receptor-binding profiles.

Table 20.3 Antipsychotic drugs		
Atypical antipsychotics[a]	**Classical antipsychotics**	
Clozapine	*Phenothiazines*	
Olanzapine	Type 1	Chlorpromazine
Quetiapine		Promazine
Risperidone	Type 2	Pericyazine
Ziprasidone[c]	Type 3	Trifluoperazine
Amisulpride[b]		Prochlorperazine
Aripiprazole		Fluphenazine
Paliperidone	*Butyrophenones*	Haloperidol
Asenapine		Benperidol
Lurasidone	*Substituted benzamide*	Sulpiride[b]
	Thioxanthines	Flupentixol Zuclopenthixol
	Other	Pimozide Loxapine

[a]No recognised classification system exists for atypical antipsychotics. Tentative terms based on receptor-binding profiles have been applied to certain drug groupings, e.g. 'broad-spectrum atypicals' for clozapine, olanzapine and quetiapine, whereas risperidone and ziprasidone have been described as 'high-affinity serotonin–dopamine antagonists'. Aripiprazole is sometimes considered to be distinct from other atypicals due to its partial agonist effect at dopamine D_2 receptors.
[b]Amisulpride and sulpiride are structurally related.
[c]Ziprasidone is not available in the UK but is listed due to prominence in other Western countries.

Indications

Antipsychotic drugs are used for the prophylaxis and acute treatment of psychotic illnesses including *schizophrenia* and *psychoses associated with depression and mania.* They also have an important role as an alternative or adjunct to benzodiazepines in the management of the *acutely disturbed patient,* for both tranquillisation and sedation. There is some evidence that quetiapine may be used for treatment-resistant anxiety disorders after other treatments (e.g. SSRIs, SNRIs, pregabalin) have failed to produce an adequate response. Certain antipsychotics have an antidepressant effect that is distinct from their ability to alleviate the psychosis associated with depression, and as such can be used to augment the effect of antidepressants or in some cases (particularly quetiapine) as monotherapy for depression. Some antipsychotics have also proved useful in the tic disorder Tourette's syndrome, and for recurrent self-harming behaviour.

Mechanism of action

The common action of conventional antipsychotics is to decrease brain dopamine function by blocking the *dopamine D_2 receptors* (Fig. 20.3). However, the atypical drugs act on numerous receptors and modulate several interacting transmitter systems. All atypicals (except sulpiride/amisulpride) exhibit affinity for *$5HT_2$ receptors* similar to or higher than that for D_2 receptors, unlike the classical agents. Also some 'atypical' drugs (e.g. sertindole) that do antagonise dopamine D_2 receptors appear to have some selectivity of effect for those in the *mesolimbic system* (producing antipsychotic effect) rather than the *nigrostriatal system* (associated with unwanted motor effects). Clozapine and risperidone

Table 20.4 Symptoms of schizophrenia

Positive symptoms	Negative symptoms
Hallucinations: most commonly auditory (i.e. voices) in the third person, which patients may find threatening. The voices may also give commands. Visual hallucinations are rare	*Affective flattening* manifest by unchanging facial expression with lack of communication through expression, poor eye contact, lack of responsiveness, psychomotor slowing
Delusions: most commonly persecutory. 'Passivity phenomen a' include delusions of thought broadcasting, thought insertion or thought withdrawal, made actions, impulses or feelings	*Alogia* (literally 'absence of words'), manifesting clinically as a lack of spontaneous speech (poverty of speech)
Bizarre behaviours including agitation, sexual disinhibition, repetitive behaviour, wearing of striking but inappropriate clothing	*Anhedonia* (inability to derive pleasure from any activity) and *associality* (narrowing of repertoire of interests and impaired relationships)
Thought disorder manifest by failure in the organisation of speech such that it drifts away from the point (tangentiality), never reaches the point (circumstantiality), moves from one topic to the next illogically (loosened associations, knight's move thinking), breaks off abruptly only to continue on an unrelated topic (derailment) or moves from one topic to the next on the basis of a pun or words that sound similar (clang association)	*Apathy/avolution* involving lack of energy, lack of motivation to work, participate in activities or initiate any goal-directed behaviour, and poor personal hygiene *Attention problems* involving an inability to focus on any one issue or engage fully with communication

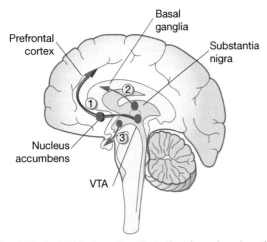

Fig. 20.3 Sagittal brain section illustrating dopaminergic pathways. (1) Mesolimbic pathway (thought to be overactive in psychotic illness according to the dopamine hypothesis of schizophrenia). (2) Nigrostriatal pathway (involved in motor control, underactive in Parkinson's disease and associated with extrapyramidal motor symptoms). (3) Tuberoinfundibular pathway (moderates prolactin release from the hypothalamus). VTA, ventrotegmental area.

exert substantial antagonism of α_2-*adrenoceptors*, a property that may explain their benefits against negative symptoms. Blockade of *muscarinic* acetylcholine receptors as with chlorpromazine and clozapine reduces the occurrence of extrapyramidal effects. Aripiprazole is a unique drug because it is a partial dopamine D_2-receptor agonist that acts conversely as an antagonist in regions where dopamine is overactive, such as the limbic system. It increases dopamine function where this is low (such as in the frontal cortex) and has little motor effect.

Pharmacokinetics

Antipsychotics are well absorbed after oral administration and distribute widely. They are metabolised mainly by hepatic cytochrome P450 isoenzymes, e.g. CYP 2D6 (risperidone, perphenazine; see Table 20.2A), CYP 3A4 (lurasidone, quetiapine; see Table 20.2B), CYP 1A2 (olanzapine, clozapine). Metabolism of some compounds is complex, e.g. zuclopenthixol and haloperidol are metabolised by both CYP 2D6 and CYP 3A4, which means that co-prescription of inhibitors of either enzyme can cause raised plasma concentrations of these antipsychotics. Amisulpride is an exception to the general rule as it is mainly eliminated unchanged by the kidneys with little hepatic metabolism. Elimination $t_{1/2}$ values range from quetiapine 7 h, clozapine 12 h, haloperidol 18 h to olazapine 33 h. Depot preparations usefully release drug over 2–4 weeks after intramuscular injection (see below).

Efficacy

Symptoms in schizophrenia are defined as *positive* and *negative* (see Table 20.4). Although a classical antipsychotic drug should provide adequate treatment of positive symptoms including hallucinations and delusions, at least 60% of patients may have unresolved negative symptoms such as apathy, flattening of affect and alogia. Evidence suggests that *clozapine* may have a significant advantage against negative symptoms. This drug has a further advantage over all other antipsychotics, whether classical or atypical, in that it is the most effective agent for 'resistant' schizophrenia, i.e. where other antipsychotics prescribed at adequate doses fail to produce improvement or are not tolerated.

Schizophrenia often runs a chronic relapsing and remitting course. Less than one-fourth of patients avoid further episodes, with the most common reason for relapse being the stopping of medication against medical advice.

Mode of use

Atypical antipsychotics are all licensed for use in schizophrenia and are now recommended as the first-line treatment for newly diagnosed cases. Some also have licences for treatment and recurrence prevention in mania and for control of agitated or disturbed behaviour in the context of a psychotic illness. In the UK, quetiapine additionally has a license for treatment of depression in bipolar disorder and for adjunctive treatment of unipolar depression, while risperidone is licensed additionally for short-term treatment of persistent aggression in Alzheimer's dementia unresponsive to non-pharmacological treatment.

The longer a psychosis is left untreated, the less favourable is the outcome, and drug treatment should be instigated as soon as an adequate period of assessment has allowed a provisional diagnosis to be established. Patients who are 'neuroleptic naïve', i.e. have never previously taken any antipsychotic agent, should start at the lowest available dose (Table 20.5). For most atypical agents, a period of dose titration by protocol from the starting dose up to a stated lowest therapeutic dose is usual, e.g. risperidone 4 mg/day, quetiapine 300 mg/day. Dose increases are indicated when there is no response until the desired effect on psychotic symptoms or calming of disturbed behaviour is achieved, the urgency of the situation determining the interval between increments until the maximum licensed dose is achieved. Conservative dose titration is advisable for the elderly and patients with learning disabilities (who may require antipsychotics for psychosis or severe behavioural disturbance).

Prescription of conventional antipsychotics follows similar rules to those for atypical drugs, starting at low doses in neuroleptic-naïve patients, e.g. haloperidol 0.5 mg/day in case

the patient is particularly susceptible to adverse, especially extrapyramidal, motor side-effects. There is a wide range of effective doses for many classical agents (e.g. chlorpromazine, once the most prescribed antipsychotic but now rarely used, has a dose range from 25 to 1000 mg/day). As the potency (therapeutic efficacy in relation to dose) of antipsychotic agents varies markedly between compounds, it is useful to think of the effective antipsychotic dose of classical agents in terms of 'chlorpromazine equivalents' (see Table 20.5). For example, haloperidol has a relatively high antipsychotic potency, such that 2–3 mg is equivalent to chlorpromazine 100 mg, whereas 200 mg sulpiride (low potency) is required for equivalent antipsychotic effect. Prescribing in excess of this requires specialist involvement. With co-prescribed antipsychotics, their total maximum antipsychotic dose should not exceed 1000 mg chlorpromazine equivalents per day, except under specialist supervision.

Clozapine may be initiated only under specialist supervision and usually after at least one other antipsychotic has failed through lack of efficacy or unacceptable adverse effects. Additionally, monitoring of leucocyte count is mandatory (danger of agranulocytosis) and blood pressure checking is required (for hypotensive effect). Patients are most vulnerable to agranulocytosis on initiation of therapy, with 75% of cases occurring in the first 18 weeks. The dose titration schedule must be followed strictly, starting with clozapine 12.5 mg at night and working up over a period of 4 weeks to a target therapeutic dose of 450 mg/day.

Alternative administration strategies in acute antipsychotic use

Preparations of antipsychotics for intramuscular injection are advantageous in patients who are unable or unwilling to swallow tablets, a common situation in psychosis or severe behavioural disturbance. Intramuscular preparations of the atypical antipsychotics *olanzapine* and *aripiprazole* are suitable for acute behavioural disturbance in schizophrenia, but the conventional agent *haloperidol* is widely used. Formulations of *risperidone* and *olanzapine* that dissolve rapidly on contact with the tongue are available. These can be rapidly absorbed even by a disturbed and uncooperative patient.

Long-acting depot injections

The classical antipsychotics haloperidol, zuclopenthixol, fluphenazine, flupentixol, and pipotiazine, and the atypicals aripiprazole, olanzapine, risperidone and its metabolite paliperidone are available as long-acting (2–4 weeks) depot intramuscular injections for maintenance treatment of patients with schizophrenia and other chronic psychotic disorders. The manufacturers of paliperidone have recently introduced a preparation which once established

Table 20.5 Relative frequency of selected adverse effects of antipsychotic drugs

Drug	CPZ equivalent dose (mg)	Maximum dose (mg/day)	Extrapyramidal effects	Anticholinergic effects	Hyperprolactinaemia	Weight gain	Cardiotoxicity	Blood dyscrasias	Diabetes/Dyslipidaemia	Sedation
Classical										
Chlorpromazine	100	1000	++	++	+++	++	+	+	–	+++
Trifluoperazine	5	50	+++	+	+++	++	+	+	–	+
Haloperidol	3	30	+++	+	+++	+	+	+	–	+
Sulpiride	200	2400	+	+	+++	+	–	+	–	–
Zuclopenthixol	25	150	++	++	+++	++	+	+	–	++
	Minimum effective dose (mg/day)	Maximum dose (mg/day)								
Atypical										
Clozapine[a]	300	900	–	+++	–	+++	+	+++	++	+++
Olanzapine[b]	5–10	20	–	++	+	+++	–	+	++	++
Quetiapine	300	800	–	+	–	++	–	+	+	++
Risperidone	2–4	16	+	+	++	++	–	+	+	+
Amisulpride[c]	400[c]	1200	+	–	++	+	–	+	–	–
Aripiprazole[d]	10	30	–	–	–	+	–	–	–	+
Paliperidone[e]	3–6	12	+	–	+	++	–	+	+	+
Lurasidone	37	148	++	–	++	+	–	–	–	+
Asenapine	10	20	+	–	+	+	–	–	–	++

CPZ, chlorpromazine. The CPZ equivalent dose concept is of value in comparing the potency of classical antipsychotics. Dose ranges are not specified as they are extremely wide, and drugs are normally increased from low starting doses, e.g. chlorpromazine 25 mg or equivalent, until an adequate antipsychotic effect is achieved or the maximum dose reached. The CPZ equivalent dose concept is of less value for atypical antipsychotics because minimum effective doses and narrower therapeutic ranges have been defined. Maximum dose should be exceeded only under specialist supervision.

[a]Dose of clozapine 50 mg is considered equivalent to chlorpromazine 100 mg.

[b]Lower doses of amisulpride, e.g. 100 mg/day, are indicated only for patients with negative symptoms of schizophrenia.

[c]Aripiprazole appears to be free of most unwanted effects characteristically associated with antipsychotics, but may cause nausea, lightheadedness, somnolence and akathisia.

[d]Paliperidone is 9-hydroxy risperidone.

requires injections only once every 3 months. Use of depot preparations improves compliance, and there is less risk of relapse from ceasing to take medication. In view of the prolonged effect, it is prudent to administer a small initial test dose and review 5–10 days later for unwanted effects.

Rapid tranquillisation

Rapid tranquillisation protocols address the problem of severely disturbed and violent patients who have not responded to non-pharmacological approaches. The risks of administering psychotropic drugs (notably cardiac arrhythmia with high-dose antipsychotics) then greatly outweigh those of non-treatment.

A first step is to offer oral medication, usually haloperidol, olanzapine or risperidone with or without the benzodiazepine, lorazepam. If this is not accepted or fails to achieve control despite repeated doses, the intramuscular route is used to administer a benzodiazepine (e.g. lorazepam or midazolam) or an antipsychotic (e.g. haloperidol or olanzapine), or both (but intramuscular olanzapine should not be given with a benzodiazepine as excess sedation may ensue). After emergency use of an intramuscular antipsychotic or benzodiazepine, pulse, blood pressure, temperature and respiration are monitored, and pulse oximetry (for oxygen saturation) if consciousness is lost.

Intramuscular zuclopenthixol acetate was previously used for patients who do not respond to two doses of intramuscular haloperidol. This usually induces a calming effect within 2 h, persisting for 2–3 days. Clinicians have become reluctant to use this heavily sedating preparation other than for patients who have previously responded well to it, and never use it for neuroleptic-naïve patients. Patients must be observed with care following administration. Some will require a second dose within 1–2 days.

Amobarbital and paraldehyde have a role in emergencies only when antipsychotic and benzodiazepine options have been exhausted.

Adverse effects (see Table 20.5)

Active psychotic illnesses often cause patients to have poor insight into their condition. Adverse drug effects can be the final straw in compromising already fragile compliance, leading to relapse. When atypical antipsychotics first came to prominence in the mid-1990s, much was made of their lower propensity to cause several of the most troublesome side-effects of classical antipsychotics, especially extrapyramidal motor effects. However, while these problems are encountered less frequently, atypical drugs have a range of troublesome metabolic side-effects which had not been reported in the previous era of classic antipsychotics. Thus, to understand the current position relating to the pros and cons of atypical antipsychotics, it is necessary first to describe the side-effect profile of classical antipsychotic drugs.

Classical antipsychotics

It is rare for any patient taking classical antipsychotic agents to escape their adverse effects completely. Thus it is essential to discuss with patients the possibility of unwanted effects and regularly to review this aspect of their care.

Extrapyramidal symptoms. All classical antipsychotics produce these effects because they act by blocking dopamine receptors in the nigrostriatal pathway. Consequently some 75% of patients experience extrapyramidal symptoms shortly after starting the drug or increasing its dose (acute effects), or sometime after a particular dose level has been established (tardive effects).

Acute extrapyramidal symptoms. Dystonias are manifest as abnormal movements of the tongue and facial muscles with fixed postures and spasm, including torticollis and bizarre eye movements ('oculogyric crisis'). *Parkinsonian symptoms* result in the classical triad of bradykinesia, rigidity and tremor. Both dystonias and parkinsonian symptoms are believed to result from a shift in favour of cholinergic rather than dopaminergic neurotransmission in the nigrostriatal pathway (see p. 338). Anticholinergic (antimuscarinic) agents, e.g. procyclidine, orphenadrine or benztropine, act to restore the balance in favour of dopaminergic transmission but are liable to provoke antimuscarinic effects (dry mouth, urinary retention, constipation, exacerbation of glaucoma and confusion) and they offer no relief for tardive dyskinesia, which may even worsen. They should be used only to treat established symptoms and not for prophylaxis. Benzodiazepines are an alternative.

Akathisia is a state of motor and psychological restlessness, in which patients exhibit persistent foot tapping, moving of legs repetitively and being unable to settle or relax. A strong association has been noted between its presence in treated schizophrenics and subsequent suicide. A β-adrenoceptor blocker, e.g. nadolol, is the best treatment, although anticholinergic agents may be effective where akathisia coexists with dystonias and parkinsonian symptoms. Differentiating symptoms of psychotic illness from adverse drug effects is often difficult: drug-induced akathisia may be mistaken for agitation induced by psychosis.

Tardive dyskinesia affects about 25% of patients taking classical antipsychotic drugs, the risk increasing with length of exposure. It was originally thought to be a consequence of up-regulation or supersensitivity of dopamine receptors, but a more recent view is that oxidative damage leads to increases in glutamate transmission. Patients display a spectrum of abnormal movements from minor tongue protrusion, lip-smacking, rotational tongue movements and facial grimacing, choreoathetoid movements of the head and neck, and even to twisting and gyrating of the whole body. Remission on discontinuing the causative agent is less likely than are simple dystonias and parkinsonian symptoms. Any anticholinergic agent should be withdrawn immediately. Reduction of the dose of classical antipsychotic is an option, but psychotic symptoms may then worsen or be 'unmasked'. Alternatively, an atypical antipsychotic can provide rapid improvement while retaining control of psychotic symptoms. Atypicals, particularly at high doses, can cause extrapyramidal effects, so this strategy is not always helpful. Clozapine, which does not appear to cause tardive dyskinesia, may be used in severe cases where continuing antipsychotic treatment is required and symptoms have not responded to other medication strategies.

If the classical antipsychotic is continued, tardive dyskinesia remits spontaneously in around 30% of patients within 1 year, but the condition is difficult to tolerate and patients may be keen to try other medications even where evidence suggests that the success rates for remission are limited. These include vitamin E, benzodiazepines, β-blockers, bromocriptine and tetrabenazine.

Cardiovascular effects. Postural hypotension may result from blockade of α_1-adrenoceptors; it is dose related. Prolongation of the QTc interval in the cardiac cycle may rarely lead to ventricular arrhythmias and sudden death. This observation led to the withdrawal from the market of thioridazine and droperidol, restrictions on the use of pimozide and general warnings regarding the use of several other antipsychotics including haloperidol.

Prolactin increase. Classical antipsychotics raise plasma prolactin concentration by blocking dopamine receptors in the tuberoinfundibular pathway, causing gynaecomastia and galactorrhoea in both sexes, and menstrual disturbances in women. A change to an atypical agent such as aripiprazole, quetiapine or olanzapine (but not risperidone or amisulpride) should minimise the effects. If continuation of the existing classical antipsychotic is obligatory, dopamine agonists such as bromocriptine and amantadine that reduce prolactin secretion may help.

Sedation. This may be a highly desirable property in the acute treatment of psychotic illness, but it may be undesirable as the patient seeks to resume work, study or relationships.

Classical antipsychotics may also be associated with:

- *Weight gain* (a problem with almost all classical antipsychotics with the exception of loxapine; most pronounced with fluphenazine and flupentixol, while haloperidol carries a lesser risk).
- *Seizures* (chlorpromazine is especially likely to lower the convulsion threshold).
- *Interference with temperature regulation* (hypothermia or hyperthermia, especially in the elderly).
- *Skin problems* (phenothiazines, particularly chlorpromazine, may provoke photosensitivity necessitating advice about limiting exposure to sunlight); rashes and urticaria may also occur.
- *Sexual dysfunction* (ejaculatory problems through α-adrenoceptor blockade).
- *Retinal pigmentation* (chlorpromazine can cause visual impairment if the dose is prolonged and high).
- *Corneal and lens opacities*.
- *Blood dyscrasias* (agranulocytosis and leucopenia).
- *Osteoporosis* (associated with increased prolactin levels).
- *Jaundice* (including cholestatic).

'Atypical' antipsychotics

Having considered the side-effect profile of classical antipsychotic agents, the adverse effects of atypical antipsychotics can be viewed as those shared with classical agents and those unique to one or more atypical agents.

Extrapyramidal effects occur less frequently than with classical agents (there is less blockade of dopamine D_2 receptors in the nigrostriatal pathway) but do occur with high doses of risperidone and olanzapine. Tardive dyskinesia is much less common with all of the atypical agents than with classical drugs. *Anticholinergic (antimuscarinic) effects* are most likely with clozapine and olanzapine. Sexual dysfunction and skin problems are rare with atypical antipsychotics. Adverse effects relating to prolactin stimulation are also rare, with the exception of risperidone and amisulpride (for which galactorrhea is as common as with classical drugs).

One of the most problematic side-effects with atypical antipsychotics, especially with olanzapine and clozapine, is these drugs' propensity to cause weight gain. The effect appears to be dose dependent for olanzapine but is often greater than 10 kg after 1 year's treatment with the 15 mg/day dose. Lurasidone, asenapine and amisulpride have a lesser propensity to cause weight gain. Atypicals have also been implicated as causing metabolic disorders, especially *diabetes mellitus* and *hyperlipidaemia*. Olanzapine, clozapine and quetiapine appear to be the most problematic. Obesity, impaired glucose tolerance and hyperlipidaemia, along with hypertension, are all features of *metabolic syndrome*. Hypertension can occur gradually with antipsychotics, most frequently as a consequence of weight gain. In a small number of cases, hypertension may result from α_2-adrenoceptor blockade. However, hypertension is less commonly an antipsychotic side-effect than the other manifestations of metabolic syndrome, and some atypical antipsychotics (notably clozapine) are associated with postural hypotension.

'Atypical' antipsychotics are associated with other important cardiovascular effects. QTc prolongation is most likely to occur with sertindole (which is restricted for this reason), but quetiapine is associated with a lower level of risk than classical antipsychotics haloperidol and pimozide. Both classical and atypical antipsychotics are associated with a small but significantly elevated risk of death when used for behavioural and psychological symptoms of dementia such as agitation and aggression, although this risk must be weighed against the dangers and distress associated with not providing adequate treatment.

Atypicals can also cause sedation. Clozapine is the most sedative followed by zotepine, quetiapine and olanzapine.

Clozapine warrants separate mention, given its value for patients with treatment-resistant schizophrenia or severe treatment-related extrapyramidal symptoms. Most important is the risk of *agranulocytosis* in up to 2% of patients (compared with 0.2% for classical antipsychotics). When clozapine was first licensed without requirement for regular blood counts, this problem caused appreciable mortality. With the introduction of strict monitoring, there have been no recorded deaths in the UK from agranulocytosis since clozapine was reintroduced, and internationally the death rate from agranulocytosis is now considerably less than 1 in 1000. In addition to postural hypotension, clozapine may cause tachycardia and provoke seizures in 3–5% of patients at doses above 600 mg/day. Finally, there are reported associations between clozapine use and cardiomyopathy and myocarditis, although both are very rare outcomes.

Neuroleptic malignant syndrome

The syndrome may develop in up to 1% of patients using antipsychotics, both classical and atypical; it is more prevalent with high doses. The elderly and those with organic brain disease, hyperthyroidism or dehydration are thought to be most susceptible. Clinical features include fever, confusion or fluctuating consciousness, rigidity of muscles which may become severe, autonomic instability manifest by labile blood pressure, tachycardia and urinary incontinence or retention.

Raised plasma creatine kinase concentration and white cell count are suggestive (but not conclusive) of neuroleptic malignant syndrome. There is some clinical overlap with the 'serotonin syndrome' (see p. 332), and concomitant use of SSRIs (or possibly TCAs) with antipsychotics may increase the risk.

When the syndrome is suspected, it is essential to discontinue the antipsychotic, and to be ready to undertake rehydration and body cooling. A benzodiazepine is indicated for sedation, tranquillising effect and may be beneficial where active psychosis remains untreated. Dopamine agonists (bromocriptine, dantrolene) are helpful in some cases. Even

when recognised and treated, the condition carries a mortality rate of 12–15%, through cardiac arrhythmia, rhabdomyolysis or respiratory failure. The condition usually lasts for 5–7 days after the antipsychotic is stopped but may continue longer when a depot preparation has been used. Fortunately those who survive tend to have no long-lasting physical effects from their ordeal, though care is required if, as is usual, they need further antipsychotic treatment.

Efficacy of conventional vs atypical antipsychotics

It was originally thought that all atypicals had an advantage over conventional agents at least for negative symptoms. More recently, evidence has emerged that for overall efficacy in schizophrenia, olanzapine, risperidone and amisulpride, in addition to clozapine, have an advantage over the other atypicals and the conventional antipsychotics. Note that clozapine is normally only used when at least two atypical antipsychotics have been tried without adequate response.

In some countries finance may be the overriding factor in favour of retaining classical agents rather than atypicals as first choice in schizophrenia. The basis for any such decision must extend beyond crude drug costs and take account of the capacity of atypicals to lessen extrapyramidal symptoms, improve compliance, and thus prevent relapse of psychotic illness and protect patients from the lasting damage of periods of untreated psychosis. Additionally, greater efficacy affords schizophrenic patients the opportunity to reintegrate into the community and make positive contributions to society, when the alternative is long-term residence in hospital. Recognising drugs as therapeutic entities as well as units of cost is an important element in deciding between classical and atypical drugs, and indeed about decision-making in the purchase of all drugs by institutions or countries.

Mood stabilisers

In bipolar affective disorder, patients suffer episodes of mania, hypomania and depression, classically with periods of normal mood in between. *Manic episodes* involve greatly elevated mood, often associated with irritability, loss of social inhibitions, irresponsible behaviour and grandiosity accompanied by biological symptoms (increased energy, restlessness, decreased need for sleep, and increased sex drive). Psychotic features may be present, particularly disordered thinking manifested by grandiose delusions and 'flight of ideas' (acceleration of the pattern of thought with rapid speech). *Hypomania* is a less dramatic and less dangerous presentation, but retains the features of elation or irritability and the biological symptoms, abnormalities in speech being limited to increased talkativeness and in social conduct to over-familiarity and mild recklessness. *Depressive episodes* may include any of the depressive symptoms described above, and may include psychotic features.

Lithium

Lithium salts were known anecdotally to have beneficial psychotropic effects as long ago as the middle of the 19th century, but scientific evidence of their efficacy was not obtained until 1949, when lithium carbonate was tried in manic patients; it was found to be effective in the acute state and, later, to prevent recurrent attacks.[4]

The mode of action is not fully understood. Its main effect is probably to inhibit hydrolysis of inositol phosphate, so reducing the recycling of free inositol for synthesis of phosphatidylinositides, which if present in excess may interfere with cell homeostasis by promoting uncontrolled cell signalling. Other putative mechanisms involve the cyclic AMP 'second messenger' system, and monoaminergic and cholinergic neurotransmitters.

Pharmacokinetics. The therapeutic and toxic plasma concentrations are close (low therapeutic index). Lithium is a small cation and, given orally, is rapidly absorbed throughout the gut. High peak plasma concentrations are avoided by using sustained-release formulations which deliver the peak plasma lithium concentrations in about 5 h. At first, lithium is distributed throughout the extracellular water, but with continued administration it enters the cells and is eventually distributed throughout the total body water with a somewhat higher concentration in brain, bones and thyroid gland. Lithium is easily dialysable from the blood, but the concentration gradient from cell to blood is relatively small and the intracellular concentration (which determines toxicity) falls slowly. Being a metallic ion it is not metabolised, nor is it bound to plasma proteins.

The kidneys eliminate lithium. Like sodium, it is filtered by the glomerulus and 80% is reabsorbed by the proximal tubule, but it is not reabsorbed by the distal tubule. Intake of sodium and water are the principal determinants of its elimination. In sodium deficiency, lithium is retained in the body, and thus concomitant use of a diuretic can reduce lithium clearance by as much as 50%, and precipitate toxicity. Sodium chloride and water are used to treat lithium toxicity.

With chronic use, the plasma $t_{1/2}$ of lithium is 15–30 h. It is usually given 12–24-hourly to avoid unnecessary fluctuation (peak and trough) and maintain plasma concentrations

just below the toxic level. A steady-state plasma concentration will be attained after about 5–6 days (i.e. $5 \times t_{1/2}$) in patients with normal renal function. Elderly patients and patients with impaired renal function will have a longer $t_{1/2}$ so that steady state will be reached later and dose increments must be adjusted accordingly.

Indications and use. Lithium carbonate is effective *treatment* in more than 75% of episodes of acute mania or hypomania. Because its therapeutic action takes 2–3 weeks to develop, lithium is generally used in combination with a benzodiazepine such as lorazepam or diazepam (or with an antipsychotic agent where there are also psychotic features).

For *prophylaxis*, lithium is indicated when there have been two episodes of mood disturbance in 2 years, although in severe cases prophylactic use is indicated after one episode. When an adequate dose of lithium is taken consistently, around 65% of patients achieve improved mood control.

Patients who start lithium only to discontinue it within 2 years have a significantly poorer outcome than matched patients who are not given any pharmacological prophylaxis. The existence of a 'rebound effect' (recurrence of manic symptoms) during withdrawal dictates that long-term treatment with the drug is of great importance.

Lithium salts are ineffective for prophylaxis of bipolar affective disorder in around 35% of patients. The search for alternatives has centered on anticonvulsants, notably carbamazepine and sodium valproate and lamotrigine, and more recently the atypical antipsychotics.

Lithium is also used to augment the action of antidepressants in treatment-resistant depression (see p. 332).

Pharmaceutics. The dose of lithium ions (Li^+) delivered varies with the pharmaceutical preparation; thus it is vital for patients to adhere to the same pharmaceutical brand. For example, *Camcolit* 250-mg tablets each contain 6.8 mmol Li^+, *Liskonum* 450-mg tablets contain 12.2 mmol Li^+ and *Priadel* 200-mg tablets contain 5.4 mmol Li^+. The proprietary name must be stated on the prescription.

Some patients cannot tolerate slow-release preparations because release of lithium distally in the intestine causes diarrhoea; they may be better served by the liquid preparation, lithium citrate, which is absorbed proximally. Patients who are naive to lithium should be started at the lowest dose of the preparation selected. Any change in preparation demands the same precautions as does initiation of therapy.

Monitoring. Dose is guided by monitoring the plasma concentration once steady state has been reached. Increments are made at weekly intervals until the concentration lies within the range 0.4–1 mmol/L (maintenance at the lower level is preferred for elderly patients). The timing of blood

---

[4]Cade J F 1970 The story of lithium. In: Ayd F J, Blackwell B (eds) Biological Psychiatry. Philadelphia, Lippincott.

sampling is important, and by convention a blood sample is taken prior to the morning dose, as close as possible to 12 h after the evening dose. Once the plasma concentration is at steady state and in the therapeutic range, it should be measured every 3 months. For toxicity monitoring, thyroid function (especially in women) and renal function (plasma creatinine and electrolytes) should be measured before initiation and every 3–6 months during therapy.

Patient education about the role of lithium in the prophylaxis of bipolar affective disorder is particularly important to achieve compliance with therapy; treatment cards, information leaflets and, where appropriate, video material are used.

Adverse effects are encountered in three general categories:

- Those occurring at plasma concentrations within the therapeutic range (0.4–1 mmol/L), which include fine tremor (especially involving the fingers; a β blocker may benefit), constipation, polyuria, polydipsia, metallic taste in the mouth, weight gain, oedema, goitre, hypothyroidism, acne, rash, diabetes insipidus and cardiac arrhythmias. Mild cognitive and memory impairment also occur.
- Signs of intoxication, associated with plasma concentrations greater than 1.5 mmol/L, are mainly gastrointestinal (diarrhoea, anorexia, vomiting) and neurological (blurred vision, muscle weakness, drowsiness, sluggishness and coarse tremor, leading on to giddiness, ataxia and dysarthria).
- Frank toxicity, due to severe overdosage or rapid reduction in renal clearance, usually associated with plasma concentrations over 2 mmol/L, constitutes a medical emergency. Hyperreflexia, hyperextension of limbs, convulsions, hyperthermia, toxic psychoses, syncope, oliguria, coma and even death may result if treatment is not instigated urgently.

Overdose. Acute overdose may present without signs of toxicity but with plasma concentrations well exceeding 2 mmol/L. This requires only measures to increase urine production, e.g. by ensuring adequate intravenous and oral fluid intake while avoiding sodium depletion (and a diuretic is contraindicated; see above). Treatment is otherwise supportive, with special attention to electrolyte balance, renal function and control of convulsions. Where toxicity is chronic, haemodialysis may be needed, especially if renal function is impaired. Plasma concentration may rise again after acute reduction, because lithium leaves cells slowly, and also due to continued absorption from sustained-release formulations. Whole bowel irrigation may be an option for significant ingestion, but specialist advice should be sought.

Interactions. Drugs that interfere with lithium excretion by the renal tubules cause the plasma concentration to rise. They include diuretics (thiazides more than loop type), angiotensin-converting enzyme (ACE) inhibitors and angiotensin-II antagonists, and non-steroidal anti-inflammatory analgesics. Theophylline and sodium-containing antacids reduce plasma lithium concentration. These effects can be important because lithium has a low therapeutic ratio. Diltiazem, verapamil, carbamazepine and phenytoin may cause neurotoxicity without affecting the plasma lithium level.

Carbamazepine

Carbamazepine is licensed as an alternative to lithium for prophylaxis of bipolar affective disorder, although clinical trial evidence is actually stronger to support its use in the treatment of acute mania. While lithium monotherapy is more effective than carbamazepine for prophylaxis of classical bipolar affective disorder, carbamazepine appears to be more effective than lithium for rapidly cycling bipolar disorders, i.e. with recurrent swift transitions from mania to depression. It is also effective in combination with lithium. (See also Epilepsy, p. 366.)

Valproate

Three forms of valproate are available: valproic acid, sodium valproate and semisodium valproate. The latter two are metabolised to valproic acid which exerts the pharmacological effect. It is the semisodium valproate preparation (Depakote) which is licensed in the UK for acute treatment of mania, underpinned by a reasonably strong evidence base. Valproate has become the drug of first choice for prophylaxis of bipolar affective disorder in the USA, despite the lack of robust supporting clinical trial evidence. Treatment with valproic acid is easy to initiate (especially compared to lithium) with no requirement for plasma concentration monitoring needed, although baseline and periodic checks of full blood count and liver function are recommended following reports of occasional blood dyscrasias or hepatic failure. It is generally well tolerated, but weight gain can be a problem, so body mass index should be recorded and evaluated at intervals. Other potential side-effects include gastric irritation, lethargy, confusion, tremor and hair loss.

Treatment with carbamazepine or valproic acid appears not to be associated with the 'rebound effect' of relapse into manic symptoms that may accompany early withdrawal of lithium therapy.

'Atypical' antipsychotics

Another drug class which is developing increasing importance in bipolar affective disorder is the atypical antipsychotics.

Antipsychotic agents (both conventional and atypical) have long been used for control of acute manic symptoms, including both the grandiose delusions and thought disorder associated with manic psychosis and the acute behavioural disturbance which can occur in an extremely agitated patient. Most atypicals can be used to treat acute manic episodes, the most recent addition being asenapine. However, a selection of atypical antipsychotics such as olanzapine, quetiapine, risperidone (by long-acting injection) and aripiprazole are now known to be useful alternatives to conventional mood stabilisers in long-term prevention of manic relapse. Quetiapine appears to be particularly useful in preventing depressive relapse. Quetiapine and lurasidone may be used in treating depressive episodes in the context of bipolar disorder.

Other drugs

Evidence is emerging for the efficacy of lamotrigine in prophylaxis of bipolar affective disorder, especially when depressive episodes predominate. Another drug class which is developing increasing importance in bipolar affective disorder is the atypical antipsychotics. Antipsychotic agents (both conventional and atypical) have long been used for control of acute manic symptoms, including both the grandiose delusions and thought disorder associated with manic psychosis and the acute behavioural disturbance which can occur in an extremely agitated patient. However, atypical antipsychotics such as olanzapine, quetiapine and aripiprazole are now known to be useful alternatives to conventional mood stabilisers in long-term prevention of manic relapse. Quetiapine appears to be particularly useful in preventing depressive relapse.

Other drugs that have been used in augmentation of existing agents include the anticonvulsants oxcarbazepine and gabapentin, the benzodiazepine clonazepam, and the calcium channel–blocking agents verapamil and nimodipine.

Drugs used in anxiety and sleep disorders

The disability and health costs caused by anxiety are high and comparable with those of other common medical conditions such as diabetes, arthritis or hypertension. People with anxiety disorders experience impaired physical and role functioning, more workdays lost due to illness, increased impairment at work and high use of health services. Our understanding of the nature of anxiety has increased greatly from advances in research in psychology and neuroscience. It is now possible to distinguish different types of anxiety with distinct biological and cognitive symptoms, and clear criteria have been accepted for the diagnosis of various anxiety disorders. The last decade has seen developments in both drug and psychological therapies such that a range of treatment options can be tailored to individual patients and their condition.

Anxiety does not manifest itself only as a psychic or mental state: there are also somatic or physical concomitants, e.g. consciousness of the action of the heart (palpitations), tremor, diarrhoea, which are associated with increased activity of the sympathetic autonomic system. These symptoms are not only caused by anxiety, they also add to the feeling of anxiety (positive feedback loop). Anxiety symptoms exist on a continuum, and many people with a mild anxiety, perhaps of recent onset and associated with stressful life events but without much disability, tend to improve without specific intervention. The chronic nature and associated disability of many anxiety disorders means that most patients who fulfil diagnostic criteria for a disorder are likely to benefit from some form of treatment.

Classification of anxiety disorders

The diagnostic criteria of the *DSM-5 (Diagnostic and Statistical Manual of Mental Disorders)* or *ICD-10 (International Classification of Diseases)* are generally used. Both divide anxiety into a series of subsyndromes with clear operational criteria to assist in distinguishing them. At any one time, many patients may have symptoms of more than one syndrome, but making the primary diagnosis is important as this can markedly influence the choice of treatment (Table 20.6). Note that DSM-5 has placed Obsessive-Compulsive disorder into a separate category outside the Anxiety Disorders grouping, but nevertheless we will consider it under 'anxiety disorders' here as remains the case in ICD-10.

The key features of each anxiety disorder follow, with a practical description of the preferred choice of medication, its dose and duration.

Panic disorder (PD)

The main feature is recurrent, unexpected panic attacks. These are discrete periods of intense fear accompanied by characteristic physical symptoms such as skipping or pounding heart, sweating, hot flushes or chills, trembling/shaking, breathing difficulties, chest pain, nausea, diarrhoea and other gastrointestinal symptoms, dizziness or lightheadedness. The first panic attack often occurs without warning but may subsequently become associated with specific situations, e.g. in a crowded shop, driving. Anticipatory anxiety and avoidance behaviour develop in response to this chain of events. The condition must be distinguished from alcohol

Table 20.6 Evidence-based drug treatments for anxiety disorders

	GAD	Panic	Social anxiety disorder	PTSD[a]	OCD
First-line treatment	SSRI (SNRIs and pregabalin are alternative first-line treatments)	SSRI venlafaxine	SSRI	Some SSRIs (sertraline or paroxetine) venlafaxine	SSRI
Monotherapy[b] Antidepressants	Most SSRIs,	All SSRIs	All SSRIs	Some SSRIs (fluoxetine, fluvoxamine, paroxetine, sertraline)	All SSRIs
	SNRIs (venlafaxine, duloxetine)	SNRI (venlafaxine)	SNRIs (venlafaxine, duloxetine)	SNRI (venlafaxine)	SNRI (venlafaxine)
	TCA imipramine	TCAs clomipramine imipramine lofepramine		some TCAs (amitriptyline, imipramine)	TCA clomipramine
	Others agomelatine trazodone vortioxetine	Others mirtazapine reboxetine moclobemide phenelzine	Others moclobemide phenelzine	Others phenelzine mirtazapine reboxetine	Others
Monotherapy[b] (benzodiazepines)	alprazolam diazepam lorazepam	alprazolam clonazepam diazepam lorazepam	bromazepam clonazepam		Clonazepam
Monotherapy[b] (others)	pregabalin buspirone hydroxyzine quetiapine	gabapentin valproate	pregabalin gabapentin topiramate tiagabine olanzapine	lamotrigine topiramate risperidone olanzapine	
Duration of drug treatment	Up to 18 months if response at 12 weeks	Further 6 months if response at 12 weeks	Further 6 months if response at 12 weeks	Further 12 months if response at 12 weeks	Further 12 months if response at 12 weeks

Continued

Table 20.6 Evidence-based drug treatments for anxiety disorders—cont'd

	GAD	Panic	Social anxiety disorder	PTSD[a]	OCD
Higher doses associated with better response	SSRIs venlafaxine pregabalin	SSRIs (limited evidence)	Individual patients may benefit	Individual patients may benefit	SSRIs
Evidence-based augmentation Strategies[c]	SSRI/SNRI + pregabalin, or antipsychotic (e.g. quetiapine, risperidone, olanzapine, aripiprazole)	SSRI + pindolol or clonazepam	SSRI + buspirone	Antidepressant + olanzapine, risperidone, prazosin	SSRI/clomipramine + antipsychotic or ondansetron/granisetron, SSRI + topiramate or lamotrigine
Relapse prevention	SSRIs duloxetine venlafaxine agomelatine pregabalin quetiapine	SSRIs imipramine venlafaxine	SSRIs pregabalin clonazepam	SSRIs	SSRIs

Notes: The above table considers drug treatment only; psychotherapy, especially cognitive behavioural therapy, is also effective and is also considered a first-line treatment in all disorders. General considerations for treatment of anxiety disorders include the need to discuss the benefits and risks of specific treatments with patients before treatment and take account of clinical features, patient needs and preference and local service availability when choosing treatments. SSRIs are usually effective in anxiety disorders and are generally suitable for first-line treatment. The SNRI venlafaxine is effective across all disorders. Pregabalin has a good evidence base in GAD and one successful trial in social anxiety disorder. TCAs, MAOIs, antipsychotics and anticonvulsants need to be considered in relation to their evidence base for specific conditions and their individual risks and benefits. Benzodiazepines are effective in many anxiety disorders, but their use should be short term except in treatment-resistant cases.
With all antidepressants, there should be specific discussion and monitoring of possible adverse effects early in treatment, especially initial 'jitteriness' or activation syndromes. For paroxetine, venlafaxine and benzodiazepines, prescribers should also discuss the dangers of stopping the drugs abruptly. Antidepressant treatment is often slow, and it is advisable to wait 12 weeks to assess efficacy. When initial treatments fail, one should consider switching to another evidence-based treatment (including psychotherapy such as CBT), combining evidence-based treatments, and referring to regional or national specialist services in refractory patients.
[a]For acute prevention, if feasible consider propranolol after major trauma. Routine debriefing is not indicated.
[b]All drugs listed have randomized trial evidence for monotherapy in the corresponding anxiety disorder.
[c]Given the limited number of studies examining specific drug combinations for adjunctive therapy, most guidelines recommend first combining treatments which both have evidence of being effective in monotherapy provided there are no contraindications.

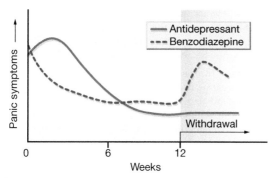

Fig. 20.4 Schematic representation of the time course of panic treatments.

withdrawal, caffeinism, hyperthyroidism and (rarely) phaeochromocytoma.

Patients experiencing panic attacks often do not know what is happening to them, and because the symptoms are similar to those of cardiovascular, respiratory or neurological conditions, often present to non-psychiatric services, e.g. casualty departments, family doctors, medical specialists, where they may either be extensively investigated or given reassurance that there is nothing wrong. A carefully taken history reduces the likelihood of this occurrence.

Treatment. The choice lies between antidepressants, (e.g. SSRIs such as sertraline or the SNRI venlafaxine) which may require some weeks to exert their clinical effect but are unlikely to be associated with dependence and withdrawal, and benzodiazepines (e.g. lorazepam) which are faster acting but present several issues in terms of tolerance, difficult withdrawal and in older patients increased risk of falls. The different time course of these two classes of agent in panic disorder is depicted in Fig. 20.4 (see also Table 20.6).

Benzodiazepines rapidly reduce panic frequency and severity and continue to be effective for months; significant tolerance to the therapeutic action is uncommon. On withdrawal of the benzodiazepine, even when it is gradual, increased symptoms of anxiety and panic attacks may occur, reaching a maximum when the final dose is stopped. Indeed, some patients find they are unable to withdraw and remain long-term on a benzodiazepine. For this reason most guidelines see benzodiazepines as less preferable than antidepressants in panic disorder.

Antidepressants (SSRIs, SNRIs and TCAs) have a slower onset of action and may cause an initial increase in both anxiety and panic frequency, such that a patient may discontinue medication, even after a single dose. This provoking reaction usually lasts for no more than 2–3 weeks after which panic frequency and severity improve quickly, but patients need help to stay on treatment in the first weeks. The doctor needs to give a clear explanation of the likely course of events, and the antidepressant should be started at one-half the usual initial dose to reduce the likelihood of exacerbation. The dose of antidepressant required to treat panic disorder is generally as high as, or higher than, that for depression, and maximal benefit may not emerge for 8–12 weeks. Patients should therefore receive as large a dose as can be tolerated for this length of time.

Social anxiety disorder

The essential feature of social phobia is a marked and persistent fear of performance situations when patients feel they will be the centre of attention and will do something humiliating or embarrassing. The situations that provoke this fear can be quite specific, for example public speaking, or be of a much more generalised nature involving fear of most social interactions, for example initiating or maintaining conversations, participating in small groups, dating, speaking to anyone in authority. Exposure to the feared situation almost invariably provokes anxiety with similar symptoms to those experienced by patients with panic attacks, but some seem to be particularly prominent and difficult, i.e. blushing, tremor, sweating and a feeling of 'drying up' when speaking.

Treatment. The antidepressant drugs with established efficacy are the SSRIs (especially *sertraline, paroxetine* and *escitalopram*), the SNRIs venlafaxine and duloxetine, the novel compound mirtazapine, the MAOI *phenelzine* and the RIMA *moclobemide* in the same doses as for depression. These achieve equivalent degrees of improvement; *phenelzine* has a slightly faster onset of action but produces more adverse effects. Some benzodiazepines are reported to provide benefit, but evidence for their therapeutic efficacy is less conclusive. *Pregabalin* has been shown to be effective in a trial in social anxiety disorder, although higher doses are required than for generalised anxiety disorder. Evidence also exists for gabapentin, olanzapine and the anticonvulsants topiramate and the β-adrenoceptor blockers continue to be widely used despite their having no proven efficacy in social phobia. But they have a place in the treatment of specific performance anxiety, e.g. in musicians, when management of the tremor is crucial.

The duration of treatment is as for depression or longer, for this can be a lifelong condition.

Post-traumatic stress disorder (PTSD)

Symptoms characteristically follow exposure to an extreme traumatic stressor event. These include persistent re-experiencing of the traumatic event, persistent avoidance of stimuli associated with the trauma and numbing of general responsiveness, and persistent symptoms of increased arousal.

In taking a history, the association with the event is usually obvious. PTSD is differentiated from acute stress disorder (below) by its persistence – the symptoms of the latter resolve within about 4 weeks. Depression quite commonly coexists with PTSD and should be enquired for in the history.

The preferred treatment immediately following the incident should probably be a short course of a hypnotic (or sedating antidepressant, e.g. *mirtazapine*) to promote sleep and help minimise mental rehearsal of the trauma that may lead to its perpetuation. Long-term therapy with antidepressants appears to be indicated at doses in the same range as for other anxiety disorders. Evidence for efficacy of several antidepressants has been reported in randomised placebo-controlled trails. These include SSRIs (fluoxetine, fluvoxamine, paroxetine, sertraline), the SNRI venlafaxine, tricyclics (amitriptyline, imipramine), as well as mirtazapine and phenelzine, while reboxetine has evidence of having a comparable effect to fluvoxamine. There is also evidence for the antipsychotics risperidone and olanzapine and the anticonvulsants topiramate and lamotrigine.'

Acute stress disorder/ adjustment disorder

Acute stress disorder is anxiety in response to a recent extreme stress. Although in some respects it is a normal and under-standable reaction to an event, the problems associated with it are not only the severe distress the anxiety causes but also the risk that it may evolve into a more persistent state.

Treatment. A benzodiazepine used for a short time is the preferred approach for treating overwhelming anxiety that needs to be brought rapidly under control. It particularly relieves the accompanying anxiety and sleep disturbance. A drug with a slow onset of action such as *oxazepam* (60–120 mg/day) causes less dependence and withdrawal, and is preferred to those that enter the brain rapidly, e.g. diazepam, lorazepam. Some patients find it hard to discontinue the benzodiazepine, so its use should be reserved for those in whom extreme distress disrupts normal coping strategies.

Generalised anxiety disorder (GAD)

The essential feature of this condition is chronic anxiety and worry. To the non-sufferer the focus of the worry often seems to be trivial, e.g. getting the housework done or being late for appointments, but to the patient it is insurmountable. The anxiety is often associated with other symptoms, which include restlessness, difficulty in concentrating, irritability, muscle tension and sleep disturbance. The course of the disorder is typically chronic with exacerbations at times of stress, and is often associated with depression. Its chronic nature with worsening at times of stress helps to distinguish GAD from anxiety in the form of episodic panic attacks with associated anticipatory anxiety (panic disorder). Hyperthyroidism and caffeinism should also be excluded.

Treatment. In modern times the drugs recommended as first-line treatments for GAD include SSRIs (escitalopram, sertraline and paroxetine having the strongest evidence), SNRIs (both venlafaxine and duloxetine) and the calcium channel modulator drug pregabalin. Among these, paroxetine, escitalopram, venlafaxine, duloxetine and pregabalin have licenses for this disorder in the UK. Other drugs having evidence for efficacy include agomelatine, trazodone, vortioxetine, the tricyclic imipramine, as well as several benzodiazepines, the antipsychotic quetiapine, and other anxiolytics such as hydroxyzine and buspirone.

Pregabalin has several randomized trials which support its efficacy in GAD, including one exclusively in the elderly. It is thought to act through the glutamate system although its mechanism is not fully understood. It works more slowly than the benzodiazepines, though faster than SSRIs. Despite its name, it does not have any effect on the neurotransmitter GABA. Its most prominent side-effects are dizziness and somnolence. Pregabalin can be combined effectively with SSRIs or SNRIs in GAD, and is also associated with allowing a reduction in benzodiazepine intake.

Historically *benzodiazepines* have been seen as an effective treatment for GAD as they rapidly reduce anxiety and improve sleep and somatic symptoms. Consequently, patients like taking them, but the chronic nature of GAD raises issues of duration of treatment, tolerance, dependence and withdrawal reactions. See recent benzodiazepine prescribing guidelines.[5]

Another sedative drug, the antihistamine *hydrozyzine*, is also used in GAD, but excessive sedation can be an issue.

Buspirone is structurally unrelated to other anxiolytics and was the first non-benzodiazepine to demonstrate efficacy in GAD. While its mode of action is not well understood, it is a $5HT_{1A}$-receptor partial agonist and over time produces anxiolysis without undue sedation. Buspirone is generally less effective and slower in action than benzodiazepines and does not improve sleep; it does not benefit benzodiazepine withdrawal symptoms but has the advantages that it does not seem to cause dependence or withdrawal reactions and does not interact with alcohol. It is less effective in patients who have previously received benzodiazepines and is therefore probably best reserved for benzodiazepine-naïve patients. A disadvantage is that useful anxiolytic effect is delayed for 2 weeks or longer.

---

[5]Baldwin D S, Aitchison K, Bateson A et al 2013 Benzodiazepines: Risks and benefits. A reconsideration. Journal of Psychopharmacology 27:967-971.

A delayed response in GAD is not as problematic as with acute situational anxiety. A sensible approach is to start with an antidepressant (SSRI or *venlafaxine*) for 6–8 weeks at least, increasing over 2–3 weeks to minimise unwanted actions; patients should be warned not to expect an immediate benefit. Those who do not respond should receive pregabalin (as monotherapy or an augmentation), with agomelatine, *buspirone*, quetiapine and vortioxetine being further alternatives. There remain some patients, including those with a long history of benzodiazepine use, who yet fail to respond despite extensive medication trials. A benzodiazepine may be the only medication that provides relief for such resistant cases, and in these circumstances can be used as the sole treatment provided there is adequate supervision with attempts to reduce benzodiazepine intake at regular intervals.

The *duration of therapy* depends on the nature of the underlying illness. If symptoms are intermittent, i.e. triggered by anxiety-provoking situations, then intermittent use of a *benzodiazepine* (for a few weeks) may be sufficient. More typically GAD requires treatment over 6–18 months with gradual withdrawal of medication thereafter.

Simple phobia

A specific phobia is a fear of a circumscribed object or situation, for instance fear of spiders, of flying, of heights. The diagnosis is not usually in doubt. A course of treatment by a trained therapist, involving graded exposure to the feared stimulus is the treatment of choice and can be very effective. By its nature such therapy generates severe anxiety, and a *benzodiazepine* (or prior treatment with an SSRI, e.g. *paroxetine*) may be necessary to allow patients to engage in therapy.

Obsessive–compulsive disorder (OCD)

Obsessive–compulsive disorder has two main components:

- The repetition of acts or thoughts which are involuntary, recognised by the sufferer to be generated by their own brain but unwanted, irrational, and out of keeping with their morals or values, and so very distressing.
- Anxiety provoked by the occurrence of such thoughts, or by prevention of the compulsive acts.

OCD on its own often starts in adolescence and has a chronic and pervasive course unless treated. OCD starting later in life is often associated with affective or anxiety disorders. Symptoms often abate briefly if the individual is taken to a new environment.

Drug treatments are *SSRIs*, venlafaxine or *clomipramine* (i.e. antidepressants that enhance serotonergic function), used at higher doses and for much longer periods than for depressive disorders. *Atypical antipsychotics* or *haloperidol* in low dose and *benzodiazepines* can be used successfully to augment the SSRIs if they are not wholly effective, especially in patients with tics. Psychosurgery is still occasionally used for severe and treatment-resistant cases, though deep brain stimulation techniques are superseding it. Interestingly the brain pathway targeted is one that recent neuroimaging studies of OCD have revealed as overactive, namely the basal ganglia/orbitofrontal pathway.

General comments about treating anxiety disorders (Table 20.7)

- There is a need to discuss the benefits and risks of specific treatments with patients before treatment and take account of their clinical features, needs, preferences and availability of local services when choosing treatments.
- SSRIs are usually effective in anxiety disorders and are generally suitable for first-line treatment.
- Benzodiazepines are effective in many anxiety disorders, but their use should be short term except in treatment-resistant cases.
- SNRIs, TCAs, MAOIs, pregabalin and antipsychotics need to be considered in relation to their evidence base for specific conditions and their individual risks and benefits.
- With all antidepressants, especially SSRIs and SNRIs, there should be specific discussion and monitoring of possible adverse effects early in treatment, and also on stopping the drugs after 1 week of treatment; this latter also applies to benzodiazepines.
- SSRI/SNRI treatment is often slow to produce the therapeutic effect, and it is advisable to allow 6–12 weeks to assess efficacy.
- In a first episode, patients may need medication for at least 6–12 months, and up to 18 months in GAD, withdrawing over a further 4–8 weeks if they are well. Those with recurrent illness may need treatment for longer periods of up to two years to enable them to learn and put into place psychological approaches to their problems. In many cases the illness is lifelong, and chronic maintenance treatment is justified if it significantly improves their well-being and function.
- Specific psychological treatments are also effective in treatment.
- When initial treatments fail, consider switching to another evidence-based treatment, combining evidence-based treatments (only when there are no contraindications), and referring to regional or national specialist services in refractory patients.

Table 20.7 Properties of anti-anxiety drugs

	Benzodiazepines	Buspirone	Pregabalin	Antidepressants (SSRIs/SNRIs)
Onset	Fast	Medium	Medium	Slow
Initial worsening of symptoms	No	Rarely	No	Sometimes
Withdrawal symptoms	Sometimes	No	Rarely	Sometimes (mostly paroxetine and venlafaxine)
Abuse potential	Yes	Zero	Sometimes	Zero
Interactions with alcohol	Marked	Slight	Slight	Slight
Sedation	Yes	Slight	Sometimes	No
Amnesia	Yes	No	Rare	No
Cardiovascular	No	Rare (reports of chest pain, tachycardia)	Rare (reports of worsening of congestive cardiac failure)*	Sometimes (e.g. citalopram, QTC prolongation, venlafaxine, hypertension)
Gastrointestinal	No	Slight	No	Yes – diarrhoea
Sexual	No	No	No	Delay orgasm

*There have been some reports of worsening of pre-existing congestive cardiac failure with pregabalin.

Drugs for insomnia

Insomnia has many potential precipitants, including psychological factors, psychiatric disorders, drug effects and physical problems (Box 20.1). Sleep–wake function involves a complex balance between arousing and sleep-inducing physiological systems. Current research suggests that arousal and wakefulness are promoted by parallel neurotransmitter systems whose cell bodies are located in brainstem or midbrain centres, with projections to the thalamus and forebrain. These activating neurotransmitters are noradrenaline/norepinephrine, serotonin, acetylcholine, dopamine and histamine. In addition, the newly discovered orexin system with cell bodies in the hypothalamus promotes wakefulness through regulating arousal 'pathways' (and inhibiting sedative ones). For all these arousal neurotransmitters, sleep can be promoted by blocking their post-synaptic actions, leading to reduced arousal. For example, many over-the-counter sleep-promoting agents contain antihistamines, which block the histamine H_1-receptor and so decrease arousal. The relatively low efficacy of these compounds may be explained by the

fact that they target only one of the parallel arousal systems. The same is true for any drug which blocks one of the other arousal systems; they produce a degree of sedation but are not generally effective hypnotics.

The promotion of sleep is regulated by a number of other neurotransmitters; primary among these is γ-aminobutyric acid (GABA), the major inhibitory neurotransmitter in the brain. The majority of brain cells are inhibited by GABA, so increasing its function reduces arousal and produces sleep, and eventually anaesthesia. There are many subsets of GABA neurones distributed throughout the brain, but a particular cluster in the hypothalamus (ventrolateral preoptic nucleus) can be considered to be the sleep 'switch'.[6] These neurones switch off brain arousal systems at the level of the cell bodies and therefore promote sleep. GABA receptors in the cortex can also promote sedation and sleep by inhibiting the target

[6]Saper C B, Scammell T E, Lu J 2005 Hypothalamic regulation of sleep and circadian rhythms. Nature 437:1257–1263.

Box 20.1 **Precipitating factors for insomnia**

Psychological

- Hyperarousal due to: *stress*
- The need to be *vigilant* at night because of sick relatives or young children
- Being *'on call'*.

Psychiatric

- Patients with *depressive illnesses* often have difficulty falling asleep at night and complain of restless, disturbed and unrefreshing sleep, and early morning waking. When their sleep is analysed by polysomnography, time to sleep onset is indeed prolonged, and there is a tendency for more REM sleep to occur in the first part of the night, with reduced deep quiet sleep in the first hour or so after sleep onset, and increased awakenings during the night. They may wake early in the morning and fail to get back to sleep again.
- *Anxiety* disorders may cause patients to complain about their sleep, either because there is a reduction in sleep continuity or because normal periods of nocturnal waking are somehow less well tolerated. Nocturnal panic attacks can make patients fearful of going off to sleep.
- *Bipolar* patients in the hypomanic or manic phase will sleep less than usual, and often changes in sleep pattern give early warning that an episode is imminent.

Pharmacological

- Non-prescription drugs such as *caffeine* or *alcohol*. Alcohol reduces the time to onset of sleep, but disrupts sleep later in the night. Regular and excessive consumption disrupts sleep continuity; insomnia is a key feature of alcohol withdrawal. Excessive intake of caffeine and theophylline, in tea, coffee or cola drinks, also contributes to sleeplessness, probably because caffeine acts as an antagonist to adenosine,

the endogenous sleep-promoting neurotransmitter.
- Starting treatment with certain *antidepressants,* especially selective serotonin reuptake inhibitors (e.g. fluoxetine, fluvoxamine) or monoamine uptake inhibitors; sleep disruption is likely to resolve after 3–4 weeks.
- Other drugs that increase central noradrenergic and serotonergic activity include stimulants, such as amfetamine, cocaine and methylphenidate, and *sympathomimetics,* such as the β-adrenergic agonist salbutamol and associated substances.
- *Withdrawal* from hypnotic drugs; this is usually short lived.
- Treatment with *β-adrenoceptor blockers* may disrupt sleep, perhaps because of their serotonergic action; a β-blocking drug that crosses blood–brain barrier less readily is preferred, e.g. atenolol.

Physical

- *Pain,* in which case adequate analgesia will improve sleep.
- *Pregnancy*.
- *Coughing* or wheezing: adequate control of asthma with stimulating drugs as above, may paradoxically improve sleep by reducing waking due to breathlessness.
- *Respiratory and cardiovascular disorders*.
- *Need to urinate;* this may be affected by timing of diuretic medication.
- *Neurological disorders,* e.g. stroke, movement disorders.
- *Periodic leg movements of sleep* (frequent jerks or twitches during the descent into deeper sleep); rarely reduce subjective sleep quality but are more likely to cause them in the subject's sleeping partner.
- *Restless legs syndrome* (irresistible desire to move the legs), which is usually worse in the evening and early night and can prevent sleep.

---

neurones of the arousal system. Most drugs used in insomnia act by increasing the effects of GABA at the GABA$_A$ receptor.

The GABA$_A$–benzodiazepine receptor complex

γ-Aminobutyric acid (GABA) is the most important inhibitory transmitter in the central nervous system, comprising up to 40% of all synapses. GABAergic neurones are distributed widely in the CNS, and GABA controls the state of neuronal excitability in all brain areas. The balance between *excitatory* inputs (mostly glutamatergic) and *inhibitory* GABAergic activity determines neuronal activity. If the balance swings

in favour of GABA, then sedation, amnesia, muscle relaxation and ataxia appear and nervousness and anxiety are reduced. The mildest reduction of GABAergic activity (or increase in glutamate) elicits arousal, anxiety, restlessness, insomnia and exaggerated reactivity.

When GABA binds with the GABA$_A$ receptor, the permeability of the central pore of the receptor complex opens, so allowing more chloride ions into the neurone and decreasing excitability. Classical benzodiazepines (BZDs) in clinical use bind to another receptor on the complex (the benzodiazepine receptor) and enhance the effectiveness of GABA, producing a larger inhibitory effect (Fig. 20.5). These drugs are agonists at the receptor and an antagonist,

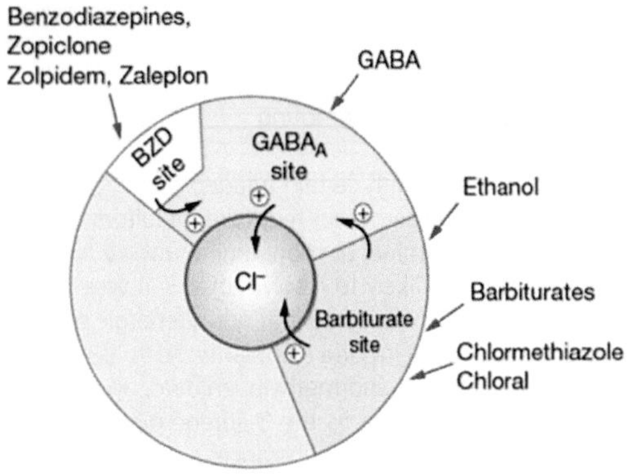

Fig. 20.5 Schematic representation of the binding sites on the GABA$_A$-benzodiazepine receptor complex. Note that drugs binding to the benzodiazepine (BZD) receptor site do not open the chloride channel directly, but rather augment the capacity of GABA to do so. Conversely, agents such as the barbiturates both potentiate GABA and at higher concentrations have a direct effect on the chloride channel. This explains why barbiturates and alcohols are more toxic in overdose than the benzodiazepines.

flumazenil, prevents agonists from binding at the receptor site; it is used clinically to reverse benzodiazepine actions.

Benzodiazepines

A general account of the benzodiazepines is appropriate here, although their indications extend beyond use as hypnotics. All *benzodiazepines,* and newer *benzodiazepine-like* drugs such as zopiclone and zolpidem, are safe and effective for insomnia if the substance with the right timing of onset of action and elimination is chosen. They should not be used for patients with sleep-related breathing disorders such as obstructive sleep apnoea (see below), which is exacerbated by benzodiazepines. Objective measures of sleep show that they decrease time to sleep onset and waking during the night. They also improve subjective sleep. Other changes in sleep architecture are to some extent dependent on duration of action, with the very short-acting compounds having the least effect. Most commonly very light (stage 1) sleep is decreased, and stage 2 sleep is increased. Higher doses of longer-acting benzodiazepines partially suppress slow wave sleep.

Pharmacokinetics. Benzodiazepines are effective after administration by mouth but enter the circulation at very different rates that are reflected in the speed of onset of action, e.g. *alprazolam* is rapid, *oxazepam* is slow (Table 20.8). Hepatic breakdown produces metabolites, some with long $t_{1/2}$ which greatly extend drug action, e.g. *chlordiazepoxide, clorazepate* and *diazepam* all form demethyldiazepam ($t_{1/2}$ 80 h).

Uses. Oral benzodiazepines are used for insomnia, anxiety, alcohol withdrawal states, muscle spasm due to a variety of causes, including tetanus and cerebral spasticity. Injectable preparations are used for rapid tranquillisation in psychosis (see previous section), anaesthesia and sedation for minor surgery and invasive investigations (see Index). The choice of drug as hypnotic and anxiolytic is determined by pharmacokinetic properties (see before, and Table 20.7).

Doses. Oral doses appear in Table 20.8.

Tolerance to the anxiolytic effects does not seem to be a problem. In *sleep disorders* the situation is not so clear; studies of subjective sleep quality show enduring efficacy, and the necessity for dose escalation in sleep disorders is rare, but the objective sleep effects have not been studied systematically over weeks and months.

Dependence. Both animal and human research has shown that brain GABA$_A$ receptors do change in function during chronic treatment with benzodiazepines, and therefore will take time to return to pre-medication status after cessation. Features of withdrawal and dependence vary. Commonly there is a kind of psychological dependence based on the fact that the treatment works to reduce patients' anxiety or sleep disturbance, and therefore they are unwilling to stop. If they do stop, there can be *relapse,* where original symptoms return. There can also be a *rebound of symptoms,* particularly after stopping hypnotics, with a worsening of sleep disturbance for one or two nights, longer sleep onset latency and increased waking during sleep – this is common. In anxiety disorders there may be a few days of increased anxiety and edginess which then resolves, probably in 10–20% of patients. More rarely, there is a *longer withdrawal syndrome* that is characterised by the emergence of symptoms not previously experienced, e.g. agitation, headache, dizziness, dysphoria, irritability, fatigue, depersonalisation, hypersensitivity to noise and visual stimuli. Physical symptoms include nausea, vomiting, muscle cramps, sweating, weakness, muscle pain or twitching and ataxia. After prolonged high doses, abrupt withdrawal may cause confusion, delirium, psychosis and convulsions. The syndrome is ameliorated by resuming medication but resolves in weeks; in a very few patients it persists, and these people have been the subject of much research, mainly focusing on their personality and cognitive factors.

Withdrawal of benzodiazepines should be gradual after as little as 3 weeks' use, but for long-term users it should be very slow, e.g. about ⅛ of the dose every 2 weeks, aiming to complete it in 6–12 weeks. Withdrawal should be slowed if marked symptoms occur, and it may be useful to substitute a drug with a long $t_{1/2}$ (*diazepam*) to minimise rapid fluctuations in plasma concentrations. Abandonment of the final dose may be particularly distressing. In difficult cases, withdrawal may be assisted by concomitant use of an antidepressant.

Table 20.8 Properties of drugs used for insomnia

	Works selectively to enhance GABA	Rapid onset	$t_{1/2}$ (h)	Usual oral dose	Daytime (hangover) effects	Safety
Zopiclone	✓	+	3.5–6	7.5 mg	?Yes	✓
Zolpidem	✓	++	1.5–3	10 mg	No	✓✓
Zaleplon*	✓	++	1–2	10 mg	No	✓
Temazepam	✓		5–12	20 mg	?Yes	✓
Loprazolam	✓		5–13	1 mg	?Yes	✓
Lormetazepam	✓	+	8–10	1 mg	?Yes	✓
Nitrazepam	✓	+	20–48	5–10 mg	Yes	✓
Lorazepam	✓	+	10–20	0.5–1 mg	Yes	✓
Diazepam	✓	+	20–60	5–10 mg	Yes	✓
Oxazepam	✓		5–20	15–30 mg	Yes	✓
Alprazolam	✓	+	9–20	0.5 mg	Yes	✓
Clonazepam	✓	+	18–50	0.5–1 mg	Yes	✓
Prolonged-release melatonin (patients older than 55)	X		3–4	2 mg	No	✓
Ramelteon	X		1–1.5	8 mg	No	✓
Chloral hydrate/chloral betaine	X	+	8–12	0.7–1 g	?Yes	X
Clomethiazole	X	+	4–8	192 mg	?Yes	X
Barbiturates	X	+			Yes	X
Promethazine	X		7–14	25 mg	?Yes	X/✓

*Can be taken during the night, until 5 h before needing to drive etc.

Adverse effects. In addition to the above, benzodiazepines affect memory and balance. Hazards with car driving or operating machinery can arise from sedation, amnesia and impaired psychomotor function. Amnesia for events subsequent to administration occurs with high doses given i.v., e.g. for endoscopy, dental surgery (with local anaesthetic), cardioversion. Paradoxical behaviour effects and perceptual disorders, e.g. hallucinations occur occasionally. Headache, giddiness, alimentary tract upsets, skin rashes and reduced libido can occur.

Benzodiazepines in pregnancy. Benzodiazepines should be avoided in early pregnancy as far as possible as their safety is not established with certainty. Safety in pregnancy is not only a matter of avoiding prescription during an established pregnancy, for individuals may become pregnant on long-term therapy. Benzodiazepines cross the placenta and can cause fetal cardiac arrhythmia, muscular hypotonia, poor suckling, hypothermia and respiratory depression in the newborn.

Interactions. The benzodiazepines offer scope for adverse interaction with numerous agents, but the underlying mechanisms can be summarised. The principal *pharmacodynamic* interaction of concern is exacerbation of *sedation* with other centrally depressant drugs, H_1-receptor antihistamines, antipsychotics, opioids, alcohol and general anaesthetics. All are likely to exacerbate breathing difficulties where this is already compromised, e.g. in obstructive sleep apnoea. Unexpected *hypotension* may occur with any co-prescribed antihypertensive drug, and vasodilators, e.g. nitrates.

Pharmacokinetic interactions occur with drugs that slow metabolism by *enzyme inhibition*, e.g. ritonavir, indinavir, itraconazole, olanzapine, cimetidine, fluvoxamine, erythromycin, increasing benzodiazepine effect. By contrast, acceleration of metabolism, lowering of plasma concentration and reduced effect occur with *enzyme inducers*, e.g. rifampicin.

Overdose. Benzodiazepines are remarkably safe in acute overdose, and even 10 times the therapeutic dose only produces deep sleep from which the subject is easily aroused. It is said that there is no reliably recorded case of death from a benzodiazepine taken alone by a person in good physical (particularly respiratory) health, which is a remarkable tribute to their safety (high therapeutic index); even if the statement is not absolutely true, death must be extremely rare. But deaths have occurred in combination with alcohol (which combination is quite usual in those seeking to end their own lives) and opiates, e.g. buprenorphine and methadone. Flumazenil selectively reverses benzodiazepine effects and is useful in diagnosis, and in treatment (see below).

Benzodiazepine antagonist. *Flumazenil* is a highly selective competitive antagonist at benzodiazepine receptors so does not oppose sedation due to non-benzodiazepines, e.g. barbiturates, alcohol.

Clinical uses include reversal of benzodiazepine sedation after endoscopy, dentistry and in intensive care. Heavily sedated patients become alert within 5 minutes. The $t_{1/2}$ of 1 h is much shorter than that of most benzodiazepines (see Table 20.7), so that repeated i.v. administration may be needed to maintain the effect. Thus the recovery period needs supervision lest sedation recurs; if used in day surgery, it is important to tell patients that they may not drive a car home. The dose is 200 µg by i.v. injection given over 15 s, followed by 100 µg over 60 s if necessary, to a maximum of 300–600 µg. Flumazenil is useful for diagnosis of self-poisoning, and also for treatment, when 100–400 µg are given by continuous i.v. infusion and adjusted to the degree of wakefulness.

Adverse effects can include brief anxiety, seizures in epileptics treated with a benzodiazepine and precipitation of withdrawal syndrome in dependent subjects.

Non-benzodiazepine hypnotics that act at the GABA$_A$-benzodiazepine receptor

Although structurally unrelated to the benzodiazepines, these drugs act on the same receptor, so their effects can be blocked by flumazenil, the receptor antagonist. Those described below are all effective in insomnia and have low propensity for tolerance, rebound insomnia, withdrawal symptoms and abuse potential. Data from long-term studies suggest these agents are safe and effective over at least 12 months. Withdrawal effects similar to the benzodiazepines hypnotics occur but to a lesser extent.

Zopiclone, a cyclopyrrolone, has an onset of action that is relatively rapid (~1 h) and that lasts for 6–8 h, making it suitable for both initial and maintenance treatment of insomnia. It may cause fewer problems on withdrawal than benzodiazepines. The duration of action is prolonged in the elderly, and in hepatic insufficiency. About 40% of patients experience a metallic aftertaste (genetically determined). People who take zopiclone have been shown to be at increased risk of road traffic accidents. Care should be taken with concomitant medication that affects its metabolic pathway (see Table 20.2A).

Zolpidem, an imidazopyridine, has a faster onset (30–60 min) and shorter duration of action. In patients over 80 years of age, clearance is slower and action longer lasting.

Zaleplon, a pyrazolopyrimidine, has a fast onset and short duration of action. In volunteers, it appeared to have no effect on psychomotor (including driving) skills when taken at least 5 h before testing. It may be taken during the night when the patient has awoken and cannot get back to sleep, as long as this is at least 5 h before having to drive.

Other drugs that act on the GABA$_A$-benzodiazepine receptor

Chloral hydrate, clomethiazole and barbiturates also enhance GABA function, but at high doses have the additional capacity directly to open the membrane chloride channel; this may lead to potentially lethal respiratory depression and explains their low therapeutic ratio. These drugs also have a propensity for abuse/misuse and thus are very much second-line treatments.

Chloral hydrate has a fast (30–60 min) onset of action and 6–8 h duration of action. Chloral hydrate, a prodrug, is rapidly metabolised by alcohol dehydrogenase into the active hypnotic *trichloroethanol* ($t_{1/2}$ 8 h). Chloral hydrate is dangerous in serious hepatic or renal impairment, and aggravates peptic ulcer. Interaction with ethanol is to be expected since both are metabolised by alcohol dehydrogenase. Alcohol (ethanol) also appears to induce the formation of trichloroethanol which attains higher concentrations if alcohol is taken, increasing sedation. Triclofos and chloral betaine are related compounds.

Clomethiazole is structurally related to vitamin B$_1$ (thiamine) and is a hypnotic, sedative and anticonvulsant. When taken orally, it is subject to extensive hepatic first-pass metabolism (which is defective in the elderly and in liver-damaged alcoholics who exhibit higher peak plasma concentrations); the $t_{1/2}$ is 4 h. It may also be given i.v. It is comparatively free from hangover, but it can cause nasal irritation and sneezing. Dependence occurs, and use should always be brief.

Barbiturates are hardly ever used as they have a low therapeutic index, i.e. relatively small overdose may endanger life; they also cause dependence and have been popular drugs of abuse.

Other drugs used in insomnia

Antihistamines. Most proprietary (over-the-counter) sleep remedies contain H_1-receptor antihistamines with sedative action (see Ch. 9). Promethazine (Phenergan) has a slow (1–2 h) onset and long duration of action ($t_{1/2}$ 12 h). It reduces sleep onset latency and awakenings during the night after a single dose, but there have been no studies showing enduring action. It is sometimes used as a hypnotic in children. There are no controlled studies showing improvements in sleep after other antihistamines. Alimemazine (trimeprazine) is used for short-term sedation in children. Most antihistamine sedatives have a relatively long action and may cause daytime sedation.

Antidepressants. In the depressed patient, improvement in mood is almost always accompanied by improvement in subjective sleep, and therefore choice of antidepressant should not usually involve additional consideration of sleep effects. Nevertheless, some patients are more likely to continue with medication if there is a short-term improvement, in which case *mirtazapine* or *trazodone* may provide effective antidepressant together with sleep-promoting effects. Antidepressant drugs, particularly those with $5HT_2$-blocking effects, may occasionally be effective in long-term insomnia (but see Table 20.7). Paradoxically, paroxetine, an SSRI, has proved to be particularly useful for insomnia in patients older than 55 years of age, probably due to its anxiolytic effect by reducing nighttime ruminations. Agomelatine, technically an antidepressant, is both a $5HT_{2C}$ antagonist and a melatonin MT_1 and MT_2 receptor agonist. It improves sleep quality in patients with depression with no increase in diurnal sedation. It may increase liver enzymes, and rarely serious liver adverse effects have been reported. Periodic monitoring of transaminases is recommended.

Antipsychotics have been used to promote sleep in resistant insomnia occurring as part of another psychiatric disorder, probably because of the combination of $5HT_2$-antagonism, α_1-adrenoceptor antagonism and histamine H_1-receptor antihistamine effects in addition to their primary dopamine antagonist effects. Antipsychotics olanzapine, quetiapine, and ziprasidone both as monotherapy and as augmentation agents improve sleep patterns and promote continuation of sleep in patients with major depression and bipolar disorder. Their long action leads to daytime sedation, and extrapyramidal movement disorders may result from their blockade of dopamine receptors (see above, Antipsychotics). They therefore should be used with great care in the context of insomnia. Nevertheless, modern antipsychotics, e.g. *quetiapine*, are being used for intractable insomnia, usually

at a dose well below the one required to treat psychosis, e.g. 25–50 mg/day.

Melatonin, the hormone produced by the pineal gland during darkness, has been investigated for insomnia. A prolonged release formulation is licensed for insomnia characterised by poor quality of sleep in people older than 55 years of age, whose melatonin rhythm is thought to be reduced. Melatonin may also be used therapeutically to reset circadian rhythm to prevent jet lag on long-haul flights, and for blind or partially sighted people who cannot use daylight to synchronise their natural rhythm. Slow-release formulations of melatonin are particularly useful in patients older than 55 years of age, as melatonin production declines with age.

Melatonin is metabolised mainly by CYP 1A enzymes and may interact with other active substances that affect these enzymes. For this reason, it should not be taken with fluvoxamine, 5- or 8-methoxypsoralen, or cimetidine, and caution should be exercised in patients on oestrogens (e.g. contraceptive or hormone replacement therapy).

Ramelteon is a melatonin agonist targeting sleep-onset problems. It promotes sleep via MT_1 receptors and synchronizing the circadian clock through MT_2 receptors. It has a short $t_{1/2}$ (~90 min).

Suvorexant is an orexin receptor antagonist (for orexin 1 and orexin 2 receptor). It is indicated for problems with sleep onset and sleep maintenance. It blocks the effects of the peptide orexin, which maintains wakefulness and regulates the sleep-wake cycle.

Herbal preparations. Randomised trials have shown some effect of valerian in mild to moderate insomnia.

Summary of pharmacotherapy for insomnia
- Drug treatment is usually effective for a short period (2–4 weeks).
- Some patients may need long-term medication.
- Intermittent medication which is taken only on nights that symptoms occur is desirable and may often be possible with modern, short-acting compounds.
- Discontinuing hypnotic drugs is usually not a problem if the patient knows what to expect. There will be a short period (usually 1–2 nights) of rebound insomnia on stopping hypnotic drugs, which can be ameliorated by phased withdrawal.

Hypersomnia

Sleep-related breathing disorders causing excessive daytime sleepiness are rarely treated with drugs. Sleepiness caused by the nighttime disruption of sleep apnoea syndrome is sometimes not completely abolished by the standard treatment of continuous positive airway pressure overnight, and wake-promoting drugs, e.g. modafinil, may have a role in these patients.

Narcolepsy is a chronic neurological disorder, characterised by excessive daytime sleepiness (EDS) and sleep attacks, usually accompanied by **cataplexy** (attacks of muscle weakness on emotional arousal). These symptoms are often associated with the intrusion into wakefulness of other elements of REM sleep, such as sleep paralysis and hypnagogic hallucinations, i.e. in a transient state preceding sleep.

Stimulants are effective in the treatment of EDS due to narcolepsy. *Modafinil* is usually preferred as it is not a controlled drug, failing which methylphenidate or dexamfetamine are added or substituted. In *narcolepsy*, patients usually need a stimulant for their hypersomnia and an antidepressant for their cataplexy. Combining an SSRI antidepressant with modafinil has been shown to be safe, but dexamfetamine and methylphenidate must not be given with MAOIs. *Cataplexy* is most effectively treated with 5HT uptake–blocking drugs such as clomipramine or fluoxetine, or other antidepressant drugs, e.g. reboxetine, or the MAOI selegiline.

Modafinil is a wake-promoting agent whose specific mechanism of action is not properly known; it does not appear to be overtly stimulant like the amfetamines. Its onset of action is slow and lasts 8–12 h. Potential for abuse is low. Modafinil is used in narcolepsy and other hypersomnias (e.g. that with sleep apnoea) and also promotes wakefulness in normal patients who need to stay awake for long periods, e.g. military personnel. Its use is associated with a wide variety of gastrointestinal, CNS and other unwanted effects; contraindications to its use include moderate to severe hypertension, a history of left ventricular hypertrophy or cor pulmonale. Modafinil accelerates the metabolism of oral contraceptives, reducing their efficacy.

Amfetamines release dopamine and noradrenaline/norepinephrine in the brain. This causes a behavioural excitation, with increased alertness, elevation of mood, increase in physical activity and suppression of appetite. *Dexamfetamine*, the dextrorotatory isomer of amfetamine, is about twice as active in humans as the levo-isomer and is the main prescribed amfetamine. It is rapidly absorbed orally and acts for 3–24 h; most people with narcolepsy find twice-a-day dosing optimal to maintain alertness during the day. About 40% of narcoleptic patients find it necessary to increase their dose, suggesting some tolerance. Although physical dependence does not occur, mental and physical depression may develop following withdrawal.

Unwanted effects include edginess, restlessness, insomnia, appetite suppression, weight loss, and increase in blood pressure and heart rate. Amfetamines are commonly abused because of their stimulant effect, but this is rare in narcolepsy. Contraindications to its use include moderate to severe hypertension, hyperthyroidism, and a history of drug or alcohol abuse.

Methylphenidate also promotes dopamine release, but its principal action is to inhibit uptake of central neurotransmitters. Its effects and adverse effects resemble those of the amfetamines. Methylphenidate has a low systemic availability and slow onset of action, making it less liable to abuse. It is also used in attention deficit/hyperactivity disorder (see below). *Unwanted effects* include anxiety, anorexia, hypertension, increase in pulse rate and difficulty sleeping; these usually subside. Methylphenidate reduces expected weight gain and has been associated with slight growth retardation. Monitoring of therapy should include height (in children) and weight, also blood pressure and blood counts (thrombocytopenia and leucopenia occur). It should not be used in patients with hyperthyroidism, severe angina, or cardiac arrhythmias.

Parasomnias

Nightmares arise out of REM sleep and are reported by the patient as structured, often stereotyped dreams that are very distressing. Usually the patient wakes up fully and remembers the dream. Psychological methods of treatment may be appropriate, e.g. a programme of rehearsing the dream and inventing a different pleasant ending. Nightmares of a particularly distressing kind are a feature of post-traumatic stress disorder. Case reports indicate benefit from various pharmacological agents, but no particular drug emerges as superior.

Night terrors and sleep-walking arise from slow-wave sleep, and they are often coexistent. There is usually a history dating from childhood, and often a family history. Exacerbations commonly coincide with periods of stress, and alcohol increases their likelihood. In a night terror, patients usually sit or jump up from deep sleep (mostly in the first few hours of sleep) with a loud cry, look terrified and move violently, sometimes injuring themselves or others. They appear asleep and uncommunicative, often returning to sleep without being aware of the event. These terrors are thought to be a welling up of anxiety from deep centres in the brain which is normally inhibited by cortical mechanisms. If the disorder is sufficiently frequent or disabling, night terrors respond to the SSRI paroxetine (also effective in sleepwalkers) or the benzodiazepine clonazepam.

REM behaviour disorder first described in 1986, consists of lack of paralysis during REM sleep which results in brief acting out of dreams, often vigorously with injury to self or others. Rarely, it can occur acutely as a result of drug or alcohol withdrawal, or in patients taking high doses of antidepressants such as clomipramine, venlafaxine or mirtazapine. More commonly it is chronic and either idiopathic or associated with neurological disorder. It is much commoner among older patients, and approximately 90% are male. It may be a very early prodrome to the onset of Parkinson's disease, Lewy body dementia or multiple system atrophy. Successful symptomatic relief has been described with clonazepam or clonidine.

Other sleep disorders

Restless legs syndrome (RLS) is a disorder characterised by disagreeable leg sensations usually prior to sleep onset, and an almost irresistible urge to move the legs. The sensation is described as 'crawling', 'aching', 'tingling' and is partially or completely relieved with leg motion returning after movement ceases. Most, if not all, patients with this complaint also have *periodic limb movements of sleep* (PLMS), which may occur independently of RLS. These periodic limb movements consist of highly stereotyped movements, usually of the legs, that occur repeatedly (typically every 20–40 s) during the night. They may wake the patient, in which case there may be a complaint of daytime sleepiness or occasionally insomnia, but often only awaken the sleeping partner, who is usually kicked. RLS may respond to formulations of levodopa or dopamine agonists.

Sleep scheduling disorders. Circadian rhythm disorders are often confused with insomnia, and both can be present in the same patient. With such sleep scheduling disorders, sleep occurs at the 'wrong' time, i.e. at a time that does not fit with work, social or family commitments. A typical pattern may be a difficulty in initiating sleep for a few nights due to stress, whereupon once asleep the subject continues sleeping well into the morning to 'catch up' the lost sleep. Thereafter the 'time since last sleep' cue for sleep initiation is delayed, and the sleep period gradually becomes more delayed until the subject is sleeping in the day instead of at night. A behavioural programme with strategic light exposure is appropriate, with pharmacological treatment as an adjunct, e.g. melatonin, to help reset the sleep–wake schedule.

Drugs for Alzheimer's[7] disease (dementia)

Dementia is described as a syndrome 'due to disease of the brain, usually of chronic or progressive nature, in which there is disturbance of multiple higher cortical functions, including memory, thinking, orientation, comprehension,

calculation, learning capacity, language and judgement, without clouding of consciousness'.[8]

Deterioration in emotional control, social behaviour or motivation may accompany or precede cognitive impairment. Alzheimer's and vascular (multi-infarct) disease are the two most common forms of dementia, accounting for about 80% of presentations. Alzheimer's disease is associated with deposition of β-amyloid in brain tissue and abnormal phosphorylation of the intracellular tau (τ) proteins causing abnormalities of microtubule assembly and collapse of the cytoskeleton. Pyramidal cells of the cortex and subcortex are particularly affected.

In Western countries, the prevalence of dementia is less than 1% in those 60–64 years of age, but doubles with each 5-year cohort to a figure of around 16% in those 80–84 years of age. The emotional impact of dementia on relatives and carers and the cost to society in social support and care facilities are great. Hence the impetus for an effective form of treatment is compelling.

Evidence indicates that *cholinergic transmission* is diminished in Alzheimer's disease. The first three drugs available for use in Alzheimer's each act to enhance *acetylcholine* activity by inhibiting the enzyme *acetylcholinesterase* which metabolises and inactivates synaptically released acetylcholine. Consequently, acetylcholine remains usable for longer. Individual drugs are categorised by the type of enzyme inhibition they cause. *Donepezil* is classed as a 'reversible' agent, as binding to the acetylcholinesterase enzymes lasts only minutes, whereas *rivastigmine* is considered 'pseudo-irreversible' as inhibition lasts for several hours. *Galantamine* is associated both with reversible inhibition and with enhanced acetylcholine action on nicotinic receptors.[9] Clinical trials show that these agents produce an initial increase in patients' cognitive ability. There also may be associated global benefits, including improvements in non-cognitive aspects such as depressive symptoms. But the drugs do not alter the underlying process, and the relentless progress of the disease is paralleled by a reduction in acetylcholine production with a decline in cognition.

A fourth drug licensed for use in Alzheimer's disease is *memantine*. Overactive glutamate signalling has been linked to cell death, and this drug is known to be a glutamine modulator through antagonism of NMDA receptors. Initially thought to have an entirely novel mode of action related to its effects on dampening excess glutamate neurotransmission, subsequent work suggests that memantine does have additional activity as an acetylcholine stimulant.

---

[7]Alois Alzheimer (1864–1915), German psychiatrist who studied the brains of demented and senile patients and correlated histological findings with clinical features.

[8]International Classification of Diseases, 10th edition, Diagnostic System.
[9]Irreversible antagonists exist but, not surprisingly, are not used in therapeutics (e.g. sarin nerve gas).

The beneficial effects of drugs are therefore to:

- *stabilise* the condition initially and sometimes improve cognitive function
- *delay* the overall pace of decline (and therefore the escalating levels of support required)
- *postpone* the onset of severe dementia.

The severity of cognitive deficits in patients suffering from, or suspected of having, dementia can be quantified by a simple 30-point schedule, the mini mental state examination (MMSE) of Folstein. A score of 21–26 denotes mild, 10–20 moderate and less than 10 severe Alzheimer's disease. The MMSE can also be used to monitor progress.

In 2001 the view of the UK National Institute for Health and Clinical Excellence (NICE) was that, subject to certain conditions, the drugs available at that time should be available as adjuvant therapy for those with an MMSE score above 12 points. Subsequent guidelines first suggested that the cost:benefit ratio for the three anticholinesterase inhibitor drugs was favourable only in those with moderate dementia (MMSE score between 10 and 20 points), only for this limitation to be subsequently removed. Guidelines for prescribing anticholinesterase inhibitors also advise the following:

- Alzheimer's disease must be diagnosed and assessed in a specialist clinic; the clinic should also assess cognitive, global and behavioural functioning, activities of daily living, and the likelihood of compliance with treatment.
- Treatment should be initiated by specialists but may be continued by family practitioners under a shared-care protocol.
- The carers' views of the condition should be sought before and during drug treatment.
- The patient should be assessed every 6 months, and drug treatment should continue only if the MMSE score remains at or above 10 points and if treatment has had a worthwhile effect on global, behavioural and functional parameters.

Use of memantine in dementia is now supported by good quality evidence, and it has been widely prescribed in the UK and many other countries. It enabled a reduction in the co-prescription of antipsychotic medication previously used for behavioural symptoms such as agitation and aggression. A small evidence base also suggests the hypothesis that the combination of memantine with an acetylcholinesterase inhibitor may be more effective than the acetylcholinesterase inhibitor alone, such that in severe Alzheimer's the combination of memantine with donepezil is now seen as a preferred option.

Doses are:

- Donepezil 5–10 mg nocte increasing to 10 mg nocte after 1 month.

- Galantamine 4 mg twice daily increasing to 8–12 mg twice daily at 4-week intervals.
- Rivastigmine 1.5 mg twice daily increasing to 3–6 mg twice daily at 2-week intervals.
- Memantine 5 mg daily increasing weekly by 5 mg to a maximum of 20 mg daily.

Adverse effects of the three anticholinesterse inhibitors inevitably include cholinergic symptoms, with nausea, diarrhoea and abdominal cramps appearing commonly. There may also be bradycardia, sinoatrial block, or atrio-ventricular block. Additionally, urinary incontinence, syncope, convulsions and psychiatric disturbances occur. Rapid dose increase appears to make symptoms more pronounced. Hepatotoxicity is a rare association with donepezil.

Memantine has a different side-effect profile with constipation, hypertension, headache, dizziness and drowsiness being highlighted as the most common adverse effects. Memantine has been reported as having an association with seizures, which may be a consideration in patients who have had previous fits.

The deterioration of function in dementia of Alzheimer's disease is often accompanied by acute behavioural disturbance. Memantine and the acetylcholinesterase inhibitors may be helpful in controlling this, but treatment with antipsychotics may be required in severe cases where agitation or aggression are a feature, or where psychotic symptoms are present. Be aware that if a person with dementia has Lewy body disease rather than Alzheimer's, antipsychotics may worsen the situation. Beyond antipsychotics, alternative drugs with randomized trial evidence for agitation or aggression in Alzheimer's dementia include the SSRI citalopram, the anticonvulsant carbamazepine and the central α-adrenoceptor–blocking agent prazosin, while the receptor-blocking agent trazodone has the strongest evidence in fronto-temporal dementia.

Drugs in attention deficit/ hyperactivity disorder

Attention deficit/hyperactivity disorder (ADHD) affects 5% of children and between 2% and 3% of adults in the UK (NICE 2008).[10] ADHD is characterised by inattention, impulsivity and motor overactivity. For diagnostic purposes, symptoms should be present before 12 years of age and cause pervasive impairment across situations, mostly (but not exclusively)

[10]National Institute for Health and Clinical Excellence, 2008. Attention Deficit Hyperactivity Disorder: Diagnosis and Management of ADHD in Children, Young People and Adults. NICE clinical guideline 72. Attention Deficit Hyperactivity Disorder: Diagnosis and Management of ADHD in Children, Young People and Adults. NICE clinical guideline 72. http://www.nice.org.uk/CG72. (Accessed 5 June 2015).

school and home in children, and work and relationships in adults. Treatment of ADHD should be initiated only by a specialist and form part of a comprehensive treatment programme of psychological, educational and social measures.

Stimulant drugs are the first-choice treatment for ADHD in both children and adults (Table 20.9). *Methylphenidate, dexamfetamine* and *lisdexamfetamine* increase synaptic dopamine and noradrenaline/norepinephrine; dexamfetamine and lisexamfetamine also block the reuptake of both neurotransmitters. Methylphenidate is the first-line treatment in the UK for ADHD; it is available both in conventional and extended-release formulations which can be combined to obtain maximum therapeutic effect. Treatment in children is frequently restricted to school terms, giving the child a 'drug holiday' when out of school. Drug holidays are necessary to determine efficacy of treatment, adjust or change dosage and avoid tolerance effects. Treatment in adults is more complex as attentional requirements are often continuous, so drug holidays may not be possible. Dosage tends to be slightly higher and combinations of different psychotropic drugs are more common. Dexamfetamine is an alternative that has similar efficacy to methylphenidate in ADHD and is the preferred drug in children with epilepsy. It has a greater potential for abuse than methylphenidate. Lisdexamfetamine is a compound of dexamfetamine and the amino acid l-lysine; it acts as a prodrug which becomes active only after hydrolysis in the blood, reducing potential for abuse.

Unwanted effects of stimulants include some slowing of growth, loss of appetite and sleep, irritability, increased blood pressure and rarely other cardiovascular problems. Weight, blood pressure and pulse should be monitored in both adults and children. In children, height should also be monitored to assess growth. Stimulants in instant-release formulations can be abused, and some have been diverted to intravenous injection; prodrug and slow-release formulations have recently been introduced to combat this problem. Both methylphenidate and dexamfetamine are controlled drugs in the UK (class B schedule 2 of the Misuse of Drugs Act), so prescribing restrictions apply.

Atomoxetine, a noradrenaline/norepinephrine reuptake inhibitor (like reboxetine), is now licenced for ADHD. It is thought to act by increasing noradrenaline/norepinephrine and dopamine availability in the frontal cortex (where dopamine is taken up into noradrenergic nerve terminals). It has no known abuse liability and is not a controlled drug. Guanfacine is an α_{2a}-adrenoceptor agonist available in a slow-release formulation for the treatment of ADHD in children and can be used on its own or as an add-on to other ADHD medications.

Table 20.9 Summary of the main pharmacological treatments of ADHD in children and adults

Drugs	Important side-effects	Parameters to monitor	Controlled Drug?
Methylphenidate/ Dexamfetamine	Weight loss Insomnia Irritability Tics Increased blood pressure Cardiac arrhythmias	Weight/height Pulse/blood pressure Tics Agitation/anxiety Drug misuse	Yes
Atomoxetine	Weight loss Constipation Fatique Increased blood pressure Postural hypotension	Weight/height Pulse/blood pressure Suicidal ideation	No
Guanfacine	Syncope Hypotension Bradycardia, Sedation Weight gain QT–interval prolongation	Pulse/blood pressure Weight	No
Bupropion	Seizures Insomnia Excessive sweating Increased blood pressure Hepatic impairment	Blood pressure Liver enzymes (if history of hepatic problems)	No

Table 20.10 Summary of indications for psychotropic drugs

	Anti-depressants	Lithium and mood stabilisers	Anti-psychotics	Benzodia-zepines	Other hypnotic and anxiolytic drugs	Other drug groups
Depressive disorders	*	*(1)	* (2)			
Depressive disorders with psychotic symptoms	*	*(1)	*			
Bipolar affective disorder (prophylaxis)		*	*			
Bipolar affective disorder (acute manic episode)		*	*	*		
Anxiety disorders	*		*(3)	*	*(4)	
Schizophrenia			*			
Acute behavioural disturbance	*(5)	* (5)	*	*		
Alcohol withdrawal				*	*(6)	*(7)
Insomnia	*(8)		* (8)	*	*	
Eating disorders	*(9)					
Dementia of Alzheimer's disease						*(10)
Attention deficit/ hyperactivity disorder			*(11)			*(12)

*Recognised indication; where numbers appear in the table, see notes below:

(1)Lithium augmentation may be used in depression. Lithium is given in combination with tricyclic, SSRI or novel antidepressants, usually when the symptoms have proved resistant to adequate trials of two or more antidepressants.

(2)Certain atypical antipsychotics are effective in depression, either as monotherapy (quetiapine) or as augmenting agents (e.g. quetiapine, aripiprazole, risperidone).

(3) Antipsychotics may be used for management of anxiety disorders, usually as augmentation of antidepressant treatments. Quetiapine has evidence as monotherapy in generalised anxiety disorder.

(4)Pregabalin and buspirone may be used in generalised anxiety disorder. Some evidence supports the use of pregabalin in other anxiety disorders. β-Adrenoceptor blockers may be helpful for performance anxiety, combating tremor and other symptoms of autonomic overactivity.

(5)While antipsychotics and benzodiazepines are most commonly used for rapid tranquillization in acute behavioural disturbance, in certain circumstances other drugs may be relevant, for example citalopram, carbamazepine and prazosin have evidence for use in agitation and aggression in Alzheimer's disease.

(6)Clomethiazole was an alternative to a benzodiazepine for alcohol withdrawal, but is now rarely used due to concerns over respiratory suppression and abuse potential.

(7)Drugs for alcohol dependence and withdrawal are discussed in Chapter 11.

(8)When a patient complaining of insomnia also has depression, a sedative antidepressant such as trazodone, mirtazapine, agomelatine or trimipramine should be considered. SSRIs do not provide direct sedation in such patients but may improve the quality of sleep over a longer period as mood improves. Quetiapine may also be used to promote sleep, but prescribers should be aware of its side-effect profile as an atypical antipsychotic.

(9)Fluoxetine is licensed for the treatment of bulimia nervosa.

(10)Acetylcholinesterase inhibitors and memantine provide transient improvement in cognitive and global functioning in dementia of Alzheimer's disease. They delay the onset of severe illness but cannot ultimately halt or change the course of the disease.

(11)The CNS stimulants methylphenidate and dexamfetamine are drugs of choice for attention deficit/hyperactivity disorder. Atomoxetine is an alternative. Second-line treatment options include clonidine and the antipsychotic agents, risperidone, haloperidol and sulpiride.

Clonidine (another α_2-adrenoceptor agonist), tricyclic antidepressants (TCAs), bupropion and the stimulant modafinil may have a role in ADHD, where methylphenidate, dexamfetamine and atomoxetine are contraindicated or have failed to produce benefit.

Drugs for psychiatric illness in childhood

Children do suffer psychiatric illnesses. Many drugs used in childhood psychiatric illness are not properly tested in young people. Now there are regulatory pressures for drugs (in general) to have safety tests in children subsequent to their licensing in adults. Some drugs are deemed not to have adequate risk:benefit ratios in children, e.g. in depression

most SSRI drugs are not recommended (an exception is fluoxetine for which evidence of efficacy and safety in children does exist). Similar caveats apply to the use of TCAs in childhood. By contrast, there are good efficacy data for several SSRIs in obsessive–compulsive disorder and social anxiety disorder, and for benefit of risperidone for aggression in children with autism.

Summary

Table 20.10 summarises indications of the major groups of psychotropic drugs. Remember that psychiatric illnesses are often associated with co-morbid conditions, which may themselves require treatment; for example, schizophrenia may be associated with depression, so both antipsychotics and antidepressants may be required.

Guide to further reading

Azermaia, M., Petrovica, M., Elseviersa, M.M., et al., 2012. Systematic appraisal of dementia guidelines for the management of behavioural and psychological symptoms. Ageing Res. Rev. 11, 78–86.

Baldwin, D.S., Aitchison, K., Bateson, A., et al., 2013. Benzodiazepines: risks and benefits. A reconsideration. J. Psychopharmacol. 27, 967–971.

Baldwin, D.S., Anderson, I.M., Nutt, D.J., et al., 2014. Evidence-based pharmacological treatment of anxiety disorders, post-traumatic stress disorder and obsessive-compulsive disorder: a revision of the 2005 guidelines from the British Association for Psychopharmacology. J. Psychopharmacol. 28, 403–439.

Barnes, T.E., the Schizophrenia Consensus Group of the British Journal of Psychopharmacology, 2011. Evidence-based guidelines for the pharmacological treatment of schizophrenia: recommendations from the British Association for Psychopharmacology. J. Psychopharmacol. 25, 567–620.

Bolea-Alamanac, B.M., Nutt, D.J., Adamou, M., 2014. Evidence-based

guidelines for the pharmacological management of attention deficit hyperactivity disorder: update on recommendations from the British Association for Psychopharmacology. J. Psychopharmacol. 28, 179–203.

Caddy, C., Amit, B.H., McCloud, T.H., et al., 2015. Ketamine and other glutamate receptor modulators for depression in adults. Cochrane Database Syst. Rev. (9), Art. No.: CD011612.

Cleare, A., Pariante, C.M., Young, A.H., et al., 2015. Evidence-based guidelines for treating depressive disorders with antidepressants: a revision of the 2008 British Association for Psychopharmacology guidelines. J. Psychopharmacol. 29, 459–525.

Cooper, S.J., Reynolds, G., Barnes, T., et al., 2016. BAP guidelines on the management of weight gain, metabolic disturbances and cardiovascular risk associated with psychosis and antipsychotic drug treatment. J. Psychopharmacol. 30, 717–748.

Davies, S.J.C., Nash, J., Nutt, D.J., 2017. Management of panic disorder in primary care. Prescriber 28, 19–26.

Fink, M., 2001. Convulsive therapy: a review of the first 55 years. J. Affect. Disord. 63, 1–15.

Fitzgerald, P.B., Daskalakis, Z.J., 2012. A practical guide to the use of repetitive transcranial magnetic stimulation in the treatment of depression. Brain Stimul. 5, 287–296.

Flockhart, D., 2016. P450 Drug Interaction Table, The Flockhart table. http://medicine.iupui.edu/clinpharm/ddis/main-table. (Accessed February 2017).

Goodwin, G.M., Haddad, P.M., Ferrier, I.N., 2009. Evidence-based guidelines for treating bipolar disorder: revised second edition – recommendations from the British Association for Psychopharmacology. J. Psychopharmacol. 23, 346–388.

Heyman, I., Mataix-Cols, D., Fineberg, N.A., 2006. Obsessive–compulsive disorder. Br. Med. J. 333, 424–429.

Katzman, M.A., Bleau, P., Blier, P., et al., 2014. Canadian clinical practice guidelines for the management of anxiety, posttraumatic stress and obsessive-compulsive disorders. BMC Psychiatry 14 (Suppl. 1), S1.

Leucht, S., Corves, C., Arbter, D., et al., 2009. Second-generation versus first-generation antipsychotic drugs for schizophrenia: a meta-analysis. Lancet 373, 31–41.

Lieberman, J.A., Mataix-Cols, D., Fineberg, N.A., for the Clinical Antipsychotic Trials of Intervention Effectiveness (CATIE) Investigators, 2005. Effectiveness of antipsychotic drugs in patients with chronic schizophrenia. N. Engl. J. Med. 353, 1209–1223.

Mann, J.J., 2005. The medical management of depression. N. Engl. J. Med. 353, 1819–1834.

Ryan, N.D., 2005. Treatment of depression in children and adolescents. Lancet 366, 933–940.

Wilson, S.J., Nutt, D.J., Alford, C., et al., 2010. British Association for Psychopharmacology consensus statement on evidence-based treatment of insomnia, parasomnias and circadian rhythm disorders. J. Psychopharmacol. 24, 1577–1601.

Wong, I.C.K., Besag, F.M.C., Santosh, P.J., Murray, M.L., 2004. Use of selective serotonin reuptake inhibitors in children and adolescents. Drug Saf. 27, 991–1000.

Chapter 21

Neurological disorders – epilepsy, Parkinson's disease and multiple sclerosis

Paul Bentley, Pankaj Sharma

SYNOPSIS

This chapter focuses on several common neurological disorders, each of which has a wide range of therapeutic strategies available. These disorders are epilepsy, Parkinson's disease and multiple sclerosis. The treatments of other common neurological disorders are covered in other sections – namely, headaches (Pain section: Ch. 18), stroke (Ch. 24) and dementia (Ch. 20). As the number of treatment types increases for many of these disorders – often with the concomitant need for close monitoring – so there is an increasing trend for these disorders to be managed in specialty clinics, wards or day-case treatment centres, run by professionals with disease-specific expertise. It also touches on the pharmacological principles of other neurological disorders, including movement disorders other than Parkinson's disease; spasticity (a physical sign indicating damage to upper motor neurons, characteristic of certain diseases such as stroke or multiple sclerosis); peripheral neuropathy; motor neurone disease; and tetanus.

Epilepsy

Definitions

A *seizure* is a distinct episode of clinical symptoms or signs caused by abnormal electrical discharges within the cerebral cortex.[1] For example, a tonic-clonic seizure refers to the clinical syndrome of abrupt loss of consciousness, generalised stiffness (tonic) and subsequent rhythmic jerks in all limbs (clonus). A different type are complex partial seizures, which are characterized by the constellation of impaired consciousness, déjà vu sensations, epigastric rising sensation, olfactory hallucinations and motor automatisms, e.g. lip smacking.[2]

By contrast, *epilepsy* refers to the clinical syndrome of recurrent seizures and implies a pathological state that predisposes to further future seizures. Hence having one, or even a single cluster of seizures (i.e. over a few days), does not in itself qualify as epilepsy, since these seizures may have been due to a febrile illness or drug intoxication that themselves later resolve. By contrast, having at least two seizures, separated by at least a few weeks, is usually sufficient to signify epilepsy. Only one-third of people having seizures develop chronic epilepsy.

Pathology and seizure types

Epilepsy affects 0.5–1% of the general population, while the lifetime risk of having a seizure is 3–5 %. There are both

---

[1] Epilepsy has been recognised since early times. A Babylonian medical text dated about 650 BC gives the following description: 'while he is sitting down, his left eye moves to the right, a lip puckers, saliva flows from his mouth, and his hand, leg and trunk on the left side jerk like a slaughtered sheep …'. Because of its unusual manifestations epilepsy was known as the 'sacred disease'. Wilson J V K, Reynolds E H 1990 Medical History 34:192.

[2] For a first-hand description of what it is like to experience a seizure, the reader is referred to many passages in the works of a lifelong epilepsy sufferer, Fyodor Dostoevsky, e.g. in *The Idiot* (1869): 'all at once everything seemed to open up before him: an extraordinary inner light flooded his soul. That lasted half a second … he clearly remembered the beginning, the first sound of a dreadful scream which burst from his chest of its own accord and which no effort of his could have suppressed.'

multiple causes and multiple seizure types.[3] Approximately one-half of adult epilepsy is believed to be due to genetic or early developmental causes, although the exact nature of these – e.g. sodium channel mutations or cerebral palsy – is determined in only a small minority. The other half of adult epilepsy is due to acquired causes, such as alcohol, stroke, traumatic head injury or brain tumours.

The cause of epilepsy determines the seizure type. Genetic causes (i.e. 'primary') predispose to generalised seizures[4] characterised by tonic-clonic or absence seizures (lapses of consciousness lasting seconds), myoclonus (random limb jerk at other times), photosensitivity (seizures triggered by flashing lights), EEG showing a 3-Hz spike-and-wave pattern and a normal MRI brain. Conversely, where focal brain injury has occurred, e.g. brain tumour or stroke, and the brain scan is abnormal, focal epileptic discharges occur within the brain leading to a partial seizure – i.e. when only a narrow set of brain functions are disturbed, e.g. causing single limb jerking (implying motor cortex involvement). Importantly, partial seizures can propagate very quickly to become a 'secondary generalised seizure'. Another common cause of adult-onset partial epilepsy is maldevelopment of the medial temporal lobes ('mesial temporal sclerosis') believed to be due to injury, e.g. hypoxia or infection, during fetal or early childhood life, and sometimes apparent as atrophic hippocampi and amygdala on high-resolution MRI.

Principles of management

- Identification of underlying cause and treatment of this where possible, e.g. cerebral neoplasm or arteriovenous malformation.
- Educate the patient about the disease, duration of treatment and need for compliance.
- Counselling the patient about avoiding harm from seizures, e.g. driving regulations, swimming or bathing alone and climbing, as well as other dangerous pursuits to be avoided.
- Avoid precipitating factors, e.g. alcohol, sleep deprivation, stroboscopic light.
- Anticipate natural variation, e.g. fits may occur particularly or exclusively around menstruation in women (catamenial[5] epilepsy).

---

[3]Some people with epilepsy make pilgrimages to Terni (Italy) to seek intercession from Saint Valentine to relieve their condition. There was more than one Saint Valentine, and it is unclear whether he was also the patron saint of lovers.
[4]So-called 'primary' or 'idiopathic' generalised epilepsies that reflect the fact that the specific cause is usually undetermined, although presumed to be developmental (e.g. in utero) or genetic.
[5]Greek *katamenios*, monthly.

- For most cases with recurrent seizures, an antiepileptic drug is prescribed with subsequent monitoring and adjustment of dosage or drug type (see below).
- Consider surgical therapies in patients with refractory seizures, e.g. vagal nerve stimulation, temporal lobectomy. For childhood refractory epilepsy, a ketogenic diet – i.e. high fat:carbohydrate ratio – is useful, as ketone bodies are antiepileptogenic.
- Acute treatment of generalised convulsive seizures consists of ensuring the patient lies on the floor away from danger, and is postictally manoeuvred into the recovery position. If a seizure continues for more than a few minutes, rectal or buccal diazepam or intranasal midazolam can be given. If convulsive seizures last for more than 5 min, patients should be transferred to hospital for consideration of intravenous benzodiazepine and phenytoin.

Practical guide to antiepilepsy drugs

1. *When to initiate.* Following a single seizure, the chance of a further seizure is approximately 25% over the following 3 years. Furthermore, only 33% of single-seizure patients develop chronic epilepsy. Hence the majority of first seizures are provoked by a reversible, and often recognisable, factor, e.g. infection, drug toxicity, surgery. For these reasons, following a *single* seizure[6] anticonvulsants are not generally prescribed, whereas after *two or more* distinct seizure episodes (i.e. with more than a few weeks apart between episodes), they generally are prescribed. Immediate treatment of single or infrequent seizures does not affect long-term remission but introduces the potential for adverse effects. Patients need to be made aware that anticonvulsant therapy reduces harm caused by generalised seizures, and may also reduce the risk of sudden death in epilepsy (SUDEP), which usually occurs during sleep.

2. *Monotherapy.* Although the choice of anticonvulsants is large (~20), first-line therapy is generally restricted to one of only a few drugs that have a good track record and are relatively safe and well-tolerated. Initial therapy is confined to a single drug (i.e. monotherapy) that is usually effective in stopping seizures or at least significantly decreasing their frequency. The majority of epilepsy patients (70%) can remain on monotherapy for adequate control,

---

[6]Or single cluster of seizures, i.e. if they all occurred on one day or over a few consecutive days, without any recurrence.

although sometimes the choice of monotherapy may need to be switched to allow for tolerance or optimisation of seizure control. As the number of single anticonvulsants tried increases, the incremental likelihood that any new one will offer a significant reduction in seizures decreases: from 50% response to a first drug, to an additional 30% to a second drug, to an extra 10% to a third drug, and less than 5% for any subsequent drug tried.

3. *What drug to initiate*. For older types of anticonvulsants, knowing the seizure type – i.e. whether partial or primary generalised – mattered, because in certain cases the spectrum of seizure efficacy is limited, and, moreover, certain seizure types can be *worsened* by ill-chosen drugs. For example, carbamazepine is an effective first-line therapy for partial seizures but may worsen primary generalised, absence or myoclonic seizures; similarly, phenytoin can worsen absence and myoclonic seizures. Ethosuximide, by contrast, is only effective in primary generalised, and not partial, seizures.

4. More modern anticonvulsants, by contrast, are in general effective over a much broader range of seizure types allowing for more confidence of use even when seizure type is uncertain. Thus sodium valproate, lamotrigine and levetiracetam are active against both primary and secondary generalised epilepsy, and being relatively well tolerated, account for most first-line prescriptions. In one head-to-head study comparing popular first-line therapies for generalised and partial seizures, lamotrigine was generally tolerated better than other drugs, while valproate was the most efficacious; carbamazepine and topiramate were more likely to cause unwanted effects.[7]

5. *Women of reproductive age and children*. These categories of patients prompt selection of particular drugs and avoidance of others (see below for more detail).

6. *Polytherapy*. If a trial of three or so successive anticonvulsants (i.e. taken as monotherapy at adequate dosage for at least several months) does not control a patient's epilepsy, it may be worthwhile trying dual therapy. Polytherapy offers the theoretical advantage of controlling neuronal hyperexcitability by more than one mechanism, which can be synergistic. In reality, increasing polytherapy often adheres to the law of diminishing returns, viz. the proportion of uncontrolled patients who show a positive response decreases at each addition of drug number. And at the same time, adverse effects become more likely.

7. *Abrupt withdrawal*. Effective therapy must never be stopped suddenly, as this is a well-recognised trigger for status epilepticus, which may be fatal. But if rapid withdrawal is required by the occurrence of toxicity, e.g. due to a severe rash or significant liver dysfunction, a new drug ought to be started simultaneously. The speed by which the dose of a new drug can be raised varies according to drug type and urgency.

8. *Circumstantial seizures*. In cases where fits are liable to occur at a particular *time*, e.g. the menstrual period, adjust the dose to achieve maximal drug effect at this time or confine drug treatment to this time. For example, in catamenial epilepsy, clobazam can be useful given only at period time.

Once treatment is stable, patients should keep to a particular proprietary brand as different brands of the same generic agent (e.g. carbamazepine) may exhibit varying pharmacokinetics.

Dosage and administration

The manner in which drug dosing is initiated depends on: (1) the drug type, and (2) the frequency and severity of the patient's seizures (i.e. the relative urgency with which therapeutic levels are reached). Phenytoin and phenobarbital allow for a rapid loading (within 24 h); valproate, levetiracetam and oxcarbazepine allow for escalation over days or a few weeks, whilst lamotrigine and carbamazepine require gradual escalations over many weeks. If seizures are infrequent at the time of presentation, e.g. every few weeks, antiepileptics should generally be started at their lowest dose, with small increments made every 1–2 weeks. In this way, the risk of unwanted effects, especially dizziness or 'feeling drunk' are minimised. A slow introduction of lamotrigine is also essential to reduce the risk of rash or more severe hypersensitivity reactions. Most drugs have a generally recognised maintenance dose range; the lowest dose within this range that achieves a reasonable degree of seizure control should be established. Monitoring of blood concentrations is helpful in guiding dosage of carbamazepine, phenytoin and phenobarbital, but not other anticonvulsants.

Failure to respond

In patients who continue fitting in spite of the recommended maintenance dose range having been reached, there are numerous possible explanations:

- Non-compliance, diarrhoea and vomiting, patients instructed to be 'nil by mouth' (revealed by measuring blood concentrations of drug).
- Inadequate dosing, including the possibility of drug interaction, e.g. another drug reducing the effective

---

[7]SANAD Study.

dose of the anticonvulsant by hepatic enzyme induction.

- Pregnancy also causes hepatic induction, and reduces the effective dose of lamotrigine.
- Increase in the severity of an underlying disease, e.g. enlargement of a brain tumour, or new disease.
- Drug resistance, e.g. genetic polymorphisms in hepatic cytochromes (such as CYP 2 C9) that metabolise drugs, sodium channel subunit SCN1A, or the P glycoprotein drug transporter (ABCB1 gene) that expels drugs from neurones.

Drug withdrawal

If patients have remained seizure-free for more than a few years, it is reasonable to consider withdrawal of antiepilepsy drug therapy.[8,9] The prognosis of a seizure disorder is determined by:

- Type of seizure disorder – benign rolandic epilepsy, solely petit mal or grand mal seizures confer a high chance of full remission, whereas juvenile myoclonic epilepsy, temporal or frontal lobe epilepsies often require lifelong treatment.
- Time to remission – early remission carries a better outlook.
- Number of drugs required to induce remission – rapid remission on a single drug is a favourable indicator for successful withdrawal.
- MRI brain scan findings – presence of an underlying lesion predicts difficult control.
- EEG findings – epileptogenic activity is a predictor of poor outcome for drug withdrawal.
- Associated neurological deficit or learning difficulty – control is often difficult.
- Length of time of seizure freedom on treatment – the longer the period, the better the outlook.

Discontinuing antiepilepsy medication is associated with about 20% relapse during withdrawal and a further 20% relapse over the following 5 years; after this period, relapse is unusual. A general recommendation is to withdraw the antiepilepsy drug over a period of 6 months. If a fit occurs during this time, full therapy must recommence until the patient has been free from seizures for several years.

Driving regulations and epilepsy

Multiple driving regulations exist that relate epilepsy (and neurological conditions predisposing to epilepsy, e.g. brain surgery) to stipulations regarding driving (according to the UK Driving Vehicle Licensing Authority). These rules are based upon statistical data relating specific diagnoses or clinically described events (e.g. blackouts without warning) with the risk of future blackout and/or car accidents. Epileptic patients who wish to continue driving therefore need to contact their national driving licensing body so that each case can be judged on its merits; while waiting for a decision, patients must not drive.

In general in the UK, patients suffering seizures, or blackouts of undetermined cause, are not permitted to drive a car for 1 year from their last attack. Exceptions include: patients who have had exclusively nocturnal seizures for at least 3 years, or patients in whom a single seizure has occurred more than 6 months earlier, providing they have a normal brain scan and EEG; these groups are usually permitted to drive.

Pregnancy and epilepsy

Pregnancy worsens epilepsy in about one-third of patients, but also improves epilepsy in another third. One of the main concerns in this patient group is that all anticonvulsants increase the chance of teratogenicity slightly, with valproate, phenytoin and phenobarbital carrying most risk. The toxicological hazard must be weighed against the risk of seizures which themselves can be harmful to mother and unborn baby, and are likely to worsen if anticonvulsants are discontinued. For instance, the risk of major congenital anomalies in the fetus is 1% for healthy mothers, 2% in untreated epileptic mothers (in observational studies, so generally not severe epileptics), and 2–3% in mothers on epilepsy monotherapy. Valproate, by contrast, has been associated with a malformation rate of approximately 10%,[10] while 20–30% of children are subsequently found to have mild learning disabilities or require 'special needs' education. The UK maintains a national drug monitoring register of all pregnant women taking antiepileptic drugs.

Doctor–patient discussions about what antiepileptic drug, if any, and at what dose, are required *pre-conception*. Advance planning is preferred because:

- neural tube defects are related to deficiencies in folic acid stores before pregnancy, so that antiepileptic drugs that affect stores, e.g. valproate, can be avoided, and folic acid 5 mg/day given for several months in advance, and

---

[8]Medical Research Council 1991 Antiepileptic Drug Withdrawal Study Group. Lancet 337:1175–1180.
[9]Medical Research Council 1993 Antiepileptic Drug Withdrawal Study Group. British Medical Journal 306:1374–1378.

[10]As well as spina bifida, cleft palates, cardiac and urogenital anomalies in the fetus, valproate during early pregnancy or pre-conception is associated with a particular dysmorphic appearance of the newborn ('fetal valproate syndrome') characterised by wide, flat nasal bridge, long philtrum, thin lip, widely spaced eyes (hypertelorism) and epicanthic folds.

- adjustments in dose and type of drug can be avoided in the early stages of pregnancy as there is a higher risk of toxicity and seizure breakthrough during this critical phase of fetal development. In general, patients having seizures with blackouts should be on an effective dose of an anticonvulsant, because of the risk of anoxia, lactic acidosis and trauma.

During pregnancy, liver enzymes become induced, which has implications in epilepsy. Firstly, patients on lamotrigine before conception require a gradually increased dose during the pregnancy, to cope with enhanced catabolism (lowering lamotrigine plasma concentration). Secondly, enzyme-inducing drugs often aggravate a relative deficiency of vitamin K that occurs in the final trimester, predisposing the patient to postpartum haemorrhage; vitamin K is therefore given by mouth during the last 2 weeks of pregnancy.

Breast feeding

Antiepilepsy drugs pass into breast milk: phenobarbital, primidone and ethosuximide in significant quantities, phenytoin and sodium valproate less so. There is a risk that the baby will become sedated or suckle poorly, but provided there is awareness of these effects, the balance of advantage favours breast feeding while taking antiepilepsy drugs.

Epilepsy and oral contraceptives

Many antiepileptic drugs induce steroid-metabolising enzymes and so can cause hormonal contraception to fail. This applies to: carbamazepine, oxcarbazepine, phenytoin, barbiturates, and topiramate. Patients receiving any of these drugs and wishing to remain on the combined contraceptive pill need a higher dose of oestrogen (at least 50 μg/day), which they should take back-to-back for three cycles ('tri-cycling'), before stopping for 3 days, and then repeating the pattern. Even this method offers a suboptimal level of contraception, and a non-oestrogenic form of contraception is preferred. Lamotrigine is not an enzyme inducer but can decrease levonorgestrel plasma concentration through other mechanisms.

Epilepsy in children

Seizures in children tend to arise from different sets of causes (usually genetic or cerebral palsy) from those arising in adults, and can carry either very good long-term outcomes, e.g. spontaneous resolution, or, less commonly, bad outcomes, e.g. gradual deterioration. Treatments are similar to those used in adults, but certain seizure types necessitate drugs that are rarely used in adults, e.g. ethosuximide for absence seizures, or vigabatrin for refractory partial seizures (partly

because children may become irritable or more cognitively impaired with drugs such as valproate and phenobarbital).

Febrile convulsions. Seizures triggered by fever due to any cause (typically viral infection) are common in young children (3 months – 5 years of age). Two-thirds of such children will have only one attack, and in total only 2% will progress to adult epilepsy. For this reason, continuous prophylaxis is seldom given, except for those cases where atypical febrile seizures occur, e.g. lasting for more than 15 min, have focal features or recur within the same febrile illness. Long-term antiepileptic therapy is avoided where possible in children due to recognised adverse effects of most such drugs on learning and social development. Febrile convulsions may be treated on an ad hoc basis by issuing parents with a specially formulated solution of diazepam for rectal administration (absorption from a suppository is too slow) that allows for easy and early administration. Febrile convulsions may be prevented by treating febrile children with paracetamol and cooling with sponge soaks.

Status epilepticus

Status epilepticus refers to continuous or repeated epileptic seizures for more than 30 min. It often arises in patients already known to have epilepsy, in whom antiepileptic drug therapy has been inappropriately withdrawn or not taken. It can be the first presentation of epilepsy, due to an acquired brain insult, e.g. viral encephalitis.

Status epilepticus is a medical emergency. In the first instance, general resuscitation (airway control, oxygen, intravenous saline, etc.) is required. Hypoglycemia needs to be rapidly excluded with finger-prick testing, and if present, addressed by immediate intravenous thiamine (100 mg) followed by 50 mL 50% dextrose.

First-line pharmacological treatment of seizures is with the intravenous benzodiazepine *lorazepam* (0.5–4 mg). Lorazepam is preferred to diazepam because it has a longer effective $t_{1/2}$ and is less lipophilic and so accumulates less in fat, causing less delayed toxicity (hypotension and respiratory depression). The speed of action of lorazepam and diazepam are both rapid.

Second-line treatment of status epilepticus (typically, when seizures have been progressing for 20–40 minutes) is with intravenous *phenytoin*. Phenytoin is given as a loading dose (15–20 mg/kg body-weight) over 1 h and requires ECG and blood pressure monitoring for arrhythmias, conduction block and hypotension. Subsequently, a maintenance dose of approximately 300 mg/day is given and adjusted according to plasma levels (corrected for albumin). Fosphenytoin is sometimes preferred because being water-soluble it has more predictable pharmacokinetics. It can be administered more quickly, by either the intramuscular or intravenous route, and avoids the danger of tissue injury due to inadvertent

369

fluid extravasation (which can occur with intravenous phenytoin due to the need to dissolve it in a basic solution with ethylene glycol).

Alternatives to intravenous phenytoin are a single large dose of intravenous valproate (40 mg/kg; max. 3000 mg), intravenous levetiracetam (60 mg/kg; max 4500 mg), or intravenous phenopharbitone (15 mg/kg), followed by regular daily doses (for all). Increasing evidence suggests that intravenous valproate or intravenous levetiracetam are as effective as intravenous phenytoin, while being safer. Phenobarbitone has the disadvantage of causing more profound sedation, and so may require airway protection or intubation. Second-line treatments result in termination of status epilepticus in up to 80% of patients.

The third-line treatment for status epilepticus, or at an earlier stage if airway or breathing appears compromised, is general anaesthesia, e.g. with midazolam, propofol, thiopental or pentobarbital. These require concomitant intubation, mechanical ventilation and intensive care management. Pharmacologically induced sedation is removed periodically to allow for assessment of seizure activity (both from clinical observations and using EEG).

If resuscitation facilities are not immediately available, diazepam by rectal solution is a useful option. In some cases, midazolam (nasally) may be preferred, e.g. in children or those with severe learning disability. *Intravenous benzodiazepines should not be used if resuscitation facilities are unavailable as there is risk of respiratory arrest.*

Always investigate and treat the cause of a generalised seizure. Give intravenous aciclovir if viral encephalitis is suspected, or, if status is triggered by removing an antiepileptic drug, it must be re-instituted. Magnesium sulphate is the treatment of choice for seizures related to eclampsia (see also p. 440).[11]

Details of further management appear in Table 21.1.

Pharmacology of individual drugs

Modes of action (Fig. 21.1)

Antiepilepsy (anticonvulsant) drugs aim to inhibit epileptogenic neuronal discharges and their propagation, while not interfering significantly with physiological neural activity. They act by one of five different mechanisms given below. It is generally recommended that when more than one drug is needed to control seizures, then drugs chosen should be selected from different classes of action, both to target epileptogenesis at more than one control point (resulting in synergistic effects) and to reduce unwanted effects.

Table 21.1 Treatment of status epilepticus in adults

Status	Treatment
Early	Lorazepam 4 mg i.v., repeat once after 10 min if necessary, or clonazepam 1 mg i.v. over 30 s, repeat if necessary, or diazepam 10–20 mg over 2–4 min, repeat once after 30 min if necessary
Established	Phenytoin 15–18 mg/kg i.v. at a rate of 50 mg/min, and/or phenobarbital 10–20 mg/kg i.v. at a rate of 100 mg/min
Refractory	Thiopental or propofol or midazolam with full intensive care support

Decreases electrical excitability. *Examples: phenytoin, carbamazepine, lamotrigine, lacosamide.* These drugs reduce cell membrane permeability to ions, particularly fast, voltage-dependent sodium channels which are responsible for the inward current that generates an action potential. Receptor blockage is typically use-dependent, meaning that only cells firing repetitively at high frequency are blocked, which permits discrimination between epileptic and physiological activity. A further potential avenue for reducing neuronal depolarisation is to use a potassium channel opener, e.g. retigabine.

Decreases synaptic vesicle release. *Examples: calcium channel blockers: e.g. gabapentin; levetiracetam.* Calcium channel activation is required for synaptic vesicle release, and so calcium channel blockers may act by decreasing synaptic transmission, and therefore activity propagation, especially during periods of high burst activity. Calcium channel blockade may also reduce excitotoxicity – a pathological process by which repetitive neuronal depolarisation leads to calcium entry into neurones, with resultant cell death. Gabapentin and pregabalin bind specifically to the $\alpha_2\delta$ subunit of the high-voltage–activated L-type calcium channels (i.e. long-activating current). Ethosuximide is specific for low-voltage–gated T-type calcium channels. Other drugs such as lamotrigine, valproate and topiramate block calcium channels as just one of many cellular actions.

Levetiracetam uniquely inhibits synaptic vesicle protein 2A (SV2A), thereby reducing synaptic vesicle recycling.

Enhancement of gamma-aminobutyric acid (GABA) transmission. *Examples: benzodiazepines, phenobarbital, valproate, vigabatrin, tiagabine.*[12] By enhancing GABA, the

---

[11]Eclampsia Trial Collaborative Group 1995 Which anticonvulsant for women with eclampsia? Evidence from the Collaborative Eclampsia Trial. Lancet 345:1455–1463.

[12]The last two of these examples have names that help to recall their mechanisms: vigabatrin (as well as valproate) being a GABA TRansamine INhibitor, and TiaGABINe being an INhibitor of GABA Transporter.

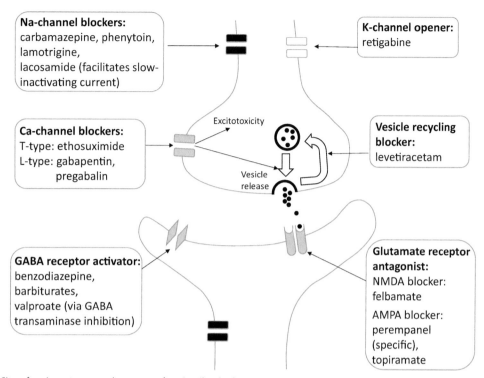

Fig. 21.1 Site of action at neuronal synapse of anti-epileptic drugs

principal inhibitory transmitter of the brain, neuronal membrane permeability to chloride ions is increased, which secondarily reduces cell excitability. Benzodiazepines and barbiturates activate the GABA receptor via specific benzodiazepine and barbiturate binding sites.

Inhibition of excitatory neurotransmitters, e.g. glutamate. *Examples: topiramate, perampanel, felbamate.* Topiramate and perampanel both inhibit glutamate activation of the ionotropic glutamate receptor AMPA (perampanel is unique in being a specific non-competitive AMPA receptor antagonist, whereas topiramate has pleiotropic actions). Felbamate inhibits the NR2B-type of NMDA ionotropic glutamate receptor (as well as positively modulating GABAA receptors). Felbamate is only used for severe refractory epilepsy, e.g. Lennox-Gastaut syndrome, because of its association with aplastic anaemia and liver failure. Glutamate inhibition both stops neuronal excitation in the short term, and excitotoxicity and cell death in the long term.

Other actions. *Example: lacosamide,* which as well as inhibiting sodium channel conductance, also targets a neuronal protein called 'collapsin-response mediator protein 2' (CRMP2).

The drugs used in the treatment of various forms of epilepsy are shown in Table 21.2.

Sodium channel blockers

Carbamazepine

Carbamazepine (Tegretol) acts predominantly as a voltage-dependent sodium channel blocker, thereby reducing membrane excitability.

Pharmacokinetics. Carbamazepine is metabolised to an epoxide; both compounds possess antiepileptic activity, but the epoxide may cause more adverse effects. The $t_{1/2}$ of carbamazepine falls from 35 h to 20 h over the first few weeks of therapy due to autoinduction of hepatic enzymes. For this reason, the dose of carbamazepine is gradually increased, over many weeks, with the expectation that plasma levels will remain within a therapeutic range over this time. Other drugs relying on hepatic metabolism may also have their effective plasma level decreased due to induction secondary to carbamazepine, e.g. glucocorticosteroids, contraceptive pill, theophylline, warfarin, as well as other anticonvulsants, e.g. phenytoin. The metabolism of carbamazepine itself may be inhibited by valproate and to a lesser extent, by lamotrigine and levetiracetam (thereby raising carbamazepine plasma levels).

Uses. Carbamazepine is effective for partial seizures with or without secondary generalisation. It is also first-line

Table 21.2 Drugs of choice for the treatment of epilepsy

Seizure disorder	Drug	Usual daily oral dose	
		Adult	**Child**
Generalised seizures			
Primary generalised	*Drugs of choice:*	1–2 g	15–40 mg/kg
Tonic–clonic (grand mal)	Sodium valproate Lamotrigine *Alternatives:* Clonazepam	^a 2–6 mg	^a <1 year: 0.5–1 mg 1–5 years: 1–3 mg 5–12 years: 3–6 mg
	Topiramate Carbamazepine[b]	200–400 mg 0.8–1.2 g	5–9 mg/kg (2–16 years) <1 year: 100–200 mg 1–5 years: 200–400 mg 5–10 years: 400–600 mg 10–15 years: 0.6–1 g
	Phenytoin	200–400 mg	4–8 mg/kg
Absence (petit mal)	*Drugs of choice:* Ethosuximide Sodium valproate *Alternatives:* Clonazepam Lamotrigine	 1–1.5 g As above As above ^a	 >6 years: 1–1.5 g As above As above ^a
Atypical absence, myotonic, atonic	*Drugs of choice:* Sodium valproate Clonazepam Lamotrigine[c] Phenytoin Ethosuximide Phenobarbital	 As above As above ^a As above As above 60–90 mg	 As above As above ^a As above As above 5–8 mg/kg
Myoclonic	*Drugs of choice:* Sodium valproate[d] Clonazepam *Alternatives:* Lamotrigine	 As above As above ^a	 As above As above ^a
Partial and/or secondary generalised seizures	*Drugs of choice:* Levetiracetam	 1–3 g	
	Sodium valproate Lamotrigine *Alternatives:* Phenytoin Gabapentin	As above As above 0.9–1.2 g	As above As above 0.9 g (26–36-kg body-weight) 1.2 g (37–50-kg body-weight)
	Vigabatrin[e]	2–3 g	0.5–1 g (10–15-kg body-weight) 1–1.5 g (15–30-kg body-weight) 1.5–3 g (30–50-kg body-weight) 2–3 g (>50-kg body-weight)

Table 21.2 Drugs of choice for the treatment of epilepsy—cont'd

Seizure disorder	Drug	Usual daily oral dose	
		Adult	**Child**
	Topiramate	As above	As above
	Oxcarbazepine	0.6–2.4 g	
	Levetiracetam	1–3 g	
	Lacosamide		
	Zonisamide		
	Pregabalin		

[a]Varies with mono or adjunctive therapy; see manufacturer's recommendations.
[b]Avoid if major seizures are accompanied by absence seizures or myoclonic jerks.
[c]Lamotrigine may be effective, particularly if used with sodium valproate.
[d]Alone or in combination with clonazepam, which may be synergistic.
[e]In adults, used as a last resort; in children, used for infantile spasms (West's syndrome). Regular visual field monitoring is mandatory.

treatment for trigeminal neuralgia. It is not recommended for primary generalised seizures (especially myoclonic epilepsy), which can be worsened by it.

Adverse effects follow from the fact that it depresses electrical excitability. In the central nervous system (CNS), this results in cerebellar and brainstem dysfunction (causing dizziness, diplopia, ataxia, nausea and reversible blurring of vision), as well as drowsiness; in the heart this can result in depression of cardiac atrioventricular (AV) conduction. Rashes, including serious reactions such as Stevens–Johnson syndrome, tend to be more of a problem for this drug than other anticonvulsants. A further set of issues arise from the hepatic induction property of carbamazepine: both osteomalacia and folic acid deficiency may occur due to enhanced metabolism of vitamin D and folic acid, respectively. Elderly patients receiving any enzyme-inducing drug should be screened for osteoporosis with bone-density scanning, and treated with bisphosphonates if necessary. Other unwanted effects can include gastrointestinal symptoms, headache, blood disorders, e.g. leucopenia, syndrome of inappropriate antidiuretic hormone (causing hyponatraemia), liver and thyroid dysfunction. Carbamazepine impairs cognitive function less than phenytoin.

Oxcarbazepine

Oxcarbazepine, like its analogue carbamazepine, acts by blocking voltage-sensitive sodium channels. It is rapidly and extensively metabolised in the liver; the $t_{1/2}$ of the parent drug is 2 h, but that of its principal metabolite (which also has therapeutic activity) is 11 h. Unlike carbamazepine, it does not form an epoxide, which may explain its lower frequency of unwanted effects; these include dizziness,

headache and hyponatraemia, and selective cytochrome enzyme induction (potentially causing failure of oestrogen contraception). Monitoring of plasma sodium may be necessary in the elderly and patients on diuretics.

Oxcarbazepine is used either as monotherapy or as add-on therapy for partial seizures. The speed with which the dose can be escalated is generally quicker than that for carbamazepine.

Eslicarbazepine

This drug is an enantiomer of a hydroxyl derivative of oxcarbazepine and has an efficacy spectrum similar to carbamazepine and oxcarbazepine, i.e. it is effective for partial epilepsy with or without secondary generalisation. It appears to have fewer of the unwanted effects of its parent drugs, and its dose can be raised to an effective range more quickly (within 1–2 weeks); only two doses are available.

Phenytoin

Phenytoin (diphenylhydantoin, Epanutin, Dilantin) acts principally by blocking neuronal voltage-dependent sodium ion channels; this action is described as membrane stabilising, and discourages the spread (rather than the initiation) of seizure discharges.

Pharmacokinetics. Phenytoin provides a good example of the application of pharmacokinetics for successful prescribing.

Saturation kinetics. Phenytoin is hydroxylated extensively in the liver, a process that becomes saturated at about the doses needed for therapeutic effect. Thus phenytoin at low doses exhibits first-order kinetics, but saturation or zero-order kinetics develop as the therapeutic plasma concentration range (10–20 mg/L) is approached, i.e. dose increments of equal size produce a *disproportional rise in steady-state plasma concentration*. Thus dose increments should become smaller as the dose increases (which is why there is a 25-mg capsule), and plasma concentration monitoring is advisable. Phenytoin given orally is well absorbed, allowing for achievement of therapeutic range concentrations within 24 h (as may be required in patients with frequent seizures).

Enzyme induction and inhibition. Phenytoin is a potent inducer of hepatic enzymes that metabolise other drugs (carbamazepine, warfarin), dietary and endogenous substances (including vitamin D and folate), and phenytoin itself. This latter causes a slight fall in steady-state phenytoin concentration over the first few weeks of therapy, though this may not be noticeable with progressive dose increments. Drugs that inhibit phenytoin metabolism (causing its plasma concentration to rise) include sodium valproate, isoniazid and certain non-steroidal anti-inflammatory drugs.

Uses. The main role of phenytoin in modern practice is in the emergency control of seizures, including status epilepticus, because of its reliable antiepileptic effect, and because an effective treatment dose can be loaded rapidly. It may also be used to prevent partial seizures with or without secondary generalisation, but is not generally used first line in this regard because of its adverse-effect profile (see below). It may worsen primary generalised epilepsies, such as absence or myoclonic seizures, and so is not used for these conditions unless status epilepticus occurs.

Other uses. The membrane-stabilising effect of phenytoin finds use in cardiac arrhythmias, trigeminal neuralgia and myotonic dystrophy (an inherited disorder in which skeletal muscle becomes over-excitable).

Adverse effects. Adverse effects of phenytoin are multitudinous, especially with years of therapy, which fact, together with its narrow therapeutic range, is why phenytoin is not favoured for long-term therapy. Unwanted effects related to the nervous system include cognitive impairment, cerebellar ataxia, dyskinesias, tremor and peripheral neuropathy. Cutaneous reactions include rashes (dose related), coarsening of facial features, hirsutism, lupus-like syndrome, gum hyperplasia (due to inhibition of collagen catabolism), and Dupuytren's contracture (caused by free-radical formation). Haematological effects include: macrocytic anaemia due to increased folate metabolism (treatable with folate supplementation), IgA hypergammaglobulinaemia, lymphadenopathy and pseudolymphoma. Osteomalacia due to increased metabolism of vitamin D occurs after years of therapy and calls for bone-density scanning.

Intravenous phenytoin is associated with cardiac depression, distal ischaemia ('purple-glove syndrome') and, if drug extravasation occurs, local but severe ulceration.

Overdose causes cerebellar symptoms and signs, coma, apnoea or even paradoxically, seizures. The patient may remain unconscious for a long time because of saturation kinetics, but will recover with standard care.

Fosphenytoin is a prodrug of phenytoin, is soluble in water, and easier and safer to administer. Its conversion in the blood to phenytoin is rapid, and it may be used as an alternative to phenytoin for status epilepticus.

Lamotrigine

Lamotrigine (Lamictal) stabilises pre-synaptic neuronal membranes by blocking voltage-dependent sodium and calcium channels, and reduces the release of excitatory amino acids, such as glutamate and aspartate. The $t_{1/2}$ of 24 h allows for a single daily dose.

Lamotrigine is a favoured first-line drug for partial and generalised epilepsy, being both effective and well tolerated. It is also used in bipolar disorder as a mood stabiliser. It has few cognitive or sedating effects relative to other antiepileptic drugs.

It causes rash in about 10% of patients, including, rarely, serious reactions such as Stevens–Johnson syndrome and toxic epidermal necrolysis (potentially fatal). The risk of rash lessens if treatment begins with a low dose and escalates slowly, whereas concomitant use of valproate, which inhibits lamotrigine metabolism, adds to the hazard. Carbamazepine, phenytoin and barbiturates accelerate the metabolic breakdown of lamotrigine, thereby prompting an increase in the prescribed lamotrigine dose. Other specific unwanted effects of lamotrigine include insomnia and headache, the latter effect distinguishing it from valproate and topiramate that are used for migraine prevention. Insomnia may respond to lamotrigine taken once daily in the morning.

Lacosamide

Lacosamide (Vimpat) selectively facilitates a 'slow-inactivating' component of the voltage-gated sodium channel, which predominates under high-frequency neural activity (e.g. seizures), without affecting 'fast-inactivating' sodium channel states that characterise more standard patterns of neural firing frequency. This offers seizure control while reducing common antiepileptic unwanted effects such as sedation or cognitive impairment. Lacosamide also targets a neuronal protein called 'collapsin-response mediator protein 2' that is involved in neuronal differentiation, axonal outgrowth and gene expression. Whether this property confers additional disease-modifying properties to lacosamide (as distinct from its antiseizure property) is unknown.

Lacosamide is effective in refractory partial epilepsy, and has the advantage of being available as a syrup and intravenous formulation. The $t_{1/2}$ is 13 h, and unwanted effects include dizziness, nausea, headache and prolongation of the PR interval on the ECG.

GABA-potentiators

Sodium valproate

Sodium valproate (valproic acid, Epilim) acts on sodium and calcium channels, as well as GABA$_A$ receptors, the latter action by virtue of inhibiting GABA transaminase (thereby increasing GABA levels, and hence neuronal inhibition).

Sodium valproate is metabolised extensively in the liver ($t_{1/2}$ 13 h). It is a non-specific metabolic inhibitor, both of its own metabolism, and that of other anticonvulsants including lamotrigine, phenytoin and carbamazepine. To avoid toxicity, patients taking valproate and starting such drugs as second-line therapy should receive lower doses of the second anticonvulsant. By contrast, the metabolism of valproate is accelerated by enzyme-inducing drugs, e.g. carbamazepine.

Sodium valproate is effective for both generalised and partial epilepsies, as well as for migraine prevention and mania (for which it acts as a mood stabiliser).

Adverse effects. The main concerns, particularly to women, are weight gain, impaired glucose tolerance, teratogenicity (see p. 123), polycystic ovary syndrome and loss of hair, which grows back curly.[13] Nausea and dyspepsia may be a more general problem, ameliorated by using an enteric-coated formulation. Some patients exhibit a rise in liver enzymes, which is usually transient and without sinister import, but patients should be closely monitored until the biochemical tests return to normal as, rarely, liver failure occurs (risk maximal at 2–12 weeks); this is often indicated by anorexia, malaise and a recurrence of seizures. Other reactions include pancreatitis, coagulation disorder due to inhibition of platelet aggregation or thrombocytopenia, and hyperammonaemia that can present with acute confusion.

Barbiturates

Some of the earliest effective antiepileptic drugs came from the barbiturate family: namely, *phenobarbital* ($t_{1/2}$ 100 h), and *primidone* (Mysoline), the latter being metabolised largely to phenobarbital, i.e. it is a prodrug. The main use of phenobarbital is for status epilepticus because of its potent antiepileptic effect and the ability to give it intravenously. It is also used as an adjunct for long-term control of refractory partial seizures, but suffers from a high level of unwanted effects (especially sedation), including cardiac or respiratory arrest if overdosed, and dependency/addiction, and interactions (enzyme induction). Withdrawal from barbiturates must be performed very slowly (typically over months) because of a high risk of inducing seizures.

Benzodiazepines

Lorazepam and *diazepam* are first-line drugs for rapid control of acute seizures, but are not recommended for long-term prophylaxis due to unwanted effects: mainly sedation, tolerance and addiction. *Clonazepam* (Rivotril) ($t_{1/2}$ 25 h) is used mainly as an adjunct in myoclonic epilepsy due to its additional effects as a muscle relaxant. *Clobazam* finds use as an oral method for establishing rapid seizure control, e.g. in patients with a first presentation of frequent symptomatic seizures, and may be effective for drug-resistant partial seizures. Its effectiveness may wane after a few months due to tolerance. Both clonazepam and clobazam should be avoided in patients with anxiety or a history of drug addiction, due to risk of addiction or misuse.

Vigabatrin

Vigabatrin (Sabril) ($t_{1/2}$ 6 h) is structurally related to the inhibitory CNS neurotransmitter GABA, and acts by irreversibly inhibiting GABA-transaminase so that GABA accumulates. GABA-transaminase is resynthesised over 6 days. The drug is not metabolised and does not induce hepatic drug-metabolising enzymes.

Vigabatrin is effective in partial and secondary generalised seizures that are not satisfactorily controlled by other anticonvulsants, and in infantile spasms, as monotherapy. It worsens absence and myoclonic seizures.

Unwanted effects from drugs sometimes become apparent only following prolonged use, and vigabatrin is a case in point. Vigabatrin had been licensed for a number of years before there were reports of visual field constriction (up to 40% of patients), an effect that is insidious and leads to irreversible tunnel vision. Consequently, it is now indicated only for refractory epilepsy, and patients taking it require 6-monthly visual field monitoring. Other adverse effects include confusion, psychosis and weight gain.

Calcium channel blockers

Gabapentin

Gabapentin (Neurontin) is a lipid-soluble analogue of GABA that crosses the blood–brain barrier. It acts as an antagonist to the L-type (long-activating) high-voltage–gated activated

---

[13] 'We thought the change might be welcomed by the patients, but one girl preferred her hair to be long and straight, and one boy was mortified by his curls and insisted on a short hair cut' (Jeavons P M, Clark J E, Harding G F 1977 Valproate and curly hair. Lancet i:359).

calcium channels, via interactions with the $\alpha_2\delta$ subunit. This has the effect of inhibiting synaptic vesicle fusion with the plasma membrane, and thus neurotransmitter release. It also facilitates GABAergic transmission, as its name suggests. It is excreted unchanged and has the advantage of not inducing or inhibiting hepatic metabolism of other drugs.

Gabapentin is effective only for partial seizures and secondary generalised epilepsy. It is also used for neuropathic pain, restless legs syndrome and anxiety.

Gabapentin may cause somnolence, unsteadiness, dizziness and fatigue, although the likelihood of these decreases if dosing is started very low (e.g. 100 mg three times per day) and increased gradually (e.g. to 900 mg three times per day).

Pregabalin

Pregabalin (Lyrica) acts similarly to gabapentin, and is sometimes used in place of gabapentin when the latter has been ineffective for refractory partial seizures. Its main adverse effects are confusion, dizziness and weight gain. As well as being an antiepileptic, it is commonly used against neuropathic pain, and it possesses anxiolytic properties.

Ethosuximide

Ethosuximide (Zarontin) ($t_{1/2}$ 55 h) is a member of the succinimide family that differs from other antiepilepsy drugs in that it blocks a particular type of calcium channel that is active in primary generalised epilepsies – especially absence seizures (petit mal) and myoclonic epilepsy. For this reason, its main use is among children. Adverse effects include gastric upset, CNS effects, and allergic reactions including eosinophilia and other blood disorders, and lupus erythematosus.

Carbonic anhydrase inhibitors

Carbonic anhydrase inhibition reduces central nervous excitability, and is a property shared by topiramate, zonisamide and acetazolamide. Acetazolamide is rarely used now as an antiepileptic, but the other two find roles as adjuncts in partial epilepsy, as well as migraine. They also share common unwanted effects, namely weakness, anorexia, weight loss, depression, paraesthesia and renal stones (due to alkalosis).

Topiramate

Topiramate (Topamax), acts via various mechanisms, including carbonic anhydrase inhibition, voltage-gated sodium channel blockade, glutamate receptor blockade and enhancement of GABA activity. The $t_{1/2}$ of 21 h allows once-daily dosing; it is excreted in the urine, mainly as unchanged drug.

Topiramate is used for partial seizures, as well as for migraine prevention (a property it shares with valproate). Unlike valproate, which causes weight gain, topiramate causes weight loss (considered an advantage by many women). Other unwanted effects include cognitive impairment, e.g. naming difficulty, acute myopia and raised intraocular pressure.

Zonisamide

Zonisamide (Zomig) is a sulphonamide analogue that acts as a carbonic anhydrase inhibitor as well as blocking both sodium and T-type calcium channels. Its sodium channel-blocking effect increases latency for neuronal recovery following inactivation. It may cause cognitive impairment, and carries a small risk of renal stones (<1%). It generally finds use as an adjunct for refractory partial epilepsy, and may benefit patients with migraine.

Levetiracetam

Levetiracetam (Keppra) is unique in inhibiting synaptic vesicle protein 2A (SV2A), which secondarily reduces synaptic vesicle recycling. It is effective for both partial and generalised seizures, is relatively well tolerated, and appears not to interact with other drugs. It is also rapidly and completely absorbed after oral administration, and can reach maintenance dose relatively quickly. For these reasons, it has become increasingly popular as a first-line agent for many seizure types. Its therapeutic index appears to be high, with the commonest adverse effects being weakness, dizziness and drowsiness. Relatively specific unwanted effects of levetiracetam are emotional lability, behavioural disturbance and psychosis, and it should be used with caution in patients with prior mood disturbance, learning disability or head injury. It is metabolised predominantly in the kidney, making it a drug of choice in liver disease, but use at lower dose in renal impairment.

A more recently developed variant of this drug – brivaracetam – acts more specifically on SV2A, allowing for greater seizure control.

Perampanel

Perampanel, recently introduced, is effective in many cases of refractory, generalised tonic-clonic seizures, as well as partial seizures. It has a novel drug action, being a specific, non-competitive antagonist of the AMPA receptor, thus blocking excitatory, glutamate transmission. Its main side-effects are drowsiness (requiring evening dosage), and psychiatric or behavioural disturbance (including suicidality, psychosis and euphoria; requiring monitoring of mental state in all patients). It reduces the effect of the oestrogen contraceptive pill.

Parkinson's disease and parkinsonism

Definitions

Parkinson's disease[14] refers to a specific neurodegenerative *disease* characterised pathologically by intracellular accumulation of Lewy bodies and subsequent neuronal loss, predominantly within the substantia nigra pars compacta (SNpc)[15] (see Fig. 20.3, p. 338). This midbrain nucleus normally provides dopaminergic input to the neostriatum (caudate and putamen), a critical aspect to motor control; one cardinal feature of Parkinson's disease is that motor symptoms are reversible by administration of dopaminergic drugs. By contrast, *parkinsonism* refers to the *clinical* symptoms and signs of Parkinson's disease (tremor, rigidity, bradykinesia and postural imbalance) that may arise either from Parkinson's disease or one of its mimics; the latter include extensive small-vessel cerebral ischaemia due to hypertension, neuroleptic drugs or other neurodegenerative disease such as multiple-systems atrophy (MSA) or Huntington's disease. Note that parkinsonism due to conditions other than Parkinson's disease generally responds poorly to dopaminergic therapies. Another distinguishing feature is that symptoms and signs of Parkinson's disease, but not other causes, are often asymmetric.

Pathophysiology of Parkinson's disease

Parkinson's disease[16] is the second commonest neurodegenerative disease after Alzheimer's disease. Both diseases show an exponentially increasing risk with age, with the risk of Parkinson's disease rising from approximately 0.2% in those younger than 60 years to 1% in those older than 60 years and 4% in those older than 85 years of age. At the time that a clinical diagnosis first becomes apparent, radioactive dopamine uptake scans (sensitive to dopaminergic neurones) reveal that approximately 70% of the patient's nigrostriatal dopaminergic neurones have already been lost. The implication of this finding is that treatments which might actually halt neuronal death ('disease-modifying drugs' as opposed to 'symptomatic treatments') should ideally be used in pre-symptomatic cases, e.g. as identified by dopamine scanning of the elderly, or relatives of affected individuals. In only about 15% of Parkinson's cases is there a clear family history, and not more than 10% of cases are caused by a recognised gene mutation.[17] Furthermore, no current treatment strategies have been shown to prevent disease progression, with the possible exception of rasagiline (see below). Rather, existing drug therapies primarily serve to enhance dopaminergic neurotransmission, whose deficiency underlies the main symptoms of Parkinson's disease.

The pathophysiology of Parkinson's disease, and its critical dependency upon dopamine, arises from an imbalance between two striatal–thalamic–cerebral cortical circuits (Fig. 21.2). To understand this, it is useful to remember that under normal circumstances the globus pallidus INternus (GPi) INhibits thalamic communication with the frontal cortex, thereby braking voluntary movements. Since dopaminergic input to the striatum itself suppresses GPi (via a 'direct' pathway), loss of dopaminergic input allows the GPi to be overactive, thereby favouring inhibition of motor cortex, and so causing slowness of movement (bradykinesia) or freezing. Loss of dopamine also encourages an indirect pathway between striatum, subthalamic nucleus and GPi, which has the net effect of increasing GPi braking of movement. Therefore replacing dopamine can increase the relative contribution of the 'direct' relative to 'indirect' pathway. Furthermore, inducing neurosurgical stereotactic against the globus pallidus or subthalamus can offer a reduction in bradykinesia (see Neurosurgery section below).[18]

Objectives of therapy

The main goal of treatment in Parkinson's disease is to manage symptoms for as long as possible while minimising treatment-associated complications. The following principles motivate pharmacological strategies:

---

[14]Sometimes referred to as idiopathic Parkinson's disease (IPD) – a name that is likely to move out of favour as its pathophysiology becomes increasingly elucidated.
[15]*Substantia nigra* is (Latin) black substance. A coronal section at this point in the brain shows the distinctive black areas, visible with the naked eye in the normal brain, but absent from the brains of patients with Parkinson's disease.
[16]James Parkinson (1755–1824), physician; he described *paralysis agitans* in 1817.

---

[17]The commonest mutations associated with Parkinson's disease (including sporadic disease – i.e. not apparently inherited) are leucine-rich repeat kinase (LRRK) and glucocerebrosidase (GBA), the latter of which in homozygous form causes the severe childhood disorder Gaucher's disease.
[18]Deep brain stimulation, a more popular neurosurgical technique, causes functional inactivity (i.e. 'virtual lesion') of either of these same target brain regions.

377

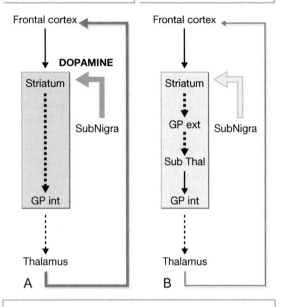

Normal dopamine levels; DIRECT pathway favoured (D1 receptor predominant) Thalamo-cortical – Motor Output	Dopamine deficiency (e.g. Parkinson's disease); INDIRECT pathway favoured (D2 receptor predominant) Thalamo-cortical – Motor Output

→ Activation (glutamate)
- - -▶ Inhibition (GABA)
Thickness of line represents relative strength of connection

Fig. 21.2 Schematic diagramme of principal 'volitional' motor pathways, and their interaction with dopaminergic input in health (A) and in Parkinson's disease (B). In A, normal dopaminergic tone favours the direct pathway which involves two sequential inhibitions, and so overall motor activation (i.e. a '–' and '–' making a '+'). In B, inadequate dopaminergic input favours the indirect pathway which involves three sequential inhibitions, and so overall motor inhibition (i.e. a '–' and '–' and '–', making a '–'). *(Adapted from Hauser R A 2009 Levodopa: past, present, and future. European Neurology 62:1–8).*

Enhancement of dopaminergic neurotransmission. This can be achieved by:

- administering the dopamine precursor levodopa.
- decreasing endogenous clearance and breakdown of dopamine by inhibiting monoamine oxidase (selegiline, rasagiline) or catechol-O-methyltransferase (entacapone, tolcapone).
- stimulating dopamine receptors with agonists (ropinirole, pramipexole, cabergoline, rotigotine, apomorphine).

- increasing pre-synaptic dopamine release (amantadine – this mechanism being only one of many by which this drug may be effective).
- avoiding dopamine antagonists (especially traditional neuroleptics such as haloperidol, and antiemetics such as prochlorperazine).[19]

Note that the most seemingly obvious treatment strategy – ingesting or infusing dopamine – is ineffective because dopamine is rapidly metabolised in the gut, blood and liver by monoamine oxidase and catechol-O-methyltransferase (COMT). Furthermore, intravenously administered dopamine, or dopamine formed in peripheral tissues, is insufficiently lipid soluble to penetrate the CNS.

Pre-empting and treating levodopa-induced motor complications. Although levodopa is the most effective symptomatic treatment at all stages of the disease, its main drawback is that it usually results in treatment-induced fluctuations in motor control ('on–off' phenomena) and dyskinesias (i.e. excessive purposeless movements appearing as restlessness or rocking) by about 5–10 years from treatment initiation. One of the main factors associated with this complication is the total previous exposure to levodopa. Hence, in patients younger than approximately 70 years of age, it is preferable to begin therapy with drugs other than levodopa, typically dopamine agonists or a monoamine oxidase inhibitor (MAOI). As the disease progresses, and symptoms become more severe in spite of non-levodopa therapies,[20] levodopa is introduced, albeit in small doses, and increasing only very gradually so that only the smallest dose providing reasonable symptom relief is used. In patients older than 70 years of age, long-term dyskinesias are not so relevant, and moreover alternatives to levodopa, namely dopamine agonists, anticholinergics and amantadine, are more prone to cause confusion in this age group.

One of the theories for why motor fluctuations occur is related to the pulsatile nature by which levodopa is traditionally administered, which results in brain concentrations of levodopa (and dopamine) that rise and fall several times over a typical day. This is in contrast to the 'physiological mode' of dopamine release that is to a large extent tonic. Pulsatile, rather than smooth, administration of levodopa or dopamine agonists has been found in animal models to result in a gradual shortening of treatment response and

---

[19]Atypical neuroleptics such as quetiapine or olanzapine, and antiemetics that only minimally cross the blood–brain barrier, such as domperidone, can be used relatively safely.
[20]The CALM-PD study, for example, randomised 300 early PD patients to levodopa or pramipexole, where either group could subsequently have the other drug added in if clinically required. At 6 years the pramipexole group had less wearing off and dyskinesias than the levodopa group, but more oedema and sleepiness. Overall quality of life was no different between groups.

dyskinesias. Consequently, methods which 'smooth' circulating levodopa concentrations may protect against eventual development of motor complications. Furthermore, a more sustained and steady supply of levodopa compared to conventional levodopa preparations can be achieved by using COMT inhibitors (entacapone or tolcapone) taken at the same time as levodopa, which has the effect of inhibiting dopamine catabolism, and so increasing dopamine availability. Using this strategy from the outset of Parkinson's disease is controversial, with one study[21] showing that levodopa-COMT inhibitors started as first-line therapy result in the *sooner* development of dyskinesias relative to standard levodopa therapy, possibly due to the fact that patients are exposed to higher effective concentrations of levodopa from early on.

Use of cholinergic drugs. One model of Parkinson's disease conceptualises its pharmacology in terms of a relative imbalance between dopamine levels (too low) and acetylcholine levels (too high). This model explains the fact that cholinergic (muscarinic-type receptor) antagonists are also effective for tremor and rigidity (but not bradykinesia). More recently, cholinesterase inhibitors (especially rivastigmine) that increase acetylcholine levels have been used successfully for psychosis and dementia in Parkinson's disease, without generally worsening the patient's motor symptoms. This observation challenges any simplistic relationship between acetylcholine excess and Parkinson's disease symptomatology.

Treatment of non-motor symptoms of Parkinson's disease. Consultations with patients should include enquiry into non-motor symptoms that are associated with Parkinson's disease, and, if present, treatments prescribed appropriately. These include: antidepressants for depression; laxatives for constipation; NSAIDs for pain (especially frozen shoulder); benzodiazepines for REM-sleep disorder; fludrocortisone for postural hypotension; cholinesterase inhibitors for psychosis or dementia; and salivary gland injections of botulinum toxin for sialorrhoea.

Recognition of conservative, surgical and co-morbidity therapies. Patients should be encouraged to keep mobile and exercise within their capabilities. Patients may need to be offered physiotherapy, speech therapy and occupational therapy, the latter of which will involve evaluation of potential risks in the environment, e.g. loose carpet, stairs. Patients with advanced disease who are not demented but suffer severe fluctuations may benefit from functional neurosurgery, the commonest procedure of which is bilateral deep brain electrical stimulation (DBS) of the subthalamic nucleus. Finally, coexisting morbidities, such as hypertension, diabetes and stroke, should be treated optimally, e.g. with antihypertensives, aspirin and statins, so as to reduce cerebral vascular injury, itself a cause of parkinsonism and dementia.

Drugs for Parkinson's disease

Dopaminergic drugs

Levodopa and dopa decarboxylase inhibitors

Levodopa ('dopa' stands for dihydroxyphenylalanine) is the natural amino acid precursor of dopamine.[22,23] It is readily absorbed from the upper small intestine[24] by active amino acid transport, and traverses the blood–brain barrier by a similar active transport mechanism. Within the brain, levodopa is decarboxylated (by dopa decarboxylase) to *dopamine.*

A major disadvantage is that levodopa is also extensively decarboxylated to dopamine in peripheral tissues, such that only 1–5% of an oral dose of levodopa reaches the brain. This means that large quantities of administered levodopa would be required for a meaningful antiparkinsonian effect. Such high doses cause a high rate of adverse effects caused by peripheral actions of levodopa and dopamine, notably nausea, cardiac arrhythmia and postural hypotension. Furthermore, high-dose levodopa inhibits gastric emptying and results in erratic delivery to the absorption site and fluctuations in plasma concentration. This problem has been largely circumvented by the development of *peripheral decarboxylase inhibitors,* which do not enter the CNS, and so selectively prevent peripheral conversion of levodopa to dopamine. Thus by combining levodopa with a peripheral decarboxylase inhibitor, unwanted effects due to peripheral dopamine production are minimised,[25] while the proportion of ingested levodopa available for export into the CNS is maximised. Decarboxylase inhibitors are given in combination with levodopa in one of several formulations:

---

[21]STRIDE-PD.

[22]Levodopa is derived from the fava bean *(Vicia faba)*; compare this with the prototypical drug for Alzheimer's disease, physostigmine, which is derived from the calabar bean. The discoverer of natural levodopa, Marcus Guggenheim, explored its physiological effects by ingesting 2.5 g of the compound. He subsequently became violently ill with vomiting – a fact not too surprising given that the recommended starting dose now is one-tenth this amount.
[23]The reason why the levo form of dopa is used is because racemic (d/l) mixtures of dopa were found to cause agranulocytosis in up to 25% of patients.
[24]Explaining why nasoduodenal tube insertion for continuous levodopa instillation (Duodopa) can be effective.
[25]For example, nausea frequency is reduced from 80% with levodopa alone to less than 15% with a decarboxylase inhibitor, for the same dopamine brain concentration achieved.

- Co-careldopa (carbidopa plus levodopa in respective proportions 12.5/50, 25/100 and 50 mg/200 mg[26]) (Sinemet).
- Co-beneldopa (benserazide plus levodopa in proportions 12.5/50, 25/100, 50 mg/200 mg) (Madopar).
- Co-careldopa with entacapone (carbidopa plus levodopa plus entacapone in same proportions as co-careldopa plus entacapone 200 mg with each tablet) (Stalevo).

These combinations produce similar brain concentrations of dopamine as achievable by levodopa alone, but with only 25% of the levodopa dose given.

The $t_{1/2}$ of levodopa given with a decarboxylase inhibitor is 90 min, but its acute motor benefit lasts for 6 h or so, while there is also a lesser effect that lasts for approximately 2 weeks. The acute motor response to levodopa gradually reduces with long-term therapy, which may be related to a progressively diminishing reserve of healthy dopaminergic neurones which store levodopa and allow gradual conversion to dopamine.

Dose management. Levodopa preparations are introduced gradually and titrated according to individual response. Compliance is important. Abrupt discontinuation of therapy can lead to relapse, that when extreme can resemble the neuroleptic malignant syndrome. A controlled-release preparation of levodopa/carbidopa is occasionally used for patients with nocturnal symptoms or akinesia on awakening, when it is prescribed for use before bedtime. This preparation has not proven to be useful for daytime fluctuations, as it increases levodopa levels slowly, and so either controls symptoms too slowly to be useful, or increases the likelihood of end-of-dose dyskinesias. A soluble form of co-beneldopa is also available which can help provide rapid relief of akinesia, e.g. on awakening, and may be more appropriate in patients with dysphagia.

Adverse effects. As mentioned above, the main drawback to levodopa use is the eventual development of *motor complications*, with about 50% of treated patients developing them within 5 years (although they can occur after only a few months with high doses, especially in young patients), and nearly all patients developing some by 10 years. These take the form of *motor fluctuations*, e.g. 'wearing off', when the duration of clinical response shortens with chronicity of treatment, or 'on-off fluctuations', when the patient's response to each levodopa dose consists of swinging abruptly between violent dyskinesias (during which the patient can move to a degree voluntarily, and so is 'on') and freezing (i.e. 'off'). *Dyskinesias* typically take the form of continual writhing, rocking or fidgeting movements (also termed 'chorea') of the limb, trunk, neck, lips or tongue. These are believed to arise from both pre-synaptic (e.g. diminution of dopa decarboxylase reserves) and post-synaptic (e.g. receptor down-regulation) mechanisms. Dyskinesias can occur coincident with both the peak levodopa blood concentration (e.g. mid-dose), or at the onset and offset of each dose's clinical effect (i.e. biphasic pattern).

Levodopa-induced dyskinesias are dose-related, so that in general the lowest dose of levodopa is used that achieves a reasonable degree of symptom relief. Further strategies that can be used against motor fluctuations/dyskinesias include: avoiding taking levodopa with meals;[27] using small doses more often; slow-release levodopa preparations taken before sleep,[28] and using adjunctive medications such as dopamine agonists;[29] amantadine,[30] and COMT inhibitors (taken together with levodopa). In advanced cases, a nasoduodenal feeding tube can be placed that allows for continuous enteric infusion of levodopa gel (Duodopa), or patients can be offered deep brain stimulation. All these methods, in enhancing the effectiveness of dopamine or providing alternative antiparkinsonian methods, enable a reduction in levodopa dose, and so provide strategies in cases where dyskinesias are prominent.

In the short term, the main unwanted effect is *nausea*, which can be minimised by increasing dosage gradually, and offering patients a safe antiemetic such as domperidone (a peripherally confined dopamine antagonist) or cyclizine (an antihistamine), taken half an hour before levodopa. This is usually only required for the first few weeks. *Postural hypotension* may occur,[31] although this can develop as a feature of advanced Parkinson's disease due to degeneration of noradrenergic nuclei within the brainstem and cord. *Agitation and confusion, including visual hallucinations*, may occur, but it may be difficult to decide whether these are due to drug or to disease. Mental changes are particularly likely in the elderly, especially when there is pre-existing dementia. If acute confusion occurs, other Parkinson's drugs that cause confusion – antimuscarinics, amantadine or dopamine agonists should be progressively withdrawn before levodopa.

---

[26]The dosage commonly referred to is the sum of both drugs – hence, 62.5 mg, 125 mg and 250 mg.

[27]Amino acids compete for levodopa uptake, and so absorption may vary depending on meal size and type.
[28]Slow-release preparations are not preferable during the day as they are generally insufficient in achieving peak levels required for normal motor activity.
[29]Dopamine agonists enable a reduction in the total levodopa dose and, in the cases of long-acting formulations, e.g. rotigotine, provide a relatively continuous and smooth level of dopaminergic stimulation.
[30]Which has an independent antidyskinesia effect.
[31]Note that dopamine causes hypotension, whereas further metabolism of levodopa to adrenaline/epinephrine and noradrenaline/ norepinephrine causes hypertension – that is not seen with levodopa therapy.

Alternatively, the anticholinesterase rivastigmine, or atypical neuroleptics such as quetiapine or clozapine, may be of benefit.

Interactions. With *non-selective* monoamine oxidase inhibitors (MAOIs), the monoamine dopamine formed from levodopa is protected from destruction; it accumulates and also follows the normal path of conversion to noradrenaline/norepinephrine, by dopamine β-hydroxylase; *severe hypertension results*. This is not generally seen with the *selective* MAO-B inhibitors, selegiline or rasagiline, used as adjuncts in Parkinson's disease.

Levodopa antagonises the effects of antipsychotics (dopamine receptor blockers). Tricyclic antidepressants are safe.

Dopamine agonists

These mimic the effects of dopamine, the endogenous agonist, which stimulates both of the main types of dopamine receptor, D_1 and D_2 (coupled respectively to adenylyl cyclase stimulation and inhibition). The D_2 receptor is the principal target in Parkinson's disease, although chronic D_1-receptor stimulation potentiates response to the D_2 receptor. The main advantage of dopamine agonists relative to levodopa is that they do not result in significant motor fluctuations or dyskinesias, which may relate to their longer $t_{1/2}$, and to the fact that they are not dependent upon pre-synaptic conversion. Whether they also protect dopaminergic neurones by sparing the levodopa dose, and therefore reducing levodopa-induced oxidative damage, has been theorised but not proven. Conversely, dopamine agonists are not as effective as levodopa, and are limited by a higher rate of confusion and psychosis in the elderly. On the other hand, the problems of developing synthetic alternatives are:

- Reproducing the right balance of D_1 and D_2 stimulation (dopamine itself is slightly D_1 selective, in test systems, but its net effect in vivo is determined also by the relative amounts and locations of receptors – which differ in parkinsonian patients from normal).
- Avoiding the undesired effects of peripheral, mainly gastric, D_2 receptors.
- Synthesising a full, not partial, agonist.

Ergot derivatives (cabergoline, pergolide, lisuride, bromocriptine). These first-generation dopamine agonists are now not preferred because of their high rate of unwanted effects. In particular, the ergotamine component can cause fibrosis of internal organs after chronic exposure, leading to serious complications (below).

Cabergoline and *pergolide* are the best known drugs of this class; the former has the advantage of being very long acting (a $t_{1/2}$ of more than 80 h), allowing a once-daily (or even twice-weekly) administration. The $t_{1/2}$ of pergolide is 6 h,

longer than that of levodopa. Both drugs therefore allow for a more enduring 'on' phase, and can relieve parkinsonian symptoms through the night and on awakening. The ergotamine property of these drugs can cause Raynaud's phenomenon (painful cold extremities due to vasospasm), while their additional properties as 5-hydroxytryptamine (5HT) type 2 receptor agonists can cause pleural effusions, pulmonary or retroperitoneal fibrosis (the latter causing renal failure due to ureteric obstruction). Additionally, cardiac valve fibrosis may result in valvular incompetency, e.g. aortic regurgitation or pulmonary valve regurgitation (the latter a very rare valvular abnormality otherwise). These effects are also seen with chronic amfetamine use, e.g. dexfenfluramine (antiobesity drugs), possibly through effects on similar receptors. Consequently, patients who previously received ergot derivatives are now treated with non-ergot derivatives. In those patients who require ergotamine dopamine agonists (because non-ergotamine equivalents may be less effective), screening for potential complications is required, e.g. by measuring plasma creatinine and performing echocardiograms 6-monthly.

Bromocriptine is a D_2-receptor agonist and a weak α-adrenoceptor antagonist. It is commonly used to suppress the production of prolactin in patients with prolactinomas (pituitary tumours) but now only rarely for Parkinson's disease because nausea, vomiting and postural hypotension are more prominent than with more modern dopamine agonists. Pleural effusions and retroperitoneal fibrosis may also occur with prolonged use.

Non-ergot dopamine agonists (ropinirole, pramipexole, rotigotine). These drugs are currently preferred as first-line therapy in newly diagnosed patients younger than 70 years of age. Beyond this age group, the long-term complications of levodopa are not felt to be so relevant (and are milder in older-onset Parkinson's patients) allowing for levodopa use from the outset. Furthermore, psychosis[32] or confusion (unwanted effects of all dopamine agonists) are more likely in elderly patients taking these drugs.

Both ropinirole and pramipexole are relatively selective D_2-receptor agonists, and are generally more effective against tremor than other symptoms. Both drugs are started at low dose and increased over weeks or months, to a maintenance dose (e.g. ropinirole starts at 0.75 mg/day and typically is increased to 9 mg/day over 9 weeks). The relatively short $t_{1/2}$ of these drugs necessitates thrice-daily administration, but formulations that allow once-daily administration are available. The dopamine agonist rotigotine can be used daily as a transdermal patch, and is particularly convenient in Parkinson's patients with dysphagia.

---

[32]This unwanted effect can be predicted from the fact that dopamine *antagonists* are used as *anti*psychotics.

Apart from psychosis in elderly patients, the other notable unwanted effects of the non-ergot dopamine agonists are: postural hypotension, ankle oedema, daytime somnolence (including sudden sleep attacks in a minority of patients[33]), and impulse-control disorders in about 15%, including punding,[34] hypersexuality, gambling, eating binges and compulsive shopping. Some of these behaviours may be more likely in Parkinson's disease patients, independent of a treatment effect, due to a dysregulated dopamine-prefrontal reward system. Where obsessionality develops on dopamine agonist therapy, this usually occurs in patients already taking a high daily levodopa dose, and indeed can lead to addiction and patient-initiated escalation of drug doses. The approach in these cases is gradually to withdraw the dopamine agonist.

Apomorphine is a derivative of morphine with structural similarities to dopamine; it is a full agonist at D_1 and D_2 receptors, as well as having ergotamine-like properties. Its main use is in patients with advanced disease who are younger than 70 years of age and have severe motor fluctuations (i.e. on–off cycles), especially when freezing is common or levodopa provides little benefit, or in patients with severe dyskinesias, in whom reducing the levodopa dose is the aim. The rapid onset of action by the subcutaneous route avoids the 'off' component without the patient waiting for 45–60 min to absorb another oral dose of levodopa. Patients can be taught to inject themselves, but because the need is greatest during 'off' periods it is more convenient for a carer to administer injections. Alternatively, patients can receive apomorphine by continuous subcutaneous infusion from a portable syringe driver in a pouch. Continuous infusion is also the preferred administration method for dyskinetic patients.

Adverse effects of apomorphine follow from the fact that it is both a dopamine agonist and a morphine derivative. An antiemetic, e.g. domperidone,[35] should accompany initial dosing as nausea is almost a universal accompaniment, at least initially. Overdose causes respiratory depression, while naloxone antagonises its action. Apomorphine can also cause confusion, psychosis and dysphoria, induce penile erection (without causing sexual excitement[36]), Raynaud's phenomenon and yawning. Autoimmune-mediated haemolytic anaemia is a rare complication in patients taking concurrent levodopa, and their blood counts should be monitored.

Inhibition of dopamine metabolism: MAO-inhibitors and COMT inhibitors

Monoamine oxidase (MAO) enzymes have an important function in modulating the intraneuronal content of neurotransmitters. The enzymes exist in two principal forms, A and B, defined by specific substrates, some of which cannot be metabolised by the other form (Table 21.3). The therapeutic importance of recognising these two forms arises because they are to some extent present in different tissues, and the enzyme at these different locations can be selectively inhibited by the individual inhibitors: *moclobemide* for MAO-A (used for depression, see p. 325) and *selegiline* or *rasagiline* for MAO-B (used in Parkinson's disease; see Table 21.3).

Selegiline is a selective, irreversible inhibitor of MAO type B. The problem with non-selective MAO inhibitors is that they prevent degradation of dietary amines, especially tyramine, which may then act systemically as sympathomimetics (causing the so-called hypertensive 'cheese reaction'[37]). Selegiline does not cause the cheese reaction, because MAO-A in the liver and sympathetic nerve endings is unaffected, allowing tyramine to be metabolised. In the CNS, selegiline reduces intraneuronal degradation of dopamine, but has no effect on synaptic cleft concentrations of other neuromodulatory amines, such as serotonin and noradrenaline/norepinephrine. The effects of these amines can be enhanced by MAO-A inhibitors used as antidepressants.

Rasagiline[38] is another MAO type B inhibitor, but has an advantage over selegiline in not producing amfetamine metabolites, which are believed to be part of the reason for confusion in susceptible patients. Furthermore, two trials[39] of rasagiline have suggested that patients who take this early in their disease course show an enduring benefit (of up to 6 years), relative both to patients on placebo, and to those who are treated with rasagiline only after a delay of 9 months. While potentially evidence for a 'disease-modifying' effect rather than merely a symptomatic treatment effect, longer-term follow-up of these patients and further independent trials will be required to confirm this.

Entacapone inhibits COMT, one of the principal enzymes responsible for the metabolism of dopamine, and so prolongs the action of levodopa. It is most effective for patients who experience only short-lived 'on' periods with levodopa, and in whom frequent levodopa doses are used (typically at 3–4-hourly intervals), by providing a more predictable and

---

[33]Patients who drive, or engage in other potentially dangerous pursuits, need to be warned about this (and to stop driving etc. if they were to experience this).
[34]Punding refers to behaviours such as sorting or hoarding objects to an extreme degree; the phrase was first coined to describe similar behaviour in chronic amfetamine abusers.
[35]Domperidone is preferred as it does not cross the blood–brain barrier, unlike metoclopramide or prochlorperazine.
[36]It also enhances the penile response to visual erotic stimulation, allegedly.

---

[37]Tyramine is an indirectly acting amine which displaces noradrenaline/norepinephrine from nerve terminals.
[38]This drug is unique in PD for having a very easy dosing schedule: 1 mg per day with no titration upwards necessary.
[39]TEMPO and ADAGIO trials with approximately 400 and 1100 mild PD patients enrolled, respectively.

Table 21.3 Isoforms of monoamine oxidase: MAO-A and MAO-B, an explanation[a]

Enzyme	MAO-A	MAO-A and B	MAO-B
Substrate	Serotonin[b]	Noradrenaline/norepinephrine[b] Adrenaline/epinephrine Dopamine Tyramine	Phenylethylamine
Inhibitors	Moclobemide	Tranylcypromine Phenelzine Iproniazid	Selegiline
Tissues	Liver CNS (neurones) Sympathetic neurones	See MAO-A and MAO-B	Gut CNS (glial cells)

[a] The table shows the definition of the isoforms by their specific substrates, and then their selectivity (or non-selectivity) towards a number of other substrates and inhibitors. Determination of therapeutic and adverse effects is a function of selectivity of the inhibitor and the tissue location of the enzyme.

[b] *Explanation:* The specific substrate for MAO-A is serotonin, whereas that for MAO-B is the non-endogenous amine, phenylethylamine (present in many brands of chocolate). Noradrenaline/norepinephrine, tyramine and dopamine can be metabolised by both isoforms of MAO. MAO-A is the major form in liver and in neurones (both CNS and peripheral sympathetic); MAO-B is the major form in the gut, but is also present in the liver, lungs and glial cells of the CNS.

stable response. It is taken at the same time as levodopa, usually as part of the same drug formulation (Stalevo). Entacapone is preferred to long-acting preparations of levodopa, whose main disadvantage is their slow onset of action. The adverse effects of entacapone include increased dyskinesias (by increasing the effective brain levodopa concentration), bodily fluids, e.g. urine, turning orange and diarrhoea.

Tolcapone is a COMT inhibitor that can be more effective than entacapone; it is taken three times per day, not necessarily at the same time as levodopa. Its main drawback is hepatotoxicity, resulting in liver failure in approximately 1 in 13 000 cases, thereby necessitating fortnightly screening blood tests.

Antimuscarinic (anticholinergic) drugs (see also p. 399)

Antimuscarinic drugs benefit parkinsonism by blocking acetylcholine receptors in the CNS, thereby partially redressing the imbalance created by decreased dopaminergic activity. Their use originated when hyoscine was given to parkinsonian patients in an attempt to reduce sialorrhoea by peripheral effect, and it then became apparent that they had other beneficial effects in this disease. Synthetic derivatives are now used orally. These include benzhexol (trihexyphenidyl), orphenadrine, benzatropine, procyclidine and biperiden. There is little to choose among these. Antimuscarinics produce modest improvements in tremor, rigidity, sialorrhoea, muscular stiffness and leg cramps, but do not generally help with bradykinesia. They are also effective intramuscularly or intravenously in acute drug-induced dystonias.

Unwanted effects include dry mouth, blurred vision, constipation, urine retention, acute glaucoma, hallucinations, memory defects and acute confusional states (which, once again, are more likely in elderly patients).

Other drugs

Amantadine antedates the discovery of dopamine receptor subtypes, and its discovery as an antiparkinsonian drug was an example of serendipity. It is an antiviral drug which, given for influenza to a parkinsonian patient, was noticed to be beneficial. The two effects are probably unrelated. It appears to act by increasing synthesis and release of dopamine, and by diminishing neuronal reuptake. It also has a slight antimuscarinic effect. The drug is much less effective than levodopa, whose action it enhances slightly, but it has the advantage of reducing levodopa-induced dyskinesias. It is more effective than the standard antimuscarinic drugs, with which it has an additive effect. Amantadine is relatively free from adverse effects, but there do occur ankle oedema (probably a local effect on blood vessels), postural hypotension, livedo reticularis and CNS disturbances, e.g. insomnia, hallucinations and, rarely, fits. It is more likely to cause confusion in the elderly and so is preferred for younger patients.

Adenosine A-2A receptor antagonists

Low doses of caffeine (100 mg/day) have been found to exert an anti-parkinsonian effect. The mechanism appears to arise from its effects as an adenosine A-2A receptor antagonist, given that these receptors are co-localized on striato-pallidal inhibitory (GABAergic) output neurons alongside dopaminergic D_2 receptors. The adenosine receptors stimulate these inhibitory neurons, as opposed to dopamine receptors that inhibit them. In light of this, more specific A-2A receptor antagonists have been trialled – tozadenant, istradefylline, and preladenant – with evidence that they reduce off-time. Similarly to levodopa though, they can cause dyskinesia, nausea and dizziness. Caffeine is not recommended as therapy because it induces tolerance, and causes stimulatory effects, e.g. insomnia, that are seen less with specific adenosine antagonists.

Neurosurgery

For patients with severe on-off fluctuations, treatment-induced dyskinesias, or refractory tremor, neurosurgical strategies can offer significant symptom relief and/or reduction in doses of levodopa (thereby reducing disability due to dyskinesias). The commonest neurosurgical approaches are Deep Brain Stimulation (DBS) of globus pallidus internus (that exerts an antidyskinetic effect), subthalmus (that allows for a reduction in levodopa dosage), or ventral intermedialis (Vim) nucleus (that reduces tremor). The most suitable patients for surgery are those with no cognitive or psychiatric impairment; young age; and those who show a good response to levodopa on at least some part of the day, with no freezing during on-periods. The main disadvantage is a risk of behavioural or cognitive disturbance, especially in verbal fluency and executive function; as well as stroke, dysarthria and depression.

Drug-induced parkinsonism

The classical antipsychotic drugs (see p. 341) block dopamine receptors, and their antipsychotic activity relates closely to this action, which notably involves the D_2 receptor, the principal target in Parkinson's disease. It comes as no surprise, therefore, that these drugs, as well as certain calcium antagonists, e.g. flunarizine (used for migraine) and valproate, can induce a state with clinical features very similar to those of idiopathic Parkinson's disease. An important distinguishing measure between drug-induced parkinsonism and Parkinson's disease is that the former shows a normal dopamine-transporter binding using a DAT scan, since the nigrostriatal terminals (on which the transporter is located) are intact; in Parkinson's disease there is typically a (asymmetric) reduction in transporter binding. The piperazine phenothiazines, e.g.

trifluoperazine, and the butyrophenones, e.g. haloperidol, are most commonly involved, whereas neuroleptics with high antimuscarinic blocking activity, e.g. thioridazine, are less likely to cause this.

Treatment of drug-induced parkinsonism firstly involves consideration of whether the offending drug can be withdrawn, or replaced, e.g. by an atypical antipsychotic such as quetiapine, olanzapine or clozapine, that provokes fewer extrapyramidal effects (see p. 341). After withdrawal of the offending drug, most cases resolve completely within 7 weeks. When drug-induced parkinsonism is troublesome, an antimuscarinic drug, e.g. trihexyphenidyl, is beneficial, while levodopa and dopamine agonists are not (and risk provoking psychosis).

Tardive dyskinesias, such as repetitive orofacial or lingual movements, that come on *after* neuroleptics have been withdrawn, are distinct from drug-induced parkinsonism, can be worsened by anticholinergics, and so are instead treated with reinstatement of the offending drug if appropriate, switching to an atypical neuroleptic, e.g. quetiapine, and addition of either tetrabenazine (which depletes presynaptic dopamine) or clonazepam.

Other movement disorders

Essential tremor is often, and with justice, called benign, but a few individuals may be incapacitated by it. Alcohol, through a central action, helps about 50% of patients but is plainly unsuitable for long-term use, and a non-selective β-adrenoceptor blocker, e.g. propranolol 120 mg/day, will benefit about 50%. Alternatives such as the benzodiazepines clonazepam or alprazolam, or the barbiturate primidone are sometimes beneficial but predispose to sedation and dependency, necessitating episodic breaks in treatment. Botulinum toxin injected into affected muscle groups can also provide benefit in certain circumstances, e.g. injection into forearm flexors and extensors for primary writing tremor, but may cause weakness of the affected part (see below). For refractory essential tremor, an increasingly popular treatment is High-Energy MR-Guided Focused Ultrasound of the ventral intermedius nucleus of the thalamus, that offers a less-invasive means of thalamotomy than stereotactic neurosurgery.

Drug-induced dystonic reactions are seen:

- As an acute reaction, often of the torsion type, and occur following administration of dopamine receptor–blocking antipsychotics, e.g. haloperidol, and antiemetics, e.g. metoclopramide. An antimuscarinic drug, e.g. biperiden or benzatropine, given i.m. or i.v. and repeated as necessary, provides relief.

- In some patients who are receiving levodopa for Parkinson's disease.
- In younger patients on long-term antipsychotic treatment, who develop tardive dyskinesia (see p. 341).

Wilson's disease. Here, there is a genetic failure to eliminate copper absorbed from food so that it accumulates in the liver, brain, cornea and kidneys. Chelating copper in the gut with penicillamine or trientine can establish a negative copper balance (with some clinical improvement if treatment is started early). The patients may also develop cirrhosis, and the best treatment for both may be liver transplantation.

Chorea of any cause may be alleviated by dopamine receptor–blocking antipsychotics, and also by tetrabenazine, which inhibits neuronal storage of dopamine and serotonin.

Dystonia. The term covers a variety of clinical syndromes characterised by abnormal postures, or tremor, due to abnormal muscle tone. Examples include cervical dystonia (e.g. torticollis), blepharospasm, hemifacial spasm, or genetic disorders such as primary generalised dystonia. Parkinson's disease, especially with young onset, Huntington's disease or Wilson's disease can also present with dystonia. The mainstay of treatment for these disorders is botulinum toxin (below), although anticholinergics or benzodiazepines can be effective.

Spasticity results from disruption of the corticospinal tract, which causes disinhibition of local spinal reflex circuits. Spasticity limited to well-defined muscle groups is best treated with botulinum toxin. Otherwise, systemic drugs can be given, including the GABA agonist baclofen, diazepam and tizanidine (an α_2-adrenoceptor agonist).

Myotonia, in which voluntary muscle fails to relax after contraction, may be symptomatically benefited by drugs that increase muscle refractory period, e.g. procainamide, phenytoin, quinidine.

Restless legs syndrome (RLS) is a condition in which patients have an urge to move their legs because of an unpleasant sensation, especially in the evening. Movement of the legs can provide temporary relief; some claim that it occurs in 5–10% of the general population. The disorder occurs from a deficiency in *descending* dopaminergic input to the spinal cord (as opposed to the deficiency of *ascending* dopaminergic fibres in Parkinson's disease); the descending opioidergic neuromodulatory system is also affected. Most cases are primary (i.e. with no associated disease), but it may also accompany iron deficiency (because of low brain ferritin levels), pregnancy, peripheral neuropathy and dopamine antagonists. Treatment consists of a dopamine agonist, e.g. pramipexole or ropinirole, either taken 1 or 2 h before symptoms develop, or taken as a long-acting preparation, e.g. rotigotine patch, in patients who experience symptoms throughout the day. Levodopa is also effective but can aggravate symptoms with chronic use. Opioids or valproate provide alternative therapies.

Botulinum toxin (Botox)

Botulinum toxin benefits many clinical states characterised by muscle overactivity, especially dystonia and spasticity, from various causes, e.g. stroke, multiple sclerosis. It is also effective for bladder overactivity (injected intravesically), achalasia (injected endoscopically), anal fissure, spasmodic dysphonia, excessive saliva production (parotid injection), and even migraine (multiple scalp and face injections). The toxin consists of metalloproteinases that prevent docking of acetylcholine vesicles at the pre-synaptic membrane, and hence effectively block the neuromuscular junction or autonomic ganglia. Type A Botox cleaves synaptosome-associated protein (SNAP-25), whereas Type B Botox cleaves a vesicle-associated membrane protein (VAMP), also called synaptobrevin.

Although the enzymes within Botox act irreversibly, new enzymes are produced by the neurones and transported gradually from cell body to pre-synaptic membrane. Thus the effect of Botox is limited typically to no more than 3 months, at which time further injections are needed. Nevertheless, Botox is at least partially effective in up to 90% of patients with dystonia or spasticity, and unwanted effects are generally limited to discomfort or weakness at the site of injection (as compared to systemic antidystonia or antispasticity drugs that typically will have CNS effects such as sedation). Injections in the anterior neck, e.g. for torticollis, run a small risk of dysphagia, while periorbital injections for blepharospasm may cause ptosis. If Botox is used to excess, generalised weakness (similar to myasthenia gravis) may occur temporarily, as may antimuscarinic effects, due to its action on postganglionic parasympathetic nerve endings, e.g. dry mouth, dizziness.

Multiple sclerosis

Multiple sclerosis (MS) is the archetypal neuroinflammatory disease and the commonest cause of neurodisability in young adults. It is important to distinguish the inflammatory component of MS, which usually manifests itself as self-terminating relapses, from a more insidious neurodegenerative component that is the cause of long-term 'progressive' disability. Most drug therapies target the former process without appearing to have significant impact on the latter.

In recent years there has been a rapid expansion in the number of available *disease-modifying* immunomodulatory

385

therapies, all of which are normally given within specialist MS centres, where close supervision of treatment response and potential adverse effects can be conducted. Intravenous therapies are increasingly prescribed, and in a similar fashion to oncology treatments, are administered in specialist day-case centres, and require close monitoring of blood counts, brain imaging, ECG, etc.

Traditional injectable disease-modifying drugs

Interferon (IFN) β was the first treatment consistently to show a reduction in the number of symptomatic relapses, and demyelinating lesions observable on MRI. IFNβ also delays disability by 12–18 months in relapsing/remitting disease, probably by reducing relapses (rather than because of an effect on progression). Clinical trials show that in ambulant MS patients with relapsing/remitting disease, IFNβ produces a relative reduction in risk of relapse of approximately one-third. Furthermore, in previously healthy patients who present with a 'clinically isolated syndrome', i.e. a single episode of neurological disturbance associated with MRI white matter lesions, IFNβ delays the occurrence of a second episode. Thus the drug may suppress the *onset* of MS (taken as the point at which more than one neurological episode has occurred).

IFNβ is a polypeptide, normally produced by fibroblasts, whose natural purpose is probably as an effector of an antiviral response. It has multiple immunological effects, including suppression of antibody production, cytokine modulation (e.g. increasing interleukin-10 while decreasing tumour necrosis factor-α and interleukin-1), and inhibition of antigen presentation, T-cell proliferation, differentiation and migration into the brain. As a therapy it is produced as a human recombinant product within either mammalian cells (type 1a; Avonex or Rebif) or modified *E. coli* bacteria (type 1b: Betaferon or Betaseron) formulations, with only the Rebif formulation available in more than one dose. It is not indicated for patients with purely progressive forms of disease, although it may still be effective at reducing relapses in patients who have entered a relapsing, progressive phase (i.e. continuous disability progression with superimposed temporary exacerbations).

IFNβ is usually self-injected either subcutaneously three times per week, or intramuscularly once per week. Unwanted effects of IFNβ are usually minor, with some patients experiencing flulike symptoms, nausea, mildly deranged liver or thyroid function tests, mood disturbance (it is thus relatively contraindicated in patients with a history of depression or suicidal thoughts) and less commonly, seizures. With IFNβ, especially type 1b preparations, some patients develop neutralising antibodies, resulting in a clear decrease in therapeutic efficacy in approximately one-third of patients. The finding of raised antibody levels may prompt change in therapy.

Glatiramer acetate (co-polymer) is an oligopeptide that suppresses various components of the MS-immune response. Like IFNβ, it is self-administered, albeit in daily subcutaneous injections, and has the advantage of not inducing neutralising antibodies. The range of patients in which it is effective, and its level of efficacy, matches that of IFNβ.

Oral disease-modifying drugs

Oral disease-modifying therapies are fast becoming first-line therapies for relapsing-remitting multiple sclerosis patients, offering both greater convenience and efficacy than interferons – which pre-2010 had been the commonest MS disease-modifying therapy. Trials suggest that the effectiveness of these therapies is superior to that of IFNβ, with relative reductions in relapse rate approaching 50% and relative reductions in new MRI lesions of 50–80%. However, there is a slightly higher risk of adverse-effects including (rarely) serious infections such as progressive multifocal leukoencephalopathy (PML; associated more with injectable therapies, see below), and so some patients may wish to use more conservative interferon therapies.

Fumarate (Tecfidera) is a citric acid cycle intermediate that acts on T-helper lymphocytes to reduce patterns of gene expression seen in relapses. One possible mechanism is that it shifts the immunophenotype of T-helper lymphocytes to a Th2 pattern (characterised by IL-4 secretion), and away from a Th1 pattern (characterised by interferon-γ secretion), the latter of which favours MS relapses. A further mechanism of action is up-regulation of antioxidant enzymes via the Nrf2 signalling pathway. It can cause flushing, diarrhoea, nausea, abdominal pain and pruritus. A few case reports of PML have been described, albeit in patients with severe lymphopenia and in whom the drug was being used for psoriasis. Lymphocyte count should therefore be monitored. *Laquinimod*, a quinolone-3-carboxamide, may work in a similar way, but appears to act on CNS immunity separately from peripheral immunity.

Fingolimod (Gilenya) is sphingolipid, with high-affinity agonism at the sphingosine-1-phosphate (S1P) receptor, causing receptor down-regulation. This receptor is normally required to allow T and B lymphocyte egress from lymph nodes, and so the drug suppresses trafficking of autoreactive T cells into the blood. Efficacy data are slightly higher for fingolimod than other oral drugs for MS, but at the price of more significant adverse effects. ECG monitoring is required as it can cause dose-dependent bradycardia or heart block (5%), although this usually only occurs upon treatment initiation, by S1P receptor expression in heart tissue. Other adverse effects include lymphopenia (requiring treatment cessation if lymphocyte count drops to <0.2 g/L), reversible macular edema in ~1%, paradoxical MS lesion worsening and, in case-reports, life-threatening disseminated herpes infections (in patients treated concomitantly with corticosteroids).

Cladribine acts as a purine nucleotide antagonist that suppresses DNA replication necessary for lymphocyte and monocyte division (indeed its original use was for the treatment of leukaemia). It has the advantage that only two 5-day courses per year need be taken to produce a significant MS-treatment effect. Thus adverse effects seen with high doses of this drug used for cancer, e.g. nephrotoxicity and neuropathy, can mostly be avoided in MS treatment. A small excess of bone marrow suppression and opportunistic infection is still observed.

Teriflunomide (Aubagio) is the active metabolite of leflunomide (used in rheumatoid arthritis) that inhibits DHODH (dihydro-orotate dehydrogenase) thereby blocking pyrimidine and, consequently, DNA synthesis. As with any chemotherapy, it is associated with mild myelosuppression, hair thinning, nausea and diarrhoea. Upper respiratory tract infections occur more commonly, as well TB reactivation, necessitating pre-treatment screening.

Intravenous therapies

Monoclonal antibodies targeted against critical steps of the cell-mediated immune reactions that underlie MS are among the most effective immunomodulatory therapies in MS. But these drugs also carry the potential for serious unwanted effects (notably opportunistic infections) and are therefore reserved for patients with rapid deterioration who have failed to respond to less intensive immunomodulatory therapies such as IFNβ.

Natalizumab (Tysabri) targets the α_4-β_1-integrin receptor VCAM-1 (vascular cell adhesion molecule) that is required for T lymphocytes to enter the CNS from the blood. Typically administered every 4 weeks, it decreases relapse rate by up to 70%. A real concern is that approximately 1 in 1000 treated patients (predominantly those taking additional immunosuppressants) develop PML. This is an aggressive cerebral white-matter disease caused by reactivation of the Creutzfeldt-Jakob virus, previously seen only in diseases characterised by immunocompromise, such as advanced HIV infection or lymphoma. Unlike PML in these diseases which are nearly always fatal, PML associated with natalizumab can be reversed if therapy discontinues soon after its development (MRI scans are necessary every few months while on treatment).

Alemtuzumab (Lemtrada, or MabCampath) comprises monoclonal antibodies against CD52 – a marker of mature lymphocytes (it is also used for chronic lymphocytic leukaemia). The overall rate of relapse reduction is two-thirds, which makes this the most effective pharmacological therapy for MS. In certain patients with frequent relapses, it has been able to completely suppress their future occurrence. This occurs at the risk of provoking new organ-based autoimmune diseases, especially thyroid disease (in 40%), immune thrombocytopenic purpura (ITP) and Goodpasture's disease, which can cause life-threatening bleeding and renal failure, respectively. Infections relating to CMV reactivation are also recognised. It is delivered as two single infusions only, 12 months apart. These infusions are associated with hypotension, rigors and rarely pulmonary oedema.

Ocrelizumab (Ocrevus) is a chimeric humanised monoclonal anti-CD20 antibody that depletes B cells, and is the first drug to retard both clinical and imaging-marker progression in primary progressive MS.[40] Unwanted effects to date have been minor (upper respiratory infection, herbes labialis) or uncommon (neoplasms in 2% more than placebo), although longer follow-up is required.

Other intravenous therapies used in advanced cases of MS include mitoxantrone (a cytotoxic drug that decreases interleukin-10 production but can cause infertility, cardiomyopathy and promyelocytic leukaemia), rituximab (an anti-CD20 monoclonal antibody), intravenous immunoglobulin, cyclophosphamide and bone-marrow ablation with subsequent autologous stem-cell transplantation.

Symptomatic therapies

Corticosteroid therapy is often used for acute, disabling attacks of MS. The drugs decrease the length of an attack but do not reduce the number of recurrent attacks or the final disability. *Methylprednisolone* (0.5–1 g) is given intravenously or by mouth over a 3–5-day period. Intravenous treatment appears to benefit relapses of optic neuritis more than do oral steroids but usually requires hospital admission.[41]

Urinary frequency and urgency (spastic bladder) is common, for which the antimuscarinics propantheline or oxybutynin can be useful by acting as a detrusor relaxant. Constipation is treated with laxatives, while impotence may respond to sildenafil. In progressive disease, muscle spasticity can be severe and disabling. Oral baclofen or tizanidine, or

---

[40]Hauser S L, Comi G, Hartung H-P et al 2017 Ocrelizumab versus Interferon Beta-1 in relapsing multiple sclerosis. New England Journal of Medicine 376:221–234.).

[41]Some MS centres have arrangements in place for patients to receive intravenous corticosteroids in their own home, e.g. by employing community nurses who can monitor the hourly infusion. This is often preferred by patients, and reduces overall medical costs.

locally injected toxin can reduce spasticity, but over-treatment may lead to flaccid weakness. Intranasal cannabinoid is a more recent treatment for spasticity. Very occasionally, baclofen given intrathecally by an implanted pump can relieve severe spasticity. Fatigue is common in MS and may respond to amantadine or modafinil. Depression or psychosis, features of MS, require specific treatments. Finally, the role of general supportive measures, such as ramps, wheelchairs, stairlifts, prevention of bedsores, cannot be overstated.

Miscellaneous neurological disorders

Peripheral neuropathies

A large number of disease processes affect peripheral nerves causing one of several clinical syndromes. For example, such diseases can be classified according to whether sensory, motor or both types of nerve fibre are affected, or divided, depending upon whether it is the myelin sheath that is damaged primarily (peripheral demyelination) or the axon (axonopathy).

One important set of causes are the inflammatory demyelinating polyneuropathies, which can be either acute (AIDP, also called Guillain–Barré syndrome) or chronic (CIDP). Both diseases are treated with *intravenous immunoglobulin* or *plasma exchange*, so as to suppress production of antibodies against gangliosides, a glycosphingolipid present in the lipid membrane. CIDP is also responsive to *glucocorticoids*; this is not the case for Guillain–Barré syndrome. Other types of inflammatory demyelinating polyneuropathy associated with plasma cell dyscrasia and paraproteinaemia, must be sought. These are treated in similar ways, although increasingly use is also made of the monoclonal anti-CD20 drug *rituximab*. Autoimmune mechanisms can also cause an axonopathy pattern of neuropathy, usually in association with a systemic vasculitis, e.g. Churg–Strauss syndrome. These conditions require a *corticosteroid* and, often, immunosuppressants such as *azathioprine, mycophenolate* or *cyclophosphamide*.

A separate group of polyneuropathies arise from metabolic derangements, commonly diabetes mellitus (which can improve or at least stabilise with rigorous glycaemic control) and alcoholism (which can respond partially to high-dose parenteral *niacin*, vitamin B_1). Others in this category include deficiency of vitamin B_{12}, or vitamin B_6 (the latter may arise as an unwanted effect of the antituberculous drug isoniazid). Multiple other types of polyneuropathy exist, a fraction of which will have their specific treatments, e.g. HIV infection (HAART therapy), Lyme disease (ceftriaxone or doxycycline), diphtheria (antitoxin, penicillin), acute intermittent porphyria (heme arginate and high-carbohydrate diet), amyloidosis (chemotherapy, e.g. melphalan), Fabry's disease (α-galactosidase gene replacement).

Motor neurone disease

The cause of the progressive destruction of upper and lower motor neurones is unknown. The only drug available, riluzole, acts by inhibiting accumulation of the neurotransmitter, glutamate. *Riluzole* prolongs survival time from 13 to 16 months, with no effect on motor function.[42] It may cause neutropenia. Its use in the UK is limited to neurologists.

Tetanus

Tetanus remains a potentially fatal disease among underprivileged people in parts of the world where immunisation programmes are inadequate. Management involves:

- Immediate neutralisation of any toxin that has not yet become attached irreversibly to the CNS. Human tetanus immunoglobulin 150 units/kg is given intramuscularly at multiple sites to neutralise unbound toxin.
- Wound debridement and destruction of *Clostridium tetani* with metronidazole.
- Control of convulsions while maintaining respiratory function. Midazolam or diazepam is given for spasms and rigidity, and tracheal intubation and mechanical ventilation for prolonged spasms with respiratory dysfunction (in severe cases, a neuromuscular blocking drug, e.g. intermittent doses of pancuronium, may be required).
- Control of cardiovascular function (tetanus toxin often causes disturbances in autonomic control, with sympathetic overactivity). First-line treatment is by sedation with a benzodiazepine and opioid; infusion of the short-acting β-blocker esmolol, or the $α_2$-adrenergic agonist clonidine, helps to control episodes of hypertension.
- Severe cases generally require admission to an intensive care unit for fluid and electrolyte management; enteral nutrition (weight loss is universal in tetanus); and monitoring for infection (usually aspiration pneumonia), thromboembolism, and pressure sores.

[42]Lacomblez L, Bensimon G, Leigh P N et al 1996 A controlled trial of riluzole in ALS. Lancet 347:1425–1431.

Guide to further reading

Baker, G.A., Lane, S., Benn, E.K., et al., 2011. Adverse antiepileptic drug effects in new-onset seizures: a case-control study. Neurology 76, 273–279.

Chong, D.J., Lerman, A.M., 2016. Practice update: review of anticonvulsant therapy. Curr. Neurol. Neurosci. Rep. 16, 39.

Drivers Medical Group, 2016. At a glance guide to the current medical standards of fitness to drive. DVLA, Swansea. Available at: http://www.dft.gov.uk/dvla/medical/ataglance.aspx (Accessed February 2011).

Fahn, S., Oakes, D., Shoulson, I., Parkinson Study Group, 2004. Levodopa and the progression of Parkinson's disease. N. Engl. J. Med. 351, 2498–2508.

Marson, A.G., Al-Kharusi, A.M., Alwaidh, M., SANAD Study Group, et al., 2007. The SANAD study of effectiveness of valproate, lamotrigine, or topiramate for generalised and unclassifiable epilepsy: an unblinded randomised controlled trial. Lancet 369, 1016–1026.

Marson, A.G., Al-Kharusi, A.M., Alwaidh, M., et al., The SANAD Study Group, 2007. The SANAD study of effectiveness of carbamazepine, gabapentin, lamotrigine, xcarbazepine, or topiramate for treatment of partial epilepsy: an unblinded randomised controlled trial. Lancet 369, 1000–1015.

Meador, K.J., Baker, G.A., Browning, N., et al., The NEAD Study Group, 2010. Effects of breastfeeding in children of women taking antiepileptic drugs. Neurology 75, 1954–1960.

Rascol, O., Fitzer-Attas, C.J., Hauser, R., et al., 2011. A double-blind, delayed-start trial of rasagiline in Parkinson's disease (the ADAGIO study): prespecified and post-hoc analyses of the need for additional therapies, changes in UPDRS scores, and non-motor outcomes. Lancet Neurol. 10, 415–423.

Siddiqui, A., Kerb, R., Weale, M.E., et al., 2003. Association of multidrug resistance in epilepsy with a polymorphism in the drug-transporter gene ABCB1. N. Engl. J. Med. 348, 1442–1448.

Section | 5 |

Cardiorespiratory and renal systems

Chapter 22

Cholinergic and antimuscarinic (anticholinergic) mechanisms and drugs

Morris J. Brown, Fraz A. Mir

SYNOPSIS

Acetylcholine is a widespread chemotransmitter in the body, mediating a broad range of physiological effects. The two classes of receptor for acetylcholine are defined on the basis of their preferential activation by the alkaloids *nicotine* and *muscarine*.

Cholinergic drugs (acetylcholine receptor agonists) mimic acetylcholine at all sites, although the balance of nicotinic and muscarinic effects is variable.

Acetylcholine antagonists that block the nicotine-like effects (neuromuscular blockers and autonomic ganglion blockers) are described elsewhere (Ch. 19).

Acetylcholine antagonists that block the muscarine-like effects, e.g. atropine, are often imprecisely called 'anticholinergics'. The more specific term 'antimuscarinic' is preferred here.

- Cholinergic drugs.
  - Classification
  - Sites of action
  - Pharmacology
  - Choline esters
  - Alkaloids with cholinergic effects
  - Anticholinesterases; organophosphate poisoning
  - Disorders of neuromuscular transmission: myasthenia gravis.
- Drugs that oppose acetylcholine action.
  - Antimuscarinic drugs.

Cholinergic drugs (cholinomimetics)

These drugs act on post-synaptic acetylcholine receptors (cholinoceptors) at all sites in the body where acetylcholine is the effective neurotransmitter. They initially stimulate and usually later block transmission. In addition, like acetylcholine, they act on the non-innervated receptors that relax peripheral blood vessels.

Uses of cholinergic drugs

- For myasthenia gravis, both to diagnose (edrophonium) and to treat symptoms (neostigmine, pyridostigmine, distigmine).
- To lower intraocular pressure in chronic simple glaucoma (pilocarpine).
- To bronchodilate patients with airflow obstruction (ipratropium, tiotropium).
- To improve cognitive function in Alzheimer's disease (rivastigmine, donepezil).

Classification

Direct-acting (receptor agonists)

- Choline esters (bethanechol, carbachol), which act at all sites, like acetylcholine, but are resistant to degradation by acetylcholinesterases (AChE;

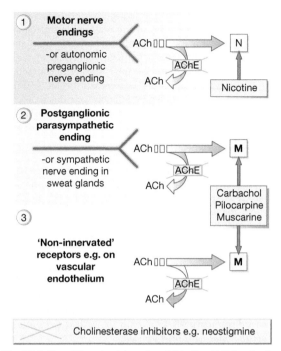

(1) **Motor nerve endings**
-or autonomic preganglionic nerve ending

(2) **Postganglionic parasympathetic ending**
-or sympathetic nerve ending in sweat glands

(3)

'Non-innervated' receptors e.g. on vascular endothelium

Cholinesterase inhibitors e.g. neostigmine

Fig. 22.1 The different origins of acetylcholine (ACh) activating nicotinic (N) versus muscarinic (M) cholinergic receptors. The three sites (numbered 1–3) are referred to in the text.

Fig. 22.1). Muscarinic effects are much more prominent than nicotinic (see p. 394).

- Alkaloids (pilocarpine, muscarine) act selectively on end-organs of postganglionic, cholinergic neurones. Effects are exclusively muscarinic.

Indirect-acting

Cholinesterase inhibitors, or anticholinesterases (physostigmine, neostigmine, pyridostigmine, distigmine, galantamine, rivastigmine, donepezil), block *acetylcholinesterase* (AChE), the enzyme that destroys acetylcholine, allowing endogenous acetylcholine to persist and produce intensified effects.

Sites of action (see Fig. 22.1)

- Autonomic nervous system (see Fig. 22.1, sites 1 and 2).
- Neuromuscular junction (see Fig. 22.1, site 1).
- Central nervous system (CNS).
- Non-innervated sites: blood vessels, chiefly arterioles (see Fig. 22.1, site 3).

Acetylcholine is released from nerve terminals to activate a post-synaptic receptor, except on blood vessels, where the action of cholinergic drugs is unrelated to cholinergic 'vasodilator' nerves. It is also produced in tissues unrelated to nerve endings, e.g. placenta and ciliated epithelial cells, where it acts as a local hormone (autacoid) on local receptors.

A list of principal effects is given below. Not all occur with every drug, and not all are noticeable at therapeutic doses. For example, CNS effects of cholinergic drugs are best seen in cases of anticholinesterase poisoning. Atropine antagonises all the effects of cholinergic drugs except nicotinic actions on autonomic ganglia and the neuromuscular junction, i.e. it has antimuscarinic but not antinicotinic effects (see below).

Pharmacology

Autonomic nervous system

There are two distinct classes of receptor for acetylcholine, defined on the basis of their preferential activation by the alkaloids *nicotine* (from tobacco) and *muscarine* (from a toxic mushroom, *Amanita muscaria*).

It was Henry Dale who, in 1914, first made this functional division, which remains a robust and useful way of classifying cholinergic drug effects. He noted that the actions of acetylcholine and substances acting like it at autonomic ganglia and the neuromuscular junction mimic the stimulant effects of nicotine (hence nicotinic). In contrast, the actions at postganglionic cholinergic endings (parasympathetic endings plus the cholinergic sympathetic nerves to the sweat glands) and non-innervated receptors on blood vessels resembled the alkaloid, muscarine (hence muscarinic).

Parasympathetic division. Stimulation of cholinoceptors in autonomic ganglia and at postganglionic endings affects chiefly the following organs:

- *Eye:* miosis and spasm of the ciliary muscle occur so that the eye is accommodated for near vision. Intraocular pressure falls.
- *Exocrine glands:* there is increased secretion most noticeably from salivary, lachrymal, bronchial and sweat glands. The last are cholinergic, but anatomically part of the sympathetic system; some sweat glands, e.g. axillary, may be adrenergic.
- *Heart:* bradycardia occurs with atrioventricular block, and eventually cardiac arrest.
- *Bronchi:* there is bronchoconstriction and mucosal hypersecretion that may be clinically serious in asthmatic subjects, in whom cholinergic drugs should be avoided if possible.

- *Gut:* motor activity is increased and may cause colicky pain. Exocrine secretion is also increased. Tone in sphincters falls, which may cause defaecation (anal sphincter) or acid reflux/regurgitation (oesophageal sphincter).
- *Urinary bladder and ureters* contract, and the drugs promote micturition.

Sympathetic division. Only the ganglia are stimulated and cholinergic nerves to the adrenal medulla. These effects are overshadowed by effects on the parasympathetic system and are usually seen only if atropine has been given to block the latter, when tachycardia, vasoconstriction and hypertension occur.

Neuromuscular (voluntary) junction

The neuromuscular junction has cholinergic nerve endings and so is activated when anticholinesterases allow acetylcholine to persist, causing muscle fasciculation. Prolonged activation leads to a secondary depolarising neuromuscular block.

Central nervous system

There is usually stimulation followed by depression, but considerable variation among drugs is observed, possibly due to differences in CNS penetration. In overdose, mental excitement occurs, with confusion and restlessness, insomnia (with nightmares during sleep), tremors and dysarthria, and sometimes even convulsions and coma. Nicotinic receptor activation in the CNS is also thought to be important for cognitive processing, which appears to be impaired in schizophrenic subjects.

Blood vessels

There is stimulation of cholinergic vasodilator nerve endings in addition to the more important dilating action on arterioles and capillaries mediated through non-innervated muscarinic receptors. Activation of these receptors stimulates nitric oxide production from the vascular endothelium that relaxes the underlying smooth muscle.

Choline esters

Acetylcholine

As acetylcholine has such importance in the body, it is not surprising that attempts have been made to use it therapeutically. But a substance with such a huge variety of effects and rapid destruction in the body is unlikely to be useful when given systemically, as its use in psychiatry illustrates.

Acetylcholine was first injected intravenously as a therapeutic convulsant in 1939, in the reasonable expectation that the fits would be less liable to cause fractures than those following therapeutic leptazol (pentylenetetrazole) convulsions. Recovery rates of up to 80% were claimed in various psychotic conditions. Enthusiasm began to wane, however, when it was shown that the fits were due to anoxia resulting from cardiac arrest and not to pharmacological effects on the brain.[1]

The following description is typical:

> *A few seconds after the injection (which was given as rapidly as possible, to avoid total destruction in the blood) the patient sat up 'with knees drawn up to the chest, the arms flexed and the head bent forward. There were repeated violent coughs, sometimes with flushing. Forced swallowing and loud peristaltic rumblings could be heard'. Respiration was laboured and irregular. 'The coughing abated as the patient sank back in the bed. Forty seconds after the injection the radial and apical pulse were zero and the patient became comatose.' The pupils dilated, and deep reflexes were hyperactive. In 45 seconds the patient went into opisthotonos with brief apnoea.*
>
> *Lachrymation, sweating and borborygmi were prominent. The deep reflexes became diminished. The patient then relaxed and 'lay quietly in bed – cold moist and gray. In about 90 seconds, flushing of the face marked the return of the pulse'. The respiratory rate rose and consciousness returned in about 125 seconds. The patients sometimes micturated but did not defaecate. They 'tended to lie quietly in bed after the treatment'. 'Most of the patients were reluctant to be retreated.'[2]*

Other choline esters

Carbachol is not destroyed by cholinesterase; its actions are most pronounced on the bladder and gastrointestinal tract, so that the drug was used to stimulate these organs, e.g. after surgery. These uses are now virtually obsolete, e.g. catheterisation is preferred for bladder atony. It is occasionally applied topically (3% solution) to the eye as a miotic.

Bethanechol resembles carbachol in its actions but is some 10-fold less potent (it differs by a single β-methyl group) and has no significant nicotinic effects at clinical doses.

[1]Harris M et al 1943 Archives of Neurology and Psychiatry 50:304.
[2]Cohen L H et al 1944 Archives of Neurology and Psychiatry 51:171.

Alkaloids with cholinergic effects

Nicotine (see also p. 155) is a social drug that lends its medicinal use as an adjunct to stopping its own abuse as tobacco. It is available as gum to chew, dermal patches, a nasal spray or an inhalator. These deliver a lower dose of nicotine than cigarettes and appear to be safe in patients with ischaemic heart disease. The patches are slightly better tolerated than the gum, which releases nicotine in a more variable fashion depending on the rate at which it is chewed and the salivary pH, which is influenced by drinking coffee and carbonated drinks. Nicotine treatment is reported to be nearly twice as effective as placebo in achieving sustained withdrawal from smoking (18% versus 11% in one review).[3] Treatment is much more likely to be successful if it is used as an aid to, not a substitute for, continued counselling. *Bupropion* is possibly more effective than the nicotine patch[4] (see also p. 156) and the partial nicotinic agonist, varenicline, slightly more effective still. The efficacy of varenicline is tempered by its ability to cause suicidal ideation and behaviour.

Pilocarpine, from a South American plant (*Pilocarpus* spp.), acts directly on muscarinic receptors (see Fig. 22.1); it also stimulates and then depresses the CNS. The chief clinical use of pilocarpine is to lower intraocular pressure in primary open-angle glaucoma (also called 'chronic simple' or 'wide-angle' glaucoma), as an adjunct to a topical β-blocker; it produces miosis, opens drainage channels in the trabecular network and improves the outflow of aqueous humour. Oral pilocarpine is available for the treatment of xerostomia (dry mouth) in Sjögren's syndrome, or following irradiation of head and neck tumours. The commonest adverse effect is sweating, an effect actually exploited in a diagnostic test for cystic fibrosis.

Arecoline is an alkaloid in the betel nut, which is chewed extensively throughout India and Southeast Asia. Presumably the lime mix in the 'chews' provides the necessary alkaline pH to maximise its buccal absorption. It produces a mild euphoric effect, like many cholinomimetic alkaloids.

Muscarine is of no therapeutic use but it has pharmacological interest. It is present in small amounts in the fungus *Amanita muscaria* (fly agaric), named after its capacity to kill the domestic fly *(Musca domestica)*; muscarine was so named because it was thought to be the insecticidal principle, but it is relatively non-toxic to flies (orally administered). The fungus may contain other antimuscarinic substances and γ-aminobutyric acid (GABA) receptor agonists (such as muscimol) in amounts sufficient to be psychoactive

in humans. The antimuscarinic components may explain why the dried fungus was used previously to treat excessive sweating, especially in patients with tuberculosis.

Poisoning with these fungi may present with antimuscarinic, cholinergic or GABAergic effects. All have CNS actions. Happily, poisoning by *Amanita muscaria* is seldom serious, but species of *Inocybe* contain substantially larger amounts of muscarine (see Ch. 10). The lengths to which humans are prepared to go in taking 'chemical vacations' when life is hard are shown by the inhabitants of eastern Siberia, who used *Amanita muscaria* recreationally for its cerebral stimulant effects. They were apparently prepared to put up with the autonomic actions to escape briefly from reality – so much so that when the fungus was scarce in winter they were even prepared to drink their own urine to prolong the experience. Sometimes, in generous mood, they would even offer their urine to others as a treat.

Anticholinesterases

At cholinergic nerve endings and in erythrocytes, there is a specific enzyme that destroys acetylcholine, true cholinesterase or *acetylcholinesterase*. In various tissues, especially plasma, there are other esterases that are not specific for acetylcholine but that also destroy other esters, e.g. suxamethonium, procaine (and cocaine) and bambuterol (a prodrug that is hydrolysed to terbutaline). Hence, they are called *pseudocholinesterases*. Chemicals that inactivate these esterases (anticholinesterases) are used in medicine and in agriculture as pesticides. They act by allowing naturally synthesised acetylcholine to accumulate instead of being destroyed. Their effects are explained by this accumulation in the CNS, neuromuscular junction, autonomic ganglia, postganglionic cholinergic nerve endings (which are principally in the parasympathetic nervous system) and in the walls of blood vessels, where acetylcholine has a paracrine[5] role not necessarily associated with nerve endings. Some of these effects oppose one another, e.g. the effect of anticholinesterase on the heart will be the result of stimulation at sympathetic ganglia and the opposing effect of stimulation at parasympathetic (vagal) ganglia and at postganglionic nerve endings.

Physostigmine is an alkaloid, obtained from the seeds of the West African Calabar bean (spp. *Physostigma*), which has had long use both as a weapon and as an ordeal poison.[6] It acts for a few hours. It has been shown to have some efficacy in improving cognitive function in Alzheimer-type dementia.

---

[3]Drug and Therapeutics Bulletin 1999; 37 (July issue).
[4]Jorenby D E, Leischow S J, Nides M A et al 1999 A controlled trial of sustained-release bupropion, a nicotine patch, or both for smoking cessation. New England Journal of Medicine 340:685–692.

[5]A hormone function that is restricted to the local environment.
[6]To demonstrate guilt or innocence according to whether the accused died or lived after the judicial dose. The practice had the advantage that the demonstration of guilt provided simultaneous punishment.

Neostigmine ($t_{1/2}$ 2 h) is a synthetic reversible anticholinesterase whose actions are more prominent on the neuromuscular junction and the alimentary tract than on the cardiovascular system and eye. It is therefore used principally in myasthenia gravis and as an antidote to competitive neuromuscular blocking agents; its use to stimulate the bowels or bladder after surgery is now obsolete. Neostigmine is effective orally, and by injection (usually subcutaneous). But higher doses may be used in myasthenia gravis, often combined with atropine to reduce the unwanted muscarinic effects.

Pyridostigmine is similar to neostigmine but has a less powerful action that is slower in onset and slightly longer in duration, and perhaps with fewer visceral effects. It is used in myasthenia gravis.

Distigmine is a variant of pyridostigmine (two linked molecules as the name implies).

Edrophonium is structurally related to neostigmine, but its action is brief and autonomic effects are minimal except at high doses. The drug is used to diagnose myasthenia gravis and to differentiate a myasthenic crisis (weakness due to inadequate anticholinesterase treatment or severe disease) from a cholinergic crisis (weakness caused by over-treatment with an anticholinesterase). Myasthenic weakness is substantially improved by edrophonium, whereas cholinergic weakness is aggravated but the effect is transient; the action of 3 mg i.v. is lost in 5 min.

Carbaryl (carbaril) is another reversible carbamoylating anticholinesterase that closely resembles physostigmine in its actions. It is used widely as a garden insecticide and, clinically, to kill head and body lice. Sensitive insects lack cholinesterase-rich erythrocytes and succumb to the accumulation of acetylcholine in the synaptic junctions of their nervous system. Effective and safe use in humans is also probably due to the very limited absorption of carbaryl after topical application. The anticholinesterase *malathion* is effective against scabies, head lice and crab lice.

A more recent use of anticholinesterase drugs has been to improve cognitive function in patients with Alzheimer's disease (see p. 359), where both the degree of dementia and amyloid plaque density correlate with the impairment of brain cholinergic function. *Donepezil, galantamine* (which has additional nicotinic agonist properties) and *rivastigmine* are licensed in the UK for this indication. They are all reversible inhibitors that are orally active and cross the blood–brain barrier readily (see p. 83).

Anticholinesterase poisoning

The anticholinesterases used in therapeutics are generally of the carbamate type that reversibly inactivates cholinesterase only for a few hours. This contrasts markedly with the very long-lived inhibition caused by inhibitors of the organophosphate (OP) type. In practice, the inhibition is so long that clinical recovery from organophosphate exposure is usually dependent on synthesis of new enzyme. This process may take weeks to complete, although clinical recovery is usually evident in days. Cases of acute poisoning are usually met outside therapeutic practice, e.g. after agricultural, industrial or transport accidents.

Substances of this type have also been developed and used in war, especially the three G agents: GA (tabun), GB (sarin) and GD (soman). Although called nerve 'gas', they are actually volatile liquids, which facilitates their use.[7] Where there is known risk of exposure, prior use of *pyridostigmine*, which occupies cholinesterases reversibly for a few hours (the lesser evil), competitively protects them from access by the irreversible warfare agent (the greater evil); soldiers during the Gulf Wars expecting attack were provided with preloaded syringes (of the same design as the Epipen) for delivering adrenaline/epinephrine as antidote therapy (see below). Organophosphate agents are absorbed through the skin, the gastrointestinal tract and by inhalation. Diagnosis depends on observing a substantial part of the list of actions below.

Typical features of acute poisoning involve the gastrointestinal tract (salivation, vomiting, abdominal cramps, diarrhoea, involuntary defaecation), the respiratory system (bronchorrhoea, bronchoconstriction, cough, wheezing, dyspnoea), the cardiovascular system (bradycardia), the genitourinary system (involuntary micturition), the skin (sweating), the skeletal system (muscle weakness, twitching) and the nervous system (miosis, anxiety, headache, convulsions, respiratory failure). Death is due to a combination of the actions in the CNS, to paralysis of the respiratory muscles by peripheral depolarising neuromuscular block, and to excessive bronchial secretions and constriction causing respiratory failure. At autopsy, ileal intussusceptions are commonly found.

Quite frequently and typically 1–4 days after resolution of symptoms of acute exposure, the *intermediate syndrome* may develop, characterised by a proximal flaccid limb paralysis that may reflect muscle necrosis. Even later, after a gap of 2–4 weeks, some exposed persons exhibit *delayed polyneuropathy*, with sensory and motor impairment usually of the lower limbs. Claims of chronic effects (subtle cognitive defects, peripheral neuropathy) following recurrent, low-dose exposure, as with organophosphate used as sheep dip, continue to be the subject of investigation but, as yet, there is no conclusive proof.

---

[7]In recent times, there have been major instances of use against populations by both military and terrorist bodies (in the field and in an underground transport system).

Treatment. As the most common circumstance of accidental poisoning is exposure to pesticide spray or spillage, contaminated clothing should be removed and the skin washed. Attendants should take care to ensure that they themselves do not become contaminated.

- *Atropine* is the mainstay of treatment; 2 mg is given i.m. or i.v. as soon as possible and repeated every 15–60 min until dryness of the mouth and a heart rate exceeding 70 beats per minute indicate that its effect is adequate. A poisoned patient may require 100 mg or more for a single episode. Atropine antagonises the muscarinic parasympathomimetic effects of the poison, i.e. due to the accumulated acetylcholine stimulating postganglionic nerve endings (excessive secretion and vasodilatation), but has no effect on the neuromuscular block, which is nicotinic.
- *Mechanical ventilation* may therefore be needed to assist the respiratory muscles; special attention to the airway is vital because of bronchial constriction and excessive secretion.
- *Diazepam* may be needed for convulsions.
- *Atropine eye drops* may relieve the headache caused by miosis.
- *Enzyme reactivation.* The organophosphate (OP) pesticides inactivate cholinesterase by irreversibly phosphorylating the active centre of the enzyme. Substances that reactivate the enzyme hasten the destruction of the accumulated acetylcholine and, unlike atropine, they have both antinicotinic and antimuscarinic effects. The principal agent is *pralidoxime,* which should be given by slow intravenous injection (diluted) over 5–10 min, initially 30 mg/kg repeated every 4–6 h or by intravenous infusion, 8 mg/kg/h; usual maximum 12 g in 24 h. Its efficacy is greatest if administered within 12 h of poisoning, then falls off steadily as the phosphorylated enzyme is further stabilised by 'ageing'. If significant reactivation occurs, muscle power improves within 30 min.

Poisoning with *reversible* anticholinesterases is appropriately treated by atropine and the necessary general support; it lasts only hours.

In poisoning with *irreversible* agents, erythrocyte or plasma cholinesterase content should be measured if possible, both for diagnosis and to determine when a poisoned worker may return to the task (should he or she be willing to do so). Return should not be allowed until the cholinesterase exceeds 70% of normal, which may take several weeks. Recovery from the intermediate syndrome and delayed polyneuropathy is slow and is dependent on muscle and nerve regeneration.

Disorders of neuromuscular transmission

Myasthenia gravis

In myasthenia gravis, synaptic transmission at the neuromuscular junction is impaired; most cases have an autoimmune basis, and some 85% of patients have a raised titre of autoantibodies to the muscle acetylcholine receptor. The condition is probably heterogeneous, as about 15% do not have receptor antibodies, or have antibodies to another neuromuscular junction protein (muscle-specific kinase, MuSK) and, rarely, it occurs with D-penicillamine used for rheumatoid arthritis.

Neostigmine was introduced in 1931 for its stimulant effects on intestinal activity. In 1934 it occurred to Dr Mary Walker that, as the paralysis of myasthenia had been (erroneously) attributed to a curare-like substance in the blood, physostigmine (eserine), an anticholinesterase drug known to antagonise curare, might be beneficial. It was, and she reported this important observation in a short letter.[8] Soon after this she used neostigmine by mouth, with greater benefit. The sudden appearance of an effective treatment for a hitherto untreatable chronic disease must always be a dramatic event for its victims. One patient described the impact of the discovery of the action of neostigmine, as follows:

> *My myasthenia started in 1925, when I was 18. For several months it consisted of double vision and fatigue … An ophthalmic surgeon … prescribed glasses with a prism. However, soon more alarming symptoms began. [Her limbs became weak and she] was sent to an eminent neurologist. This was a horrible experience. He … could find no physical signs … declared me to be suffering from hysteria and asked me what was on my mind. When I answered truthfully, that nothing except anxiety over my symptoms, he replied 'my dear child, I am not a perfect fool …', and showed me out. [She became worse and at times she was unable to turn over in bed. Eating and even speaking were difficult. Eventually, her fiancé, a medical student, read about myasthenia gravis and she was correctly diagnosed in 1927.] There was at that time no known treatment and therefore many things to try. [She had gold injections, thyroid, suprarenal extract, lecithin, glycine and ephedrine. The last had a slight effect.] Then in February 1935, came the day that I shall always*

---

[8]Walker M B 1934 Lancet i:1200.

remember. I was living alone with a nurse … It was one of my better days, and I was lying on the sofa after tea … My fiancé came in rather late saying that he had something new for me to try. My first thought was 'Oh bother! Another injection, and another false hope'. I submitted to the injection with complete indifference and within a few minutes began to feel very strange … when I lifted my arms, exerting the effort to which I had become accustomed, they shot into the air, every movement I attempted was grotesquely magnified until I learnt to make less effort … it was strange, wonderful and at first, very frightening … we danced twice round the carpet. That was my first meeting with neostigmine, and we have never since been separated.[9]

Pathogenesis. The clinical features of myasthenia gravis are caused by specific autoantibodies to the nicotinic acetylcholine receptor. These antibodies accelerate receptor turnover, shortening their typical lifetime in the skeletal muscle membrane from around 7 days, to 1 day in a myasthenic. This process results in marked depletion of receptors from myasthenic skeletal muscle (about 90%), explaining its fatigability. The frequent finding of a specific human leucocyte antigen (HLA) haplotype (A1-B8-Dw3) in myasthenics and concurrent hyperplasia or tumours of the thymus support the autoimmune basis for the disease.

Diagnosis. Edrophonium dramatically and transiently (5 min) relieves myasthenic muscular weakness. A syringe is loaded with edrophonium 10 mg; 2 mg is given i.v., and if there is no improvement in weakness in 30 s, the remaining 8 mg is injected. Adults without suitable veins may receive 10 mg by i.m. injection. Atropine should be at hand to block severe cholinergic autonomic (muscarinic) effects, e.g. bradycardia, should they occur.

Titres of acetylcholine receptor antibodies should also be measured to confirm the diagnosis.

Treatment involves immunosuppression, thymectomy (unless contraindicated) and symptom relief with drugs:

- *Immunosuppressive treatment* is directed at eliminating the acetylcholine receptor autoantibody. *Prednisolone* induces improvement or remission in 80% of cases. The dose should be increased slowly using an alternate-day regimen until the minimum effective amount is attained; an immunosuppressive improvement may take several weeks. *Azathioprine* may be used as a steroid-sparing agent. Prednisolone is effective for ocular myasthenia, which is fortunate,

for this variant of the disease responds poorly to thymectomy or anticholinesterase drugs. Some acute and severe cases respond poorly to prednisolone with azathioprine and, for these, intermittent plasmapheresis or immunoglobulin i.v. (to remove circulating anti-receptor antibody) can provide dramatic short-term relief.

- *Thymectomy* should be offered to those with generalised myasthenia gravis younger than 40 years of age, once the clinical state allows and unless there are powerful contraindications to surgery. Most cases benefit, and about 25% can discontinue drug treatment. Thymectomy should also be undertaken in all myasthenic patients who have a thymoma, but the main reason is to prevent local infiltration, as the procedure is less likely to relieve the myasthenia.

- *Symptomatic* drug treatment is decreasingly used. Its aim is to increase the concentration of acetylcholine at the neuromuscular junction with anticholinesterase drugs. The mainstay is usually *pyridostigmine*, starting with 60 mg by mouth 4-hourly. It is preferred because its action is smoother than that of neostigmine, but the latter is more rapid in onset and can with advantage be given in the mornings to get the patient mobile. Either drug can be given parenterally if bulbar paralysis makes swallowing difficult. An antimuscarinic drug, e.g. propantheline (15–30 mg t.i.d.), should be added if muscarinic effects are troublesome.

Excessive dosing with an anticholinesterase can actually worsen the muscle weakness in myasthenics if the accumulation of acetylcholine at the neuromuscular junction is sufficient to cause depolarising blockade *(cholinergic crisis)*. It is important to distinguish this type of muscle weakness from an exacerbation of the disease itself *(myasthenic crisis)*. The dilemma can be resolved with a test dose of edrophonium 2 mg i.v. (best before next dose of anticholinesterase), which relieves a myasthenic crisis but worsens a cholinergic one. The latter may be severe enough to precipitate respiratory failure and should be attempted only with full resuscitation facilities, including mechanical ventilation, at hand.

A cholinergic crisis should be treated by withdrawing all anticholinesterase medication, providing mechanical ventilation if required, and administering intravenous atropine for muscarinic effects of the overdose. The neuromuscular block is a nicotinic effect and will be unchanged by atropine. A resistant myasthenic crisis may be treated by withdrawal of drugs and mechanical ventilation for a few days. Plasmapheresis or intravenous immunoglobulin may be beneficial by removing anti-receptor antibodies (see above).

---

[9]Disabilities and How to Live with Them. (1952) Lancet Publications, London.

Lambert–Eaton syndrome

Separate from myasthenia gravis is the Lambert–Eaton syndrome, in which symptoms similar to those of myasthenia gravis occur in association with a carcinoma; in 60% of patients this is a small-cell lung cancer. The defect here is pre-synaptic with a deficiency of acetylcholine release due to an autoantibody directed against L-type voltage-gated calcium channels.

Patients with the Lambert–Eaton syndrome do not usually respond well to anticholinesterases. The drug 3,4-diaminopyridine (3,4-DAP) increases neurotransmitter release and also the action potential (by blocking potassium conductance), producing a non-specific enhancement of cholinergic neurotransmission. It should be taken orally, four or five times a day. Adverse effects due to CNS excitation (insomnia, seizures) can occur. An example of an orphan drug without a product licence, 3,4-DAP is available in the UK on a 'named patient' basis.

Drug-induced disorders of neuromuscular transmission

Quite apart from the neuromuscular blocking agents used in anaesthesia, a number of drugs possess actions that impair neuromuscular transmission and, in appropriate circumstances, give rise to:

- postoperative respiratory depression in people with otherwise normal neuromuscular transmission.
- aggravation or unmasking of myasthenia gravis.
- a drug-induced myasthenic syndrome.

These drugs include:

Antimicrobials. Aminoglycosides (neomycin, streptomycin, gentamicin), polypeptides (colistimethate sodium, polymyxin B) and perhaps the quinolones (e.g. ciprofloxacin) may cause postoperative breathing difficulty if they are instilled into the peritoneal or pleural cavity. It appears that the antibiotics both interfere with the release of acetylcholine and also have a competitive curare-like effect on the acetylcholine receptor.

Cardiovascular drugs. Those that possess local anaesthetic properties (quinidine, procainamide, lidocaine) and certain β-blockers (propranolol, oxprenolol) interfere with acetylcholine release and may aggravate or reveal myasthenia gravis.

Other drugs. *Penicillamine* causes some patients, especially those with rheumatoid arthritis, to form antibodies to the acetylcholine receptor and a syndrome indistinguishable from myasthenia gravis results. Spontaneous recovery occurs in about two-thirds of cases when penicillamine is withdrawn. Phenytoin may rarely induce or aggravate myasthenia gravis, or induce a myasthenic syndrome, possibly by depressing release of acetylcholine. Lithium may impair pre-synaptic neurotransmission by substituting for sodium ions in the nerve terminal.

Drugs that oppose acetylcholine

These may be divided into:

- *Antimuscarinic drugs,* which act principally at postganglionic cholinergic (parasympathetic) nerve endings, i.e. atropine-related drugs (see Fig. 22.1). Muscarinic receptors can be subdivided according to their principal sites, namely in the brain (M_1), heart (M_2) and glandular, gastric parietal cells and smooth muscle cells (M_3). As with many receptors, the molecular basis of the subtypes has been defined together with two further cloned subtypes M_4 and M_5, the precise functional roles of which remain to be clarified.
- Antinicotinic drugs: ganglion-blocking drugs (see Ch. 24)
- Neuromuscular blocking drugs (see Fig. 22.1 and Ch. 19).

Antimuscarinic drugs

Atropine is the prototype drug of this group and will be described first. Other named agents will be mentioned only in so far as they differ from atropine. All act as non-selective and competitive antagonists of the various muscarinic receptor subtypes (above). Atropine is a simple tertiary amine; certain others (see Summary) are quaternary nitrogen compounds, a modification that increases antimuscarinic potency in the gut, imparts ganglion-blocking effects and reduces CNS penetration.

Atropine

Atropine is an alkaloid from the deadly nightshade, *Atropa belladonna.*[10] It is a racemate (DL-hyoscyamine), and almost

---

[10]The first name commemorates its success as a homicidal poison, for it is derived from the senior of three legendary Fates, Atropos, who cuts with shears the thread of life spun out by her sister Clothos, of a length determined by her other sister, Lachesis (there is a minor synthetic atropine-like drug called lachesine). The notion that the name derives from a once fashionable female practice of using an extract of the plant to dilate the pupils to improve attractiveness has been comprehensively debunked. Atropa belladonna is "named for the bringer of death and for the Bellonaria, priestesses of Bellona the goddess of war, and for their uses of it as 'war + gifts' – *bella* + *dona*." The full account appears in: Oakley H, Knowles J, de Swiet M, Dayan A. A garden of medicinal plants. London: Royal College of Physicians; Little Brown. 2015, pp 24–18.

all of its antimuscarinic effects are attributable to the L-isomer alone. Atropine is more stable chemically as the racemate, which is the preferred formulation. In general, the effects of atropine are inhibitory, but in large doses it stimulates the CNS (see poisoning, below). Atropine also blocks the muscarinic effects of injected cholinergic drugs, both peripherally and on the CNS. The clinically important actions of atropine at parasympathetic postganglionic nerve endings are listed below; they are mostly the opposite of the activating effects on the parasympathetic system produced by cholinergic drugs.

Exocrine glands. All secretions except milk are diminished. Dry mouth and dry eye are common. Gastric acid secretion is reduced but so also is the total volume of gastric secretion, so that pH may be little altered. Sweating is inhibited (sympathetic innervation but releasing acetylcholine). Bronchial secretions are reduced and may become viscid, which can be a disadvantage, as removal of secretion by cough and ciliary action is rendered less effective.

Smooth muscle is relaxed. In the gastrointestinal tract there is reduction of tone and peristalsis. Muscle spasm of the intestinal tract induced by morphine is reduced, but such spasm in the biliary tract is not significantly affected. Atropine relaxes bronchial muscle, an effect that is useful in some asthmatics. Micturition is slowed, and urinary retention may be induced, especially when there is pre-existing prostatic enlargement.

Ocular effects. Mydriasis occurs with a rise in intraocular pressure due to the dilated iris blocking drainage of the intraocular fluid from the angle of the anterior chamber. An attack of glaucoma may be induced in eyes predisposed to primary angle (also called 'acute closed-angle' or 'narrow-angle') closure and is a medical emergency. There is no significant effect on pressure in normal eyes. The ciliary muscle is paralysed, and so the eye is accommodated for distant vision. After atropinisation, normal pupillary reflexes may not be regained for 2 weeks. Atropine use is a cause of unequally sized and unresponsive pupils.[11]

Cardiovascular system. Atropine reduces vagal tone, thus increasing the heart rate and enhancing conduction in the bundle of His. As efficacy depends on the level of vagal tone, full atropinisation may increase heart rate by 30 beats/min in a young subject, but has little effect in the elderly.

Atropine has no significant effect on peripheral blood vessels in therapeutic doses, but in overdose there is marked vasodilatation.

Central nervous system. Atropine is effective against both the tremor and rigidity of parkinsonism. It prevents or abates motion sickness.

Antagonism to cholinergic drugs. Atropine opposes the effects of muscarinic agonists on the CNS, at postganglionic cholinergic nerve endings and on peripheral blood vessels. It does not block cholinergic effects at the neuromuscular junction or significantly at the autonomic ganglia, i.e. atropine opposes the muscarine-like but not the nicotine-like effects of acetylcholine.

Pharmacokinetics. Atropine is readily absorbed from the gastrointestinal tract and may also be injected by the usual routes, including intratracheal instillation in an emergency setting. The occasional cases of atropine poisoning following use of eye drops are due to the solution running down the lachrymal ducts into the nose and being swallowed. Atropine is in part destroyed in the liver and in part excreted unchanged by the kidney ($t_{1/2}$ 2 h).

Dose. 0.6–1.2 mg by mouth at night or 0.6 mg i.v., repeated as necessary to a maximum of 3 mg/day; for chronic use atropine has largely been replaced by other antimuscarinic drugs.

Poisoning with atropine (and other antimuscarinic drugs) presents with the more obvious peripheral effects: dry mouth (with dysphagia); mydriasis; blurred vision; hot, flushed, dry skin; and, in addition, hyperthermia (CNS action plus absence of sweating); restlessness; anxiety; excitement; hallucinations; delirium; and mania. The cerebral excitation is followed by depression and coma or, as it has been described with characteristic American verbal felicity, 'hot as a hare, blind as a bat, dry as a bone, red as a beet and mad as a hen'.[12] Poisoning is typically seen (especially in children) following ingestion of the rather attractive berries of solanaceous plants, e.g. deadly nightshade and henbane. Treatment involves activated charcoal to adsorb the drug, sponging to cool the patient and diazepam for the central excitement.

Other antimuscarinic drugs

In the following accounts, the peripheral atropine-like effects of the drugs may be assumed; only differences from atropine are described.

---

[11]A doctor, after working in his garden greenhouse, was alarmed to find that the vision in his left eye was blurred and the pupil was grossly dilated. Physical examination failed to reveal a cause, and the pupil gradually and spontaneously returned to normal, suggesting that the explanation was exposure to some exogenous agent. The doctor then recalled that his greenhouse contained flowering plants called angel's trumpet (sp. *Brugmansia,* syn. *Datura,* of the nightshade family), and he may have brushed against them. Angel's trumpet is noted for its content of scopolamine (hyoscine), and is very toxic if ingested. The plant is evidently less angelic than the name suggests (Merrick J, Barnett S 2000 Fillers. Not such an angel. British Medical Journal 321:219).

[12]Cohen H L et al 1944 Acetylcholine treatment of schizophrenia. Archives of Neurology and Psychiatry 51:171–175.

Uses of antimuscarinic drugs

- **For their central actions** – some (trihexyphenidyl (benzhexol) and orphenadrine) are used against the rigidity and tremor of *parkinsonism,* especially drug-induced parkinsonism, where doses higher than the usual therapeutic amounts are often needed and tolerated. They are used as *antiemetics* (principally hyoscine, promethazine). Their sedative action is used in anaesthetic premedication (hyoscine).

- **For their peripheral actions** – atropine, homatropine and cyclopentolate are used in *ophthalmology* to dilate the pupil and to paralyse ocular accommodation. Patients should be warned of a transient, but unpleasant, stinging sensation, and that they cannot read or drive (at least without dark glasses) for at least 3–4 h. Tropicamide is the shortest acting of the mydriatics. If it is desired to dilate the pupil and to spare accommodation, a sympathomimetic, e.g. phenylephrine, is useful.

  In anaesthesic premedication, atropine, and hyoscine[13] block the vagus and reduce mucosal secretions; hyoscine also has useful sedative effects. Glycopyrronium[13] is frequently used during anaesthetic recovery to block the muscarinic effects of neostigmine given to reverse a non-depolarising neuromuscular blockade.

  In the respiratory tract, ipratropium[13] is a useful bronchodilator in chronic obstructive pulmonary disease and acute asthma.

- **For their actions on the gut,** against muscle spasm and hypermotility, e.g. against colic (pain due to spasm of smooth muscle), and to reduce morphine-induced smooth muscle spasm when the analgesic is used against acute colic.

- **In the urinary tract,** flavoxate, oxybutynin, propiverine, tolterodine, trospium, solifenacin, darifenacin and propantheline[13] are indicated to relieve any urinary frequency, urgency, or incontinence, whether transient accompanying infection in cystitis, or for more chronic causes. Solifenacin was the first of the 'bladder-specific' M3 receptor antimuscarinics which may improve efficacy and patient compliance by achieving greater blockade of the receptor on bladder muscle, without similar increase in blockade of muscarinic receptors on salivary glands. The 'STAR' study demonstrated non-inferiority of solfenacin compared to tolteridine, comparing the primary outcome of micturitions per 24 h.[14]

- **In disorders of the cardiovascular system,** atropine is useful in bradycardia following myocardial infarction.

- **In cholinergic poisoning,** atropine is an important antagonist of both central nervous, parasympathomimetic and vasodilator effects, though it has no effect at the neuromuscular junction and will not prevent voluntary muscle paralysis. It is also used to block muscarinic effects when cholinergic drugs, such as neostigmine, are used for their effect on the neuromuscular junction in myasthenia gravis.

  Disadvantages of the antimuscarinics include glaucoma and urinary retention, where there is prostatic hypertrophy.

---

[13]Quaternary ammonium compounds (see text).

[14]Robinson D, Cardozo L 2009 Solifenacin: pharmacology and clinical efficacy. Expert Rev Clin Pharmacol. 2:239–253.

Hyoscine (scopolamine) is structurally a close relative of atropine. It differs chiefly in being a CNS depressant, although it may sometimes cause excitement. Elderly patients are often confused by hyoscine and so it is avoided in their anaesthetic premedication. Mydriasis is also briefer than with atropine.

Hyoscine butylbromide (strictly *N*-butylhyoscine bromide; Buscopan) also blocks autonomic ganglia. If injected, it is an effective relaxant of smooth muscle, including the cardia in achalasia, the pyloric antral region and the colon, properties utilised by radiologists and endoscopists. It may sometimes be useful for colic.

Homatropine is used for its ocular effects (1% and 2% solutions as eye drops). Its action is shorter than that of atropine, and it is therefore less likely to cause serious increases in intraocular pressure; the effect wears off in 1 or 2 days. Complete cycloplegia cannot always be obtained unless repeated instillations are made every 15 min for 1–2 h.

Its effects are especially unreliable in children, in whom cyclopentolate or atropine is preferred. The pupillary dilatation may be reversed by physostigmine eye drops.

Tropicamide (Mydriacyl) and *cyclopentolate* (Mydrilate) are useful (as 0.5% or 1% solutions) for mydriasis and cycloplegia. They are quicker and shorter acting than homatropine. Both cause mydriasis in 10–20 min and cycloplegia shortly thereafter. The duration of action is 4–12 h.

Ipratropium (Atrovent) is used as an inhaled bronchodilator for both acute asthma and chronic obstructive pulmonary disease (COPD), and in chronic COPD. It has very limited efficacy in most chronic asthmatics.

Tiotropium (Spiriva) is a long-acting (>24 h) alternative to ipratropium, but only for patients with chronic COPD. It is not licensed for acute bronchoconstriction because of its slow onset of action.

Flavoxate (Urispas) is used for urinary frequency, tenesmus and urgency incontinence because it increases bladder capacity and reduces unstable detrusor contractions (see p. 492).

Oxybutynin is also used for detrusor instability, but antimuscarinic adverse effects may limit its value.

Glycopyrronium is used in anaesthetic premedication to reduce salivary secretion; given intravenously it causes less tachycardia than atropine.

Propantheline (Pro-Banthine) also has ganglion-blocking properties. It may be used as a smooth muscle relaxant, e.g. for irritable bowel syndrome and diagnostic procedures.

Dicyclomine (Merbentyl) is an alternative.

Benzhexol *(trihexyphenidyl)* and *orphenadrine*: see parkinsonism (p. 378).

Solifenacin, darifenacin are indicated for overactive bladder symptoms in women, and as an adjunct to alpha-blockade in the treatment of benign prostatic hyperplasia.

Promethazine. See p. 357.

Propiverine, *tolterodine* and *trospium* diminish unstable detrusor contractions and are used to reduce urinary frequency, urgency and incontinence.

Oral antimuscarinics have occasional use in the treatment of hyperhidrosis.

Summary

- Acetylcholine is the most important receptor agonist neurotransmitter in both the brain and the peripheral nervous system.
- It acts on neurones in the CNS and at autonomic ganglia, on skeletal muscle at the neuromuscular junction, and at a variety of other effector cell types, mainly glandular or smooth muscle.
- The effector response is terminated rapidly through enzymatic destruction by acetylcholinesterase.
- Outside the CNS, acetylcholine has two main classes of receptor: those on autonomic ganglia and skeletal muscle responding to stimulation by nicotine, and the rest which respond to stimulation by muscarine.
- Drugs that mimic or oppose acetylcholine have a wide variety of uses. For instance, the muscarinic agonist pilocarpine lowers intraocular pressure, and antagonist atropine reverses vagal slowing of the heart.
- The main use of drugs at the neuromuscular junction is to relax muscle in anaesthesia, or to inhibit acetylcholinesterase in diseases where nicotinic receptor activation is reduced, e.g. myasthenia gravis.

Guide to further reading

Cohen, L.H., Thale, T., Tissenbaum, M.J., 1944. Acetylcholine treatment of schizophrenia. Arch. Neurol. Psychiatry 51, 171–175.

Costa, L.G., 2006. Current issues in organophosphate toxicology. Clin. Chim. Acta 366, 1–13.

De Nunzio, C., Tubaro, A., 2015. Benign prostatic hyperplasia in 2014: Innovations in medical and surgical treatment. Nat. Rev. Urol. 12, 76–78.

Hawkins, J.R., Tibbetts, R.W., 1956. Intravenous acetylcholine therapy in neurosis. A controlled clinical trial. J. Ment. Sci. 102, 43–51. (In the same issue see also: Carbon dioxide inhalation therapy in neurosis. A controlled clinical trial. p. 52; The placebo response, p. 60).

Medical Manual of Defence Against Chemical Agents, 1987. (no. 0117725692) (JSP 312). HMSO, London.

Meriggioli, M.N., Sanders, D.B., 2009. Autoimmune myasthenia gravis: emerging clinical and biological heterogeneity. Lancet Neurol. 8, 475–490.

Morita, H., Yanigasawa, T., Shimizu, M., et al., 1995. Sarin poisoning in Matsumoto, Japan. Lancet 346, 290–293.

Morton, H.G., 1939. Atropine intoxication: its manifestation in infants and children. J. Pediatr. 14, 755–760.

Weitz, G., 2003. Love and death in Wagner's Tristan und Isolde – an epic anticholinergic crisis. Br. Med. J. 327, 1469–1471. (and the Commentary by Jeff Aronson, pp. 1471–1472).

Chapter | 23 |

Adrenergic mechanisms and drugs

Morris J. Brown

SYNOPSIS

Anyone who administers drugs acting on cardiovascular adrenergic mechanisms requires an understanding of how they act in order to use them to the best advantage and with safety.

- Adrenergic mechanisms.
- Classification of sympathomimetics: by mode of action and selectivity for adrenoceptors.
- Individual sympathomimetics.
- Mucosal decongestants.
- Shock.
- Chronic orthostatic hypotension.

Adrenergic mechanisms

The discovery in 1895 of the hypertensive effect of adrenaline/epinephrine was initiated by Dr Oliver, a physician in practice, who conducted a series of experiments on his young son, into whom he injected an extract of bovine suprarenal and detected a 'definite narrowing of the radial artery'.[1] The effect was confirmed in animals and led eventually to the isolation and synthesis of adrenaline/epinephrine in the early 1900s. Many related compounds were examined and, in 1910, Barger and Dale invented the word 'sympathomimetic'[2] and also pointed out that noradrenaline/norepinephrine mimicked the action of the sympathetic nervous system more closely than did adrenaline/epinephrine.

Adrenaline/epinephrine, noradrenaline/norepinephrine and dopamine are synthesised in the body and are used in therapeutics. The pathway is: tyrosine → dopa → dopamine → noradrenaline/norepinephrine → adrenaline/epinephrine. The final step to adrenaline/epinephrine only occurs in the adrenal medulla.

Classification of sympathomimetics

By mode of action

Noradrenaline/norepinephrine is synthesised and stored in vesicles within adrenergic nerve terminals (Fig. 23.1). The vesicles can be released from these stores by stimulating the nerve or by drugs (ephedrine, amfetamine). The noradrenaline/norepinephrine stores can also be replenished by intravenous infusion of noradrenaline/norepinephrine, and abolished by reserpine or by cutting the sympathetic nerve. Sympathomimetics may be classified on the basis of their sites of action (see Fig. 23.1) as acting:

1. *Directly*: *adrenoceptor agonists*, e.g. adrenaline/epinephrine, noradrenaline/norepinephrine, isoprenaline (isoproterenol), methoxamine,

---

[1] Dale H 1938 Edinburgh Medical Journal 45:461.

[2] 'Compounds which … simulate the effects of sympathetic nerves not only with varying intensity but with varying precision … a term … seems needed to indicate the types of action common to these bases. We propose to call it "sympathomimetic". A term which indicates the relation of the action to innervation by the sympathetic system, without involving any theoretical preconception as to the meaning of that relation or the precise mechanism of the action' (Barger G, Dale H H 1910 Chemical structure and sympathomimetic action of amines. Journal of Physiology 41:19–59.

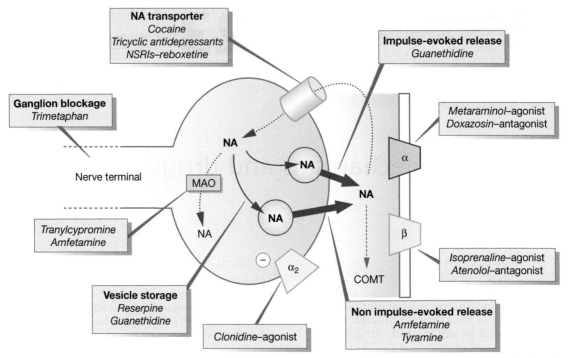

Fig. 23.1 Noradrenergic nerve terminal releasing noradrenaline/norepinephrine (NA) to show the sites of action of drugs that impair or mimic adrenergic function. α and β refer to adrenergic receptor subtypes; MAO, monoamine oxidase.

xylometazoline, metaraminol (entirely); and dopamine and phenylephrine (mainly).

2. *Indirectly*: by causing a release of preformed *noradrenaline/norepinephrine* from stores in nerve endings,[3] e.g. amfetamines, tyramine and ephedrine (largely).

3. *By both mechanisms* (1 and 2, though one usually predominates): *other synthetic agents*.

All of the above mechanisms operate in both the central and peripheral nervous systems, but discussion below will focus on agents that influence peripheral adrenergic mechanisms.

Tachyphylaxis (rapidly diminishing response to repeated administration) is a particular feature of group 2 drugs. It reflects depletion of the 'releasable' pool of noradrenaline/norepinephrine from adrenergic nerve terminals that makes

these agents less suitable as, for example, pressor agents than drugs in group 1. Longer-term tolerance (see p. 80) to the effects of direct sympathomimetics is much less of a clinical problem and reflects an alteration in adrenergic receptor density or coupling to second-messenger systems.

Interactions of sympathomimetics with other vasoactive drugs are complex. Some drugs block the reuptake mechanism for noradrenaline/norepinephrine in adrenergic nerve terminals and potentiate the pressor effects of noradrenaline/norepinephrine, e.g. cocaine, tricyclic antidepressants or highly noradrenaline/norepinephrine-selective reuptake inhibitors (NSRIs) such as reboxetine (see Fig. 23.1). Others deplete or destroy the intracellular stores within adrenergic nerve terminals (e.g. reserpine and guanethidine) and thus block the action of indirect sympathomimetics.

Sympathomimetics are also generally optically active drugs, with only one stereoisomer conferring most of the clinical efficacy of the racemate (a 50:50 mixture of stereoisomers); for instance, L-noradrenaline/norepinephrine is at least 50 times as active as the D-form. Noradrenaline/norepinephrine, adrenaline/epinephrine and phenylephrine are all used clinically as their L-isomers.

---

[3]Fatal hypertension can occur when this class of agent is taken by a patient treated with a monoamine oxidase inhibitor. In addition, remember that large amounts of tyramine are contained in certain food items (cheese, red wine and marmite), forming the basis of the pressor 'cheese reaction' in these patients (see p. 425).

History. Up to 1948 it was known that the peripheral motor (vasoconstriction) effects of adrenaline/epinephrine were preventable and that the peripheral inhibitory (vasodilatation) and cardiac stimulant actions were not preventable by the then available antagonists (ergot alkaloids, phenoxybenzamine). That same year, Ahlquist hypothesised that this was due to two different sorts of adrenoceptors (α and β). For a further 10 years, only antagonists of α-receptor effects (α-adrenoceptor block) were known, but in 1958 the first substance selectively and competitively to prevent β-receptor effects (β-adrenoceptor block), dichloroisoprenaline, was synthesised. It was unsuitable for clinical use because it behaved as a partial agonist, and it was not until 1962 that pronethalol (an isoprenaline analogue) became the first β-adrenoceptor blocker to be used clinically. Unfortunately it had a low therapeutic index and was carcinogenic in mice; it was soon replaced by propranolol.

It is evident that the site of action has an important role in selectivity, e.g. drugs that act on end-organ receptors directly and stereospecifically may be highly selective, whereas drugs that act indirectly by discharging noradrenaline/norepinephrine indiscriminately from nerve endings, e.g. amfetamine, will have a wider range of effects.

Subclassification of adrenoceptors is shown in Table 23.1.

Consequences of adrenoceptor activation

All adrenoceptors are members of the G-coupled family of receptor proteins, i.e. the receptor is coupled to its effector protein through special transduction proteins called 'G-proteins' (themselves a large protein family). The effector protein differs among adrenoceptor subtypes. In the case of β-adrenoceptors, the effector is adenylyl cyclase and hence cyclic AMP is the second-messenger molecule. For α-adrenoceptors, phospholipase C is the commonest effector protein, and the second messenger here is inositol trisphosphate (IP_3). It is the cascade of events initiated by the second-messenger molecules that produces the variety of tissue effects shown in Table 23.1. Hence, specificity is provided by the receptor subtype, not the messengers.

Selectivity for adrenoceptors

The following classification of sympathomimetics and antagonists is based on selectivity for receptors and on use. But selectivity is relative, not absolute; some agonists act on both α and β receptors, some are partial agonists and, if sufficient drug is administered, many will extend their range. The same applies to selective antagonists (receptor blockers), e.g. a β_1-selective-adrenoceptor blocker can cause severe exacerbation of asthma (a β_2 effect), even at low dose. It is important to remember this because patients have

died in the hands of doctors who have forgotten or been ignorant of it.[4]

Adrenoceptor agonists (see Table 23.1)

$\alpha + \beta$ **effects, non-selective:** *adrenaline/epinephrine* is used as a vasoconstrictor (α) with local anaesthetics, as a mydriatic (α), and in the emergency treatment of anaphylactic shock (see p. 119).

α_1 **effects:** *noradrenaline/norepinephrine* (with slight β effect on the heart) is selectively released physiologically, but as a therapeutic agent it is used for hypotensive states, excepting septic shock where dopamine and dobutamine are preferred (for their cardiac inotropic effect). Other agents with predominantly α_1 effects are imidazolines (xylometazoline, oxymetazoline), metaraminol, phenylephrine, phenylpropanolamine, ephedrine and pseudoephedrine; some are used solely for topical vasoconstriction (nasal decongestants).

α_2 **effects in the central nervous system:** *clonidine, moxonidine.*

β **effects, non-selective (i.e. $\beta_1 + \beta_2$):** *isoprenaline* (isoproterenol). Used as a bronchodilator (β_2), positive cardiac inotrope and to enhance conduction in heart block (β_1, β_2), it has been largely superseded by more selective agents. Other non-selective β agonists (ephedrine and orciprenaline) are also obsolete.

β_1 **effects, with some α effects:** *dopamine,* used in cardiogenic shock.

β_1 **effects:** *dobutamine,* used for cardiac inotropic effect.

β_2 **effects,** used in *asthma,* or to relax the uterus, include salbutamol, terbutaline, fenoterol, pirbuterol, reproterol, rimiterol, isoxsuprine, orciprenaline and ritodrine.

Adrenoceptor antagonists (blockers)

See page 424.

Effects of a sympathomimetic

The overall effect of a sympathomimetic depends on the site of action (receptor agonist or indirect action), on receptor specificity and on dose; for instance, adrenaline/epinephrine ordinarily dilates muscle blood vessels (β_2; mainly arterioles, but veins also) but in very large doses constricts them (α). The end results are often complex and unpredictable, partly

---

[4]Although it is simplest to regard the selectivity of a drug as relative, being lost at higher doses, strictly speaking it is the benefits of the receptor selectivity of an agonist or antagonist that are dose-dependent. A 10-fold selectivity of an agonist at the β_1 receptor, for instance, is a property of the agonist that is independent of dose, and means simply that 10 times less of the agonist is required to activate this receptor compared with the β_2 subtype.

Table 23.1 Clinically relevant aspects of adrenoceptor functions and actions of agonists

α_1-Adrenoceptor effects[a]	β-Adrenoceptor effects
Eye:[b] mydriasis	**Heart** (β_1, β_2):[c] increased rate (SA node) increased automaticity (AV node and muscle) increased velocity in conducting tissue increased contractility of myocardium increased oxygen consumption; decreased refractory period of all tissues
Arterioles: constriction (only slight in coronary and cerebral)	**Arterioles:** dilatation (β_2) **Bronchi** (β_2): relaxation **Anti-inflammatory effect:** inhibition of release of autacoids (histamine, leukotrienes) from mast cells, e.g. asthma in type I allergy
Uterus: contraction (pregnant)	**Uterus** (β_2): relaxation (pregnant) **Skeletal muscle**: tremor (β_2)
Skin: sweat, pilomotor **Male ejaculation** **Blood platelet**: aggregation **Metabolic effect:** hyperkalaemia	**Metabolic effects:** hypokalaemia (β_2) hepatic glycogenolysis (β_2) lipolysis (β_1, β_2)
Bladder sphincter: contraction	**Bladder detrusor**: relaxation

Intestinal smooth muscle relaxation is mediated by α and β adrenoceptors.
α_2-adrenoceptor effects:[a] α_2 receptors on the nerve ending, i.e. presynaptic autoreceptors, mediate negative feedback which inhibits noradrenaline/norepinephrine release.
Use of the term 'cardioselective' to mean β_1-receptor selective only, especially in the case of β-receptor–blocking drugs, is no longer appropriate.
Although in most species the β_1 receptor is the only cardiac β receptor, this is not the case in humans. What is not generally appreciated is that the endogenous sympathetic neurotransmitter noradrenaline/norepinephrine has about a 20-fold selectivity for the β_1 receptor – similar to that of the antagonist atenolol – with the consequence that under most circumstances, in most tissues, there is little or no β_2-receptor stimulation to be affected by a non-selective β-blocker. Why asthmatics should be so sensitive to β-blockade is paradoxical: all the bronchial β receptors are β_2, but the bronchi themselves are not innervated by noradrenergic fibres and the circulating adrenaline levels are, if anything, low in asthma.

[a]For the role of subtypes (α_1 and α_2), see prazosin.
[b]Effects on intraocular pressure involve both α and β adrenoceptors as well as cholinoceptors.
[c]Cardiac β_1 receptors mediate effects of sympathetic nerve stimulation. Cardiac β_2 receptors mediate effects of circulating adrenaline, when this is secreted at a sufficient rate, e.g. following myocardial infarction or in heart failure. Both receptors are coupled to the same intracellular signalling pathway (cyclic AMP production) and mediate the same biological effects.

because of the variability of homeostatic reflex responses and partly because what is observed, e.g. a change in blood pressure, is the result of many factors, e.g. vasodilatation (β) in some areas, vasoconstriction (α) in others, and cardiac stimulation (β).

To block all the effects of adrenaline/epinephrine and noradrenaline/norepinephrine, antagonists for both α and β receptors must be used. This can be a matter of practical importance, e.g. in phaeochromocytoma (see p. 442).

Physiological note. The termination of action of noradrenaline/norepinephrine released at nerve endings is by:

- reuptake into nerve endings by the noradrenaline/norepinephrine transporter where it is stored in vesicles or metabolised by monoamine oxidase (MAO) (see Fig. 23.1)
- diffusion away from the area of the nerve ending and the receptor (junctional cleft)
- metabolism (by extraneuronal MAO and catechol-O-methyltransferase, COMT).

These processes are slower than the rapid destruction of acetylcholine at the neuromuscular junction by extracellular acetylcholinesterase seated alongside the receptors. This reflects the differing signalling requirements: almost instantaneous (millisecond) responses for voluntary muscle movement versus the much more leisurely contraction of arteriolar muscle to control vascular resistance.

Synthetic non-catecholamines in clinical use have a $t_{1/2}$ of hours, e.g. salbutamol 4 h, because they resist enzymatic degradation by MAO and COMT. They may be given orally, although much higher doses are then required versus parenteral routes. They penetrate the central nervous system (CNS) and may have prominent effects, e.g. amfetamine. Substantial amounts appear in the urine.

Pharmacokinetics

Catecholamines (adrenaline/epinephrine, noradrenaline/norepinephrine, dopamine, dobutamine, isoprenaline)

(plasma $t_{1/2}$ ~2 min) are metabolised by MAO and COMT. These enzymes are present in large amounts in the liver and kidney, and account for most of the metabolism of injected catecholamines. MAO is also present in the intestinal mucosa (and in peripheral and central nerve endings). COMT is present in the adrenal medulla and tumours arising from chromaffin tissue, but not in sympathetic nerves. This explains the recent discovery that the COMT product, metanephrines, is a more sensitive and specific marker of phaeochromocytoma than measurement of the parent catecholamines. Because of both enzymes, catecholamines are ineffective when swallowed (they are not *bioavailable*), but non-catecholamines, e.g. salbutamol and amfetamine, are effective orally.

Adverse effects

These may be deduced from their actions (see Table 23.1, Fig. 23.2). Tissue necrosis due to intense vasoconstriction (α) around injection sites occurs as a result of leakage from intravenous infusions. The effects on the heart (β_1) include tachycardia, palpitations, cardiac arrhythmias including ventricular tachycardia and fibrillation, and muscle tremor (β_2). Sympathomimetic drugs should be used with great caution in patients with heart disease.

The effect of the sympathomimetic drugs on the pregnant uterus is variable and difficult to predict, but serious fetal distress can occur, due to reduced placental blood flow as a result both of contraction of the uterine muscle (α) and

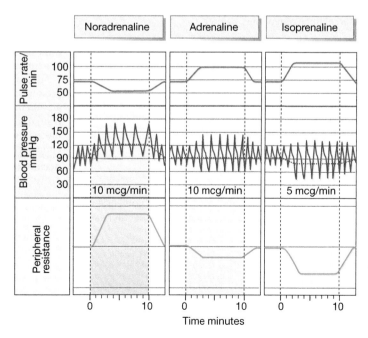

Fig. 23.2 Cardiovascular effects of noradrenaline/norepinephrine, adrenaline/epinephrine and isoprenaline (isoproterenol): pulse rate (beats/min), blood pressure in mmHg (*dotted line* is mean pressure), peripheral resistance in arbitrary units. The differences are due to the differential α- and β-agonist selectivities of these agents (see text). (*After Ginsburg J, Cobbold A F In: Vane J R, Wolstenholme G E W, O'Connor M O (eds) Adrenergic Mechanisms Churchill, London 1960.*)

arterial constriction (α). β₂ agonists are used to relax the uterus in premature labour, but unwanted cardiovascular actions (tachycardia in particular) can be troublesome for the mother. The oxytocin antagonist atosiban does not have these unwanted effects.

Sympathomimetics and plasma potassium. Adrenergic mechanisms have a role in the physiological control of plasma potassium concentration. The Na/K pump that shifts potassium into cells is activated by β₂-adrenoceptor agonists (adrenaline/epinephrine, salbutamol, isoprenaline) and can cause hypokalaemia. β₂-adrenoceptor antagonists block the effect.

The hypokalaemic effect of administered (β₂) sympathomimetics may be clinically important, particularly in patients with pre-existing hypokalaemia, e.g. due to intense adrenergic activity such as occurs in myocardial infarction,[5] in fright (admission to hospital is accompanied by transient hypokalaemia), or with previous diuretic therapy, and patients taking digoxin. In such subjects, the use of a sympathomimetic infusion or of an adrenaline/epinephrine-containing local anaesthetic may precipitate cardiac arrhythmia. Hypokalaemia may occur during treatment of severe asthma, particularly where the β₂-receptor agonist is combined with theophylline.

β-adrenoceptor blockers, as expected, enhance the hyperkalaemia of muscular exercise, and one of their benefits in preventing cardiac arrhythmias after myocardial infarction may be due to block of β₂-receptor–induced hypokalaemia.

Overdose of sympathomimetics is treated according to rational consideration of mode and site of action (see Adrenaline/epinephrine, below).

Individual sympathomimetics

The actions are summarised in Table 23.1. The classic, mainly endogenous, substances will be described first despite their limited role in therapeutics, and then the more selective analogues that have largely replaced them.

Catecholamines

Traditionally catecholamines have had a dual nomenclature (as a consequence of a company patenting the name

---

Adrenalin), broadly European and North American. The North American naming system has been chosen by the World Health Organization as recommended International Nonproprietary Names (rINNs) (see Ch. 7), and the European Union has directed member states to use rINNs. By exception, 'adrenaline' and 'noradrenaline' are the terms used in the titles of monographs in the *European Pharmacopoeia* and are thus the official names in the member states. Because uniformity has not yet been achieved, and because of the scientific literature, we use both names. For pharmacokinetics, see above.

Adrenaline/epinephrine

Adrenaline/epinephrine (α- and β-adrenoceptor effects) is used:

- as a vasoconstrictor with local anaesthetics (1 in 80 000 or weaker) to prolong their effects (about two-fold)
- as a topical mydriatic (sparing accommodation; it also lowers intraocular pressure)
- for severe allergic reactions, i.e. anaphylactic shock, intramuscularly or intravenously. The route must be chosen with care (for details, see p. 119). The subcutaneous route is not recommended as the intense vasoconstriction slows absorption.

Adrenaline/epinephrine is used in anaphylactic shock because of its mix of actions, cardiovascular and bronchial; it may also stabilise mast cell membranes and reduce release of vasoactive autacoids. Patients who are taking non-selective β-blockers may not respond to adrenaline/epinephrine (use intravenous salbutamol) and indeed may develop severe hypertension (see below).

Adrenaline/epinephrine (topical) decreases intraocular pressure in chronic open-angle glaucoma, as does dipivefrine, an adrenaline/epinephrine ester prodrug. These drugs are contraindicated in closed-angle glaucoma because they are mydriatics. Hyperthyroid patients are intolerant of adrenaline/epinephrine.

Accidental overdose with adrenaline/epinephrine occurs occasionally. It is rationally treated with propranolol to block the cardiac β effects (cardiac arrhythmia) and phentolamine or chlorpromazine to control the α effects on the peripheral circulation that will be prominent when the β effects are abolished. Labetalol (α- + β-blockade) is a good alternative. β-adrenoceptor block alone is hazardous as the then unopposed α-receptor vasoconstriction causes (severe) hypertension (see Phaeochromocytoma, p. 442). Use of other classes of antihypertensives is irrational and may even cause adrenaline/epinephrine release.

---

[5]Normal subjects, infused with intravenous adrenaline/epinephrine in amounts that approximate to those found in the plasma after severe myocardial infarction, show a fall in plasma potassium concentration of about 0.8 mmol/L (Brown M J, Brown D C, Murphy M B 1983 Hypokalemia from beta2-receptor stimulation by circulating epinephrine. New England Journal of Medicine 309:1414–1419).

Noradrenaline/norepinephrine (chiefly α and β₁ effects)

The main effect of administered noradrenaline/norepinephrine is to raise the blood pressure by constricting the arterioles and so increasing the total peripheral resistance, with reduced blood flow (except in coronary arteries, which have few α_1 receptors). Though it does have some cardiac stimulant (β_1) effect, the resulting tachycardia is masked by the profound reflex bradycardia caused by the hypertension. Noradrenaline/norepinephrine is given by intravenous infusion to obtain a controlled and sustained response; the effect of a single intravenous injection is unpredictable and would last only a minute or so. It is used where peripheral vasoconstriction is specifically required, e.g. vasodilatation of septic shock. Adverse effects include peripheral gangrene and local necrosis following accidental extravasation from a vein; tachyphylaxis occurs, and withdrawal must be gradual.

Isoprenaline (isoproterenol)

Isoprenaline (isopropylnoradrenaline) is a non-selective β-receptor agonist, i.e. it activates both β_1 and β_2 receptors. It relaxes smooth muscle, including that of the blood vessels and airways, and has negligible metabolic or vasoconstrictor effects. It causes a marked tachycardia, which is its main disadvantage in the treatment of bronchial asthma. It is still occasionally used in complete heart block, massive overdose of a β-blocker, and in cardiogenic shock (for hypotension).

Dopamine

Dopamine activates different receptors depending on the dose used. At the lowest effective dose, it stimulates specific dopamine (D_1) receptors in the CNS and the renal and other vascular beds (dilator); it also activates presynaptic autoreceptors (D_2) which suppress release of noradrenaline/norepinephrine. As the dose is increased, dopamine acts as an agonist on β_1-adrenoceptors in the heart (increasing contractility and rate); at high doses it activates α-adrenoceptors (vasoconstrictor). It is given by continuous intravenous infusion because, like all catecholamines, its $t_{1/2}$ is short (2 min). An intravenous infusion (2–5 µg/kg/min) increases renal blood flow (partly through an effect on cardiac output). As the dose rises the heart is stimulated, resulting in tachycardia and increased cardiac output. At these higher doses, dopamine is referred to as an 'inoconstrictor'.

Dopamine is stable for about 24 h in sodium chloride or dextrose. Subcutaneous leakage causes vasoconstriction and necrosis (compare with noradrenaline/norepinephrine), and should be treated by local injection of an α-adrenoceptor–blocking agent (phentolamine 5 mg, diluted). It may be mixed with dobutamine.

For CNS aspects of dopamine, agonists and antagonists, see Neuroleptics (p. 301) and Parkinsonism (p. 378).

Dobutamine

Dobutamine is a racemic mixture of D- and L-dobutamine. The racemate behaves primarily as a β_1-adrenoceptor agonist with greater inotropic than chronotropic effects on the heart; it has some α-agonist effect, but less than dopamine. It is useful in shock (with dopamine) and in low-output heart failure (in the absence of severe hypertension).

Dopexamine

Dopexamine is a synthetic catecholamine whose principal action is as an agonist for the cardiac β_2-adrenoceptors (positive inotropic effect). It is also a weak dopamine agonist (thus causing renal vasodilatation) and inhibitor of noradrenaline/norepinephrine uptake, thereby enhancing stimulation of cardiac β_1 receptors by noradrenaline/norepinephrine. It is used occasionally to optimise the cardiac output, particularly perioperatively.

Non-catecholamines

Salbutamol, fenoterol, rimiterol, reproterol, pirbuterol, salmeterol, ritodrine and terbutaline are β-adrenoceptor agonists that are relatively selective for β_2 receptors, so that cardiac (chiefly β_1-receptor) effects are less prominent. Tachycardia still occurs because of atrial (sinus node) β_2-receptor stimulation; the β_2-adrenoceptors are less numerous in the ventricle, and there is probably less risk of serious ventricular arrhythmias than with the use of non-selective catecholamines. The synthetic agonists are also longer acting than isoprenaline because they are not substrates for COMT, which methylates catecholamines in the liver. They are used principally in asthma, and to reduce uterine contractions in premature labour.

Salbutamol (see also Asthma)

Salbutamol (Ventolin) ($t_{1/2}$ 4 h) is taken orally, 2–4 mg up to four times per day; it also acts quickly by inhalation, and the effect can last for 4–6 h, which makes it suitable for both prevention and treatment of asthma. Of an inhaled dose, less than 20% is absorbed and can cause cardiovascular effects. It can also be given by injection, e.g. in asthma, premature labour (β_2 receptor) and for cardiac inotropic (β_1) effect in heart failure (where the β_2-vasodilator action is also useful). Clinically important hypokalaemia can also occur (the shift of potassium into cells). The other drugs above are similar.

409

Salmeterol (Serevent) is a variant of salbutamol that has an additional binding site adjacent to the β_2-adrenoceptor; this results in slow onset (15–30 min) and long duration of action (12–18 h) (see p. 503). This behaviour is distinct from the other widely used long-acting β_2-agonist, formoterol, which has a rapid bronchodilator effect like salbutamol (within a few minutes).

Ephedrine

Ephedrine ($t_{1/2}$ ∼6 h) is a plant alkaloid[6] with indirect sympathomimetic actions that resemble those of adrenaline/epinephrine peripherally and amfetamine centrally. Hence, (in adults) it produces increased alertness, anxiety, insomnia, tremor and nausea; children may be sleepy when taking it. In practice, central effects limit its use as a sympathomimetic in asthma.

Ephedrine is well absorbed when given orally and, unlike most other sympathomimetics, undergoes relatively little first-pass metabolism in the liver (it is not a substrate for MAO or COMT); it is excreted largely unchanged by the kidney. It differs from adrenaline/epinephrine principally in that its effects come on more slowly and last longer. Tachyphylaxis occurs on repeated dosing. It can be given by mouth for reversible airways obstruction, topically as a mydriatic and mucosal vasoconstrictor or by slow intravenous injection to reverse hypotension from spinal or epidural anaesthesia. Newer drugs that are better suited for these purposes have largely replaced it. It is sometimes useful in myasthenia gravis (adrenergic agents enhance cholinergic neuromuscular transmission). *Pseudoephedrine* is similar to ephedrine but much less active.

Phenylpropanolamine (norephedrine) is similar but with fewer CNS effects. Prolonged administration of phenylpropanolamine to women as an anorectic has been associated with pulmonary valve abnormalities and stroke, leading to its withdrawal in some countries.[6]

Amfetamine (Benzedrine) and *dexamfetamine* (Dexedrine) act indirectly. They are seldom used for their peripheral effects, which are similar to those of ephedrine, but usually for their effects on the CNS (narcolepsy, attention deficit in children). For a general account of amfetamine, see p. 358.

Phenylephrine has actions qualitatively similar to those of noradrenaline/norepinephrine but of longer duration, up to several hours. It can be used as a nasal decongestant (0.25–0.5% solution), but sometimes irritates. In the doses usually given, the CNS effects are minimal, as are the direct effects on the heart. It is also used as a mydriatic and briefly lowers intraocular pressure.

Mucosal decongestants

Nasal and bronchial decongestants (vasoconstrictors) are widely used in allergic rhinitis, colds, coughs and sinusitis, and to prevent otic barotrauma, as nasal sprays or taken orally. All of the sympathomimetic vasoconstrictors, i.e. with α effects, have been used for the purpose, with or without an antihistamine (H_1 receptor), and there is little to choose between them. Ischaemic damage to the mucosa is possible if they are used excessively (more often than 3-hourly) or for prolonged periods (more than 3 weeks), and is a common problem for regular users of cocaine. The occurrence of rebound congestion is also liable to lead to overuse.

The least objectionable drugs are ephedrine 0.5% and phenylephrine 0.5%. Xylometazoline 0.1% (Otrivine) should be used, if at all, for only a few days because longer application reduces the ciliary activity and leads to rebound congestion. Oily drops and sprays, used frequently and long term, may also enter the lungs and eventually cause lipoid pneumonia. They interact with antihypertensives and can be a cause of unexplained failure of therapy unless enquiry into patient self-medication is made. Fatal hypertensive crises have occurred when patients treated for depression with a monoamine oxidase inhibitor have taken these preparations.

Shock

Definition. Shock is a state of inadequate organ perfusion (oxygen deficiency) sufficient adversely to affect cellular metabolism, causing the release of enzymes and vasoactive substances,[7] i.e. it is a *low flow* or *hypoperfusion* state.

Typically the blood pressure is low, reflecting reduced cardiac output. The exception is septic shock, where the cardiac output is typically high, but it is maldistributed (due to constriction, dilatation, shunting), leading to poor oxygen utilisation and tissue injury (warm shock).

The essential element, hypoperfusion of vital organs, is present whatever the cause, whether pump failure (myocardial infarction), maldistribution of blood (septic shock) or loss of

---

[6]Ephedra alkaloids are found in Chinese herbal remedies (ma huang) and in guarana-derived caffeine products which are widely consumed as appetite suppressants or for energy enhancement. These have been associated with stroke and seizures only rarely. The relationship of phenylpropanolamine consumption and haemorrhagic stroke seems clearer and has led to the suspension of its sale in the USA (Fleming G A 2000 The FDA, regulation, and the risk of stroke. New England Journal of Medicine 243:1886–1887).

[7]In fact, a cocktail of substances (autacoids) – kinins, prostaglandins, leukotrienes, histamine, endorphins, serotonin, vasopressin – has been implicated. In endotoxic shock, the toxin also induces synthesis of nitric oxide, the endogenous vasodilator, in several types of cell other than the endothelial cells that are normally its main source.

intravascular volume (bleeding or increased permeability of vessels damaged by bacterial cell products, burns or anoxia). Functions of vital organs, such as the brain (consciousness), lungs (gas exchange) and kidney (urine formation) are clinical indicators of adequacy of perfusion of these organs.

Treatment may be summarised as follows:

- *Treatment of the cause:* bleeding, infection, adrenocortical deficiency.
- *Replacement of any fluid* lost from the circulation.
- *Perfusion of vital organs* (brain, heart, kidneys) and maintenance of the mean blood pressure.

Blood flow (oxygen delivery) rather than blood pressure is of the greatest immediate importance for the function of vital organs. A reasonable blood pressure is needed to ensure organ perfusion, but peripheral vasoconstriction may maintain a normal mean arterial pressure despite a very low cardiac output. Under these circumstances, blood flow to vital organs will be inadequate, and multiple organ failure will ensue unless the patient is resuscitated adequately.

The decision on how to treat shock depends on assessment of the pathophysiology:

- Whether cardiac output, and thus peripheral blood flow, is inadequate (low pulse volume, cold-constricted periphery).
- Whether cardiac output is normal or high and peripheral blood flow is adequate (good pulse volume and warm dilated periphery), but there is maldistribution of blood.
- Whether the patient is hypovolaemic or not, or needs a cardiac inotropic agent, a vasoconstrictor or a vasodilator.

Types of shock

In poisoning by a cerebral depressant or after spinal cord trauma, the principal cause of hypotension is low peripheral resistance due to reduced vascular tone. The cardiac output can be restored by infusing fluid and/or giving vasoactive drugs (e.g. noradrenaline/norepinephrine, metaraminol).

In central circulatory failure (cardiogenic shock, e.g. after myocardial infarction), the cardiac output and blood pressure are low because of pump failure; myocardial perfusion is dependent on aortic pressure. Venous return (central venous pressure) is normal or high. The low blood pressure may trigger the sympathoadrenal mechanisms of peripheral circulatory failure summarised below.

Not surprisingly, the use of drugs in low-output failure caused by acute myocardial damage is disappointing. Vasoconstriction (by an α-adrenoceptor agonist) may raise the blood pressure by increasing peripheral resistance, but the additional burden on the damaged heart can further reduce the cardiac output. Cardiac stimulation with a β1-adrenoceptor agonist may fail; it increases myocardial oxygen consumption and may cause an arrhythmia. Dobutamine or dopamine offers a reasonable choice if a drug is judged necessary; dobutamine is preferred as it tends to vasodilate, i.e. it is an 'inodilator'. If there is bradycardia (as sometimes complicates myocardial infarction), cardiac output can be increased by accelerating the heart rate by vagal block with atropine.

Septic shock[8] is severe sepsis with hypotension that is not corrected by adequate intravascular volume replacement. It is caused by lipopolysaccharide (LPS) endotoxins from Gram-negative organisms and other cell products from Gram-positive organisms; these initiate host inflammatory and procoagulant responses through the release of cytokines, e.g. interleukins, and the resulting diffuse endothelial damage is responsible for many of the adverse manifestations of shock. The procoagulant state, in particular, predisposes to the development of microvascular thrombosis that leads to tissue ischaemia and organ hypoperfusion. Activation of nitric oxide production by LPS and cytokines worsens the hypoperfusion by decreasing arterial pressure. This initiates a vigorous sympathetic discharge that causes constriction of arterioles and venules; the cardiac output may be high or low according to the balance of these influences.

There is a progressive peripheral anoxia of vital organs and acidosis. The veins (venules) dilate, and venous pooling occurs so that blood is sequestered in the periphery; effective circulatory volume decreases because of this, and fluid is lost into the extravascular space from endothelial damage caused by bacterial products.

When septic shock is recognised, appropriate antimicrobials should be given in high dose immediately after taking blood for culture (see p. 179). Beyond that, the primary aim of treatment is to restore cardiac output and vital organ perfusion by increasing venous return to the heart, and to reverse the maldistribution of blood. Increasing intravascular volume will achieve this, guided by the central venous pressure to avoid overloading the heart. Oxygen is essential as there is often uneven pulmonary perfusion.

After adequate fluid resuscitation has been established, inotropic support is usually required. *Noradrenaline/norepinephrine* is the vasoactive drug of choice for septic shock: its potent α-adrenergic effect increases the mean arterial pressure, and its modest β1 effect may raise cardiac output, or at least maintain it as the peripheral vascular resistance increases. *Dobutamine* may be added to augment cardiac output further. Some clinicians use adrenaline/epinephrine, in preference

---

[8]See also: Sepsis: recognition, diagnosis and early management, NICE https://www.nice.org.uk/guidance/ng51/chapter/recommendations

to noradrenaline/norepinephrine plus dobutamine, on the basis that its powerful α and β effects are appropriate in the setting of septic shock; it may exacerbate splanchnic ischaemia and lactic acidosis.

Hypotension in (atherosclerotic) occlusive vascular disease is particularly serious, for these patients are dependent on pressure to provide the necessary blood flow in vital organs whose supplying vessels are less able to dilate. It is important to maintain an adequate mean arterial pressure, whichever inotrope is selected.

Choice of drug in shock

On present knowledge, the best drug would be one that both stimulates the myocardium and selectively modifies peripheral resistance to increase flow to vital organs.

- *Dobutamine* is used when cardiac inotropic effect is the primary requirement.
- *Adrenaline/epinephrine* is used when a more potent inotrope than dobutamine is required, e.g. when the vasodilating action of dobutamine compromises mean arterial pressure.
- *Noradrenaline/norepinephrine* is used when vasoconstriction is the first priority, plus some cardiac inotropic effect, e.g. septic shock.

Metaraminol, an α1-adrenoceptor agonist, has become increasingly popular in recent times as the first choice sympathomimetic amine for the treatment of acute hypotension. Inflammatory conditions such as septic shock inhibit the generation of endogenous APC, which normally inactivates factors Va and VIIIa, with the result that production of these procoagulant factors is unchecked. Recombinant human APC improved survival of patients with septic shock and multi-organ failure in a large randomised controlled trial.[9]

Monitoring drug use

Modern monitoring by both invasive and non-invasive techniques is complex and is undertaken in units dedicated to, and equipped for, this activity. The present comment is an overview. Monitoring normally requires close attention to heart rate and rhythm, blood pressure, fluid balance and urine flow, pulmonary gas exchange and central venous pressure. The use of drugs in shock is secondary to accurate assessment of cardiovascular state (especially of peripheral flow) and to other essential management, treatment of infection and maintenance of intravascular volume.

Restoration of intravascular volume[10]

In an emergency, speed of replacement is more important than its nature. *Crystalloid* solutions, e.g. isotonic saline, Hartmann's, Plasma-Lyte, are immediately effective, but they leave the circulation quickly. (Note that dextrose solutions are completely ineffective because they distribute across both the extracellular and intracellular compartments.) Macromolecules *(colloids)* remain in the circulation longer. The two classes (crystalloids and colloids) may be used together.

The choice of crystalloid or colloid for fluid resuscitation remains controversial. Current NICE guidance recommends crystalloids rather than colloids. There is some evidence for the use of human albumin solution in patients with cirrhotic liver disease. A Cochrane review of over 56 clinical trials with mortality data concluded that in critically ill patients there was no evidence that colloids offered superior survival over the use of crystalloids in patients following trauma, burns or surgery.[11] Colloids are also much more expensive than crystalloids.

Artificial colloidal solutions include dextrans (glucose polymer), gelatin (hydrolysed collagen) and hydroxyethyl starch.

Dextran 70 (mol. wt. 70 000) has a plasma restoring effect lasting for 5–6 h. Dextran 40 is used to decrease blood sludging and so to improve peripheral blood flow.

Gelatin products (e.g. Haemaccel, Gelofusine) have a plasma-restoring effect of 2–3 h (at best).

Etherified starch. Several hydroxyethyl starch solutions are available, with widely differing effects on plasma volume: high molecular weight (450 000) solutions restore volume for 6–12 h, whereas the effect of medium molecular weight (200 000) starches lasts for 4–6 h.

Adverse effects include anaphylactoid reactions; dextran and hydroxyethyl starch can impair haemostatic mechanisms.

Chronic orthostatic hypotension

Chronic orthostatic hypotension occurs most commonly with increasing age, in primary progressive autonomic failure,

---

[9]Bernard G D, Vincent J L, Laterre P F et al 2001 Efficacy and safety of recombinant human activated protein C for severe sepsis. New England Journal of Medicine 344:699–709.

[10]Nolan J 2001 Fluid resuscitation for the trauma patient. Resuscitation 48:57–69.
[11]Perel P, Roberts I, Pearson M 2007 Colloids versus crystalloids for fluid resuscitation in critically ill patients. Cochrane Database of Systematic Reviews 2007, Issue 4. Art. No.: CD000567. DOI: 10.1002/14651858.CD000567.pub3. Available at: http://mrw. interscience.wiley.com/cochrane/clsysrev/articles/CD000567/frame.html (accessed 2 August 2010).

and secondary to parkinsonism and diabetes. The clinical features can be mimicked by saline depletion. The two conditions are clearly separated by measurement of plasma concentrations of noradrenaline/norepinephrine (supine and erect) and renin, which are raised in saline depletion, but depressed in most causes of hypotension due to autonomic failure.

As blood pressure can be considered a product of 'volume' and 'vasoconstriction', the logical initial treatment of orthostatic hypotension is to expand blood volume using a sodium-retaining adrenocortical steroid (fludrocortisone[12]) or desmopressin (see p. 515), plus elastic support stockings to reduce venous pooling of blood when erect.

It is more difficult to reproduce the actions of the endogenous vasoconstrictors, and especially their selective release on standing, in order to achieve erect normotension without supine hypertension. Because of the risk of hypertension when the patient is supine, only a modest increase in erect blood pressure should be sought; fortunately a systolic blood pressure of 85–90 mmHg is usually adequate to maintain cerebral perfusion in these patients. Few drugs have been formally tested or can be recommended with confidence.

Clonidine and pindolol are partial agonists at, respectively, α and β receptors, and may therefore be more effective agonists in the absence of the endogenous agonist, noradrenaline/ norepinephrine, than in normal subjects. Midodrine, an α-adrenoceptor agonist, is the only vasoconstrictor drug to receive UK regulatory approval for the treatment of postural hypotension. It is given at doses of 5–15 mg three times daily. The norepinephrine prodrug droxidopa (= dihydroxy-phenylserine) is approved in the USA for the treatment of orthostatic dizziness, lightheadedness, or the 'feeling that you are about to black out' in adults with symptomatic neurogenic orthostatic hypotension associated with primary autonomic failure (e.g. Parkinson's disease, multiple system atrophy or pure autonomic failure), dopamine β-hydroxylase deficiency or nondiabetic autonomic neuropathy. The pressor effect results from conversion of droxidopa to norepinephrine by the widely expressed enzyme dopa decarboxylase outside the central nervous system.

Postprandial fall in blood pressure (probably due to redistribution of blood to the splanchnic area) is characteristic of this condition; it occurs especially after breakfast (blood volume is lower in the morning). Substantial doses of caffeine (two large cups of coffee) can mitigate this, but they need to be taken before or early in the meal. The action may be due to block of splanchnic vasodilator adenosine receptors. Administration of the somatostatin analogue octreotide also prevents postprandial hypotension, but twice-daily subcutaneous injections are often not attractive; long-acting formulations of somatostatin (and its relative lanreotide) are available, which can be given as subcutaneous or intramuscular depots monthly – this may be more tolerable.

Some of the variation reported in drug therapy may be due to differences in adrenergic function dependent on whether the degeneration is central, peripheral, preganglionic, postganglionic or due to age-related changes in the adrenoceptors on end-organs. In central autonomic degeneration – 'multi-system atrophy' – noradrenaline/ norepinephrine is still present in peripheral sympathetic nerve endings. In these patients, an indirect-acting amine may be successful, and one patient titrated the amount of Bovril (a tyramine-rich meat extract drink) she required in order to stand up.[13]

Erythropoietin has also been used with success (it increases haematocrit and blood viscosity), but a cautionary note: increasing the haematocrit in this way is known to cause an excess of cardiovascular deaths in chronic renal failure patients and a significant thrombosis risk in cancer patients given erythropoietin.[14]

Detrusor relaxation for urinary frequency, urgency and urge incontinence

Mirabegron, a β3-adrenoceptor agonist, is being used increasingly in patients with urinary symptoms due to detrusor instability where anti-cholinergic agents are less suitable. In addition to the bladder, the β3-adrenoceptor is present in skeletal muscle and adipose tissue and has a role in both lipolysis and thermogenesis. Its use needs to be considered carefully in those with a history of hypertension, renal dysfunction or with concomitant liver enzyme inhibitor use (CYP 3A4).

---

[13]Karet F E, Dickerson J E C, Brown J et al 1994 Bovril and moclobemide: a novel therapeutic strategy for central autonomic failure. Lancet 344:1263–1265.
[14]Drüeke TB, Locatelli F, Clyne N et al 2006 Normalization of hemoglobin level in patients with chronic kidney disease and anemia. New England Journal of Medicine 355:2071–2084. And FDA advisory: http://www.fda.gov/Drugs/DrugSafety/
PostmarketDrugSafetyInformationforPatientsandProviders/ucm126485.htm (accessed 2 August 2010).

---

[12]Effective doses may not restore blood volume and may work by sensitising vascular adrenoceptors.

Summary

- The adrenergic arm of the autonomic system uses noradrenaline/norepinephrine as its neurotransmitter.
- Adrenaline/epinephrine, unlike noradrenaline/norepinephrine, is a circulating hormone.
- These two catecholamines act on the same adrenoceptors: α_1 and α_2, which are blocked by phenoxybenzamine but not by propranolol, and β_1 and β_2, which are blocked by propranolol but not phenoxybenzamine. Noradrenaline/norepinephrine is a 20-fold weaker agonist at β_2 receptors than is adrenaline/epinephrine.
- Distinction between receptor classes is made initially by defining the differing ability of two agonists (or antagonists) to mimic (or block) the effects of catecholamines.
- Often these differences correlate with a difference in receptor type on two different tissues: e.g. stimulation of cardiac contractility by β_1 receptors, and bronchodilatation by β_2 receptors.
- The distinction between α_1 and α_2 receptors corresponds to their principal location on blood vessels (causing vasoconstriction) and neurones, respectively.
- Catecholamines themselves can be used in therapy when rapid onset and offset are desired. Selective mimetics at each of the four main receptor subtypes are used for individual locations, e.g. α_1 for nasal decongestion, α_2 for systemic hypotension, α_1 for septic shock, β_2 for bronchoconstriction.
- Both α- and β-blockade are used in hypertension; selective β-blockade is used in angina and heart failure.

Guide to further reading

Ahlquist, R.P., 1948. A study of adrenotropic receptors. Am. J. Physiol. 153, 586–600.

Brown, M.J., 1995. To b-block or better block? Br. Med. J. 311, 701–702.

Brown, S.G., 2005. Cardiovascular aspects of anaphylaxis: implications for treatment and diagnosis. Curr. Opin. Allergy Clin. Immunol. 5, 359–364.

Gibbons, C.H., Schmidt, P., Biaggioni, I., et al., 2017. The recommendations of a consensus panel for the screening, diagnosis, and treatment of neurogenic orthostatic hypotension and associated supine hypertension. J. Neurol. 264, 1567–1582.

Insel, P.A., 1996. Adrenergic receptors – evolving concepts and clinical implications. N. Engl. J. Med. 334, 580–585.

Moore, F.A., McKinley, B.A., Moore, E.E., et al., 2004. The next generation in shock resuscitation. Lancet 363, 1988–1996.

Rice, T.W., Bernard, G.R., 2005. Therapeutic intervention and targets for sepsis. Annu. Rev. Med. 56, 225–248.

Russell, J.A., 2006. Management of sepsis. N. Engl. J. Med. 355, 1699–1713.

Chapter | **24** |

Arterial hypertension, angina pectoris, myocardial infarction and heart failure

Morris J. Brown

SYNOPSIS

Hypertension and coronary heart disease (CHD) are of great importance. Hypertension affects more than 20% of the total population of the USA, with its major impact on those older than 50 years of age. CHD is the cause of death in 30% of males and 22% of females in England and Wales. Management requires attention to detail, both clinical and pharmacological.

The way in which drugs act in these diseases is outlined, and the drugs are described according to class.

- Hypertension and angina pectoris: how drugs act.
- Drugs used in both hypertension and angina.
- Diuretics.
- Vasodilators: organic nitrates, calcium channel blockers, ACE inhibitors, angiotensin II receptor antagonists.
- Adrenoceptor-blocking drugs, α and β.
- Peripheral sympathetic nerve terminal.
- Autonomic ganglion-blocking drugs.
- Central nervous system.
- Treatment of angina pectoris.
- Acute coronary syndromes and myocardial infarction.
- Arterial hypertension.
- Sexual function and cardiovascular drugs.
- Phaeochromocytoma.

There is also now a better understanding of the mechanisms that sustain the failing heart. Carefully selected and monitored drugs can have a major impact on morbidity and mortality. However, much of the risk that patients with heart failure encounter is due to ventricular arrhythmias, which are minimised with implantable cardioverter defibrillators (ICDs) and cardiac resynchronisation therapy (CRT) rather than drugs. In view of the current complex range of choices for individuals with these issues, specialist referral should be considered in all cases.

- Specific treatments, including those for cardiac arrest.
- Drugs for cardiac failure.

Hypertension: how drugs act

Consider the following relationship:

Blood pressure = cardiac output × peripheral resistance

This being true, drugs can lower blood pressure by:

- Dilating arteriolar *resistance vessels;* achieved through direct relaxation of vascular smooth muscle cells, indirect relaxation by stimulating nitric oxide (NO) production, or by blocking the production or action of endogenous vasconstrictors, such as noradrenaline/norepinephrine and angiotensin.
- Dilating venous *capacitance vessels;* reduced venous return to the heart (preload) leads to reduced cardiac output, especially in the upright position.
- Reduction of cardiac *contractility* and *heart rate.*

415

- Depletion of *body sodium*. This reduces plasma volume (transiently) and reduces arteriolar response to noradrenaline/norepinephrine.

Angina pectoris: how drugs act

Angina can be viewed as a problem of supply and demand. So the drugs used in angina pectoris either increase supply of oxygen and nutrients, or reduce the demand for them, or both.

The supply of myocardial oxygen can be increased by:

- dilating coronary arteries
- slowing the heart (coronary flow, uniquely, occurs in diastole, which lengthens as heart rate falls).

Demand can be decreased by:

- reducing afterload (i.e. peripheral resistance), so reducing the work of the heart in perfusing the tissues
- reducing preload (i.e. venous filling pressure); according to Starling's law of the heart, workload and therefore oxygen demand varies with stretch of cardiac muscle fibres
- slowing the heart rate.

Drugs used in hypertension and angina

Two groups of drugs, β-adrenergic blockers and calcium channel blockers, are used in both hypertension and angina. Several drugs for hypertension are also used in the treatment of heart failure.

Diuretics (see also Ch. 27)

Diuretics, particularly the thiazides, are useful antihypertensives. They cause an initial loss of sodium with a parallel contraction of the blood and extracellular fluid volume. The effect may reach 10% of total body sodium, but it is not maintained. After several months of treatment, the main blood pressure–lowering effect appears to reflect a reduced responsiveness of resistance vessels to endogenous vasoconstrictors, principally noradrenaline/norepinephrine. Although this hyposensitivity may be a consequence of the sodium depletion, thiazides are generally more effective antihypertensive agents than loop diuretics, despite causing less salt loss, and evidence suggests an independent action of thiazides on an unidentified ion channel on vascular smooth muscle cell membranes. Maximal effect on blood pressure is delayed for several weeks, and other drugs are best added after this time.

Adverse metabolic effects of thiazides on serum potassium, blood lipids, glucose tolerance and uric acid metabolism led to suggestions that they should be replaced by newer agents without these effects. Unnecessarily high doses of thiazides were used in the past, but the pendulum then swung to inadequately low doses. Bendroflumethiazide 2.5 mg/day (equivalent to hydrochlorothiazide 25 mg or indapamide 2.5 mg) is effective and well tolerated. However, the most effective diuretic regimen for reducing blood pressure, without changing plasma K+ or glucose, is a combination of hydrochlorothiazide (12.5–25 mg) and amiloride (5–10 mg). Diuretics have been effective in several outcome trials in preventing the major complications of hypertension, myocardial infarction and stroke. The characteristic reduction in renal calcium excretion induced by thiazides may, in long-term therapy, also reduce the occurrence of hip fractures in older patients and benefit women with postmenopausal osteoporosis.

Vasodilators

Organic nitrates

Organic nitrates (and nitrite) were introduced into medicine in the 19th century.[1] De-nitration in the smooth muscle cell releases nitric oxide (NO), which is the main physiological vasodilator, normally produced by endothelial cells. *Nitrodilators* (a generic term for drugs that release or mimic the action of NO) activate the soluble guanylate cyclase in vascular smooth muscle cells and cause an increase in intracellular cyclic guanosine monophosphate (GMP) concentrations. This is the second messenger which alters calcium fluxes in the cell, decreases stored calcium and induces relaxation. The result is a generalised dilatation of venules (capacitance vessels) and to a lesser extent of arterioles (resistance vessels), causing a fall of blood pressure that is postural at first; the larger coronary arteries especially dilate. Whereas some vasodilators can 'steal' blood away from atheromatous arteries, with their fixed stenoses, to other, healthier arteries, nitrates probably have the reverse effect as a result of their supplementing the endogenous NO. Atheroma is associated with impaired endothelial function, resulting in reduced release of NO and, possibly, its accelerated destruction by the oxidised low-density lipoprotein (LDL) in atheroma (see Ch. 26).

The venous dilatation causes a reduction in venous return and a fall in left ventricular filling pressure with reduced

---

[1]Murrell W 1879 Nitroglycerin as a remedy for angina pectoris. Lancet i:80–81. Nitroglycerin was actually first synthesised by Sobrero in 1847 who noted that, when he applied it to his tongue, it caused a severe headache.

stroke volume, but cardiac output is sustained by the reflex tachycardia induced by the fall in blood pressure.

Pharmacokinetics. The nitrates are generally well absorbed across skin and the mucosal surface of the mouth or gut wall. Nitrates absorbed from the gut are subject to extensive first-pass metabolism in the liver, as shown by the substantially higher doses required by that route compared with sublingual application (and explains why swallowing a sublingual tablet of glyceryl trinitrate terminates its effect). They are first de-nitrated and then conjugated with glucuronic acid. The $t_{1/2}$ periods vary (see below), but for glyceryl trinitrate (GTN) it is 1–4 min. The de-nitration of GTN is in fact genetically determined as the enzyme responsible, a mitochondrial alcohol dehydrogenase, ALDH2, is polymorphic and in subjects carrying a common coding variant (E504K) sublingual GTN has reduced efficacy.[2]

Tolerance to the characteristic vasodilator headache comes and goes quickly (hours).[3] Ensuring that a continuous steady-state plasma concentration is avoided prevents tolerance. This is easy with occasional use of GTN, but with nitrates having longer $t_{1/2}$ (see below) and sustained-release formulations it is necessary to plan the dosing to allow a low plasma concentration for 4–8 h, e.g. overnight; alternatively, transdermal patches may be removed for a few hours if tolerance is suspected.

Uses. Nitrates are chiefly used to relieve angina pectoris and sometimes left ventricular failure. An excessive fall in blood pressure will reduce coronary flow as well as cause fainting due to reduced cerebral blood flow, so it is important to avoid accidental overdosing. Patients with angina should be instructed on the signs of overdose – palpitations, dizziness, blurred vision, headache and flushing followed by pallor – and what to do about it (see below).

The discovery that coronary artery occlusion by thrombosis is itself 'stuttering' – developing gradually over hours – and associated with vasospasm in other parts of the coronary tree has made the use of isosorbide dinitrate (Isoket) by continuous intravenous infusion adjusted to the degree of pain, a logical and effective form of analgesia for unstable angina.

Transient relief of pain due to spasm of other smooth muscle (colic) can sometimes be obtained, so that relief of

chest pain by nitrates does not prove the diagnosis of angina pectoris.

Nitrates are contraindicated in angina due to anaemia.

Adverse effects. Collapse due to fall in blood pressure resulting from overdose is the commonest side-effect. The patient should remain supine with the legs raised above the head to restore venous return to the heart. The patient should also spit out or swallow the remainder of the tablet.

Nitrate headache, which may be severe, is probably due to the stretching of pain-sensitive tissues around the meningeal arteries resulting from the increased pulsation that accompanies the local vasodilatation. If headache is severe the dose should be halved. Methaemoglobinaemia can occur with heavy dosage.

Interactions. An important footnote to the use of nitrates (and NO dilators generally) has been the marked potentiation of their vasodilator effects observed in patients taking phosphodiesterase (PDE) inhibitors, such as sildenafil (Viagra) and tadalafil (Cialis). These agents target an isoform of PDE (PDE-5) expressed in the blood vessel wall. Other methylxanthine PDE inhibitors, such as theophylline, do not cause a similar interaction because they are rather weak inhibitors of PDE-5, even at the doses effective in asthma. A number of pericoital deaths reported in patients taking sildenafil have been attributed to the substantial fall in blood pressure that occurs when used with a nitrate. This is an ironic twist for an agent in first-line use in erectile dysfunction that was originally developed as a drug to treat angina.[4]

Glyceryl trinitrate (see also above)

Glyceryl trinitrate (1879) (trinitrin, nitroglycerin, GTN) ($t_{1/2}$ 3 min) is an oily, non-flammable liquid that explodes on concussion with a force greater than that of gunpowder. Physicians meet it mixed with inert substances and made into a tablet, in which form it is both innocuous and fairly stable. But tablets more than 8 weeks old or exposed to heat or air will have lost potency by evaporation and should be discarded. Patients should also be warned to expect the tablet to cause a burning sensation under the tongue if it still contains active GTN. An alternative is to use a nitroglycerin spray (see below), which, formulated as a pressurised liquid GTN, has a shelf-life of at least 3 years.

GTN is the drug of choice in the treatment of an attack of angina pectoris. The tablets should be chewed and dissolved under the tongue, or placed in the buccal sulcus,

---

[2]Journal of Clinical Investigation 2006; 116:506–511. This same coding variant confers flushing to alcohol challenge and in parts of Southeast Asia has a prevalence of almost 50%.

[3]Explosives factory workers exposed to a nitrate-contaminated environment lost it over a weekend, and some chose to maintain their intake by using nitrate-impregnated headbands (transdermal absorption) rather than have to accept the headaches and re-acquire tolerance so frequently. A recent study has also reported that patients with angina who develop a headache with GTN are less likely to have obstructive coronary artery disease (His D H, Roshandel A, Singh N, et al. 2005 Headache response to glyceryl trinitrate in patients with and without obstructive coronary artery disease. Heart 91:1164–1166).

[4]It has been argued that deaths on sildenafil largely reflect the fact that it is used by patients at high cardiovascular risk. But post-marketing data show that death is 50 times more likely after sildenafil taken for erectile failure than alprostadil, the previous first-line agent (Mitka M 2000 Some men who take Viagra die – why? Journal of the American Medical Association 283:590–593).

where absorption is rapid and reliable. Time spent ensuring that patients understand the way to take the tablets, and that the feeling of fullness in the head is harmless, is time well spent. The action begins in 2 min and lasts for up to 30 min. The dose in the standard tablet is 300 µg, and 500- or 600-microgram strengths are also available; patients may use up to 6 mg/day in total, but those who require more than two or three tablets per week should take a long-acting nitrate preparation. GTN is taken at the onset of pain and as a prophylactic immediately before any exertion likely to precipitate the pain. Sustained-release buccal tablets are available (Suscard), 1–5 mg. Absorption from the gastro-intestinal tract is good, but extensive hepatic first-pass metabolism renders the sublingual or buccal route preferable; an oral metered-dose aerosol that is sprayed under the tongue (nitrolingual spray) is an alternative.

For prophylaxis, GTN can be given as an oral (buccal, or to swallow, Sustac) sustained-release formulation or via the skin as a patch (or ointment); these formulations can be useful for sufferers from nocturnal angina.[5]

Venepuncture. The ointment can assist difficult venipuncture, and a transdermal patch adjacent to an intravenous infusion site can prevent extravasation and phlebitis, and prolong infusion survival.

Isosorbide dinitrate (Cedocard) ($t_{1/2}$ 20 min) is used for prophylaxis of angina pectoris and for congestive heart failure (tablets sublingual, and to swallow). An intravenous formulation, 500 µg/mL (Isoket), is available for use in left ventricular failure and unstable angina.

Isosorbide mononitrate (Elantan) ($t_{1/2}$ 4 h) is used for prophylaxis of angina (tablets to swallow). Hepatic first-pass metabolism is much less than for the dinitrate so that systemic bioavailability is more reliable.

Pentaerithrityl tetranitrate (Peritrate) ($t_{1/2}$ 8 h) is less efficacious than its metabolite pentaerithrityl trinitrate ($t_{1/2}$ 11 h).

Calcium channel blockers

Calcium is involved in the initiation of smooth muscle and cardiac cell contraction, and in the propagation of the cardiac impulse. Actions on cardiac pacemaker cells and conducting tissue are described in Chapter 25.

Vascular smooth muscle cells. Contraction of these cells requires an influx of calcium across the cell membrane. This occurs through voltage-operated ion channels (VOCs), and this influx is able to trigger further release of calcium from intracellular stores in the sarcoplasmic reticulum. The VOCs have relatively long opening times and carry large fluxes; hence they are usually referred to as 'L-type channels'.[6] The rise in intracellular free calcium results in activation of the contractile proteins, myosin and actin, with shortening of the myofibril and contraction of smooth muscle. During relaxation, calcium is released from the myofibril and either pumped back into the sarcoplasm or lost through Na/Ca exchange at the cell surface.

There are three structurally distinct classes of calcium channel blocker:

- Dihydropyridines (the most numerous).
- Phenylalkylamines (principally verapamil).
- Benzothiazepine (diltiazem).

The differences among their clinical effects can be explained in part by their binding to different parts of the L-type calcium channel. All members of the group are vasodilators, and some have negative inotropic and negative chronotropic effects on the heart via effects on pacemaker cells in the conducting tissue. The attributes of individual drugs are described below.

The therapeutic benefit of the calcium channel blockers in hypertension and angina is due mainly to their action as vasodilators. Their action on the heart gives non-dihydropyridines an additional role as class 4 antiarrhythmics.

Pharmacokinetics. Calcium channel blockers in general are well absorbed from the gastrointestinal tract, and their systemic bioavailability depends on the extent of first-pass metabolism in the gut wall and liver, which varies among the drugs. All undergo metabolism to less active products, predominantly by cytochrome P450 CYP3A4, which is the source of interactions with other drugs by enzyme induction and inhibition. As their action is terminated by metabolism, dose adjustments for patients with impaired renal function are therefore either minor or unnecessary.

Indications for use

- *Hypertension:* amlodipine, lercanidipine, nicardipine, nifedipine, verapamil.
- *Angina:* amlodipine, diltiazem, nicardipine, nifedipine, verapamil.
- *Cardiac arrhythmia:* verapamil.
- *Raynaud's disease:* nifedipine.
- *Prevention* of ischaemic neurological damage following subarachnoid haemorrhage: nimodipine.

---

[5]Useful, but not always safe. Defibrillator paddles and nitrate patches make an explosive combination, and it is not always in the patient's interest to have the patch as unobtrusive as possible (see Canadian Medical Association Journal 1993; 148:790).

[6]Several calcium-selective channels have been described in different tissues, e.g. the N (present in neuronal tissue) and T (transient, found in brain, neuronal and cardiovascular pacemaker tissue); the drugs discussed here selectively target the L-channel for its cardiovascular importance.

Adverse effects. Headache, flushing, dizziness, palpitations and hypotension may occur during the first few hours after dosing, as the plasma concentration is increasing, particularly for shorter-acting dihydropyridines. Longer-acting drugs, especially amlodipine, are more likely to cause ankle oedema, which is not relieved by a diuretic but disappears after lying flat, e.g. overnight. The oedema is probably due to a rise in intracapillary pressure as a result of the selective dilatation by calcium channel blockers of the precapillary arterioles. Indeed, the oedema is less of a problem in patients already receiving an ACE inhibitor or ARB, since these classes dilate the post-capillary venules as well as the pre-capillary sphincter. Bradycardia may occur, especially when the non-dihydropyridines are combined with β-blockade. Gastrointestinal effects of verapamil include constipation.

The calcium channel blockers are at least as effective as any other class of antihypertensives in protecting against the cardiovascular complications of hypertension, with most evidence coming from trials with amlodipine, or long-acting formulations of nifedipine.[7]

Interactions are numerous. Generally, the drugs in this group are extensively metabolised, and there is risk of decreased effect with enzyme inducers, e.g. rifampicin, and increased effect with enzyme inhibitors, e.g. ketoconazole or cimetidine. Conversely, calcium channel blockers decrease the plasma clearance of several other drugs by mechanisms that include delaying their metabolic breakdown. The consequence, for example, is that diltiazem and verapamil cause increased exposure to carbamazepine, quinidine, statins, ciclosporin, metoprolol, theophylline and (HIV) protease inhibitors. Verapamil increases plasma concentration of digoxin, possibly by interfering with its biliary excretion. β-Adrenoceptor blockers may exacerbate atrioventricular (AV) block and cardiac failure. Grapefruit juice raises the plasma concentration of dihydropyridines (except amlodipine) and verapamil, while St John's wort, as an inducer of CYP3A4, can reduce bioavailability of verapamil and dihydropyridines.

Individual calcium channel blockers

Nifedipine ($t_{1/2}$ 2 h) is the prototype dihydropyridine. It selectively dilates arteries with little effect on veins; its negative myocardial inotropic and chronotropic effects are much less than those of verapamil. There are sustained-release formulations of nifedipine that permit once-daily dosing, minimising peaks and troughs in plasma concentration so that adverse effects due to rapid fluctuation of concentrations are lessened. Various methods have been used to prolong, and smooth, drug delivery, and bioequivalence between these formulations cannot be assumed; prescribers should specify the brand to be dispensed. The adverse effects of calcium channel blockers with a short duration of action may include the hazards of activating the sympathetic system each time a dose is taken. The dose range for nifedipine is 30–90 mg/day. In addition to the adverse effects listed above, gum hypertrophy may occur. Nifedipine can be taken 'sublingually', by biting a capsule and squeezing the contents under the tongue. In point of fact, absorption is still largely from the stomach after this manoeuvre, and it should not be used in a hypertensive emergency because the blood pressure reduction is unpredictable and sometimes large enough to cause cerebral ischaemia (see p. 440).

Amlodipine has a $t_{1/2}$ (40 h) sufficient to permit the same benefits as the longest-acting formulations of nifedipine without requiring a special formulation. It is the drug of choice for initial treatment of many types of hypertension, with no serious contraindication or adverse consequence, and a wealth of long-term efficacy data. Its slow association with L-channels and long duration of action render it unsuitable for emergency reduction of blood pressure where frequent dose adjustment is needed. On the other hand, an occasional missed dose is of little consequence. Amlodipine differs from all other dihydropyridines listed in this chapter in being safe to use in patients with cardiac failure (the PRAISE study).[8]

Verapamil ($t_{1/2}$ 4 h) is an arterial vasodilator with some venodilator effect; it also has marked negative myocardial inotropic and chronotropic actions. It is given thrice daily as a conventional tablet or daily as a sustained-release formulation. Because of its negative effects on myocardial conducting and contracting cells, it should not be given to patients with bradycardia, second- or third-degree heart block, or patients with Wolff–Parkinson–White syndrome to relieve atrial flutter or fibrillation. Amiodarone and digoxin increase the AV block. Verapamil increases plasma quinidine

[7]Brown M J, Palmer C R, Castaigne A et al 2000 Morbidity and mortality in patients randomised to double-blind treatment with a long-acting calcium-channel blocker or diuretic in the International Nifedipine GITS study: Intervention as a Goal in Hypertension Treatment [INSIGHT]. Lancet 356:355–372; ALLHAT Officers and Coordinators for the ALLHAT Collaborative Research Group. The Antihypertensive and Lipid-Lowering Treatment to Prevent Heart Attack Trial. 2002. Major outcomes in high-risk hypertensive patients randomized to angiotensin-converting enzyme inhibitor or calcium channel blocker vs diuretic: The Antihypertensive and Lipid-Lowering Treatment to Prevent Heart Attack Trial (ALLHAT). Journal of the American Medical Association 288: 2981–2997; Dahlöf B, Sever P S, Poulter N R et al 2005 Prevention of cardiovascular events with an antihypertensive regimen of amlodipine adding perindopril as required versus atenolol adding bendroflumethiazide as required, in the Anglo-Scandinavian Cardiac Outcomes Trial-Blood Pressure Lowering Arm (ASCOT-BPLA): a multicentre randomised controlled trial. Lancet 366: 895–906.

[8]PRAISE – Prospective Randomised Amlodipine Survival Evaluation (see Packer M, O'Connor C M, Ghali J K et al 1996 The effect of amlodipine on morbidity and mortality in severe chronic heart failure. New England Journal of Medicine 335:1107–1114).

concentration, and this interaction may cause dangerous hypotension.

Diltiazem ($t_{1/2}$ 5 h) is given thrice daily, or once or twice daily if a slow-release formulation is prescribed. It causes less myocardial depression and prolongation of AV conduction than does verapamil but should not be used where there is bradycardia, second- or third-degree heart block or sick sinus syndrome.

Nimodipine has a moderate cerebral vasodilating action. Cerebral ischaemia after subarachnoid haemorrhage may be partly due to vasospasm; clinical trial evidence indicates that nimodipine given after subarachnoid haemorrhage reduces cerebral infarction (incidence and extent). Although the benefit is small, the absence of any more effective options has led to the routine administration of nimodipine (60 mg every 4 h) to all patients for the first few days after subarachnoid haemorrhage. No benefit has been found in similar trials following other forms of stroke.

Other members include felodipine, isradipine, lacidipine, lercanidipine and nisoldipine.

Angiotensin-converting enzyme (ACE) inhibitors, angiotensin (AT) II receptor blockers (ARBs) and renin inhibitors

Renin is an enzyme produced by the kidney in response to a number of factors, but principally adrenergic (β_1 receptor) activity and sodium depletion. Renin converts a circulating glycoprotein (angiotensinogen) into the biologically inert angiotensin I, which is then changed by *angiotensin-converting enzyme* (ACE or kininase II) into the highly potent vasoconstrictor *angiotensin II*. ACE is located on the luminal surface of capillary endothelial cells, particularly in the lungs; and there are also renin–angiotensin systems in many organs, e.g. brain, heart, the relevance of which is uncertain.

Angiotensin II acts on two G-protein–coupled receptors, of which the angiotensin 'AT$_1$' subtype accounts for all the classic actions of angiotensin. As well as vasoconstriction, these include stimulation of aldosterone (the sodium-retaining hormone) production by the adrenal cortex. It is evident that angiotensin II can have an important effect on blood pressure. In addition, it stimulates cardiac and vascular smooth muscle cell growth, probably contributing to the progressive amplification in hypertension once the process is initiated. The AT$_2$-receptor subtype is coupled to inhibition of muscle growth or proliferation, but appears of minor importance in the adult cardiovascular system. The recognition that the AT$_1$-receptor subtype is the important target for drugs that antagonise angiotensin II has led, a little confusingly, to alternative nomenclatures for these drugs: angiotensin II blockers, AT$_1$-receptor blockers or the acronym, ARB. The latter abbreviation is used here for consistency.

Bradykinin (an endogenous vasodilator found in blood vessel walls) is also a substrate for ACE. Potentiation of bradykinin contributes to the blood pressure–lowering action of ACE inhibitors in patients with low-renin causes of hypertension. Either bradykinin or one of the neurokinin substrates of ACE (such as substance P) may stimulate cough (below). The ARBs differ from the ACE inhibitors in having no effect on bradykinin, and they do not cause cough. ARBs are slightly more effective than ACE inhibitors at preventing angiotensin II vasoconstriction, because angiotensin II can be generated from angiotensin I by non-ACE enzymes such as chymase. ACE inhibitors are more effective at suppressing aldosterone production in patients with normal or low plasma renin levels.

Uses

Hypertension. The antihypertensive effect of ACE inhibitors, ARBs and renin inhibitors results primarily from vasodilatation (reduction of peripheral resistance) with little change in cardiac output or rate; renal blood flow may increase (desirable). A fall in aldosterone production may also contribute to the blood-pressure–lowering action of ACE inhibitors. Both classes slow progression of glomerulopathy. Whether the long-term benefit of these drugs in hypertension exceeds that to be expected from blood pressure reduction alone remains controversial.

ACE inhibitors, ARBs and renin inhibitors are most useful in hypertension when the raised blood pressure results from excess renin production, e.g. renovascular hypertension, or where concurrent use of another drug (diuretic or calcium channel blocker) renders the blood pressure renin dependent. The fall in blood pressure can be rapid, especially with short-acting ACE inhibitors, and low initial doses of these should be used in patients at risk: those with impaired renal function or suspected cerebrovascular disease. These patients may be advised to omit any concurrent diuretic treatment for a few days before the first dose. The antihypertensive effect increases progressively over weeks with continued administration (as with other antihypertensives), and the dose may be increased at intervals of 2 weeks.

Cardiac failure (see p. 428). ACE inhibitors have a useful vasodilator and diuretic-sparing (but not diuretic-substitute) action that is critical to the treatment of all grades of heart failure. Mortality reduction here may result from their being the only vasodilator that does not reflexly activate the sympathetic system.

The ARBs are at least as effective as ACE inhibitors in patients with heart failure, and they can be substituted if patients are intolerant of an ACE inhibitor. Based on the Candesartan in Heart Failure Assessment of Reduction in Mortality and Morbidity (CHARM) trial, they may also benefit patients with heart failure and a low ejection fraction when added to treatment with a β-blocker and ACE inhibitor.[9]

Diabetic nephropathy. In patients with type I (insulin-dependent) diabetes, hypertension often accompanies the diagnosis of frank nephropathy, and aggressive blood pressure control is essential to slow the otherwise inexorable decline in renal function that follows. ACE inhibitors appear to have a specific renoprotective effect, probably because of the role of angiotensin II in driving the underlying glomerular hyperfiltration.[10] These drugs are now first-line treatment for hypertensive type I diabetics, although most patients will need a second or third agent to reach the rigorous blood pressure targets for this condition (see below). Their role in preventing the progression of the earliest manifestation of renal damage, microalbuminuria, is more complicated. Here the evidence suggests that ACE inhibitors do not slow the incidence of microalbuminuria in type I diabetics, and an ARB may actually substantially increase it.[10] In contrast, an ACE inhibitor halves the incidence of microalbuminuria in type 2 diabetics with hypertension and normal renal function on follow-up. A parallel group on verapamil did not show any protection confirming that inhibition of the renin–angiotensin–aldosterone (RAAS) axis is required for this effect, not simply lowering the blood pressure.[11] For hypertensive type 2 diabetics with established nephropathy, both ARBs and ACE inhibitors protect against a decline in renal function and reduce macroproteinuria.[10] The evidence suggests they are interchangeable in this respect. Combining the two classes of drugs ('dual block') is not recommended, even though 'dual block' does produce better urine protein sparing than either agent alone.[10]

Myocardial infarction (MI). Following a myocardial infarction, the left ventricle may fail acutely from the loss of functional tissue or in the long term from a process of 'remodelling' due to thinning and enlargement of the scarred ventricular wall (see p. 448). Angiotensin II plays a key role in both of these processes, and an ACE inhibitor given after MI markedly reduces the incidence of heart failure. The effect is seen even in patients without overt signs of cardiac failure, but who have low left ventricular ejection fractions (<40%) during the convalescent phase (3–10 days) following the MI. Such patients receiving captopril in the SAVE trial[12] had a 37% reduction in progressive heart failure over the 60-month follow-up period compared with placebo. The benefits of ACE inhibition after MI are additional to those conferred by thrombolysis, aspirin and β-blockers. ARBs also prevent remodelling and heart failure in post-MI patients, but there is no additional benefit from 'dual blockade'.[13]

Cautions

Certain constraints apply to the use of ACE inhibitors:

- *Heart failure*: severe hypotension may result in patients taking diuretics, or who are hypovolaemic, hyponatraemic, elderly, have renal impairment or with systolic blood pressure of less than 100 mmHg. A test dose of ca ptopril 6.25 mg by mouth may be given because its effect lasts for only 4–6 h. If tolerated, the preferred long-acting ACE inhibitor may then be initiated in low dose.
- *Renal artery stenosis* (RAS, whether unilateral, bilateral renal or suspected from the presence of generalised atherosclerosis): an ACE inhibitor may cause renal failure and is contraindicated. ARBs are not necessarily any safer in this situation, because angiotensin II–mediated constriction of the efferent arteriole is thought to be crucial to the maintenance of glomerular perfusion in RAS.
- *Aortic stenosis/left ventricular outflow tract obstruction*: an ACE inhibitor may cause severe, sudden hypotension and, depending on severity, is relatively or absolutely contraindicated.
- *Pregnancy* represents an absolute contraindication (see below).
- *Angioedema* may result (see below).

Adverse effects

ACE inhibitors:

- *Persistent dry cough* occurs in 10–15% of patients.
- *Urticaria and angioedema* (less than 1 in 100 patients) are much rarer, occurring usually in the first weeks of treatment. The angioedema varies from mild swelling

[9]Demers C, McMurray J J V, Swedberg K et al for the CHARM investigators 2005 Impact of candesartan on nonfatal myocardial infarction and cardiovascular death in patients with heart failure. Journal of the American Medical Association 294:1794–1798.

[10]For a review see: Ruggenenti P, Cravedi P, Remuzzi G 2010 The RAAS in the pathogenesis and treatment of diabetic nephropathy. Nature Reviews Nephrology 6:319–330. Available at: http://www.nature.com/nrneph/journal/v6/n6/full/nrneph.2010.58.html (accessed 3 August 2010).

[11]Ruggenenti P, Fassi A, Ilieva A P et al 2004 Preventing microalbuminuria in type 2 diabetes. New England Journal of Medicine 351:1941–1951. This was the BENEDICT trial comparing type 2 diabetics randomised to trandolopril, verapamil and the combination versus placebo with a 3.6 year follow-up.

[12]Pfeffer M A, Braunwald E, Moye L A et al 1992 Effect of captopril on mortality and morbidity in patients with left ventricular dysfunction after myocardial infarction. Results of the survival and ventricular enlargement trial. The SAVE Investigators. New England Journal of Medicine 327:669–677.

[13]Pfeffer M A, McMurray J V C, Velaquez E J et al for the Valsartan in Acute Myocardial Infarction Trial Investigators 2004 Valsartan, captopril, or both in myocardial infarction complicated by heart failure, left ventricular dysfunction, or both. New England Journal of Medicine 349:1893–1906.

of the tongue to life-threatening tracheal obstruction, when subcutaneous adrenaline/epinephrine should be given. The basis of the reaction is probably pharmacological rather than allergic, due to reduced breakdown of bradykinin.

- *Impaired renal function* may result from reduced glomerular filling pressure, systemic hypotension or glomerulonephritis, and plasma creatinine levels should be checked before and during treatment.
- *Hyponatraemia* may develop, especially where a diuretic is also given; clinically significant hyperkalaemia (see effect on aldosterone above) is confined to patients with impaired renal function.
- ACE inhibitors have been associated with major malformations in the first trimester and are *fetotoxic* in the second trimester, causing reduced renal perfusion, hypotension, oligohydramnios and fetal death (see Pregnancy hypertension, p. 440).
- *Neutropenia* and other blood dyscrasias occur. Other reported reactions include rashes, taste disturbance (dysguesia), musculoskeletal pain, proteinuria, liver injury and pancreatitis.

ARBs are absolutely contraindicated in the mid-trimester of pregnancy as are ACE inhibitors, and best avoided in the first. They lack the other complications of the ACE inhibitors – especially the cough and angioedema. They are, in fact, the only antihypertensive drug class for which there is no 'typical' side-effect.

Interactions. Hyperkalaemia can result from use with potassium-sparing diuretics. Renal clearance of lithium is reduced and toxic concentrations of plasma lithium may follow. Severe hypotension can occur with diuretics (above) and with chlorpromazine, and possibly other phenothiazines.

Individual drugs

Captopril (Capoten) has a $t_{1/2}$ of 2 h and is partly metabolised and partly excreted unchanged; adverse effects are more common when renal function is impaired; it is given twice or thrice daily. Captopril is the shortest acting of the ACE inhibitors, one of the few that is itself active by mouth, not requiring de-esterification after absorption.

Enalapril (Innovace) is a prodrug ($t_{1/2}$ 35 h) that is converted to the active enalaprilat ($t_{1/2}$ 10 h). Effective 24-h control of blood pressure probably requires twice-daily administration.

Other members include *cilazapril, fosinopril, imidapril, lisinopril, moexipril, perindopril, quinapril, ramipril* and *trandolapril*. Of these, lisinopril has a marginally longer $t_{1/2}$ than enalapril (it is the lysine analogue of enalaprilat), probably justifying its popularity as a once-daily ACE inhibitor. Some

of the others are longer acting, with quinapril and ramipril also having a higher degree of binding to ACE in vascular tissue. The clinical significance of these differences is disputed. In the Heart Outcomes Prevention Evaluation (HOPE) study of 9297 patients, ramipril reduced, by 20–30%, the rates of death, myocardial infarction and stroke in a broad range of high-risk patients who were not known to have a low ejection fraction or heart failure.[14] The authors considered (probably erroneously) that the results could not be explained entirely by blood pressure reduction.

Losartan was the first ARB to be licensed in the UK. It is a competitive blocker with a non-competitive active metabolite. The drug has a short $t_{1/2}$ (2 h), but the metabolite is much longer lived ($t_{1/2}$ 10 h), permitting once-daily dosing.

Other ARBs in clinical use include *candesartan, eprosartan, irbesartan, telmisartan, valsartan, olmesartan* and *azilsartan*. Some of these may be marginally more effective than losartan at lowering blood pressure, but few if any comparisons have been performed at maximal dose of each drug. Losartan is generally used in combination with hydrochlorothiazide. In a landmark study, this combination was 25% more effective than atenolol plus hydrochlorothiazide in preventing stroke.[15]

This class of drug is very well tolerated; in clinical trials the side-effect profiles are indistinguishable or even better than those of placebo. Unlike the ACE inhibitors, they do not produce cough, and are a valuable alternative for the 10–15% of patients who thereby discontinue their ACE inhibitor. ARBs are used to treat hypertension, left ventricular (LV) failure after MI and established heart failure. With the possible exception of chronic heart failure, they do not appear to be superior to ACE inhibitors.

The cautions listed for the use of ACE inhibitors (above) apply also to AT_1-receptor blockers.

Renin inhibitors share the benefit of ARBs over ACE inhibitors in terms of cough and angioedema. By implication, with other agents targeting the RAAS they should not be used in pregnancy.

Interactions. Hyperkalaemia can result from use with potassium-sparing diuretics. Severe hypotension can occur on first dosing if given after agents that increase circulating renin levels such as diuretics (especially loop diuretics) and potent vasodilators.

[14]Yusuf S, Sleight P, Pogue J et al 2000 Effects of an angiotensin-converting-enzyme inhibitor, ramipril, on cardiovascular events in high-risk patients. The Heart Outcomes Prevention Evaluation Study Investigators. New England Journal of Medicine 342:145–153.
[15]Dahlof B, Devereux R B, Kjeldsen S E et al 2002 Cardiovascular morbidity and mortality in the Losartan Intervention For Endpoint reduction in hypertension study (LIFE): a randomised trial against atenolol. Lancet 359:995–1010.

Individual drugs

Aliskiren is the only orally active non-peptide renin inhibitor licensed ($t_{1/2}$ 40 h). The agent is well tolerated apart from dose-dependent diarrhoea; it is not clear if this is a class side-effect. It produces additive effects on blood pressure with ACE inhibitors, ARBs, calcium channel blockers and thiazide diuretics. There are no outcome data in terms of preventing hypertension-related cardiovascular events, so it should be reserved for inhibiting the RAAS where an ACE inhibitor or ARB is not tolerated.[16]

Other vasodilators

Several older drugs are powerfully vasodilating, but precluded from routine use in hypertension by their adverse effects. Minoxidil and nitroprusside still have special indications.

Minoxidil is a vasodilator selective for arterioles rather than for veins, similar to diazoxide and hydralazine. Like the former, it acts through its sulphate metabolite as an adenosine triphosphate (ATP)-dependent potassium channel opener. It is highly effective in severe hypertension, but in common with all potent arterial vasodilators its hypotensive action is accompanied by a compensatory baroreceptor-mediated sympathetic discharge, causing tachycardia and increased cardiac output. There is also renin release with secondary salt and water retention, which antagonises the hypotensive effect (so-called 'tolerance' on long-term use). Therefore, it is used in combination with a β-blocker and loop diuretic (as is hydralazine; see below). *Hypertrichosis* is perhaps the most notorious side-effect of minoxidil. The hair growth is generalised when taken orally and, although a cosmetic problem in women, it has been exploited as a 2–5% topical solution for the treatment of male-pattern baldness (Regaine).

Sodium nitroprusside is a highly effective antihypertensive agent when given intravenously. Its effect is almost immediate and lasts for 1–5 min. Therefore it must be given by a precisely controllable infusion. It dilates both arterioles and veins, which would cause collapse were the patient to stand up, e.g. for toilet purposes. There is a compensatory sympathetic discharge with tachycardia and tachyphylaxis to the drug.

The action of nitroprusside is terminated by metabolism within erythrocytes. Specifically, electron transfer from haemoglobin iron to nitroprusside yields methaemoglobin and an unstable nitroprusside radical. This breaks down, liberating cyanide radicals capable of inhibiting cytochrome oxidase (and thus cellular respiration). Fortunately, most of the cyanide remains bound within erythrocytes, but a small fraction does diffuse out into the plasma and is converted to thiocyanate. Hence, monitoring plasma thiocyanate concentrations during prolonged (days) nitroprusside infusion is a useful marker of impending systemic cyanide toxicity. Poisoning may be obvious as a progressive metabolic acidosis, or may manifest as delirium or psychotic symptoms. Intoxicated subjects are also reputed to have the characteristic bitter almond smell of hydrogen cyanide. Clearly nitroprusside infusion must be used with caution, and outside specialist units it may be safer overall to choose another more familiar drug.

Sodium nitroprusside is used in hypertensive emergencies, refractory heart failure and for controlled hypotension in surgery. An infusion[17] may begin at 0.3–1 microgram/kg/min, and control of blood pressure is likely to be established at 0.5–6 µg/kg/min; close monitoring of blood pressure is mandatory, usually by direct arterial monitoring; rate changes of infusion may be made every 5–10 min.

Hydralazine is now little used for hypertension except for that related to pregnancy (owing to its established lack of teratogenicity), but it may have a role as a vasodilator (plus nitrates) in heart failure. It reduces peripheral resistance by directly relaxing arterioles, with negligible effect on veins; the mechanism of vasorelaxation is unclear. The $t_{1/2}$ is 1 h.

In most hypertensive emergencies (except for dissecting aneurysm), hydralazine 5–20 mg i.v. may be given over 20 min, when the maximum effect will be seen in 10–80 min; it can be repeated according to need and the patient transferred to oral therapy within 1–2 days.

Prolonged use of hydralazine at doses above 50 mg/day may cause a systemic lupus-like syndrome, more commonly in white than in black races, and in those with the slow acetylator phenotype.

Three other vasodilators find a role outside hypertension:

Nicorandil is effective through two actions: it acts as a nitrate by activating cyclic GMP (see above) but also opens the ATP-dependent potassium channel to allow potassium efflux and hyperpolarisation of the membrane, which reduces calcium ion entry and induces muscular relaxation. It is indicated for use in angina, where it has similar efficacy to β-blockade, nitrates or calcium channel blockade. It is administered orally and is an alternative to nitrates when tolerance is a problem, or to the other classes when these are contraindicated by asthma or cardiac failure. Adverse effects to nicorandil are similar to those of nitrates, with

---

[16]An outcome study ('Altitude') was stopped early because futility analysis showed no chance of demonstrating the hypothesised benefit of adding aliskiren to ACE inhibitors or ARBs in patients with diabetes. The fall in GFR and rise in serum K+ in the aliskiren group led guidelines to discourage the use of 'dual RAS blockade' (Parving HH, Brenner BM, McMurray JJ et al. Cardiorenal end points in a trial of aliskiren for type 2 diabetes. New England Journal of Medicine 367:2204–2213)

[17]Light causes sodium nitroprusside in solution to decompose; hence solutions should be made fresh and immediately protected by an opaque cover, e.g. aluminium foil. The fresh solution has a faint brown colour; if the colour intensifies, then it should be discarded.

headache reported in 35% of patients. It is the only antianginal drug for which at least one trial has demonstrated a beneficial influence on outcome.[18]

Papaverine is an alkaloid present in opium, but is structurally unrelated to morphine. It inhibits phosphodiesterase, and its principal action is to relax smooth muscle throughout the body, especially in the vascular system. It is occasionally injected into an area where local vasodilatation is desired, especially into and around arteries and veins to relieve spasm during vascular surgery and when setting up intravenous infusions. It is also used to treat male erectile dysfunction (see p. 493).

Alprostadil is a stable form of prostaglandin E_1. It is effective in psychogenic and neuropathic penile erectile dysfunction by direct intracorporeal injection (see p. 493) and is used intravenously to maintain patency of the ductus arteriosus in the newborn with congenital heart disease.

Vasodilators in heart failure

See page 416.

Vasodilators in peripheral vascular disease

The aim has been to produce peripheral arteriolar vasodilatation without a concurrent significant drop in blood pressure, so that an increased blood flow in the limbs will result. Drugs are naturally more useful in patients in whom the decreased flow of blood is due to spasm of the vessels (Raynaud's phenomenon) than where it is due to organic obstructive changes that may make dilatation in response to drugs impossible (arteriosclerosis, intermittent claudication, Buerger's disease).

Intermittent claudication. Patients should 'stop smoking and keep walking', i.e. take frequent exercise within their capacity. Other risk factors should be treated vigorously, especially hypertension and hyperlipidaemia. Patients should also receive low-dose aspirin (75 mg/day) as an antiplatelet agent. Most patients with intermittent claudication succumb to ischaemic or cerebrovascular disease, and therefore a major objective of treatment should be prevention of such outcomes. Vasodilators such as naftidrofuryl (Praxilene) and pentoxifylline (Trental) increase blood flow to skin rather than muscle; they have been used successfully in the treatment of venous leg ulcers (varicose and traumatic). A trial of these drugs for intermittent claudication is worthwhile, but they should be withdrawn if there is no benefit within a few weeks.

Naftidrofuryl has several actions. It is classed as a metabolic enhancer because it activates the enzyme succinate dehydrogenase, increasing the supply of ATP and reducing lactate concentrations in muscle. It also blocks $5HT_2$ receptors and inhibits serotonin-induced vasoconstriction and platelet aggregation.

Pentoxifylline is thought to improve oxygen supply to ischaemic tissue by improving erythrocyte deformability and reducing blood viscosity, in part by reducing plasma fibrinogen. Neither of these drugs is a direct vasodilator, as is the third drug used for intermittent claudication, *inositol nicotinate*. The evidence in favour of any benefit is stronger for the first two, for which meta-analyses provide some evidence of efficacy (increase in walking distance). Most vasodilators act selectively on healthy blood vessels, causing a diversion ('steal') of blood from atheromatous vessels.

Night cramps occur in the disease, and quinine has a somewhat controversial reputation in their prevention. Nevertheless, meta-analysis of six double-blind trials of nocturnal cramps (not necessarily associated with peripheral vascular disease) shows that the number, but not severity or duration of episodes, is reduced by a nighttime dose.[19] The benefit may not be seen for 4 weeks.

Raynaud's phenomenon may be helped by nifedipine, and also by topical glyceryl trinitrate; other vasodilators are worth trying in resistant cases. In severe cases, especially patients with ulceration, intermittent infusions over several hours of the endogenous vasodilator, epoprostenol (prostacyclin), achieve long-lasting improvements in symptoms.

β-Adrenoceptor blockers exacerbate peripheral vascular disease and Raynaud's phenomenon by reducing perfusion of a circulation that is already compromised. Switching to a $β_1$-selective blocker is unhelpful, because the adverse effect is due to reduced cardiac output rather than unopposed α-receptor–induced vasoconstriction.

Adrenoceptor-blocking drugs

Adrenoceptor-blocking drugs occupy the adrenoceptor in competition with adrenaline/epinephrine and noradrenaline/norepinephrine (and other sympathomimetic amines) whether released from stores in nerve terminals or injected.

---

[18] The Impact Of Nicorandil in Angina (IONA) study was a double-blind, randomised, placebo-controlled trial conducted in the UK, in which high-risk patients with stable angina were assigned placebo or nicorandil 10–20 mg. Over a mean follow-up of 1.6 years, significantly more placebo-treated patients suffered an acute coronary syndrome or coronary death (15.5% vs. 13.1%, $P = 0.01$) (IONA Study Group 2002 Effect of nicorandil on coronary events in patients with stable angina: the Impact Of Nicorandil in Angina (IONA) randomised trial. Lancet 359:1269–1275).

[19] Man-Son-Hing M, Wells G 1995 Meta-analysis of efficacy of quinine for treatment of nocturnal cramps in elderly people. British Medical Journal 310:13–17.

There are two principal classes of adrenoceptor, α and β: for details of receptor effects, see Table 23.1.

α-Adrenoceptor–blocking drugs

There are two main subtypes of α adrenoceptor:

- 'Classic' α_1 adrenoceptors, on the effector organ (post-synaptic), mediate vasoconstriction.
- α_2 Adrenoceptors are present both on some effector tissues (post-synaptic) and on the nerve ending (pre-synaptic). The pre-synaptic receptors (or autoreceptors) inhibit release of chemotransmitter (noradrenaline/norepinephrine), i.e. they provide negative feedback control of transmitter release. They are also present in the CNS.

The first generation of α-adrenoceptor blockers were imidazolines (e.g. phentolamine), which blocked both α_1 and α_2 receptors. When subjects taking such a drug stand from the lying position or take exercise, the sympathetic system is physiologically activated (via baroreceptors). The normal vasoconstrictive (α_1) effect (to maintain blood pressure) is blocked by the drug, and the failure of this response causes further sympathetic activation and the release of additional transmitter. This would normally be restrained by negative feedback through α_2 autoreceptors, but these are blocked too.

The β adrenoceptors, however, are not blocked, and the excess transmitter released at adrenergic endings is free to act on them, causing a tachycardia that may be unpleasant. Hence, non-selective α-adrenoceptor blockers are not used on their own in hypertension.

An α_1-adrenoceptor blocker that spares the α_2 receptor, so that negative feedback inhibition of noradrenaline/norepinephrine release is maintained, is more useful in hypertension (less tachycardia and postural and exercise hypotension); prazosin is such a drug (see below).

For use in prostatic hypertrophy, see page 492.

> ### Uses of α-adrenoceptor–blocking drugs
>
> - Hypertension
>   - essential: doxazosin, labetalol
>   - phaeochromocytoma: phenoxybenzamine; phentolamine (for crises).
> - Peripheral vascular disease.
> - Benign prostatic hypertrophy (to relax capsular smooth muscle that may contribute to urinary obstruction).
> - Ureteric stones[20]

---

[20]Hollingsworth J M, Canales B K, Rogers M A M et al 2016 Alpha blockers for treatment of ureteric stones: systematic review and meta-analysis. British Medical Journal 355:i6112.

Adverse effects. The converse of the benefit in the treatment of prostatism is the adverse effect of urinary incontinence in women. Other adverse effects of α-adrenoceptor blockade are postural hypotension, nasal stuffiness, red sclerae and, in the male, failure of ejaculation. They may also exacerbate symptoms of angina.[21]

Effects peculiar to each drug are mentioned below.

Notes on individual drugs

Prazosin blocks postsynaptic α_1 receptors but not presynaptic α_2 autoreceptors. It has a curious adverse 'first-dose effect': within 2 h of the first dose (rarely after another), there may be a brisk fall in blood pressure sufficient to cause loss of consciousness. Hence the first dose should be small (0.5 mg) and given before going to bed. This unwanted effect, together with a rather short duration of action ($t_{1/2}$ 3 h) has led to a sharp decline in its use.

Doxazosin ($t_{1/2}$ 8 h) was the first α-adrenoceptor blocker suitable for once-daily prescribing. The first-dose effect is also much less marked, although it is still advisable to start patients at a lower dose than is intended for maintenance. It is convenient, for instance, to prescribe 1 mg/day, increasing after 1 week to double this dose without repeating the blood pressure measurement at this stage. A slow-release formulation, doxazosin XL, can be started at the maintenance dose of 4 mg/day. Other α-adrenoceptor blockers used for prostatic symptoms are *alfuzosin* and *terazosin*.

Indoramin is an older α_1-blocker, which is a less useful antihypertensive but still used for prostatic symptoms. It is taken twice or thrice daily.

Phentolamine is a non-selective α-adrenoceptor blocker. It is given intravenously for brief effect in adrenergic hypertensive crises, e.g. phaeochromocytoma or the monoamine oxidase inhibitor–sympathomimetic interaction ('cheese reaction'). In addition to α-receptor block, it has direct vasodilator and cardiac inotropic actions. The dose for hypertensive crisis is 2–5 mg i.v. repeated as necessary (in minutes to hours). This is not a reliable diagnostic test for phaeochromocytoma!

Phenoxybenzamine is an irreversible non-selective α-adrenoceptor–blocking drug whose effects may last for 2 days or longer. The daily dose must therefore be increased slowly. It is impossible to reverse the circulatory effects by secreting noradrenaline/norepinephrine or other sympathomimetic drugs because its effects are insurmountable. This makes it the preferred α-blocker for treating phaeochromocytoma (see p. 442).

---

[21]It can be the reflex sympathetic activation, as much as hypotension itself, that causes problems. Many cardiologists have had their efforts at controlling angina in elderly patients sabotaged when the patient visits a urologist for his prostatic symptoms, and is treated with a powerful α_1-blocker.

425

It is wise to observe the effects of a single test dose closely before starting regular administration.

Indigestion and nausea can occur with oral therapy, which is best given with food.

Moxisylyte (thymoxamine) is a non-selective α-blocker for which Raynaud's phenomenon is the only extant indication.

Labetalol has both α- and β-receptor–blocking actions that are due to different isomers (see β-adrenoceptor block, below). Its parenteral preparation is valuable in the treatment of hypertension emergencies (see p. 439).

Chlorpromazine and amitriptyline, among their other actions, can both produce clinically significant α-blockade, which may be sufficient to cause postural hypotension and falls in the elderly.

β-Adrenoceptor–blocking drugs

Actions

These drugs selectively block the β-adrenoceptor effects of noradrenaline/norepinephrine and adrenaline/epinephrine. They may be pure antagonists or may have some agonist activity in addition (when they are described as partial agonists).

Intrinsic heart rate. Sympathetic activity (through β_1 adrenoceptors) accelerates, and parasympathetic activity (through muscarinic M_2 receptors) slows, the heart. If the sympathetic and the parasympathetic drives to the heart are simultaneously and adequately blocked by a β-adrenoceptor blocker plus atropine, the heart will beat at its 'intrinsic' rate. The intrinsic rate at rest is usually about 100 beats/min, as opposed to the usual rate of 80 beats/min, i.e. normally there is parasympathetic vagal 'tone', which decreases with age.

The *cardiovascular* effects of β-adrenoceptor block depend on the amount of sympathetic tone present. The chief effects result from reduction of sympathetic drive:

- Reduced automaticity (heart rate).
- Reduced myocardial contractility (rate of rise of pressure in the ventricle).
- Reduced renin secretion from the juxtaglomerular apparatus in the renal cortex.

With reduced rate, the cardiac output per minute is reduced and the overall cardiac oxygen consumption falls. The results are more evident on the response to exercise than at rest. With acute administration of a pure β-adrenoceptor blocker, i.e. one with no intrinsic sympathomimetic activity (ISA), *peripheral vascular resistance* tends to rise. This is probably a reflex response to the reduced cardiac output, but also occurs because the β-adrenoceptor (vasoconstrictor) effects are no longer partially opposed by β_2-adrenoceptor (dilator) effects; peripheral flow is reduced. With chronic use, peripheral resistance returns to about pre-treatment levels or a little

below, varying according to presence or absence of ISA. But peripheral blood flow remains reduced. The cold extremities that accompany chronic therapy are probably due chiefly to reduced cardiac output with reduced peripheral blood flow, rather than to the blocking of peripheral (β_2) dilator receptors.

Hepatic blood flow may be reduced by as much as 30%, prolonging the $t_{1/2}$ of the lipid-soluble drugs whose metabolism is limited by hepatic blood flow, i.e. whose first-pass metabolism is so extensive that it is actually limited by the rate of blood delivery to the liver; these include propranolol, verapamil and lidocaine, which may be used concomitantly for cardiac arrhythmias.

Effects

Within hours of starting treatment with a β-blocker, blood pressure starts to fall. This reflects the acute effect on cardiac output (heart rate and contractility), but this is not sustained, and on chronic administration the blockade of renin secretion appears to be the main cause of blood pressure reduction. An additional contributor may be the two- to three-fold increase in natriuretic peptide secretion caused by β-blockade.

A substantial advantage of β-blockade in hypertension is that physiological stresses such as exercise, *upright posture* and *high environmental temperature* are not accompanied by hypotension, as they are with agents that interfere with α-adrenoceptor–mediated homeostatic mechanisms. With β-blockade, these necessary adaptive α-receptor constrictor mechanisms remain intact.

At first sight, the cardiac effects might seem likely to be disadvantageous rather than advantageous, and indeed maximum exercise capacity is reduced. But the heart has substantial functional reserves so that use may be made of the desired properties in the diseases listed below, e.g. angina, without inducing heart failure. Indeed, β-blockade is now routine practice in patients with established mild to moderate heart failure and usually safe provided uptitration is slow. But heart failure can occur in patients with seriously diminished cardiac reserve.

For the effect on plasma potassium concentration, see p. 408.

β-Adrenoceptor selectivity

Some β-adrenoceptor blockers have higher affinity for cardiac β_1 receptors than for cardiac and peripheral β_2 receptors (Table 24.1). The ratio of the amount of drug required to block the two receptor subtypes is a measure of the *selectivity* of the drug. (See note to Table 23.1, p. 406, regarding the use of the terms 'β_1 selective' and 'cardioselective'.) The question is whether the differences between selective and non-selective β-blockers confer clinical advantages. In theory, β_1-blockers are less likely to cause bronchoconstriction, but

Table 24.1 β-Adrenoceptor–blocking drugs: properties at therapeutic doses

Drug		Partial agonist effect (intrinsic sympathomimetic effect)	Membrane stabilising effect (quinidine-like effect)
Division I: non-selective (β₁ + β₂) blockade			
Group I	Oxprenolol	+	+
Group II	Propranolol	−	+
Group III	Pindolol	+	−
Group IV	Sotalol	−	−
	Timolol	−	−
	Nadolol	−	−
Division II: β₁-('cardio')ª-selective blockadeᵇ			
Group I	Acebutolol	+	+
Group III	Esmolol	+	+
Group IV	Atenolol	−	−
	Bisoprolol	−	−
	Metoprolol	−	−
	Nebivolol	−	−
	Betaxolol	−	−
	Celiprololᶜ	−	−
Division III: non-selective β-blockade + α₁ blockade			
Group II	Carvedilol	−	+
Group IV	Labetalolᶜ	−	−

ªSee Table 23.1, page 406 regarding use of the term 'cardioselective'. *Note:* hybrid agents having β-receptor block plus vasodilation unrelated to adrenoceptor have been developed, e.g. nebivolol releases nitric oxide.
ᵇβ₁-selective drugs are considered to be up to 300 times (nebivolol) as effective against β₁-receptors compared with β₂-receptors. What selectivity really means is that 300 times more of the blocker is required to achieve the same blockade of the β₂-receptor as for the β₁-receptor. Therefore, as the dose (concentration at receptors) rises, the benefit of selectivity is gradually lost.
ᶜCeliprolol and labetalol both have partial β₂-selective agonist activity.

in practice few available β₁-blockers are sufficiently selective to be safely recommended in asthma. Bisoprolol and nebivolol may be exceptions that can be tried at low doses in patients with mild asthma and a strong indication for β-blockade. There are unlikely ever to be satisfactory safety data to support such use. The main practical use of β₁-selective blockade is in diabetics, where β₂ receptors mediate both the symptoms of hypoglycaemia and the counterregulatory metabolic responses that reverse the hypoglycaemia.

Some β-blockers (antagonists) also have agonist action or ISA, i.e. they are *partial agonists*. These agents cause less fall in resting heart rate than do the pure antagonists and may thus be less effective in severe angina pectoris, where reduction of heart rate is particularly important. The fall in cardiac output may be less, and fewer patients may experience unpleasantly cold extremities. Intermittent claudication may be worsened by β-blockade whether or not there is partial agonist effect. Both classes of drug can *precipitate* heart failure, and indeed no important difference is to be expected because patients with heart failure already have high sympathetic drive (but note that β-blockade can be used to *treat* cardiac failure, p. 429).

Abrupt withdrawal may be less likely to lead to a rebound effect if there is some partial agonist action, as there may be less up-regulation of receptors, such as occurs with prolonged receptor block.

Some β-blockers have a membrane-stabilising (quinidine-like or local anaesthetic) effect, a property that is unimportant at clinical doses but relevant in overdose (see below). Additionally, agents having this effect will anaesthetise the eye (undesirable) if applied topically for glaucoma (timolol is used in the eye and does not have this action).

The ankle jerk relaxation time is prolonged by β_2-adrenoceptor block, which may be misleading if the reflex is being relied on in diagnosis and management of hypothyroidism.

Pharmacokinetics

The plasma concentration of a β-adrenoceptor blocker may have a complex relationship with its effect, for several reasons. First-order kinetics usually apply to elimination of drug from plasma, but the decline in receptor block is zero order. The practical application is important: within 4 h of giving propranolol 20 mg i.v., the plasma concentration falls by 50%, but the receptor block (as measured by exercise-induced tachycardia) falls by only 35%. The relationship between the concentration of the parent drug in plasma and its effect is further obscured if pharmacologically active metabolites are also present. Additionally, for some of the lipid-soluble β-blockers, especially timolol, plasma $t_{1/2}$ may not reflect the duration of β-blockade, because the drug remains bound to the tissues near the receptor when the plasma concentration is negligible.

Most β-adrenoceptor blockers can be given orally once daily in either ordinary or sustained-release formulations because the $t_{1/2}$ of the pharmacodynamic effect exceeds the elimination $t_{1/2}$ of the parent substance in the blood.

Lipid-soluble agents are extensively metabolised (hydroxylated, conjugated) to water-soluble substances that can be eliminated by the kidney. Plasma concentrations of drugs subject to extensive hepatic first-pass metabolism vary greatly between subjects (up to 20-fold) because the process itself is dependent on two highly variable factors: speed of absorption and hepatic blood flow, with the latter being the rate-limiting factor.

Lipid-soluble agents readily cross cell membranes and so have a high apparent volume of distribution. They also readily enter the central nervous system (CNS), e.g. propranolol reaches concentrations in the brain 20 times those of the water-soluble atenolol.

Water-soluble agents show more predictable plasma concentrations because they are less subject to liver metabolism, being excreted unchanged by the kidney; thus their half-lives are greatly prolonged in renal failure, e.g. atenolol $t_{1/2}$ is increased from 7 to 24 h. Drugs (of any kind) having a long $t_{1/2}$ and an action terminated by renal elimination are best avoided in patients with renal disease. Water-soluble agents are less widely distributed and may have a lower incidence of effects attributed to penetration of the CNS, e.g. nightmares.

- The most lipid-soluble agents are propranolol, metoprolol, oxprenolol and labetalol.
- The least lipid-soluble (and most water-soluble) agents are atenolol, sotalol and nadolol.
- Others are intermediate.

Classification of β-adrenoceptor–blocking drugs

- *Pharmacokinetic*: lipid soluble, water soluble, see above.
- *Pharmacodynamic* (see Table 24.1). The associated properties (partial agonist action and membrane-stabilising action) have only minor clinical importance with current drugs at doses ordinarily used and may be insignificant in most cases. But it is desirable that they be known, for they can sometimes matter and they may foreshadow future developments.

β-Adrenoceptor blockers not listed in Table 24.1 include:

- *Non-selective*: carteolol, bufuralol.
- *β_1-receptor selective*: betaxolol, esmolol (ultra-short acting: minutes).
- *β- and α-receptor block*: bucindolol.

Uses of β-adrenoceptor–blocking drugs

Cardiovascular uses: *Angina pectoris:* β-blockade reduces cardiac work and oxygen consumption.

Hypertension: β-blockade reduces renin secretion and cardiac output; there is little interference with homeostatic reflexes.

Cardiac tachyarrhythmias: β-blockade reduces drive to cardiac pacemakers: subsidiary properties (see Table 25.1, p. 454) may also be relevant.

Myocardial infarction and β-adrenoceptor blockers: there are two modes of use that reduce acute mortality and prevent recurrence: the so-called 'cardioprotective' effect.

- *Early use* within 6 h (or at most 12 h) of onset (intravenously for 24 h then orally for 3–4 weeks). Benefit has been demonstrated only for atenolol. Cardiac work is reduced, resulting in a reduction in infarct size by up to 25% and protection against cardiac rupture. Surprisingly, tachyarrhythmias are not less frequent, perhaps because the cardiac β_2 receptor is not blocked by atenolol. Maximum benefit is in the first 24–36 h, but mortality remains lower for up to 1 year. Contraindications to early use include bradycardia (<55 beats/min), hypotension (systolic <90 mmHg) and left ventricular failure. A patient already taking a β-blocker may be given additional doses.
- *Late use* for secondary prevention of another myocardial infarction. The drug is started between 4

days and 4 weeks after the onset of the infarct and is continued for at least 2 years.[22]

- *Choice of drug.* The agent should be a pure antagonist, i.e. without ISA.

Aortic dissection and after subarachnoid haemorrhage: by reducing force and speed of systolic ejection (contractility) and blood pressure.

Obstruction of ventricular outflow where sympathetic activity occurs in the presence of anatomical abnormalities, e.g. tetralogy of Fallot (cyanotic attacks): hypertrophic subaortic stenosis (angina); some cases of mitral valve disease.

Hepatic portal hypertension and oesophageal variceal bleeding: reduction of portal pressure (see p. 583).

Cardiac failure (see also Ch. 25): β-blockade is beneficial in terms of mortality for patients with all grades of moderate heart failure. Data support the use of both non-selective (carvedilol, α-blocker as well) and β₁-selective (metoprolol and bisoprolol) agents. Survival benefit exceeds that provided by ACE inhibitors over placebo. The negative inotropic effects can still be significant, so the starting dose is low (e.g. bisoprolol 1.25 mg orally daily in the morning or carvedilol 3.125 mg twice daily, with food) and may be tolerated only with additional antifailure therapy, e.g. diuretic.

Endocrine uses. *Hyperthyroidism:* β-blockade reduces unpleasant symptoms of sympathetic overactivity; there may also be an effect on metabolism of thyroxine (peripheral de-iodination from T_4 to T_3). A non-selective agent (propranolol or timolol) is preferred to counteract both the cardiac (β₁ and β₂) effects and tremor (β₂).

Phaeochromocytoma: blockade of β-agonist effects of circulating catecholamines always in combination with adequate α-adrenoceptor block. Only small doses of a β-blocker are required.

Other uses:

- Central nervous system:
  - *anxiety* with somatic symptoms (non-selective β-blockade may be more effective than β₁-selective)
  - *migraine* prophylaxis (see p. 304)
  - *essential tremor,* some cases
  - *alcohol and opioid acute withdrawal* symptoms.
- Eyes:
  - *glaucoma:* carteolol, betaxolol, levobunolol and timolol eye drops act by altering production and outflow of aqueous humour.

Adverse reactions due to β-adrenoceptor blockade

Bronchoconstriction (β₂ receptor) occurs as expected, especially in patients with asthma[23] (in whom even eye drops are dangerous[24]). In elderly chronic bronchitics, there may be gradually increasing bronchoconstriction over weeks (even with eye drops). Plainly, risk is greater with non-selective agents, but β₁-receptor–selective members can still have significant β₂-receptor occupancy and may precipitate asthma.

Cardiac failure may arise if cardiac output is dependent on high sympathetic drive (but β-blockade can be introduced at very low dose to treat cardiac failure; see above). The degree of heart block may be made dangerously worse.

Incapacity for vigorous exercise due to failure of the cardiovascular system to respond to sympathetic drive.

Hypotension when the drug is given after myocardial infarction.

Hypertension may occur whenever blockade of β receptors allows pre-existing α effects to be unopposed, e.g. phaeochromocytoma.

Reduced peripheral blood flow, especially with non-selective members, leading to cold extremities which, rarely, can be severe enough to cause necrosis; intermittent claudication may be worsened.

Reduced blood flow to liver and kidneys, reducing metabolism and biliary and renal elimination of drugs, is liable to be important if there is hepatic or renal disease.

Hypoglycaemia: β₂ receptors mediate both the symptoms of hypoglycaemia and the counterregulatory metabolic responses that restore blood glucose. Non-selective β-blockers, by blocking β₂ receptors, impair the normal sympathetic-mediated homeostatic mechanism for maintaining blood glucose levels, and recovery from hypoglycaemia is delayed; this is important in diabetes and after substantial exercise. Further, as α adrenoceptors are not blocked, hypertension

---

[22]In the first major study, sudden death occurred in 13.9% of placebo-treated and 7.7% of timolol-treated patients (Norwegian Multicentre Study Group 1981 Timolol-induced reduction in mortality and reinfarction in patients surviving myocardial infarction. New England Journal of Medicine 304:801–807).

[23]A 36-year-old patient with asthma collected, from a pharmacy, chlorphenamine for herself and oxprenolol for a friend. She took a tablet of oxprenolol by mistake. Wheezing began in 1 h and worsened rapidly; she experienced a convulsion, respiratory arrest and ventricular fibrillation. She was treated with positive-pressure ventilation (for 11 h) and intravenous salbutamol, aminophylline and hydrocortisone, and survived (Williams I P, Millard F J 1980 Severe asthma after inadvertent ingestion of oxprenolol. Thorax 35:160). There is a logical – or rather pharmacological – link between the use of timolol as eye drops and the risk of asthma. For local administration, a drug needs high potency, so that a high degree of receptor blockade is achieved using a physically small (and therefore locally administrable) dose of drug. Nevertheless, timolol is used topically as a 0.25–0.5% solution, which means the initial concentration of timolol in the tear film is up to 5 mg/mL (or >10 mmol/L). As the majority of this will be swallowed and a few milligrams orally will block systemic β₂ receptors, it is apparent why one drop of timolol down the lachrymal duct (of the wrong patient) is hazardous.
[24]Müller M E, van der Velde N, Krulder J W M, van der Cammen T J M 2006 Syncope and falls due to timolol eye drops. British Medical Journal 332:960–961.

(which may be severe) can occur as the sympathetic system discharges in an 'attempt' to reverse the hypoglycaemia. The symptoms of hypoglycaemia, in so far as they are mediated by the sympathetic nervous system (anxiety, palpitations), will not occur, except (cholinergic) sweating, and the patient may miss the warning symptoms of hypoglycaemia and slip into coma. β_1-Selective drugs are preferred in diabetes.

Plasma lipoproteins: high-density lipoprotein (HDL) cholesterol falls and triglycerides rise during chronic β-blockade with non-selective agents. β_1-Selective agents have much less impact overall. Patients with hyperlipidaemia needing a β-blocker should generally receive a β_1-selective one.

Sexual function: interference is unusual and generally not supported in placebo-controlled trials.

Abrupt withdrawal of therapy can be dangerous in angina pectoris and after myocardial infarction, and withdrawal should be gradual, e.g. reduce to a low dose and continue this for a few days. The existence and cause of a β-blocker withdrawal phenomenon is debated, but probably occurs due to up-regulation of β_2 receptors. It is particularly inadvisable to initiate an α-blocker at the same time as withdrawing a β-blocker in patients with ischaemic heart disease, because the β-blocker causes reflex activation of the sympathetic system. The β-blocker withdrawal phenomenon appears to be least common with partial agonists and most common with β_1-selective antagonists. Rebound hypertension is insignificant.

Adverse reactions not certainly due to β-adrenoceptor blockade

These include loss of general well-being, tired legs, fatigue, depression, sleep disturbances including insomnia, dreaming, feelings of weakness, gut upsets, rashes.

Oculomucocutaneous syndrome occurred with chronic use of practolol (now obsolete) and even occasionally after cessation of use.[25] Other members either do not cause it, or so rarely do so that they are under suspicion only and, properly prescribed, the benefits of their use far outweigh such a very low risk. The mechanism of the syndrome is uncertain but appears immunological.

---

[25]Practolol was developed to the highest current scientific standards; it was marketed in 1970 as the first cardioselective β-blocker, and only after independent review by the UK drug regulatory body. All seemed to go well for about 4 years, by which time there had accumulated about 200 000 patient-years of experience with the drug. It then became apparent that a small proportion of patients taking practolol could develop a bizarre syndrome that included conjunctival scarring, nasal and mucosal ulceration, fibrous peritonitis, pleurisy and cochlear damage (oculomucocutaneous syndrome). The condition was first recognised by an alert ophthalmologist who ran a special clinic for external eye diseases. (See Wright P 1975 Untoward effects associated with practolol administration: oculomucocutaneous syndrome. British Medical Journal i:595–589.)

Overdose

Overdose, including self-poisoning, causes bradycardia, heart block, hypotension and low-output cardiac failure that can proceed to cardiogenic shock; death is more likely with agents that have a membrane-stabilising action (see Table 24.1). Bronchoconstriction can be severe, even fatal, in patients subject to any bronchospastic disease; loss of consciousness may occur with lipid-soluble agents that penetrate the CNS. Receptor blockade will outlast the persistence of the drug in the plasma.

Rational treatment includes:

- *Atropine* (1–2 mg i.v. as one or two bolus doses) to eliminate the unopposed vagal activity that contributes to bradycardia. Most patients also require direct cardiac pacing.
- *Glucagon*, which has cardiac inotropic and chronotropic actions independent of the β-adrenoceptor (dose 50–150 µg/kg in glucose 5% i.v., repeated if necessary) to be used at the outset in severe cases (an unlicensed indication).
- If there is no response, intravenous injection or infusion of a β-adrenoceptor agonist is an alternative, e.g. isoprenaline (4 µg/min, increasing at 1–3-min intervals until the heart rate is 50–70 beats/min).
- Other sympathomimetics may be used as judgement counsels, according to the desired receptor agonist actions (β_1, β_2, α) required by the clinical condition, e.g. dobutamine, dopamine, dopexamine, noradrenaline/norepinephrine, adrenaline/epinephrine.
- For bronchoconstriction, salbutamol may be used; aminophylline has non-adrenergic cardiac inotropic and bronchodilator actions and should be given intravenously very slowly to avoid precipitating hypotension.
- A cardiac pacemaker may be used to increase the heart rate.

Treatment may be needed for days. With prompt treatment, death is unusual.

Interactions

Pharmacokinetic. β blockers that are metabolised in the liver exhibit higher plasma concentrations when co-administered with drugs that inhibit hepatic metabolism, e.g. cimetidine. Enzyme inducers enhance the metabolism of this class of β blockers. β-Adrenoceptor blockers themselves reduce hepatic blood flow (with a fall in cardiac output) and reduce the metabolism of β blockers and other drugs whose metabolic elimination is dependent on the rate of delivery to the liver, e.g. lidocaine, chlorpromazine.

Pharmacodynamic. The effect on the blood pressure of sympathomimetics having both α- and β-receptor agonist actions is increased by block of β receptors, leaving the α-receptor vasoconstriction unopposed (even adrenaline/epinephrine added to local anaesthetics may cause hypertension); the pressor effect of abrupt clonidine withdrawal is enhanced, probably by this action. Other cardiac antiarrhythmic drugs are potentiated, e.g. hypotension, bradycardia, heart block. Combination with verapamil (i.v.) is hazardous in the presence of atrioventricular nodal or left ventricular dysfunction because the latter has stronger negative inotropic and chronotropic effects than do other calcium channel blockers.

Most non-steroidal anti-inflammatory drugs (NSAIDs) attenuate the antihypertensive effect of β blockers (but not perhaps of atenolol), presumably due to inhibition of formation of renal vasodilator prostaglandins, leading to sodium retention.

β-Adrenoceptor blockers potentiate the effect of other antihypertensives, particularly when an increase in heart rate is part of the homeostatic response (calcium channel blockers and α-adrenoceptor blockers).

Non-selective β-receptor blockers potentiate hypoglycaemia of insulin and sulphonylureas.

Pregnancy

β-Adrenoceptor blockers are used in pregnancy-related hypertension, including pre-eclampsia. Both lipid- and water-soluble members enter the fetus and may cause neonatal bradycardia and hypoglycaemia. They are not teratogenic in pregnancy, but some studies have suggested they cause intrauterine growth restriction.

Notes on some individual β-adrenoceptor blockers

(For general pharmacokinetics, see p. 81)

Propranolol is available in standard (twice or three times daily) and sustained-release (once daily) formulations. When given i.v. (1 mg/min over 1 min, repeated every 2 min up to 10 mg) for cardiac arrhythmia or thyrotoxicosis, it should be preceded by atropine (1–2 mg i.v.) to prevent excessive bradycardia; hypotension may occur.

Atenolol has a $\beta_1:\beta_2$ selectivity of $1:15$. It is widely used for angina pectoris and hypertension, in a dose of 25–100 mg orally once a day. The tendency in the past has been to use higher than necessary doses. When introduced, atenolol was considered not to need dose ranging, unlike propranolol, but this was in part because the initial dose was already at the top of the dose–response curve. Some 90% of absorbed drug is excreted by the kidney, and the dose should be reduced when renal function is impaired, e.g. to 50 mg/day

when the glomerular filtration rate (GFR) is 15–35 mL/min. It is best avoided in patients with GFR of less than 10 mL/min. The $t_{1/2}$ is 7 h.

Bisoprolol is more β_1 selective than atenolol (ratio $50:1$). Although a relatively lipid-soluble agent, its $t_{1/2}$ (11 h) is one of the longest, and there is not the wide range of dose requirement seen with propranolol. It is worth starting at a low dose (5 mg), to avoid causing unnecessary tiredness and obtain the maximum benefit of its selectivity. There is no need to alter doses when renal or hepatic function is reduced.

Nebivolol resembles bisoprolol in terms of lipophilicity and $t_{1/2}$ (10 h) but is more β_1 selective (ratio $1:300$). Its unique feature is a direct vasodilator action (due to the D-isomer of the racemate, the L-isomer being the β_1 antagonist). The mechanism appears to be through direct activation of nitric oxide production by vascular endothelium.

Combined β₁- and α-adrenoceptor-blocking drug

Labetalol is a racemic mixture: one isomer is a β-adrenoceptor blocker (non-selective); another blocks α-adrenoceptors. Its dual effect on blood vessels minimises the vasoconstriction characteristic of non-selective β-blockade so that, for practical purposes, the outcome is similar to that of a β_1-selective β blocker (see Table 24.1). It is less effective than drugs such as atenolol or bisoprolol for the routine treatment of hypertension, but is useful for some specific indications.

The β-blockade is 4 to 10 times greater than the α-blockade, varying with dose and route of administration. Labetalol is useful as a parenterally administered drug in the emergency reduction of blood pressure. Ordinary β blockers may lower blood pressure too slowly, in part because reflex stimulation of unblocked α receptors opposes the fall in blood pressure. In most patients, even those with severe hypertension, a gradual reduction in blood pressure is desirable to avoid the risk of cerebral or renal hypoperfusion, but in the presence of a great vessel dissection or of fits, a more rapid effect is required (below).

Postural hypotension (characteristic of α-receptor blockade) is liable to occur at the outset of therapy and if the dose is increased too rapidly. But with chronic therapy when the β-receptor component is largely responsible for the antihypertensive effect, it is not a problem.

Labetalol reduces the hypertensive response to orgasm in women.

The $t_{1/2}$ is 4 h; it is extensively metabolised in the hepatic first-pass. The drug is given twice daily in a dose of 100–800 mg.

For emergency control of severe hypertension (including pregnancy), the most convenient regimen is to initiate infusion at 1 mg/min, and titrate upwards at half-hourly intervals as required. If bradycardia is a problem, then intravenous atropine should be given (as 600-microgram boluses). The labetalol infusion is stopped as blood pressure control is achieved (up to 200 mg may be required) and is re-initiated as frequently as required until regular oral therapy has been successfully introduced.

Peripheral sympathetic nerve terminal

Adrenergic neurone-blocking drugs

Adrenergic neurone-blocking drugs are taken up into adrenergic nerve endings by the active noradrenaline/norepinephrine reuptake mechanism (uptake 1) (Fig. 24.1). They are relatively ineffective in reducing blood pressure except in the erect position, and their use to control hypertension is now obsolete. Guanethidine is still licensed in the UK as an option for the rapid control of blood pressure, and may also be used for regional intravenous sympathetic blockade in patients with intractable Raynaud's disease.

Meta-iodobenzylguanidine (MIBG) is used diagnostically as a radio-iodinated tracer, to locate or confirm chromaffin tumours (phaeochromocytoma and neuroblastoma), which accumulate with drugs in this class (see p. 442).

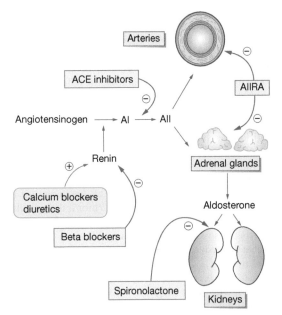

Fig. 24.1 Effects of drugs on the renin-angiotensin system. AI/II, angiotensin I/II.

Depletion of stored transmitter (noradrenaline/norepinephrine)

Reserpine is an alkaloid from plants of the genus *Rauwolfia*, used in medicine since ancient times for insanity. Reserpine depletes adrenergic nerves of noradrenaline/norepinephrine, primarily by blocking the transport of noradrenaline/norepinephrine into storage vesicles (see Fig. 23.1). Its antihypertensive action is chiefly a peripheral action, but it enters the CNS and depletes central catecholamine stores; this explains the sedation, depression and parkinsonian side-effects that can accompany its use. Reserpine is rarely used now that its low cost is matched by many superior classes.

Inhibition of synthesis of transmitter

Metirosine (α-methyl-*p*-tyrosine) is a competitive inhibitor of the enzyme *tyrosine hydroxylase*, which converts tyrosine to DOPA. It is occasionally used as an adjuvant (with phenoxybenzamine) to treat phaeochromocytomas that cannot be removed surgically. Catecholamine synthesis is reduced by up to 80% over 3 days. It also enters the CNS and depletes brain noradrenaline/norepinephrine and dopamine, causing reserpine-like adverse effects (see above). Hence, if life expectancy is threatened more by tumour invasion than hypertension, the need for the drug should be weighed carefully.

Autonomic ganglion-blocking drugs

Hexamethonium was the first orally active drug to treat hypertension, but the blockade of both sympathetic and parasympathetic systems caused severe side-effects. Its use in hypertension is long obsolete.

Trimetaphan, a short-acting agent, is given intravenously for the emergency control of hypertension; pressure may be adjusted by tilting the body to provide 'minute-to-minute' control, when the lack of selectivity is useful.

Central nervous system

α_2-Adrenoceptor agonists

Clonidine is an imidazoline that is an agonist to α_2-adrenoceptors (postsynaptic) in the brain, stimulation of which suppresses sympathetic outflow and reduces blood pressure. Drugs of this type are said to be selective for an imidazoline receptor (I_1), rather than the α_2 receptor. In fact, no such receptor has been identified at the molecular level, and genetic knockout experiments have shown that it is the α_2 receptor that is required for the blood pressure–lowering action of imidazoline drugs. At high doses, clonidine activates peripheral α_2-adrenoceptors (presynaptic autorecep-tors) on the adrenergic nerve ending; these mediate negative feedback suppression of noradrenaline/norepinephrine release.

Clonidine was discovered to be hypotensive, not by the pharmacologists who tested it in the laboratory but by a physician who used it on himself as nose drops for a common cold. The $t_{1/2}$ is 6 h. Clonidine reduces blood pressure with little postural or exercise-related drop.

Its most serious handicap is that abrupt or even gradual withdrawal causes rebound hypertension. This is characterised by plasma catecholamine concentrations as high as those seen in hypertensive attacks of phaeochromocytoma. The onset may be rapid (a few hours) or delayed for as long as 2 days; it subsides over 2–3 days. The treatment is either to reinstitute clonidine, intramuscularly if necessary, or to treat as for a phaeochromocytoma (see below). Clonidine should never be used with a β-adrenoceptor blocker that exacerbates withdrawal hypertension (see phaeochromocytoma, p. 442). Other common adverse effects include sedation and dry mouth.

Tricyclic antidepressants antagonise the antihypertensive action and increase the rebound hypertension of abrupt withdrawal. Low-dose clonidine (Dixarit 50–75 mg twice daily) also has a minor role in migraine prophylaxis, menopausal flushing and choreas.

Rebound hypertension is a less important problem with longer-acting imidazolines, e.g. moxonidine, and a single dose can be omitted without rebound.

False transmitter

Chemotransmitters and receptors in the CNS are similar to those in the periphery, and the drug in this section also has peripheral actions, as is to be expected.

Methyldopa acts in the brainstem vasomotor centres. It is a substrate (in the same manner as L-dopa) for the enzymes that synthesise noradrenaline/norepinephrine. The synthesis of α-methylnoradrenaline results in tonic stimulation of CNS α_2 receptors because α-methylnoradrenaline cannot be metabolised by monoamine oxidase, and selectively stimulates the α_2-adrenoceptor, i.e. methyldopa acts in the same way as clonidine. Methyldopa is reliably absorbed from the gastrointestinal tract and readily enters the CNS. The $t_{1/2}$ is 1.5 h.

Adverse effects include: sedation (frequent), nightmares and depression. Less common is a positive Coombs' test with haemolytic anaemia, and a rare but life-threatening adverse event is hepatitis.

For these reasons, methyldopa has long been dropped from routine management of hypertension, but remains popular with obstetricians for the hypertension of pregnancy because of its apparent safety for the fetus.

Drug treatment of angina, myocardial infarction and hypertension

Angina pectoris[26]

An attack of angina pectoris[27] occurs when myocardial demand for oxygen exceeds supply from the coronary circula-tion. The principal forms relevant to choice of drug therapy are angina of exercise (commonest) and its worsening form, unstable (preinfarction or crescendo) angina (see below), which occurs at rest. Variant (Prinzmetal) angina (very uncommon) results from spasm of a large coronary artery.

Antiangina drugs act as follows:

* *Organic nitrates* reduce preload and afterload and dilate the main coronary arteries (rather than the arterioles).
* *β-Adrenoceptor blockers* reduce myocardial contractility and slow the heart rate. They may increase coronary artery spasm in variant angina.
* *Calcium channel blockers* reduce cardiac contractility, dilate the coronary arteries (where there is evidence of spasm) and reduce afterload (dilate peripheral arterioles).

These classes of drug complement one another and can be used together. The combined nitrate and potassium channel activator *nicorandil* is an alternative when any of the other drugs is contraindicated.

Summary of treatment

* Any contributory cause is treated when possible, e.g. anaemia, arrhythmia.
* Lifestyle is changed so as to reduce the number of attacks. Weight reduction can be very helpful; stop smoking.
* For immediate pre-exertional prophylaxis: glyceryl trinitrate sublingually or nifedipine (bite the capsule and hold the liquid in the mouth or swallow it).
* For an acute attack: glyceryl trinitrate (sublingual) or nifedipine (bite capsule, as above).

For long-term prophylaxis:

* A *β₁-adrenoceptor-blocking drug*, e.g. bisoprolol, is given regularly (not merely when an attack is expected).

---

[26]Angina pectoris: *angina*, a strangling; *pectoris*, of the chest.
[27]For a personal account by a physician of his experiences of angina pectoris, coronary bypass surgery, ventricular fibrillation and recovery, see Swyer G I M 1986 Personal view. British Medical Journal 292:337. Compelling and essential reading.

Dosage is adjusted by response. Warn the patient of the risk of abrupt withdrawal.

- A *calcium channel blocker*, e.g. nifedipine or diltiazem, is an alternative to a β-adrenoceptor blocker; use especially if coronary spasm is suspected or if the patient has myocardial insufficiency or any reversible airflow obstruction. It can also be used with a β blocker, or
- A *long-acting nitrate*, isosorbide dinitrate or mononitrate: use so as to avoid tolerance (see p. 416).
- *Nicorandil*, a long-acting potassium channel activator, does not cause tolerance like the nitrates.
- Drug therapy may be adapted to the time of attacks, e.g. nocturnal (transdermal glyceryl trinitrate, or isosorbide mononitrate orally at night).
- Antiplatelet therapy (aspirin or clopidogrel) reduces the incidence of fatal and non-fatal myocardial infarction in patients with unstable angina, used alone or with low-dose heparin.
- Revascularisation in selected cases (largely by percutaneous coronary intervention (PCI) and stenting).

Newer therapies

Ivabradine blocks the cardiac pacemaker I_f ('funny') current that controls the spontaneous diastolic depolarisation in the sinus node and regulates heart rate. The cardiac effects are specific to the sinus node with no effect on intra-atrial, atrioventricular or intraventricular conduction times, nor on myocardial contractility or ventricular repolarisation.

Blockade of I_f causes bradycardia and hence a reduction in myocardial work by slowing the sinus node. It offers an advantage over β blockers in being safe to use in asthmatics. Ivabradine can interact also with the retinal current I_h, which closely resembles cardiac I_f, leading in occasional patients to a transient enhanced brightness in a limited area of the visual field. *Ranolazine* blocks the late sodium current and prevents calcium overload in ischaemic cardiac tissue. It also has antiarrhythmic properties and by an unknown mechanism reduces fasting blood glucose and HbA1c levels in diabetics. Nevertheless, the exact role of this agent remains to be determined.

In treating angina, it is important to remember not only the objective of reducing symptoms but also that of preventing complications, particularly myocardial infarction and sudden death. This requires vigorous treatment of all risk factors (hypertension, hyperlipidaemia, diabetes mellitus) and, of course, cessation of smoking. There is little evidence that the symptomatic treatments, medical or surgical, themselves affect outcome except in patients with stenosis of the main stem of the left coronary artery, who require surgical intervention. Although aspirin has not been studied specifically in patients with stable angina, it is now reasonable therapy, by extrapolation from the studies of aspirin in other patient groups.

Myocardial infarction (MI)

(See also Ch. 29.)

An overview

The *acute coronary syndromes* (ACSs) are now classified on the basis of the ECG and plasma troponin measurements into: (1) patients with ST elevation myocardial infarction (STEMI); (2) non-ST elevation myocardial infarction (non-STEMI, by ECG and a positive troponin test); or (3) unstable angina (by ECG and negative troponin test). The present account recognises that this is a rapidly evolving field, but therapeutic strategies are likely to evolve according to these forms of ACS.

A general practitioner or paramedic can administer the initial treatment appropriately before a definite diagnosis is established or the patient reaches hospital, namely:

- Morphine or diamorphine (2.5 or 5 mg i.v. because of the certainty of haematoma formation when intramuscular injections are followed by thrombolytic therapy).
- Aspirin 150–300 mg orally.
- 60% oxygen.

The immediate objectives are relief of pain and initiation of treatment demonstrated to reduce mortality. Subsequent management of proven MI is concerned with treatment of complications, *arrhythmias, heart failure* and *thromboemboli*, and then *prevention* of further infarctions.

When STEMI is diagnosed, instituting myocardial reperfusion as early as possible provides the greatest benefit. Previously this was achieved pharmacologically, but primary coronary angioplasty (PCI), with or without stenting, is now the preferred option. If thrombolysis is used, it is initiated after arrival at hospital and provided there are no contraindications to thrombolysis (see below). Patients with non-STEMI may still benefit, especially those with left bundle branch block, but several trials have shown that patients without ECG changes (especially ST elevation) and patients with unstable angina benefit only slightly, if at all, from thrombolytic therapy.

The choice of thrombolytic is in most places dictated first by a wealth of comparative outcome data from well-designed trials, and second by relative costs. So, for a first MI, patients should receive streptokinase 1 500 000 units infused over 1 h, unless they are in cardiogenic shock. For subsequent infarcts, the presence of antistreptokinase antibodies dictates the use of the recombinant tissue plasminogen activator (rtPA), *alteplase* (or *reteplase*). Both alteplase and streptokinase bind plasminogen and convert it to plasmin, which lyses fibrin. Alteplase has a much higher affinity for plasminogen bound to fibrin than in the circulation. This selectivity does not confer any therapeutic advantage as was originally anticipated, as severe haemorrhage following thrombolysis is almost always due to lysis of an appropriate clot at previous sites of bleeding or trauma. Indeed, the tendency for some lysis of circulating fibrinogen as well as fibrin gives streptokinase anticoagulant activity, which is lacking with alteplase, use of which needs to be accompanied and followed by heparin (for further details of thrombolytics, see p. 521).

For a discussion about the role of *aspirin*, see p. 254.

A third treatment reduces mortality in MI, namely *β-blockade*. In the ISIS-1 study,[28] atenolol 5 mg was given intravenously, followed by 50 mg orally. The reduction in mortality is due mainly to prevention of cardiac rupture, which appears interestingly to remain the only complication of MI that is not reduced by thrombolysis. The usual contraindications to *β*-blockade apply, but most patients with a first MI should be able to receive this treatment.

Other antiplatelet agents. The final common pathway to platelet aggregation and thrombus formation involves the expression of the glycoprotein IIb/IIIa receptor at the cell surface. This receptor binds fibrinogen with high affinity and can be blocked using either a specific monoclonal antibody (*abciximab*) or one of a rapidly expanding class of specific antagonists, e.g. *eptifibatide* and *tirofiban*. Another agent, *clopidogrel*, acts by inhibiting ADP-dependent platelet aggregation. It is more effective than aspirin for the prevention of ischaemic stroke, cardiovascular death in patients at high risk (see p. 522) or following a STEMI or non-STEMI event.

These drugs are useful adjuncts for the treatment of unstable angina, and in the prevention of thrombosis following percutaneous revascularisation procedures such as angioplasty and coronary artery stenting (especially with coated stents).

> **Principal contraindications to thrombolysis**
>
> - Haemorrhagic diathesis.
> - Pregnancy.
> - Recent symptoms of peptic ulcer or gastrointestinal bleeding.
> - Recent stroke (previous 3 months).
> - Recent surgery (previous 10–14 days), especially neurosurgery.
> - Prolonged cardiopulmonary resuscitation (during current presentation).

> - Proliferative diabetic retinopathy.
> - Severe, uncontrolled hypertension (diastolic blood pressure >120 mmHg).

Unstable angina necessitates admission to hospital, the objectives of therapy being to relieve pain, and avert progression to MI and sudden death. Initial management is with aspirin 150–300 mg chewed or dispersed in water, followed by heparin or one of the low molecular weight preparations, e.g. dalteparin or enoxaparin. Nitrate is given preferably as isosorbide dinitrate by intravenous infusion until the patient has been pain-free for 24 h. A *β*-adrenoceptor blocker, e.g. metoprolol, should be added orally or intravenously unless it is contraindicated, when a calcium channel blocker is substituted, e.g. diltiazem or verapamil. Patients perceived to be at high risk may also receive a glycoprotein IIb/IIIa inhibitor, e.g. eptifibatide or tirofiban.

Secondary prevention

(See also Ch. 29.)

The best predictor of the risk of MI is to have had previous infarction. After the measures instituted in the first few hours, the principal objective of treatment therefore becomes prevention of future infarcts. Patients should receive advice about exercise and diet before discharge, and most enter a formal rehabilitation programme after leaving hospital. In particular, patients need to reduce saturated fat intake, and there is increasing evidence of the benefit of increased intake of fish and olive oil.

Drugs for secondary prevention

All patients should receive *aspirin* (see Ch. 4, Fig. 4.3), an ACE inhibitor and a *β blocker* for at least 2 years, unless contraindicated. The commonest contraindications to *β*-blockade after MI are *transient* heart failure, which should now be uncommon after a first MI, and various degrees of heart block or bradyarrhythmias. These are, however, usually transient, so the β blocker can be introduced during convalescence.

Any of these agents, aspirin, a β blocker or an ACE inhibitor,[29] will reduce the incidence of reinfarction by 20–25%, although their benefit has not been shown to be additive.

---

[28]First International Study of Infarct Survival Collaborative Group 1986 Randomised trial of intravenous atenolol among 16027 cases of suspected acute myocardial infarction: ISIS-1. Lancet ii:57–66.

[29]In the SAVE (Survival and Ventricular Enlargement) study, captopril 50 mg three times daily or placebo was started 3–16 days after MI in 2231 patients without overt cardiac failure but with a left ventricular ejection fraction of less than 40%. The captopril group had a lower incidence of recurrent myocardial infarction (133) and death (228) than the placebo group (170 and 275, respectively) (Rutherford J D, Moye L A, Pfeffer M A et al for the SAVE investigators 1994 Effects of captopril on ischemic events after myocardial infarction. Results of the Survival and Ventricular Enlargement trial. SAVE Investigators. Circulation 90:1731–1738). Several other trials of ACE inhibitors have provided similar results.

In addition to these drugs, most patients should receive a statin, regardless of their plasma cholesterol concentration. Long-term benefit from LDL reduction after MI has been shown for simvastatin (20–40 mg/day) and pravastatin (40 mg/day).[30]

There is no place for routine antiarrhythmic prophylaxis, and long-term anticoagulation is similarly out of place, except when indicated by arrhythmias or poor left ventricular function.

Arterial hypertension

Clinical evaluation of antihypertensive drugs seeks to answer two types of question:

1. Whether long-term reduction of blood pressure benefits the patient by preventing complications and prolonging life; these studies take years, require enormous numbers of patients and are extremely costly.
2. Whether a drug is capable of effective, safe and comfortable control of blood pressure for about 1 year. There is now sufficient evidence of the benefit of reducing raised blood pressure that regulatory authorities do not demand trials of the first kind for all new drugs. Shorter studies are therefore deemed sufficient to allow the introduction of a new drug.

Aims of treatment

The long-term aim is the prevention of stroke, MI and (especially in older patients) heart failure; prevention also requires attention to other risk factors such as smoking and plasma cholesterol. The more immediate aim of treatment is to reduce the blood pressure as near to normal as possible without causing symptomatic hypotension or otherwise impairing well-being (quality of life).

When this aim is achieved in severe cases, there is great symptomatic improvement: retinopathy clears and vision improves; headaches are abolished. A variable amount of irreversible damage has often been done by the high blood pressure before treatment is started; so renal failure may progress despite treatment, left ventricular hypertrophy may not fully reverse, and arterial damage leads to ischaemic events (stroke and MI).

It is desirable to start treatment before irreversible changes occur, and in mild and moderately severe cases this usually means advising treatment for symptom-free people whose hypertension was revealed by screening.

Threshold and targets for treatment

The joint NICE/British Hypertension Society guidelines[31] require that antihypertensive drug therapy be *initiated*:

- when sustained blood pressure exceeds 160/100 mmHg, or
- when blood pressure is in the range 140–159/90–99 mmHg and there is evidence of target organ damage, cardiovascular disease or a 10-year cardiovascular risk greater than 20%
- for diabetics when blood pressure exceeds 140/90 mmHg.

The optimal *target* is to lower blood pressure to 140/90 mmHg or less in all patients. Some guidelines require a lower target of less than 130/80 mmHg in patients with renal impairment or diabetes mellitus, while recognising that there is a dearth of prospective randomized data to support the lower target. Ironically, the best data for a lower target now comes from a study, SPRINT, which randomized patients without diabetes to systolic targets of 120 mmHg or 140 mmHg.[32]

Effective treatment reduces the risk of all complications: strokes and MI, but also heart failure, renal failure and possibly dementia. It is easier in individual trials to demonstrate the benefits of treatment in preventing stroke, because the curve relating risk of stroke to blood pressure is almost twice as steep as that for MI. This raises issues of relative and absolute risk.

Relative risk refers to the increased likelihood of a patient having a complication, compared with a normotensive

---

[30]In the Heart Protection Study of 20 536 high-risk patients (one-third had previous MI), those randomly assigned to simvastatin 40 mg/day (compared with placebo) had a 12% reduction in all-cause mortality, and a 24% reduction in strokes and coronary heart disease. The authors estimated that 5 years of statin treatment will prevent 100 major vascular events in every 1000 patients with previous MI, or 70 to 80 events in patients with other forms of coronary heart disease or diabetes. There was no upper age limit to this benefit, and no lower limit to the level of LDL at which benefit was seen (Heart Protection Study Collaborative Group 2002 MRC/BHF Heart Protection Study of cholesterol lowering with simvastatin in 20 536 high-risk individuals. Lancet 360:7–22).

[31]The British Hypertension Society Guidelines (BHS-IV) are summarised in British Medical Journal 2004; 328:634–640 or online at http://www. bhsoc.org. Joint guidance with the National Institute of Clinical Excellence (NICE) was issued in 2006. The update of 2011 is flawed, and the editors advise following the 2006 recommendations (see Brown MJ et al 2012, in Guide to Further Reading). Revised NICE guidance will be issued in 2018.
[32]SPRINT Research Group, Wright J T Jr, Williamson J D, et al 2015 A randomized trial of intensive versus standard blood-pressure control. New England Journal of Medicine 373:2103–2116. This trial studied 9361 patients with CV disease and SBP >130 mmHg. The initial enthusiasm for its finding of 25% lower mortality in the more intensively treated patients has given way to uncertainties about interpretation, arising from an unusual method of blood pressure measurement, the withdrawal of diuretic from many patients in the less intensive arm, and predominance of heart failure among the endpoints reduced by intensive treatment. Unusually for a blood pressure trial, stroke incidence was not significantly affected.

patient of the same age and sex. *Absolute* risk refers to the number of patients out of 100, with the same age, sex and blood pressure, predicted to have a complication over the next 10 years (see p. 51). So, the *relative* risk of MI due to hypertension is fixed, but substantial reduction in the *absolute* risk of MI is possible by reducing the level of cholesterol and blood pressure, i.e. both factors contribute independently to the risk of MI, whereas hypertension is a more important risk factor for stroke than hypercholesterolaemia.

Treatment will almost always be lifelong for essential hypertension, because discontinuation of therapy leads to prompt restoration of pre-treatment blood pressures. If it does not, one should suspect the original diagnosis of hypertension, which should not be made unless blood pressure is increased on at least three occasions over 3 months.

The relative risk of hypertension and the benefits of treating the condition in the elderly are less than in those younger than 65 years of age, but the absolute risks and benefits are greater. Given the large choice of treatments available, doctors cannot cite improved quality of life as an excuse for not treating hypertension in the elderly. Starting doses should often be halved, and, pending further evidence, less challenging targets for blood pressure reduction may be acceptable.

It is obvious that adverse effects of therapy are important in that very large numbers of patients must be treated with antihypertensives so that a few may gain (in terms of numbers needed to treat, this is several hundreds); this is a salient feature of the use of drugs to prevent disease.

Principles of antihypertensive therapy

General measures may be sufficient to control mild cases as follows:

- Obesity: reduce it.
- Alcohol: stay within recommended limits, e.g. 14 units/week for women, 21 units/week for men.
- Smoking: stop it.
- Diet: of proven value for the short-term reduction in blood pressure is reduction in fat content, and increase in fruit, vegetables and fibre. There is additional benefit from reducing intake of salt (<6 g/day): avoidance of highly salted foods, and omission of added salt from freshly prepared food.[33]
- Relaxation therapy: worth considering for highly motivated borderline patients.

---

[33]DASH-Sodium Collaborative Research Group 2001 Effects on blood pressure of reduced dietary sodium and the Dietary Approaches to Stop Hypertension (DASH) diet. New England Journal of Medicine 344:3–10.

Drug therapy

Blood pressure may be reduced by any one or more of the actions listed at the beginning of this chapter (see p. 415). The large number of different drug classes for hypertension reduces, paradoxically, the likelihood of a randomly selected drug being the best for an individual patient. Patients and drugs can be divided broadly into two groups depending on their renin status and drug effect on this (see Fig. 24.1).

- Type 1, or *high-renin* patients, are the younger, non-black patients (<55 years of age); they respond better to an ACE inhibitor, ARB, or β blocker.
- Type 2, or *low-renin* patients, in whom diuretics or calcium channel blockers are more likely to be effective as single agents.

As each drug acts on only one or two of the blood pressure control mechanisms, the factors that are uninfluenced by monotherapy are liable to adapt (homeostatic mechanism), to oppose the useful effect and to restore the previous state. There are two principal mechanisms of such adaptation or tolerance:

1. *Increase in blood volume*: this occurs with any drug that reduces peripheral resistance (increases intravascular volume) or cardiac output (reduces glomerular flow) due to activation of the renin–angiotensin system. The result is that cardiac output and blood pressure rise. Adding a diuretic in combination with the other drug can prevent this compensatory effect.
2. *Baroreceptor reflexes*: a fall in blood pressure evokes reflex activity of the sympathetic system, causing increased peripheral resistance and cardiac activity (rate and contractility).

Therefore, whenever high blood pressure is proving difficult to control and whenever a number of antihypertensives are used in combination, the drugs chosen should between them act on all three main determinants of blood pressure, namely:

- blood volume
- peripheral resistance
- cardiac output.

Such combinations will:

- maximise antihypertensive efficacy by exerting actions at three different points in the cardiovascular system
- minimise the opposing homeostatic effects by blocking the compensatory changes in blood volume, vascular tone and cardiac function
- minimise adverse effects by permitting smaller doses of each drug each acting at a different site and having different unwanted effects.

First-dose hypotension is now uncommon and occurs mainly with drugs having an action on veins (α-adrenoceptor blockers, ACE inhibitors) when baroreflex activation is

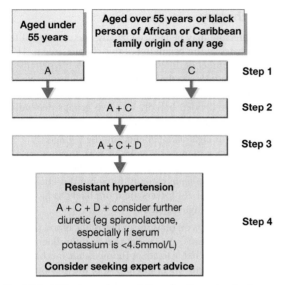

Aged under 55 years

Aged over 55 years or black person of African or Caribbean family origin of any age

| A | | C | Step 1 |

A + C — Step 2

A + C + D — Step 3

Resistant hypertension

A + C + D + consider further diuretic (eg spironolactone, especially if serum potassium is <4.5mmol/L)

Consider seeking expert advice — Step 4

Fig. 24.2 ACD schema for escalation of antihypertensive therapy. A, ACE inhibitor; C, calcium channel blocker; D, diuretic (see text). *(From Williams B W, Poulter N R, Brown M J et al 2004 British Hypertension Society guidelines for hypertension management 2004 (BHS-1 V): summary. British Medical Journal 328: 634–640, with permission).*

impaired, e.g. old age or with a contracted intravascular volume following diuretics.

Treating hypertension

A simple stepped regimen in keeping with the 2006 revision of the National Institute for Health and Clinical Excellence (NICE)/British Hypertension Society guidelines[34] is the 'A/CD' schema illustrated in Fig. 24.2.[35]

1. If the patient is young (<55 years of age) or non-black, use either an *A*CE inhibitor (or ARB) (**A**). For older patients start with either a *C*alcium channel blocker or thiazide *D*iuretic as first-line therapy (C or

D). If a drug is effective but not tolerated, switch to the other member of the pair.
2. If the blood pressure is not controlled at 4 weeks, a second agent should be added, using the opposite pair to the first drug, e.g. if the patient is on an ACE inhibitor add a calcium channel blocker or thiazide diuretic (A + C or A + D), as either vasodilatation or diuresis will stimulate the renin–angiotensin system and turn non–renin-dependent hypertension into renin-dependent hypertension.
3. If blood pressure control is still inadequate on dual therapy, A + C + D is the ideal triple regimen.
4. Patients whose blood pressure remains substantially above target on triple therapy should have either escalated diuretic therapy, e.g. by addition of spironolactone; or addition of α- or β-blockade. There is some evidence that a trial-and-error approach at this point can be avoided by measurement of plasma renin, with low plasma renin indicating the need for further diuretic.

Treatment and severity

A single drug may adequately treat mild hypertension, and a few patients with hypertension due to pure vasoconstriction or pure sodium excess. In most patients, the target systolic blood pressure of <140 mmHg recommended by most guidelines requires two or more drugs. While convention until recently has been to 'step-care' from single to combination therapy, the risks of adverse effects from treatment, and of early complications from uncontrolled hypertension, may be diminished by starting with combination therapy.[36]

Monitoring

The blood pressure must be monitored by a doctor or specialist nurse (particularly important in the elderly) and also sometimes by the patient. A 24-h ambulatory blood pressure monitoring (ABPM) system is the 'gold standard', but the devices are too expensive to be recommended for most patients. Nevertheless, the 24-h blood pressure profile does predict outcome better than clinic blood pressure and can indicate whether a difficult or high-risk patient does need additional medication. Home monitoring is a cheaper alternative, provided the sphygmomanometer is validated. The easy-to-use wrist monitors are unfortunately unreliable in patients receiving drug treatment.

Diuretics and potassium. The potassium-losing (kaliuretic) diuretics used in hypertension can deplete body potassium

[34]Available online, as the 2011 revision, at: https://www.nice.org.uk/guidance/CG127.
[35]The original schema included β-blockers, i.e. four drug groups AB/CD (Dickerson J E C, Hingorani A D, Ashby M J et al 1999 Optimisation of anti-hypertensive treatment by crossover rotation of four major classes. Lancet 353:2008–2013). This was revised in the light of clinical trial evidence that β-blockers are usually less effective than other antihypertensives at reducing major cardiovascular events, particularly stroke, and are associated with an unacceptably high risk of diabetes especially in combination with diuretics. Hence they are no longer recommended either as monotherapy (B in the original schema) or in combination with diuretics (B + D) unless there is a second indication for prescribing the β-blocker, e.g. angina, or in women planning to have children. In 2011, D(iuretics) were also dropped from first-line options. This was probably an error, and D is retained in all other international guidelines as a first-choice option.

[36]Brown M J, McInnes G T, Papst C C et al 2011 Aliskiren and the calcium channel blocker amlodipine combination as an initial treatment strategy for hypertension control (ACCELERATE): a randomised, parallel-group trial. Lancet 377:312–320.

by up to 10–15%. However, at low doses, e.g. bendroflume-thiazide 2.5 mg/day, significant hypokalaemia is unusual, and should raise suspicion of Conn's syndrome (see p. 443). Vulnerable patients, e.g. the elderly, should be monitored for potassium loss at 3 months and thereafter every 6–12 months. If required, for correction of hypokalaemia, a potassium-sparing diuretic (amiloride) in a fixed-dose combination with a thiazide (co-amilozide) is preferred over the use of fixed-dose diuretic/potassium chloride formulations (most supplements, typically 8 mmol KCl, are in any case inadequate).

A potassium-sparing diuretic should be used with caution in patients who have reduced renal function or diabetes, especially if they are also receiving an ACE inhibitor or ARB.

Compliance. Multi-drug therapy poses a substantial problem of compliance. As treatment will be lifelong, it is worthwhile finding the most convenient regimen for each individual and transferring to a fixed-dose combination where possible. A single daily dose is available for most antihypertensive drugs, where necessary by using sustained-release formulations. Where non-compliance is suspected, this is readily checked by measuring the prescribed drugs in a spot sample of the patient's urine.[37]

Resistant hypertension

Although many patients with resistant hypertension are simply resistant to taking their antihypertensive medicines, an estimated 3–10% of patients fail to achieve target blood pressure despite use of three drugs – 'A+C+D'. Most of these patients can be controlled by addition of the aldosterone receptor antagonist, spironolactone 25–50 mg/day. It is likely indeed that at least 25% of patients with apparently resistant hypertension have undiagnosed primary aldosteronism.[38]

Treatment of hypertensive emergencies

It is important to distinguish three circumstances that may exist separately or together; see the Venn diagram (Fig. 24.3)[39] which emphasises the following:

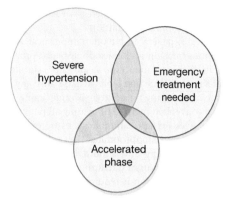

Fig. 24.3 Venn diagram illustrating intersections of three overlapping clinical states defined in the text.

- *Severe hypertension* is not on its own an indication for urgent (or large) reductions in blood pressure.
- Blood pressure can occasionally require urgent (emergency) reduction even when the hypertension is not severe, especially where the blood pressure has risen rapidly.
- *Accelerated phase* (malignant) *hypertension* rarely requires urgent reduction, and should instead be regarded as an indication for slow reduction in blood pressure during the first few days.
- The indications for *emergency reduction* of blood pressure are rare. They are:
  - Hypertensive encephalopathy (including eclampsia).
  - Acute left ventricular failure (due to hypertension).
  - Dissecting aortic aneurysm.

In these conditions, blood pressure should be reduced over the course of 1 hour. In patients with a dissecting aneurysm, where the blood pressure may have been completely normal prior to dissection, the target is a blood pressure of about 110/70 mmHg. Otherwise even small reductions will usually remove the emergency.

Accelerated-phase hypertension was previously called 'malignant' hypertension because the lack of treatment heralded death within 1 year of diagnosis. It is characterised pathologically by fibrinoid necrosis of the small arteries. An important consequence is the loss of autoregulation of the cerebral and renal circulation, so that any reduction in blood pressure causes a proportional fall in perfusion of these organs. It is therefore vital not to reduce diastolic blood pressure by more than 20 mmHg on the first day of treatment. To ignore this is to risk cerebral infarction.

Treatment. Unless contraindicated, the best treatment for all circles in the Venn diagram is β-blockade, e.g. atenolol

[37]Tomaszewski M, White C, Patel P et al 2014 High rates of non-adherence to antihypertensive treatment revealed by high-performance liquid chromatography-tandem mass spectrometry (HP LC-MS/MS) urine analysis. Heart 100:855–861.

[38]Williams B, McDonald T, Morant S, et al 2015 Spironolactone versus placebo, bisoprolol, and doxazosin to determine the optimal treatment for drug-resistant hypertension (PATHWAY-2): a randomised, double-blind, crossover trial. Lancet 386:2059–2068.

[39]J Venn (1834–1923), an English logician who 'adopted the diagrammatic method of illustrating propositions by inclusive and exclusive circles' (Dictionary of National Biography). A medical pilgrimage to Cambridge, where Venn worked, should take in Gonville and Caius College (named after its founder, Dr Caius, physician to the Tudor court and early president of the London College of Physicians in the 16th century); as well as stained glass windows celebrating Venn's circles, the visitor can see a portrait of the most famous medical Caian, William Harvey.

25 or 50 mg orally. In emergencies, a vasodilator should be given intravenously in addition.

A theoretically preferable, but often impractical, alternative is intravenous infusion of the vasodilator, nitroprusside (see p. 423). In dissecting aneurysm, vasodilators should not be used unless patients are first β-blocked, because any increase in the rate of rise of the pulse stroke is undesirable. *Labetalol* provides a convenient method of treating all patients within the three circles (except asthmatics), using either oral or parenteral therapy as appropriate. That said, it is not the most effective therapy and should be combined with a long-acting formulation of nifedipine, orally, where further blood pressure reduction is required.

Low doses of all drugs should be used if other antihypertensive drugs have recently been taken or renal function is impaired.

Oral maintenance treatment for severe hypertension should be started at once if possible; parenteral therapy is seldom necessary for more than 48 h.

Pregnancy hypertension

Effective treatment of pregnancy-induced hypertension improves fetal and perinatal survival. There is a lack of good clinical trial evidence on which to base recommendations. Instead, drug selection reflects longevity of use without obvious harm to the fetus, and methyldopa is still the drug of choice for many obstetricians. Calcium channel blockers (especially nifedipine) are common second-line drugs; parenteral hydralazine is reserved for emergency reduction of blood pressure in late pregnancy, preferably in combination with a β-blocker to avoid unpleasant tachycardia.

β-Blockers (labetalol and atenolol) are often effective and are probably the drugs of choice in the third trimester; there is anecdotal evidence to suggest growth retardation with β-blockade used in the first and second trimesters. Diuretics reduce the chance of developing pre-eclampsia, but are avoided in pre-eclampsia itself because these patients already have a contracted circulatory volume.

ACE inhibitors and angiotensin II receptor blockers (ARBs) 'should be avoided in pregnancy unless essential' (advice given in the British National Formulary). They have been associated with major malformations after first-trimester exposure[40] and fetal death, typically mid-trimester. For this reason, they are probably best avoided in women of child-bearing age, especially where there is no effective contraception, since it is not uncommon for women to discover their pregnancy late into its first trimester. If they are used, women should be counselled to stop an ACE or ARB as soon as they suspect they are pregnant.

Raised blood pressure and proteinuria (pre-eclampsia) complicates 2–8% of pregnancies and may proceed to fitting (eclampsia), a major cause of mortality in mother and child. Magnesium sulphate halves the risk of progress to eclampsia (typically 4 g i.v. over 5–10 min followed by 1 g/h by i.v. infusion for 24 h after the last seizure).[41] Additionally, if a woman has one fit (treat with diazepam), then the magnesium regimen is superior to diazepam or phenytoin in preventing further fits.[42]

Aspirin, in low dose, was reported in early studies to reduce the incidence of pre-eclampsia in at-risk patients, but a more recent meta-analysis has not supported this. Consequently, it is not routinely recommended.

Unwanted interactions with antihypertensive drugs

Specific interactions are described in the accounts of individual drugs. The following are general examples for this diverse group of drugs.

Alcohol intake is the commonest contributing factor, or even cause, of hypertension, and should always be considered as a cause of erratic or failed responses to treatment (measurement of the γ-glutamyl transpeptidase and red cell mean corpuscular volume may be useful).

Prostaglandin synthesis. NSAIDs, e.g. indometacin, attenuate the antihypertensive effect of β-adrenoceptor blockers and of diuretics, perhaps by inhibiting the synthesis of vasodilator renal prostaglandins. This effect can also be important when a diuretic is used for severe left ventricular failure.

Enzyme inhibition. Ciprofloxacin and cimetidine inhibit hepatic metabolism of lipid-soluble β-adrenoceptor blockers, e.g. metoprolol, labetalol, propranolol, increasing their effect. Methyldopa plus a monoamine oxidase inhibitor (MAOI) may cause excitement and hallucinations.

Pharmacological antagonism. Sympathomimetics, e.g. amfetamine, phenylpropanolamine (present in anorectics and cold and cough remedies), may lead to loss of antihypertensive effect, and indeed to a *hypertensive reaction* when taken by a patient already on a β-adrenoceptor blocker, due to unopposed α-adrenergic stimulation.

Surgical anaesthesia may lead to a brisk fall in blood pressure in patients taking antihypertensives. Antihypertensive

[40]Cooper W O, Hernandez-Diaz S, Arbogast P G et al 2006 Major congenital malformations after first-trimester exposure to ACE inhibitors. New England Journal of Medicine 354:2443–2451.

[41]Magpie Trial Collaborative Group 2002 Do women with pre-eclampsia, and their babies, benefit from magnesium sulphate? The Magpie Trial: a randomised placebo-controlled trial. Lancet 359:1877–1890.
[42]Eclampsia Trial Collaborative Group 1995 Which anticonvulsant for women with eclampsia? Evidence from the Collaborative Eclampsia Trial. Lancet 345:1455–1463.

therapy should not be routinely altered before surgery, although it obviously can complicate care both during and after the operation. Anaesthetists must be informed.

Sexual function and cardiovascular drugs

All drugs that interfere with sympathetic autonomic activity can potentially interfere with male sexual function, expressed as a failure of ejaculation or difficulty in sustaining an erection. Nevertheless, placebo-controlled trials have emphasised how common a symptom this is in the untreated male population (sometimes approaching 20–30%). It is also likely that hypertension itself is associated with an increased risk of sexual dysfunction, since loss of nitric oxide production by the vascular endothelium is an early feature of the pathophysiology of this disease.

Laying the blame on antihypertensive medication is incorrect in most instances. Calcium channel blockers, ACE inhibitors and angiotensin II (AT_1) receptor blockers (ARBs) all have reported rates of sexual dysfunction that do not differ from placebo. If symptoms persist with these drugs, other causes should be sought. Sildenafil (Viagra) can be used safely in patients receiving any of the commonly used antihypertensive drugs.

As well as the concerns about sexual performance in treated hypertensives, there may be concerns about fitness per se to attempt intercourse. The real possibility that it is hazardous is compounded often by their age and concurrent coronary artery disease.

Sexual intercourse and the cardiovascular system

Normal sexual intercourse with orgasm is accompanied by transient but brisk physiological changes, e.g. tachycardia up to 180 beats/min, with increases of 100 beats/min over less than 1 min. Systolic blood pressure may rise by 120 mmHg and diastolic by 50 mmHg. Orgasm may be accompanied by transient pressure of 230/130 mmHg, even in normotensive individuals. Electrocardiographic abnormalities may occur in healthy men and women. Respiratory rate may rise to 60 breaths/min.

Such changes in the healthy might bode ill for the unhealthy (with hypertension, angina pectoris or after myocardial infarction). Sudden deaths do occur during or shortly after sexual intercourse (ventricular fibrillation or subarachnoid haemorrhage), usually in clandestine circumstances such as the bordello or the mistress's bed, especially when an older man and a younger woman are involved – although this may just reflect reporting bias in the press. In one series, 0.6% of all sudden deaths were (reportedly) attributable to sexual intercourse, and cardiac disease was present in about one-half of these. Clearly, the older patient with coronary heart disease should aspire cautiously to the haemodynamic heights attainable in youth.

There are few, if any, records of sudden cardiovascular death among these women under these circumstances.

If there is substantial concern about cardiovascular stress (hypertension or arrhythmia) during sexual intercourse in either sex, a dose of labetalol about 2 h before the event may well be justified (taking account of other therapy already in use). But patients taking a β-blocker long term for angina prophylaxis have shown reductions in peak heart rate during coitus from 122 to 82 beats/min.

Patients subject to angina pectoris should also use glyceryl trinitrate or isosorbide dinitrate as usual for pre-exertional prophylaxis 10 min before intercourse. *But they should be aware of the potentially fatal interaction of sildenafil (Viagra) and other PDE_5 inhibitors with nitrates* (see p. 417).

Summary

- The treatment of both hypertension and angina requires drugs that reduce the work of the heart either directly or by lowering peripheral vascular resistance.
- β-Blockade, which acts mainly through reduced cardiac output, and calcium channel blockade, acting by selective arterial dilatation, may be used in either condition.
- Other vasodilators are suited preferentially to hypertension (ACE inhibitors, angiotensin (AT_1) receptor blockers (ARBs) and α-adrenoceptor blockers) or to angina (nitrates).
- The treatment of myocardial infarction requires thrombolysis, aspirin and β-adrenoceptor blockade acutely, with the latter two continued for at least 2 years as secondary prevention of a further infarction.
- Other important steps in secondary prevention include ACE inhibitors for cardiac failure and statins for hypercholesterolaemia in selected patients.

Pulmonary hypertension

Therapy is determined by the underlying cause. When the condition is secondary to hypoxia accompanying chronic obstructive pulmonary disease, *long-term oxygen therapy* improves symptoms and prognosis; anticoagulation is essential when the cause is multiple pulmonary emboli.

Idiopathic (primary) pulmonary arterial hypertension (PAH). Verapamil may give symptomatic benefit. Prostanoid formulations used to treat PAH include intravenous epoprostenol (prostacyclin) and inhaled ilo-prost.[43] The prostanoid formulations have the limitations of a short half-life and a heterogeneous response to therapy. Evidence suggests that endothelin, a powerful endogenous vasoconstrictor, may play a pathogenic role; the antagonists, *bosentan, ambrisentan* and *Sitaxsentan*, improve symptoms and haemodyamic measurements, but dose is limited by hepatic toxicity. The PDE$_5$ inhibitors, sildenafil, tadalafil, and vardenafil, are an alternative. Only tadalafil has been shown to improve survival, although in a comparison of the three drugs only sildenafil increased exercise tolerance. Heart and lung transplantation is recommended for younger patients.

Treatment of secondary hypertension

In at least 5% of patients, it is possible to identify a single cause of the hypertension, and some of these can be cured by a surgical or endovascular intervention. In some of these cases, either the diagnostic workup, preparation for surgery, or long-term management requires some clinical pharmacology different from the management of essential hypertension. This is particularly true for adrenal causes of hypertension.

Phaeochromocytoma

This tumour of chromaffin tissue, usually arising in the adrenal medulla, secretes principally noradrenaline/norepinephrine, but often also variable amounts of adrenaline/epinephrine. Symptoms are related to this. Hypertension may be sustained or intermittent. If the tumour secretes only noradrenaline/norepinephrine, which stimulates α- and β_1-adrenoceptors, rises in blood pressure are accompanied by reflex bradycardia due to vagal activation; this is sufficient to overcome the chronotropic effect of β_1-receptor stimulation. The recognition of *bradycardia* at the time of catecholamine-induced symptoms (e.g. anxiety, tremor or sweating) is useful in alerting the physician to the possibility of this rare syndrome, as physiological sympathetic nervous activation is coupled to vagal withdrawal and causes *tachycardia*. If the tumour also secretes adrenaline/epinephrine, which stimulates α-, β_1- and β_2-adrenoceptors, blood pressure and heart rate change in parallel. This is because stimulation of the vasodilator β_2 receptor in resistance arteries attenuates the rise in diastolic pressure, and vagal activation is insufficient then to oppose the chronotropic effect of combined β_1 and β_2 receptor stimulation in the heart.

Diagnosis is made by measurement of the *O*-methylated metabolite of catecholamines, namely normetanephrine (from noradrenaline/norepinephrine) and metanephrine (from adrenaline/epinephrine) in blood or 24-h urine. Because the enzyme catechol-*O*-methyltransferase is present in phaeochromocytoma but not sympathetic nerve endings, the measurement of 'fractionated metanephrines' (i.e. normetanephrine and metanephrine separated from each other) provides > 90% specificity and sensitivity – higher than older diagnostic tests – and even modest elevations should not be ignored. Biochemical evidence for a phaeochromocytoma should usually precede the imaging hunt for a tumour. The finding of elevated metaphrine secretion (as well as normetanephrine) indicates an adrenal location since only the adrenal tumours are exposed to the high concentration of cortisol required to induce phenylethanolamine *N*-methyltransferase (PNMT) – the enzyme which catalyses methylation of noradrenaline/norepinephrine to adrenaline/epinephrine. However, the portocapillary circulation from cortex to medulla is progressively disrupted as a tumour grows, so that very large adrenal tumours may cease to secrete adrenaline/epinephrine.

In cases of borderline biochemistry, pharmacological suppression tests are useful. Either the ganglion-blocking drug pentolinium or centrally acting α_2-agonist clonidine suppresses physiological elevations of metaphrines, but not autonomous secretion from a tumour.[44,45]

Provocation tests should not be deliberately employed; but the initial search for phaeochromocytoma may be prompted by a history of hypertensive crisis induced by dopamine antagonists (e.g. metoclopramide) or any drug that releases histamine (opioids, curare, trimetaphan).

Control of blood pressure before surgery or when the tumour cannot be removed is achieved by α-adrenoceptor blockade, which reverses peripheral vasoconstriction. An important function of the α-blockade is not just blood pressure control, but expansion of intravascular volume. Phaeochromocytoma is the best example of pure vasoconstrictor hypertension, with compensatory pressure natriuresis.

[43]Barst R J, Rubin L J, Long W A et al 1996 A comparison of continuous intravenous epoprostenol (prostacyclin) with conventional therapy for primary pulmonary hypertension. New England Journal of Medicine 334:296–302. In a trial of 81 patients with severe PAH, a 12-week infusion of epoprostenol improved quality of life, mean pulmonary arterial pressure (–8 versus +3%), pulmonary vascular resistance (–21 versus +9%), and exercise capacity, as measured by a 6-min walk test (+47 versus –66 meters). Eight patients died during the trial, all of whom were in the standard therapy group.

[44]Brown M J, Allison D J, Jenner D A et al 1981 Increased sensitivity and accuracy of phaeochromocytoma diagnosis achieved by plasma adrenaline estimations and a pentolinium suppression test. Lancet ii:174–177.
[45]Bravo E L, Tarazi R C, Fouad F M et al 1981 Clonidine-suppression test: a useful aid in the diagnosis of pheochromocytoma. New England Journal of Medicine 305:623–626.

Consequently, patients are usually volume depleted, often severely, and this must be corrected before it is safe to proceed to surgery.

Not infrequently, the pressure natriuresis completely compensates for vasoconstriction, and patients present with features other than hypertension – even hypotension after an episode of fluid depletion. Such patients need α-blockade prior to surgery in order to volume expand, being at risk of postoperative hypotension if not adequately prepared. β-Blockade may also be required to control tachycardia in patients with adrenaline/epinephrine-secreting tumours. Since adrenaline/epinephrine secretion, as explained above, tends to fall as tumours enlarge, tachycardia is not usually a major problem. Initiation of α-blocker treatment can unmask tachycardia, because there is no longer baroreceptor-induced vagal activation to oppose β-receptor stimulation of the heart. A β-receptor blocker should never be given alone, because abolition of the peripheral vasodilator effects of adrenaline/epinephrine leaves the powerful α effects unopposed. A low dose of a β_1-selective agent (e.g. bisoprolol 5 mg) is safe in the presence of α-blockade. Occasionally, non-selective β-blockade is required, once α-blockade is established, in order to treat β_2-effects (tremor, tachycardia) of an atypical adrenaline/epinephrine-secreting phaeochromoctyoma.

For phaeochromocytoma, the preferred α-blocker is not one of the selective α_1-blockers, as in essential hypertension, but the irreversible α-blocker, *phenoxybenzamine 10–80 mg/day*, whose blockade cannot be overcome by a catecholamine surge, e.g. during tumour manipulation at surgery. Titration of the dose requires inspection of the jugular venous pressure, as index of volume replacement, as well as measurement of blood pressure in the supine and erect position.

During surgical removal – which is usually by laparoscopic adrenalectomy – *phentolamine* (or sodium nitroprusside) should be at hand to control rises in blood pressure when the tumour is handled. When the adrenal veins have been clamped, volume expansion is often required to maintain blood pressure even after adequate preoperative α-blockade. If a pressor infusion is still needed, isoprenaline is more use than the usual α agonists, to which the patient will be insensitive due to existing α-receptor blockade.

Metirosine (α-methyltyrosine) has been used with some success to block catecholamine synthesis in malignant phaeochromocytomas.

Meta-iodobenzylguanidine (MIBG, an analogue of guanethidine) is actively taken up by adrenergic tissue and is concentrated in phaeochromocytomas. Radio-iodinated MIBG ($[^{123}I]$MIBG) allows localisation of tumours and detection of metastases, and selective therapeutic irradiation of functioning metastases or other tumours of chromaffin tissue, e.g. carcinoid.

Primary aldosteronism (Conn's syndrome)

This refers to autonomous secretion of the sodium-retaining hormone aldosterone by the outer zone ('zona glomerulosa') of the adrenal cortex. The condition is potentially curable when due – in about one-half of affected patients – to a benign unilateral adenoma. This is present in 5–10% of patients with hypertension. The uncertainty arises from the small size of many such tumours, often <1 cm in diameter, leading to their being overlooked in most cases. Conn's adenomas are diagnosed by finding a suppressed plasma renin, without suppression of aldosterone, and an adrenal adenoma on CT or MRI. Since 5% of adults have incidental non-functional adrenal adenomas, the key step in diagnosis is lateralisation: the demonstration that the adenoma is responsible for excess aldosterone secretion. Conventionally this is done by adrenal venous sampling. An alternative, in specialist centres, is a PET-CT using a tracer dose of the anaesthetic drug metomidate labelled with C^{11}, which has high affinity binding to the steroid synthases (Fig. 24.4).

Definitive treatment of a proven aldosteronoma is by laparoscopic adrenalectomy. This is recommended in younger patients, who are the ones most likely to have their hypertension cured, and in older patients uncontrolled by, or intolerant of, multiple drugs. Prior to surgery, or longer-term when surgery is not selected, the hypertension (and hypokalaemia present in ~25% of patients) should be treated by the mineralocorticoid receptor antagonists spironolactone or eplerenone, or by the diuretic amiloride, which inhibits Na^+ transport through the epithelial Na^+ channel stimulated by aldosterone. Spironolactone 25–100 mg/day is the most effective, but causes gynaecomastia on chronic dosing. A useful strategy is to combine eplerenone or low-dose spironolactone with amiloride 5–10 mg/day, although regular electrolyte monitoring is necessary to avoid hyperkalaemia and hyponatraemia.

Heart failure and its treatment

Some physiology and pathophysiology

Cardiac output (CO) depends on the rate of contraction of the heart, heart rate (HR), and the volume of blood that is ejected with each beat, the stroke volume (SV); it is expressed by the relationship:

$$CO = HR \times SV$$

The three factors that regulate the stroke volume are preload, afterload and contractility:

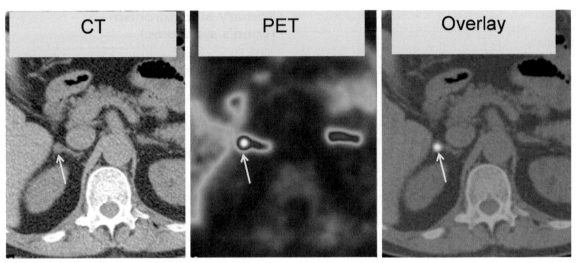

Fig. 24.4 PET-CT of a 0.5-cm right adrenal adenoma. The radio-tracer is 11 C-metomidate *(From Burton T J, MacKenzie I S, Balan K et al 2012 Evaluation of the sensitivity and specificity of 11C-metomidate positron emission tomography (PET)-CT for lateralizing aldosterone secretion by Conn's adenomas. J Clin Endocrinol Metab 97:100–109, with permission).*

- Preload is the load on the heart created by the volume of blood received into the left ventricle from the left atrium (at the end of ventricular diastole) and that it must eject with each contraction. It can also be viewed as the amount of stretch to which the left ventricle is subject. As the preload rises, so also do the degree of stretch and the length of cardiac muscle fibres. Preload is thus a volume load and can be excessive, e.g. when there is valvular incompetence.
- Afterload refers to the load on the contracting ventricle created by the resistance to the blood projected by the ventricle into the arterial system, i.e. the total peripheral resistance. Afterload is thus a pressure load and is excessive, e.g. in arterial hypertension.
- Contractility refers to the capacity of the myocardium to generate the force necessary to respond to preload and to overcome afterload.

Definition of chronic heart failure

As the population ages and the treatment of acute myocardial infarction improves, this condition is becoming increasingly common, and there is talk of an 'epidemic' of heart failure. Chronic heart failure is present when the heart cannot provide all organs with the blood supply appropriate to demand. This definition incorporates two elements: firstly, cardiac output may be normal at rest, but secondly, when demand is increased, perfusion of the vital organs (brain and kidneys)

continues at the expense of other tissues, especially skeletal muscle. Overall, systemic arterial pressure is sustained until the late stages. These responses follow neuroendocrine activation when the heart begins to fail.

The therapeutic importance of recognising this patho-physiology is that many of the neuroendocrine abnormalities of heart failure – particularly the increased renin output and sympathetic activity – can be a consequence of drug treatment, as well as the disease. Renal perfusion is normal in early heart failure, whereas diuretics and vasodilators stimulate renin and noradrenaline/norepinephrine production through actions at the juxtaglomerular apparatus in the kidney and on the arterial baroreflex, respectively. The earliest endocrine abnormality in almost all types of cardiac disease is increased release of the heart's own hormones, the natriuretic peptides ANP and BNP (A for atrial, B for brain, where it was first discovered). The concentration in plasma of BNP provides a strong prognostic indicator for patients with all stages of heart failure. These peptides normally suppress renin and aldosterone production, but heart failure overrides this control, and measurement of BNP now aids the diagnosis of heart failure, with a raised plasma concentration being a sensitive indicator of the disease.[46]

---

[46]Braunwald E 2008 Biomarkers in heart failure. New England Journal of Medicine 358:2148–2159.

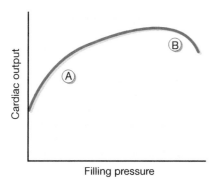

Fig. 24.5 The Starling curve of the relationship between cardiac filling pressure and cardiac output. In phase A, the curve shows that lowering the blood volume (by diuretics) will reduce the filling pressure, but the cardiac output will fall. In phase B, lowering the blood volume will reduce the filling pressure, but the cardiac output will increase (see text).

The Starling curve and heart failure

The Starling[47] curve originally described increased contractility of cardiac muscle fibres in response to increased stretch, but, applied to the whole ventricle, it can explain the normal relationship between filling pressure and cardiac output (Fig. 24.5). Most patients with heart failure present in phase 'A' of the relationship, and before the 'decompensated' phase (B), in which there is gross dilatation of the ventricle. Diuretic therapy improves the congestive symptoms of heart failure, which are due to the increased filling pressure (preload), but actually reduces cardiac output in most patients. Depending on whether their predominant symptom is dyspnoea (due to pulmonary venous congestion) or fatigue (due to reduced cardiac output), patients feel better or worse. It is likely that a principal benefit of using angiotensin-converting enzyme (ACE) inhibitors in heart failure is their diuretic sparing effect.

Natural history of chronic heart failure

Injury to the heart, e.g. myocardial infarction, hypertension, leads to adaptive ('compensatory') molecular, cellular and interstitial changes that alter its size, shape and function. Myocardial hypertophy and 'remodelling' takes place over weeks or months in response to haemodynamic load, neurohormonal activation and other factors, and the resulting pattern differs according to whether the stimulus is a pressure or volume overload. With the passage of time, and with maladaption, the heart 'decompensates' and heart failure worsens. The process is outlined in Fig. 24.6.

The degree of activity that the patient can undertake without becoming dyspnoeic provides one useful classification of the severity of heart failure. The New York Heart Association (NYHA) classification[48] offers also an approximate prognosis, with that of the worst grade (Class IV) being as bad as most cancers. Many patients with heart failure die from an arrhythmia, rather than from terminal decompensation, and drugs that avoid increasing the heart's exposure to increased catecholamine concentrations, as do some vasodilators (but see below), appear best for improving prognosis.

Objectives of treatment

As for cardiac arrhythmias, these are to reduce morbidity (relief of symptoms, avoid hospital admission) and mortality.

There is some tension between these two objectives in that the condition is both disabling and deadly, and the action of diuretic and some vasodilator drugs, which temporarily improve symptoms, can jeopardise survival. There is a further tension between the needs of treating the features of forwards failure, or low output, and backwards failure, or the congestive features. The principal symptom of a low cardiac output, fatigue, is difficult to quantify, and patients have tended to have their treatment tailored more to the consequences of venous congestion.

Haemodynamic aims of drug therapy

Acute or chronic failure of the heart usually results from disease of the myocardium itself, mainly ischaemic, or an excessive load imposed on it by arterial hypertension, valvular disease or an arteriovenous shunt. The management of chronic heart failure requires both the relief of any treatable underlying or aggravating cause, and therapy directed at the failure itself.

Distinguishing between the capacity of the myocardium to pump blood and the load against which the heart must work is useful in therapy. The failing myocardium is so strongly stimulated to contract by increased sympathetic drive that therapeutic efforts to induce it to function yet more vigorously are in themselves alone unlikely to be of benefit. Despite numerous candidate drugs introduced over recent years, digoxin remains the only inotropic drug suitable for chronic oral use.

By contrast, agents that reduce preload or afterload can be very effective, especially where the left ventricular volume is increased (less predictably so for failure of the right

---

[47]Ernest Henry Starling, 1866–1927, Professor of Physiology, University College, London. He also coined the word 'hormone'.

[48]NYHA Class I, minimal dyspnoea (except after moderate exercise); Class II, dyspnoea while walking on the flat; Class III, dyspnoea on getting in/out of bed; Class IV, dyspnoea while lying in bed.

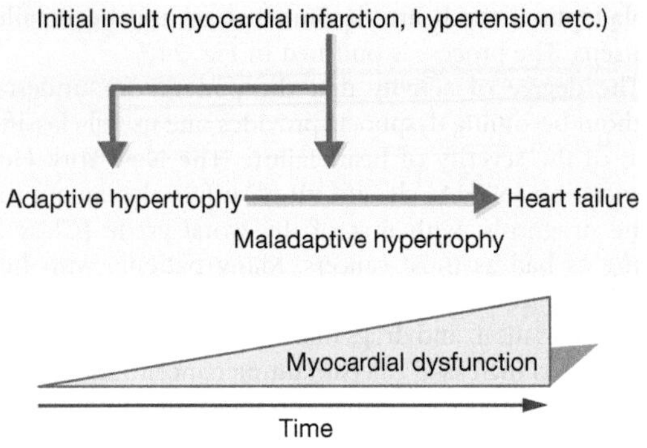

Fig. 24.6 Progression of ventricular disease from hypertrophy through to failure following the initial insult. The process is generically referred to as 'cardiac remodelling', and the aim of much drug therapy in heart failure treatment is to try to place a brake on this process.

ventricle). The main hazard of their use is a drastic fall in cardiac output in those occasional patients whose output is dependent on a high left ventricular filling pressure, e.g. who are volume depleted by diuretic use or have severe mitral stenosis.

Classification of drugs

Reduction of preload

Diuretics increase salt and water loss, reduce blood volume and lower excessive venous filling pressure (see Ch. 27). They are almost invariably required to relieve the congestive features of oedema, in the lungs and the periphery; when the heart is grossly enlarged, cardiac output will also increase (see discussion of Starling curve, above). They are used flexibly, starting with a low dose; the usual sequence would be to begin with a thiazide, then move to furosemide, and in the most extreme cases then judiciously add metolazone.

Nitrates (see also Ch. 24) dilate the smooth muscle in venous capacitance vessels; increase the volume of the venous vascular bed (which normally may compose 80% of the whole vascular system); reduce ventricular filling pressure, thus decreasing heart wall stretch; and reduce myocardial oxygen requirements. Their arteriolar dilating action is relatively slight. Glyceryl trinitrate provides benefit in acute left ventricular failure sublingually or by intravenous infusion. For chronic left ventricular failure, nitrates have fallen out of favour, because the ACE inhibitors are more effective.

Reduction of afterload

Hydralazine (see also Ch. 24) relaxes arterial smooth muscle and reduces peripheral vascular resistance. Reflex tachycardia

limits its usefulness, and lupus erythematosus is a risk usually only if the dose exceeds 100 mg/day.

Reduction of preload and afterload

ACE inhibitors and angiotensin receptor II blockers (ARBs) (see also Ch. 24) act in the following manner:

- Reduction of afterload, by preventing the conversion of angiotensin I to the active form, angiotensin II, or by blocking the effects of angiotensin II, which is a powerful arterioconstrictor and is present in the plasma in high concentration in heart failure.
- Reduction of preload, because the formation of aldosterone, and thus retention of salt and water (increased blood volume), is prevented by reducing the effects of angiotensin II.
- ACE inhibitors are the only drugs that reduce peripheral resistance (afterload) without causing a reflex activation of the sympathetic system. The landmark CONSENSUS study compared enalapril with placebo in patients with NYHA class IV heart failure; after 6 months, 26% of the enalapril group had died, compared with 44% in the control group. The reduction in mortality occurred among patients with progressive heart failure.[49] There is now strong evidence from long-term studies that ACE inhibitors[50] and ARBs[51] improve survival in and reduce hospital admissions for heart failure.

A common practice has been to give a test dose of a short-acting ACE inhibitor (e.g. ramipril 1.25 mg by mouth) to patients who are in heart failure or on diuretic therapy for another reason, e.g. hypertension. Maintenance of blood pressure in such individuals may depend greatly on an activated renin–angiotensin–aldosterone system, and a standard dose of an ACE inhibitor or ARB can cause a sudden fall in blood pressure. That said, some of the many ACE inhibitors now available (see p. 421) have a sufficiently prolonged action that the initial doses have a cumulative effect on blood pressure over several days. Long-acting ACE inhibitors such as lisinopril ($t_{1/2}$ 12 h) and perindopril ($t_{1/2}$ 31 h) avoid the risk of sudden falls in blood pressure or

[49]Cooperative North Scandinavian Enalapril Survival Study (CONSENSUS) Trial Study Group 1987 Effects of enalapril on mortality in severe congestive heart failure. New England Journal of Medicine 316:1430–1435.
[50]Flather M D, Yusuf S, Kober L et al for the ACE-Inhibitor Myocardial Infarction Collaborative Group 2000 Long-term ACE-inhibitor therapy in patients with heart failure or left-ventricular dysfunction: a systematic overview of data from individual patients. Lancet 355:1575–1587.
[51]Demers C, McMurray J J V, Swedberg K et al for the CHARM investigators 2005 Impact of candesartan on nonfatal myocardial infarction and cardiovascular death in patients with heart failure. Journal of the American Medical Association 294:1794–1798.

renal function (glomerular filtration) after the first dose. Such drugs can be initiated outside hospital in patients who are unlikely to have a high plasma renin (absence of gross oedema or widespread atherosclerotic disease), although it is prudent to arrange for the first dose to be taken just before going to bed. Therapy begins with an ACE inhibitor, and an ARB is substituted if there is intolerance, or added if symptoms continue.

β-**Adrenoceptor blockers.** The realisation that activation of the renin–angiotensin–aldosterone and sympathetic nervous systems can adversely affect the course of chronic heart failure led to exploration of the possible benefits in heart failure from blockade of β-adrenoceptors. Clinical trials have, indeed, shown that bisoprolol, carvedilol or metoprolol lower mortality and decrease hospitalisation when added to conventional treatment that is likely to include diuretics, digoxin and an ACE inhibitor (see below).

Spironolactone. Plasma aldosterone levels are raised in heart failure. Spironolactone acts as a diuretic by competitively blocking the aldosterone receptor, but in addition it has a powerful effect on outcome in heart failure (see below). Eplerenone, an alternative mineralocorticoid antagonist, also has beneficial effects including in mild to moderate heart failure.

Stimulation of the myocardium

Digoxin improves myocardial contractility (positive inotropic effect) most effectively in the dilated, failing heart and, in the longer term, after an episode of heart failure has been brought under control. This effect occurs in patients in sinus rhythm and is distinct from its (negative chronotropic) action of reducing ventricular rate and thus improving ventricular filling in atrial fibrillation. Over 200 years after the first use of digitalis for dropsy, the DIG trial provided relief for doctors seeking evidence of long-term benefit.[52] Unlike all other positive inotropes, digoxin does not increase overall mortality or arrhythmias.

The phosphodiesterase inhibitors enoximone and milrinone have positive inotropic effects due to selective myocardial enzyme inhibition and may be used for short-term treatment of severe congestive heart failure. Evidence from longer-term use indicates that these drugs reduce survival.

Drug management of heart failure

Chronic heart failure

A schema for the stepwise drug management of chronic heart failure appears in Fig. 24.7. Points to emphasise in this schema are that all patients, even those with mild heart failure, should receive an ACE inhibitor or ARB as first-line therapy. Several long-term studies have demonstrated improved survival, even when cardiac failure is mild.[53] Further improvement in survival is obtained by using the combination drug sacubitril valsartan.[54] Sacubitril inhibits the enzyme which inactivates natriuretic peptides, so potentiating the actions of atrial and brain natriuretic peptides. It also inhibits metabolism of bradykinin, and hence should never be combined with an ACE inhibitor – a combination previously found to cause angioneurotic oedema in 4% of patients.

Black patients have a less activated renin system than other ethnic groups. In a landmark study, following subgroup analyses of earlier trials, 1050 black patients who had New York Heart Association class III or IV heart failure with dilated ventricles were randomly assigned to receive a combination of isosorbide dinitrate 120 mg/day plus hydralazine 225 mg/day or placebo in addition to standard therapy for heart failure. The study was terminated early owing to a significantly higher mortality rate in the placebo group, 10.2%, than in the group receiving the active combination, 6.2%, $P = 0.02$.[55]

Diuretic therapy is very useful for symptom management but has no impact on survival. For most patients, the choice will be a loop diuretic, e.g. furosemide starting at 20–40 mg/day. Because of the potassium-sparing effect of ACE inhibition, amiloride (also potassium sparing) is often not required, at least with low doses of a loop diuretic.

There is now overwhelming evidence for the benefit of β-blockers in chronic heart failure, despite the long-held belief that their negative inotropic effect was a contraindication.

---

[52]This prospective randomised trial compared digoxin with placebo in 7788 patients in NYHA Class II–III heart failure and sinus rhythm, most of whom also received an ACE inhibitor and a diuretic. Overall mortality did not differ between the groups, but patients who took digoxin had fewer episodes of hospitalisation for worsening heart failure (Digitalis Investigation Group 1997 The effect of digoxin on mortality and morbidity in patients with heart failure. New England Journal of Medicine 336:525–532).

[53]In the Studies of Left Ventricular Dysfunction (SOLVD, enalapril was compared with placebo in patients with either clinical features of heart failure or reduced left ventricular function in the absence of symptoms. Treatment reduced serious events (myocardial infarction and unstable angina) by approximately 20% and hospital admissions with progressive heart failure by up to 40%. (SOLVD Investigators 1991 Effect of enalapril on survival in patients with reduced left ventricular ejection fractions and congestive heart failure. New England Journal of Medicine 325:293–302).

[54]McMurray J J, Packer M, Desai A S et al 2014 Angiotensin-neprilysin inhibition versus enalapril in heart failure. New England Journal of Medicine 371:993–1004. 8442 patients with class II, III, or IV heart failure and an ejection fraction of 40% or less were randomly assigned to receive either sacubitril valsartan (at a dose of 200 mg twice daily) or enalapril (at a dose of 10 mg twice daily), in addition to recommended therapy. A total of 711 patients (17.0%) receiving sacubitril valsartan and 835 patients (19.8%) receiving enalapril died (hazard ratio for death from any cause, 0.84; 95% CI, 0.76 to 0.93; P <0.001)

[55]Taylor A L, Ziesche S, Yancy C et al 2004 Combination of isosorbide dinitrate and hydralazine in blacks with heart failure. New England Journal of Medicine 351:2049–2057.

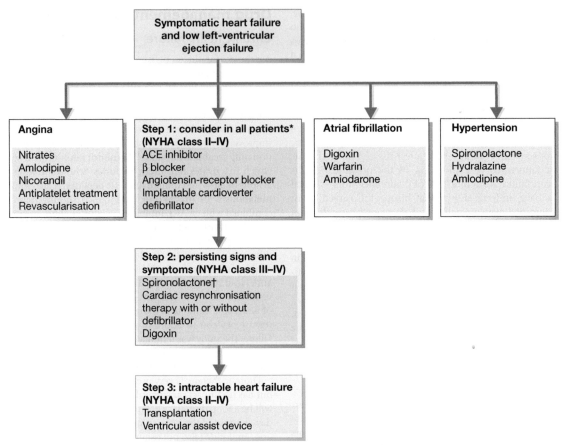

Fig. 24.7 Treatment algorithm for patients with heart failure and reduced left ventricular systolic function. *These treatments generally supplement existing diuretic drugs, with flexible dosing to maintain dry weight; consider hydralazine plus isosorbide dinitrate for black patients, as clinical trials indicate a favourable response in this subgroup. † The safety and efficacy of the combination of an ACE inhibitor, an ARB, and an aldosterone antagonist are unknown. NYHA, New York Heart Association. *(From McMurray J J, Pfeffer M A 2005 Heart failure. Lancet 365:1877–1889 with permission.)*

Early trials were underpowered, but a meta-analysis did suggest a 31% reduction in the mortality rate. Subsequently, the CIBIS-2 and MERIT-HF trials have independently confirmed that chronic β-blockade has a survival effect of this size in moderate to severe (NHYA III/IV) heart failure.[56] Both studies confirmed the one-third reduction in mortality. In the MERIT-HF trial, a life was saved for just 27 patient-years

of treatment, i.e. it was unusually cost effective – more so than ACE inhibitor therapy. The action is probably a class effect of β-blockade, given the divergent pharmacology of the drugs used to date. Indeed, a similar benefit is achieved by slowing the heart rate with ivrabidine, prescribed at 5 to 7.5 mg b.d.

The reduction in mortality is additive to ACE inhibition, and the survival benefit is largely through a decrease in sudden deaths as opposed to a reduction in progressive pump failure seen with ACE inhibitors. The only cautionary note is that patients must be β-blocked very gradually from low starting doses (e.g. bisoprolol 1.25 mg/day or carvedilol 3.125 mg twice daily) with regular optimisation of the dose of other drugs, especially the loop diuretic, to prevent decompensation of heart failure control.

---

[56]Until 1997, 24 trials of β-blockade in heart failure provided just 3141 patients. MERIT-HF (1999 Effect of metoprolol CR/XL in chronic heart failure: Metoprolol CR/XL Randomised Intervention Trial in Congestive Heart Failure [MERIT-HF]. Lancet 353:2001–2007) alone contained 3991 patients and CIBIS-2 (1999 The Cardiac Insufficiency Bisoprolol Study II [CIBIS-II]: a randomised trial. Lancet 353:9–13) provided a further 2467.

The use of spironolactone has received considerable support from the RALES trial,[57] which implies that ACE inhibition even at high dose does not effectively suppress hyperaldosteronism in heart failure. The benefit occurs at a surprisingly low dose of spironolactone (25 mg/day); it probably reflects both improved potassium and magnesium conservation (both are antiarrhythmic) and reversal of fibrosis in the myocardium by aldosterone.

None of the available oral phosphodiesterase inhibitors is established in routine therapy, because the short-term benefit of the increased contractility is offset by an increased mortality rate (presumably due to arrhythmias) on chronic dosing. Their use is restricted to short-term symptom control prior to, for example, transplantation.

Acute left ventricular failure

This is a common medical emergency, despite possible lessening in frequency with the advent of thrombolysis for myocardial infarction. The approach should be to reassure the anxious patient, who should sit upright with his or her legs dependent to reduce systemic venous return. A loop diuretic, e.g. furosemide 40–80 mg i.v., is the mainstay of therapy and provides benefit both by a rapid and powerful venodilator effect, reducing preload, and by the subsequent diuresis. Oxygen should be given, if the patient can tolerate a face mask, and diamorphine or morphine i.v. which, in addition to relieving anxiety and pain, have valuable venodilator effects.

Although there may be a case for short-term use of inotropic drugs (see Ch. 25) for heart failure where low output is a dominating feature, most such drugs substantially increase the risk of arrhythmias when the heart is hypoxic. The pharmacokinetics of digoxin does not favour emergency use. The possibility of assisted ventilation should be considered; where pulmonary oedema is the main problem, ventilation is likely to be both safer and more effective than inotropic drugs.

Surgery for heart failure

Although these options lie outside the scope of clinical pharmacology, an important element in meeting the objectives of treatment (see p. 445) is to recognise when further drug treatment is unlikely to improve symptoms or prognosis. Then, the physician must consider the possibility of a surgical intervention. Increasingly this may involve procedures short of transplantation itself, e.g. bypass grafting or stenting where stenosed vessels contribute to the heart failure or even a left ventricular assist device (LVAD) or totally artificial heart. On occasion, it can help to make the patient aware that failure of both the heart and the drugs is not necessarily the end of the road.

---

[57]The RALES trial randomised 1663 patients with stable heart failure to either placebo or spironolactone. All patients maintained their 'optimised' therapy, which included ACE inhibitors. After 2 years of follow-up, the trial terminated prematurely following the demonstration of a 30% reduction in the mortality rate of spironolactone-treated patients, from sudden death as well as progressive pump failure. Gynaecomastia or breast discomfort occurred in 10% of patients receiving spironolactone (1% in controls), but significant hyperkalaemia occurred in surprisingly few patients. RALES was not adequately powered to decide whether the action of spironolactone was additive to that of a β-blocker (Pitt B, Zannad F, Remme W J et al 1999 The effect of spironolactone on morbidity and mortality in patients with severe heart failure. Randomized Aldactone Evaluation Study Investigators. New England Journal of Medicine 341:709–717).

> **Summary**
>
> - Heart failure is present when the heart cannot provide all organs with the blood supply appropriate to demand.
> - Stroke volume is regulated by preload, afterload and contractility.
> - In chronic heart failure, diuretics and nitrates reduce preload and provide symptomatic relief without affecting outcome.
> - ACE inhibitors reduce both preload and afterload, and reduce morbidity and mortality by about one-third in all patients.
> - β-Adrenoceptor blockers, gradually introduced, have an effect equivalent to that of ACE inhibitors in patients with moderate or severe heart failure (NYHA III or IV).
> - Spironolactone, in low dose, adds further benefit.
> - Digoxin improves myocardial contractility most effectively in the dilated, failing heart but also in the longer term, including in patients in sinus rhythm.
> - The principal agents for treating acute left ventricular failure are furosemide, diamorphine and oxygen.

Guide to further reading

Armstrong, P.W., 2011. Aldosterone antagonists – last man standing? N. Engl. J. Med. 364, 79–80.

Ashrafian, H., Williams, L., Frenneaux, M.P., 2008. The pathophysiology of heart failure: a tale of two paradigms revisited. Clin. Med. (Northfield Il) 8, 192–197.

Braunwald, E., 2009. Biomarkers in heart failure. N. Engl. J. Med. 358, 2148–2159.

Brown, M.J., 2006. Hypertension and ethnic group. Br. Med. J. 332, 833–836.

Brown, M.J., 2007. Renin: friend or foe? Heart 93, 1026–1033.

Brown, M.J., 2010. Secondary hypertension. In: Warrell, D., Cox, T., Firth, J. (Eds.), Oxford Textbook of Medicine, fifth ed. Oxford University Press, Oxford, (Chapter 16.17.3).

Brown, M.J., 2008. Aliskiren. Circulation 118, 773–784.

Brown, M.J., Cruickshank, J.K., Macdonald, T.M., 2012. Navigating the shoals in hypertension: discovery and guidance. Br. Med. J. 344, 23–26.

Camm, A.J., Kirchhof, P., Lip, G.Y., et al., 2010. Guidelines for the management of atrial fibrillation: the Task Force for the Management of Atrial Fibrillation of the European Society of Cardiology (ESC). Eur. Heart J. 31, 2369–2429.

Crystal, E., Connolly, S.J., 2004. Role of oral anticoagulation in management of atrial fibrillation. Heart 90, 813–817.

Delacretaz, E., 2006. Clinical practice. Supraventricular tachycardia. N. Engl. J. Med. 354, 1039–1051.

Dobrev, D., Nattel, S., 2010. New antiarrhythmic drugs for treatment of atrial fibrillation. Lancet 375, 1212–1223.

Duley, L., Meher, S., Abalos, A., 2006. Clinical review: management of preeclampsia. Br. Med. J. 332, 463–468.

Dworkin, L.D., Cooper, C.J., 2009. Clinical practice: renal artery stenosis. N. Engl. J. Med. 361, 1972–1978.

Gaziano, T.A., Opie, L.H., Weinstein, M.S., et al., 2006. Cardiovascular disease prevention with a multidrug regimen in the developing world: a cost-effectiveness analysis. Lancet 368, 679–686.

Hansson, G.K., 2005. Inflammation, atherosclerosis, and coronary artery disease. N. Engl. J. Med. 352, 1685–1695.

Hillis, L.D., Lange, R.A., 2009. Optimal management of acute coronary syndromes. N. Engl. J. Med. 360, 2237–2239.

Huikuri, H.V., Castellanos, A., Myerburg, R.J., et al., 2001. Sudden death due to cardiac arrhythmias. N. Engl. J. Med. 345, 1473–1482.

James, P.A., Oparil, S., Carter, B.L., et al., 2014. 2014 Evidence-based guideline for the management of high blood pressure in adults. Report from the panel members appointed to the Eighth Joint National Committee (JNC 8). JAMA 311, 507–520.

Jarcho, J.A., 2005. Resynchronizing ventricular contraction in heart failure. N. Engl. J. Med. 352, 1594–1597.

Joint British Societies' consensus recommendations for the prevention of cardiovascular disease (JBS3). Available at: http://dx.doi.org/10.1136/heartjnl-2014-305693.

Kaplan, N.M., Opie, L.H., 2006. Controversies in hypertension. Lancet 367, 168–176.

Krum, H., Abraham, W.T., 2009. Heart failure. Lancet 373, 41–955.

Lip, G.Y., Halperin, J.L., 2010. Improving stroke risk stratification in atrial fibrillation. Am. J. Med. 123, 484–488.

McMurray, J.J., 2010. Systolic heart failure. N. Engl. J. Med. 362, 228–238.

Messerli, F.H., 1995. This day 50 years ago. N. Engl. J. Med. 332, 1038–1039. [an account of the hypertension and stroke suffered by US President F D Roosevelt].

Morady, F., 2004. Catheter ablation of supraventricular arrhythmias: state of the art. J. Cardiovasc. Electrophysiol. 15, 124–139.

Neubauer, S., 2007. The failing heart – an engine out of fuel. N. Engl. J. Med. 356, 1140–1151.

Page, R.L., 2004. Newly diagnosed atrial fibrillation. N. Engl. J. Med. 351, 2408–2416.

Page, R.L., Roden, D.M., 2005. Drug therapy for atrial fibrillation: where do we go from here? Nat. Rev. Drug Discov. 4, 899–910.

Piccini, J.P., Fauchier, L., 2016. Rhythm control in atrial fibrillation. Lancet 388, 829–840.

Pickering, T.G., Shimbo, D., Haas, D., et al., 2006. Ambulatory blood-pressure monitoring. N. Engl. J. Med. 354, 2368–2374.

Redfield, M.M., 2016. Heart failure with preserved ejection fraction. N. Engl. J. Med. 375, 1868–1877.

Staessen, J.A., Li, Y., Richart, T., 2006. Oral renin inhibitors. Lancet 368, 1449–1456.

Torp-Pedersen, C., Pedersen, O.D., Kober, L., 2010. Antiarrhythmic drugs: safety first. J. Am. Coll. Cardiol. 55, 1577–1579.

Turnbull, F., 2003. Effects of different blood-pressure-lowering regimens on major cardiovascular events: results of prospectively-designed overviews of randomised trials. Lancet 362, 1527–1535.

Van Gelder, I.C., Rienstra, M., Crijns, H.J., Olshansky, B., 2016. Rate control in atrial fibrillation. Lancet 388, 818–828.

Vaughan, C.J., Delanty, N., 2000. Hypertensive emergencies. Lancet 356, 411–417.

Williams, B., MacDonald, T.M., Morant, S., et al., 2015. British Hypertension Society's PATHWAY Studies Group. Spironolactone versus placebo, bisoprolol, and doxazosin to determine the optimal treatment for drug-resistant hypertension (PATHWAY-2): a randomised, double-blind, crossover trial. Lancet 386, 2059–2068.

Wicks, E.C., Davies, L.C., 2016. Heart failure – what the general physician needs to know. Clin. Med. 16, 25–33.

Williams, B., Poulter, N.R., Brown, M.J., et al., 2004. British Hypertension Society guidelines for hypertension management 2004 (BHS-IV): summary. Br. Med. J. 328, 634–640.

Zimetbaum, P., 2007. Amiodarone for atrial fibrillation. N. Engl. J. Med. 356, 935–941.

Chapter 25

Cardiac arrhythmia

Andrew Grace

SYNOPSIS

The pathophysiology of cardiac arrhythmias is complex, and the actions of drugs that are useful in stopping or controlling them may seem equally so. Nevertheless, many patients with arrhythmias respond well to therapy with drugs, and a working knowledge of their effects and indications pays dividends, for disturbance of the heartbeat is at least inconvenient and at worst can be fatal. Drug therapy for arrhythmias has a place beside radiofrequency ablation and the use of implanted devices, e.g. pacemakers or implantable cardioverter defibrillators (ICDs), which may often provide better treatment options. In view of the current complex range of choices for individuals with heart rhythm problems, specialist referral should be considered in all cases.

We still have few drug options for patients with cardiac arrhythmias, and new often-novel approaches are being developed. Carefully selected and monitored drugs may have useful impacts, but newer agents, e.g. dronedarone, have generally proven difficult to use and clinically disappointing. Patients with heart disease die of either pump failure or arrhythmia, and much of the risk they encounter is due to ventricular arrhythmias, which in selected cases can be minimised with implantable devices such as ICDs rather than with drugs.

- Drugs for cardiac arrhythmias.
- Principal drugs by class.
- Specific treatments, including those for cardiac arrest.

Objectives of treatment

In almost no other set of conditions is it so clearly obvious to remember the dual objectives, which are to reduce *morbidity* and *mortality*.

Arrhythmias are frequently asymptomatic but may be fatal even at first presentation. Indeed, an estimated 70 000 deaths per year are ascribed to ventricular arrhythmias just in the UK. Antiarrhythmic drugs themselves are also capable of generating arrhythmias (see below) and find use only in the presence of clear indications. In addition, antiarrhythmic agents are to a variable degree negatively inotropic (except for digoxin and possibly amiodarone). These observations provide important primary reasons for caution in the use of these drugs.

A background reason for a careful approach to antiarrhythmic treatment is the gulf between knowledge of their mechanism of action and their clinical uses. On the side of normal physiology, we can see the spontaneous generation and propagation of the cardiac impulse requiring a combination of specialised conducting tissue and inter-myocyte conduction. The heart also has backstops in case of problems with a sequential hierarchy of intrinsic pacemakers. By contrast, the available drugs are at an early stage of evolution, and useful antiarrhythmic actions are yet discovered by chance.

Doctors and drugs have historically generally interfered with cardiac electrophysiology at their peril. In emergencies, the most junior doctor in the team often needs to take action, and some rote recommendations are clearly necessary. The diagnosis and elective treatment of chronic or episodic arrhythmias require experience to achieve the best balance between risk and benefit, and this realisation has led to the development of *cardiac electrophysiology* as a distinct therapeutically effective subspecialty of cardiology.

451

Antiarrhythmic drugs in general have had a hard time proving superior safety or efficacy over other therapeutic (non-drug) options.

Some physiology and pathophysiology

There are broadly two types of cardiac tissue.

The *first type* is ordinary myocardial (atrial and ventricular) muscle, responsible for the pumping action of the heart.

The *second type* is specialised conducting tissue that initiates the cardiac electrical impulse and determines the order in which the muscle cells contract. The important property of being able to form impulses spontaneously (*automaticity*) is a feature of certain parts of the conducting tissue, e.g. the sinoatrial (SA) and atrioventricular (AV) nodes. The SA node has the highest frequency of spontaneous discharge, usually around 70 times per minute, and thus controls the contraction rate of the whole heart, making the cells more distal in the system fire more rapidly than they would do spontaneously, i.e. it is the pacemaker. If the SA node fails to function, the next fastest component takes over. This is often the AV node (~45 discharges per min) or sites in the His–Purkinje system (discharge rate about 25 per min).

Altered rates of automatic discharge or an abnormality in the mechanism by which an impulse is generated from a centre in the nodes or conducting tissue, is one cause of cardiac arrhythmia, e.g. atrial fibrillation, atrial flutter or atrial tachycardia.

Ionic movements into and out of cardiac cells

Nearly all cells in the body exhibit a difference in electrical voltage between their interior and exterior, the membrane potential. Some cells, including the conducting and contracting cells of the heart, are excitable. An appropriate stimulus alters the properties of the cell membrane; ions flow across it and thereby elicit an action potential. This spreads to adjacent cells, i.e. it is conducted as an electrical impulse and, when it reaches a muscle cell, causes it to contract; this is excitation–contraction coupling.

In the resting state, the interior of the cell (conducting and contracting types) is electrically negative with respect to the exterior, owing to the disposition of ions (mainly sodium, potassium and calcium) across its membrane, i.e. it is *polarised*. The ionic changes of the action potential first result in a rapid redistribution of ions such that the potential alters to positive within the cell (*depolarisation*); subsequent and slower flows of ions then restore the resting potential

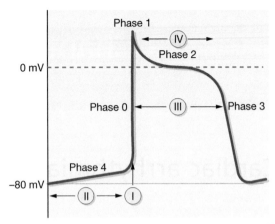

Fig. 25.1 The action potential of a cardiac cell that is capable of spontaneous depolarisation (SA or AV nodal, or His–Purkinje) indicating phases 0–4. The gradual increase in transmembrane potential (mV) during phase 4 is shown; cells that are not capable of spontaneous depolarisation do not exhibit increased voltage during this phase (see text). The modes of action of antiarrhythmic drugs of classes I, II, III and IV are indicated in relation to these phases.

(*repolarisation*). These ionic movements separate into phases, which are briefly described here and in Fig. 25.1, as they help to explain the actions of antiarrhythmic drugs.[1]

Classification of antiarrhythmic drugs

The classification still used partially relates to the phases of the cardiac cycle depicted in Fig. 25.1.

Phase 0 is the rapid depolarisation of the cell membrane that is associated with a fast inflow of sodium ions through channels that are selectively permeable to these ions.

Phase 1 is a short initial period of rapid repolarisation brought about mainly by an outflow of potassium ions.

Phase 2 is a period when there is a delay in repolarisation caused mainly by a slow movement of calcium ions from the exterior into the cell through channels that are selectively permeable to these ions ('long-opening' or L-type calcium channels).

[1]Dobrev D, Nattel S 2010 New antiarrhythmic drugs for treatment of atrial fibrillation. Lancet 375:1212–1223.

Phase 3 is a second period of rapid repolarisation during which potassium ions move out of the cell.

Phase 4 begins with the fully repolarised state. For cells that discharge *automatically,* potassium ions then progressively move back into, and sodium and calcium ions move out of, the cell. The result is that the interior becomes gradually less negative until a certain (threshold) potential is reached, which allows rapid depolarisation (phase 0) to occur, and the cycle is repeated; the prevailing sympathetic tone also influences automaticity. Cells that do not discharge spontaneously rely on the arrival of an action potential from another cell to initiate depolarisation.

In phases 1 and 2, the cell is in an *absolutely refractory* state and is incapable of responding further to any stimulus, but during phase 3, the *relative refractory period*, the cell will depolarise again if a stimulus is sufficiently strong. The orderly transmission of an electrical impulse (the action potential) throughout the conducting system may be retarded in an area of disease, e.g. localised ischaemia or scar tissue due to previous myocardial infarction. An impulse travelling down a normal Purkinje fibre may spread to an adjacent fibre that has transiently failed to transmit, and pass up it in the *reverse* direction. Should such a retrograde impulse in turn re-excite the cells that provided the original impulse, *re-entrant excitation* becomes established and may cause an arrhythmia, e.g. ventricular tachycardia, paroxysmal supraventricular tachycardia, atrial flutter, and so on.

Most cardiac arrhythmias are due to either:

- *slowed conduction* in part of the system leading to the formation of re-entry circuits (more than 90% of tachycardias), or
- *altered rate of spontaneous discharge* in conducting tissue. Some ectopic pacemakers appear to depend on adrenergic drive.

Classification of drugs

The Vaughan-Williams[2] classification of antiarrhythmic drugs is still commonly used despite its many peculiarities, and on occasion provides a useful shorthand for referring to particular groups or actions of drugs.

Class I: sodium channel blockade. These drugs restrict the rapid inflow of sodium during phase 0 and thus slow the maximum rate of depolarisation. Another term for this property is *membrane stabilising activity*; the action may contribute to stopping arrhythmias by limiting the responsiveness to excitation of cardiac cells. The class subdivides into drugs that:

1A. *lengthen* action potential duration and refractoriness (adjunctive class III action), e.g. quinidine, disopyramide, procainamide
1B. *shorten* action potential duration and refractoriness, e.g. lidocaine and mexiletine
1C. have *negligible effect* on action potential duration and refractoriness, e.g. flecainide, propafenone.

One value of using the classification is the knowledge that drugs in class 1B are ineffective for supraventricular arrhythmias, whereas they all have some action in ventricular arrhythmias. One feature is that it is not useful in explaining why the classes differ anatomically in their efficacy.

Class II: catecholamine blockade. Propranolol and other β-adrenoceptor antagonists reduce background sympathetic tone in the heart, reduce automatic discharge (phase 4) and protect against adrenergically stimulated ectopic pacemakers.

Class III: lengthening of refractoriness (without effect on sodium inflow in phase 0). Prolongation of the cardiac action potential and increased cellular refractoriness beyond a critical point may stop a re-entrant circuit being completed and thereby prevent or halt a re-entrant arrhythmia (see above), e.g. amiodarone, sotalol. These drugs act by inhibiting I_{Kr}, the rapidly activating component of the delayed rectifier potassium current (phase 3). The gene *hERG* (the *human ether-à-go-go related gene*) encodes a major subunit of the protein responsible for I_{Kr}. These are the most commonly used antiarrhythmic drugs, although newer agents in this class, e.g. dofetilide, azimilide, dronedarone, have not achieved wide use based on a variety of concerns.

Class IV: calcium channel blockade These drugs depress the slow inward calcium current (phase 2) and prolong conduction and refractoriness particularly in the SA and AV nodes, which helps to explain their effectiveness in terminating paroxysmal supraventricular tachycardia, e.g. verapamil.

Antiarrhythmic drugs are classified here according to a characteristic major action, but most have other effects as well. For example, quinidine (class I) has major class III effects, propranolol (class II) has minor class I effects, and sotalol (class II) has major class III effects. Amiodarone and dronedarone both have class I, II, III and IV effects but are usually placed under class III.

Principal drugs by class

For further data, see Table 25.1.

---

[2]Roden D M 2003 Antiarrhythmic drugs: past, present and future. Journal of Cardiovascular Electrophysiology 14:1389–1396.

Table 25.1 Drugs for cardiac arrhythmia

Class	Drug	Usual doses[a] and interval	Effect on ECG	Usually effective plasma concentration
1A	Disopyramide	p.o.: 300–800 mg/day in divided doses i.v.: see specialist literature	Prolongs QRS, QTc and (±) PR	2–5 mg/L
IB	Lidocaine	i.v. loading: 100 mg as a bolus over a few min i.v.; maintenance: 1–4 mg/min	No significant change	1.5–6 mg/L
	Mexiletine	p.o.: initial dose 400 mg, then after 2 h 200–250 mg × 6–8 h i.v: see specialist literature	No significant change	0.5–2 mg/L
IC	Flecainide	p.o.: 50–150 mg × 12 h: see specialist literature	Prolongs PR and QRS	0.2 mg/L
	Propafenone	p.o.: see specialist literature	Prolongs PR and QRS	Active metabolite precludes establishment
II	Propranolol	p.o.: 10–80 mg × 6 h i.v: 1 mg over 1-min intervals to 10 mg max. (5 mg in anaesthesia)	Prolongs PR (±) No change in QRS Shortens QTc Bradycardia	Not established
	Sotalol	40–160 mg × 2/day	Prolongs QTc and PR Sinus bradycardia	Not clinically useful
	Esmolol	i.v: infusion 50–200 μg/kg/min	As for propranolol	0.15–2 mg/L
III	Amiodarone Dronedarone	p.o.: loading: 200 mg × 8 h for 1 week, then 200 mg × 12 h for 1 week; maintenance 200 mg/day 400 mg b.d.	Prolongs PR, QRS and QTc Sinus bradycardia No significant change	Not established Not clinically useful
IV	Verapamil	p.o.: 40–120 mg × 8–12 h i.v: see specialist literature	Prolongs PR	Not clinically useful
Other	Digoxin	p.o.: initially 1–1.5 mg in divided doses over 24 h; maintenance: 62.5–500 μg/day	Prolongs PR Depresses ST segment Flattens T wave	1–2 μg/L
	Adenosine	i.v: 6 mg initially; if no conversion after 1–2 min, give 12 mg and repeat once if necessary. Follow each bolus with saline flush	Prolongs PR Transient heart block	Not clinically useful

[a]Doses based on *British National Formulary* recommendations. Patients with decreased hepatic or renal function may require lower doses (see text). This table is adapted from that published in the *Medical Letter on Drugs and Therapeutics* (USA) 1996. We are grateful to the Chairman of the Editorial Board for allowing us to use this material.

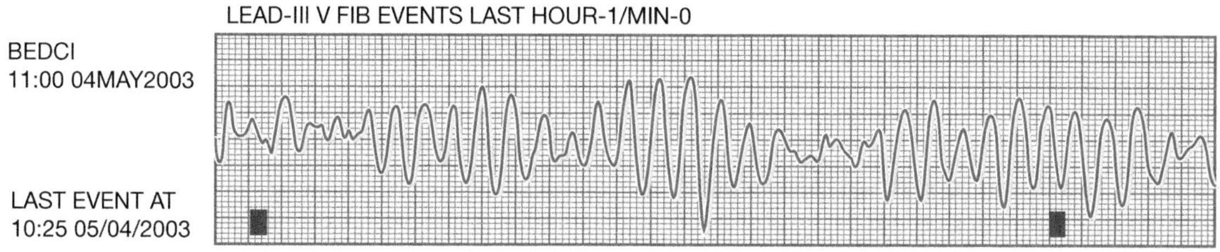

LEAD-III V FIB EVENTS LAST HOUR-1/MIN-0

BEDCI
11:00 04MAY2003

LAST EVENT AT
10:25 05/04/2003

Fig. 25.2 Torsade de pointes ventricular arrhythmia. This patient had received the potassium channel–blocking drug, amiodarone, which prolonged the QTc interval and produced this characteristic 'twisting about the points' pattern.

Class 1A (sodium channel blockade with lengthened refractoriness)

Quinidine

Quinidine is considered the prototype antiarrhythmic drug,[3] although it is now used quite rarely and indeed is not available in some jurisdictions. It has a newly identified use that is unique in that it appears to be effective in reducing the risks of sudden cardiac death in those with Brugada syndrome.[4] In addition to its class IA activity, quinidine slightly enhances contractility of the myocardium (positive inotropic effect) and reduces vagus nerve activity on the heart (antimuscarinic effect).

Pharmacokinetics. Absorption of quinidine from the gut is rapid; 75% of the drug is metabolised, and the remainder is eliminated unchanged in the urine ($t_{1/2}$ 7 h). Active metabolites may accumulate when renal function is impaired.

Adverse reactions. Quinidine must not be used alone to treat atrial fibrillation or flutter as its antimuscarinic action enhances AV conduction and the heart rate may accelerate. Other cardiac effects include serious ventricular tachyarrhythmias associated with electrocardiographic QT prolongation, i.e. *torsade de pointes* (Fig. 25.2), the cause of 'quinidine syncope'. Non-cardiac effects, called 'cinchonism', include diarrhoea and other gastrointestinal symptoms, rashes, thrombocytopenia and fever, and these have substantially limited its use.

---

[3]In 1912, K F Wenckebach, a Dutch physician (who described 'Wenckebach block') was visited by a merchant who wished to get rid of an attack of atrial fibrillation (he had recurrent attacks which, although they did not unduly inconvenience him, offended his notions of good order in life's affairs). On receiving a guarded prognosis, the merchant inquired why there were heart specialists if they could not accomplish what he himself had already achieved. In the face of Wenckebach's incredulity, he promised to return the next day with a regular pulse, which he did, at the same time revealing that he had done it with quinine (an optical isomer of quinidine). Examination of quinine derivatives led to the introduction of quinidine in 1918 (Wenckebach K F 1923 Cinchona derivates in the treatment of heart disorders. Journal of the American Medical Association 81:472–474).
[4]An inherited condition that is the major cause of sudden unexpected death syndrome (SUDS), commonly in young men.

Disopyramide

Disopyramide was the most commonly used drug in this class but is much less so now. It has significant antimuscarinic activity.

Pharmacokinetics. Disopyramide is used orally (see Table 25.1) and is well absorbed. It is in part excreted unchanged and in part metabolised. The $t_{1/2}$ is 6 h.

Adverse reactions. The antimuscarinic activity is often a significant clinical problem causing dry mouth, blurred vision, glaucoma, micturition hesitancy and retention. Gastrointestinal symptoms, rash and agranulocytosis can also occur. Effects on the cardiovascular system include hypotension and heart failure (negative inotropic effect).

Class IB (sodium channel blockade with shortened refractoriness)

Lidocaine

Lidocaine finds use principally for ventricular arrhythmias, especially those complicating myocardial infarction or occurring, e.g., after cardiothoracic surgery. Its kinetics render it unsuitable for oral administration, and its application is restricted to the treatment of acute ventricular arrhythmias.

Pharmacokinetics. Lidocaine is used intravenously and has occasionally been used intramuscularly; dosing by mouth is unsatisfactory because its $t_{1/2}$ is short (1.5 h) and the drug undergoes extensive pre-systemic (first-pass) elimination in the liver.

Adverse reactions are uncommon unless infusion is rapid or there is significant heart failure; they include hypotension, dizziness, blurred sight, sleepiness, slurred speech, numbness, sweating, confusion and convulsions.

Mexiletine is similar to lidocaine but is effective orally ($t_{1/2}$ 10 h). It has been used for ventricular arrhythmias, especially those complicating myocardial infarction, but is usually poorly tolerated and has been withdrawn in many jurisdictions.

455

Adverse reactions, almost universal and dose related, include nausea, vomiting, hiccough, tremor, drowsiness, confusion, dysarthria, diplopia, ataxia, cardiac arrhythmia and hypotension.

Class IC (sodium channel blockade with minimal effect on refractoriness)

Flecainide

Flecainide slows conduction in all cardiac cells including the accessory pathways responsible for the Wolff–Parkinson–White (WPW) syndrome.

One common indication – indeed where it is the drug of choice – is atrioventricular (AV) re-entrant tachycardia, such as AV nodal tachycardia or in the tachycardias associated with the WPW syndrome or similar conditions with anomalous pathways. This should be as a prelude to definitive treatment with radiofrequency ablation, which is the overall treatment approach of choice. Flecainide is also very useful in patients with paroxysmal atrial fibrillation, used in conjunction with an agent that blocks the AV node to protect against rapid conduction to the ventricle. Following the salutary findings of the CAST study,[5] flecainide is now restricted to patients without evidence of coronary or structural heart disease. Indeed, before it is used an echocardiogram is essential, and in patients at potential risk of coronary artery disease an exercise test or an alternative test of ischaemia is often conducted.

Pharmacokinetics. Metabolism in the liver and renal elimination of unchanged metabolites terminates its action. The $t_{1/2}$ is 14 h in healthy adults but may be over 20 h in patients with heart disease, in the elderly and in those with poor renal function.

Adverse reactions. Flecainide is contraindicated in patients with sinus node disease, heart failure, and in those with a history of myocardial infarction, especially if they have a history of ventricular arrhythmias. Minor adverse effects include blurred vision, abdominal discomfort, nausea, dizziness, tremor, abnormal taste sensations and paraesthesiae.

Propafenone

In addition to the defining properties of this class, propafenone has β-adrenoceptor–blocking activity equivalent to a low dose of propranolol. It is occasionally used to suppress non-sustained ventricular arrhythmias in patients whose left ventricular function is normal.

Pharmacokinetics. Propafenone is metabolised by the liver and is a substrate for CYP 2D6. Some 7% of Caucasian patients are poor metabolisers who, for equivalent doses, thus have higher plasma concentrations than the remainder of the population.

Adverse reactions are similar to those of flecainide and are commoner in poor metabolisers. In addition, conduction block may occur, heart failure may worsen and ventricular arrhythmias may be exacerbated, and propafenone should not be used in patients with sustained ventricular tachycardia and poor left ventricular function.

Class II (catecholamine blockade)

β-Adrenoceptor antagonists

(See also Ch. 24.)

β-Adrenoceptor blockers are effective in the prophylaxis of cardiac arrhythmia probably because they counteract the arrhythmogenic effect of catecholamines. The following actions appear to be relevant:

- The rate of automatic firing of the SA node is accelerated by β-adrenoceptor activation, and this effect is abolished by β-blockers. Some ectopic pacemakers appear to be dependent on adrenergic drive.
- β-Blockers prolong the refractoriness of the AV node, which may prevent re-entrant tachycardias that are dependent on the AV node for their perpetuation.
- Many β-Blocking drugs (propranolol, oxprenolol, acebutolol, labetalol) also possess membrane stabilising (class I) properties. Sotalol also prolongs cardiac refractoriness (class III effect) but has no class I effects; it is often preferred when a β-blocker is indicated for arrhythmias, but should be used with care. Esmolol (below) is a short-acting $β_1$-selective agent, whose sole use is in the treatment of arrhythmias. Its short duration and $β_1$ selectivity make it an option for some patients with contraindications to other β-blocking drugs.

---

[5]Flecainide, encainide and moricizine underwent clinical trial to establish whether suppression of asymptomatic premature beats with antiarrhythmic drugs would reduce the risk of death from arrhythmia after myocardial infarction. The study was terminated after preliminary analysis of 1727 patients revealed that the mortality rate in patients treated with flecainide or encainide was 7.7% compared with 3% in controls. The most likely explanation for the result was the induction of fatal ventricular arrhythmias, possibly in conjunction with ischaemia by flecainide and encainide, i.e. a proarrhythmic effect (Cardiac Arrhythmia Suppression Trial (CAST) Investigators 1989 Preliminary report: effect of encainide and flecainide on mortality in a randomised trial of arrhythmia suppression after myocardial infarction. New England Journal of Medicine 321:406–412).

- β-Adrenoceptor antagonists are effective for a range of supraventricular arrhythmias, in particular those associated with exercise, emotion or hyperthyroidism. Sotalol finds use to suppress ventricular ectopic beats and ventricular tachycardia, although care should be taken with careful monitoring of the QT interval whenever it is used.

Pharmacokinetics. For long-term use, any of the oral preparations of β-blocker are suitable. In emergencies, esmolol is used (see Table 25.1), its short $t_{1/2}$ (9 min) rendering it suitable for administration by intravenous infusion with rapid alterations in dose, according to response.

Adverse reactions. Cardiac effects from overdosage include heart block or even cardiac arrest. Heart failure may be precipitated in a patient dependent on sympathetic drive to maintain cardiac output.

Interactions. Concomitant intravenous administration of a calcium channel blocker that affects conduction (verapamil, diltiazem) increases the risk of bradycardia and AV block. In patients with depressed myocardial contractility, the combination of oral or intravenous β-blockade and calcium channel blockade (nifedipine, verapamil) may cause hypotension or heart failure.

Class III (lengthening of refractoriness due to potassium channel blockade)

Amiodarone

Amiodarone is the most powerful antiarrhythmic drug available for the treatment and prevention of both atrial and ventricular arrhythmias. Even short-term use can result in serious toxicity, and its use should always follow a consideration or a trial of alternatives. Amiodarone prolongs the effective refractory period of myocardial cells, the AV node and of anomalous pathways. It also blocks β-adrenoceptors non-competitively.

Amiodarone is used in chronic ventricular arrhythmias and in atrial fibrillation, in which condition it both slows the ventricular response and may restore sinus rhythm (chemical cardioversion). It may also be used to maintain sinus rhythm after cardioversion for atrial fibrillation or flutter. Amiodarone has been used for the management of re-entrant supraventricular tachycardias associated with the WPW syndrome, but radiofrequency ablation is now the treatment of choice and amiodarone should not in general be used.

Pharmacokinetics. Amiodarone is effective given orally; its enormous apparent distribution volume (70 L/kg) indicates that little remains in the blood. It is stored in fat and many other tissues, and the $t_{1/2}$ of 54 days after multiple dosing signifies slow release from these sites (and slow accumulation to steady state means that a loading dose is necessary; see Table 25.1). The drug is metabolised in the liver and eliminated through the biliary and intestinal tracts.

Adverse reactions. Cardiovascular effects include bradycardia, heart block and induction of ventricular arrhythmia associated with QT prolongation. Other effects include nausea, vomiting, taste disturbances and the development of corneal microdeposits, which may rarely cause visual halos, night glare and photophobia; the latter are dose related, resolve on discontinuation and do not threaten vision. Sleep disturbance and vivid dreams may be prominent and problematic. Plasma transaminase levels may rise (requiring dose reduction or withdrawal if accompanied by acute liver disorders). Amiodarone contains iodine, and both hyperthyroidism and hypothyroidism are quite common; monitoring thyroid function before and during therapy is essential (see Ch. 37).

Photosensitivity reactions are common, may be severe and patients should be warned explicitly when starting the drug. Amiodarone may also cause a bluish discoloration on exposed areas of the skin (occasionally reversible on discontinuing the drug). Less commonly, pneumonitis and pulmonary fibrosis occur and hepatitis, sometimes rapidly during short-term use of the drug; these may be fatal, so vigilance should be high. Cirrhosis is reported. Peripheral neuropathy and myopathy occur (usually reversible on withdrawal).

Interaction with digoxin (by displacement from tissue-binding sites and interference with its elimination) and with warfarin (by inhibiting its metabolism) increases the effect of both these drugs. β-Blockers and calcium channel antagonists augment the depressant effect of amiodarone on SA and AV node function.

Dronedarone

While amiodarone is less pro-arrhythmic than other conventional antiarrhythmic drugs, e.g. flecainide (possibly because it is a 'multi-channel blocker'), it has substantial non-cardiac toxic effects. Dronedarone is structurally similar to amiodarone but has no iodine component and reduced lipophilicity. Dronedarone thus has a shorter half-life and appears better tolerated, with low pro-arrhythmic risk.

Dronedarone has been shown to reduce the time to first recurrence of atrial fibrillation. In the EURIDIS and ADONIS clinical trials,[6] patients taking dronedarone had a 25%

---

[6]Singh B N, Connolly S J, Crijns H J et al; EURIDIS and ADONIS Investigators 2007 Dronedarone for maintenance of sinus rhythm in atrial fibrillation or flutter. New England Journal of Medicine 357:987–999.

reduction in the risk of AF recurrence over 1 year, compared with placebo. In the ATHENA study,[7] dronedarone also reduced the combined risk of cardiovascular hospitalisation or all-cause death by 24% in patients with current or recent AF and an additional risk factor for death, compared with placebo. A post hoc analysis found that dronedarone, compared with placebo, was associated with a significant reduction in the risk of stroke in paroxysmal and persistent AF patients. Data from the DIONYSOS trial[8] suggest that dronedarone may have an improved safety profile when compared to amiodarone, mainly driven by fewer thyroid and neurologic events and less premature discontinuation due to adverse events.

Pharmacokinetics. The absolute bioavailability of dronedarone (given with food) is 15%. It undergoes extensive first-pass metabolism through the CYP 450 3A4 system; hence strong inhibitors of this enzyme should not be co-administered with dronedarone. After oral administration in fed conditions, peak plasma concentrations of dronedarone are reached within 3–6 hours. Steady state is reached within 4–8 days. Dronedarone is mostly excreted in the faeces with only 6% excreted renally, and it has an elimination half-life of 28 h.

Contraindications. Dronedarone is contraindicated in patients with unstable haemodynamic conditions, including patients with symptoms of heart failure at rest or with minimal exertion (corresponding with NYHA class IV and unstable class III patients). Dronedarone is not recommended in stable patients with recent (1–3 months) NYHA class III heart failure, or left ventricular ejection fraction <35%. Patients should consult their doctor if they experience worsening heart failure symptoms.

Due to pharmacokinetic and possible pharmacodynamic interactions, both β-blockers and calcium channel blockers with depressant effects on the sinus and atrioventricular nodes (such as verapamil and diltiazem) should be used with caution when prescribed with dronedarone. They should be initiated at low dose, which should only be increased after ECG assessment. In patients already taking β-blockers or calcium channel blockers, an ECG should be performed and the β-blocker/calcium channel blocker dose should be adjusted if needed.

Unwanted effects. Common side-effects include diarrhoea, abdominal discomfort, nausea, vomiting and prolonged QT interval. Supportive symptomatic treatment should be provided, and attention should be paid to hydration in those most severely affected. In a proportion of patients, dronedarone may need to be discontinued because of intolerance. There is an increased incidence of skin rash and bradycardia.

Plasma creatinine should be measured 7 days after starting dronedarone, as an increase of approximately 10 micromol/L has been observed with dronedarone 400 mg twice daily in both healthy controls and in patients. This occurs early after treatment initiation and reaches a plateau after 7 days.

Recently released European Society of Cardiology guidelines have included dronedarone as a treatment option for non-permanent AF for rhythm and rate control (see below, Fig. 25.6).

Class IV (calcium channel blockade)

Calcium is involved in the contraction of cardiac and vascular smooth muscle cells, and in the automaticity of cardiac pacemaker cells. Actions of calcium channel blockers on vascular smooth muscle cells appear with the main account of these drugs in Chapter 24. Although the three classes of calcium channel blocker have similar effects on vascular smooth muscle in the arterial tree, their cardiac actions differ. The phenylalkylamine, verapamil, depresses myocardial contraction more than the others, and both verapamil and diltiazem slow conduction in the AV node.

Calcium and cardiac cells

Cardiac muscle cells are normally depolarised by the fast inward flow of sodium ions, following which there is a slow inward flow of calcium ions through the L-type calcium channels (phase 2 in Fig. 25.1); the consequent rise in free intracellular calcium ions activates the contractile mechanism.

Pacemaker cells in the SA and AV nodes rely heavily on the slow inward flow of calcium ions (phase 4) for their capacity to discharge spontaneously, i.e. for their automaticity.

Calcium channel blockers inhibit the passage of calcium through the membrane channels; the result in myocardial cells is to depress contractility, and in pacemaker cells to suppress their automatic activity. Members of the group therefore may have negative cardiac inotropic and chronotropic actions, which can be separated: nifedipine, at therapeutic concentrations, acts almost exclusively on non-cardiac ion channels and has no clinically useful antiarrhythmic activity, whereas verapamil is an effective rate control agent.

[7]Hohnloser S H, Crijns H J, van Eickels M et al; ATHENA Investigators 2009 Effect of dronedarone on cardiovascular events in atrial fibrillation. New England Journal of Medicine 360:668–678.
[8]Le Heuzey J Y, De Ferrari G M, Radzik D et al 2010 A short-term, randomised, double-blind, parallel-group study to evaluate the efficacy and safety of dronedarone versus amiodarone in patients with persistent atrial fibrillation: the DIONYSOS study. Journal of Cardiovascular Electrophysiology 21:597–605.

Verapamil

Verapamil (see also p. 419) prolongs conduction and refractoriness in the AV node and depresses the rate of discharge of the SA node. If adenosine is not available, verapamil is a very attractive and, with due care, safe alternative for terminating narrow complex paroxysmal supraventricular tachycardia. Verapamil should not be given intravenously to patients with broad complex tachyarrhythmias whatever the presumptive mechanism, for it may prove lethal.

Adverse effects include nausea, constipation, headache, fatigue, hypotension, bradycardia and heart block.

Other arrhythmia modifying agents

Digoxin and other cardiac glycosides[9]

Crude digitalis is a preparation of the dried leaf of the foxglove plants *Digitalis purpurea* or *lanata*. Digitalis contains a number of active glycosides (digoxin, lanatosides) whose actions are qualitatively similar, differing principally in rapidity of onset and duration of action; the pure individual glycosides are used. The following account refers to all the cardiac glycosides, but digoxin is the principal one.

Mode of action. Cardiac glycosides affect the heart both directly and indirectly in a series of complex actions, some of which oppose one another. The *direct* effect is to inhibit the membrane-bound sodium–potassium adenosine triphosphatase (Na$^+$, K$^+$-ATPase) enzyme that supplies energy for the system that pumps sodium out of and transports potassium into contracting and conducting cells. By reducing the exchange of extracellular sodium with intracellular calcium, digoxin raises the store of intracellular calcium, which facilitates muscular contraction. The *indirect* effect is

to enhance vagal activity by complex peripheral and central mechanisms. The clinically important consequences are on:

- the contracting cells: increased contractility and excitability
- SA and AV nodes and conducting tissue: decreased impulse generation and propagation.

Uses. Digoxin is not strictly an antiarrhythmic agent, but rather it modulates the response to arrhythmias. Its most useful property, in this respect, is to slow conduction through the AV node. The main uses are in the following:

- *Atrial fibrillation*, benefiting chiefly by the vagal effect on the AV node, reducing conduction through it and thus slowing the ventricular rate. Its use in this setting is limited, and treatment with β-blockers and calcium channel blockers is generally preferred as they are more effective and less likely to cause adverse effects.
- *Atrial flutter*, benefiting by the vagus nerve action of shortening the refractory period of the atrial muscle so that flutter may occasionally be converted to fibrillation (in which state the ventricular rate is more readily controlled). Electrical cardioversion followed by referral for radiofrequency ablation is the preferred option when ablation is available.
- *Heart failure*, benefiting chiefly by the direct action to increase myocardial contractility. Digoxin is still used occasionally in chronic heart failure due to ischaemic, hypertensive or valvular heart disease, especially in the short term. This is no longer a major indication following the introduction of other groups of drugs.

Pharmacokinetics. Digoxin is eliminated 85% unchanged by the kidney, and the remainder is metabolised by the liver. The $t_{1/2}$ is 36 h. Digoxin is usually administered by mouth.

Dose and therapeutic plasma concentration (see Table 25.1). *Reduced* dose of digoxin is necessary in: renal impairment (see above); the elderly (probably due to the decline in renal clearance with age); electrolyte disturbances (hypokalaemia accentuates the potential for adverse effects of digoxin, as does hypomagnesaemia); and hypothyroid patients (who are intolerant of digoxin).

Adverse effects. Abnormal cardiac rhythms due to digoxin usually take the form of ectopic arrhythmias (ventricular ectopic beats, ventricular tachyarrhythmias, paroxysmal supraventricular tachycardia) and heart block. Gastrointestinal effects include anorexia, which usually precedes vomiting and is a warning that dosage is excessive. Diarrhoea may also occur. Visual effects include disturbances of colour vision, e.g. yellow discolouration (xanthopsia) but also red or green vision, photophobia and blurring. Gynaecomastia in men and breast enlargement in women is seen with

---

[9]In 1775 Dr William Withering was making a routine journey from Birmingham (England), his home, to see patients at the Stafford Infirmary. While the carriage horses were being changed half-way, he was asked to see an old dropsical (oedematous) woman. He thought she would die and so some weeks later, when he heard of her recovery, was interested enough to enquire into the cause. Recovery was attributed to a herb tea containing some 20 ingredients, among which Withering, already the author of a botanical textbook, found it 'not very difficult … to perceive that the active herb could be no other than the foxglove'. He began to investigate its properties, trying it on the poor of Birmingham, whom he used to see without fee each day. The results were inconclusive and his interest flagged until one day he heard that the principal of an Oxford College had been cured by foxglove after 'some of the first physicians of the age had declared that they could do no more for him'. This put a new complexion on the matter and, pursuing his investigation, Withering found that foxglove extract caused diuresis in some oedematous patients. He defined the type of patient who might benefit from it and, equally importantly, he standardised his foxglove leaf preparations and was able to lay down accurate dosage schedules. His advice, with little amplification, served until relatively recently (Withering W 1785 An Account of the Foxglove. Robinson, London).

long-term use (cardiac glycosides have structural resemblance to oestrogen). Mental effects include confusion, restlessness, agitation, nightmares and acute psychoses.

Acute digoxin poisoning causes initial nausea and vomiting and hyperkalaemia because inhibition of the Na^+, K^+-ATPase pump prevents intracellular accumulation of potassium. The ECG changes (see Table 25.1) of prolonged use of digoxin may be absent. There may be exaggerated sinus arrhythmia, bradycardia and ectopic rhythms with or without heart block.

Treatment of overdose. For severe digoxin poisoning, infusion of the digoxin-specific binding (Fab) fragment of an antibody to digoxin (Digibind) neutralises digoxin in the plasma and is an effective treatment. Because it lacks the Fc segment, this fragment is relatively non-immunogenic and is sufficiently small to be eliminated as the digoxin–antibody complex in the urine. Intravenous phenytoin has been used for ventricular arrhythmias, although formal efficacy has not been established, with atropine used for bradycardia. Temporary electrical pacing may be needed.

Interactions. Verapamil, nifedipine and amiodarone raise steady-state plasma digoxin concentrations (see above), and the digoxin dose should be lowered when any of these is added. The likelihood of AV block due to digoxin is increased by verapamil and by β-adrenoceptor blockers.

Adenosine

Adenosine is an endogenous purine nucleotide that slows atrioventricular conduction and dilates coronary and peripheral arteries. It is rapidly metabolised by circulating adenosine deaminase and is also taken up by cells; hence its residence in plasma is brief ($t_{1/2}$ <2 s), and it must be given rapidly intravenously.

Administered as a bolus injection, adenosine is effective for terminating paroxysmal supraventricular (re-entrant) tachycardias, including episodes in patients with Wolff–Parkinson–White syndrome. The initial dose in adults is 6 mg over 2 s with continuous ECG monitoring, with doubling increments every 1–2 min. The average total dose is 125 µg/kg.

Adenosine is an alternative to verapamil for supraventricular tachycardia and possibly safer because adenosine is short acting and not negatively inotropic; verapamil is dangerous if used mistakenly in a ventricular tachycardia.

Adverse effects from adenosine are usually not serious because of the brevity of its action, but it may cause distressing dyspnoea, facial flushing, chest pain and transient arrhythmias, e.g. bradycardia. Adenosine should not be given to asthmatics or to patients with second- or third-degree AV block or sick sinus syndrome (unless a pacemaker is in place).

Cardiac effects of the autonomic nervous system

Some drugs used for arrhythmias exert their actions through the autonomic nervous system by mimicking or antagonising the effects of the sympathetic or parasympathetic nerves that supply the heart. The neurotransmitters in these two branches of the autonomic system, noradrenaline/norepinephrine and acetylcholine, are functionally antagonistic by having opposing actions on cyclic AMP production within the cardiomyocyte. Their receptors are coupled to the two trimeric GTP-binding proteins, G_s and G_i, which stimulate and inhibit adenylyl cyclase, respectively.

The sympathetic division (adrenergic component of the autonomic nervous system), when stimulated, has the following (receptor) effects on the heart:

- Tachycardia due to increased rate of discharge of the SA node.
- Increased automaticity in the AV node and His–Purkinje system.
- Increase in conductivity in the His–Purkinje system.
- Increased force of contraction.
- Shortening of the refractory period.

Isoprotenerol, a β-adrenoceptor agonist, has been used to accelerate the heart when there is extreme bradycardia due to heart block, prior to the insertion of an implanted pacemaker, although this is now rarely used. It is also used by interventional cardiac electrophysiologists to induce cardiac arrhythmias both for diagnosis and both before and after ablation procedures. Adverse effects are those expected of β-adrenoceptor agonists and include tremor, flushing, sweating, palpitation, headache and diarrhoea.

The vagus nerve (*cholinergic, parasympathetic*), when stimulated, affects the heart in ways that are useful in the therapy of arrhythmias, by causing:

- bradycardia due to depression of the SA node
- slowing of conduction through and increased refractoriness of the AV node
- shortening of the refractory period of atrial muscle cells
- decreased myocardial excitability.

There is also reduced *force of contraction* of atrial and ventricular muscle cells.

Vagal stimulation can slow or terminate supraventricular arrhythmias, reflexly by physical manoeuvres (under ECG control, if possible).

Carotid sinus massage activates stretch receptors: external pressure is applied gently to one side at a time (but not to both sides at once). Some individuals are very sensitive to the procedure and develop severe bradycardia and hypotension.

Other methods include the *Valsalva manoeuvre* (deep inspiration followed by expiration against a closed glottis, which both stimulates stretch receptors in the lung and reduces venous return to the heart); *the Müller procedure* (deep expiration followed by inspiration against a closed glottis); production of nausea and retching by inviting patients to put their own fingers down their throat.

The effects of vagus nerve activity are blocked by *atropine* (antimuscarinic action), an action that is used to accelerate the heart during episodes of sinus bradycardia as may occur after myocardial infarction. The dose is 600 µg i.v. and repeated as necessary to a maximum of 3 mg.

Adverse effects are those of muscarinic blockade, namely dry mouth, blurred vision, urinary retention, confusion and hallucination.

Proarrhythmic drug effects

All antiarrhythmic drugs can also cause arrhythmia; they should be used with care and almost invariably following advice from a specialist (heart rhythm specialist/electrophysiologist). Such proarrhythmic effects most commonly occur with drugs that prolong the QTc interval or QRS complex of the ECG; hypokalaemia aggravates the danger. Quinidine may cause tachyarrhythmias, *torsade de pointes* (see Fig. 25.2) in an estimated 4–6% of patients. The Cardiac Arrhythmia Suppression Trial (CAST) revealed a probable pro-arrhythmic effect of flecainide resulting in fatalities (see p. 456). Digoxin can induce a variety of bradyarrhythmias and tachyarrhythmias (see above).

Choice between drugs and electroconversion

Direct current (DC) electric shock applied externally is often the best way to convert cardiac arrhythmias to sinus rhythm. Many atrial or ventricular arrhythmias start from transiently operating factors but, once they have begun, the abnormal mechanisms are self-sustaining. With a successful electric shock, the heart is depolarised, the ectopic focus is extinguished and the SA node, the part of the heart with the highest automaticity, resumes as the dominant pacemaker.

Electrical conversion has the advantage that it is immediate, unlike drugs, which may take days or longer to act; also, the effective doses and adverse effects of drugs are largely unpredictable and can be serious.[10]

Uses of electrical conversion: in supraventricular and ventricular tachycardia, ventricular fibrillation and atrial fibrillation and flutter. Drugs can be useful to prevent a relapse, e.g. sotalol, amiodarone. See also the UK Resuscitation Council's guidelines (Figs 25.3–25.5).

Specific treatments[11]

Sinus bradycardia

Acute sinus bradycardia requires treatment if it is symptomatic, e.g. where there is hypotension or escape rhythms; extreme bradycardia may allow a ventricular focus to take over and lead to ventricular tachycardia. The foot of the bed should be raised to assist venous return, and atropine should be given intravenously. Chronic symptomatic bradycardia is an indication for the insertion of a permanent pacemaker.

Atrial ectopic beats

Reduction in the use of tea, coffee and other methylxanthine-containing drinks, and of tobacco, may suffice for ectopic beats not due to organic heart disease. For persistent symptoms, a small dose of a β-adrenoceptor blocker may be effective.

Paroxysmal supraventricular (AV re-entrant or atrial) tachycardia

For acute attacks, if vagal stimulation (by carotid sinus massage, or swallowing ice) is unsuccessful, adenosine has the dual advantage of being effective in most such tachycardias, while having no effect on a ventricular tachycardia. The response to adenosine is therefore also of diagnostic value. Intravenous verapamil is an alternative for the acute management of a narrow complex tachycardia. If the patient is in circulatory shock from the tachycardia, or drug treatment fails, DC conversion delivers immediate effects. Flecainide and sotalol are the drugs of choice for prophylaxis, but patients should also be referred to heart rhythm

---

[10]To the layperson, 'shock' treatment could be interpreted as frights (which stimulate the vagus, as described above), or as the electrical sort. Dr James Le Fanu quotes a Belfast doctor who reported a farmer with a solution that covered both possibilities. He had suffered from episodes of palpitations and dizziness for 30 years. When he first got

them, he would jump from a barrel and thump his feet hard on the ground at landing. This became less effective with time. His next 'cure' was to remove his clothes, climb a ladder and jump from a considerable height into a cold water tank on the farm. Later, he discovered the best and simplest treatment was to grab hold of his high-voltage electrified cattle fence – although if he was wearing Wellington (rubber) boots he found he had to earth the shock, so besides grabbing the fence with one hand he simultaneously shoved a finger of the other hand into the ground.

[11]See also UK Resuscitation Council guidelines (Figs 25.3–25.5).

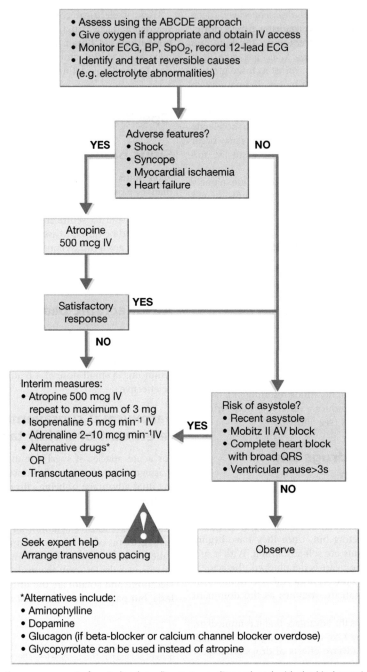

- Assess using the ABCDE approach
- Give oxygen if appropriate and obtain IV access
- Monitor ECG, BP, SpO$_2$, record 12-lead ECG
- Identify and treat reversible causes
  (e.g. electrolyte abnormalities)

Adverse features?
- Shock
- Syncope
- Myocardial ischaemia
- Heart failure

YES   NO

Atropine
500 mcg IV

Satisfactory response   YES

NO

Interim measures:
- Atropine 500 mcg IV
  repeat to maximum of 3 mg
- Isoprenaline 5 mcg min^{-1} IV
- Adrenaline 2–10 mcg min^{-1}IV
- Alternative drugs*
  OR
- Transcutaneous pacing

YES

Risk of asystole?
- Recent asystole
- Mobitz II AV block
- Complete heart block
  with broad QRS
- Ventricular pause>3s

NO

Seek expert help
Arrange transvenous pacing

Observe

*Alternatives include:
- Aminophylline
- Dopamine
- Glucagon (if beta-blocker or calcium channel blocker overdose)
- Glycopyrrolate can be used instead of atropine

Fig. 25.3 Algorithm for the management of acute bradycardia. mcg, μg. *(Reproduced with the kind permission of the Resuscitation Council (UK). The latest version can be found at:* http://www.resus.org.uk).

Tachycardia algorithm
(with pulse)

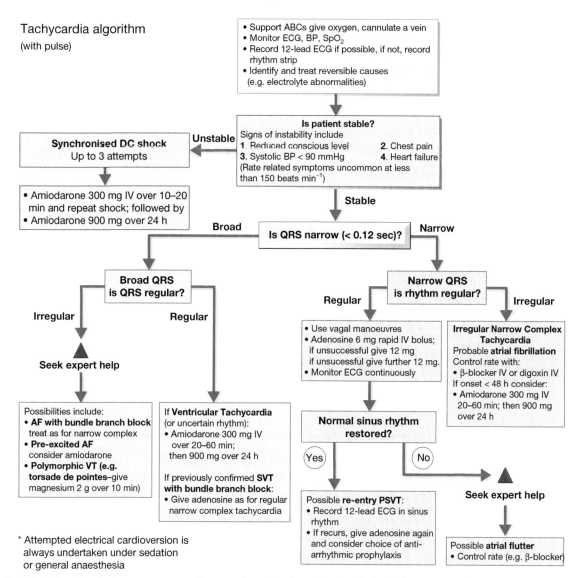

- Support ABCs give oxygen, cannulate a vein
- Monitor ECG, BP, SpO₂
- Record 12-lead ECG if possible, if not, record rhythm strip
- Identify and treat reversible causes (e.g. electrolyte abnormalities)

Is patient stable?
Signs of instability include
1. Reduced conscious level   **2.** Chest pain
3. Systolic BP < 90 mmHg   **4.** Heart failure
(Rate related symptoms uncommon at less than 150 beats min⁻¹)

Unstable

Synchronised DC shock
Up to 3 attempts

- Amiodarone 300 mg IV over 10–20 min and repeat shock; followed by
- Amiodarone 900 mg over 24 h

Stable

Is QRS narrow (< 0.12 sec)?

Broad

Narrow

**Broad QRS
is QRS regular?**

**Narrow QRS
is rhythm regular?**

Irregular   **Regular**

Regular   **Irregular**

Seek expert help

- Use vagal manoeuvres
- Adenosine 6 mg rapid IV bolus; if unsuccessful give 12 mg if unsuccessful give further 12 mg.
- Monitor ECG continuously

Irregular Narrow Complex Tachycardia
Probable **atrial fibrillation**
Control rate with:
- β-blocker IV or digoxin IV
If onset < 48 h consider:
- Amiodarone 300 mg IV 20–60 min; then 900 mg over 24 h

Possibilities include:
- **AF with bundle branch block** treat as for narrow complex
- **Pre-excited AF** consider amiodarone
- **Polymorphic VT (e.g. torsade de pointes**–give magnesium 2 g over 10 min)

If **Ventricular Tachycardia** (or uncertain rhythm):
- Amiodarone 300 mg IV over 20–60 min; then 900 mg over 24 h

If previously confirmed **SVT with bundle branch block**:
- Give adenosine as for regular narrow complex tachycardia

Normal sinus rhythm restored?

(Yes)   (No)

Possible **re-entry PSVT**:
- Record 12-lead ECG in sinus rhythm
- If recurs, give adenosine again and consider choice of anti-arrhythmic prophylaxis

Seek expert help

Possible **atrial flutter**
- Control rate (e.g. β-blocker)

* Attempted electrical cardioversion is always undertaken under sedation or general anaesthesia

Fig. 25.4 Algorithm for the management of acute tachycardia. *(Reproduced with the kind permission of the Resuscitation Council (UK). The latest version can be found at:* http://www.resus.org.uk).

specialists for the definitive treatment of their arrhythmia with radiofrequency ablation.

Atrial fibrillation (AF)

Atrial fibrillation (AF) is the most commonly encountered arrhythmia. Its incidence increases with age and is estimated to affect approximately 6% of people older than 65 years of age. AF increases the risk of stroke by four- to five-fold and death by around two-fold. The health-care costs associated with AF are substantial.

What management options are available? Treatment can be divided into rhythm or rate control, utilising pharmacological and/or non-pharmacological therapies. Thromboembolic prevention is strongly advocated in all patients, the level of risk determining the degree to which

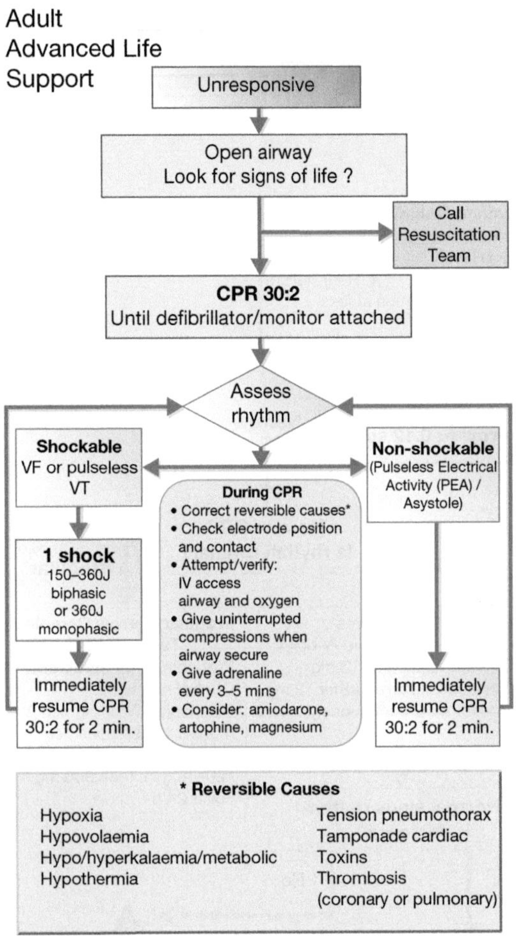

Adult
Advanced Life
Support

| Unresponsive |

Open airway
Look for signs of life ?

Call
Resuscitation
Team

CPR 30:2
Until defibrillator/monitor attached

Assess
rhythm

Shockable
VF or pulseless
VT

Non-shockable
(Pulseless Electrical
Activity (PEA) /
Asystole)

During CPR
• Correct reversible causes*
• Check electrode position
  and contact
• Attempt/verify:
  IV access
  airway and oxygen
• Give uninterrupted
  compressions when
  airway secure
• Give adrenaline
  every 3–5 mins
• Consider: amiodarone,
  artophine, magnesium

1 shock
150–360J
biphasic
or 360J
monophasic

Immediately
resume CPR
30:2 for 2 min.

Immediately
resume CPR
30:2 for 2 min.

* Reversible Causes

Hypoxia	Tension pneumothorax
Hypovolaemia	Tamponade cardiac
Hypo/hyperkalaemia/metabolic	Toxins
Hypothermia	Thrombosis (coronary or pulmonary)

Fig. 25.5 Adult advanced life support. *(Reproduced with the kind permission of the Resuscitation Council (UK). The latest version can be found at:* http://www.resus.org.uk).

this is pursued. Rhythm control should theoretically be superior to rate control, as the former maintains the physiological, sequential and coordinated pumping actions of the atria and ventricles. At the same time, it should reduce the risk of thrombus formation in the atria. Clinical trials fail to support these arguments, although the use of differing anticoagulation regimens complicates interpretation of results. The potential side-effects of currently available anti-arrhythmic agents may negate any benefit conferred by maintenance of sinus rhythm (see below).

The therapeutic options for the management of atrial fibrillation are therefore complex and include asking questions that concern:

• Treatment or no treatment?
• Conversion or rate control?

• Immediate or delayed conversion?
• Drugs, DC conversion or radiofrequency ablation?

The information that should be considered is extensive and includes:

• Ventricular rate ('normal' or high).
• Haemodynamic state ('normal' or compromised).
• Atrial size ('normal' or enlarged).

In many patients, AF is an incidental finding on the background of some existing cardiovascular disease, and with a large atrium. With a prolonged history of symptoms, *rate-controlling medication* such as a β-blocker, digoxin or calcium antagonist may suffice.

If the history appears shorter, and the atrium is of normal size, i.e. is unlikely to contain thrombus, or there has been recent onset of heart failure or shock, cardioversion should be considered. Electrical (DC) conversion is often favoured where treatment is either urgent or likely to be successful in holding the patient in sinus rhythm. Amiodarone can often provide pharmacological conversion over hours to days, and is also effective for patients who revert rapidly to AF after DC conversion. In cases in which the AF duration exceeds 48 h, cardioversion should be delayed for at least 1 month to permit anticoagulation with a NOAC or warfarin, which should be continued for 4 weeks thereafter. If cardioversion is deemed urgent, then transoesophageal echocardiography should be used to show there is no thrombus visible in the left atrium.

In patients who have reverted to AF after previous conversions, amiodarone is the drug of choice prior to further attempts at cardioversion. Amiodarone may also be used to suppress episodes of paroxysmal atrial fibrillation, but dronedarone, sotalol or flecainide are preferred[12] (Fig. 25.6). Radiofrequency ablation is now established as the treatment of choice in many patients with both paroxysmal and persistent atrial fibrillation, and patients with symptomatic atrial fibrillation should ideally be referred to heart rhythm specialists for advice on further management.

Additional treatments in persistent atrial fibrillation. Long-term thromboprophylaxis with a NOAC or warfarin is almost mandatory to reduce embolic complications. The efficacy of aspirin as an antithrombotic agent is questionable and most likely adverse and is little used in those not having a vascular indication. Specifically whilst warfarin or NOACs provide protection against stroke aspirin does not but all carry similar risks of bleeding.

---

[12]The Task Force for the Management of Atrial Fibrillation of the European Society of Cardiology (ESC) has issued guidance preferring these agents to amiodarone depending on the characteristics of the patient (see Fig. 25.6). European Heart Rhythm Association; European Association for Cardio-Thoracic Surgery, Camm A J et al 2010 Guidelines for the management of atrial fibrillation: the Task Force for the Management of Atrial Fibrillation of the European Society of Cardiology (ESC). European Heart Journal 31:2369–2429.

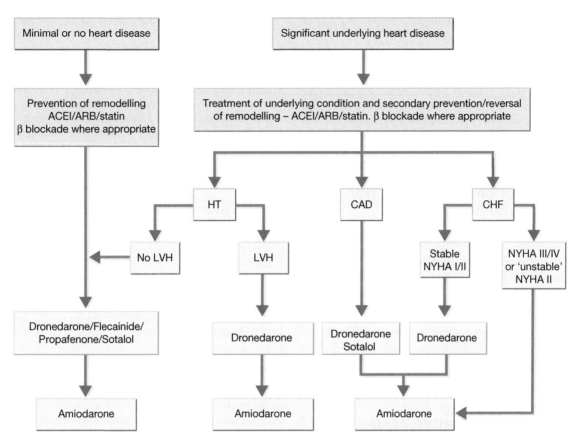

Fig. 25.6 Choice of antiarrhythmic drug for atrial fibrillation according to underlying pathology. ACEI, angiotensin-converting enzyme inhibitor; ARB, angiotensin receptor blocker; CAD, coronary artery disease; CHF, congestive heart failure; HT, hypertension; LVH, left ventricular hypertrophy; NYHA, New York Heart Association; unstable, cardiac decompensation within the prior 4 weeks. Antiarrhythmic agents are listed in alphabetical order within each treatment box. ? = evidence for 'upstream' therapy for prevention of atrial remodelling still remains controversial. *Taken from the Task Force for the Management of Atrial Fibrillation of the European Society of Cardiology (ESC) guidance. European Heart Rhythm Association; European Association for Cardio-Thoracic Surgery, Camm A J et al 2010 Guidelines for the management of atrial fibrillation: the Task Force for the Management of Atrial Fibrillation of the European Society of Cardiology (ESC). European Heart Journal 31:2369–249. With permission.*

Atrial flutter

It is doubtful whether this differs in any important way in its origins or sequelae from atrial fibrillation. The ventricular rate is usually faster (typically, one-half an atrial rate of 300 beats/min, where 2 : 1 block is present), which is too fast to leave without treatment. Previously, conversion without prior anticoagulation was undertaken occasionally, but transoesphageal echocardiography or anticoagulation is now mandatory. Patients should not remain in chronic atrial flutter, and DC conversion will usually either restore sinus rhythm or result in atrial fibrillation (treated as above). Patients who fail to convert, or who revert to atrial flutter,

should be referred for radiofrequency ablation, which is highly effective and removes the cause of the atrial flutter in nearly all patients. The potential later recurrence of atrial fibrillation is much more readily managed than atrial flutter.

Atrial tachycardia with variable AV block

The atrial rate varies, and commonly there is AV block. Digoxin is a possible cause of the arrhythmia and should be withdrawn. If the patient is not taking digoxin, it may be introduced to control the ventricular rate. These patients should be referred to a heart rhythm specialist and be considered for radiofrequency ablation.

Heart block

In an emergency, antimuscarinic vagal block with atropine 600 µg i.v. or the β-adrenoceptor agonist, isoprenaline (0.5–10 µg/min i.v.) can improve AV conduction, but advanced heart block always requires implantation of a permanent pacemaker, possibly preceded by a temporary pacing wire.

Pre-excitation (Wolff–Parkinson–White) syndromes

These occur in otherwise healthy individuals who possess an anomalous (accessory) atrioventricular (AV) pathway; they often experience attacks of paroxysmal AV re-entrant tachycardia or atrial fibrillation. Drugs that both suppress the initiating ectopic beats and delay conduction through the accessory pathway are used to prevent attacks, e.g. flecainide, sotalol or amiodarone. Do not use verapamil or digoxin, which may *increase* conduction through the anomalous pathway. Electrical conversion restores sinus rhythm when the ventricular rate is very rapid. Radiofrequency ablation of aberrant pathways provides a cure and is the treatment of choice.

Ventricular premature beats

These are common after myocardial infarction. One particular significance in those with ischaemic heart disease is that the R-wave (ECG) of an ectopic beat, superimposed upon the early or peak phases of the T-wave of a normal beat, may precipitate ventricular tachycardia or fibrillation (the 'R-on-T' phenomenon). About 80% of patients with myocardial infarction who proceed to ventricular fibrillation have preceding ventricular premature beats. Lidocaine effectively suppresses ectopic ventricular beats but is not often used, as its addition increases overall risk.

Ventricular tachycardia

Ventricular tachycardia demands urgent treatment because it frequently leads to ventricular fibrillation and circulatory arrest. A powerful thump of the fist on the mid-sternum or praecordium may very occasionally stop a tachycardia. If there is rapid haemodynamic deterioration, electrical conversion is the treatment of choice. When the patient is in good cardiovascular condition, treatment may begin with intravenous lidocaine, failing which, intravenous amiodarone may be used. For recurrent ventricular tachycardia, amiodarone or sotalol is preferred. Patients should be referred to a heart rhythm specialist and be considered for the insertion of an implantable cardioverter defibrillator (ICD) that will often be combined with radiofrequency ablation directed at the arrhythmogenic substrate.

Ventricular fibrillation and cardiac arrest

Ventricular fibrillation is usually caused by myocardial infarction or ischaemia, or serious organic heart disease and is the main cause of *cardiac arrest*. Guidelines for the management of peri-arrest arrhythmias and cardiac arrest are issued by the UK Resuscitation Council and appear in Figs 25.3–25.5. Patients suffering 'failed' sudden cardiac death (SCD) should be considered for the insertion of an ICD.

Long QT syndromes

These are caused by malfunction of ion channels, leading to impaired ventricular repolarisation (expressed as prolongation of the QT interval) and a characteristic ventricular tachycardia, *torsade de pointes* (see Fig. 25.2).[13] The symptoms range from episodes of syncope to cardiac arrest. Several drugs are responsible for the acquired form of the condition including antiarrhythmic drugs (see above), antimicrobials, histamine H_1-receptor antagonists and serotonin receptor antagonists; predisposing factors are female sex, recent heart rate slowing, and hypokalaemia.[14] Congenital forms of the long QT syndrome are due to mutations of the genes encoding ion channels, and exposure to drugs reveals some of these.

---

[13]French: *torsade,* twist; *pointe,* point. 'Twisting of the points', referring to the characteristic sequence of 'up' followed by 'down' QRS complexes. The appearance has been called a 'cardiac ballet'.
[14]Roden D M 2004 Drug-induced prolongation of the QT interval. New England Journal of Medicine 350:1013–1022.

Summary

- The treatment of cardiac arrhythmias has advanced enormously and can be directly physical, electrical, pharmacological or surgical. Radiofrequency ablation and devices such as permanent pacemakers and ICDs increasingly provide the preferred approaches. The use of drugs alone is declining, but they often constitute adjunctive treatments.

- The choice among drugs follows partly from theoretical predictions of their action on the cardiac cycle but substantially from short- and long-term observations of their efficacy and safety.

- All antiarrhythmics can be potentially dangerous, and should be used only in patients who have been properly and fully assessed.

- Adenosine is the treatment of choice for diagnosis and reversal of supraventricular arrhythmias. Verapamil is an alternative for the management of narrow complex tachycardias.

- Amiodarone is the most effective drug for reversing and preventing atrial fibrillation, and for preventing ventricular arrhythmias, but it has notable adverse effects. Dronedarone has been designed to provide the actions of amiodarone without the side-effects but is not so effective.

- New drugs are needed, but very few are in the pipeline. In view of the increasing complexity and range of treatment options, all patients should be considered for referral to a heart rhythm specialist for a full discussion of the options available.

Guide to further reading

Delacretaz, E., 2006. Clinical practice. Supraventricular tachycardia. N. Engl. J. Med. 354, 1039–1051.

Dobrev, D., Nattel, S., 2010. New antiarrhythmic drugs for treatment of atrial fibrillation. Lancet 375, 1212–1223.

Freedman, B., Potpara, T.S., Lip, G.Y., 2016. Stroke prevention in atrial fibrillation. Lancet 388, 806–817.

Groeneveld, P.W., Dixit, S., 2017. Cardiac pacing and defibrillation devices: cost and effectiveness. Annu. Rev. Med. 68, 1–13.

Kirchhof, P., Benussi, S., Kotecha, D., et al., 2016. 2016 ESC Guidelines for the management of atrial fibrillation developed in collaboration with EACTS. Eur. Heart J. 37, 2893–2962.

Piccini, J.P., Fauchier, L., 2016. Rhythm control in atrial fibrillation. Lancet 388, 829–840.

Van Gelder, I.C., Rienstra, M., Crijns, H.J., Olshansky, B., 2016. Rate control in atrial fibrillation. Lancet 388, 818–828.

Zimetbaum, P., 2007. Amiodarone for atrial fibrillation. N. Engl. J. Med. 356, 935–941.

Chapter | 26 |

Hyperlipidaemias

John P. D. Reckless

SYNOPSIS

Correction of blood lipid abnormalities offers scope for a major impact on cardiovascular disease. Drugs play a significant role and have a variety of modes of action. Dietary and lifestyle adjustment are essential components of overall risk prevention.

- **Pathophysiology.**
- **Primary (inherited) and secondary hyperlipidaemias.**
- **Management: risk assessment, secondary and primary prevention, drugs, diet, lifestyle.**
- **Drugs used in treatment: statins; ezetimibe; anion-exchange resins; modulators of PCSK9 (proprotein convertase subtilisin/kexin type 9). Nicotinic acid and derivatives now have a minimal or no role. Fibric acid derivatives have modest indications.**

Some physiology and pathophysiology

The normal function of lipoproteins is to distribute and recycle cholesterol and triglycerides. The pathways of lipid metabolism and transport and their *primary* (inherited) disorders are shown in Fig. 26.1 and can be summarised thus:

- Chylomicrons transport dietary triglyceride from the gut to peripheral tissues. Cholesterol is absorbed from the *intestine* within chylomicrons. These are catabolised by lipoprotein lipase (LPL) to remnants, which are taken up by the hepatic low-density lipoprotein (LDL)-receptor–related protein (LRP).
- Most cholesterol in the body is synthesised de novo within the *liver* and *peripheral tissues* where, for example, it is converted to steroid hormones or used to form cell walls and membranes. Much of the

hepatic cholesterol enters the circulation as very-low-density lipoprotein (VLDL) which carry triglycerides. In tissues, VLDL is metabolised to remnant lipoproteins after LPL removes triglyceride. The remnant lipoproteins are removed by the liver through apolipoprotein E receptors or LDL receptors (LDL-R) or further metabolised to LDL and then removed by peripheral tissues or the liver by LDL-R.

- The quantity of cholesterol transported from the liver to peripheral tissues greatly exceeds its catabolism there, and mechanisms exist to return cholesterol to the liver. Through this 'reverse transport', cholesterol is carried by high-density lipoprotein (HDL) from peripheral cells to the liver, where it is taken up by a process involving hepatic lipase. Cholesterol in the plasma is also recycled to LDL and VLDL by cholesterol-ester transport protein (CETP). Cholesterol also returns to the liver through hepatic LDL uptake.
- LDL-R, carrying LDL, are internalised into hepatic and peripheral tissue cells. After catabolism of the LDL, the LDL-R are either recycled back to the plasma membrane or are directed to catabolism through the action of PCSK9. Low activity levels of PCSK9 (either naturally or through pharmacological inhibition) therefore lead to increased cell LDL uptake and lower plasma LDL.
- Cholesterol in the liver is reassembled into lipoproteins, or secreted in bile then recycled by absorption at the terminal ileum or excreted in the faeces.

Lipid disorders

Disorders of lipid metabolism are manifest by elevation of the plasma concentrations of the various lipid and lipoprotein

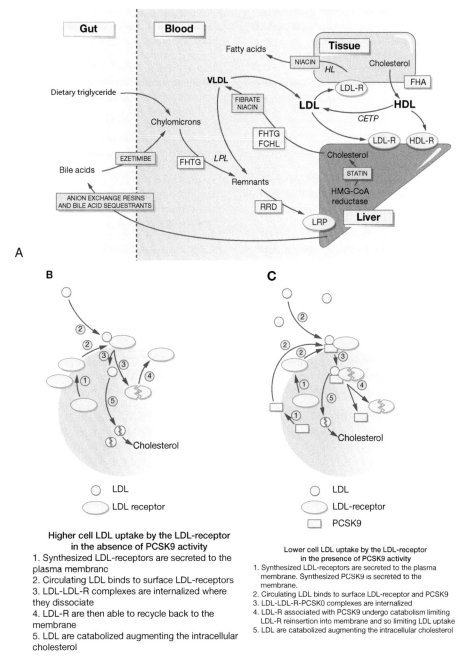

Fig. 26.1 (A) Pathway of lipid transport and sites of drug action. (nicotinic acid (niacin) usage is no longer indicated.) (B) Higher cell LDL uptake by the LDL receptor in the absence of PCSK9 activity. (C) Lower cell LDL uptake by the LDL receptor in the presence of PCSK9 activity. LPL, lipoprotein lipase; CETP, cholesterol ester transfer protein; HL, hormone-sensitive lipase.

fractions (total and LDL cholesterol, VLDL, triglycerides, chylomicrons), and they result, predominantly, in cardiovascular disease. This chapter addresses approaches (non-drug as well as drug) to correct abnormal lipid profiles and diminish vascular disease and its consequences.

Additionally, hypertriglyceridaemia is associated with fatty liver disease, which may progress to steatohepatitis and cirrhosis. Severe hypertriglyceridaemia can lead to acute pancreatitis.

Deposition of cholesterol in the arterial wall is central to the atherosclerotic process. Carriage of all the apoprotein-B–containing lipoproteins (VLDL, remnant lipoproteins, LDL) to arteries can thus be viewed as potentially *atherogenic*. In the reverse process, HDL can carry cholesterol away from the arterial wall and in most circumstances can be regarded as *protective* against atherogenesis.

Overproduction of VLDL in the liver raises plasma VLDL, remnant lipoproteins and LDL if the capacity to metabolise these lipoproteins is compromised either by a primary (inherited) and/or secondary (environmental) abnormality.

Elevation of *LDL cholesterol* is associated particularly with risk of coronary heart disease, but it is increasingly clear that moderate elevations of triglycerides, and of VLDL, IDL and LDL, are also atherogenic, particularly when HDL cholesterol is low. Therefore, consideration of non-HDL cholesterol is likely to be a better marker of cardiovascular risk than LDL cholesterol, does not require a fasting sample, and is recommended by the National Institute for Health and Care Excellence (NICE).[1]

While the epidemiological relationship between LDL cholesterol and stroke is quite weak, the lowering of cholesterol significantly reduces stroke risk.

Primary inherited lipoprotein disorders

There are five *primary inherited lipoprotein disorders* which disturb lipid metabolism at the points indicated in Fig. 26.1. These are:

- *Familial hypertriglyceridaemia* (FHTG) (uncommon), including lipoprotein lipase (LPL) deficiency (rare), in which low LPL activity results in decreased removal of, and thus increase in, plasma *triglyceride*; there is increased hepatic secretion and thus raised plasma concentration of *triglyceride-rich VLDL*. Patients are at risk of recurrent acute pancreatitis when plasma triglyceride exceeds 10 mmol/L, and especially when >20 mmol/L.
- *Familial combined hyperlipidaemia* (FCHL) (more common) in which there is increased hepatic

secretion of apolipoprotein B–containing VLDL, and conversion to LDL; in consequence, plasma *LDL and VLDL* are raised. Patients exhibit macrovascular disease (coronary heart, peripheral and cerebral).
- *Remnant removal disease* (RRD, also called 'remnant lipaemia', 'familial dysbetalipoproteinaemia') (uncommon) in which there is a defect of apolipoprotein E. This is the major ligand that allows internalisation and subsequent metabolism of remnant particles derived from VLDL and chylomicrons. Often manifest when environmental factors are also in play, the consequence is accumulation of VLDL remnants called 'intermediate density lipoprotein (IDL)' with cholesterol and triglycerides usually in the range 6–9 mmol/L. Patients experience severe macrovascular disease (as above) often in middle age.
- *Familial hypoalphalipoproteinaemia* (FHA, Tangier disease) (rare) in which the serum concentration of (protective) HDL is very low. Coronary heart and peripheral vascular disease result.
- *Familial hypercholesterolaemia* (FH) (common) is characterised by elevation of *total* and *LDL cholesterol* in plasma. In the less severe heterozygous form, it affects about 1:250 of the population (most often one copy of the LDL receptor protein is absent or defective, while in some cases there is an abnormal apolipoprotein-B, or PCSK9 activity excess). LDL cholesterol is elevated from childhood. If untreated, one-half of the males will die by 60 years of age, and half the females 10 years later. The principal consequence is coronary heart disease, but occasionally also peripheral and cerebrovascular disease. Homozygosity is rare and would be 4 per million at a heteozygosity rate of 1:250. Untreated such individuals are unlikely to survive into adulthood.

Secondary lipoprotein disorders

Secondary hyperlipidaemias result from: liver and biliary disease, obesity, hypothyroidism, diabetes, diet, alcohol excess, renal disease (nephrotic syndrome) and drugs (including etretinate, HIV protease inhibitors, thiazide diuretics, oral contraceptive steroids, glucocorticoids, β-adrenoceptor antagonists, ciclosporin).

Most commonly, patients present with more modest elevations of total and LDL cholesterol which results from overproduction of VLDL in the liver due to a combination of high dietary fat, obesity and individual (genetic) susceptibility; it is thus called polygenic, manifests in adult life, with atherosclerosis occurring early but not as early as in FH.

---

[1]National Institute for Health and Care Excellence. Clinical Guidance (CG) 181. Cardiovascular disease: risk assessment and reduction, including lipid modification, July 2014.

The most severe hyperlipidaemias usually occur in patients with concurrent conditions, e.g. diabetes mellitus with one of the primary hyperlipidaemias.

Sites of drug action

In general, most drugs act directly or indirectly to reduce the concentration of cholesterol within hepatocytes, causing a compensatory increase in LDL receptors (LDL-R) on their surface, and increased uptake of cholesterol-rich LDL particles from the bloodstream (see Fig. 26.1).

Statins decrease the synthesis of cholesterol and hence secretion of VLDL and increase the surface expression of hepatic LDL receptors.

Bile-acid–binding (anion exchange) resins increase bile acid faecal excretion, thus depleting the bile acid and thus the cholesterol pool.

Fibrates decrease the secretion of VLDL and increase the activity of LPL, thereby increasing the removal of triglycerides. *Nicotinic acid* decreases fatty acid production in the tissues and the secretion of VLDL and the clearance of HDL. It also enhances LPL. However it is not clinically effective.

Ezetimibe blocks the uptake of cholesterol from the gut by targeting a specific cholesterol transporter.

PCSK9 inhibition increases recycling of LDL receptors back to the plasma membrane while reducing their degradation, so leading to more removal of plasma LDL.

Management

The management of hyperlipidaemias should be viewed against the background of the following observations.

- Hyperlipidaemias are common; 66% of the adult UK population have a plasma cholesterol concentration in excess of 5.2 mmol/L. Randomised controlled trial evidence has shown mortality reduction benefit when LDL cholesterol is reduced to no more than 1.6 mmol/L, and down to <1.0 mmol/L in certain high-risk groups.
- Investigation of hyperlipidaemia must be directed initially at excluding contributory causes, i.e. secondary hyperlipidaemias (see above). None of these should be assumed to be the sole cause, even if present. NICE (CG181)[1] advises at least one lipid sample to measure a full lipid profile (total cholesterol, HDL cholesterol, non-HDL cholesterol and triglyceride concentrations) before starting lipid modification therapy for the primary prevention of CVD. A fasting sample is not needed.
- All patients (and their spouses/partners, as appropriate) should receive advice on lifestyle, and on diet and weight control, for these are important components of overall macrovascular risk prevention.

Dietary treatment of hypercholesterolaemia has a modest effect at best (around 8% reduction in LDL cholesterol is possible), but diet and weight reduction are more effective for hypertriglyceridaemia. Total fat, especially saturated fat should be reduced (and partially replaced with mono- and poly-unsaturated fats). Foods with significant hydrogenated fats should be avoided.

- Spreads containing plant stanols and sterols (e.g. Benecol and Flora Proactiv) can reduce plasma cholesterol by up to 10% when taken with a mixed meal as part of a healthy diet. Although they are lipid-modifying, as stanols and sterols do not have hard outcome evidence for CVD reduction, they have not been recommended by NICE (CG181).[1]
- In some individuals, especially those with mixed hyperlipidaemia (elevated cholesterol and triglycerides), often due to secondary factors on a polygenic background, successful adherence to dietary advice, and weight loss, may produce very significant improvements. Patients with remnant lipaemia (RRD hyperlipidaemia) may respond excellently to diet, weight loss (and possibly the addition of a fibrate or statin).
- Much of the work of lipid clinics is taken up with attending to multiple interacting risk factors such as hypertension, diabetes, thyroid disease, alcohol and smoking, as well as to the lipid abnormality. Lipid clinics can also help overcome perceived statin intolerance in high-risk patients. Perceived intolerance is considerably more common than the true incidence of myopathy, and concordance encouragement is important.

The non-pharmacological matters that should be considered include appropriate diet, physical activity, weight management, alcohol consumption, and smoking cessation. Potential dyslipidaemic effects of other pharmacological therapies being taken should be considered.

- The decision to use lipid-lowering drugs is made on the basis of the overall absolute cardiovascular risk.
- Since the landmark Scandinavian 4S study,[2] meta-analysis of data from 174 000 individuals in 27 randomised primary and secondary prevention statin trials have demonstrated CVD reduction,[3] with

[2]Scandinavian Simvastatin Survival Study Group 1994 Randomised trial of cholesterol lowering in 4444 patients with coronary heart disease: the Scandinavian Simvastatin Survival Study (4S). Lancet 344:1383–1389.
[3]Fulcher J, O'Connell R, Voysey M et al 2015 The Cholesterol Treatment Trialists' (CTT) Collaboration. Efficacy and safety of LDL-lowering therapy among men and women: meta-analysis of individual data from 174,000 participants in 27 randomised trials. Lancet 385:1397–1405.

more intensive therapy also showing benefit over less intensive statin regimens. For each LDL cholesterol reduction of 1 mmol/L, there was about a 20% reduction in CVD events and a 10% reduction in all-cause mortality. Benefit was seen in low-risk individuals (<10% risk/5 years) and down to achieved LDL cholesterol value of around 1.6 mmol/L. Previous concerns about cancer risk and violent deaths have not been substantiated.

- Individuals with any form of atherosclerotic cardiovascular disease (previous myocardial infarction, angina pectoris, stroke, transient ischaemic attack, peripheral vascular disease) will almost all require statin treatment.
- Individuals with diabetes (type 1 and type 2) are at high CVD risk and should be considered for treatment.
- For primary prevention, risk calculation is required. Previously the absolute CVD risk has been computed using risk equations based on longitudinal cohorts such as Framingham often using a simple colour-coded chart to input the patient's age, sex, smoking status, pre-treatment blood pressure and plasma total cholesterol/HDL cholesterol ratio. With the availability of data from very large cohorts of millions of patients in UK National Health Service primary care, a more appropriate calculation using the Q-RISK2 programme can be made.[4] NICE's CG181[1] recommends offering primary prevention treatment to individuals with a CVD risk of ≥10%/10 years. NICE does not recommend routine monitoring of statin treatment in this group, but a follow-up result is likely to encourage treatment concordance.
- There is evidence that statins protect against stroke.
- For secondary prevention, drug treatment should be initiated at the time of the event but it should be emphasised that this is in addition to the need for lifestyle change. Lifestyle management including dietary modification should be offered for both primary and secondary prevention subjects. It is recognised that the effect of the dietary changes that individuals can make and maintain may be modest.
- The decision to offer a patient primary prophylaxis is influenced by the absolute risk for the individual, the potential risks from the statin therapy, costs to the

health provider, and the view of the individual. As statins have an excellent safety record over a long period, costs will escalate with a decision to treat lower levels of absolute risk, the costs offset by the very substantial reduction in price of generic products. Current UK recommendations suggest treating all patients with a CVD risk of at least 10% over 10 years (this is the composite risk of non-fatal MI or stroke, fatal MI or stroke or new-onset angina); all diabetics should be assumed to be in this highest-risk category.

Management may proceed as follows:

1. *Any medical disorder* that may be causing hyperlipidaemia, e.g. diabetes, hypothyroidism, should be treated first.
2. *Dietary adjustment.* The following applies to all patients:
   a. Those who are overweight should reduce their total caloric intake, ideally aiming to approach a weight more appropriate for their height. This will include reduced intake of alcohol and of total (especially animal) fat. Elevated triglyceride concentrations may respond particularly well to alcohol withdrawal.
   b. Those who fail to achieve adequate weight reduction or who are already at an appropriate weight should reduce their total fat intake; poly- and monounsaturated fats or oils may be taken partially to substitute for the reduction in animal fats. Reduction in dietary cholesterol is a much less important element of the diet. Taking Benecol or Flora Proactiv with a mixed meal can reduce LDL cholesterol by up to 10%. Without hard CVD outcome evidence, this treatment was not recommended by NICE, but individuals may choose to provide this for themselves.
3. Specific types of hyperlipidaemia are treated thus:
   a. Familial hypertriglyceridaemia responds best to dietary modification and weight reduction (above) together with a fibrate; nicotinic acid is now used rarely. For the rare very severe forms (such as with LPL deficiency), dietary fat intake needs to be reduced to ≤10% of calories which is not that palatable.
   b. Familial combined hyperlipidaemia should be treated with dietary modification and weight reduction (above) together with a statin. A fibrate may be added in resistant cases.
   c. Remnant removal disease (remnant lipaemia) will often respond to dietary modification and weight reduction. Drug therapy with a fibrate or a statin

---

[4]Hippisley-Cox J, Coupland S, Vinogradova Y et al 2008 Predicting cardiovascular risk in England and Wales: prospective derivation and validation of QRISK2. British Medical Journal 336:1475–1482. Also QRISK2-2016 risk calculator at: https://qrisk.org.

may be added to non-pharmacological measures where there is insufficient response.

d. Familial or polygenic hypercholesterolaemia is treated by dietary modification, lifestyle changes, and a statin in the first place. Ezetimibe may be added, which has effectively largely replaced anion-exchange resins.

e. In single-gene defect familial hypercholesterolaemia (FH), LDL cholesterol is particularly raised, and the advice is to lower the untreated LDL cholesterol by at least 50%; this is likely to require statin plus ezetimibe therapy. From an identified proband, cascade screening of relatives is required. PCSK9-inhibitors may be indicated in limited circumstances.

f. Individuals with homozygous familial hypercholesterolaemia require LDL apheresis. In familial hypercholesterolaemia, apheresis should also be considered for very-high-risk patients who are compound heterozygotes, and in secondary prevention for severely affected heterozygous patients failing to reach adequately low levels of LDL cholesterol.

g. Familial hypoalphalipoproteinaemia may respond to exercise and weight loss. Statin therapy may be required (to lower LDL rather than increasing HDL) if overall CVD risk warrants. To date, therapies to increase HDL cholesterol have been disappointing. Nicotinic acid has been shown to be ineffective with increased adverse effects compared to placebo. Inhibition of the enzyme CETP does increase HDL cholesterol and may reduce LDL cholesterol, but trials of such inhibitors have had side effects, been ineffective, or had just modest effect (see below).[5]

Drugs used in treatment

Statins

These drugs block the rate-limiting enzyme for endogenous cholesterol synthesis, *hydroxy-methyl-glutaryl coenzyme A* (HMG CoA) reductase. This results in increased synthesis of LDL receptors (up-regulation) in the liver and increased clearance of LDL from the circulation; plasma total cholesterol and LDL cholesterol fall with a maximum effect within 1 month of commencing therapy. All statins cause a dose-dependent reduction in total and LDL cholesterol, although there are differences in their therapeutic efficacy.

Simvastatin at 10 mg daily may reduce LDL cholesterol by around 28%, while at the same dose pravastatin and fluvastatin are around 5–6% lower, atorvastatin 5–6% higher, and rosuvastatin somewhat higher still. Across the statins, each doubling of a statin dose will reduce LDL cholesterol by around a further 5–6%.

There is no tolerance to continued administration of a statin, and because of a circadian rhythm to LDL receptor synthesis, some statins with a shorter half-life are slightly more effective if given in the evening rather than in the morning. Efficacy in both primary and secondary treatment of hypercholesterolaemia is probably a class effect, without long-term outcome studies showing any clear differentiation between the drugs. Choice of agent is influenced by acquisition cost, the likely ability to achieve an intended lower LDL cholesterol (or non-HDL cholesterol) level, and any potential interaction with other pharmacological interventions an individual may be requiring. In the UK currently NICE in CG181[1] recommends generic atorvastatin at 20 mg in primary prevention and at full dose of 80 mg for secondary prevention.

On current information, with no clear advantages or disadvantages among the different statins, the choice of agent to achieve the suggested total or LDL cholesterol levels (see above) is heavily influenced by their relative cost, and the dose likely to achieve the target cholesterol concentration.

Statins are well absorbed by mouth, and are metabolised in the liver. Except for pravastatin, they are metabolised through CYP pathways (usually 3A4), which are an important source of drug interactions (see below). They are well tolerated, the commonest adverse effect being transient, and usually minor, elevation of serum transaminases in some 1% of patients. Asymptomatic elevation of muscle enzymes (creatine phosphokinase, CPK) and myositis (with a generalised muscle discomfort) occurs more rarely,[3] but is more frequent when statins are combined with other antihyperlipidaemic drugs such as fibrates (gemfibrozil). Interactions with other drugs vary somewhat for each statin, and potential should be checked when prescribing. They are more likely at high statin dose. As an example, myositis is more likely when statins are co-administered with anti-HIV protease inhibitors (such as ritonavir), although such patients have increased CVD risk. Examples of other agents are ciclosporin, amiodarone, amlodipine, diltiazem and some antibiotics. With an acute short antibiotic course, it may be reasonable just to briefly omit the statin.

Patients should be counselled about myositis when statins are prescribed and when there is co-administration of significant drugs. Muscle symptoms are common in the population, and few will be statin-related. When considering a statin-treated patient presenting with musculoskeletal symptoms, a generalised muscle discomfort, pain, tenderness or weakness should raise the possibility of the uncommon

---

[5]The HPS3/TIMI55–REVEAL Collaborative Group. Effects of Anacetrapib in Patients with Atherosclerotic Vascular Disease. N Engl J Med 2017; 377: 1217

side-effect of drug-related myositis. Localised muscle symptoms are not likely to be statin-related, and joint symptoms are unrelated.

Statin treatment is associated with a modest increased incidence of new-onset diabetes, often in individuals with other risk factors for diabetes. At a ≥10%/10 year CVD risk, statin benefit persists.

Fibric acid derivatives (fibrates)

The class includes *bezafibrate, ciprofibrate, fenofibrate* and *gemfibrozil*; the original fibrate, clofibrate, is obsolete. Gemfibrozil has higher side-effects, and fenofibrate is the more commonly used. The drugs partly resemble short-chain fatty acids and increase the oxidation of these acids in both liver and muscle. In the liver, secretion of triglyceride-rich lipoproteins falls, and in muscle the activity of lipoprotein lipase and fatty acid uptake from plasma are both increased. Fibrates act through a nuclear transcription factor (PPARα) which up-regulates expression of LDL cholesterol and apolipoprotein A-1 genes, and down-regulates expression of the apolipoprotein C-11 gene. The result is that plasma triglyceride declines by 20–30% and cholesterol by 10–15%; associated with this is a rise in the 'protective' HDL cholesterol.

It has been postulated that these effects may have contributed to the reduction in nonfatal myocardial infarction with gemfibrozil in the Helsinki Heart Study[6] and the VA-HIT[7] trials. In the FIELD trial of a large diabetes cohort, fenofibrate did not produce a significant change in CVD outcome, although some diabetes microvascular complications were modified.[8] There was significant statin 'drop-in' during the trial. Addition of a fibrate is likely to be considered in individuals on statin treatment who have persisting hypertriglyceridaemia and a low HDL cholesterol. Fibrate treatment may also be used in severe hypertriglyceridaemia.

Fibric acid derivatives are well absorbed from the gastrointestinal tract, extensively bound to plasma proteins and excreted mainly by the kidney as unchanged drug or metabolites. They are contraindicated where hepatic or renal function is severely impaired. Rarely, fibric acid derivatives may induce a myositis-like syndrome; the risk is greater in patients with poor renal function, and in those who are also receiving a statin. Fibrates enhance the effect of co-administered oral anticoagulants. Creatinine may rise with fibrate treatment but is reversible.

Anion-exchange resins (bile acid sequestrants)

Colestyramine is an oral anion-exchange resin, which binds bile acids in the intestine. Bile acids are formed from cholesterol in the liver, pass into the gut in the bile and are largely reabsorbed at the terminal ileum. The total bile acid pool is only 3–5 g, but, because such *enterohepatic recycling* takes place 5–10 times per day, on average 20–30 g of bile acids are delivered into the intestine every 24 h. Bile acids bound to colestyramine are lost in the faeces, and the depletion of the bile acid pool stimulates conversion of cholesterol to bile acid: the result is a fall in intracellular cholesterol in hepatocytes, and an increase (up-regulation) in both LDL receptors and cholesterol synthesis. The former has the predominant influence on plasma LDL cholesterol, which falls by 20–25%. In many patients, there is some compensatory increase in hepatic triglyceride output. Anion exchange resins therefore may be used first line for *hypercholesterolaemia*, but not when there is significant hypertriglyceridaemia, which may be aggravated in such patients. It is not particularly palatable, and the powder is taken mixed with water or orange juice and shaken in a closed container.

Colestyramine can be poorly tolerated with up to 50% of patients experiencing constipation; some complain of anorexia, abdominal fullness and occasionally of diarrhoea. These effects are dose-related but may limit or prevent its use. Because the drug binds anions, drugs such as warfarin, digoxin, thiazide diuretics, phenobarbitone and thyroid hormones should be taken 1 h before or 4 h after colestyramine to avoid impairment of their absorption. It also binds fat-soluble vitamins in the gut, which may be sufficient to cause clinical deficiency, e.g. vitamin-K–responsive prolongation of the prothrombin time.

Colestipol, in capsule form, is similar in effects to colestyramine.

Colesevelam is a bile acid sequestrant (not an anion exchange resin) that binds bile acids and forms an insoluble complex that passes out in the faeces. It has the same effects on hepatic metabolism as the resins.

Because of the tolerance issues, and in relation to cost, ezetimibe is preferred as additional therapy to statins.

[6]Frick M H, Elo O, Haapa K et al 1987 Helsinki Heart Study: primary-prevention trial with gemfibrozil in middle-aged men with dyslipidemia. Safety of treatment, changes in risk factors, and incidence of coronary heart disease. New England Journal of Medicine 317:1237–1245.
[7]Rubins H B, Robins S J, Collins D et al for the Veterans Affairs High-Density Lipoprotein Cholesterol Intervention Trial Study Group 1999 Gemfibrozil for the secondary prevention of coronary heart disease in men with low levels of high-density lipoprotein cholesterol. New England Journal of Medicine 341:410–418.
[8]The FIELD study investigators 2005 Effects of long-term fenofibrate therapy on cardiovascular events in 9795 people with type 2 diabetes mellitus (the FIELD study): randomised controlled trial. Lancet 366:1849–1861.

Ezetimibe

Some 30–70% of serum cholesterol is attributable to cholesterol absorbed from the gut. Ezetimibe selectively blocks intestinal cholesterol absorption by inhibition of the Niemann-Pick C1-Like 1 (NCPC1L1) transporter, which interrupts the enterohepatic cycling of cholesterol (see above). It is effective when used as monotherapy with a 10-mg dose producing a 17% fall in LDL cholesterol when used alone or when added to a statin. Ezetimibe is actually a pro-drug, and metabolism in the liver produces the more effective blocker of cholesterol transport, ezetimibe glucuronide ($t_{1/2}$ 22 h) which is secreted in bile.

Tolerability is similar to placebo, and the drug has largely displaced resins and sequestrants.

In Technology Appraisal 385, NICE[9] (which TA is to be considered in conjunction with CG181[1]) has recommended defined uses for ezetimibe.

It is recommended for primary hypercholesterolaemia (familial or non-familial) where statins are contraindicated or are not tolerated at all or not in sufficient dose, in familial hypercholesterolaemia where LDL reduction of 50% has not been achieved, and added to generic statin rather than changing to a non-generic statin of high acquisition cost.

PCSK9 inhibitors

After LDL-R with attached LDL are internalised, the LDL is catabolised while the LDL-R are either degraded or are recycled back into the cell membrane. PCSK9 is a protein that binds to the internalised LDL-R and directs the complex to intracellular degradation, so that fewer LDL-R are available to reduce extra-cellular levels of LDL. Epidemiologically, individuals with loss-of-function mutations in the *PCSK9* gene have lower plasma LDL levels and have reduced CVD rates. Since the discovery of PCSK9, it is just a period of a decade for the development of inhibitors to be taken to clinical use.

Two agents, *alirocumab* and *evolocumab*, are currently available, licensed in Europe and the USA for use in selected high-risk populations. These agents are monoclonal antibodies and are given by patient-administered subcutaneous injection on a 2–4 weekly basis. Current cost is much higher, compared to those for ezetimibe and for statins. The companies have been required to have agreed discounted patient access schemes. Other monoclonal antibodies, peptide

mimics and gene silencing approaches have been in development.

The NICE technology appraisal guidance recommended alirocumab (75–150 mg fortnightly) and evolocumab (140 mg fortnightly) as a treatment option for treating primary hypercholesterolaemia or mixed dyslipidaemia, only if LDL remained above specified thresholds despite maximal tolerated lipid-lowering therapy.[10,11] For secondary prevention, LDL-C should be >4.0 mmol/L (>3.5 mmol/L in FH or in very high risk non-familial), and for primary prevention (only for FH) >5.0 mmol/L. Recently the European Commission has agreed to a 420-mg-monthly option for evolocumab.

A meta-analysis in 2015 of study-level data from over 10 000 patients in 24 randomised controlled trials has suggested effective reduction of CVD and total mortality,[12] without major adverse events.

A secondary-prevention randomised controlled trial of evolocumab in 27 564 statin-treated patients with baseline LDL cholesterol ≥1.8 mmol/L (published 16 March 2017)[13] demonstrated a 59% lower LDL cholesterol from 2.4 mmol/L to 0.78 mmol/L. Over just 2.2 years, CVD events (CVD death, myocardial infarction, stroke, unstable angina hospitalisation, coronary revascularisation) were reduced by 15% (CI 0.79–0.92, P <0.001). The key secondary efficacy composite (CVD death, myocardial infarction, stroke) was reduced by 20% (CI 0.73–0.88, P <0.001). There were no significant adverse events except increased injection site reactions for evolocumab (2.1%:1.6%). The study was too short to assess total mortality.

More information on total mortality, and on long-term safety, is still required.

Nicotinic acid and derivatives

Nicotinic acid acts as an antilipolytic agent in adipose tissue, reducing the supply of free fatty acids and hence the availability of substrate for hepatic triglyceride synthesis and

---

[9]National Institute for Health and Care Excellence. Technology Appraisal (TA) 385. Ezetimibe for treating primary heterozygous-familial and non-familial hypercholesterolaemia, February 2016.

[10]National Institute for Health and Care Excellence. Technology Appraisal Guidance 393. Evidence-based recommendations on alirocumab for treating primary hypercholesterolaemia or mixed dyslipidaemia in adults. NICE June 2016.
[11]National Institute for Health and Care Excellence. Technology Appraisal Guidance 394. Evolocumab for treating primary hypercholesterolaemia and mixed dyslipidaemia. NICE June 2016.
[12]Navarese E P, Kolodziejczak M, Schulze V et al 2015 Effects of Proprotein Convertase Subtilisin/Kexin Type 9 antibodies in adults with hypercholesterolemia: a systematic review and meta-analysis. Annals of Internal Medicine 163:40–51.
[13]Sabatine M S, Giugliano R P, Keech A C et al for the FOURIER Steering Committee and Investigators 2017 Evolocumab and clinical outcomes in patients with cardiovascular disease. New England Journal of Medicine 376:1713–1722.

the secretion of VLDL. It lowers plasma triglyceride and cholesterol concentrations, and raises HDL cholesterol. It produces modest reduction in plasma lipoprotein Lp(a) which is potentially pro-atherogenic.

However, nicotinic acid and derivatives now have no role in management of lipid disorders for the prevention of CVD. This follows the very large trial (>25 000 patients for 5 years) of an extended-release nicotinic acid, HPS2-THRIVE.[14] This trial also included laropiprant to substantially block the flushing caused by nicotinic acid. There was no reduction in CVD, and cancer was not affected. Known side-effects of skin irritation and gastrointestinal irritation occurred, and new recognition of bleeding and infection-risk side-effects.

Possible limited use may remain in unresponsive severe hypertriglyceridaemia with pancreatitis but would be by lipid specialists only.

Other drugs

Omega-3 marine triglycerides (Maxepa) contain the triglyceride precursors of two polyunsaturated fatty acids (eicosapentaenoic acid and docosahexaenoic acid) derived from oily fish. A related product, Omacor, contains omega 3-acid ethyl esters instead of triglycerides. They have no role in treating hypercholesterolaemia, but patients with more severe hypertriglyceridaemia may respond to either agent.

In CG181, NICE[1] has stated that patients should be informed that there is no outcome evidence that omega-3 fatty acid compounds help to prevent CVD.

Orlistat, a weight-reducing agent, lowers the glycaemia of diabetes mellitus to a degree that accords with the weight loss, and improves hyperlipidaemia to an extent greater than would be expected (see p. 468). Since it is a lipase inhibitor, there is a risk of steatorrhoea and malabsorption of the fat-soluble vitamins A, D and E; hence it is licensed only for a maximum of 2 years of continuous use. The UK advisory body NICE further recommends its use only if patients show a 2.5-kg fall in body weight by dieting alone in the month before treatment commences, and use beyond 3 and 6 months only with further 5% and 10% falls, respectively, in body weight.

Orlistat increases the rate of weight loss achieved by a calorie-restricted, low-fat diet. It is not absorbed and it works by inhibiting gut lipase and reducing the absorption of residual dietary fat by about 30%. Retribution occurs with side-effects of bloating and fatty diarrhoea if a high fat meal is inappropriately taken. A half-dose preparation 'Alli' is available over the counter.

In the rare case of familial hypertriglyceridaemia with pancreatitis, orlistat may be used as an adjunct to the *very-low-fat diet* ($\leq$10% of calories) that is required.

CETP inhibitors elevate HDL cholesterol and lower triglycerides and LDL cholesterol. Use of torcetrapib resulted in an increased mortality rate, while dalcetrapib and evacetrapib did not have significant efficacy despite increased HDL cholesterol, which appears not to have been functionally active.

In the large TIMI55/REVEAL trial anacetrapib reduced CVD by a modest 9 percent.[15] Obicetrapib remains in development.

Lomitapide is an 'orphan' drug for treatment of homozygous familial hypertriglyceridaemia. It has been licensed in the USA and in the European Union. It inhibits the microsomal triglyceride transfer protein (MTP or MTTP) which is necessary for very-low-density lipoprotein (VLDL) assembly and secretion in the liver. A low-fat diet is appropriate. Transaminases rise, and hepatic fat accumulation occur. These patients are likely also to require LDL apheresis.

Mipomersen is an antisense oligonucleotide which binds to the messenger RNA that codes for hepatic apolipoprotein B-100, the structural protein for VLDL and LDL. The RNA is degraded, and apolipoprotein B-100 is not translated.

As an 'orphan' drug, mipomersen has been licensed by the US Food and Drug Administration under a strict 'risk evaluation & mitigation strategy programme for homozygous familial hypercholesterolaemia'. It is given by injection. Substantial transaminase elevation and fatty liver disease are major complications.

Volanesorsen is a chimeric antisense therapeutic oligonucleotide targeting the messenger RNA for apolipoprotein C3 (apo-CIII). It is in phase III trials as an 'orphan' drug for a very rare group of patients with the severe hypertriglyceridaemia of familial chylomicronaemia syndrome, and familial partial lipodystrophy. Triglycerides can fall by 70%, but long-term outcomes are not yet known.

[14]The HPS2-THRIVE Collaborative Group 2014 Effects of extended-release niacin with laropiprant in high-risk patients. New England Journal of Medicine 371:203–212.

[15] The HPS3/TIMI55–REVEAL Collaborative Group. Effects of Anacetrapib in Patients with Atherosclerotic Vascular Disease. N Engl J Med 2017; 377: 1217.

Summary

- The commonest and most important hyperlipidaemia is hypercholesterolaemia, which is one of the major risk factors for cardiovascular disease.
- Most treatment works by reducing the intracellular concentration of cholesterol in hepatocytes, leading to compensatory increase in low-density lipoprotein (LDL) receptors on their surface, and increased uptake of cholesterol-rich LDL particles from the bloodstream.
- With a long history of use, the most effective cholesterol-reducing drugs for the great majority of individuals are the statins, which inhibit the rate-limiting step in cholesterol synthesis.
- Additional agents may be required for mixed or severe hyperlipidaemia.
- In outcome studies of around 5 years, each 1 mmol/L LDL cholesterol reduction led to a 20% CVD reduction and a 10% reduction in all-cause mortality. With treatment concordance and longer use, benefits will be higher.
- The main indications for their use are patients with even modest elevations of cholesterol (>5 mmol/L) after any macrovascular event, in familial hypercholesterolaemia, with diabetes, and in patients with an absolute CVD risk ≥10%/10 years.

Guide to further reading

FIELD study investigators, 2005. Effects of long-term fenofibrate therapy on cardiovascular events in 9795 people with type 2 diabetes mellitus (the FIELD study): randomised controlled trial. Lancet 366, 1849–1861.

Frick, M.H., Elo, O., Haapa, K., et al., 1987. Helsinki Heart Study: primary-prevention trial with gemfibrozil in middle-aged men with dyslipidemia. Safety of treatment, changes in risk factors, and incidence of coronary heart disease. N. Engl. J. Med. 317, 1237–1245.

Fulcher, J., O'Connell, R., Voysey, M., et al., 2015. The Cholesterol Treatment Trialists' (CTT) Collaboration. Efficacy and safety of LDL-lowering therapy among men and women: meta-analysis of individual data from 174,000 participants in 27 randomised trials. Lancet 385, 1397–1405.

Hippisley-Cox, J., Coupland, S., Vinogradova, Y., et al., 2008. Predicting cardiovascular risk in England and Wales: prospective derivation and validation of QRISK2. Br. Med. J. 336, 1475–1482. Also QRISK2-2016 risk calculator at:https:// qrisk.org.

HPS2-THRIVE Collaborative Group, 2014. Effects of extended-release niacin with laropiprant in high-risk patients. N. Engl. J. Med. 371, 203–212.

The HPS3/TIMI55–REVEAL Collaborative Group, 2017. Effects of Anacetrapib in Patients with Atherosclerotic Vascular Disease. N. Engl. J. Med. 377, 1217.

National Institute for Health and Care Excellence, February 2016. Technology Appraisal (TA) 385. Ezetimibe for treating primary heterozygous-familial and non-familial hypercholesterolaemia.

National Institute for Health and Care Excellence, June 2016. Technology Appraisal Guidance 393. Evidence-based recommendations on alirocumab for treating primary hypercholesterolaemia or mixed dyslipidaemia in adults.

National Institute for Health and Care Excellence, June 2016. Technology Appraisal Guidance 394. Evolocumab for treating primary hypercholesterolaemia and mixed dyslipidaemia.

National Institute for Health and Care Excellence, July 2014. Clinical Guidance (CG) 181. Cardiovascular disease: risk assessment and reduction, including lipid modification.

Navarese, E.P., Kolodziejczak, M., Schulze, V., et al., 2015. Effects of Proprotein Convertase Subtilisin/ Kexin Type 9 antibodies in adults with hypercholesterolemia: a systematic review and meta-analysis. Ann. Intern. Med. 163, 40–51.

Rubins, H.B., Robins, S.J., Collins, D., et al. for the Veterans Affairs High-Density Lipoprotein Cholesterol Intervention Trial Study Group, 1999. Gemfibrozil for the secondary prevention of coronary heart disease in men with low levels of high-density lipoprotein cholesterol. N. Engl. J. Med. 341, 410–418.

Sabatine, M.S., Giugliano, R.P., Keech, A.C., et al. for the FOURIER Steering Committee and Investigators, 2017. Evolocumab and clinical outcomes in patients with cardiovascular disease. N. Engl. J. Med. 376, 1713–1722.

Scandinavian Simvastatin Survival Study Group, 1994. Randomised trial of cholesterol lowering in 4444 patients with coronary heart disease: the Scandinavian Simvastatin Survival Study (4S). Lancet 344, 1383–1389.

Chapter | **27** |

Kidney and genitourinary tract

Thomas F. Hiemstra

SYNOPSIS

The kidneys compose only 0.5% of body-weight, yet they receive 25% of the cardiac output. Drugs that affect renal function have important roles in cardiac failure and hypertension. Disease of the kidney must be taken into account when prescribing drugs that are eliminated by it.

- Diuretic drugs: their sites and modes of action, classification, adverse effects and uses in cardiac, hepatic, renal and other conditions.
- Carbonic anhydrase inhibitors.
- Cation-exchange resins and other cation binders.
- Alteration of urine pH.
- Drugs and the kidney.
- Adverse effects.
- Drug-induced renal disease: by direct and indirect biochemical effects and by immunological effects.
- Prescribing for renal disease: adjusting the dose according to the characteristics of the drug and to the degree of renal impairment.
- Nephrolithiasis and its management.
- Pharmacological aspects of micturition.
- Benign prostatic hyperplasia.
- Erectile dysfunction.

Diuretic drugs

(See also Ch. 24.)

Definition. A diuretic is any substance that increases water and solute excretion, usually with the objective of reducing extracellular volume in oedematous states. Since a saline infusion or a water load both induce a diuresis while expanding total body water and or solute, a more clinically useful definition of a diuretic is a substance that increases water and solute excretion *and reduces extracellular volume.*

Diuretics are among the most commonly used drugs, perhaps because the evolutionary advantages of sodium retention have left an ageing population without salt-losing mechanisms of matching efficiency. Each day the body produces 180 L of glomerular filtrate which is modified in its passage down the renal tubules to appear as approximately 1.5 L of urine. Thus, if reabsorption of tubular fluid falls by 1%, urine output doubles. Most clinically useful diuretics are organic anions, which enter the renal tubular lumen through glomerular filtration. The following brief account of tubular function with particular reference to sodium transport will help to explain where and how diuretic drugs act; it should be read with reference to Fig. 27.1.

Sites and modes of action

Proximal convoluted tubule

The proximal tubule actively reabsorbs 60% of the filtered sodium through the sodium pump (Na^+, K^+-ATPase), with chloride following through passive transport. Filtered bicarbonate is also reabsorbed, through an action involving carbonic anhydrase. These solute shifts give rise to the iso-osmotic reabsorption of water, with the result that more than 70% of the glomerular filtrate is returned to the blood from this section of the nephron.

Osmotic diuretics such as *mannitol* have their action in the proximal tubule. These agents are non-resorbable solutes which retain water in the tubular fluid (Site 1, Fig. 27.1), increasing water rather than sodium loss. This is reflected in

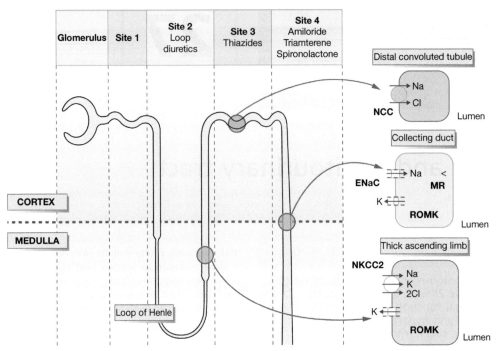

Fig. 27.1 Sites of action of diuretic drugs. Inset cartoons show the transporters and ion channels targeted in tubular cells at these sites. ENaC, epithelial sodium channel; NCCT, thiazide-sensitive Na–Cl co-transporter; NKCC2, Na–K–2Cl co-transporter; ROMK, rectifying outer medullary potassium channel.

their special use acutely to reduce intracranial or intraocular pressure and not states associated with sodium overload.

Loop of Henle

The tubular fluid now passes into the loop of Henle, where 25% of the filtered sodium is reabsorbed. There are two populations of nephron: those with short loops that are confined to the cortex, and the juxtamedullary nephrons whose long loops penetrate deep into the medulla and are concerned principally with *water* conservation;[1] the following discussion refers to the latter.

The physiological changes are best understood by considering first the *ascending* limb. In the thick segment (Site 2, Fig. 27.1), sodium and chloride ions are transported from the tubular fluid into the interstitial fluid by the three-ion co-transporter system (i.e. Na⁺/K⁺/2Cl⁻ called 'NKCC2') driven by the sodium pump. The co-transport of these ions is dependent on potassium returning to the lumen through the rectifying outer medullary potassium (ROMK) channel; otherwise potassium would be rate limiting. As the tubule

epithelium is impermeable to water here, the tubular fluid becomes dilute, the interstitium becomes hypertonic, and fluid in the adjacent *descending* limb, which is permeable to water, becomes more concentrated as it approaches the tip of the loop, because the hypertonic interstitial fluid sucks water out of this limb of the tubule. The 'hairpin' structure of the loop thus confers on it the property of a *countercurrent multiplier*, i.e. by active transport of ions a small change in osmolality laterally across the tubular epithelium is converted into a steep vertical osmotic gradient.

The high osmotic pressure in the medullary interstitium is sustained by the descending and ascending vasa recta, long blood vessels of capillary thickness that lie close to the loops of Henle and act as *countercurrent exchangers*, for the incoming blood receives sodium from the outgoing blood.[2] *Furosemide, bumetanide, piretanide, torasemide* and

---

[1]Beavers and other freshwater-adapted mammals typically have nephrons with short loops, whereas desert-adapted mammals have long loops.

[2]The most easily comprehended countercurrent exchange mechanism (in this case for heat) is that in wading birds in cold climates whereby the veins carrying cold blood from the feet pass closely alongside the arteries carrying warm blood from the body and heat exchange takes place. The result is that the feet receive blood below body temperature (which does not matter) and the blood from the feet, which is often very cold, is warmed before it enters the body so that the internal temperature is maintained more easily. The principle is the same for maintaining renal medullary hypertonicity.

ethacrynic acid act principally at Site 2 by inhibiting the three-ion transporter, thus preventing sodium ion reabsorption and lowering the osmotic gradient between cortex and medulla; this results in the formation of large volumes of dilute urine. Hence, these drugs are called 'loop' diuretics.

Distal convoluted tubule

The ascending limb of the loop then re-enters the renal cortex where its morphology changes into the thin-walled distal convoluted tubule (Site 3, Fig. 27.1). Here uptake is still driven by the sodium pump, but sodium and chloride are taken up through a different transporter, the Na–Cl co-transporter, called 'NCC' (formerly 'NCCT'). Both ions are rapidly removed from the interstitium because cortical blood flow is high and there are no vasa recta present; the epithelium is also water impermeable at Site 3, and consequently the urine becomes more dilute. *Thiazides* act principally at this region of the cortical diluting segment by blocking the NCC transporter.

Collecting duct

In the collecting duct (Site 4), sodium ions are exchanged for potassium and hydrogen ions. The sodium ions enter through the epithelial Na channel (called ENaC), which is stimulated by aldosterone. The aldosterone (mineralocorticoid) receptor is inhibited by the competitive receptor antagonist *spironolactone*, whereas the sodium channel is inhibited by *amiloride* and *triamterene*. All three of these diuretics are potassium sparing because potassium is normally secreted through the potassium channel, ROMK (see Fig. 27.1), down the potential gradient created by sodium reabsorption.

All other diuretics, acting proximal to Site 4, cause potassium loss, because they increase delivery of sodium into the collecting duct. Removal of this sodium through ENaC increases the potential gradient for potassium secretion through ROMK. The potassium-sparing diuretics are normally considered weak diuretics because Site 4 is normally responsible for 'only' 2–3% of sodium reabsorption, and they usually cause less sodium loss than thiazides or loop diuretics. Nevertheless, patients with genetic abnormalities of ENaC show salt wasting or retention to a degree that significantly affects their blood pressure, depending on whether the mutation causes, respectively, loss or gain of channel activity. Although ENaC clearly does not have the capacity to compensate for large sodium losses, e.g. during loop diuretic usage, it is the main site of physiological control (via aldosterone) over sodium loss.

The collecting duct then travels back through the medulla to reach the papilla; in doing so it passes through a gradient of increasing osmotic pressure which draws water out of tubular fluid. This final concentration of urine is under the influence of *vasopressin* (also known as 'antidiuretic hormone', ADH) whose action is to increase water permeability by increasing the expression of specific water channels (or aquaporins); in its absence water remains in the collecting duct. The vasopressin receptor antagonist *tolvaptan* acts by competitive binding of collecting duct V_2 receptors. *Ethanol* causes diuresis by inhibiting the release of ADH from the posterior pituitary gland.

Diuresis may also be achieved by extrarenal mechanisms, by raising the cardiac output and increasing renal blood flow, e.g. with dobutamine and dopamine.

Classification

The maximum efficacy in removing salt and water that any drug can achieve is dependent on its site of action, and it is appropriate to rank diuretics according to their natriuretic capacity, as set out below. The percentages refer to the highest fractional excretion of filtered sodium under carefully controlled conditions and should not be taken to represent the average fractional sodium loss during clinical use.

High efficacy

Furosemide and the other 'loop' diuretics can cause up to 25% of filtered sodium to be excreted. Their action impairs the powerful urine-concentrating mechanism of the loop of Henle and confers higher efficacy compared with drugs that act in the relatively hypotonic cortex (see below). Progressive increase in dose is matched by increasing diuresis, i.e. they have a high 'ceiling' of effect. In fact, they are so effective that over-treatment can readily dehydrate the patient. Loop diuretics remain effective at a glomerular filtration rate (GFR) below 10 mL/min (normal 120 mL/min).

Moderate efficacy

The thiazide family, including *bendroflumethiazide* and the related *chlortalidone, clopamide, indapamide, mefruside, metolazone* and *xipamide,* cause 5–10% of filtered sodium load to be excreted. Increasing the dose produces relatively little added diuresis compared to loop diuretics, i.e. they have a low 'ceiling' of effect. Such drugs cease to be effective once the GFR has fallen below 20 mL/min (except *metolazone*).

Low efficacy

Triamterene, amiloride and spironolactone cause 2–3% of the filtered sodium to be excreted. They are potassium sparing and combine usefully with more efficacious diuretics to prevent the potassium loss, which other diuretics cause.

Osmotic diuretics, e.g. *mannitol,* also fall into this category.

Individual diuretics

High-efficacy (loop) diuretics

Furosemide

Furosemide acts on the thick portion of the ascending limb of the loop of Henle (Site 2) to produce the effects described above. Because more sodium is delivered to Site 4, exchange with potassium leads to urinary potassium loss and hypokalaemia. Magnesium and calcium loss are increased by furosemide to about the same extent as sodium; the effect on calcium is utilised in the emergency management of hypercalcaemia (see p. 485).

Pharmacokinetics. Absorption of furosemide from the gastrointestinal (GI) tract is subject to considerable intra- and inter-individual variation and it is highly bound to plasma proteins. The $t_{1/2}$ is 2 h, but this rises to over 10 h in renal failure.

Uses. Furosemide is very successful for the relief of oedema. Urine production rises progressively with increasing dose. Taken orally it acts within 1 h, and diuresis lasts up to 6 h. Enormous urine volumes can result, and over-treatment may lead to hypovolaemia and circulatory collapse. Given intravenously, it acts within 30 min and can relieve acute pulmonary oedema, partly by a venodilator action which precedes the diuresis. An important feature of furosemide is that it retains efficacy even at a low GFR (10 mL/min or less). The adult dose is 20–120 mg/day p.o. i.m., or i.v. 20–40 mg is given initially. For use in renal failure, high-dose tablets (500 mg) are available, and a solution of 250 mg in 25 mL, which should be infused intravenously at a rate not greater than 4 mg/min. In patients with heart failure, absorption from the gut is prolonged, the dose–response curve for furosemide is shifted to the right and downward, i.e. the response to any given dose is reduced; this should be borne in mind when dosing these patients.

Adverse effects are uncommon, apart from excess of therapeutic effect (electrolyte disturbance and hypotension due to low plasma volume) and those mentioned in the general account for diuretics (below). They include nausea, pancreatitis and, rarely, deafness, which is usually transient and associated with rapid intravenous injection in renal failure. Non-steroidal anti-inflammatory drugs (NSAIDs), notably indometacin, reduce furosemide-induced diuresis, probably by inhibiting the formation of vasodilator prostaglandins in the kidney.

Bumetanide, piretanide and *ethacrynic acid* are similar to furosemide. Bumetanide may be preferred over furosemide in heart failure because of its more predictable oral absorption. Ethacrynic acid is less widely used as it is more prone to cause adverse effects, especially nausea and deafness. *Torasemide* is an effective antihypertensive agent at lower (non-natriuretic) doses (2.5–5 mg/day) than those used for oedema (5–40 mg/day).

Moderate-efficacy diuretics

(See also Hypertension, Ch. 24.)

Thiazides

Thiazides depress salt reabsorption in the distal convoluted tubule (at Site 3), i.e. upstream of the region of sodium–potassium exchange at Site 4. Hence these drugs have the important effect of raising potassium excretion. Thiazides lower blood pressure, initially due to a reduction in intravascular volume but chronically by a reduction in peripheral vascular resistance. The latter is accompanied by diminished responsiveness of vascular smooth muscle to noradrenaline/norepinephrine; they may also have a direct action on vascular smooth muscle membranes, acting on an as yet unidentified ion channel.

Uses. Thiazides are given for mild cardiac failure and mild hypertension, or for more severe degrees of hypertension, in combination with other drugs.

Pharmacokinetics. Thiazides are generally well absorbed orally, and most begin to act within 1 h. Differences among the numerous derivatives lie principally in duration of action. The relatively water-soluble, e.g. *cyclopenthiazide, chlorothiazide, hydrochlorothiazide,* are most rapidly eliminated, their peak effect occurring within 4–6 h and passing off by 10–12 h. They are excreted unchanged in the urine, and active secretion by the proximal renal tubule contributes to their high renal clearance and $t_{1/2}$ of less than 4 h.

The relatively lipid-soluble members of the group, e.g. *polythiazide, hydroflumethiazide,* distribute more widely into body tissues and act for >24 h, which can be problematic if the drug is used for diuresis, but there is no evidence this property makes them more effective at controlling hypertension. With the exception of *metolazone,* thiazides are not effective when renal function is moderately impaired (GFR <20 mL/min), because they are not filtered in sufficient concentration to inhibit the NCC.

Adverse effects in general are discussed below. Rashes (sometimes photosensitive), thrombocytopenia and agranulocytosis occur. Thiazide-type drugs increase total plasma cholesterol concentration, but in long-term use this is less than 5%, even at high doses. The questions about the appropriateness of thiazides for mild hypertension, of which ischaemic heart disease is a common complication, are laid to rest by their proven success in randomised outcome comparisons (see Ch. 24).

Bendroflumethiazide is a satisfactory member for routine use. For a diuretic effect, the oral dose is 5–10 mg, which usually lasts less than 12 h, so that it should be given in the morning. As an antihypertensive, 2.5 mg is commonly prescribed. However, this dose does not achieve maximal blood pressure reduction in patients with salt-dependent hypertension (which includes most patients receiving a blocker of the renin–angiotensin system), and has not been shown to prevent strokes or heart attacks. Higher doses (5 mg) are recommended if the plasma potassium concentration is >4.5 mmol/L. Important potassium depletion is uncommon, but plasma potassium concentration should be checked in potentially vulnerable groups such as the elderly (see Ch. 25). If marked hypokalaemia occurs, hyperaldosteronism should be excluded.

Hydrochlorothiazide is a satisfactory alternative. Other members of the group include benzthiazide, chlorothiazide, cyclopenthiazide, hydroflumethiazide and polythiazide.

Diuretics related to the thiazides. Several compounds, although not strictly thiazides, share structural similarities with them and probably act at the same site on the nephron; they therefore exhibit moderate therapeutic efficacy. Overall, these substances have a longer duration of action, are used for oedema and hypertension, and their profile of adverse effects is similar to that of the thiazides. They are listed below.

Chlortalidone acts for 48–72 h after a single oral dose.

Indapamide is structurally related to chlortalidone but lowers blood pressure at subdiuretic doses, perhaps by altering calcium flux in vascular smooth muscle. It has less apparent effect on potassium, glucose or uric acid excretion (see below).

Metolazone is effective when renal function is impaired. It potentiates the diuresis produced by furosemide, and the combination can be effective in resistant oedema, although the risk of hypokalaemia is very high.

Xipamide is structurally related to chlortalidone and to furosemide. It induces a diuresis for about 12 h that is brisker than with thiazides; this may trouble the elderly.

Low-efficacy diuretics

Spironolactone (Aldactone) is structurally similar to aldosterone and competitively inhibits its action in the distal tubule (Site 4; exchange of potassium for sodium); excessive secretion of aldosterone contributes to fluid retention in hepatic cirrhosis, nephrotic syndrome, congestive heart failure (see specific use in Ch. 25) and primary hypersecretion (Conn's syndrome). Spironolactone is also the treatment of choice for many patients with resistant hypertension, where increased aldosterone sensitivity is increasingly recognised as a contributory factor.

Spironolactone itself has a short $t_{1/2}$ (1.6 h), being extensively metabolised, and its prolonged diuretic effect is due to the most significant active product, canrenone ($t_{1/2}$ 17 h). Spironolactone is relatively ineffective as a diuretic when used alone but is more efficient when combined with a drug that reduces sodium reabsorption proximally in the tubule, i.e. a loop diuretic. Spironolactone (and amiloride and triamterene; see below) usefully reduces the potassium loss caused by loop diuretics, but its combination with another potassium-sparing diuretic must be avoided as hyperkalaemia will result. Dangerous potassium retention is possible if spironolactone is given to patients with impaired renal function. As a diuretic, it is given orally in one or more doses totalling 100–200 mg/day. Maximum diuresis may not occur for up to 4 days. If after 5 days the response is inadequate, the dose may be increased to 300–400 mg/day. Lower doses (0.5–1 mg/kg) are required to treat hypertension.

Adverse effects. Oestrogenic effects are the major limitation to its long-term use. They are dose dependent, but in the Randomized Aldactone Evaluation Study (RALES)[3] (see Ch. 25) even 25 mg/day caused breast tenderness or enlargement in 10% of men. Women may also report breast discomfort or menstrual irregularities, including amenorrhoea. Minor GI upset also occurs, and there is increased risk of gastroduodenal ulcer and bleeding. These are reversible on stopping the drug. Spironolactone is reported to be carcinogenic in rodents, but many years of clinical experience suggest that it is safe in humans. Nevertheless, the UK licence for its use in essential hypertension was withdrawn (i.e. possible use long term in a patient group that includes the relatively young), but is retained for other indications.

Eplerenone is a spironolactone analogue licensed for use in heart failure that appears to be free of the oestrogenic effects; probably because of its lower affinity for the oestrogen receptor. It is useful in patients who need an aldosterone-receptor–blocking agent, but are intolerant of the endocrine effects of spironolactone.

Amiloride blocks the ENaC sodium channels in the distal tubule. This action complements that of the thiazides with which it is frequently combined to increase sodium loss and limit potassium loss. One such combination, co-amilozide (Moduretic; amiloride 2.5–5 mg plus hydrochlorothiazide 25–50 mg) is used for hypertension or oedema. The maximum effect of amiloride occurs about 6 h after an oral dose, with a duration of action greater than 24 h ($t_{1/2}$ 21 h). The oral dose is 5–20 mg daily.

---

[3]Pitt B, Zannad F, Remme W J et al 1999 The effect of spironolactone on morbidity and mortality in patients with severe heart failure. Randomized Aldactone Evaluation Study Investigators. New England Journal of Medicine 341:709–717.

Triamterene (Dytac) is a potassium-sparing diuretic with an action and use similar to that of amiloride. The diuretic effect extends over 10 h. Gastrointestinal upsets occur. Reversible, non-oliguric renal failure may occur when triamterene is used with indometacin (and presumably other NSAIDs). It may also give the urine a blue coloration.

Indications for diuretics

- *Oedema states* associated with sodium overload, e.g. cardiac, renal or hepatic disease, and also without sodium overload, e.g. acute pulmonary oedema following myocardial infarction. Note that oedema may also be localised, e.g. angioedema over the face and neck or around the ankles with some calcium channel blockers, or due to low plasma albumin, or immobility in the elderly; in none of these circumstances is a diuretic indicated.
- *Hypertension*, by reducing intravascular volume and probably by other mechanisms too, e.g. reduction of sensitivity to noradrenergic vasoconstriction.
- *Hypercalcaemia*. Furosemide reduces calcium reabsorption in the ascending limb of the loop of Henle, which action may be utilised in the emergency reduction of raised plasma calcium levels in addition to rehydration and other measures.
- *Idiopathic hypercalciuria*, a common cause of renal stone disease, may be reduced by thiazide diuretics.
- The *syndrome of inappropriate secretion of antidiuretic hormone secretion* (SIADH) may be treated with furosemide if there is a dangerous degree of volume overload (see also p. 446).
- *Nephrogenic diabetes insipidus*, paradoxically, may respond to thiazide diuretics. Hydrochlorothiazide restores aquaporine abundance in animal models of lithium-induced nephrogenic DI.[4] The antidiuretic effect may also result from contracted intravascular volume, with a secondary increase in salt and water reabsorption in the proximal tubule.

Therapy

Congestive cardiac failure

The main account appears in Chapter 24, where the emphasis is now on early use of angiotensin-converting enzyme (ACE) inhibitors and β-adrenoceptor antagonists that are specifically diuretic sparing. But oral diuretics are easily given repeatedly, and lack of supervision can result in insidious over-treatment. Relief at disappearance of the congestive features can mask exacerbation of the low-output symptoms of heart failure, such as tiredness and postural dizziness due to reduced blood volume. A rising blood urea level is usually evidence of reduced glomerular blood flow consequent on a fall in cardiac output, but does not distinguish whether the cause of the reduced output is over-diuresis or worsening of the heart failure itself. The simplest guide to the success or failure of diuretic regimens is to monitor *body-weight*, which the patient can do equipped with just bathroom scales. Fluid intake and output charts are more demanding of nursing time, and often less accurate.

Acute pulmonary oedema: left ventricular failure

(See p. 448.)

Renal oedema

The chief therapeutic aims are to reduce dietary sodium intake and to prevent excessive sodium retention using diuretic drugs. Reduction of sodium reabsorption in the renal tubule by diuretics is most effective where glomerular filtration has not been seriously reduced by disease. Furosemide and bumetanide are effective even when the filtration rate is very low; furosemide may usefully be combined with metolazone, but the resulting profound diuresis requires careful monitoring. Secondary hyperaldosteronism complicates the nephrotic syndrome because albumin loss causes plasma colloid pressure to fall, and the resulting diversion of intravascular volume to the interstitium activates the renin–angiotensin–aldosterone system; spironolactone may then be added usefully to potentiate a loop diuretic and to conserve potassium, loss of which can be severe.

Hepatic ascites

(See also p. 585.)

Ascites and oedema are due to portal venous hypertension together with decreased plasma colloid osmotic pressure causing hyperaldosteronism as with nephrotic oedema (above). Furthermore, diversion of renal blood flow from the cortex to the medulla favours sodium retention. In addition to dietary sodium restriction, spironolactone is the preferred diuretic to produce a gradual diuresis; too vigorous depletion of sodium with added potassium loss and hypochloraemic alkalosis may worsen hepatic

---

[4]Kim G-H, Lee J W, Oh Y K et al 2004 Antidiuretic effect of hydrochlorothiazide in lithium-induced nephrogenic diabetes insipidus is associated with upregulation of aquaporin-2, Na-Cl cotransporter and epithelial sodium channel. Journal of the American Society of Nephrology 15: 2836–2843.

encephalopathy. Abdominal paracentesis can be very effective if combined with human albumin infusion to prevent further aggravating hypoproteinaemia.

Adaptation to diuretic therapy

Inhibition of sodium reabsorption in one nephron segment results in important adaptations in another nephron segment. Although the initial dose of a diuretic usually induces a brisk diuresis, this is followed by a new steady state, where fluid and solute excretion matches intake, and subsequent doses of diuretic result in a reduced response. Periods in between dosing may be characterised by avid sodium and fluid retention, particularly when diuretics with a short $t_{1/2}$ are used. This may be circumvented by using longer-acting diuretics, more frequent dosing, or combination treatment with 'sequential nephron blockade', i.e. combining a loop diuretic with a thiazide.

Adverse effects characteristic of diuretics

Potassium depletion

Diuretics that act at Sites 1, 2 and 3 (see Fig. 27.1) cause more sodium to reach the sodium–potassium exchange site in the distal tubule (Site 4) and so increase potassium excretion. This subject warrants discussion because hypokalaemia may cause cardiac arrhythmia in patients at risk (e.g. receiving digoxin). The safe lower limit for plasma potassium concentration is normally quoted as 3.5 mmol/L. Whether or not diuretic therapy causes significant lowering of serum potassium levels depends both on the drug and on the circumstances in which it is used:

- *The loop diuretics* produce a smaller fall in serum potassium concentration than do the thiazides, for equivalent diuretic effect, but have a greater capacity for diuresis, i.e. higher efficacy especially in large dose, and so are associated with greater decline in potassium levels. If diuresis is brisk and continuous, clinically important potassium depletion is likely to occur.
- *Low dietary intake* of potassium predisposes to hypokalaemia; the risk is particularly notable in the elderly, many of whom ingest less than 50 mmol/day (the dietary normal is 80 mmol).
- Hypokalaemia may be aggravated by other drugs, e.g. β_2-adrenoceptor agonists, theophylline, corticosteroids, amphotericin.
- Hypokalaemia during diuretic therapy is also more likely in *hyperaldosteronism,* whether primary or more commonly secondary to severe liver disease,

congestive cardiac failure or nephrotic syndrome.
- Potassium loss occurs with diarrhoea, vomiting or small bowel fistula, and may be aggravated by diuretic therapy.
- When a thiazide diuretic is used for hypertension, there is probably no case for routine prescription of a potassium supplement if no predisposing factors are present (see Ch. 25).
- Potassium depletion can be minimised or corrected by:
  - maintaining a good dietary potassium intake (fruits, fruit juices, vegetables)
  - combining a potassium-depleting with a potassium-sparing drug
  - intermittent use of potassium-losing drugs, i.e. drug holidays
  - potassium supplements: KCl is preferred because chloride is the principal anion excreted along with sodium when high-efficacy diuretics are used. Potassium-sparing diuretics generally defend plasma potassium more effectively than potassium supplements. All forms of potassium are irritant to the GI tract, and in the oesophagus may even cause ulceration. The elderly, in particular, should be warned never to take such tablets dry but always with a large cupful of liquid and sitting upright or standing.

Hyperkalaemia may occur, especially if a potassium-sparing diuretic is given to a patient with impaired renal function. ACE inhibitors and angiotensin II receptor antagonists can also cause a modest increase in plasma potassium levels. They may cause dangerous hyperkalaemia if combined with KCl supplements or other potassium-sparing drugs, in the presence of impaired renal function. These may not be obvious, for example, to the patient who is using an unprescribed 'low-sodium' salt substitute to reduce salt (NaCl) intake.[5] However, with suitable monitoring the combination can be used safely, as was well illustrated by the RALES trial.[6] Ciclosporin, tacrolimus, indometacin and possibly other NSAIDs may cause hyperkalaemia with the potassium-sparing diuretics.

---

[5]These typically contain equal proportions by weight of NaCl and KCl, so 1 g could contain 7 mmol of KCl, and consuming the recommended 6 g/d of salt as the 'low sodium' form could provide >40 mmol/d of KCl!

[6]Pitt B, Zannad F, Remme W J et al 1999 The effect of spironolactone on morbidity and mortality in patients with severe heart failure. Randomized Aldactone Evaluation Study Investigators. New England Journal of Medicine 341:709–717.

Treatment of hyperkalaemia

Depends on the severity, and the following measures are appropriate:

- Any potassium-sparing diuretic should be discontinued.
- A cation-exchange resin, e.g. polystyrene sulphonate resin (Resonium A, Calcium Resonium, see below) can be used orally (more effective than rectally), to remove body potassium by the gut:
  - glucose, 50 mL 50% solution, plus 10 units soluble insulin by i.v. infusion
  - nebulised β_2-agonist, salbutamol 5–10 mg, is effective in stimulating the pumping of potassium into skeletal muscle.
- Hypertonic sodium bicarbonate (50 mL 8.4% via a central line) may reduce plasma potassium, although the effect is small and this strategy is generally not recommended.
- In the presence of ECG changes, calcium gluconate, 10 mL of 10% solution, should be given i.v. and repeated if necessary in a few minutes; it has no effect on the serum potassium but opposes the myocardial effect of a raised serum potassium level. Calcium may potentiate digoxin and should be used cautiously, if at all, in a patient taking this drug. Sodium bicarbonate and calcium salt must not be mixed in a syringe or reservoir because calcium precipitates.
- Dialysis may be needed in refractory cases and is highly effective.

Newer oral potassium-binding compounds such as patiromer and sodium zirconium cyclosilicate (ZS-9) are also effective in lowering plasma potassium. Patiromer is a non-absorbed polymer which binds intestinal potassium in exchange for calcium, predominantly in the distal colon.[7] ZS-9 traps potassium in exchange for sodium and hydrogen. It is effective proximally in the GI tract and therefore has a more rapid onset of action than patiromer. Their utility in the treatment of acute hyperkalaemia is currently unknown.

Hypovolaemia can result from over-treatment. Acute loss of excessive fluid leads to postural hypotension and dizziness. A more insidious state of chronic hypovolaemia can develop, especially in the elderly. After initial benefit, the patient becomes sleepy and lethargic. Blood urea concentration rises, and sodium concentration may be low. Renal failure may result.

[7]Weir M R, Bakris G L, Bushinsky D A 2015 Patiromer in patients with kidney disease and hyperkalemia receiving RAAS inhibitors. New England Journal of Medicine 372:211–221.

Urinary retention. Sudden vigorous diuresis can cause acute retention of urine in the presence of bladder neck obstruction, e.g. due to prostatic enlargement.

Hyponatraemia may result if sodium loss occurs in patients who drink a large quantity of water when taking a diuretic. Other mechanisms are probably involved, including enhancement of antidiuretic hormone release. Such patients have reduced total body sodium and extracellular fluid and are oedema free. Discontinuing the diuretic and restricting water intake are effective. The condition should be distinguished from hyponatraemia with oedema, which develops in some patients with congestive cardiac failure, cirrhosis or nephrotic syndrome. Here salt and water intake should be restricted because extracellular fluid volume is expanded.

The combination of a potassium-sparing diuretic and ACE inhibitor can also cause severe hyponatraemia – more commonly than life-threatening hyperkalaemia.

Urate retention with hyperuricaemia and, sometimes, clinical gout occurs with thiazides and loop diuretics. The effect is unimportant or negligible with the low-efficacy diuretics, e.g. amiloride and spironolactone. Two mechanisms appear to be responsible. First, diuretics cause volume depletion, reduction in glomerular filtration and increased absorption of almost all solutes in the proximal tubule, including urate. Second, diuretics and uric acid are organic acids and compete with urate for the transport mechanism that pumps such substances from the blood into the tubular fluid. Diuretic-induced hyperuricaemia can be prevented by allopurinol or probenecid (which also antagonises diuretic efficacy by reducing their transport into the urine).

Magnesium deficiency. Loop and thiazide diuretics cause significant urinary loss of magnesium; potassium-sparing diuretics probably also cause magnesium retention. Magnesium deficiency brought about by diuretics is rarely severe enough to induce the classic picture of neuromuscular irritability and tetany, but cardiac arrhythmias, mainly of ventricular origin, do occur and respond to repletion of magnesium (2 g or 8 mmol of Mg^{2+} is given as 4 mL 50% magnesium sulphate infused i.v. over 10–15 min followed by up to 72 mmol infused over the next 24 h).

Carbohydrate intolerance is caused by those diuretics that produce prolonged hypokalaemia, i.e. the loop and thiazide type. This may affect the depolarisation and entry of calcium into islet cells which is necessary to stimulate formation and release of insulin, so glucose intolerance is probably due to secondary insulin deficiency. Insulin requirements thus increase in established diabetics, and the disease may become manifest in latent diabetics. The effect is generally reversible over several months.

Calcium homeostasis. Renal calcium loss is increased by the loop diuretics; in the short term this is not a serious disadvantage, and indeed *furosemide* may be used in the management of hypercalcaemia after rehydration has been achieved. In the long term, hypocalcaemia may be harmful, especially in elderly patients, who tend in any case to be in negative calcium balance. *Thiazides,* by contrast, decrease renal excretion of calcium, and this property may influence the choice of diuretic in a potentially calcium-deficient or osteoporotic individual, as thiazide use is associated with a reduced risk of hip fracture in the elderly. The hypocalciuric effect of the thiazides has also been used effectively in patients with idiopathic hypercalciuria, the commonest metabolic cause of renal stones.

Interactions

Loop diuretics (especially as intravenous boluses) potentiate ototoxicity of aminoglycosides and nephrotoxicity of some cephalosporins. NSAIDs tend to cause sodium retention, which counteracts the effect of diuretics; the mechanism may involve inhibition of renal prostaglandin formation. Diuretic treatment of a patient taking lithium can precipitate toxicity from this drug (the increased sodium loss is accompanied by reduced lithium excretion). Other drugs that may induce hyperkalaemia, hypokalaemia, hyponatraemia or glucose intolerance with diuretics are described above.

Abuse of diuretics

Psychological abnormality sometimes takes the form of abuse of diuretics and/or purgatives. The subject usually desires to slim to become more attractive, or may have anorexia nervosa. There can be severe depletion of sodium and potassium, with renal tubular damage due to chronic hypokalaemia.

Osmotic diuretics

Osmotic diuretics are low-molecular-weight substances that are filtered by the glomerulus but not reabsorbed by the renal tubule, and thus increase the osmolarity of the tubular fluid. Thus they prevent reabsorption of water (and also, by more complex mechanisms, of sodium) principally in the proximal convoluted tubule and probably also the loop of Henle. The result is that urine volume increases according to the load of osmotic diuretic.

Mannitol, a polyhydric alcohol (mol. wt. 452), is used most commonly; it is given intravenously. In addition to its effect on the kidney, mannitol encourages the movement of water from inside cells to the extracellular fluid, which is thus transiently expanded before diuresis occurs. These properties define its uses, which are for rapid reduction of intracranial or intraocular pressure, and to maintain urine flow to prevent renal tubular necrosis. Because it increases circulatory volume, mannitol is contraindicated in congestive cardiac failure and pulmonary oedema.

Methylxanthines

The general properties of the methylxanthines (theophylline, caffeine) are discussed elsewhere (see p. 159). Their mild diuretic action probably depends in part on smooth muscle relaxation in the afferent arteriolar bed increasing renal blood flow, and in part on a direct inhibitory effect on salt reabsorption in the proximal tubule. Their uses in medicine depend on other properties.

Carbonic anhydrase inhibitors

The enzyme carbonic anhydrase facilitates the reaction between carbon dioxide and water to form carbonic acid (H_2CO_3), which then breaks down to hydrogen (H^+) and bicarbonate (HCO_3^-) ions. This process is fundamental to the production of either acid or alkaline secretions, and high concentrations of carbonic anhydrase are present in the gastric mucosa, pancreas, eye and kidney. Because the number of H^+ ions available to exchange with Na^+ in the proximal tubule is reduced, sodium loss and diuresis occur. But HCO_3^- reabsorption from the tubule is also reduced, and its loss in the urine leads within days to metabolic acidosis, which attenuates the diuretic response to carbonic anhydrase inhibition. Consequently, inhibitors of carbonic anhydrase are obsolete as diuretics, but still have specific uses. *Acetazolamide* is the most widely used carbonic anhydrase inhibitor.

Reduction of intraocular pressure. This action is not due to diuresis (thiazides actually raise intraocular pressure slightly). The formation of aqueous humour is an active process requiring a supply of bicarbonate ions which depends on carbonic anhydrase. Inhibition of carbonic anhydrase reduces the formation of aqueous humour and lowers intraocular pressure. This is a local action and is not affected by the development of acid–base changes elsewhere in the body, i.e. tolerance does not develop. In patients with acute glaucoma, acetazolamide can be taken either orally or intravenously. Acetazolamide is not recommended for long-term use because of the risk of hypokalaemia and acidosis, but *brinzolamide* or *dorzolamide* are effective as eye drops, well tolerated, and thus suitable for chronic use in glaucoma.

High-altitude (mountain) sickness may affect unacclimatised people at altitudes over 3000 metres, especially after rapid ascent; symptoms range from nausea, lassitude and headache to pulmonary and cerebral oedema. The initiating cause is hypoxia: at high altitude, the normal hyperventilatory response to falling oxygen tension is inhibited because alkalosis is also induced. Acetazolamide induces metabolic acidosis, increases respiratory drive, notably at night when apnoetic attacks may occur, and thus helps to maintain arterial oxygen tension. The usual dose is 125–250 mg twice daily, given orally on the day before the ascent and continued for 2 days after reaching the intended altitude; 250 mg twice daily is used to treat established high-altitude sickness, combined with a return to a lower altitude. (Note that this is an unlicensed indication in the UK.) As an alternative or in addition to acetazolamide, dexamethasone may be used: 2 mg 6-hourly for prevention, and 4 mg 6-hourly for treatment.

The drug has two other uses. In *periodic paralysis*, where sudden falls in plasma K^+ concentration occur due to its exchange with Na^+ in cells, the rise in plasma H^+ caused by acetazolamide provides an alternative cation to K^+ for exchange with Na^+. Acetazolamide may be used occasionally as a second-line drug for *tonic-clonic* and *partial epileptic seizures*.

Adverse effects. High doses of acetazolamide may cause drowsiness and fever; rashes (it is a sulfonamide-type drug) and paraesthesiae may occur (from the acidosis). Blood disorders have been reported. Renal calculi may develop, because the urine calcium is in less soluble form, owing to low citrate content of the urine, a consequence of metabolic acidosis.

Dichlorphenamide is a similar, but a more potent, inhibitor of carbonic anhydrase.

Cation-exchange compounds

Cation-exchange resins are used to treat hyperkalaemia by accelerating potassium loss through the gut, especially in the context of poor urine output or before dialysis (the most effective means of treating hyperkalaemia). The resins consist of aggregations of big insoluble molecules carrying fixed negative charges, which loosely bind positively charged ions (cations); these readily exchange with cations in the fluid environment to an extent that depends on their affinity for the resin and their concentration.

Resins loaded with sodium or calcium exchange these cations preferentially with potassium cations in the intestine (about 1 mmol potassium per g resin); the freed cations (calcium or sodium) are absorbed, and the resin plus bound potassium is passed in the faeces. The resin does not merely prevent absorption of ingested potassium, but it also takes up the potassium normally secreted into the intestine and ordinarily reabsorbed.

In hyperkalaemia, oral administration or retention enemas of a polystyrene sulphonate resin may be used. A sodium-phase resin (Resonium A) should obviously not be used in patients with renal or cardiac failure as sodium overload may result. A calcium-phase resin (Calcium Resonium) may cause hypercalcaemia and should be avoided in predisposed patients, e.g. those with multiple myeloma, metastatic carcinoma, hyperparathyroidism and sarcoidosis. Orally they are very unpalatable, and as enemas patients rarely manage to retain them for as long as necessary (at least 9 h) to exchange potassium at all available sites on the resin. Their use may be complicated by colonic ulceration.

Patiromer is a cation exchange compound that comes in powder form, made up of non-absorbed spherical beads that exchange calcium for potassium when dissolved in a small amount of water. Patiromer does not appear to bind any potassium in the small intestine, with its action confined to the colon. Its use is associated with constipation, and it results in a gradual decline in potassium, which makes it unsuited to the acute situation. The amount of calcium released from patiromer and absorbed is very small.

Sodium zirconium cyclosilicate (ZS-9) is a compound with a molecular lattice structure which binds potassium preferentially, in exchange for sodium and hydrogen. It remains in the intestine during transit, and in vitro, it binds at least 10 times as much potassium as calcium resins do. ZS-9 is active proximally in the GI tract, and has a rapid onset of action with reductions in plasma potassium evident after as little as 1 hour.

The safety of patiromer and ZS-9 with long-term use is unknown.

Alteration of urine pH

Alteration of urine pH by drugs is sometimes desirable. The most common reason is in the treatment of poisoning (a fuller account is given on p. 129). A summary of the main indications appears below.

Alkalinisation of urine:

- increases the elimination of salicylate, phenobarbital and chlorophenoxy herbicides, e.g. 2,4-D, MCPA
- treats crystal nephropathy by increasing drug solubility, e.g. of methotrexate, sulphonamides and triamterene. NB indinavir requires acidification
- reduces irritation of an inflamed urinary tract
- discourages the growth of certain organisms, e.g. *Escherichia coli.*

The urine can be made alkaline by intravenous sodium bicarbonate or by oral potassium citrate. Sodium overload may exacerbate cardiac failure, and sodium or potassium excess are dangerous when renal function is impaired.

Acidification of urine:

- is used as a test for renal tubular acidosis
- increases elimination of amfetamine, methylene dioxymethamfetamine (MDMA or 'Ecstasy'), dexfenfluramine, quinine and phencyclidine, although it is very rarely needed.

Oral NH_4Cl, taken with food to avoid vomiting, acidifies the urine. It should not be given to patients with impaired renal or hepatic function. Other means include arginine hydrochloride, ascorbic acid and calcium chloride by mouth.

Drugs and the kidney

Adverse effects

The kidneys compose only 0.5% of body-weight, yet they receive 25% of the cardiac output. It is hardly surprising that drugs can damage the kidney and that disease of the kidney affects responses to drugs.

Drug-induced renal disease

Drugs and other chemicals damage the kidney by the following:

1. *Direct biochemical effect.* Substances that cause such toxicity include:
   - heavy metals, e.g. mercury, gold, iron, lead
   - antimicrobials, e.g. aminoglycosides, amphotericin, cephalosporins
   - iodinated radiological contrast media, e.g. agents for visualising the biliary tract
   - analgesics, e.g. NSAID combinations and paracetamol (actually its metabolite, NABQI, in overdose, see p. 292)
   - solvents, e.g. carbon tetrachloride, ethylene glycol.
2. *Indirect biochemical effect:*
   - cytotoxic drugs and uricosurics may cause urate to be precipitated in the tubule
   - calciferol may cause renal calcification by inducing hypercalcaemia
   - diuretic and laxative abuse can cause tubular damage secondary to potassium and sodium depletion
   - anticoagulants may cause haemorrhage into the kidney.
3. *Immunological effect.* A wide range of drugs produces a wide range of injuries:
   - drugs include phenytoin, gold, penicillins, hydralazine, isoniazid, rifampicin, penicillamine, probenecid, sulphonamides

   - injuries include arteritis, glomerulitis, interstitial nephritis, systemic lupus erythematosus.

A drug may cause damage by more than one of the above mechanisms, e.g. gold. The sites and pathological types of injury are as follows:

Glomerular damage. The large surface area of the glomerular capillaries renders them susceptible to damage from circulating immune complexes; glomerulonephritis, proteinuria and nephrotic syndrome may result, e.g. following treatment with penicillamine when the patient has made an immune response to the drug. The degree of renal impairment is best reflected in the creatinine clearance, which measures the GFR because creatinine is eliminated entirely by this process.

Tubule damage. By concentrating 180 L glomerular filtrate into 1.5 L urine each day, renal tubule cells are exposed to much greater amounts of solutes and environmental toxins than are other cells in the body. The proximal tubule, through which most water is reabsorbed, experiences the greatest concentration and so suffers most drug-induced injury. Specialised transport processes concentrate acids, e.g. salicylate (aspirin), cephalosporins and bases, e.g. aminoglycosides, in renal tubular cells. Heavy metals and radiographic contrast media also cause damage at this site. Proximal tubular toxicity is manifested by leakage of glucose, phosphate, bicarbonate and amino acids into the urine.

The countercurrent multiplier and exchange systems of urine concentration (see p. 480) cause some drugs to accumulate in the renal medulla. Analgesic nephropathy is often first evident at this site, partly because of high tissue concentration and partly, it is believed, because of ischaemia through inhibition of locally produced vasodilator prostaglandins by NSAIDs. The distal tubule is the site of lithium-induced nephrotoxicity; damage to the medulla and distal nephron is manifested by failure to concentrate the urine after fluid deprivation and by failure to acidify urine after ingestion of ammonium chloride.

Tubule obstruction. Given certain physicochemical conditions, crystals can deposit within the tubular lumen. Methotrexate, for example, is relatively insoluble at low pH and can precipitate in the distal nephron when the urine is acid, typically in high dose for chemotherapy. Similarly the uric acid produced by the metabolism of nucleic acids released during rapid tumour cell lysis can cause a fatal urate nephropathy. This was a particular problem with the introduction of chemotherapy for leukaemias until the introduction of allopurinol, which is now routinely given before the start of chemotherapy to block xanthine oxidase so that the much more soluble uric acid precursor, hypoxanthine, is excreted instead. A recent and highly effective alternative to allopurinol for high-risk patients is recombinant uric acid oxidase (Rasburicase), which catalyses conversion

489

of uric acid to the more soluble allantoin. Crystal nephropathy is also reported with agents as diverse as indinavir, orlistat, ciprofloxacin, aciclovir, sulfadiazine and triamterene.

Other drug-induced lesions of the kidney include:

- Vasculitis, caused by allopurinol, isoniazid, sulphonamides.
- Allergic interstitial nephritis, caused by penicillins (especially), thiazides, allopurinol, phenytoin, sulphonamides.
- Drug-induced lupus erythematosus, caused by hydralazine, procainamide, sulfasalazine.
- Drugs may thus induce any of the common clinical syndromes of renal injury, namely:
  - *Acute renal failure*, e.g. aminoglycosides, cisplatin.
  - *Nephrotic syndrome*, e.g. penicillamine, gold, captopril (only at higher doses than now recommended).
  - Chronic renal failure, e.g. NSAIDs.
  - *Functional impairment*, i.e. reduced ability to dilute and concentrate urine (lithium), potassium loss in urine (loop diuretics), acid–base imbalance (acetazolamide).

Prescribing in renal disease

Drugs may:

- exacerbate renal disease (see above)
- be ineffective, e.g. thiazide diuretics in moderate or severe renal failure; uricosurics
- be potentiated by accumulation due to failure of renal excretion.

Clearly, the first option is to seek an alternative drug that does not depend on renal elimination. Problems of safety arise for patients with impaired renal function who must be treated with a drug that is potentially toxic and that is wholly or largely eliminated by the kidney.

A knowledge of, or at least access to, sources of pharmacokinetic data is essential for safe therapy for such patients, e.g. manufacturers' data, formularies and specialist journals.

The profound influence of impaired renal function on the elimination of some drugs is illustrated in Table 27.1.

The $t_{1/2}$ of other drugs, where activity is terminated by metabolism, is unaltered by renal impairment, but many such drugs produce *pharmacologically active metabolites* that are more water soluble than the parent drug, rely on the kidney for their elimination, and accumulate in renal failure, e.g. acebutolol, diazepam, warfarin, pethidine.

The majority of drugs fall into an intermediate class and are partly metabolised and partly eliminated unchanged by the kidney.

Table 27.1 Drug $t_{1/2}$ (h) in normal and severely impaired renal function

	Normal	Severe renal impairment[a]
Captopril	2	25
Amoxicillin	2	14
Gentamicin	2.5	>50
Atenolol	6	100
Digoxin	36	90

[a]Glomerular filtration rate <5 mL/min (normal value is 120 mL/min). These values illustrate the major effect of impaired renal function on the elimination of certain drugs. Depending on the circumstances, alternative drugs must be found or special care exercised when prescribing drugs that depend significantly on the kidney for elimination.

Administering the correct dose to a patient with renal disease must therefore take into account both the extent to which the drug normally relies on renal elimination and the degree of renal impairment; the best guide to the latter is the *creatinine clearance* and not the serum creatinine level itself,[8] which can be notoriously misleading in the elderly and at extremes of body mass.

Dose adjustment for patients with renal impairment

- Adjustment of the *initial* dose (or where necessary the *priming* or *loading* dose, see p. 99) is generally unnecessary, as the volume into which the drug has to distribute should be the same in the uraemic as in the healthy subject. There are exceptions to this rule of thumb; for example, the volume of distribution of digoxin is contracted in uraemic patients due to altered tissue binding of the drug.
- Adjustment of the *maintenance* dose involves either reducing each dose given or lengthening the time between doses.
- Special caution is needed when the patient is *hypoproteinaemic* and the drug is usually extensively plasma protein bound, or in advanced renal disease

---

[8]The creatinine clearance can be predicted from the serum creatinine concentration, sex, age and weight using formulae such as the Cockcroft–Gault or MDRD formulae. A number of free online calculators are available, e.g. from http://www.medical-calculator.nl/calculator/GFR/. Free apps are also available for smartphones, e.g. from www.qxmd.com.

when accumulated metabolic products may compete for protein-binding sites. Careful observation is required in the early stages of dosing until response to the drug can be gauged.

General rules

1. Drugs that are *completely* or *largely* excreted by the kidney, or drugs that produce *active, renally eliminated metabolites:* give a normal or, if there is special cause for caution (see above), a slightly reduced initial dose, and lower the maintenance dose or lengthen the dose interval in proportion to the reduction in creatinine clearance.
2. Drugs that are *completely* or *largely metabolised* to inactive products: give normal doses. When the note of special caution (see above) applies, a modest reduction of initial dose and the maintenance dose rate are justified while drug effects are assessed.
3. Drugs that are *partly* eliminated by the kidney and partly metabolised: give a normal initial dose, and modify the maintenance dose or dose interval in the light of what is known about the patient's renal function and the drug, its dependence on renal elimination and its inherent toxicity.

Recall that the time to reach steady-state blood concentration (see p. 88) is dependent only on drug $t_{1/2}$, and a drug reaches 97% of its ultimate steady-state concentration in 5 $\times t_{1/2}$. Thus, if $t_{1/2}$ is prolonged by renal impairment, so also will be the time to reach steady state.

Schemes for modifying drug dosage for patients with renal disease diminish but do not remove their increased risk of adverse effects; such patients should be observed particularly carefully throughout a course of drug therapy. Where the service is available, dosing should be monitored by drug plasma concentration measurements.

Nephrolithiasis

Calcareous stones result from hypercalciuria, hyperoxaluria and hypocitraturia. Hypercalciuria and hyperoxaluria render urine supersaturated in respect of calcium salts; citrate makes calcium oxalate more soluble and inhibits its precipitation from solution.

Non-calcareous stones occur most commonly in the presence of urea-splitting organisms, which create conditions in which magnesium ammonium phosphate (struvite) stones form. Urate stones form when urine is unusually acid (pH <5.5).

Management. Recurrent stone-formers should maintain a urine output exceeding 2.5 L/day. Some benefit from restricting dietary calcium or reducing the intake of oxalate-rich foods (rhubarb, spinach, tea, chocolate, peanuts).

- Thiazide diuretics reduce the excretion of calcium and oxalate in the urine, and reduce the rate of stone formation.
- Sodium cellulose phosphate (Calcisorb) binds calcium in the gut, reduces urinary calcium excretion and may benefit calcium stone-formers.
- Allopurinol is effective in those who have high excretion of uric acid in the urine.
- Potassium citrate, which alkalinises the urine, should be given to prevent formation of pure uric acid stones.

Pharmacological aspects of micturition

Some physiology

The detrusor, whose smooth muscle fibres comprise the body of the bladder, is innervated mainly by parasympathetic nerves, which are excitatory and cause the muscle to contract. The internal sphincter, a concentration of smooth muscle at the bladder neck, is well developed only in the male, and its principal function is to prevent retrograde flow of semen during ejaculation. It is rich in α_1 adrenoceptors, activation of which causes contraction. There is an abundant supply of oestrogen receptors in the distal two-thirds of the female urethral epithelium, which degenerates after the menopause causing loss of urinary control.

When the detrusor relaxes and the sphincters close, urine is stored; this is achieved by central inhibition of parasympathetic tone accompanied by a reflex increase in α-adrenergic activity. Voiding requires contraction of the detrusor, accompanied by relaxation of the sphincters. These acts are coordinated by a micturition centre, probably in the pons.

Functional abnormalities

The main abnormalities that require treatment are:

- *Unstable bladder* or detrusor instability, characterised by uninhibited, unstable contractions of the detrusor which may be of unknown aetiology or secondary to an upper motor neurone lesion or bladder neck obstruction.
- *Decreased bladder activity* or hypotonicity due to a lower motor neurone lesion or over-distension of the bladder, or both.
- *Urethral sphincter dysfunction* which is due to various causes including weakness of the muscles and ligaments around the bladder neck, descent of the

urethrovesical junction and periurethral fibrosis; the result is stress incontinence.

- Atrophic change affecting the distal urethra in females.

Drugs that may be used to alleviate abnormal micturition

Antimuscarinic drugs such as *oxybutynin* and *flavoxate* are used to treat urinary frequency; they increase bladder capacity by diminishing unstable detrusor contractions. Both drugs may cause dry mouth and blurred vision, and may precipitate glaucoma. Oxybutynin has a high level of unwanted effects; the dose needs to be carefully assessed, particularly in the elderly. Flavoxate has less marked side-effects but is also less effective. *Propiverine*, *tolterodine* and *trospium* are also antimuscarinic drugs used for urinary frequency, urgency and incontinence. Propantheline was formerly used widely in urinary incontinence but had a low response rate and a high incidence of adverse effects; it is now used mainly for adult enuresis. The need for continuing antimuscarinic drug therapy should be reviewed after 6 months.

Tricyclic antidepressants. Imipramine, amitriptyline and nortriptyline are effective, especially for nocturnal but also for daytime incontinence. Their parasympathetic blocking (antimuscarinic) action is probably in part responsible, but imipramine may also benefit by altering the patient's sleep profile.

Oestrogens, either applied locally to the vagina or taken by mouth, may benefit urinary incontinence due to atrophy of the urethral epithelium in post-menopausal women.

Parasympathomimetic drugs, e.g. bethanechol, carbachol and distigmine, may be used to stimulate the detrusor when the bladder is hypotonic, e.g. due to an upper motor neurone lesion. Distigmine, which is an anticholinesterase, is preferred, but, as its effect is not sustained, intermittent catheterisation is also needed when the hypotonia is chronic.

Benign prostatic hyperplasia (BPH)

One of the commonest problems in men older than 50 years of age, BPH was for a long time helped only by surgical intervention. The prostate gland is a mixture of capsular and stromal tissue, rich in α_1 adrenoceptors, and glandular tissue under the influence of androgens. Both these, the α receptors and androgens, are targets for drug therapy. Because the bladder itself has few α receptors, it is possible to use selective α_1-blockade without affecting bladder contraction.

α-**Adrenoceptor antagonists.** Prazosin, alfuzosin, indoramin, terazosin and doxazosin are all α-adrenoceptor

blockers with selectivity for the α_1 subtype. They cause significant increases (compared to placebo) in objective measures such as maximal urine flow rate, and drugs also improve semi-objective symptom scores. In normotensive men, falls in blood pressure are generally negligible; in hypertensive patients, the decline in pressure can be regarded as an added bonus (provided concurrent treatment is adjusted). These drugs can cause dizziness and asthenia, even in the absence of marked changes in blood pressure. Nasal stuffiness can be a problem – especially in patients who resort to α-agonists (e.g. pseudoephedrine) for rhinitis.

These adverse events are avoided by using *tamsulosin*, which selectively blocks the α_{1A} subclass[9] of adrenoceptors and is therefore less likely to affect blood pressure, provided the single 400-microgram daily dose of tamsulosin is not exceeded.

Finasteride. An alternative drug for such prostatic symptoms is the type II 5α-reductase inhibitor, finasteride, which inhibits conversion of testosterone to its more potent metabolite, dihydrotestosterone. Finasteride does not affect serum testosterone, or most non-prostatic responses to testosterone. It reduces prostatic volume by about 20% and increases urinary flow rates by a similar degree. These changes translate into modest clinical benefits, which are generally inferior to those of an α_1 antagonist.

Finasteride ($t_{1/2}$ 6 h) is taken as a single 5-mg tablet each day. The improvement in urine flow appears over 6 months (as the prostate shrinks in size), and in 5–10% of patients may be at the cost of some loss of libido. The serum concentration of prostate-specific antigen is approximately halved. Although this may reflect a real reduction in risk of prostatic cancer, in patients receiving finasteride it is safer to regard values of the antigen in the upper half of the usual range as abnormal. Lower doses of finasteride have also been used successfully to halt the development of baldness.[10] *Dutasteride* is an alternative 5α-reductase inhibitor.

Other antiandrogens, such as the gonadorelin agonists, are used in the treatment of prostatic cancer, but the need for parenteral administration makes them less suitable for BPH.

---

[9]There are three cloned subtypes for the α_1-adrenoceptor: α_{1A}, α_{1B} and α_{1D}. The α_{1A} is the predominant subtype in the bladder base and prostatic urethra, whereas contraction of vascular smooth muscle is largely mediated by the α_{1B} subtype. Hence, α_{1A} selectivity would confer, at least in principle, 'prostatic' selectivity. But selectivity determined in vitro against cloned α_1 receptors only poorly predicts in vivo 'uroselectivity', which also diminishes as dose is increased (compare the discussion of β-adrenoceptor selectivity with β-blocking drugs, Ch. 24, p. 426).

[10]It has also been used as a treatment for hirsutism in women. Scalp follicles (of both sexes) contain type II 5α-reductase, and the levels are increased in balding scalps (Tartagni M, Schonauer M, Cicinelli E et al 2004 Intermittent low-dose finasteride is as effective as daily administration for the treatment of hirsute women. Fertility and Sterility 82:752–755).

Erectile dysfunction

Erectile dysfunction (ED), the inability to achieve or maintain a penile erection sufficient to permit satisfactory sexual intercourse, is estimated to affect over 100 million men worldwide, with a prevalence of 39% in those 40 years of age.[11]

Its numerous causes include cardiovascular disease, diabetes mellitus and other endocrine disorders, alcohol and substance abuse, and psychological factors (14%). Although the evidence is not conclusive, drug therapy is thought to underlie 25% of cases, reputedly from antidepressants (selective serotonin-reuptake inhibitors (SSRIs) and tricyclics), phenothiazines, cyproterone acetate, fibrates, levodopa, histamine H_2-receptor blockers, phenytoin, carbamazepine, allopurinol, indometacin and, possibly, β-adrenoceptor blockers and thiazide diuretics.

Sexual arousal releases from the endothelial cells of penile blood vessels neurotransmitters that relax the smooth muscle of the arteries, arterioles and trabeculae of its erectile tissue, greatly increasing penile blood flow and facilitating rapid filling of the sinusoids and expansion of the corpora cavernosa. The venous plexus that drains the penis thus becomes compressed between the engorged sinusoids and the surrounding and firm tunica albuginea, causing the near-total cessation of venous outflow. The penis becomes erect, with an intracavernous pressure of 100 mmHg. The principal neurotransmitter is nitric oxide, which acts by raising intracellular concentrations of cyclic guanosine monophosphate (cGMP) to relax vascular smooth muscle. The isoenzyme phosphodiesterase type 5 (PDE5) is selectively active in penile smooth muscle and terminates the action of cGMP by converting it to the inactive non-cyclic GMP.

Sildenafil (Viagra) is a highly selective inhibitor of PDE5 (70-fold more so than isoenzymes 1, 2, 3 and 4 of PDE), prolonging the action of cGMP, and thus the vasodilator and erectile response to normal sexual stimulation. Its emergence as an agent for erectile dysfunction is an example of serendipity in drug development. Sildenafil was originally being developed for another indication, but when the clinical trials ended the volunteers declined to return surplus tablets for they had discovered that the drug conferred unexpected benefits on their sexual lives. Its development for erectile dysfunction followed.

Sildenafil is well absorbed orally, reaches a peak in the blood after 30–120 min and has a $t_{1/2}$ of 4 h. The drug should be taken 1 h before intercourse in an initial dose of 50 mg (25 mg in the elderly); thereafter 25–100 mg may be taken according to response, with a maximum of one 100-mg dose per 24 h. Food may delay the onset and offset of effect. Sildenafil is effective in 80% of patients with erectile dysfunction.

Adverse effects are short lived, dose related, and comprise headache, flushing, nasal congestion and dyspepsia. High doses can inhibit PDE6, which is needed for phototransduction in the retina, and some patients report a transient blue coloration to their vision.[12] Some patients experience non-arteritic anterior ischaemic optic neuropathy (NAION), consisting of blurred vision and/or visual field loss generally within 24 h of taking sildenafil. Priapism[13] has been reported.

Interactions Sildenafil is *contraindicated* in patients who are taking organic nitrates, for their metabolism is blocked and severe and acute hypotension result. Patients with recent stroke or myocardial infarction, or whose blood pressure is known to be less than 90/50 mmHg, should not use it. Sildenafil is a substrate for the P450 isoenzyme CYP 3A4 (and to a lesser extent CYP2C9, which gives scope for drug–drug interactions). The metabolic inhibitors erythromycin, saquinavir and ritonavir (protease inhibitors used for AIDS), and cimetidine produce substantial rises in the plasma level of sildenafil. More selective PDE5 inhibitors now available include vardenafil, which has a kinetic profile similar to that of sildenafil, and taladafil, which has a very long $t_{1/2}$ (17 h). This latter could be viewed as a mixed blessing in erectile dysfunction, but is important for the use of this drug class in pulmonary hypertension.

Alprostadil is a stable form of prostaglandin E_1, a powerful vasodilator (see p. 424), and is effective for psychogenic and neuropathic erectile dysfunction. Alprostadil increases arterial inflow and reduces venous outflow by contracting the corporal smooth muscle that occludes draining venules. It can be administered either as a urethral suppository (0.125–1 mg) or injected directly into the dorsolateral aspect of the proximal third of the penis (so-called 'intracavernosal' injection). The duration and grade of erection are dose related. The patient package insert from the manufacturer provides some helpful drawings. The dose (5–20 μg) is titrated initially in the doctor's surgery, aiming for an erection lasting for not more than 1 h. Painful erection is the commonest adverse effect.

[11]Feldman H A, Goldstein I, Hatzichristou D G et al 1994 Impotence and its medical and psychological correlates: results of Massachusetts male aging study. Journal of Urology 151:54–61.

[12]The problem is reported much less frequently with the newer and more PDE5-specific taladafil and vardenafil. This very unusual drug effect is reminiscent of the disturbed colour perception caused by digoxin (in overdose), except here patients report yellowed vision (xanthopsia). This may not be an adverse effect in all cases, as it has been suggested that xanthopsia is the explanation for the predominance of yellow in Van Gogh's art.
[13]Persistent erection (>4 h) of the penis, with pain and tenderness. In Greek mythology, Priapus was a god of fertility. He was also a patron of seafarers and shepherds.

Papaverine, an alkaloid (originally extracted from opium but devoid of narcotic properties[14]), is also a non-specific phosphodiesterase inhibitor. It is effective (up to 80%) for psychogenic and neurogenic erectile dysfunction by intracavernosal self-injection shortly before intercourse (efficacy may be increased by also administering the α-adrenoceptor blocker phentolamine),[15] although its use has waned with the availability of orally active selective PDE5 inhibitors such as sildenafil. Papaverine used in this way can cause priapism requiring aspiration of the corpora cavernosa and injection of an α-adrenoceptor agonist, e.g. metaraminol.

---

[14]Papaveretum, whose actions are principally those of its morphine content, has occasionally been supplied in error, to the surprise, distress and hazard of the subject.

[15]Brindley G S 1986 Pilot experiments on the actions of drugs injected into the human corpus cavernosum penis. British Journal of Pharmacology 87:495 – an account of self-experimentation with 17 drugs.

Summary

- The actions of drugs on the kidney are of an importance disproportionate to the low prevalence of kidney disorders.
- The kidney is the main site of loss, or potential loss, of all body substances. It is among the functions of drugs to help reduce losses of desirable substances and increase losses of undesired substances.
- The kidney is also at increased risk of toxicity from foreign substances because of the high concentrations these can achieve in the renal medulla.
- Diuretics are among the most commonly used drugs, perhaps because the evolutionary advantages of sodium retention have left an ageing population without salt-losing mechanisms of matching efficiency.
- Loop diuretics, acting on the ascending loop of Henle, are the most effective, and are used mainly to treat the oedema states. Potassium is lost as well as sodium.
- Thiazides, acting on the cortical diluting segment of the tubule, have lower natriuretic efficacy, but slightly greater antihypertensive efficacy than loop diuretics. Potassium loss is rarely a significant problem with thiazides, and thiazides reduce loss of calcium.
- Potassium retention with hyperkalaemia can occur with potassium-sparing diuretics, which block sodium transport in the last part of the distal tubule, either directly (e.g. amiloride) or by blocking aldosterone receptors (spironolactone).
- Drugs have little ability to alter the filtering function of the kidney when this is reduced by nephron loss.
- Prostatic enlargement is the main disease of the lower urinary tract; drugs can be used to postpone, or avoid, surgery. The symptoms of benign prostatic hyperplasia are partially relieved either by α_1-adrenoceptor blockade or by inhibiting synthesis of dihydrotestosterone in the prostate.
- Drugs are effective for the relief of erectile dysfunction, notably sildenafil, a highly specific phosphodiesterase inhibitor.

Guide to further reading

Basnyat, B., Murdoch, D.R., 2003. High-altitude illness. Lancet 361, 1967–1974.

Brown, M.J., 2011. The choice of diuretic in hypertension: saving the baby from the bathwater. Heart 97, 1547–1551.

Ernst, M.E., Moser, M., 2009. Use of diuretics in patients with hypertension. N. Engl. J. Med. 361, 2153–2164.

Hood, S.J., Taylor, K.P., Ashby, M.J., et al., 2007. The Spironolactone, Amiloride, Losartan and Thiazide (SALT) double-blind crossover trial in patients with low-renin hypertension and elevated aldosterone/renin ratio. Circulation 116, 268–275.

Lameire, N., Van Biesen, W., Vanholder, R., et al., 2005. Acute renal failure. Lancet 365, 417–430.

McMahon, C.N., Smith, C.J., Shabsigh, R., et al., 2006. Treating erectile dysfunction when PDE5 inhibitors fail. Br. Med. J. 332, 589–592.

Moe, O.W., 2006. Kidney stones: pathophysiology and medical management. Lancet 367, 333–344.

Moynihan, R., 2005. The marketing of a disease: female sexual dysfunction. Br. Med. J. 330, 192–194.

Ouslander, J.G., 2004. Management of overactive bladder. N. Engl. J. Med. 350, 786–799.

Quaseem, A., Snow, V., Denberg, T.D., et al., 2009. Hormonal testing and pharmacologic treatment of erectile dysfunction: a clinical practice guideline from the American College of Physicians. Available at: http://annals.org/aim/fullarticle/745155/hormonal-testing-pharmacologic-treatment-erectile-dysfunction-clinical-practice-guideline-from (accessed 18 November 2011).

Thorpe, A., Neal, D., 2003. Benign prostatic hyperplasia. Lancet 361, 1359–1367.

Vidal, L., Shavit, M., Fraser, A., et al., 2005. Systematic comparison of four sources of drug information regarding adjustment of dose for renal function. Br. Med. J. 331, 263–266.

Chapter | **28** |

Respiratory system

Lucinda Kennard

SYNOPSIS

- **Cough: modes of action and uses of antitussives.**
- **Respiratory stimulants: their place in therapy.**
- **Pulmonary surfactant.**
- **Oxygen therapy: its uses and dangers.**
- **Histamine, antihistamines and allergies.**
- **Bronchial asthma: types, modes of prevention, agents used for treatment and their use in asthma of varying degrees of severity.**
- **Infections (see Ch. 14).**

Cough

There are two sorts of cough: the useful and the useless. Cough is useful when it effectively expels secretions or foreign objects from the respiratory tract, i.e. when it is *productive;* it is useless when it is unproductive and persistent. Useful cough should be allowed to serve its purpose and suppressed only when it is exhausting the patient or is dangerous, e.g. after eye surgery. Useless persistent cough should be stopped. Asthma, rhinosinusitis (causing postnasal drip) and oesophageal reflux are the commonest causes of persistent cough. Recently, *eosinophilic bronchitis* has been recognised as a possibly significant cause; it responds well to an inhaled or oral corticosteroid. Clearly the overall approach to persistent cough must involve attention to underlying factors. The British Thoracic Society publishes guidelines on cough and its management that are available online.[1]

---

[1]https://www.brit-thoracic.org.uk/document-library/clinical-information/cough/cough-guidelines/recommendations-for-the-management-of-cough-in-adults/ (accessed 15 Jan 2017).

Sites of action for treatment

Peripheral sites

On the *afferent* side of the cough reflex: by reducing input of stimuli from throat, larynx, trachea, a warm moist atmosphere has a demulcent effect on the pharynx.

On the *efferent* side of the cough reflex: measures to render secretions more easily removable (mucolytics, postural drainage) will reduce the amount of coughing needed, by increasing its efficiency.

The best antitussive of all is removal of the cause of the cough itself, i.e. treatment of underlying conditions (above). In patients with hypertension or cardiac failure, a common cause of a dry cough is treatment with an angiotensin-converting enzyme (ACE) inhibitor. This can be stopped by switching to an angiotensin II receptor blocker (ARB), e.g. losartan.

Central nervous system

Agents may act on the:

- medullary paths of the cough reflex (opioids)
- cerebral cortex
- subcortical paths (opioids and sedatives in general).

Cough is also under substantial voluntary control and can be inducible by psychogenic factors (e.g. the anxiety not to cough during the quiet parts of a musical concert) and reduced by a placebo. Considerations such as these are relevant to practical therapeutics.

Cough suppression

Antitussives that act peripherally

Smokers should stop smoking.

Cough originating above the larynx often benefits from syrups and lozenges that glutinously and soothingly coat the pharynx (demulcents[2]), e.g. simple linctus (mainly sugar-based syrup). Small children are prone to swallow lozenges, so a sweet on a stick may be preferred.

Linctuses are demulcent preparations that can be used alone and as vehicles for other specific antitussive agents. Their exact constitution is not critical, and medical students in 1896 were taught the following:

> Many of you know that this (simple) linctus used to be very much thicker than it is now, and very likely the thicker linctus was more efficacious. The reason why it was made thinner was this. It was discovered that a large number of children came to the surgery complaining of cough, and they were given the linctus, but instead of their using it as a medicine, they took it to an old woman out in Smithfield, who gave them each a penny, took their linctus, and made jam tarts with it.[3]

Cough originating below the larynx is often relieved by water aerosol inhalations and a warm environment – the archetypal 'steam' inhalation. Compound benzoin tincture[4] may be used to give the inhalation a therapeutic smell (aromatic inhalation). This manoeuvre may have more than a placebo effect by promoting secretion of a dilute mucus that gives a protective coating to the inflamed mucous membrane. Menthol and eucalyptus are alternatives. Transient receptor potential channels are responsible for the effect of menthol. Menthol induces a cool sensation via activation of TRPM8. TRPV1-mediated currents induced by capsaicin (the hot chilli component of capsicum and cough trigger) can be inhibited by menthol in a dose-dependent manner, and TRPM8 currents induced by menthol can be inhibited by capsaicin also in a dose-dependent manner, suggesting a complex relationship and mutually inhibitory effects of agonists to these channels.[5]

Local anaesthetics can also be used topically in the airways to block the mucosal cough receptors (modified stretch receptors and C-fibre endings) directly. Nebulised lidocaine, for example, reduces coughing during fibreoptic bronchoscopy and is also effective in the intractable cough that may accompany bronchial carcinoma. There may be increased risk of aspiration of food and airway secretions due to local anaesthesia.

Antitussives that act centrally

The most consistent means of suppressing cough irrespective of its cause is blockade of the *medullary cough centre* itself. *Opioids*, such as methadone and codeine, are very effective, although part of this antitussive effect could reflect their sedatory effect on higher nervous centres; nevertheless antitussive potency of an opiate is generally poorly correlated with its potency at causing respiratory depression.

As *dextromethorphan* (the D-isomer of the codeine analogue levorphanol) and *pholcodine* also have an antitussive effect that is not blocked by naloxone, non–μ-type opiate receptors are probably involved (and dubbed σ-type) and dextromethorphan is also an NMDA receptor antagonist. It is not surprising, then, that these opiates also have no significant analgesic or respiratory-depressant effects at the doses required for their antitussive action.

Opioids are usually formulated as *linctuses* for antitussive use. Deciding on which agent to use depends largely on whether sedation and analgesia may be useful actions of the linctus. Hence methadone or diamorphine linctus may be preferred in patients with advanced bronchial carcinoma. In contrast, dextromethorphan, being non-sedating and non-addictive, is widely incorporated into over-the-counter linctuses (see Table 4 in footnote 1).

Sedation generally reduces the sensitivity of the cough reflex. Hence older sedating antihistamines, e.g. diphenhydramine, can suppress cough by non–H_1-receptor actions; often the doses needed cause substantial drowsiness so that combination with other drugs, such as pholcodine and dextromethorphan, is common in over-the-counter cough remedies. They may be useful in nocturnal cough.

Mucolytics and expectorants

Normally about 100 mL of fluid is produced from the respiratory tract each day, and most of it is swallowed. Respiratory mucus consists largely of water, and its slimy character is due to glycoproteins cross-linked together by disulphide bonds. In pathological states, much more mucus may be produced; an exudate of plasma proteins that bond with glycoproteins and form larger polymers results in the mucus becoming more viscous. Patients with chest diseases such as cystic fibrosis (CF) and bronchiectasis have difficulty in clearing their chest of viscous sputum by cough because the bronchial cilia are rendered ineffective. Drugs that liquefy mucus can provide benefit.

Mucolytics

Carbocisteine and *mecysteine* have free sulphydryl groups that open disulphide bonds in mucus and reduce its viscosity. They are given orally or by inhalation (or instillation) and

---

[2]Latin: *demulcere*, to caress soothingly.
[3]Brunton L 1897 Lectures on the action of medicines. Macmillan, London.
[4]Friar's Balsam.
[5]Takaishi M, Uchida K, Suzuki Y et al 2016 Reciprocal effects of capsaicin and menthol on thermosensation through regulated activities of trpv1 and trpm8. Journal of Physiological Sciences 66:143–155.

may be useful chiefly where particularly viscous secretion is a problem (cystic fibrosis, care of tracheostomies). Mucolytics may cause gastrointestinal irritation and allergic reaction.

Water inhalation via an aerosol (breathing over a hot basin) is a cheap and effective expectorant therapy in bronchiectasis. Simply hydrating a dehydrated patient can also have a beneficial effect in lowering sputum viscosity.

Dornase α is phosphorylated glycosylated recombinant human deoxyribonuclease. It is given daily by inhalation of a nebulised solution containing 2500 units (2.5 mg). It is of modest value only in patients with cystic fibrosis, whose genetic defect in chloride transport causes particularly viscous sputum. The blocked airways, as well as the sputum itself, are a trap for pathogens, and the lysis of invading neutrophils leads to substantial levels of free and very viscous DNA within the CF airways.

Expectorants

These are said to encourage productive cough by increasing the volume of bronchial secretion; there is little clinical evidence to support this, and they may be of no more value than placebo. The group includes squill, guaiphenesin, ipecacuanha, creosotes and volatile oils.

Cough mixtures

Every formulary is replete with combinations of antitussives, expectorants, mucolytics, bronchodilators and sedatives. Although choice is not critical, knowledge of the active ingredients is important, as some contain sedative antimuscarinic antihistamines or phenylpropanolamines (which may antagonise antihypertensives). Use of glycerol or syrup as a demulcent cough preparation, or of simple linctus (citric acid), is probably defensible.

Choice of drug therapy for cough

As always, it is necessary to have a clear idea of the underlying problem before starting any therapy. For example, the approach to cough due to invasion of a bronchus by a neoplasm differs from that due to postnasal drip from chronic sinusitis or to that due to chronic bronchitis. The following are general recommendations.

Simple suppression of useless cough

Codeine, pholcodine, dextromethorphan and methadone linctuses can be used in large, infrequent doses. In children, cough is nearly always useful and sedation at night is more effective to give rest. A sedative antihistamine is convenient (e.g. promethazine), although

---

sputum thickening may be a disadvantage. In pertussis infection (whooping cough), codeine and atropine methonitrate may be tried.

To increase bronchial secretion slightly and to liquefy what is there

Water aerosol with or without menthol and benzoin inhalation, or menthol and eucalyptus inhalation may provide comfort harmlessly.

Carbocysteine or another mucolytic orally may occasionally be useful.

Preparations containing any drug with antimuscarinic action are undesirable because this thickens bronchial secretions. Oxygen inhalation dries secretions, so rendering them even more viscous; oxygen must be bubbled through water, and patients having oxygen may need measures to liquefy sputum.

Cough originating in the pharyngeal region

Glutinous sweets or lozenges (demulcents), incorporating a cough suppressant or not, as appropriate, are used.

Respiratory stimulants

The drugs used (analeptics) are central nervous system (CNS) stimulants capable of causing convulsions in doses just above those used therapeutically. Hence, their use must be monitored carefully.

Doxapram increases the rate and depth of respiration by stimulating the medullary respiratory centres both directly and reflexly through the carotid body. A continuous i.v. infusion of 1.5–4 mg/min is given according to the patient's response. Coughing and laryngospasm that develop after its use may represent a return of normal protective responses. Doxapram is also an effective inhibitor of shivering following general anaesthesia.

Adverse effects include restlessness, twitching, itching, vomiting, flushing, bronchospasm and cardiac arrhythmias, and in addition doxapram causes patients to experience a feeling of perineal warmth; in high doses it raises blood pressure.

Aminophylline (a complex of theophylline and EDTA) in addition to its other actions (see also p. 462) is a respiratory stimulant and may be infused slowly i.v.

Uses

Respiratory stimulants have a considerably reduced role in the management of acute ventilatory failure, following the increased use of non-invasive nasal positive-pressure ventilation for respiratory failure. Situations where they may still be encountered are:

- Acute exacerbations of chronic lung disease with hypercapnia, drowsiness and inability to cough or to tolerate low (24%) concentrations of inspired oxygen (air is 21% oxygen). A respiratory stimulant can arouse the patient sufficiently to allow effective physiotherapy and, by stimulating respiration, can improve ventilation–perfusion matching. This should only be used when non-invasive ventilation (NIV) is unavailable or inappropriate.
- Used for respiratory depression post-anaesthesia to stimulate ventilation in the post-operative period.
- Apnoea in premature infants; aminophylline and caffeine may benefit some cases.
- The manufacturer's data sheet suggests the use of doxapram for buprenorphine overdoses where the respiratory depression is not responsive to naloxone.

Avoid respiratory stimulants in patients with epilepsy (risk of convulsions), ischaemic heart disease, acute severe asthma ('status asthmaticus'), pulmonary embolism, mechanical obstruction of airways, severe hypertension and thyrotoxicosis.

Irritant vapours, to be inhaled, have an analeptic effect in fainting, especially if it is psychogenic, e.g. aromatic solution of ammonia (Sal Volatile). No doubt they sometimes 'recall the exorbitant and deserting spirits to their proper stations'.[6]

Pulmonary surfactant

The endogenous surfactant system produces stable low surface tension in the alveoli, preventing their collapse. Failure of production of natural surfactant occurs in respiratory distress syndrome (RDS), including that in the neonate. Synthetic phospholipids are now available for intratracheal instillation to act as surfactants: *colfosceril palmitate, poractant-α* and *beractant*. These need to be stored chilled, and the manufacturers' instructions followed carefully, because on reaching body temperature their physicochemical properties change rapidly. Their function is to coat the surface of the alveoli and maintain their patency, and their administration to premature neonates with RDS is a key part in reducing mortality and long-term complications in this condition.

---

[6]Thomas Sydenham (1624–1689). He is called the 'English Hippocrates' for his classic description of diseases, based on observation and recording.

Oxygen therapy

Oxygen used in therapy should be prescribed with the same care as any drug, including its specific inclusion on the patient's drug chart; there should be a well-defined purpose, and its effects should be monitored objectively.

The absolute indication to supplement inspired air is *inadequate tissue oxygenation*. As clinical signs may be imprecise, arterial blood gases should be measured whenever suspicion arises. An elevated serum lactate is also a useful marker. Nevertheless, tissue hypoxia should be assumed when the PaO_2 falls below 6.7 kPa (50 mmHg) in a previously normal acutely ill patient, e.g. with myocardial infarction, acute pulmonary disorder, drug overdose, musculoskeletal or head trauma. Chronically hypoxic patients may maintain adequate tissue oxygenation with a PaO_2 below 6.7 kPa by compensatory adaptations, including an increased red cell mass and altered haemoglobin–oxygen binding characteristics. Oxygen therapy is used as follows:

- *High-concentration* oxygen therapy is reserved for a state of low PaO_2 in association with *normal* or *low* $PaCO_2$ *(type I respiratory failure)*, as in: pulmonary embolism, pneumonia, pulmonary oedema, myocardial infarction and young patients with acute severe asthma. Concentrations of oxygen up to 100% may be used for short periods, as there is little risk of inducing hypoventilation and carbon dioxide retention.
- *Low-concentration* oxygen therapy is reserved for a state of low PaO_2 in association with a raised $PaCO_2$ *(type II failure)*, typically seen during exacerbations of chronic obstructive pulmonary disease. The normal stimulus to respiration is an increase in $PaCO_2$, but this control is blunted in chronically hypercapnic patients whose respiratory drive comes from *hypoxia*. Increasing the PaO_2 in such patients by giving them high concentrations of oxygen removes their stimulus to ventilate, exaggerates carbon dioxide retention and may cause fatal respiratory acidosis. The objective of therapy in such patients is to provide just enough oxygen to alleviate hypoxia without exaggerating the hypercapnia and respiratory acidosis; normally the inspired oxygen concentration should not exceed 28%, and in some 24% may be sufficient.
- *Continuous long-term domiciliary oxygen therapy* (LTOT) is given to patients with severe persistent hypoxaemia (see below). Patients are provided with an oxygen concentrator. Clinical trial evidence indicates that taking oxygen for more than 15 h per day improves survival.

Histamine, antihistamines and allergies

Histamine is a naturally occurring amine that has long fascinated pharmacologists and physicians. It is found in most tissues in an inactive bound form, within granules in basophils and mast cells, and pharmacologically active free histamine, released in response to stimuli such as physical trauma or immunoglobulin (Ig) E–mediated activation, is an important component of the acute inflammatory response.

The physiological functions of histamine are suggested by its *distribution in the body*, in:

- *body epithelia* (the gut, the respiratory tract and in the skin), where it is released in response to invasion by foreign substances
- *glands* (gastric, intestinal, lachrymal, salivary), where it mediates part of the normal secretory process
- *mast cells* near blood vessels, where it plays a role in regulating the microcirculation.

Actions. Histamine acts as a local hormone (autacoid) similarly to serotonin or prostaglandins, i.e. it functions within the immediate vicinity of its site of release. With gastric secretion, for example, stimulation of receptors on the histamine-containing cell causes release of histamine, which in turn acts on receptors on parietal cells which then secrete hydrogen ions (see Gastric secretion, Ch. 32). The actions of histamine that are clinically important are those on the following:

Smooth muscle. In general, histamine causes smooth muscle to contract (excepting arterioles, but including the larger arteries). Stimulation of the pregnant human uterus is insignificant. A brisk attack of bronchospasm may be induced in subjects who have any allergy, particularly asthma.

Blood vessels. Arterioles are dilated, with a consequent fall in blood pressure. This action is due partly to nitric oxide release from the vascular endothelium of the arterioles in response to histamine receptor activation. Capillary *permeability* also increases, especially at postcapillary venules, causing oedema. These effects on arterioles and capillaries represent the *flush* and the *wheal* components of the triple response described by Thomas Lewis.[7] The third part, the *flare*, is arteriolar dilatation due to an axon reflex releasing neuropeptides from C-fibre endings.

---

[7] Lewis T, Grant R T 1924 Vascular reactions of the skin to injury. Part 11. The liberation of histamine-like substance in the injured skin, the underlying cause of factitious urticaria and of wheals produced by burning: and observations upon the nervous control of certain skin reactions. Heart 11:209–265.

Skin. Histamine release in the skin can cause itch.

Gastric secretion. Histamine increases the acid and pepsin content of gastric secretion.

As may be anticipated from the above actions, *anaphylactic shock*, which is due in large part to histamine release, is characterised by circulatory collapse and bronchoconstriction. The most rapidly effective antidote is adrenaline/epinephrine (see below), and an antihistamine (H_1 receptor) may be given as well.

Various chemicals can cause release of histamine. The more powerful of these (proteolytic enzymes and snake venoms) have no place in therapeutics, but a number of useful drugs, such as D-tubocurarine and morphine, and even some antihistamines, cause histamine release. This *anaphylactoid* (i.e. IgE-independent) effect is usually clinically mild with a transient reduction in blood pressure or a local skin reaction, but significant bronchospasm may occur in asthmatics.

Metabolism. Histamine is formed from the amino acid histidine and is inactivated largely by deamination and methylation. In common with other local hormones, this process is extremely rapid.

Histamine receptors. Histamine binds to H_1, H_2 and H_3 receptors, all of which are G-protein coupled. The H_1 receptor is largely responsible for mediating its pro-inflammatory effects, including the vasomotor changes, increased vascular permeability and up-regulation of adhesion molecules on vascular endothelium (see p. 422), i.e. it mediates the oedema and vascular effects of histamine. H_2 receptors mediate release of gastric acid (see p. 562). Blockade of histamine H_1 and H_2 receptors has substantial therapeutic utility.

H_3 receptors are expressed in a wide range of tissues including brain and nerve endings, and function as feedback inhibitors for histamine and other neurotransmitters. More recently identified is the H_4 receptor, which is involved in leucocyte chemotaxis.

Histamine antagonism

The effects of histamine can be opposed:

- *By using a drug with opposing effects.* Histamine constricts bronchi, causes vasodilatation and increases capillary permeability; adrenaline/epinephrine, by activating α- and β$_2$-adrenoceptors, produces opposite effects – referred to as 'physiological antagonism'.
- *By blocking histamine binding to its site of action* (receptors), i.e. using competitive H_1- and H_2-receptor antagonists.
- *By substances that produce effects that are specifically opposed to those of the H_1-receptor agonist,* i.e. inverse agonists, see p. 78.

- *By preventing the release of histamine from storage cells.*
Glucocorticoids and sodium cromoglicate can suppress IgE-induced release from mast cells; β_2 agonists have a similar effect.

H_1 antihistamines were traditionally thought to act as competitive antagonists at the H_1 receptor. However, we now know the H_1 receptor, a g-protein coupled receptor, can have constitutive activity, and H_1 antihistamines are actually inverse agonists.[8] They stabilise the H_1 receptor into an inactive state and in doing so produce the opposite effect to histamine. H_1 antihistamines effectively inhibit the components of the triple response and partially prevent the hypotensive effect of histamine, but they have no effect on histamine-induced gastric secretion, which is suppressed by blockade of histamine H_2 receptors.

Thus drugs opposing histamine include:

- H_1 antihistamines – chlorpheniramine, cetirizine, loratadine, fexofenadine
- H_2 antihistamines – cimetidine, famotidine, nizatidine, ranitidine.

Furthermore the selectivity implied by the term 'antihistamine' is unsatisfactory because the older first-generation H_1 antihistamines (see below) show considerable blocking activity against muscarinic receptors, and often serotonin and α-adrenergic receptors as well. These features are a disadvantage when H_1 antihistamines are used specifically to antagonise the effects of histamine, e.g. for allergies. Hence the appearance of second-generation H_1 antihistamines that are more selective for H_1 receptors and largely free of antimuscarinic and sedative effects (see below) has been an important advance. They can be discussed together.

Actions. H_1 antihistamines oppose, to varying degrees, the effects of liberated histamine. They strongly block all components of the triple response (a pure H_1-receptor effect), but only partially counteract the hypotensive effect of high-dose histamine (a mixed H_1- and H_2-receptor effect). H_1 antihistamines are of negligible use in asthma, in which non-histamine mediators, such as the cysteinyl-leukotrienes, are the predominant constrictors. They are more effective if used before histamine has been liberated, and reversal of effects of free histamine is more readily achieved by physiological antagonism with adrenaline/epinephrine, which is used first in life-threatening allergic reactions.

The older *first-generation* H_1 antihistamines such as chlorpheniramine cause drowsiness, and patients should be warned of this, e.g. about driving or operating machinery, and about additive effects with alcohol. Paradoxically, they

---

[8]Church D S, Church M K 2011 Pharmacology of antihistamines. World Allergy Organization Journal 4(Suppl 3):252.

can increase seizure activity in epileptics, especially children, and can cause seizures in non-epileptic subjects if taken in overdose. The *second-generation* H_1 antihistamines such as cetirizine and loratadine penetrate the blood–brain barrier less readily and are largely devoid of such central effects.

Antimuscarinic effects of first-generation H_1 antihistamines are sometimes put to therapeutic advantage in parkinsonism and motion sickness. The newest antihistamines sometimes referred to as 'third generation' were designed to use the therapeutically active metabolites (e.g. fexofenadine, desloratadine) or (levocetirizine) active enantiomer of the second generation cetirizine with the intention of minimising adverse effects.

Pharmacokinetics. H_1 antihistamines taken orally are readily absorbed. They are metabolised mainly in the liver. Excretion in the breast milk may be sufficient to cause sedation in infants. They are generally administered orally and can also be given intramuscularly or intravenously.

Uses. The H_1 antihistamines are used for symptomatic relief of allergies such as hay fever and urticaria (see below). They are of broadly similar therapeutic efficacy.

Individual H_1-receptor antihistamines

Non-sedative second-generation drugs including the 'third-generation' antihistamines

These newer drugs are relatively selective for H_1 receptors, enter the brain less readily than do the earlier antihistamines, and lack the unwanted antimuscarinic effects. Differences lie principally in their duration of action.

Loratadine ($t_{1/2}$ 15 h) and *terfenadine* ($t_{1/2}$ 20 h) are effective taken once daily and are suitable for general use. *Acrivastine* ($t_{1/2}$ 2 h) is so short acting that it is best reserved for intermittent therapy, e.g. when breakthrough symptoms occur in a patient using topical therapy for hay fever. Other non-sedating antihistamines are fexofenadine, levocetirizine and mizolastine.

Adverse effects. The second-generation antihistamines are well tolerated, but an important adverse effect occurs with terfenadine. This drug can prolong the QTc interval on the surface ECG by blocking a potassium channel in the heart (the rapid component of delayed rectifier potassium current, I_{Kr}), which triggers a characteristic ventricular tachycardia (*torsade de pointes*, see p. 466) and probably explains the sudden deaths reported during early use of terfenadine (and prompted its withdrawal from North American markets). It is associated with either high doses of terfenadine or inhibition of its metabolism. Terfenadine depends solely on the 3A4 isoform of cytochrome P450, and inhibiting drugs include erythromycin, ketoconazole and even grapefruit juice. Fexofenadine, the active metabolite, has a much lower affinity for the I_{Kr} channel and does not cause QTc prolongation.

Sedative first-generation agents

Chlorphenamine ($t_{1/2}$ 20 h) is effective when urticaria is prominent, and its sedative effect is then useful.

Diphenhydramine ($t_{1/2}$ 9 h) is strongly sedative and has antimuscarinic effects; it is also used in parkinsonism and motion sickness.

Promethazine ($t_{1/2}$ 12 h) is so strongly sedative that it is used as a hypnotic in adults and children.

Alimemazine, azatadine, brompheniramine, clemastine, cyproheptadine, diphenylpyraline, doxylamine, hydroxyzine and triprolidine are similar.

Adverse effects. Apart from sedation, these include: dizziness, fatigue, insomnia, nervousness, tremors and antimuscarinic effects, e.g. dry mouth, blurred vision and gastrointestinal disturbance. Dermatitis and agranulocytosis can occur. Severe poisoning due to overdose results in coma and sometimes in convulsions.

Drug management of some allergic states

Histamine is released in many allergic states, but it is not the sole cause of symptoms; other chemical mediators, e.g. leukotrienes and prostaglandins, are also involved. Hence the usefulness of H_1-receptor antihistamines in allergic states is variable, depending on the extent to which histamine, rather than other mediators, is the cause of the clinical manifestations.

Note also that H_2-receptor antagonists (separate from their role in reducing gastric acid secretion) are occasionally used to reduce the effects of a type I hypersensitivity response, e.g. rhinitis, urticaria and conjunctivitis, but their clinical effectiveness is less than H_1 antihistamines.

Hay fever. If symptoms are limited to rhinitis, a glucocorticoid (beclometasone, betamethasone, budesonide, flunisolide or triamcinolone), ipratropium or sodium cromoglicate applied topically as a spray or insufflation is often all that is required. Ocular symptoms alone respond well to sodium cromoglicate drops. When both nasal and ocular symptoms occur, or there is itching of the palate and ears as well, a systemic non-sedative H_1-receptor antihistamine is used. Sympathomimetic vasoconstrictors, e.g. ephedrine, are immediately effective when applied topically, but rebound swelling of the nasal mucous membrane occurs when medication is stopped ('rhinitis medicamentosa'), and therefore they should be only used for up to 7 days. Rarely, a systemic glucocorticoid, e.g. prednisolone, is justified for a severely affected patient to provide relief for a short period, e.g. during academic examinations.[9]

Desensitisation, by subcutaneous injection of graded and increasing amounts of grass and tree pollen extracts, is an option for seasonal allergic hay fever due to pollens (which has not responded to antiallergy drugs), and of bee and wasp allergen extracts for people who exhibit allergy to these venoms (exposure to which can be life-threatening). If desensitisation is undertaken, facilities for immediate cardiopulmonary resuscitation must be available because of the risk of anaphylaxis. A sublingual tablet containing a very-low-dose grass pollen extract (Grazax) is also now available to effect similar desensitisation. It has to be taken daily before and throughout the grass pollen season. Immunotherapy is also available for other allergens such as house-dust mite.

In severe allergic asthma, a monocloncal antibody against IgE (Omalizumab), which causes a rapid, dose-related and sustained fall in plasma IgE concentrations is used. The antibody is designed to bind to the part of the IgE molecule that interacts with the high-affinity IgE receptor (FcRI) on mast cells and basophils, thus preventing the activation of these cells by cross-linking of bound IgE.

In severe eosinophilic asthma, mepolizumab is used it is a monoclonal antibody that binds IL-5 and prevents IL-5 from binding to the IL 5 receptor alpha subunit on eosinophils. IL-5 is a key driver of eosinophil recruitment and asthma.

Urticaria. See page 283.

Anaphylactic shock. See page 118.

Bronchial asthma

Asthma affects 10–15% of the UK population; this figure is increasing.

Some pathophysiology

The bronchi become hyperreactive as a result of a persistent *inflammatory* process in response to a number of stimuli that include biological agents, e.g. allergens, viruses, and environmental chemicals such as ozone and glutaraldehyde.

---

[9]A man with severe hay fever who received at least one depot injection of corticosteroid each year for 11 years developed avascular necrosis of both femoral heads, an uncommon but serious complication of exposure to corticosteroid (Nasser S M S, Ewan P W 2001 Lesson of the week: depot corticosteroid treatment for hay fever causing avascular necrosis of both hips. British Medical Journal 322:1589–1591).

Inflammatory mediators are liberated from mast cells, eosinophils, neutrophils, monocytes and macrophages. Some mediators such as histamine are preformed, and their release causes an immediate bronchial reaction. Others are formed after activation of cells and produce more sustained bronchoconstriction; these include metabolites of arachidonic acid from both the cyclo-oxygenase, e.g. prostaglandin D_2 and lipo-oxygenase, e.g. cysteinyl-leukotrienes C_4 and D_4, pathways.

The relative importance of many of the mediators is not defined precisely, but they interact to produce mucosal oedema, mucus secretion and damage to the ciliated epithelium. Breaching of the protective epithelial barrier allows hyperreactivity to be maintained by bronchoconstrictor substances or by local axon reflexes through exposed nerve fibres. Wheezing and breathlessness result. The bronchial changes also obstruct access of inhaled drug to the periphery, which is why they can fail to give full relief.

Asthma, like many of the common chronic disorders (hypertension, diabetes mellitus), is a polygenic disorder, and already genetic loci linked to either increased production of IgE or bronchial hyperreactivity have been reported in some families with an increased incidence of asthma.

Early in an attack, there is hyperventilation so that Pao_2 is maintained and $Paco_2$ is lowered, but with increasing airways obstruction the Pao_2 declines and $Paco_2$ rises, signifying a serious asthmatic episode.

Types of asthma

Asthma is increasingly being recognised as having both specific phenotypes and endotypes.[10] An endotype is a subtype of a disease with a specific pathophysiology. In the future, it is likely this disease characterization process will be further defined.

Allergic asthma

This is the commonest and occurs in patients who develop allergy to inhaled antigenic substances. They are also frequently atopic, showing positive responses to skin prick testing with the same antigens. The hypersensitivity reaction in the lung (and skin) is of the immediate type (type I) involving IgE-mediated mast cell activation. Allergen avoidance is particularly relevant to managing this type of asthma. Corticosteroids, montelukast and omalizumab are useful.

Severe asthma with fungal sensitization and allergic bronchopulmonary aspergillosis (ABPA) are two further allergic groups of patients. These patients get a severe inflammatory response to non-invasive aspergillus fumigatus. Antifungal agents such as itraconazole are used.

Late-onset eosinophilic asthma

These patients have a lack of an identifiable allergen. This group of patients have eosinophilia, and IL-5 is a key disease driver. The condition is steroid responsive. Mepolizumab is used for severe cases. Mepolizumab is designed for this group of patients.

Neutrophilic asthma

These patients can have a sputum neutrophilia, and the Th17 pathway is involved.

Obesity-related asthma

These patients have a female preponderance, lack of atopy and late onset. They are often very symptomatic and lack Th2 markers. Weight loss is important in their management.

Other types of asthma

Exercise-induced asthma

Some patients develop wheeze that regularly follows within a few minutes of exercise. A similar response occurs following the inhalation of cold air, as the common mechanism appears to be airway drying. Inhalation of a β_2-adrenoceptor agonist prior to exercise is the drug of choice. However, if a patient is on inhaled corticosteroids and is otherwise well controlled except exercise, then this may represent poorly controlled asthma, and drugs – for example sodium cromoglicate (see below) or one of the newer leukotriene receptor antagonists (see below) – can be used.

Aspirin-sensitive asthma

This is often accompanied with severe rhinosinusitis and nasal polyposis and life-threatening reactions to aspirin/non-steroidal anti-inflammatories.

Asthma associated with chronic obstructive pulmonary disease

A number of patients with persistent airflow obstruction exhibit substantial variation in airways resistance and in the extent to which they benefit from bronchodilator drugs. It is important to recognise that asthma may coexist with chronic obstructive pulmonary disease, and to assess their responses to bronchodilators or glucocorticoids over a period of time (as formal tests of respiratory function may not reliably predict clinical response in this setting).

[10]Wenzel S E 2012 Asthma phenotypes: the evolution from clinical to molecular approaches. Nature Medicine 18:716–725.

Approaches to treatment

With the foregoing discussion in mind, the following approaches to treatment are logical:

- Prevention of exposure to allergen(s).
- Reduction of the bronchial inflammation and hyperreactivity.
- Dilatation of narrowed bronchi.

These objectives may be achieved as follows:

Prevention of exposure to allergen(s)

This approach is appropriate for allergic asthma. Identification of an allergen may be aided by the patient's history (wheezing in response to contact with pollens, animals), by skin prick testing or intra-dermal injection of selected allergen or by demonstrating specific IgE antibodies in the patient's serum, i.e. via ImmunoCAP (a sandwich immunoassay). Avoiding an allergen may be feasible when it is related to some specific situation, e.g. occupation, but is less easy if widespread, as with house-dust mite.

Reduction of the bronchial inflammation and hyperreactivity

As persistent inflammation is central to bronchial hyperreactivity, the use of anti-inflammatory drugs is logical.

Glucocorticoids (see p. 250) bring about a gradual reduction in bronchial hyperreactivity. They are the mainstay of asthma treatment. The mechanisms are complex involving binding to the intracellular glucocorticoid receptor and permitting translocation to the nucleus acting on glucocorticoid response elements and other transcriptions factors modulating pro- and anti-inflammatory gene transcription. This results in inhibition of the influx of inflammatory cells into the lung after allergen exposure; inhibition of the release of mediators from macrophages and eosinophils; and reduction of the microvascular leakage that these mediators cause. Glucocorticoids used in asthma include *prednisolone* (orally), and *beclometasone, fluticasone, budesonide* and *ciclesonide* (by inhalation) (see Ch. 35).

Sodium cromoglicate (cromolyn, Intal) impairs the immediate response to allergen and was formerly thought to act by inhibiting the release of mediators from mast cells. Evidence now suggests that the late allergic response and bronchial hyperreactivity are also inhibited, and points to effects of cromoglicate on other inflammatory cells and also on local axon reflexes. Cromoglicate is poorly absorbed from the gastrointestinal tract but well absorbed from the lung, and it is given by inhalation (as powder, aerosol or nebuliser); it is eliminated unchanged in the urine and bile.

As it does not antagonise the bronchoconstrictor effect of the mediators after they have been released, cromoglicate is not effective at terminating an existing attack, i.e. it *prevents* bronchoconstriction rather than inducing bronchodilation. Special formulations are used for *allergic rhinitis* and *allergic conjunctivitis.*

Sodium cromoglicate is effective in extrinsic (allergic) asthma, including asthma in children and exercise-induced asthma, but its use has declined since the efficacy and safety of low-dose inhaled corticosteroid have become apparent.

It is remarkably non-toxic. Apart from cough and bronchospasm induced by the powder, it may rarely cause allergic reactions. Application to the eye may produce a local stinging sensation, and the oral form may cause nausea.

Nedocromil sodium (Tilade) is structurally unrelated to cromoglicate but has a similar profile of actions and can be used by metered aerosol in place of cromoglicate.

Other drugs. Ketotifen is a histamine H_1-receptor blocker that may also have some anti-asthma effects, but its benefit has not been demonstrated conclusively. In common with other antihistamines, it causes drowsiness.

Dilatation of narrowed bronchi

This is achieved most effectively by *physiological antagonism* of bronchial muscle contraction, namely by stimulation of adrenergic bronchodilator mechanisms. Pharmacological antagonism of specific bronchoconstrictors is less effective, either because individual mediators are not on their own responsible for a large part of the bronchoconstriction (acetylcholine, adenosine, leukotrienes) or because the mediator is not even secreted during asthma attacks (histamine).

β_2-Adrenoceptor agonists. The predominant adrenoceptors in bronchi are of the β_2 type, and their stimulation causes bronchial muscle to relax. β_2-Adrenoceptor activation also stabilises mast cells. Agonists in widespread use include *salbutamol, terbutaline,* and *salmeterol,* and are discussed in Chapter 23. Salmeterol is longer acting because its lipophilic side-chain anchors the drug in the membrane adjacent to the receptor, slowing tissue washout.

Less selective adrenoceptor agonists such as adrenaline/ epinephrine, ephedrine, isoetharine, isoprenaline and orciprenaline are less safe, being more likely to cause cardiac arrhythmias. α-Adrenoceptor activity contributes to bronchoconstriction, but α-adrenoceptor antagonists have not proved effective in practice.

Theophylline, a methylxanthine, relaxes bronchial muscle, although its precise mode of action is still debated. Inhibition of phosphodiesterase (PDE), especially its type 4 isoform, now seems the most likely explanation for its bronchodilating and more recently reported anti-inflammatory effects.

Theophylline is also an adenosine receptor antagonist. Other actions of theophylline include chronotropic and inotropic effects on the heart and a direct effect on the rate of urine production (diuresis).

Absorption of theophylline from the gastrointestinal tract is usually rapid and complete. Some 90% is metabolised by the liver, and there is evidence that the process is saturable at therapeutic doses. The $t_{1/2}$ is 8 h, with substantial variation. It is prolonged in patients with severe cardiopulmonary disease and cirrhosis; obesity and prematurity are associated with reduced rates of elimination; tobacco smoking enhances theophylline clearance by inducing hepatic P450 enzymes. These pharmacokinetic factors and the low therapeutic index render necessary the therapeutic monitoring of the plasma theophylline to achieve the best outcome; the desired concentration range is 10–20 mg/L (55–110 micromol/L).

Theophylline is relatively insoluble and is formulated either as a salt with choline (choline theophyllinate) or complexed with EDTA (aminophylline). *Aminophylline* is sufficiently soluble to permit intravenous use of theophylline in acute severe asthma (status asthmaticus). Rapid intravenous injection will induce unwanted effects (below) by exposing the heart and brain to high concentrations before distribution is complete. Intravenous injection must be slow (a loading dose of 5 mg/kg over 20 min followed by an infusion of 0.5 mg/kg/h, adjusted according to subsequent plasma theophylline concentrations). The loading dose should be avoided in any patient who is already taking a methylxanthine preparation (always enquire about this before injecting the loading dose!).

There are numerous sustained-release oral forms for use in chronic asthma, but because they are not bioequivalent patients should not switch between them once they are stabilised on a particular preparation.

Adverse effects. At high therapeutic doses, some patients experience nausea and diarrhoea, and plasma concentrations above the recommended range risk cardiac arrhythmia and seizures. Enzyme inhibition by erythromycin, ciprofloxacin, allopurinol or oral contraceptives increases the plasma concentration of theophylline; enzyme inducers such as carbamazepine, phenytoin and rifampicin reduce the concentration.

Overdose with theophylline has assumed greater importance with the advent of sustained-release preparations that prolong toxic effects, with peak plasma concentrations being reached 12–24 h after ingestion. Vomiting may be severe, but the chief dangers are cardiac arrhythmia, hypotension, hypokalaemia and seizures. Activated charcoal should be given every 2–4 h until the plasma concentration is below 20 mg/L. Potassium replacement is important to prevent arrhythmias, and a benzodiazepine (e.g. diazepam) is used to control convulsions.

Antimuscarinic bronchodilators. Release of acetylcholine from vagal nerve endings in the airways activates muscarinic (M_3) receptors on bronchial smooth muscle causing bronchoconstriction. Blockade of these receptors with atropine causes bronchodilatation, although the preferred antimuscarinics in clinical practice are inhaled *ipratropium*, *oxitropium* or the long-acting *tiotropium* (its effects last for up to 24 h). These synthetic compounds, unlike atropine, are permanently charged molecules that resist significant absorption after inhalation and thus minimise antimuscarinic effects outside of the lung. They are used mostly in older patients with chronic obstructive pulmonary disease, but are useful in acute severe asthma when combined with β_2-adrenoceptor agonists.

Leukotriene receptor antagonists, e.g. *montelukast* and *zafirlukast*, competitively prevent the bronchoconstrictor effects of cysteinyl-leukotrienes (C_4, D_4 and E_4) by blocking their common cysLT1 receptor. They are normally used as add on therapy in asthma (Fig. 28.1). There are no studies to justify their use as steroid-sparing (far less, replacement) therapy. When used occasionally in this way in patients unwilling or unable to use metered-dose inhalers, serial monitoring of spirometry is essential.

Montelukast is given once per day and zafirlukast twice daily. Leukotriene receptor antagonists are generally well tolerated, although Churg–Strauss syndrome has been reported rarely with their use. This may represent unmasking of the disease as glucocorticoids are withdrawn following addition of the leukotriene receptor antagonist. Alerting features to this development are vasculitic rash, eosinophilia, worsening respiratory symptoms, cardiac complications and peripheral neuropathy. Zafirlukast can rarely cause hepatic failure. Patients must be advised to look for nausea, vomiting, malaise and jaundice whilst on this drug.

Drug therapy by inhalation

The inhaled route has been developed to advantage because the undesirable effects of systemic exposure to drugs, especially glucocorticoids, are substantially reduced. The pharmacokinetic advantages of using the inhaled versus the oral route are apparent from the substantially reduced dose requirement: salbutamol 100 µg from an aerosol inhaler will provide bronchodilatation similar to 2000 µg by mouth.

Before a drug can be inhaled, it must first be converted into particulate form; the optimum particle size to reach and be deposited in the small bronchi is around 2 µm. Such particles are delivered to the lung as an aerosol, i.e. dispersed in a gas, which can be produced in a number of different ways:

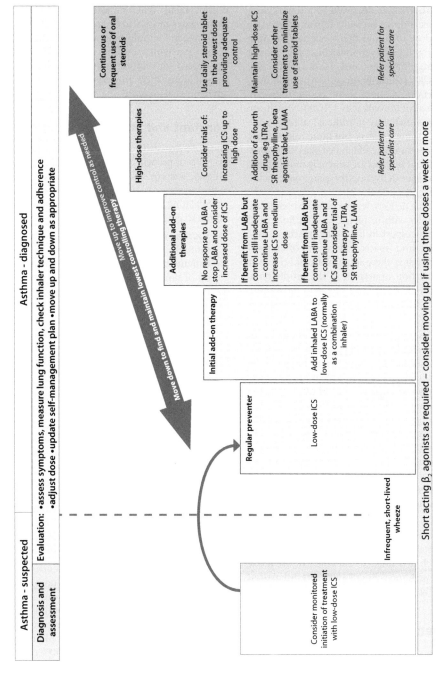

Fig. 28.1 A five-step management scheme for chronic asthma. β₂, β_2-Adrenoceptor agonist; GCC, glucocorticoid, e.g. beclometasone, budesonide or fluticasone. (*From British Thoracic Society BTS/SIGN British guideline on the management of asthma (BTS 2016) with permission.*)

Pressurised aerosol. Drug is dissolved in a low boiling point liquid in a canister under pressure. Opening the valve releases a metered dose of liquid that is ejected into the atmosphere; the carrier liquid evaporates instantly, leaving an aerosol of the drug that is inhaled. Until recently the vehicle has been a CFC (chlorofluorocarbon), but due to concerns over depletion of atmospheric ozone these are being replaced by hydrofluoroalkanes (HFAs), which are ozone-friendly. This switch has introduced a noticeable change in the taste of some inhalers, but more importantly it has changed the bioequivalence of inhaled glucocorticoids. HFA-based glucocorticoid inhalers are generally more potent than a CFC-based inhaler delivering the same dose at the lips (typically the efficacy is doubled).

To ensure optimal drug delivery, it is necessary to coordinate activation of the inhaler with inspiration and a final hold of breath. Many patients, especially the young and the elderly, find this very difficult, and 'spacer' devices are often used between the inhaler and lips; these act as an aerosol reservoir and also reduce impaction of aerosol in the oropharynx. Topical deposition can cause local side-effects in the mouth, particularly candida with inhaled glucocorticoids; a spacer abolishes this problem.

Nebulisers convert a solution or suspension of drug into an aerosol. Jet nebulisers require a driving gas, usually air from a compressor unit for home use, or oxygen in hospital; the solution in the nebulising chamber is broken into droplets by the jet, and the larger droplets are filtered off leaving the smaller ones to be inhaled. Ultrasonic nebulisers convert a solution into particles of uniform size by vibrations created by a piezoelectric crystal (which converts electricity into mechanical vibration). With either method, the aerosol is delivered to the patient by a mouthpiece or facemask, so no coordination is called for, and the dose can be altered by changing the strength of the solution. Much larger doses can be administered by nebuliser than by pressurised aerosol.

Dry-powder inhalers. The drug is formulated as a micronised powder and placed in a device, e.g. a spin-haler or diskhaler, from which it is inhaled. Patients can often use these when they fail with metered-dose aerosols. Inhalation of powder occasionally causes transient bronchoconstriction.

Drug treatment

This varies with the severity and type of asthma. It is a general rule that the effectiveness of changes in drug and dose should be monitored by serial measurements of the simple respiratory function tests such as peak expiratory flow rate (PEFR) or forced expiratory volume in 1 s (FEV_1). Neither the patient's feelings nor physical examination are alone sufficient to determine whether there is still room for improvement. When an asthmatic attack is severe, arterial blood gases must also be measured.

All patients should have a personalised asthma management plan which outlines their medication regime and how based on symptoms and peak flow monitoring they should adjust their drug regime and when to seek medical advice.

Constant and intermittent asthma

The 2016 British Thoracic Society guidelines recommend a five-step approach[11] to the drug management of chronic asthma (see Fig. 28.1). The scheme starts with a patient requiring an occasional β_2-adrenoceptor agonist and follows an escalating plan of add-on anti-inflammatory treatment. Points to emphasise are:

1. Short-acting β_2-adrenoceptor agonists are used throughout as rescue therapy for acute symptoms.
2. Patients must be reviewed regularly as they can move up or down the scheme.
3. Particular attention should be paid to inhaler technique, as this is an important cause of treatment failure. Patients who cannot manage inhaled therapy, even with the addition of a spacer device or use of a dry-powder device, can be given oral therapy, although this will be accompanied by more systemic side-effects.

An inhaled β_2-adrenoceptor agonist should be used initially. *Salbutamol* or *terbutaline* (1–2 puffs up to four times daily) are typical short-acting β_2-adrenoceptor agonists whose bronchodilator effect is prompt in onset (within a few minutes) and lasts 4–6 h. *Salmeterol* and *formoterol* have a much longer duration of effect (12–24 h), making them useful for nocturnal symptoms; they should not be used as 'rescue' bronchodilator (salmeterol in particular, because its bronchodilating action takes 15–30 min to emerge) or as a replacement for inhaled glucocorticoid (see Step 3). β_2-Adrenoceptor agonists all cause dose-dependent tremor, especially if given orally rather than inhaled.

Anti-inflammatory agents commence low-dose inhaled glucocorticoid (Step 1). The inhaled glucocorticoids in current use (*beclometasone, budesonide, fluticasone* and *ciclesonide*) are characterised by low oral bioavailability because of high first-pass metabolism in the liver (almost 100% for fluticasone). This property is important, as it minimises the systemic effects of inhaled glucocorticoid, 80–90% of which is actually swallowed. Precisely for this reason, prednisolone or

---

[11]British Thoracic Society. 2016. Guidelines on the management of asthma. Available at: https://www.brit-thoracic.org.uk/document-library/clinical-information/asthma/btssign-asthma-guideline-2016/.

hydrocortisone would have less advantage (over oral administration) if inhaled, because they are absorbed from the gut and enter the circulation with relatively little pre-systemic metabolism. Inhaled glucocorticoids also exhibit higher lipid solubility and potency than those usually administered orally. Potency (the physical mass of drug in relation to its effect, see p. 79) is generally unimportant in comparisons of oral drugs, but is essential for locally administered drugs.

Inhaled glucocorticoids are generally safe at low doses. Topical effects (oral candida and hoarseness) are reduced by using a spacer device or rinsing the mouth. High doses (>2000 µg/day) are reported to carry a slightly increased risk of cataract and glaucoma; this may reflect local aerosol deposition rather than a true systemic effect. Bone turnover is also increased in adults, suggesting a long-term risk of accelerated osteoporosis, and bone growth may be reduced in children (although evidence indicates that normal adult height can be attained[12]). Therefore, it is important that patients are maintained on the minimum dose of inhaled glucocorticoid necessary for symptom control. Ciclesonide has a special drug delivery, and the particles are in a much smaller size, permitting better delivery to the lung, and less risk of oral candidiasis.

Oral prednisolone is very effective for severe exacerbations, and short courses (e.g. at least 40 mg for 5 days) are frequently given. Provided symptoms and peak flows respond promptly, more prolonged courses or prolonged reduction of dose are unnecessary. When oral glucocorticoids are used long term (Step 5), doses should be adjusted much more slowly. Adverse corticosteroid effects may also be minimised by administering a single morning dose to coincide with the normal peak cortisol concentration (and thus the least suppression of feedback to the hypothalamic–adrenal axis). This is possible because of the long duration of their biological effect (18–36 h) compared with plasma $t_{1/2}$ (3 h for prednisolone). Morning dosing with inhaled glucocorticoid may also have a prednisolone-sparing effect. Some patients may get further prednisolone-sparing by addition of nebulised high-dose budesonide, 1–2 mg twice daily or fluticasone 500 µg twice daily.

Chest infections in asthma

Antimicrobials are over-prescribed for exacerbations of asthma. Respiratory tract infections do cause increased airflow obstruction and bronchial hyperresponsiveness, but viral not bacterial pathogens are the commonest culprits.

Antimicrobials should be prescribed only if there is high suspicion of a bacterial respiratory tract infection, e.g. purulent sputum. Note that macrolide antibiotics, such as erythromycin and clarithromycin, interfere with theophylline metabolism.

Acute severe asthma ('status asthmaticus')

This is a life-threatening emergency requiring rapid aggressive treatment. The airways may become refractory to β₂-adrenoceptor agonists after 36–48 h, partly for pharmacological reasons (possibly receptor desensitisation) and partly due to the prolonged respiratory acidosis. The mucous plugs, which are the hallmark of the condition, may also prevent inhaled drugs from reaching the distal airways.

The following lists, with some explanation, the recommendations of the British Thoracic Society[9] for managing acute severe asthma:

Immediate treatment

- *Oxygen* by mask (humidified, to help liquefy mucus). Carbon dioxide narcosis is rare in asthma, and 60% can be used if the diagnosis is not in doubt. In older patients, or when there is any concern about chronic carbon dioxide retention, start with 28% oxygen and check that the Pa_{CO_2} has not risen before delivering 35% oxygen.
- *Salbutamol* by nebuliser in a dose of 2.5–5 mg over about 3 min, repeated in 15 min. Terbutaline 5–10 mg is an alternative. Nebuliser must be driven through oxygen to avoid desaturation.
- *Prednisolone* 40–50 mg by mouth or hydrocortisone 100–200 mg i.v.
- *Avoid sedation* of any kind.
- Chest radiography is required to exclude pneumothorax.
- If not improving, add nebulised ipratropium 0.5 mg driven through oxygen with the nebulised beta-2 agonist.

If life-threatening features are present (absent breath sounds, cyanosis, bradycardia, exhausted appearance, PEFR <33% predicted or best, arterial oxygen saturation of <92%):

- Consider i.v. magnesium sulphate (1.2–2 g over 20 min).[13]
- Alert the intensive care unit.

---

[12]Agertoft L, Pedersen S 2000 Effect of long-term treatment with inhaled budesonide on adult height in children with asthma. New England Journal of Medicine 343:1064–1069.

[13]This intervention is generally safe but not proven to affect outcome. The British Thoracic Society guideline no longer recommends intravenous aminophylline without consultation with a senior physician. Doubtless, this reflects an equal lack of evidence base for benefit and the very clear potential for harm if given to patients already taking oral theophyllines.

Subsequent management. If the patient is *improving,* continue:

- 40–60% oxygen.
- Prednisolone 40–50 mg daily or hydrocortisone 100–200 mg 6-hourly.
- Nebulised salbutamol or terbutaline 4-hourly.

If the patient is *not improving* after 15–30 min:

- Continue oxygen and glucocorticoid.
- Give *nebulised* β_2-adrenoceptor agonist more frequently, e.g. salbutamol up to 10 mg/h.
- Add ipratropium 0.5 mg to nebuliser and repeat 6-hourly until patient is improving.

If the patient is *still not improving*:

- Consider intravenous infusion of aminophylline or see p. 503 (already discussed dosing there)
- Consider as an alternative intravenous β_2-adrenoceptor agonist salbutamol
- Contact the intensive care unit to discuss intubation and mechanical ventilation.

Monitoring response to treatment

- By peak expiratory flow rate (PEFR) every 15–30 min.
- Oxygen saturation: aim 94–98%. Repeat blood gas measurements if initial PaO_2 <8 kPa (60 mmHg) and/or initial $PaCO_2$ is normal or raised (the tachypnoea is expected to reduce $PaCO_2$ in most patients).

Treatment in intensive care unit. Transfer (accompanied by doctor with facilities for intubation) is required if:

- any of the above deteriorates, despite maximal treatment
- the patient becomes exhausted, drowsy, or confused
- coma or respiratory arrest occurs.

Treatment at discharge from hospital. Patients should:

- continue high-dose inhaled glucocorticoid and complete course of oral prednisolone
- be instructed to monitor their own PEFR and not to reduce dose if the PEFR falls, or there is a recurrence of early morning dipping in the reading (patients should not generally be discharged until there is less than 25% diurnal variation in PEFR readings).

Warnings

Asthma may be precipitated by β-adrenoceptor blockade, and the use of β-adrenoceptor antagonists is *contraindicated* in asthmatics; fatal asthma has been precipitated by β-blocker eye drops, even allegedly β_1-selective agents.

Overuse of β_2-adrenergic agonists is dangerous. In the mid-1960s, there was an epidemic of sudden deaths in young asthmatics outside hospital. It was associated with the introduction of a high-dose, metered aerosol of isoprenaline (β_1 and β_2 agonist); it did not occur in countries where the high concentration was not marketed.[14] The epidemic declined in Britain when the profession was warned, and the aerosols were restricted to prescription only. Though the relationship between the use of β_2-receptor agonists and death is presumed to be causal, the actual mechanism of death is uncertain; overdose causing cardiac arrhythmia is not the sole factor. The subsequent development of selective β_2-receptor agonists was a contribution to safety, but a review in New Zealand during the 1980s found that the use of fenoterol (β_2 selective) by metered-dose inhalation was associated with increased risk of death in severe asthma,[15] and later analysis concluded that it was the most likely cause.[16] A further cause for concern comes from a meta-analysis of 19 clinical trials which concluded that *long-acting β_2 agonists* (LABAs) increased severe and life-threatening asthma exacerbations, as well as asthma-related deaths.[17] The US Food and Drug Administration has recently confirmed their belief that the benefits of LABAs still outweigh these risks but have opted for a more cautious labelling policy.[18]

A recent multicenter, randomised, double-blind trial of over 11 000 patients compared fluticasone plus salmeterol versus fluticasone alone and found that those with a combination inhaler had fewer severe asthma exacerbations than the fluticasone-alone group and did not have significantly higher risk of serious asthma-related events.[19] The BTS guidelines recommend that LABAs are not prescribed alone, but in combination inhalers.

[14]Stolley P D 1972 Why the United States was spared an epidemic of deaths due to asthma. American Review of Respiratory Diseases 105:833–890.
[15]Crane J, Pearce N, Flatt A et al 1989 Prescribed fenoterol and death from asthma in New Zealand: case control study. Lancet i:917–922.
[16]Pearce N, Beasley R, Crane J et al 1995 End of the New Zealand asthma mortality epidemic. Lancet 345:41–44.
[17]Salpeter S R, Buckley N S, Ormiston T M et al 2006 Meta-analysis: effect of long-acting β agonists on severe asthma exacerbations and asthma-related deaths. Annals of Internal Medicine 144:901–912.
[18]Chowdhury B A, Dal Pan G 2010 The FDA and safe use of long-acting beta-agonists in the treatment of asthma. New England Journal of Medicine 362:1169–1171.
[19]Stempel D A, Raphiou I H, Kral K M for the AUSTRI Investigators et al 2016 Serious asthma events with fluticasone plus salmeterol versus fluticasone alone. New England Journal of Medicine 374:1822–1830.

Chronic obstructive pulmonary disease (COPD)

Whereas asthma is characterised by *reversible* airways obstruction and bronchial hyperreactivity, COPD is characterised by *incompletely reversible* airways obstruction and *mucus hypersecretion;* it is predominantly a disease of the smaller airways. Nevertheless, distinguishing the two can be difficult in some patients, and one view is that asthma predisposes smokers to COPD (the Dutch hypothesis). In practice, even though – indeed precisely because – most of the airway obstruction is fixed in COPD, it is important to maximise the reversible component. To differentiate asthma from COPD: COPD will have **limited or absent reversibility** i.e FEV1 (forced expiratory volume in 1 s) <400 ml response after 30 mg daily oral prednisolone for 2 weeks or bronchodilators.[20]

Drugs used to treat COPD are exactly as for asthma, except that antimuscarinics, such as *ipratropium* or the longer-acting *tiotropium*, are often more effective bronchodilators than β_2 agonists. Patients with reversible airways obstruction should also receive an inhaled glucocorticoid, and its combination with a LABA may improve control, especially in moderate or severe disease (FEV$_1$ <50% predicted), e.g. fluticasone + salmeterol (Seretide). This strategy is designed to reduce the frequency of disease exacerbations rather than affect the decline in lung function per se.[21]

A recent randomised, double-blind double-dummy clinical trial showed that a fixed-dose long-acting beta-agonist (LABA)/long acting muscarinic antagonist (LAMA) had fewer COPD exacerbations than LABA/inhaled corticosteroid (ICS).[22]

A theophylline may also be effective in patients with severe disease, but requires special care in the elderly, including monitoring of plasma theophylline. Mucolytic drugs reduce acute episodes of COPD and days of illness; they are best reserved for patients with recurrent, prolonged or severe exacerbations of the disease. Quitting smoking remains the only action of proven benefit in preserving lung function in COPD.

Long-term oxygen therapy improves survival in hypoxic patients. It is indicated when:

- PaO_2 is less than 7.3 kPa (56 mmHg) when stabilised on optimal medical treatment.
- PaO_2 is 7.3–8.0 kPa, and there is evidence of right-sided cardiac failure (cor pulmonale), polycythaemia or pulmonary hypertension.

Summary

- Asthma is characterised by hypersensitivity to the endogenous bronchoconstrictors, acetylcholine and histamine, and by reversible obstruction of the airways.
- Asthma is increasingly being divided into phenotypes and endotypes with a targeted treatment approach.
- Most anti-asthma treatment is currently aimed either at reducing release of inflammatory cytokines (glucocorticoids and sodium cromoglicate) or at direct bronchodilatation by stimulation of the bronchial β_2-adrenoceptors.
- Aggressive use of glucocorticoids, especially by the inhaled route, is the keystone of the modern stepped approach to asthma management.
- New asthma treatments include monoclonal antibodies such as omalizumab and mepolizumab.
- H$_1$ antihistamines have a wide range of applications in treatment of allergic disorders and anaphylaxis.
- The principal adverse effect of older first-generation antihistamines, sedation, is avoided by use of newer second-generation drugs which do not enter the CNS.
- Smoking cessation and long-term treatment with oxygen are the only interventions that are known to improve survival in chronic obstructive pulmonary disease.

---

[20]National Institute for Health and Care Excellence 2010 Chronic obstructive pulmonary disease in over 16s: diagnosis and management. London: National Clinical Guideline Centre. Available at https://www.nice.org.uk/guidance/cg101/chapter/1-Guidance #diagnosing-copd.
[21]A trial in patients without reversibility found that inhaled glucocorticoid had no effect on the decline in their lung function (Pauwels R A, Lofdahl C G, Laitinen L A et al 1999 Long-term treatment with inhaled budesonide in persons with mild chronic obstructive pulmonary disease who continue smoking. New England Journal of Medicine 340:1948–1953).
[22]Wedzicha J A, Banerji D, Chapman K R et al; FLAME Investigators 2016 Indacaterol-glycopyrronium versus salmeterol-fluticasone for COPD. New England Journal of Medicine 347:2222–2234.

Guide to further reading

British Thoracic Society, 2016. BTS/ SIGN British guideline on the management of asthma. Available at: https://www.brit-thoracic.org.uk/ standards-of-care/guidelines/btssign-british-guideline-on-the-management-of-asthma/.

Devereux, G., 2006. ABC of chronic obstructive pulmonary disease. Definition, epidemiology, and risk factors. Br. Med. J. 332, 1142–1144 (the first in a series of 12 weekly articles on the subject).

Hendeles, L., Colice, G.L., Meyer, R.J., 2007. Withdrawal of albuterol inhalers containing chlorofluorocarbon propellants. N. Engl. J. Med. 356, 1344–1351.

Holgate, S.T., Polosa, R., 2006. The mechanisms, diagnosis and management of severe asthma in adults. Lancet 368, 780–793.

Irwin, R.S., Madison, J.M., 2000. The diagnosis and treatment of cough. N. Engl. J. Med. 343, 1715–1721.

Kay, A.B., 2001. Allergy and allergic diseases. N. Engl. J. Med. 344, 30–37 (part I); 109–113 (part 2).

Murray, L.A., Grainge, C., Wark, P.A., Knight, D.A., 2017. Use of biologics to treat acute exacerbations and manage disease in asthma, COPD and IPF. Pharmacol. Ther. 169, 1–12.

National Institute for Health and Care Excellence, 2010a. Chronic obstructive pulmonary disease in over 16s: diagnosis and management. Available at: https://www.nice.org.uk/guidance/cg101.

National Institute for Health and Care Excellence, 2010b. Chronic obstructive pulmonary disease: management of chronic obstructive pulmonary disease in adults in primary and secondary care (partial update). London: National Clinical Guideline Centre; 2010. Available at: http://www.nice.org.uk/CG101. (Accessed 15 January 2017).

Newoehner, D., 2010. Outpatient management of severe COPD. N. Engl. J. Med. 362, 1407–1416.

O'Byrne, P.M., Parameswaran, K., 2006. Pharmacological management of mild or moderate persistent asthma. Lancet 368, 794–803.

Plaut, M., Valentine, M.D., 2005. Allergic rhinitis. N. Engl. J. Med. 353, 1934–1944.

Reynolds, S.M., Mackenzie, A.J., Spina, D., Page, C.P., 2004. The pharmacology of cough.

Trends Pharmacol. Sci. 25, 569–576.

Stempel, D.A., Raphiou, I.H., Kral, K.M., et al.; for the AUSTRI Investigators, 2016. Serious asthma events with fluticasone plus salmeterol versus fluticasone alone. N. Engl. J. Med. 374, 1822–1830. (Accessed 15 January 2017).

Takaishi, M., Uchida, K., Suzuki, Y., et al., 2016. Reciprocal effects of capsaicin and menthol on thermosensation through regulated activities of trpv1 and trpm8. J. Physiol. Sci. 66, 143–155.

Weir, E.K., López-Barneo, J., Buckler, K.J., Archer, S.L., 2005. Acute oxygen-sensing mechanisms. N. Engl. J. Med. 353, 2042–2055.

Wenzel, S.E., 2012. Asthma phenotypes: the evolution from clinical to molecular approaches. Nat. Med. 18, 716–725.

Wedzicha, J.A., Banerji, D., Chapman, K.R., FLAME Investigators, et al., 2016. Indacaterol-glycopyrronium versus salmeterol-fluticasone for COPD. N. Engl. J. Med. 347, 2222–2234.

Section | 6 |

Blood and neoplastic disease

Chapter | 29 |

Drugs and haemostasis

Mike Laffan, Trevor Baglin

SYNOPSIS

Occlusive vascular disease is a major cause of morbidity and mortality. There is now a better understanding of the mechanisms by which the haemostatic system maintains blood in a fluid state within vessels yet forms a solid plug when a vessel is breached, and of the ways in which these processes may be altered by drugs to prevent or reverse (lyse) thrombosis.

- **Coagulation system: the mode of action of drugs that promote coagulation and that prevent it (anticoagulants) and their uses.**
- **Fibrinolytic system: the mode of action of drugs that promote fibrinolysis (fibrinolytics) and their uses to lyse arterial and venous thrombi (thrombolysis).**
- **Platelets: the ways that drugs that inhibit platelet activity benefit arterial disease.**

Introduction

It is essential that blood remains fluid within the circulation but clots at sites of vascular injury. The haemostatic system maintains the integrity of the vascular tree through a complex network of cellular, ligand–receptor and enzymatic interactions. In normal circumstances there is an equilibrium between the natural coagulant–anticoagulant and fibrinolytic–antifibrinolytic systems. In response to endothelial damage, there is rapid molecular switching to thrombin generation and antifibrinolysis at the site of injury, and enhanced natural anticoagulant activity and fibrinolytic activity at areas of adjacent healthy intact endothelium. Regulation of the haemostatic network in such a way results in localised thrombus formation with minimal loss of vascular patency.

Pathological disruption of the network results in thrombosis or bleeding, or both; the extreme example of haemostatic pathology is a complete breakdown as occurs in disseminated intravascular coagulation (DIC). Drugs that modulate the haemostatic system are valuable in the management of bleeding and thrombotic disorders. Drugs can be classified according to the component of the system they affect and their perceived primary mode of action.

The coagulation system

Coagulation initiates with *tissue factor* (TF), a cell membrane protein that binds activated factor VII (indicated by adding the letter 'a', i.e. factor VIIa). Although there is a small fraction of circulating factor VII in the activated state, it has little or no enzymatic activity until it is bound to TF. Most non-vascular cells express TF in a constitutive[1] fashion, whereas de novo TF synthesis can be induced in monocytes and damaged endothelial cells. Injury to the arterial or venous wall exposes extravascular TF-expressing cells to blood. Lipid-laden macrophages in the core of atherosclerotic plaques are particularly rich in TF, thereby explaining the propensity for thrombus formation at sites of plaque disruption. Once bound to TF, factor VIIa activates factor IX and factor X (to IXa and Xa, respectively), leading to thrombin generation and clot formation (Fig. 29.1).

The classical view of blood coagulation with separate 'extrinsic' and 'intrinsic' pathways initiated by either TF or contact with an anionic surface does not reflect physiological coagulation. It is now evident that coagulation does not occur as linear sequential enzyme activation pathways but

---

[1]Genetically controlled by an active promoter and constantly produced rather than depending on the presence of an inducer.

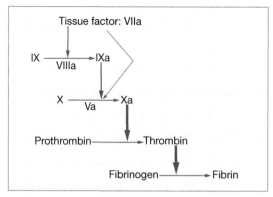

Fig. 29.1 The blood coagulation network (see text).

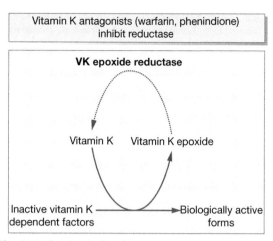

Fig. 29.2 The vitamin K cycle.

rather by a network of simultaneous interactions, which undergo regulation and modulation during the thrombin generation process itself.

In the current model, blood coagulation starts with exposure of *tissue factor* following endothelial damage, resulting in the formation of sub-nanomolar amounts of *thrombin* via TF/VIIa-driven Xa formation (extrinsic-tenase). The initial thrombin activity is necessary to prime the system for a full thrombin explosion. Tissue factor pathway inhibitor (TFPI) rapidly shuts down this priming pathway, and the full thrombin explosion is then dependent on factor IXa–driven Xa formation. Factor IXa–driven Xa formation (intrinsic-tenase) is amplified by the thrombin explosion itself, as thrombin forms a positive feedback loop by activating cofactors V and VIII as well as factor XIa (not shown in Fig. 29.1), which converts more IX to IXa.

Thrombin converts soluble fibrinogen into insoluble fibrin monomers, which spontaneously polymerise to form the fibrin mesh that is then stabilised and cross-linked by activated factor XIII (factor XIIIa), a thrombin-activated transglutaminase. Thrombin amplifies its own generation by:

- feedback activation of factor V and factor VIII
- activating platelet-bound factor XI, thereby leading to further factor Xa generation
- activating cells, including platelets, that provide the phospholipid surface required for assembly of the macromolecular enzymatic complexes.

Procoagulant drugs

Vitamin K

Vitamin K ('Koagulation' vitamin) is essential for normal coagulation. It occurs naturally in two forms. Vitamin K_1 (phylloquinone) is widely distributed in plants, and K_2 includes vitamin synthesised in the alimentary tract by bacteria, e.g. *Escherichia coli* (menaquinones). Leafy green vegetables are a good source of vitamin K_1. Bile is required for the absorption of the natural forms of vitamin K, which are fat soluble. The storage pool of vitamin K is modest and can be exhausted in 1 week, although gut flora will maintain suboptimal production of vitamin K–dependent proteins. A synthetic analogue, *menadione* (K_3), is water soluble.

Vitamin K is necessary for the final stage in the synthesis of coagulation proteins in the liver: the *procoagulant* factors II (prothrombin), VII, IX and X, and *anticoagulant* regulatory proteins, proteins C, S and Z. The vitamin allows γ-carboxylation of glutamic acid residues in their structure; this permits calcium to bind to the molecule, mediating the conformational change required for enzymatic activity, and binding to negatively charged phospholipid surfaces, e.g. platelets. Membrane binding is required for full enzymatic potential.

During γ-carboxylation of the proteins, the *reduced* and *active* form of vitamin KH_2 converts to an epoxide, an *oxidation* product. Subsequently, vitamin K epoxide reductase converts oxidised vitamin K back to the active vitamin K, i.e. there exists an interconversion cycle between vitamin K epoxide and reduced vitamin K (Fig. 29.2).

When the vitamin is deficient or where drugs inhibit its action, the coagulation proteins produced are unable to associate with calcium in order to form the necessary three-dimensional configuration and associated membrane-binding properties that are required for full enzymatic activity. Their physiologically critical binding to membrane surfaces fails to occur, and this impairs the coagulation mechanism. These proteins are called 'proteins induced in vitamin K absence' or PIVKAs.

Oral vitamin K antagonists exert an anticoagulant effect by interrupting the vitamin K cycle. There are two classes of drugs: the *coumarins*, including warfarin and acenocoumarol, and the *indanediones* such as pheneindione. The anticoagulant effect of oral vitamin K antagonists is expressed as the International Normalised Ratio (INR).

Vitamin K deficiency may arise from:

- dietary deficiency
- bile failing to enter the intestine, e.g. obstructive jaundice or biliary fistula
- malabsorption syndromes, e.g. coeliac disease, or after extensive small intestinal resection
- reduced alimentary tract flora, e.g. in newborn infants and rarely after broad-spectrum antibiotics.

The following preparations of vitamin K are available:

Phytomenadione (Konakion), the naturally occurring fat-soluble vitamin K_1, acts within about 12 h and should reduce the anticoagulant effect of warfarin within 24–48 h when given orally in a dose of 5–10 mg. The intravenous formulation will begin to reverse a vitamin K–deficient coagulopathy within 6 h in a patient with normal liver function. It should be administered slowly to reduce the risk of an anaphylactoid reaction with facial flushing, sweating, fever, chest tightness, cyanosis and peripheral vascular collapse. Phytomenadione may also be given orally using either tablet formulations or the preparation for intravenous use. Oral administration will result in a slower and often incomplete correction of coagulopathy. Otherwise phytomenadione may be given intramuscularly, subcutaneously or orally. The preferred route depends on the degree of coagulopathy and urgency of correcting the haemorrhagic tendency. The intramuscular route should not be used if the INR is increased, as local intramuscular haemorrhage may be induced; subcutaneous absorption is variable and, despite the risk of allergic reaction, the intravenous route ensures rapid effect.

Menadiol sodium phosphate (vitamin K_3), the synthetic analogue of vitamin K, being water soluble, is preferred in intestinal malabsorption or in states in which bile flow is deficient. The main disadvantage is that it takes 24 h to act, but its effect lasts for several days. The dose is 5–40 mg daily, orally. Menadiol sodium phosphate in moderate doses causes haemolytic anaemia and, for this reason, neonates should not receive it, especially those that are deficient in glucose 6-phosphate dehydrogenase; their immature livers are unable to cope with the heavy bilirubin load, and there is danger of kernicterus.

Fat-soluble analogues of vitamin K that are available in some countries include acetomenaphthone and menaphthone.

Vitamin K is used to treat the following:

- Haemorrhage or threatened bleeding due to the coumarin or indanedione anticoagulants.

Phytomenadione is preferred for its more rapid action; dosage regimens vary according to the degree of urgency and the original indication for anticoagulation.

- Haemorrhagic disease of the newborn, which develops usually between 2 and 7 days, and late haemorrhagic disease that presents at 6–7 months. Prophylaxis is recommended during the period of vulnerability with vitamin K (phytomenadione, as Konakion) 1 mg by single i.m. injection at birth. Alternatively, give vitamin K by mouth as two doses of a colloidal (mixed micelle) preparation of phytomenadione in the first week. Breast-fed babies should receive a further 2 mg at 1 month of age. Formula-fed babies do not need this last supplement as the formula contains vitamin K. Fears that intramuscular vitamin K might cause childhood cancer have been dispelled.
- Intestinal malabsorption syndromes; menadiol sodium phosphate should be used as it is water soluble.

Coagulation factor concentrates

Bleeding due to deficiency of specific coagulation factors is treated by either elevating the deficient factor, e.g. treatment of mild factor VIII deficiency with desmopressin (see below), or replacement of the missing factor. Recombinant factor VIII and IX are now available in many countries for patients with congenital deficiency of these factors. For patients with rare coagulation factor deficiencies or multiple acquired deficiencies (liver disease, massive blood loss with dilutional coagulopathy or DIC), replacement therapy requires human-derived fresh frozen plasma (FFP) or prothrombin complex concentrates (PCC) containing factors II, VII, IX and X (Beriplex, Octaplex).

Solvent–detergent virally inactivated FFP (Octaplas) is currently given to selected patients in the UK, for example those with rare bleeding disorders and patients with thrombotic thrombocytopenic purpura who require repeated exposure to FFP. Methylene blue–treated single-donor–unit FFP is also available as a virally inactivated product.

Use of coagulation factor concentrates

Management of haemophilia A and haemophilia B (deficiency of factor VIII and IX, respectively) requires special expertise, but the following points are notable:

- Superficial haemorrhage sometimes responds to local pressure.
- Minor bleeding can arrest with plasma factor concentrations of 0.25–0.30 units/mL, but severe bleeding requires at least 0.50 units/mL, and surgical

procedures or life-threatening haemorrhage require 0.75–1 units/mL by infusion of factor concentrate.

- In haemophilia A, *factor VIII concentrate* ($t_{1/2}$ 8–12 h) is used for bleeding that is more than minor. Repeat dosing is necessary to maintain haemostatic levels.
- *Factor IX* ($t_{1/2}$ 18–24 h) is used for bleeding that is more than minor in haemophilia B (Christmas disease).
- Modified recombinant *Factor VIII and IX* molecules with extended half-life are now entering clinical use.[2]
- The speed of recovery of the affected joint or resolution of a haematoma determines the duration of therapy. After surgery, 7–14 days of replacement therapy is required to ensure adequate wound healing and to prevent secondary haemorrhage.
- Primary prophylaxis with factor concentrates every 2 or 3 days at doses sufficient to keep the factor above 0.01–0.02 units/mL reduces bleeding and hence the severity of chronic haemophilic arthropathy.

FEIBA is a human donor–derived factor concentrate for patients with inhibitory antibodies to factor VIII or IX. It contains a mixture of coagulation factors and produces thrombin generation, even in the presence of antibodies (inhibitors) to factor VIII or IX.

Recombinant factor VIIa (NovoSeven) is effective for patients with inhibitory antibodies to factor VIII or IX or deficiency of factor VII. A pure synthetic activated coagulation factor, it generates thrombin, even in the presence of inhibitors to factor VIII or IX. Owing to its short duration of action, three doses (90 µg/kg) are usually necessary at 2-h intervals. Alternatively, a single large dose can be used (270 µg/kg).

Desmopressin (DDAVP)

Desmopressin is a vasopressin analogue that increases the plasma concentrations of factor VIII and von Willebrand factor, and potentiates platelet activation. Desmopressin is usually given subcutaneously or intravenously, but unwanted effects (headache, flushing and tachycardia) are less severe after subcutaneous use. A concentrated form is available for intranasal use.

Desmopressin is useful for treating patients with mild haemophilia A and von Willebrand disease, especially for short-term therapy. For dental extraction, a single subcutaneous injection or intravenous infusion of 0.3 µg/kg 1–2 h before surgery, combined with the oral antifibrinolytic drug, tranexamic acid, for 5–7 days after the procedure (see Antifibrinolytic drugs, p. 523), will often produce normal haemostasis and prevent secondary haemorrhage.

The response to desmopressin varies according to the underlying defect, and a test dose is usually given to assess this before using therapeutically. Patients with Type 3 (severe) or some forms of Type 2 von Willebrand disease (VWD) and some with Type 1 with severe haemorrhage, or patients who require major surgery, need *replacement* therapy with human-derived intermediate-purity factor VIII concentrate known to contain high molecular weight von Willebrand factor (VWF) multimers. The larger multimers are required for normal haemostatic function. Cryoprecipitate that is rich in factor VIII and VWF is not virally inactivated and should not be used for patients with VWD or mild to moderate factor VIII deficiency. A recombinant VWF concentrate containing no factor VIII has now been developed and is entering clinical use.

Desmopressin shortens the bleeding time in patients with renal or liver failure.

Adverse effects. Water retention and hyponatraemia may complicate therapy, and very young children (<1 year of age) should not receive desmopressin unless close monitoring is available. Adult fluid intake should not exceed 1 L in the 8 h following treatment, and with repeated doses the plasma sodium should be monitored. Tachyphylaxis (progressively diminishing response to the same dose) can occur.

Other agents

Adrenaline/epinephrine is effective as a topical agent for epistaxis, applied in ribbon gauze that is packed into the nostril, haemorrhage being arrested by local vasoconstriction.

Fibrin glue consists of fibrinogen and thrombin contained in two syringes, the tips of which form a common port that allows delivery of the two components to a bleeding point where fibrinogen converts to fibrin at a rate determined by the concentration of thrombin. Fibrin glue can be used to secure surgical haemostasis, e.g. on a large raw surface, and to prevent external oozing of blood in patients with haemophilia (see also above).

Sclerosing agents produce inflammation and thrombosis in veins to induce permanent obliteration, e.g. ethanolamine oleate injection, sodium tetradecyl sulphate (given intravenously for varicose veins) and oily phenol injection (given submucosally for haemorrhoids). Local reactions and tissue necrosis may occur.

Anticoagulant drugs

Anticoagulant drugs act principally to reduce the activity of *thrombin*, the enzyme that is mainly responsible for blood

---

[2]Laffan M 2016 New products for the treatment of haemophilia. British Journal of Haematology. 172:23–31.

clotting. The following discussion will show that drugs do so by:

- *limiting thrombin generation*, either as a result of inhibiting other proteases (clotting factors) involved in its generation or by reducing the activity of zymogens (the precursor inactive forms of the enzymes); or
- *inhibiting (neutralising) thrombin activity*, either directly or indirectly, depending on whether or not they activate the natural serpin-dependent anticoagulant pathway.[3]

Oral vitamin K antagonists (VKA)

Warfarin and other oral vitamin K antagonists (VKA) reduce the activity of zymogens.

Pharmacokinetics. Warfarin is readily absorbed from the gastrointestinal tract and is more than 90% bound to plasma proteins. Metabolism in the liver terminates its action. Warfarin ($t_{1/2}$ 36 h) is a racemic mixture of approximately equal amounts of two isomers, S ($t_{1/2}$ 27 h) and R ($t_{1/2}$ 40 h) warfarin, i.e. it is in effect two drugs. S warfarin is four times more potent than R warfarin. The isomers respond differently to drugs that interact with warfarin.

Pharmacodynamics. During the γ-carboxylation of factors II (prothrombin), VII, IX and X (and also the natural anticoagulant proteins C and S), active vitamin K (KH_2) is oxidised to an epoxide and must be reduced by the enzymes vitamin K epoxide reductase and vitamin K reductase to become active again (see the vitamin K cycle, p. 513). Coumarins[4] are structurally similar to vitamin K and competitively inhibit vitamin K epoxide reductase and vitamin K reductase, so limiting availability of the active reduced form of the vitamin to form coagulant (and anti-coagulant) proteins. The overall result is a shift in haemostatic balance in favour of anticoagulation because of the accumulation of clotting proteins with absent or decreased γ-carboxylation sites (PIVKAs).[5]

This shift does not take place until functioning vitamin K–dependent proteins, made before the drug was administered, have been cleared from the circulation. The process occurs at different rates for individual coagulation factors (VII $t_{1/2}$ 6 h, IX and X $t_{1/2}$ 18–24 h, prothrombin $t_{1/2}$ 72 h). The *anticoagulant* proteins C and S have a shorter $t_{1/2}$ than the *pro-coagulant* proteins, and their more rapid decline in concentration may create a *transient hypercoagulable state*. This can be dangerous in individuals with inherited protein C or S deficiency who may develop thrombotic skin necrosis during initiation of oral anticoagulant therapy with vitamin K antagonists. Anticoagulation with heparin until the effect of warfarin is well established reduces the risk of skin necrosis when rapid induction of anticoagulation is required.

The therapeutic anticoagulant effect of warfarin develops only after 4–5 days. Furthermore, the INR does not reliably reflect anticoagulant protection during this initial phase, as the vitamin K–dependent factors diminish at different rates and the INR is particularly sensitive to the level of factor VII, which is not a principal determinant of thrombotic or bleeding risk.

Because of the delay in onset of anticoagulant effect with oral VKAs, there is a need for an immediate-acting anticoagulant, such as a heparin, in the first few days of therapy if rapid anticoagulation is required.

The response to warfarin, and other coumarins, varies within and between individuals, and therefore regular monitoring of dose is essential. The pharmacokinetics (absorption and metabolism) and pharmocodynamics (haemostatic effect) are influenced by vitamin K intake and absorption, by heritable functional polymorphisms affecting metabolism such as P450 CYP 2 C9 polymorphisms, by rates of synthesis and clearance of coagulation proteins, and by drugs. The effectiveness of anticoagulant therapy with oral VKAs is determined by the INR, a standardised method derived from the prothrombin time that permits comparison between different laboratories.

Dose. There is much inter-individual variation in dose requirements. It is usual to initiate therapy with 10-mg doses, depending on the daily INR, with the maintenance dose then adjusted according to the INR using an established protocol. Several well-studied protocols are available for this purpose.[6]

---

[3]Serpin: serine protease inhibitors. Antithrombin is the principal serpin involved in regulating coagulation.

[4]Coumarins are present in many plants and are important in the perfume industry; the smell of new mown hay and grass is due to coumarins. Yellow sweet clover (King's clover) is rich in coumarins and was used as a herbal medicine to reduce inflammation. It was a constituent of an ointment to 'cool and dry and comfort the Membre' of King Henry VIII of England, who enjoyed a particularly active sexual life (Cutler T 2003 College Commentary, May/June. Royal College of Physicians, London, p. 23). The discovery of coumarins as anticoagulants dates from investigation of an unexplained haemorrhagic disease of cattle that had eaten mouldy sweet clover. Subsequent research at the University of Wisconsin, USA, culminated in the isolation of the causative agent, dicoumarol (Stahmann M A, Huebner C F, Link K P 1941 Journal of Biological Chemistry 138:513–527).

[5]Warfarin is 10 times more potent than dicoumarol and was originally used as a rodenticide. Its name is derived from the patent holder, Wisconsin Alumni Research Foundation, and the suffix comes from 'coumarin'.

[6]Crowther M A, Ginsberg J B, Kearon C et al 1999 A randomized trial comparing 5-mg and 10-mg warfarin loading doses. Archives of Internal Medicine 159:46–48.

The level of anticoagulation matches the perceived risk of thrombosis (see below). The target INR for deep vein thrombosis (DVT) is 2.5 (typical range 2.0–3.0).

Adverse effects. The major complication of treatment with warfarin is *bleeding*. As well as a risk of haemorrhage after trauma or surgery, spontaneous bleeding may occur. Each year a patient is on treatment there is a 1 in 20 (5%) risk of minor haemorrhage. The annual risk of major bleeding is 1 in 100, of which one-quarter are fatal. The risk of bleeding relates to the INR, not the dose of warfarin: the higher the INR, the greater the chance of bleeding. The risk of over-anticoagulation increases with intercurrent illness and interaction with other drugs, and is more likely in patients whose anticoagulant control is unstable. Therefore, it is essential to:

- maintain as stable a level of anticoagulation as possible
- adopt the lowest effective target INR
- educate patients about risk, particularly that associated with additional drug use.

Warfarin is a small molecule that crosses the placenta and can produce harmful effects in the developing fetus.

Warfarin embryopathy develops only after exposure to oral anticoagulant during the first trimester of pregnancy. The most common feature is chondrodysplasia punctata, characterised by abnormal cartilage and bone formation (with stippling of epiphyses visible on radiography) in vertebrae and femur, and the bones of the hands and feet during infancy and early childhood; these disappear with age (warfarin is not the only cause of this abnormality). Other less common skeletal abnormalities include nasal hypoplasia and hypertelorism (wide-set eyes).

Bleeding into the central nervous system is a danger throughout pregnancy but particularly at the time of delivery.

As a consequence of the above, warfarin is contraindicated in the first 6–12 weeks of pregnancy and should be replaced by heparin before the anticipated date of delivery, as the action of the latter drug can be terminated rapidly prior to the birth.

Withdrawal of oral anticoagulant therapy. The balance of evidence is that abrupt, as opposed to gradual, withdrawal of oral anticoagulant therapy does not of itself add to the risk of thromboembolism, for renewed synthesis of functional vitamin K–dependent clotting factors takes several days.

Reversal of anticoagulation can be gradual or rapid depending on the circumstances, i.e. from undue prolongation of INR to frank bleeding. Vitamin K 5–10 mg is usually adequate for complete reversal, oral administration being less rapid than intravenous. Immediate reversal is more readily achieved with a factor concentrate than fresh frozen plasma. Detailed guidance on corrective therapy in relation to the degree of over-anticoagulation is available, e.g. from the *British National Formulary*.[7]

Drug interactions. Warfarin or VKA control must be precise for safety and efficacy. If a drug that alters the action of warfarin is essential, monitor the INR frequently and adjust the dose of warfarin during the period of institution of the new drug until a new stable therapeutic dose of warfarin results; careful monitoring is also needed on withdrawal of the interacting drug.

Analgesics. Avoid, if possible, non-steroidal anti-inflammatory drugs (NSAIDs) including aspirin because of their irritant effect on gastric mucosa and action on platelets. Paracetamol is acceptable, but doses above 1.5 g/day may raise the INR. Dextropropoxyphene inhibits warfarin metabolism, and compounds that contain it, e.g. co-proxamol, should be avoided. Codeine, dihydrocodeine and combinations with paracetamol, e.g. co-dydramol, are preferred. Concomitant use of misoprostol with an NSAID may reduce the risk of gastric bleeding, and a selective cyclo-oxygenase (COX)-2 inhibitor may be associated with a lower bleeding risk in patients taking oral anticoagulants.

Antimicrobials. Aztreonam, cefamandole, chloramphenicol, ciprofloxacin, co-trimoxazole, erythromycin, fluconazole, itraconazole, ketoconazole, metronidazole, miconazole, ofloxacin and sulphonamides (including co-trimoxazole) increase anticoagulant effect by mechanisms that include interference with warfarin or vitamin K metabolism. Rifampicin and griseofulvin induce relevant hepatic enzymes and accelerate warfarin metabolism, reducing its effect. Intensive broad-spectrum antibiotic use, e.g. eradication regimens for *Helicobacter pylori*, may increase sensitivity to warfarin by reducing the intestinal flora that provide vitamin K.

Anticonvulsants. Carbamazepine, phenobarbital and primidone accelerate warfarin metabolism (by enzyme induction); the effect of phenytoin is variable. Clonazepam and sodium valproate are safe.

Antiarrhythmics. Amiodarone, propafenone and possibly quinidine potentiate the effect of warfarin, and dose adjustment is required, but atropine, disopyramide and lidocaine do not interfere.

Antidepressants. Selective serotonin reuptake inhibitors may enhance the effect of warfarin, but tricyclics may be used.

Gastrointestinal drugs. Avoid cimetidine and omeprazole, which inhibit the clearance of R warfarin, and sucralfate, which may impair its absorption. Ranitidine may be used. Most antacids are safe.

---

[7]Makris M, Van Veen J J, Tait CR et al 2013 Guideline on the management of bleeding in patients on antithrombotic agents. British Journal of Haematology 160:35–46.

Lipid-lowering drugs. Fibrates, and some statins, enhance anticoagulant effect. Avoid colestyramine as it may impair the absorption of both warfarin and vitamin K.

Sex hormones and hormone antagonists. The hormone antagonists danazol, flutamide and tamoxifen enhance the effect of warfarin.

Sedatives and anxiolytics. Benzodiazepines may be used. Otherwise check standard reference sources, e.g. BNF.

Uses of oral VKA

Oral vitamin K antagonist drugs are used to prevent and treat venous thrombosis and pulmonary embolus, and to prevent arterial thromboemboli in patients with atrial fibrillation or cardiac disease, including mechanical heart valves. The British Society for Haematology publishes recommended target INRs and duration of therapy for different thrombotic disorders (http://www.b-s-h.org.uk/guidelines/). The following are general indications:

- *Target INR 2.5* is appropriate for treatment of DVT; pulmonary embolism (PE); systemic embolism; prevention of venous thromboembolism in myocardial infarction; mitral stenosis with embolism; transient ischaemic attacks; atrial fibrillation; mechanical prosthetic aortic valves.
- *Target INR 3.5* is preferred for recurrent DVT and PE when already on warfarin with target of 2.5, arterial disease and some mechanical prosthetic mitral valves.
- At least 6 weeks' anticoagulation is recommended after calf vein thrombosis and at least 3 months after proximal DVT or PE. For patients with temporary risk factors and a low risk of recurrence, 3 months of treatment may be sufficient. For patients with idiopathic venous thromboembolism or permanent risk factors, longer term anticoagulation is often recommended.

Surgery in patients receiving oral VKA

Elective surgery. Warfarin is withdrawn 5 days before the operation and recommenced when the patient resumes oral intake; heparin (low molecular weight heparin (LMWH) or unfractionated heparin (UFH); see below) can be used in the intervening period if the thrombotic risk is high.[8]

---

[8]Keeling D, Campbell Tait R, Watson H, and on behalf of the British Committee of Standards for Haematology 2016 Peri-operative management of anticoagulation and antiplatelet therapy. A British Society for Haematology Guideline. British Journal of Haemotology. 175: 602–613. In patients with mechanical mitral prosthetic valves, LMWH or UFH is added when the INR is subtherapeutic.

Emergency surgery. Proceed as for bleeding (above).

Dental extractions. Anticoagulation may continue for patients whose INR is less than 4.0. The INR is measured no more than 72 h before the procedure to ensure that the INR will be less than 4.0 on the day of the extraction.

Other vitamin K antagonists

Acenocoumarol (nicoumalone) is similar to warfarin but seldom used in the UK, although more commonly in mainland Europe; the kidney eliminates it mainly in unchanged form. Phenprocoumon may also be encountered in travellers to the UK.

Indanedione anticoagulants are rarely used because of allergic reactions unrelated to coagulation; phenindione is still available.

Oral direct thrombin and factor Xa inhibitors

A number of novel agents, collectively referred to as direct-acting oral anticoagulants (DOACs) have recently been developed and licensed for a variety of indications. They act as direct inhibitors of thrombin (factor IIa) or factor Xa. They are described below, and their properties are summarized in Table 29.1. Whilst they are replacing warfarin in their licensed areas, they have not been effective in all areas.

Dabigatran

Dabigatran is a small molecule (mol. wt. 471) direct thrombin inhibitor (DTI). Dabigatran etexilate is an oral prodrug of the active compound dabigatran. Dabigatran is a direct specific competitive inhibitor of free and fibrin-bound thrombin. It binds to the active site of thrombin with high affinity (Kd 7×10^{-10} M). Absorption of the prodrug is rapid (C_{max} <4 h), and the half-life of dabigatran is 12–14 h in healthy volunteers and 14–17 h in patients undergoing major orthopaedic surgery. The active compound is not metabolised and is eliminated by renal excretion with 85% of an administered dose detectable in urine. Clearance is significantly prolonged when the glomerular filtration rate is less than 50 mL/min. There is a significant potentiating drug interaction with amiodarone and other drugs.

A specific monoclonal antibody antidote for dabigatran (Idaracizumab) has recently been licensed. A single treatment effectively abolishes all dabigatran activity in the circulation[9]

---

[9]Pollack C V, Reilly P A, Eikelboom J et al 2015 Idaracizumab for dabigatran reversal. New England Journal of Medicine 373:511–520.

Table 29.1 Direct-acting oral anticoagulants (DOACs)

	Dabigatran	**Rivaroxaban**	**Apixaban**	**Edoxaban**
Target	Factor IIa	Factor Xa	Factor Xa	Factor Xa
Time to peak	2 h	2–4 h	1–3 h	1–2 h
$t_{1/2}$	12–14 h	7–11 h	12 h	10–14 h
Dosing (AF)	BD	OD	BD	OD
Metabolism	Esterase catalysed hydrolysis	CYP P450 dependent and independent mechanisms	CYP P450	Hydrolysis by carboxylesterase conjugation or oxidation by CYP3A4/5
Excretion	85% renal	33% renal	25% renal	35% renal
Dose	150 mg 110 mg (>80 y, verapamil or increased bleed risk)	20 mg 15 mg (CrCL 30–49 mL/min)	5 mg 2.5 (2 or more: >80 y, weight <60 kg, Cr >133 μm/L) or CrCl 15–39 mL/min	60 mg 2.5 (1 or more: PgP inhibitors, weight <60 kg, or CrCl 15–50 mL/min)
Indications	Orthopaedic surgery Non-valvular AF Treatment of VT and PE	Orthopaedic surgery Non-valvular AF Treatment of VT and PE Acute coronary syndrome	Orthopaedic surgery Non-valvular AF Treatment of VT and PE	Non-valvular AF Treatment of VT and PE

Rivaroxaban, apixaban and edoxaban

These three agents are all small molecules which achieve their anticoagulant effect by direct competitive inhibition of factor Xa. They are all immediate acting and reach peak concentrations 1–4 hours after oral administration. Specific details are given in Table 29.1. Although they vary somewhat in their dependence on renal function for elimination, they are all metabolised by cytochromes and all subject to interaction with P-glycoprotein inhibitors or inducers. Nonetheless, their predictable dose response means that unlike warfarin they can be given in a fixed dose without the need for monitoring. Nor do they require such attention to dietary factors as are required with warfarin. At present no specific antidote is available, and in an emergency it is recommended to attempt counterbalancing the anticoagulant using prothrombin complex concentrate or FEIBA.

The licensed indications are shown in Table 29.1. In general these agents have been shown to be at least as effective as warfarin in preventing or treating thrombosis. Most notably they are all associated with a significant reduction in intracerebral haemorrhage compared to warfarin. This, coupled with the ease of administration is resulting in their increased use. They have not proved effective for mechanical prosthetic valves and are contraindicated in pregnancy. As the number of indications increases a variety of dosing regimens are being employed for which the product literature should be consulted.

Parenteral anticoagulants

Heparin

A medical student, J McLean, working at Johns Hopkins Medical School in 1916, discovered heparin. Seeking to devote 1 year to physiological research, he was set to study 'the thromboplastic (clotting) substance in the body'. He found that extracts of brain, heart and liver accelerated clotting but that activity deteriorated during storage. To his surprise, the extract of liver that he had kept longest not only failed to accelerate but actually retarded clotting. His personal account states:

After more tests and the preparation of other batches of heparophosphatide, I went one morning to the door of Dr. Howell's office, and standing there (he was seated at his desk), I said 'Dr. Howell, I have discovered antithrombin'. He was most skeptical. So I had the Deiner, John Schweinhant, bleed a cat. Into a small beaker full of its blood, I stirred all of a proven batch of heparophosphatides, and I placed this on Dr. Howell's laboratory table and asked him to call me when it clotted. It never did clot. [It was heparin].[10]

Heparin is a sulphated mucopolysaccharide that is found in the secretory granules of mast cells and is prepared commercially from porcine intestinal mucosa to give preparations that vary in molecular weight from 3000 to 30 000 Da (average 15 000 Da). It is the strongest organic acid in the body and in solution carries an electronegative charge. The low molecular weight heparins (LMWH, mean mol. wt. 4000–6500 Da) are prepared from standard unfractionated (UF) heparin by a variety of chemical techniques. Commercial preparations contain different fractions and display different pharmacokinetics. Some currently available in the UK include *bemiparin, dalteparin, enoxaparin, reviparin* and *tinzaparin.*

Pharmacokinetics. Heparin is poorly absorbed from the gastrointestinal tract and is given intravenously or subcutaneously; once in the blood, its effect is immediate. Heparin binds to several plasma proteins, to endothelial cells, and is taken up by reticuloendothelial cells; the kidney excretes a proportion. Because of these different mechanisms, elimination of heparin from the plasma involves a combination of zero- and first-order processes. The result is that the plasma biological effect $t_{1/2}$ alters disproportionately with dose, being 60 min after 75 units/kg and increasing to 150 min after 400 units/kg.

LMWHs are less protein bound and have a predictable dose–response profile when administered subcutaneously or intravenously. They also have a longer $t_{1/2}$ than standard heparin preparations.

Pharmacodynamics. Heparin depends for its anticoagulant action on the presence in plasma of a single-chain glycoprotein called *antithrombin* (formerly antithrombin III), a naturally occurring inhibitor of activated coagulation proteases (factors) that include thrombin, factor Xa and factor IXa. Heparin binds to antithrombin, via a specific pentasaccharide sequence, inducing a conformational change that leads to rapid inhibition of the proteases of the coagulation pathway. In the presence of heparin, antithrombin becomes approximately 1000-fold more active, and inhibition is essentially instantaneous. Following destruction of the proteases, the affinity of antithrombin for heparin falls; heparin then dissociates from the antithrombin–protease complex and catalyses further antithrombin–protease interactions.

Factor Xa is critical to thrombin generation (see Fig. 29.1), and heparin has the capacity to accelerate antithrombin inhibition of factor Xa in small quantities. This provides the rationale for using low-dose subcutaneous heparin to *prevent* thrombus formation.

LMWHs inhibit factor Xa at a dose similar to that for UFH, but have much less antithrombin activity, the principal action of conventional heparin. Fibrin formed in the circulation binds to thrombin and protects it from inactivation by the heparin–antithrombin complex; this may provide a further explanation for the higher doses of heparin needed to stop *extension* of a thrombus than to *prevent* it.

Fondaparinux is a synthetic form of the heparin pentasaccharide that inhibits factor Xa by an antithrombin-dependent mechanism. Fondaparinux has a molecular weight of 1728. Its specific anti-Xa activity is higher than that of LMWH, and its half-life after subcutaneous injection is longer than that of LMWH. Based on its almost complete bioavailability after subcutaneous injection, lack of variability in anticoagulant response and long half-life, fondaparinux can be administered subcutaneously once daily in fixed doses without coagulation monitoring. Fondaparinux is contraindicated in patients with renal insufficiency (CrCl <30 mL/min). It is used for prevention and treatment of venous thromboembolism in the same way as traditional LMWHs. The risk of HIT(T) (see below) is lower, but the risk of bleeding may be greater than that associated with LMWHs.

Monitoring heparin therapy. Control of standard heparin therapy is traditionally by the activated partial thromboplastin time (APTT); the target therapeutic range is usually 1.5–2.5 times the control. The laboratory should confirm that this corresponds to an anti-Xa assay result of 0.3–0.7 IU/mL. In many circumstances, the anti-Xa assay is preferable because it is not confounded by acute-phase reactants. Therapeutic amounts of LMWH do not prolong the APTT, and, because the pharmacokinetics are predictable, a safe and effective dose can be calculated without laboratory monitoring, using an algorithm that is adjusted for body-weight.

Adverse effects. Bleeding is the main acute complication of heparin therapy. Patients with impaired hepatic or renal function, with carcinoma, and those older than 60 years of age are most at risk. An APTT ratio greater than 3 is associated with an increased risk of bleeding.

Heparin-induced thrombocytopenia (HIT), sometimes accompanied by *thrombosis* (HIT/T), is due to an autoantibody against heparin in association with platelet factor 4, which activates platelets. It occurs most commonly with heparin derived from bovine lung and is more common with UFHs than with LMWHs. Suspect HIT in any patient in whom the platelet count falls by 50% or more after starting heparin. It usually occurs after 5–14 days of heparin exposure (or sooner if the patient has previously been exposed to heparin). Thrombosis occurs in less than 1% of patients treated with

---

[10]McLean gives a fascinating account of his struggles to pay his way through medical school, as well as his discovery of heparin, in: McLean J 1959 The discovery of heparin. Circulation 19:75–78.

LMWHs but is associated with a mortality and limb amputation rate in excess of 30%. Patients with HIT/T should discontinue all heparin (UF and LMW) and receive an alternative thrombin inhibitor, such as danaparoid, agatroban or fondaparinux. Warfarin should not be commenced until there is adequate anticoagulation with one of these agents and the platelet count has returned to normal.

Osteoporosis may complicate long-term heparin exposure. It is dose related and most frequently observed during pregnancy. The relative risk between LMWHs is not yet established but it appears to be less than with UFHs.

Hypersensitivity reactions and skin necrosis (similar to that seen with warfarin) occur but are rare. Transient alopecia may occur.

Heparin reversal. Protamine, a protein obtained from fish sperm, immediately reverses the anticoagulant action of unfractionated heparin. It is as strongly basic as heparin is acidic, which explains its rapid action. The effect of UFH is short lived, and reversal with protamine sulphate is seldom required except after extracorporeal perfusion for heart surgery. Protamine sulphate, 1 mg by slow i.v. injection, neutralises 80–100 units UFH. The quantity of heparin given and its expected $t_{1/2}$ determine the amount required, but the maximum must not exceed 50 mg. Protamine itself has some anticoagulant effect, and overdosage is to be avoided. It is only partially effective against LMWH.

Use of heparin

Treatment of established venous thromboembolism. Patients with acute venous thromboembolism can be treated safely and effectively with LMWH as outpatients. Large-scale studies demonstrate that outpatient treatment of acute DVT with unmonitored, body-weight–adjusted LMWH is as safe and effective as inpatient treatment with adjusted-dose i.v. UFH. Further trials confirm the safety and efficacy of LMWH therapy in acute PE.

The traditional regimen for standard UFH is a bolus i.v. injection of 5000 units (or 10000 units in major PE) followed by a constant-rate i.v. infusion of 1000–2000 units/h. The APTT should be measured 6 h after starting therapy and the administration rate adjusted to keep it in the optimal therapeutic range of 1.5–2.5; this usually requires at least daily measurement of APTT.

Coincident with commencing heparin, patients usually start taking an oral anticoagulant, traditionally warfarin in the UK but now possibly a DOAC. If warfarin is used, then the INR is monitored and loading doses of VKA are given according to a validated loading protocol in order to minimise the risk of over-anticoagulation and bleeding. Ideally the INR should be measured daily during the first 4 days of loading with a VKA; guidance is available at http://www.b-s-h.org.uk/guidelines/.

Prevention of venous thromboembolism. LMWHs are often used for perioperative prophylaxis because of their convenience. They are as effective and safe as UFH at preventing venous thrombosis. Once-daily subcutaneous administration suffices, as their duration of action is longer than that of UFH and no laboratory monitoring is required.

If UFH is used, 5000 units should be given subcutaneously every 8 or 12 h without monitoring (this dose does not prolong the APTT), or in pregnancy 5000–10000 units subcutaneously every 12 h with monitoring (except for pregnant women with prosthetic heart valves, for whom specialist monitoring is needed).

Cardiac disease. LMWHs are at least as effective as standard heparin for unstable angina. Patients undergoing angioplasty may also receive LMWHs.

Heparin is used to reduce the risk of venous thromboembolism, and the size of emboli from mural thrombi following acute myocardial infarction.

Peripheral arterial occlusion. In the acute phase following thrombosis or arterial embolism, heparin may prevent extension of a thrombus and hasten its recanalisation. Long-term antithrombotic therapy for patients with ischaemic peripheral vascular disease generally requires specific antiplatelet therapy (see p. 525).

Other anticoagulant drugs

Danaparoid sodium is a mixture of several types of non-heparin glycosaminoglycans extracted from pig intestinal mucosa (84% heparan sulphate). It is an indirect thrombin inhibitor and effective for the treatment of DVT, prophylaxis in high-risk patients and treatment of patients with heparin-associated thrombocytopenia (HIT/T).

Bivalirudin is a bivalent direct thrombin inhibitor produced as a 20–amino-acid recombinant polypeptide. It is a relatively low-affinity inhibitor of thrombin and may thus present a lower bleeding risk, but clinical advantage remains to be shown.

Argatroban, a carboxylic acid derivative, binds non-covalently to the active site of thrombin and is an effective alternative to heparin in patients with HIT.

Anticoagulant drugs under development

Research continues to pursue thrombin and factor Xa as suitable targets for anticoagulant therapy with the aim of improving specificity, pharmacokinetics and finding binding kinetics which reduce thrombotic risk whilst having minimal effect on bleeding risk. Factor XI has emerged as a novel target because Factor XI deficiency is associated with only a mild bleeding risk but a significant reduction in thrombosis.

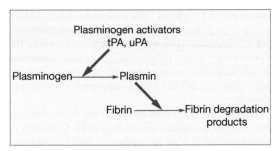

Fig. 29.3 The blood fibrinolytic system. tPA, tissue-type plasminogen activator; uPA, urokinase-type plasminogen activator.

Factor XI may be targeted by reducing plasma levels using SiRNA or by inhibitory antibodies or small molecules.[11]

Other proteases such as factor IXa are also potential targets as is the factor VII-tissue factor complex.

Fibrinolytic (thrombolytic) system

The system acts to remove intravascular fibrin, thereby restoring blood flow.

Plasminogen activators that convert plasminogen to plasmin initiate the process. The trypsin-like protease, *plasmin*, then degrades fibrin into soluble *fibrin degradation products* (Fig. 29.3).

Two immunologically distinct plasminogen activators are found in blood, namely *tissue-type* (tPA) and *urokinase-type* (uPA), both of which are synthesised and released from endothelial cells. Intravascular plasminogen activation is initiated by tPA. In this process, plasminogen and tPA bind to fibrin, and the enzymatic activity of tPA is enhanced by fibrin. The result is that plasmin formation takes place only on the *fibrin surface* and not generally in the circulation, where widespread defibrination would occur and compromise the whole coagulation mechanism. tPA is the plasminogen activator used for the treatment of cerebral vascular occlusion.

Fibrinolysis inhibitors. The most important is *endothelial cell–derived type 1 plasminogen activator inhibitor* (PAI-1), which blocks the action of tPA. Another inhibitor, α_2-antiplasmin, rapidly complexes with and inactivates *free* plasmin. Antiplasmin is cross-linked to fibrin by factor XIII and provides important protection from fibrinolysis. An enzyme, known as *thrombin-activatable fibrinolysis inhibitor* (TAFI), attenuates fibrinolysis by cleaving carboxyl-terminal lysine residues from fibrin, the removal of which decreases plasminogen and

plasmin binding to fibrin, retarding the lytic process. TAFI thus serves as a link between coagulation and fibrinolysis.

Drugs that promote fibrinolysis

An important application of fibrinolytic drugs has been to dissolve thrombi in acutely occluded arteries, thereby restoring blood flow and reducing ischaemic damage, e.g. in stroke. The approach is to give a *plasminogen activator* by intravenous infusion or bolus injection in order to increase the formation of the fibrinolytic enzyme *plasmin*.

Recombinant thrombolytic proteins can be re-engineered to prolong $t_{1/2}$ and possibly reduce the induced systemic fibrinolytic state. Current drugs possess a broadly equivalent risk of inducing bleeding. Recombinant drugs of human origin are non-antigenic, whereas those with a bacterial origin, whether purified from bacteria or produced by recombinant technology, can result in antibody formation and produce allergic reactions that preclude repeated treatment. The $t_{1/2}$ determines whether a drug is suitable for bolus i.v. injection or continuous i.v. infusion. Reteplase and tenecteplase are most appropriate for bolus injection.

Alteplase ($t_{1/2}$ 2–6 min) is a single-chain recombinant tissue-type plasminogen activator (rtPA) that is usually given by continuous i.v. infusion over 30–180 min, according to the indication, i.e. for acute myocardial infarction and acute ischaemic stroke. A bolus dose is recommended for pulmonary embolus.

Reteplase is a deletion mutant of tPA lacking a growth factor and the kringle-binding domain; it possesses a longer $t_{1/2}$ (1.6 h) than alteplase. This permits a double bolus regimen, with completion of treatment in 30 min, rather than the need for administration by infusion. It is licensed for acute myocardial infarction.

Tenecteplase is a tPA variant with amino acid substitutions that confer a longer $t_{1/2}$ (2 h), greater enzymatic efficiency and a more fibrin-specific profile. It is administered as a single i.v. injection over 5–10 s and is licensed for treatment of acute myocardial infarction.

Streptokinase, derived from culture filtrates of *Streptococcus haemolyticus*, is not an enzyme. It binds human plasminogen to produce a plasminogen activator that undergoes a time-dependent change of conformation to create an active site that auto-catalytically converts plasminogen to plasmin. The plasmin-complexed streptokinase then decays by proteolytic degradation.

Streptokinase ($t_{1/2}$ 20 min) is given by i.v. infusion, e.g. for up to 72 h when treating patients with venous thromboembolism. It finds use for acute myocardial infarction, deep vein thrombosis and pulmonary embolism, acute arterial thromboembolism, and central retinal venous or

[11]Büller HR, Gailani D, Weitz JI et al, for the FXI-ASO TKA Investigators 2015 Factor XI antisense oligonucleotide for venous thrombosis. New England Journal of Medicine 372:232–240.

arterial thrombosis. The rate of infusion may be limited by tachycardia, fever and muscle aches. Nausea and vomiting may also occur.

Uses of thrombolytic drugs

Vascular occlusion

Fibrinolytic activators such as tPA are licensed for treatment of myocardial infarction and acute ischaemic stroke. In all cases, the outcome is improved by early administration. For stroke, treatment must begin within 4.5 hours after onset of symptoms. For myocardial infarction treatment may still show benefit up to 12 hours after onset, but when available, acute coronary intervention is now preferred. Fibrinolysis is also used for massive pulmonary embolism with haemodynamic instability, limb-threatening venous thrombosis and acute peripheral arterial occlusion.

Contraindications to thrombolytic drug use are those that predispose to intracranial haemorrhage (haemorrhagic stroke, intracranial tumour, recent neurosurgery or brain trauma within the previous 10 days and uncontrolled hypertension) or massive haemorrhage (major surgery of thorax or abdomen within the previous 10 days, current major bleeding such as from the gastrointestinal tract or prolonged cardiopulmonary resuscitation).

Adverse effects. In all cases the limiting factor is the risk of haemorrhage. If bleeding occurs, thrombolytic therapy must cease. Depending on the timing of bleeding in relation to therapy, consider *antifibrinolytic* therapy with aprotonin (for longer-acting drugs) and restoring the fibrinogen and antiplasmin concentrations with fresh frozen plasma or cryoprecipitate (more likely required after streptokinase therapy). Platelet transfusion may be given to correct the platelet function defect induced by plasmin proteolysis of platelet membrane receptors.

Following thrombolytic therapy, intramuscular injections are contraindicated, any venepuncture requires at least 10 min of local compression, and arterial puncture must be avoided.

Hypotension can follow treatment with any thrombolytic drug, but febrile allergic reactions are about six times more likely with use of a thrombolytic of bacterial origin. Some milder reactions can be managed with paracetamol, an H_1-receptor antihistamine and corticosteroid.

Drugs that prevent fibrinolysis

Antifibrinolytics are useful in a number of bleeding disorders.

Tranexamic acid competitively inhibits the binding of plasminogen and tPA to fibrin and effectively blocks conversion of plasminogen to plasmin; fibrinolysis is thus retarded.

An intravenous bolus passes largely unchanged in the urine with a $t_{1/2}$ of 1.5 h. Oral and topical formulations are available.

Tranexamic acid is used principally to prevent the *hyperplasminaemic bleeding state* that results from damage to tissues rich in plasminogen activator, e.g. after prostatic surgery, tonsillectomy, uterine cervical cone biopsy and menorrhagia, whether primary or induced by an intrauterine contraceptive device. Tranexamic acid may also reduce bleeding after ocular trauma, and in von Willebrand disease and haemophilia after dental extraction. It is frequently given as an adjunct to desmopressin therapy.

Some patients with *hereditary angioedema* may benefit, presumably by prevention of plasmin-induced activation of the complement system.

Tranexamic acid may be of value in *thrombocytopenia* (idiopathic or following cytotoxic chemotherapy). The natural fibrinolytic destabilisation of small platelet plugs is inhibited, reducing the risk of haemorrhage and requirement for platelet transfusion.

Adverse effects are rare but include nausea, diarrhoea and sometimes orthostatic hypotension. Tranexamic acid is contraindicated for patients with haematuria because clot lysis in the urinary tract is prevented and clot colic results.

Aprotinin is a naturally occurring inhibitor of plasmin and other proteolytic enzymes that has been used to limit perioperative bleeding during cardiac bypass and liver transplantation surgery. In 2008, aprotinin was withdrawn from the market after studies suggested it may be associated with an increased mortality following cardiopulmonary bypass. However in 2012, a review of these data concluded that they were unreliable and the ban was lifted so that its use was approved for patients 'undergoing isolated heart bypass surgery who are at high risk of major blood loss' (http://www.ema.europa.eu/docs/en_GB/document_library/Press_release/2012/02/WC500122914.pdf).

Platelet function

Platelets have a key role in maintaining vascular integrity. They aggregate at and adhere to exposed collagen to form a physical barrier at the site of vessel injury; they accelerate the activation of coagulation proteins; they release stored granules that promote vasoconstriction and wound healing.

Platelets have rightly been termed 'pharmacological packages'. To deliver the above functions, they must first undergo a process of *activation* that involves multiple agonists through numerous intracellular second-messenger pathways and complex networks (see Fig. 29.3). These pathways converge on and activate the fibrinogen receptor, *glycoprotein IIbIIIa* (integrin αIIbβ3), inducing a conformational change that results in fibrinogen/fibrin binding. When fibrinogen occupies the receptor, outside-in signalling consolidates platelet activation by up-regulating second-messenger pathways, so providing a positive feedback loop.

In the *coagulation process*, platelets provide an anionic phospholipid surface for assembly of the macromolecular enzymatic complexes required for thrombin generation. Phospholipids in the bilayer membrane of resting platelets are distributed asymmetrically, with anionic phospholipid held in the internal leaflet. Full platelet activation results in scrambling of the membrane with exposure of negatively charged phospholipid on the external leaflet. This lipid cooperates in the assembly of the thrombin-generating enzymatic complexes.

Receptors on the *platelet membrane* that are known to result in platelet activation through intracellular second messengers include those for thrombin, adenosine diphosphate (ADP), collagen, thromboxane and adrenaline/epinephrine.

Activation is enhanced by occupancy of glycoprotein IIbIIIa (the fibrinogen receptor) and glycoprotein Ib (a component of the Ib/IX/V receptor for von Willebrand protein). The process is mediated primarily through G-coupled second messengers in response to occupancy of the thrombin, ADP and collagen receptors (at high collagen concentration), and through phospholipases and consequent thromboxane generation in response to occupancy of the thromboxane, adrenaline/epinephrine and collagen receptors (at low collagen concentration).

Both thromboxane and ADP are produced in response to platelet activation, and recruit further platelets to activation sites, so providing a positive feedback loop to their respective receptors. There are several ADP receptors on the platelet membrane. Multiple second-messenger pathways are probably involved in their mechanism of activation, not just G-protein–coupled systems. Collagen-induced platelet activation involves at least three receptors with both thromboxane-dependent and thromboxane-independent second-messenger pathways.

High 'shear forces' also activate platelets, but the mechanisms are unclear: fibrinogen and its receptor, GPIIbIIIa, are required at low shear rates, and von Willebrand factor and its receptor, GPIb, at high shear rates. ADP and adrenaline/epinephrine are synergistic at high shear and result in larger thrombi for a given rate of shear.

Drugs that inhibit platelet activity (antiplatelet drugs)

(See also Myocardial infarction, p. 525.)

Aspirin (acetylsalicylic acid) acetylates and thus inactivates COX, the enzyme responsible for the first step in the formation of prostaglandins, the conversion of arachidonic acid to prostaglandin H_2. As acetylation of COX is *irreversible* and the platelet is unable to synthesise new enzyme, COX activity is lost for the platelet lifetime (8–10 days).

Aspirin prevents formation of both thromboxane A_2 (TXA_2) and prostacyclin (PGI_2) (see Fig. 16.1, p. 249). Therapeutic interest in the antithrombotic effect of aspirin has centred on separating these actions by using a low dose. In general, 75–100 mg/day by mouth will abolish synthesis of TXA_2 without significant impairment of prostacyclin formation, i.e. amounts substantially below the 2.4 g/day used to control pain and inflammation. Laboratory testing of TXA_2 production or TXA_2-dependent platelet function can provide an assessment of the adequacy of aspirin dose. Among several causes of reduced response to aspirin are genetic polymorphisms of COX-1 and other genes involved in thromboxane biosynthesis.[12]

Low-dose aspirin is not without risk: a proportion of peptic ulcer bleeds in people older than 60 years of age occur from prophylactic low-dose aspirin.

Dipyridamole reversibly inhibits platelet phosphodiesterase, and consequently cyclic AMP concentration is increased and platelet activity reduced. Dipyridamole also inhibits the reuptake of adenosine by platelets resulting in elevated extracellular adenosine concentration. It is bound extensively to plasma proteins and has a $t_{1/2}$ of 12 h.

Clopidogrel is a thienopyridine derivative that irreversibly inhibits ADP-dependent platelet aggregation by covalently binding to the ADP P2Y12 receptor. The $t_{1/2}$ of the parent drug is 40 h, and metabolism by the liver converts it to its active form. Clopidogrel reduces the risk of the combined outcome of stroke, myocardial infarction (MI) or vascular death in patients with thromboembolic stroke. It decreases vascular death and MI in patients with unstable angina, reduces acute occlusion of coronary bypass grafts, and improves walking distance and decreases vascular complications in patients with peripheral vascular disease. Clopidogrel also finds use in the prevention of stroke in patients who are intolerant of aspirin. An initial dose of 300 mg is followed by a daily dose of 75 mg.

Prasugrel is a thienopyridine derivative like clopidogrel. It inhibits ADP-induced platelet aggregation more rapidly, more consistently, and to a greater extent than standard-dose clopidogrel. A 60-mg loading dose results in at least 50% inhibition of platelet aggregation by 1 h in 90% of patients. The subsequent daily dose is 10 mg.

Ticagrelor. Ticagrelor is another orally active inhibitor of the platelet ADP receptor. Unlike other members of this

[12]Hankey G J, Eikelboom J W. 2006. Aspirin resistance. Lancet 367:606–617.

group, it is not a prodrug and is an allosteric, reversible inhibitor of the P2Y12 receptor. It is licensed for secondary prevention of MI and for acute coronary syndromes, usually in combination with aspirin.

Epoprostenol (prostacyclin) may be given as an anticoagulant during renal dialysis, with or without heparin; it is infused intravenously and subcutaneously ($t_{1/2}$ 3 min). It is a potent vasodilator.

Glycoprotein (GP) IIb–IIIa antagonists

The platelet glycoprotein IIb–IIIa complex is the predominant platelet integrin, a molecule restricted to megakaryocytes and platelets that mediates platelet aggregation by the binding of proteins such as fibrinogen and von Willebrand factor (VWF) (Fig. 29.4). Hereditary absence of the GPIIb–IIIa complex (Glanzmann thrombasthenia) results in platelets that are incapable of aggregation by physiological agonists.

GPIIb–IIIa antagonists have been developed as antiplatelet agents. As blockers of the *final common pathway* of platelet aggregation (the binding of fibrinogen or VWF to the GPIIb–IIIa complex), they are more complete inhibitors of platelets than either aspirin or clopidogrel, which act only on the cyclo-oxygenase or ADP pathway, respectively. GPIIb–IIIa antagonists also have an anticoagulant effect by reducing availability of platelet membrane anionic phospholipid. Inhibition of platelet aggregation is dose dependent.

Abciximab is a human–murine chimeric monoclonal antibody Fab fragment that binds to the GPIIb–IIIa complex with a high affinity and slow dissociation rate. Given intravenously, it is cleared rapidly from plasma ($t_{1/2}$ 20 min). Abciximab (0.25 mg/kg bolus then 0.125 µg/kg/min infusion

for 12 h) produces immediate and profound inhibition of platelet activity that lasts for 12–36 h after termination of the infusion. The dose causes and maintains blockade of more than 80% of receptors, with a greater than 80% reduction in aggregation. Patients may also receive heparin and an antiplatelet drug, e.g. aspirin. Abciximab is effective in acute coronary syndromes, but again widespread use is limited by bleeding.

Eptifibatide is a cyclic heptapeptide based upon the Lys-Gly-Asp sequence. *Tirofiban* and *lamifiban* are non-peptide mimetics. All three are competitive inhibitors of the GPIIb–IIIa complex, with lower affinities and higher dissociation rates than abciximab and relatively short plasma $t_{1/2}$ values (2–2.5 h). Platelet aggregation returns to normal from 30 min to 4 h after discontinuation. Eptifibatide and tirofiban are effective in acute coronary syndromes.

Adverse effects. Platelet transfusion after cessation of abciximab is necessary for refractory or life-threatening bleeding. After transfusion, the antibody redistributes to the transfused platelets, reducing the mean level of receptor blockade and improving platelet function. Thrombocytopenia may occur from 1 h to days after commencing treatment in up to 1% of patients. This necessitates platelet counts 2–4 h after commencement and then daily; if severe, therapy must be stopped and, if necessary, platelets transfused. EDTA-induced pseudothrombocytopenia has been reported, and a low platelet count should prompt examination of a blood film for agglutination before therapy is stopped.

Uses of antiplatelet drugs

Antiplatelet therapy protects at-risk patients against stroke, myocardial infarction or death. A meta-analysis of 145 clinical trials of prolonged (>1 month) antiplatelet therapy versus control, and trials between antiplatelet regimens, found that the chance of non-fatal myocardial infarction and non-fatal stroke fell by one-third, and that there was a one-sixth reduction in the risk of death from any vascular cause.[13] Expressed in another way, in the first month after an acute myocardial infarction (a vulnerable period), aspirin prevents death, stroke or a further heart attack in about 4 of every 100 patients treated. Continuing treatment from the end of year 1 to year 3 conferred further benefit.

Aspirin is by far the most commonly used anti-platelet agent. The optimal dose is not certain, but one not exceeding

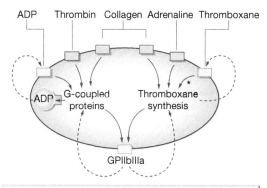

ADP Thrombin Collagen Adrenaline Thromboxane

ADP G-coupled proteins Thromboxane synthesis

GPIIbIIIa

* COX and TXA2 are required for thromboxane synthesis and are targets for antiplatelet drugs, for example aspirin

Fig. 29.4 Mechanisms for the activation of platelets. ADP, adenosine diphosphate; COX, cyclo-oxygenase; GP, glycoprotein; TXA$_2$, thromboxane A$_2$.

[13]Antiplatelet Trialists' Collaboration. 1994. Collaborative overview of randomised trials of antiplatelet therapy – I: Prevention of death, myocardial infarction and stroke by prolonged antiplatelet therapy and various categories of patients. British Medical Journal 308:81–106.

aspirin 325 mg/day is acceptable, and 75–100 mg/day may be as effective and preferred where there is gastric intolerance. Aspirin alone (mainly) or aspirin plus dipyridamole greatly reduced the risk of occlusion where vascular grafts or arterial patency were studied systematically.[14]

Many patients who take aspirin for vascular disease may also require an NSAID, e.g. for joint disease. Given their common mode of action by inhibiting prostaglandin synthesis, this raises the issue that NSAIDs may block access of aspirin to active sites on platelets, with loss of cardioprotection. Retrospective cohort[15] and case-control[16] studies suggest no adverse interaction with ibuprofen, but the issue remains unresolved, and in the meantime it seems prudent to take aspirin 2 h before an NSAID, e.g. at bedtime.

[14]Antiplatelet Trialists' Collaboration. 1994. Collaborative overview of randomised trials of antiplatelet therapy – II: Maintenance of vascular grafts or arterial patency by antiplatelet therapy. British Medical Journal 308:159–168.

[15]García Rodríguez L A, Varas-Lorenzo C, Maguire A, González-Pérez A. 2004.Nonsteroidal anti-inflammatory drugs and the risk of myocardial infarction in the general population. Circulation 109:3000–3006.
[16]Patel T N, Goldberg K C. 2004. Use of aspirin and ibuprofen compared with aspirin alone and the risk of myocardial infarction. Archives of Internal Medicine 164:852–856.

Summary

- Coagulation does not occur as a consequence of linear sequential enzyme activation pathways but by a network of simultaneous interactions, with regulation and modulation of these interactions during the thrombin generation process itself.
- Vitamin K is necessary for the final stage in the synthesis of coagulant factors II (prothrombin), VII, IX and X, and anticoagulant regulatory proteins, proteins Z, C and S.
- Vitamin K is used to treat haemorrhage or threatened bleeding due to the coumarin or indanedione anticoagulants, haemorrhagic disease of the newborn and hypoprothrombinaemia due to intestinal malabsorption syndromes.
- Desmopressin increases the plasma concentration of factor VIII and von Willebrand factor, primes platelets, and is useful in patients with mild haemophilia A and von Willebrand disease.
- The predominant effect of anticoagulant drugs is to limit thrombin generation, or to neutralise thrombin.
- Warfarin and other oral vitamin K antagonists act by reducing the activity of vitamin K–dependent clotting factors (see above); they take 4–5 days to produce a therapeutic effect.
- Oral VKA have a delayed pharmacodynamic effect relative to their pharmacokinetic profiles with both a slow on and off effect, but the anticoagulant effect can be reversed with factor concentrate (II, VII, IX and X) and vitamin K.
- Oral direct thrombin and anti-Xa inhibitors have a fast pharmacodynamic effect in parallel with their pharmacokinetic profile. A specific antidote is available for dabigatran.
- Oral anticoagulant drugs are used to prevent and treat venous thrombosis and pulmonary embolus, and to prevent arterial thromboemboli in patients with atrial fibrillation or cardiac disease. VKAs are the only choice for mechanical heart valves.
- Heparin depends for its anticoagulant action on the presence in plasma of antithrombin, a naturally occurring inhibitor of activated coagulation proteases that include thrombin, factor Xa and factor IXa.
- Patients with acute venous thromboembolism can be treated safely and effectively with low molecular weight heparin or some DOACs as outpatients.
- LMWHs and direct thrombin and Xa inhibitors are the preferred drugs for perioperative prophylaxis (according to procedure) and are at least as effective as standard heparin for unstable angina.
- Fibrinolytic drugs dissolve thrombi in acutely occluded coronary arteries, thereby restoring blood flow to ischaemic myocardium and improving prognosis. The earlier thrombolysis is given the better the outcome. Thrombolysis is also effective for massive pulmonary emboli with cardiovascular compromise.
- Aspirin acetylates and thus inactivates cyclo-oxygenase (COX), the enzyme responsible for the first step in the formation of prostaglandins, and in low dose reduces platelet activity by preventing the formation of thromboxane.
- Clopidogrel inhibits ADP-dependent platelet aggregation; it reduces the risk of stroke, myocardial infarction or vascular death.
- GPIIb–IIIa antagonists block the final common pathway of platelet aggregation (the binding of fibrinogen or VWF to the GPIIb–IIIa complex) and are more complete inhibitors of platelets than either aspirin or clopidogrel.
- Antiplatelet therapy protects at-risk patients against stroke, myocardial infarction or death.

Guide to further reading

Baglin, T., Barrowcliffe, T.W., Cohen, A., Greaves, M., 2006. Guidelines on the use and monitoring of heparin. Br. J. Haematol. 133, 19–34.

CRASH-2 trial collaborators, Shakur, H., Roberts, I., Bautista, R., et al., 2010. Effects of tranexamic acid on death, vascular occlusive events, and blood transfusion in trauma patients with significant haemorrhage (CRASH-2): a randomised, placebo-controlled trial. Lancet 376, 23–32.

De Meyer, S.F., Vanhoorelbeke, K., Broos, K., et al., 2008. Antiplatelet drugs. Br. J. Haematol. 142, 515–528.

Di Nisio, M., Middeldorp, S., Büller, H.R., et al., 2005. Direct thrombin inhibitors. N. Engl. J. Med. 353, 1028–1040.

Huntington, J.A., Baglin, T.P., 2003. Targeting thrombin: rational drug design from natural mechanisms. Trends Pharmacol. Sci. 24, 589–595.

Keeling, D.M., Baglin, T.P., Tait, C., et al., 2011. Guidelines on oral anticoagulation (warfarin), 4th ed. Br. J. Haematol. 154, 311–324.

Millar, C.M., Laffan, M.A., 2017. Drug therapy in anticoagulation: which drug for which patient? Clin. Med. (Lond.) 17, 233–244.

Patrono, C., Garcia Rodriguez, L.A., Landolfi, R., Baigent, C., 2005. Low-dose aspirin for the prevention of atherothrombosis. N. Engl. J. Med. 353, 2373–2383.

Weitz, J.I., Eikelboom, J.W., Samama, M.M., 2012. New antithrombotic drugs: American College of Chest Physicians evidence-based clinical practice guidelines, 9th ed. Chest 141, e152S–e184S.

Chapter | 30 |

Red blood cell disorders

M. Hasib Sidiqi, Wendy N. Erber

SYNOPSIS

Disorders of red blood cells may be due to reduced or excessive production in the bone marrow, premature cell destruction (haemolysis) or loss from the circulation. A precise diagnosis must be made from the blood count, blood film, biochemistry and/or bone marrow examination so that appropriate therapy can be instituted. Anaemia due to a haematinic deficiency can be treated with specific replacement therapy (e.g. iron, vitamin B_{12} or folic acid) along with management of the underlying cause. Other secondary anaemias may benefit from haemopoietic growth factor therapy such as erythropoiesis-stimulating agents (e.g. for chronic renal disease), immunosuppression (e.g. for autoimmune haemolytic or aplastic anaemia) or avoidance of specific drugs (e.g. sulfonamides or antibiotics). Inherited disorders of red cells (e.g. haemoglobinopathies) may require specific drug therapy (e.g. hydroxycarbamide for sickle cell disease), folate supplementation and blood transfusion. Over-production of red cells, as in polycythaemia vera, is managed by venesection and, for some patients, suppressing marrow erythropoiesis.

- Iron.
- Vitamin B_{12}.
- Folic acid.
- Haemolytic anaemia.
- Haemoglobinopathies.
- Aplastic anaemia.
- Polycythaemia vera.
- Haemopoietic growth factors.

Iron

Iron is a trace element that is required for oxygen transport by erythrocytes and for oxidative metabolism in all cells. Up to 75% of body iron is present in haemoglobin (Hb), and the majority of the remainder in myoglobin and enzymes. A normal daily diet contains approximately 10–20 mg iron which is present in meat (heme iron), grains and vegetables. Only 5–10% of dietary iron is absorbed, which is sufficient to compensate for the normal daily loss of iron (1 mg/day) in faeces and desquamation of skin. Iron requirements are greater during periods of growth (i.e. childhood), as a result of blood loss in menstruation (average menstrual cycle loses 10–15 mg iron) and increased requirements (e.g. pregnancy up to 3 mg/day of iron). Gastrointestinal iron absorption can increase up to five-fold with increased demand. Ascorbate increases iron absorption, whereas phytates and tannins reduce absorption.

Dietary iron is reduced to the ferrous (Fe^{2+}) state at the brush border of the duodenum. *Divalent metal transport 1* (DMT1), located on the membrane of duodenal enterocytes, then transports iron across the intestinal lumen; this is aided by an acidic environment. *Ferroportin*, facilitated by hephaestin, then releases iron into the bloodstream. *Hepcidin* is a key regulator of iron homeostasis and directly inhibits ferroportin release of iron (Fig. 30.1). In the plasma, iron binds to *transferrin* and delivers it to transferrin receptors on developing erythroblasts in the bone marrow. If not utilised, iron may be stored intracellularly, or excreted in faeces from shed mucosal cells. Red blood cells have a 120-day life span after which they die and release haemoglobin. The free haemoglobin is phagocytosed by macrophages and exported by ferroportin back to plasma transferrin. Excess iron is stored in the bone marrow, hepatocytes and spleen as *ferritin* (20–300 µg/L).

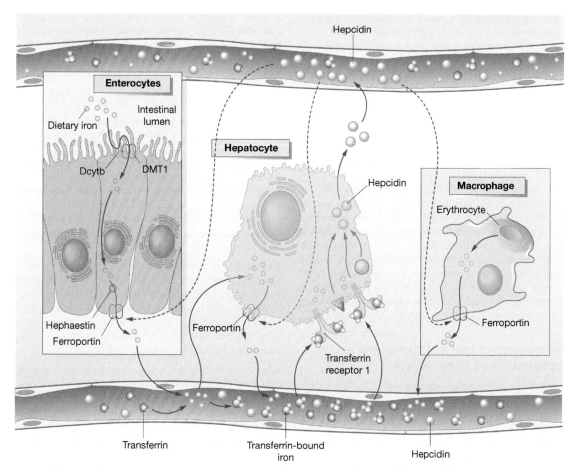

Fig. 30.1 Iron homeostasis. At the brush border, dietary iron is reduced to the ferrous state by duodenal ferric reductase (Dcytb), transported into the mucosal cell by divalent metal transporter 1 (DMT1) and released via ferroportin into the circulation facilitated by hephaestin. Most absorbed iron is delivered to erythroid precursors. Hepatocytes take up iron from the circulation either as free iron or transferrin-bound iron via transferrin receptors 1 and 2. Hepcidin secretion by hepatocytes down-regulates ferroportin-mediated release of iron from enterocytes, macrophages and hepatocytes. *(From Fleming R E, Bacon B R 2005 Orchestration of iron homeostasis. New England Journal of Medicine 352:1741–1744, with permission.)*

Iron deficiency

Case study

A 36-year-old mother of two children presents with shortness of breath on exertion, fatigue and menorrhagia. Her haemoglobin (Hb) is 64 g/L with a mean cell volume of 72 fL (normal 80–100 fL). The blood film shows hypochromic microcytic red cells. The serum ferritin is 2 µg/L (normal 20–200 µg/L). Iron-deficiency anaemia secondary to blood loss is diagnosed. Although symptomatic, she refuses blood transfusion therapy. Oral iron therapy is commenced with 200 mg ferrous sulphate (non–enteric coated) administered three times daily. She is referred to a gynaecologist for management of the menorrhagia. Iron therapy is prescribed for 3 months, or until the Hb and ferritin have normalised.

Iron deficiency is the commonest cause of anaemia worldwide. The major causes are:

- Inadequate dietary intake: young infants with inadequate intake of solids (18 months to 3 years), poverty and poor nutrition.

- Increased physiological iron requirements: increased iron demands for growth, i.e. prematurity, rapid growth in adolescence and pregnancy (especially third trimester).
- Reduced iron absorption: coeliac disease, post-gastrectomy and gluten-induced enteropathy.
- Blood loss: menstruation, menorrhagia, gastrointestinal malignancy, other causes of chronic haemorrhage (e.g. associated with salicylate and non-steroidal anti-inflammatory drugs), hookworm infection and chronic intravascular haemolysis.

The serum ferritin concentration correlates with body iron stores; serum ferritin of <15 μg/L is virtually specific for iron deficiency. As ferritin is an acute-phase reactant, a normal result does not exclude iron deficiency in the presence of infective and inflammatory conditions. In anaemia of chronic disease, a serum ferritin <50 μg/L may be associated with reduced storage iron, whereas ferritin levels of >50 μg/L generally indicate the presence of iron stores. Measurement of serum soluble transferrin receptor (increased in iron deficiency but not by inflammation) may help in differentiating iron deficiency from the anaemia of chronic disease.

Management of iron deficiency and prophylactic iron administration

Management of iron deficiency requires:

1. identification and treatment of the underlying cause, and
2. iron replacement therapy.

Oral iron preparations are the treatment of choice due to their effectiveness, safety and low cost. Iron can be administered as simple iron salts (e.g. ferrous sulphate, fumarate or gluconate) or in saccharated form (Table 30.1). Administration of 200 mg ferrous sulphate three times daily provides 180 mg elemental iron per day; up to 30% of the orally administered iron will be absorbed. The haemoglobin will increase by 1 g/dL in the first week; a rise of 2 g/dL after 3 weeks' therapy is evidence of adequate response. Daily administration for 1–3 months will correct anaemia due to iron deficiency. Therapy should be continued for a further 3 months and until the haemoglobin has normalised and iron stores replenished (i.e. serum ferritin >20 μg/L).

Liquid iron formulations can be used for small children, but they stain the teeth. Formulations include ferrous sulphate solution (5 mL contains 12 mg elemental iron), iron polymaltose solutions and polysaccharide–iron complex (5 mL contains 100 mg elemental iron). *Prophylactic oral iron* is appropriate in pregnancy, menorrhagia, following partial or complete gastrectomy, for patients with chronic renal disease receiving erythropoietin, in the early treatment of severe pernicious anaemia (rapid erythropoiesis may exhaust iron stores) and for low-birth-weight or premature infants. Lower doses of oral iron (e.g. 200 mg ferrous sulphate daily) are generally prescribed.

Sustained or slow-release iron preparations have iron bound to resins, chelates (sodium feredetate) or plastic matrices (e.g. Ferrograd, Feospan). Iron is released in the lower small intestine, and it has therefore bypassed the duodenum, the site of maximal iron absorption, before becoming available. They are therefore *relatively ineffective* sources of iron and should *not* be used to treat iron deficiency.

Adverse effects of oral iron (e.g. nausea, epigastric pain, diarrhoea and constipation) are related to the amount of available iron. These effects can generally be ameliorated by reducing the dose, using divided doses, switching to an alternative iron salt (e.g. ferrous gluconate), and/or taking the iron with food. Although these approaches reduce the amount of iron available to be absorbed, the speed of normalisation of the haemoglobin concentration is not usually critical. Sustained and slow-release iron preparations cause fewer unwanted effects, reflecting the small amount of iron absorbed. Managing the gastrointestinal disturbance is important to ensure the patient continues treatment. Failure of oral iron therapy is most commonly due to poor compliance, persistent bleeding or incorrect diagnosis. Oral iron may not be well absorbed in patients who have had a partial or complete gastrectomy or coeliac disease. Folate deficiency may be unmasked by effective iron therapy. Where there is a deficiency of both iron and folate, the latter may not be obvious until iron is administered. This is most likely in pregnancy due to high fetal requirements for both haematinics.

Parenteral iron is rarely required to treat iron deficiency and should only be administered if there is:

- proven iron deficiency and oral iron cannot be tolerated
- ongoing blood loss so severe that oral therapy is insufficient to maintain iron stores
- inadequate gastrointestinal iron absorption.

Table 30.1 Oral iron preparations			
	Tablet size (mg)	Daily dose (mg/day)	Elemental iron (mg/day)
Ferrous sulphate	200	200–600	60–180
Ferrous gluconate	300	300–1800	35–210
Ferrous fumarate	200	210–1260	68–408
Ferrous succinate	100	100–600	35–210

Parenteral iron formulations include:

- Iron dextran (ferric hydroxide complexed with dextrans, 50 mg/mL) which can be administered by deep intramuscular injection, slow intravenous injection or infusion.
- Iron sucrose (ferric hydroxide complexed with sucrose, 20 mg/mL) which is delivered by slow intravenous injection or infusion (not recommended for children).
- Ferric carboxymaltose (Ferinject) consists of an iron hydroxide carbohydrate complex (50 mg/mL of iron) and is given as an intravenous infusion over 15–30 minutes at a maximum dose of 1000 mg at a time. Patients requiring higher doses are given subsequent infusions typically at least 1 week apart. The complex enables slow, controlled systemic release of bioavailable iron to iron-binding proteins. There is little risk of release of free iron leading to few adverse side effects. It is indicated for iron-deficiency anaemia that does not respond to oral iron preparations or when these are contraindicated. The efficacy of ferric carboxymaltose in treating iron-deficiency anaemia and reducing transfusion rates has been proven in multiple trials including in patients with renal failure, congestive cardiac failure, the second and third trimester of pregnancy and perioperatively. These intravenous formulations are increasingly being used prior to major surgery (e.g. orthopaedics, gynaecology) to reduce the need for blood transfusion in the perioperative period.

The dose of parenteral iron is based on body weight and the Hb deficit, as follows:

$$\text{Dose of iron (mg)} = \{\text{Target Hb (g/dL)} - \text{Actual Hb} \\ \times \text{weight (kg)} \times 2.4\} + 500 \text{ mg}$$

The speed of haemopoietic response is no faster with parenteral therapy than with full-dose oral iron when reliably taken and normally absorbed. Parenterally administered iron is stored and utilised over months.

Adverse effects of intravenous iron include immediate, severe and potentially life-threatening anaphylactoid reactions, fever and arthropathy. Patients should therefore be closely monitored during administration, and facilities for cardiopulmonary resuscitation should be available. A history of allergic disorders including asthma, eczema and anaphylaxis is a contraindication to parenteral iron. Intramuscular iron can be painful and may permanently stain the skin.[1]

---

[1]Staining can be minimised by inserting the needle through the skin and then moving the subcutaneous tissue laterally before entering muscle, so that the needle track is disrupted when the needle is withdrawn (Z technique).

Less severe manifestations include urticaria, rashes and nausea; delayed reactions such as arthralgia, myalgia and fever can also occur. Intramuscular iron has also been associated with soft-tissue sarcomas. Oral iron preparations should not be given for 24 h prior to parenteral therapy or for 5 days after the last intravenous injection. This is to prevent adverse reactions as a result of saturation of transferrin-binding capacity leading to a high, unbound plasma iron concentration.

Drug interactions

Iron chelates a number of drugs including tetracyclines, penicillamine, methyldopa, levodopa, carbidopa, ciprofloxacin, norfloxacin and ofloxacin, thereby reducing their absorption. Iron also forms stable complexes with thyroxine, captopril and bisphosphonates. Administration of these drugs should be separated from the iron therapy by a minimum of 2 h. Ascorbic acid increases iron absorption, but its use is not clinically important in routine therapy. Antacids, tea (tannins) and bran reduce iron absorption.

Anaemia of chronic disease

> ### Case study
>
> A 54-year-old woman with active rheumatoid arthritis is noted to be anaemic (Hb 93 g/L). Apart from her swollen and painful small joints, she is asymptomatic. Her blood film shows normochromic normocytic red cells with a mild neutrophilia. Analysis of her iron status shows serum iron of 3 µmol/L (normal = 14–32 µmol/L), transferrin 1.5 g/L (normal = 2.0–3.6 g/L) and ferritin 250 µg/L (normal = 20–200 µg/L). A diagnosis of anaemia of chronic disease is made. As she is asymptomatic from the anaemia, transfusions are not required and iron therapy is not indicated.

Anaemia of chronic disease occurs in response to chronic infective or inflammatory processes and malignancies and must be distinguished from iron deficiency. Increased hepcidin expression reduces intestinal iron absorption and increases iron stored in macrophages and hepatocytes. Serum iron is therefore reduced and ferritin normal or increased. The aim of therapy is to treat the underlying disorder, which generally is the cause of the patient's symptoms and not the anaemia *per se*. If the anaemia is sufficiently severe to impair quality of life, red cell transfusions may be indicated. Erythropoiesis-stimulating agents (ESAs) generally do not give significant improvement in quality of life and can increase the risk of venous thromboembolic disease and mortality, especially in patients with malignant disease. Iron should not be given to patients with the anaemia of chronic disease as the abnormality is impaired iron utilisation and not iron deficiency.

Functional iron deficiency

Functional iron deficiency occurs when the iron demands of developing erythroblasts exceed the body's ability to deliver iron to the marrow. In the anaemia of chronic renal disease, for example, this impairment of iron delivery can limit the haemoglobin response to ESA therapy. This can be overcome with regular low-dose intravenous iron administration (e.g. 100 mg iron sucrose monthly). The serum ferritin should be monitored to ensure it does not exceed 500–1000 µg/L.

Chronic iron overload

Severe tissue iron overload can result from excessive absorption (hereditary haemochromatosis), frequent or chronic red cell transfusion therapy (>100 units as in thalassaemia or myelodysplasia[2]) leading to transfusion haemosiderosis and excessive parenteral iron therapy. Iron chelation is required to prevent irreversible end-organ (e.g. heart, liver) damage. In haemochromatosis, iron is removed by weekly venesection (450 mL blood eliminates 200–250 mg iron) until the ferritin has normalised and thereafter, as required, to maintain the ferritin at <50 µg/L.

Iron chelation therapy has been available since the 1970s and is used when venesection is contraindicated, most commonly for transfusion haemosiderosis. This is particularly for patients who are transfusion-dependent from infancy (e.g. thalassaemia major). In thalassaemia, iron chelation therapy is generally commenced after 1 year of monthly blood transfusions. In older transfusion-dependent patients with refractory anaemia (e.g. myelodysplasia), iron chelation is commenced after 20 transfusions or when the serum ferritin level is two to three times the upper limit of normal. Both parenteral and oral iron chelators are available.

Parenteral iron chelator. Desferrioxamine is administered by subcutaneous injection or intravenously (30–50 mg/kg/day) over an 8–12 h period, 5–7 nights per week. It has a half-life of 6 h. Compliance with therapy is a problem because of the slow parenteral administration. Desferrioxamine complexes with ferric iron to form ferrioxamine, which is excreted in urine and in bile. Simultaneous administration of ascorbic acid should be avoided; although ascorbic acid increases the availability of free iron for chelation, it also mobilises iron from reticuloendothelial storage sites to a potentially toxic pool in parenchymal cells. Serious *adverse effects* of desferrioxamine are uncommon but do include anaphylactic reactions. Rapid infusion can result in hypotension, shock or urticaria. There is danger of potentially fatal adult respiratory distress syndrome if infusion proceeds beyond 24 h.[3] Chronic use can result in hearing and visual disturbances (cataract and retinal damage).

Oral iron chelators. Orally absorbed iron chelators have become available in the past decade and give improved compliance and quality of life for those who require lifelong iron chelation. The two major products available are:

Deferiprone (3-hydroxy-1,2-dimethylpyridin-4-one). Deferiprone is an oral iron chelator that binds iron in a 3:1 molar ratio. It is administered 25 mg/kg three times daily. It can prevent iron accumulation but not necessarily protect against iron-induced organ damage. Deferiprone is absorbed in the upper gastrointestinal tract and is mainly excreted via the kidneys; the elimination half-life is 2–3 h. It is less effective than desferrioxamine and carries a risk of arthropathy, neutropenia and agranulocytosis. It is, however, a useful alternative for patients who are unwilling or unable to tolerate desferrioxamine. Combination therapy of deferiprone with desferrioxamine is effective in the management of cardiac siderosis.

Deferasirox. This is a tridentate oral iron chelator that mobilises stored iron by binding selectively to ferric iron. It provides 24-h chelation with a once-daily dose (20–30 mg/kg/day). It is effective in removing cellular (i.e. cardiac and hepatic) and serum iron, which it excretes in the faeces. Side-effects include gastrointestinal disturbances, skin rash, cytopenias and increased creatinine.

Iron poisoning and acute overdose

Iron poisoning is commonest in children. It is usually accidental and particularly dangerous. The phases in acute oral iron poisoning are shown in Box 30.1. Ferrous sulphate is the most toxic, whilst sustained-release iron preparations and multivitamins cause less severe poisoning. Poisoning is severe if the plasma iron concentration exceeds the total iron-binding capacity (upper limit 75 mmol/L) or plasma becomes pink due to the formation of ferrioxamine. Treatment is urgent and involves chelating iron in plasma. As an immediate measure, raw egg and milk help bind iron in the stomach. Iron chelation therapy is required for severe toxicity. Desferrioxamine is administered by intravenous

---

[2] A 26-year-old subject with β-thalassaemia major had been transfused with 404 units of blood over his lifetime. His iron stores were so high (estimated at above 100 g) that he triggered a metal detector at an airport security checkpoint Jim RT. Lancet. 1979. Nov 10;2(8150):1028.

[3] Tenenbein M, Kowalski S, Sienko A et al 1992 Pulmonary toxic effects of continuous desferrioxamine administration in acute iron poisoning. Lancet 339:699–701.

Box 30.1 **Acute iron poisoning**

Phase 1

0.5–1 h after ingestion: Abdominal pain, grey-black vomit, diarrhoea, leucocytosis and hyperglycaemia. Severe cases have acidosis and cardiovascular collapse which may proceed to coma and death.

Phase 2

Improvement occurs, lasting 6–12 h; may be sustained or may deteriorate to next phase.

Phase 3

Jaundice, hypoglycaemia, bleeding, encephalopathy, metabolic acidosis and convulsions are followed by cardiovascular collapse, coma and sometimes death 48–60 h after ingestion. Severe brain and liver damage is seen at autopsy.

Phase 4

1–2 months later: scarring and stricture may cause upper gastrointestinal obstruction.

infusion (not exceeding 15 mg/kg/h and maximum 80 mg/kg in 24 h) to chelate serum free iron.

Vitamin B$_{12}$

The cobalamins are a family of compounds (cyano-, hydroxyo-, methyl- and adenosylcobalamin) that have vitamin B$_{12}$ activity. They have the same basic structure with cobalt within a central corrin ring. Vitamin B$_{12}$ is produced only by microorganisms, and humans obtain it by ingesting foods of animal origin. Vitamin B$_{12}$ is required by all cells for DNA synthesis; it is also required for red cell production, methylation and myelin synthesis. A normal diet contains 5–30 µg/day of vitamin B$_{12}$ of which 1–3 µg is absorbed. Ingested vitamin B$_{12}$ binds to intrinsic factor (IF) synthesised by gastric parietal cells. The cobalamin–IF complex passes to the terminal ileum, where it is absorbed. Newly absorbed vitamin B$_{12}$ binds to transcobalamin to form holotranscobalamin (20–30% of plasma vitamin B$_{12}$); this is the biologically active form which is available for delivery to cells. Most vitamin B$_{12}$ (70%) in the blood is bound to haptocorrin (holohaptocorrin, formerly transcobalamin I) which is taken up by and stored in the liver. The liver stores up to 2–5 mg of vitamin B$_{12}$, which is sufficient for several years after absorption ceases. Cobalamin is not metabolised significantly and passes into bile and urine.

Vitamin B$_{12}$ deficiency

The causes of vitamin B$_{12}$ deficiency are listed in Table 30.2. The most common are:

- Inadequate dietary intake: the elderly and vegans.
- Pernicious anaemia. Autoimmune destruction of gastric parietal cells produces atrophic gastric mucosa and reduced secretion of intrinsic factor. Vitamin B$_{12}$ deficiency results from failure to absorb cobalamin in the terminal ileum.
- Malabsorption syndromes. Intestinal disease affecting the terminal ileum can interrupt the normal enterohepatic circulation of vitamin B$_{12}$ and result in vitamin B$_{12}$ deficiency. Malabsorption can also result from poor release of vitamin B$_{12}$ from food as a consequence of impaired secretion of acid and pepsin by the stomach.
- Drugs. A number of drugs can reduce vitamin B$_{12}$ absorption, including metformin, aminosalicylic acid, nicotine, phenytoin and large doses of vitamin C.

Vitamin B$_{12}$ deficiency can result in:

- subclinical disease: mild anaemia without clinical symptoms or signs
- megaloblastic anaemia (macrocytic anaemia with oval macrocytes and hypersegmented neutrophils)
- subacute combined degeneration of the brain, spinal cord and peripheral nerves
- abnormalities of epithelial tissue, particularly the alimentary tract, e.g. sore tongue and malabsorption.

Cobalamin deficiency is generally diagnosed by measuring plasma vitamin B$_{12}$ (normal 150–900 pmol/L). Most assays measure total serum B$_{12}$ levels, i.e. both the inactive and active forms. Deficiency of vitamin B$_{12}$ may be 'falsely' diagnosed when haptocorrin levels are low (e.g. during pregnancy or in patients with inherited haptocorrin deficiency) despite adequate levels of active vitamin B$_{12}$. Conversely, in some haematological malignancies the haptocorrin and serum cobalamin levels may be normal or high despite low active vitamin B$_{12}$. In vitamin B$_{12}$ deficiency, levels of methylmalonic acid (MMA) and homocysteine are both elevated. Despite their utility in assessing vitamin B$_{12}$, they are rarely measured: MMA is relatively specific for vitamin B$_{12}$ deficiency, but the test is expensive and difficult to perform. Elevated homocysteine has many causes and therefore lacks specificity for vitamin B$_{12}$ deficiency. Assessment of holotranscobalamin (HoloTC) is another approach, as this measures the 'active' portion of serum vitamin B$_{12}$. HoloTC has high sensitivity and specificity for clinically significant cobalamin deficiency and is not affected by pregnancy or haematological malignancies. 'Reflexive' HoloTC testing can be used when serum cobalamin assay measurements are borderline. In vitamin B$_{12}$ deficiency, serum folate

Table 30.2 Causes of vitamin B$_{12}$ and folate deficiency

Deficiency	Cause	Abnormality
Vitamin B$_{12}$	Inadequate dietary intake	Veganism Breast-fed infants of vegan mothers
	Reduced vitamin B$_{12}$ absorption	Pernicious anaemia Achlorhydria Gastrectomy Gastric bypass surgery Ileal disease Malabsorption syndromes Stagnant loop syndrome Tropical sprue
	Drugs	Nitrous oxide (prolonged exposure) Metformin Antacids Aminosalicylic acid Nicotine Phenytoin Zidovudine
	Congenital defects	Transcobalamin deficiency Enzyme defects
Folate	Inadequate dietary intake	Poor diet: elderly, malnourished, poverty, alcoholics Psychiatrically disturbed patients Infants fed solely on goats' milk
	Malabsorption syndromes	Gluten-sensitive enteropathy Tropical sprue Salazopyrine therapy Partial gastrectomy Jejunal resection
	Increased folate requirements	Pregnancy Prematurity Chronic haemolytic anaemia Psoriasis Exfoliative dermatitis Crohn's disease Dialysis
	Anti-folate drugs	Long-term antiepileptic use (phenytoin, primidone and phenobarbital) Methotrexate Trimethoprim Pyrimethamine

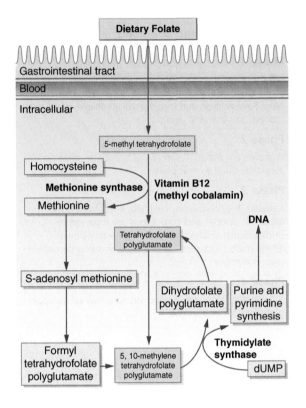

Fig. 30.2 Schematic diagram showing the link between vitamin B$_{12}$ and folate metabolism.

may be elevated and red cell folate reduced due to disturbance of normal absorption and metabolism (Fig. 30.2).

Management of vitamin B$_{12}$ deficiency and prophylactic administration

Vitamin B$_{12}$ administration is indicated for the prevention and treatment of deficiency. *Hydroxocobalamin* is the preferred form of vitamin B$_{12}$ for clinical use. In vitamin B$_{12}$ deficiency, hydroxocobalamin should be given at a dose of 1 mg i.m. three times per week for 2 weeks (6 doses) to replenish body vitamin B$_{12}$ stores. Maintenance therapy (1 mg every 3 months) is required if the underlying cause cannot be corrected, such as in pernicious anaemia, which requires lifelong vitamin B$_{12}$ therapy. After commencing therapy, there is rapid clinical improvement, there is a blood reticulocyte peak at 5–7 days, and the haemoglobin, red cell count and haematocrit rise after 1 week. The blood indices normalise within 2 months. Failure to respond implies an incorrect or incomplete diagnosis (e.g. additional haematinic deficiency). Stimulation of erythropoiesis may deplete iron and folate stores, and these may require supplementation. Hypokalaemia may occur at the height of the erythrocyte response in severe cases due to uptake of potassium by the rapidly increasing erythrocyte mass. Oral potassium should be considered prior to initiating therapy with low or borderline plasma potassium levels. Reversal of neurological damage is slow, rarely marked, and inversely related to the extent and duration of neuropathy. Adverse effects are extremely rare. Both vitamin B_{12} and folic acid should be administered in megaloblastic anaemia while plasma levels are awaited. *Prophylactic vitamin B_{12}* (e.g. for vegans) should be administered at a dose of 1 mg every 3 months.

Contraindications to cobalamin

Vitamin B_{12} should not be administered for undiagnosed anaemia. Proper haematological and biochemical workup is essential in determining the cause prior to commencement of therapy. Even a single dose of vitamin B_{12} can interfere with the haematological picture for weeks and result in a delay in diagnosis and instigation of the correct therapy.

Folic acid (pteroylglutamic acid)

Folic acid[4] is one of the B group vitamins and is widely distributed, particularly in green vegetables, fruits, yeast and liver. A normal adult diet contains approximately 400 μg of folic acid (one-third in monoglutamate and two-thirds polyglutamate form), and 100–200 μg is absorbed. Daily requirements are 50–100 μg. Folate polyglutamate is deconjugated to the monoglutamate form prior to absorption in the proximal jejunum. Within the plasma, folate is present mainly as 5-methyl tetrahydrofolate. This enters the cell and is demethylated to tetrahydrofolate, a process that requires vitamin B_{12} (see Fig. 30.2). Total folate content of the body is 6–10 mg, stores which will last for only 3–4 months on a folate-deficient diet. Folate is required for amino acid and DNA synthesis and cell division. Folate is present in both the serum and red blood cell, and assays are available to assess both. Serum folate assays are cheap, automated and available in most clinical laboratories; however, the levels can fluctuate significantly with recent dietary intake and do not reflect long-term folate status. Red cell folate gives a more accurate assessment of body folate status but is a more complex assay and prone to analytical variables.

---

[4]Latin: *folium*, a leaf.

Folic acid deficiency

Deficiency of folic acid causes megaloblastic anaemia as a result of impaired production of purines and pyrimidines, essential for DNA synthesis. The haematological features are indistinguishable from vitamin B_{12} deficiency. It is critical to determine which of these haematinics is deficient, as incorrect therapy can have severe ramifications; specifically, folic acid supplements may accelerate progression of subacute combined degeneration of the spinal cord due to vitamin B_{12} deficiency.

> ### Case study
>
> A 26-year-old woman has a routine blood count performed in the third trimester of pregnancy. She is noted to be anaemic with Hb 53 g/L, mean cell volume 102 fL (normal 80–100 fL) and have mild leucopenia (3.2 × 10⁹/L) and thrombocytopenia (87 × 10⁹/L). The blood film shows oval macrocytes, megaloblastic nucleated red blood cells and hypersegmented neutrophils. Biochemical analyses show serum folate 2.2 μg/L (normal = 3–16 μg/L), red cell folate 80 μg/L (normal >250 μg/L), vitamin B_{12} 350 pmol/L (normal = 150–900 pmol/L), mild hyperbilirubinaemia and a normal ferritin. A full dietary history shows the patient has a poor diet containing minimal folic acid. The patient is treated with oral folic acid (5 mg/day until the red cell folate has normalised) and given dietary advice.

The most common *causes* of folic acid deficiency are those listed in Table 30.2.

Specific clinical settings in which folate deficiency can occur deserve mention. In *pregnancy*, daily folate requirements increase to 400 μg/day in the third trimester to meet the demands of the developing fetus and placenta. This increase is commonly not met by a normal Western diet. The problem is even greater in developing countries where nutritional deficiency may be aggravated by increased requirements due to haemoglobinopathies and endemic malaria. *Premature neonates* require folate supplementation because they lack the buildup of folate stores that normally occurs in the last weeks of pregnancy and hence are commonly deficient. In *chronic haemolytic anaemia* (e.g. autoimmune haemolytic anaemia; sickle cell anaemia; hereditary spherocytosis), the compensatory increased bone marrow erythroid activity results in increased folate demand. *Renal dialysis* removes folate, and therefore chronic haemodialysis or peritoneal dialysis can result in folate depletion. A number of *drugs* interfere with folate absorption, inhibit the activity of folate-dependent enzymes or displace folate from transport proteins. Dihydrofolate reductase is inhibited by methotrexate, trimethoprim and pyrimethamine. The antidote to these drugs is folinic acid (5-methyl tetrahydrofolate).

Management of folic acid deficiency and prophylactic administration

Large doses of synthetic folic acid (5 mg/day p.o. for 4 months) are used to treat folate deficiency irrespective of the cause; up to 15 mg may be required if there is malabsorption. Long-term use may be required if the underlying condition cannot be controlled and/or folate deficiency is likely to recur (e.g. sickle cell disease). It is critical that vitamin B_{12} deficiency be excluded and treated prior to commencement of folic acid therapy. If not, cobalamin neuropathy may develop. *Adverse reactions* are rare; allergy occurs, and status epilepticus may be precipitated. There is no advantage in giving folinic acid instead of folic acid, except in the treatment of the toxic effects of folic acid antagonists such as methotrexate.

In many countries, foods such as flour are fortified to prevent neural tube defects. Assessment of folate status before conception should be considered and folate supplementation (400 μg/day orally) given if required. In women hoping to conceive who have had a previous neural tube defect fetus, 5 mg/day of folate is recommended.[5,6] Prophylactic folic acid (200–500 μg daily) should be taken throughout pregnancy; this is generally administered together with prophylactic iron.

Haemolytic anaemia

Haemolytic anaemia occurs where red cells survive less than 120 days and there is an inadequate bone marrow erythropoietic response. Acquired haemolytic anaemia may be due to immune (autoimmune, alloimmune or drug-induced) or non-immune (e.g. secondary to infection, mechanical trauma, drugs) causes. Inherited haemolytic anaemias may be due to defects of the red cell membrane (e.g. hereditary spherocytosis), abnormalities of red cell metabolism (e.g. glucose 6-phosphate dehydrogenase deficiency or pyruvate kinase deficiency) or defective globin chains (i.e. haemoglobinopathies). Management is determined by the underlying mechanism. In general, iron should not be given in haemolytic anaemia since iron from lysed cells is

recirculated; moreover, in chronic haemolysis there is increased iron absorption and iron supplementation can result in haemosiderosis. Iron may be required in chronic intravascular haemolysis as haemoglobinuria may result in iron deficiency. Folate supplementation is commonly required with chronic haemolysis as the compensatory erythroid hyperplasia results in increased folic acid utilisation. Some of the more common types of haemolytic anaemia are described.

Autoimmune haemolytic anaemia

Autoimmune haemolytic anaemia (AIHA) occurs as a result of autoantibodies causing premature red cell destruction. AIHA may be idiopathic or secondary to malignancy (especially lymphoid neoplasms), drugs, infection and connective tissue diseases. The autoantibodies are described as 'warm' or 'cold', based on their thermal range of activity. Warm AIHA is caused by IgG antibodies and results in extravascular haemolysis by Fc receptor–mediated immune clearance; it is characterised by spherocytes on the blood film. Corticosteroids are used (typically prednisone 1–1.5 mg/kg/day) to reduce antibody production, suppress red cell clearance and down-regulate Fc receptors; the median time to response is 7–10 days. When there is evidence of a haematological response, the corticosteroid dose is gradually reduced to minimise complications of long-term use. A lack of response by 3 weeks prompts alternative therapy, such as high-dose intravenous γ-globulin, other immunosuppressive therapies (e.g. vinca alkaloids, azathioprine and cyclophosphamide), danazol or rituximab (CD20 monoclonal antibody). Corticosteroids and alkylating agents are usually ineffective in cold AIHA. In both warm and cold AIHA, folate supplementation is commonly required (5 mg/day) to compensate for the demands from increased erythropoiesis.

Drug-induced haemolytic anaemia

Case study

A 32-year-old woman presented with severe lethargy and jaundice 10 days following caesarean section. She had received 1 g cefotetan as antibiotic prophylaxis prior to surgery. On presentation, her Hb was 5.2 g/dL, she had spherocytes on her blood film, an unconjugated hyperbilirubinaemia, elevated lactate dehydrogenase and a positive direct antiglobulin test (IgG) with drug-associated antibodies. A diagnosis of life-threatening cephalosporin-induced haemolytic anaemia was made. Due to the severity of her anaemia, she required red cell transfusion support. Folic acid (5 mg/day for 2 weeks) was administered. She made a spontaneous recovery.

[5]Hernández-Díaz S et al 1991 Prevention of neural tube defects: results of the Medical Research Council Vitamin study: MRC Vitamin Study Research Group Lancet 338:131–137.
[6]A supplement of folic acid 5 mg/day is proposed for fuller risk reduction (Wald N J, Law M R, Morris J K, Walk D S 2001 Quantifying the effect of folic acid. Lancet 358:2069–2073).

Many drugs can cause increased red cell destruction by immune or non-immune mechanisms (Table 30.3). Drug-induced immune-mediated haemolytic anaemia is most commonly secondary to penicillins, second- and third-generation cephalosporins (in particular cefotetan and ceftriaxone), quinine, quinidine and α-methyldopa. Other drugs and toxins can cause direct damage to the red cell membrane (e.g. copper, mitomycin C) or induce oxidative haemolysis (e.g. sulfonamides, dapsone). Drug withdrawal is usually sufficient but, if severe, red cell transfusions may be required.

Table 30.3 Some drugs and chemicals that can cause haemolytic anaemia

Mechanism	Drug, chemical or toxin
Immune-mediated haemolytic anaemia	Cephalosporins Chlorpropamide Diclofenac Hydralazine Ibuprofen α-Interferon Isoniazid Mefenamic acid α-Methyldopa Penicillins Probenicid Procainamide Quinine Quinidine Sulfonamides Tetracyclines
Oxidative haemolytic anaemia	Aminosalicylic acid Dapsone Methylthioninium chloride (methylene blue) Nitrofurantoin Sulfonamides (e.g. sulfasalazine) Primaquine Pyridium (phenazopyridine)
Direct red cell membrane damage	Amphotericin Arsine Chlorate Cisplatin Ciclosporin Lead Mitomycin C

Glucose-6-phosphate dehydrogenase deficiency

Case study

An 18-year-old male presented to a hospital emergency department febrile, dyspnoeic and jaundiced after eating a meal which included fava beans. He was anaemic with an Hb of 87 g/L, and the blood film showed 'bite' cells.*
A methyl violet stain for Heinz bodies was positive. Bilirubin and lactate dehydrogenase were elevated, and his G6PD was reduced (20% activity). A diagnosis of G6PD deficiency was made and classified as a 'mild deficiency'. He was managed conservatively and did not require a transfusion. He was advised to avoid foods (broad beans) and drugs (i.e. primaquine, sulfonamides) that cause oxidative haemolysis, and to present early for medical attention at times of infections.

*The profile of some red cells carries a concave defect (like a bite), an appearance that is indicative of haemolytic anaemia.

Glucose-6-phosphate dehydrogenase (G6PD) deficiency is an X-linked inherited enzyme defect that causes haemolytic anaemia following an acute febrile illness, hypoxia or intake of drugs, foods or other substances that cause oxidation of haemoglobin (Table 30.4). Diagnosis is made on a blood

Table 30.4 Drugs and substances that can cause oxidative haemolysis in G6PD deficiency

Drug type	Drug name
Analgesics	Pyridium (phenazopyridine)
Anti-bacterials	Dapsone Nitrofurantoin
Anti-malarials	Primaquine Pamaquine Pentaquine
Sulphonamides and sulphones	Sulphamethoxazole (including co-trimoxazole) Sulphasalazine Sulphacetamide Sulphanilamide Dapsone
Others	Ascorbic acid Flutemide Methylthioninium chloride (methylene blue) Naphthalene Rasburicase

film which shows 'bite' cells, resulting from splenic removal of oxidised haemoglobin, a positive Heinz body test and a G6PD enzyme assay. Treatment is supportive and includes avoidance of drugs and foods (e.g. fava beans) with oxidant potential.

Haemoglobinopathies

Sickle cell anaemia

In sickle cell disease, deoxygenated haemoglobin S (HbS) forms polymers resulting in erythrocytes becoming inflexible 'sickle-shaped' forms. Sickle red cells can obstruct blood flow and cause the clinical features of sickle cell disease, principally haemolytic anaemia, acute chest syndrome and painful crises. *Hydroxycarbamide* (hydroxyurea) can be used in sickle cell disease to increase the HbF levels in maturing erythrocytes, decrease HbS polymerisation and erythrocyte sickling, and reduce the frequency and severity of sickling complications. It also increases nitric oxide (promoting vasodilatation), causes a fall in leucocyte count and improves red cellular hydration, all of which result in a reduction in vaso-occlusive events.[7] The indications for initiating hydroxy-carbamide include frequent acute painful crises and acute chest syndrome. Beneficial effects of hydroxycarbamide have been seen in adults, children and infants, with a reduction in hospital admissions, pain, acute chest syndrome, blood transfusions and mortality. Neurological complications, e.g. stroke, may not be reduced. Long-term daily administration of hydroxycarbamide raises HbF levels to 15–20% (normally <1% in adults). Hydroxycarbamide is relatively non-toxic, its myelosuppressive effects are reversible and the long-term risk of leukaemogenesis is negligible. There is no adverse effect on growth or development in children, and it does not appear to increase the risk of malignancy.

Thalassaemia

Thalassaemias[8] vary in their severity from clinically silent to transfusion-dependent, with many being of intermediate severity. Severely affected *thalassaemia major* patients are likely to require regular red blood cell transfusions and iron chelation therapy (see p. 532). Iron chelation is usually started after 1 year of monthly blood transfusions. Patients are monitored regularly to assess growth, endocrine and

cardiac function, iron status (serum ferritin, MRI for liver iron concentration) and adverse effects related to therapy. Patients with less severe thalassaemia *(thalassaemia intermedia)* generally only require intermittent transfusions; the need for iron chelation therapy is based on iron load (ferritin). Hydroxycarbamide can be used in these patients, in the same manner as for sickle cell disease, to increase HbF and total haemoglobin levels. Individuals with *thalassaemia minor* (i.e. carriers) are typically asymptomatic and do not require therapy.

Aplastic anaemia

Case study

A 21-year-old female presented with bruising and shortness of breath. Blood tests showed pancytopenia with Hb 71 g/L, neutrophils 0.2×10^9/L and platelets 10 $\times 10^9$/L. A bone marrow examination was performed to establish the cause. This showed the marrow to be markedly hypoplastic with a reduction in all haemopoietic elements, and aplastic anaemia was diagnosed. The patient was treated with anti-thymocyte globulin, ciclosporin and prednisolone but failed to respond necessitating ongoing requirements for blood products. Treatment was commenced with the thrombopoietin receptor agonist eltrombopag in addition to the ciclosporin. This led to a haematological response with normalisation of the haemoglobin and platelet count and increase in the neutrophils to 1.5×10^9/L. The patient was referred for workup for allogeneic stem cell transplantation.

Aplastic anaemia may be idiopathic or secondary to chemicals (e.g. benzene), drugs or infection. Treatment is determined by the severity of the cytopenias, patient age, availability of a marrow donor, and, less commonly, the cause. Therapeutic choice is between immunosuppression and allogeneic bone marrow transplantation. The latter carries survival rates of 75–80%, but chronic graft-versus-host disease causes continued morbidity. Good supportive treatment is important (i.e. antibiotics and transfusions). Patients who are not candidates for transplantation due to age or lack of a donor (up to 70% of patients) receive immunosuppression. Anti-thymocyte globulin (ATG) induces haematological responses, transfusion independence and freedom from infection in 70% of patients. Addition of ciclosporin (5 mg/kg/day) to ATG improves the speed of response, with survival rates in responders up to 90%. Treatment should be initiated within 14 days of diagnosis, and responses generally occur within 4 months. Adverse effects of ATG

---

[7]Steinberg M H, Barton F, Castro O et al 2003 Effect of hydroxyurea on mortality and morbidity in adult sickle cell anaemia: risks and benefits up to 9 years of treatment. Journal of the American Medical Association 289:1645–1651.

[8]The genetic defect results in reduced rate of synthesis or absent synthesis of one of the globin chains that make up haemoglobin.

include fever, rigors and lethargy, and these are common in the first 2 days of treatment. Approximately 7–10 days post-infusion serum sickness, with rash, joint pain and fever may occur; this can be modified by giving prednisolone (1 mg/kg/day). Anaphylaxis and exacerbation of the cytopenias are rare adverse effects. Relapse occurs in 35% within 5 years, but relapsed patients may respond to further immunosuppression (rabbit anti-lymphocyte globulin after initial ATG). In refractory patients, novel therapies such as the thrombopoietin receptor agonist eltrombopag may be considered (see below). Supportive care with haemopoietic growth factors, granulocyte colony-stimulating factor (G-CSF: 5–10 mg/kg s.c.) and ESAs can improve the neutrophil count and haemoglobin, respectively.

Polycythaemia vera

Polycythaemia vera (PV) is a myeloproliferative neoplasm where there is uncontrolled over-production of erythrocytes in the bone marrow. The clinical manifestations include arterial (especially coronary and cerebral) and venous vascular events, splenic pain, pruritus, gout and constitutional symptoms such as fatigue. PV may progress to myelofibrosis or undergo leukaemic transformation to acute myeloid leukaemia (AML). The aims of treatment are to reduce the risk of thrombosis and haemorrhage, minimise the risk of transformation to myelofibrosis and AML and manage complications.

Management of PV

Venesection of 300–500 mL venous blood is performed once or twice weekly to achieve a haematocrit of less than 0.45, and thereafter every 3–6 months to maintain the haematocrit at this level. Iron deficiency may occur and requires cautious treatment. Low-dose aspirin (100 mg/day) reduces thrombotic complications. Cytoreductive therapy should be considered when venesection is poorly tolerated or there is symptomatic or progressive splenomegaly, thrombocytosis or the presence of symptoms that may indicate disease progression (e.g. night sweats; weight loss). Optimal therapy is determined by the patient's age and the adverse effects of each drug.

Hydroxycarbamide (hydroxyurea) is the most commonly used drug in PV and is given orally. It inhibits ribonucleotide reductase, an enzyme which has a rate-limiting role in the regulation of DNA synthesis. Hydroxycarbamide (1–2 g/daily) inhibits myeloproliferation, normalises the platelet count and spleen size, reduces venesection requirements, reduces the incidence of thrombosis and ameliorates hypercatabolic symptoms. It is generally good at controlling PV but requires continuous use. Hydroxycarbamide is first-line therapy for patients older than 40 years of age. Its use

should be limited in younger patients due to the (low) risk of leukaemogenesis. Complications are leucopenia and thrombocytopenia.

Interferon-α (IFN-α) is first-line therapy for PV in patients younger than 40 years of age and second-line for patients 40–75 years of age. IFN-α suppresses the proliferation of haemopoietic progenitor cells in the marrow. It is effective in controlling the platelet count, haematocrit, splenomegaly and constitutional symptoms in PV and is not leukaemogenic; it may be used in pregnant women. Treatment is continuous at doses of 3–5 mU three times per week by subcutaneous injection. Unwanted effects include flulike symptoms, fatigue and depression.

Anagrelide, a prostaglandin synthetase inhibitor, inhibits cyclic nucleotide phosphodiesterase and the release of arachidonic acid from phospholipase. It is second-line therapy for patients up to 75 years of age. Anagrelide lowers the platelet count by inhibiting megakaryocyte differentiation; it can control the thrombocytosis of venesection and can be used in combination with hydroxycarbamide. It is orally active, and the usual dose is 1–2 mg daily. Adverse effects are related to its vasodilatory properties and include headache, palpitations and fluid retention.

JAK2 inhibitors are widely used in myeloproliferative neoplasms, including PV. Mutations of JAK2, an intracellular signalling molecule coupled with cell surface growth factor receptors including the erythropoietin receptor and thrombopoietin receptor, are present in more than 95% of patients with PV. Oral JAK1/JAK2 inhibitors (e.g. ruxolitinib) can be used for PV patients with splenomegaly who are venesection dependent and is well tolerated. Among the most common adverse effects are low-grade anaemia and thrombocytopenia. Abrupt cessation of the drug can induce rapid rebound splenomegaly and a systemic inflammatory response; therefore weaning doses are recommended. Longer-term data are needed to assess the risk of secondary malignancies.

Other drugs are available for PV but are only used in specific clinical situations. *Busulfan* is an alkylating agent that reduces vascular events and delays myelofibrosis in PV. Due to its mutagenic potential, its use is restricted to older patients or when other treatments are poorly tolerated. *Pipobroman* is a bromide derivative of piperazine, which inhibits DNA and RNA polymerase and reduces the incorporation of pyrimidine nucleotides into DNA. It is effective in long-term control of PV and has low leukaemogenic potential. *Radioactive phosphorus* (^{32}P) is concentrated in bone and rapidly dividing cells; consequently, erythroid precursors receive most of the β-irradiation. ^{32}P can be used intermittently and is good at controlling PV. It increases the rate of leukaemic transformation, and therefore its use is restricted to elderly patients.

Therapy of other clinical features of PV: Pruritus generally improves with reduction in the haematocrit. In some cases paroxetine and antihistamines (H_1- and/or H_2-histamine receptor blockade) may be required. Hyperuricaemia, due to cell destruction, is corrected with allopurinol.

Haemopoietic growth factors

Haemopoietic growth factors, such as ESAs and granulocyte colony-stimulating factor (G-CSF), are produced by recombinant DNA technology. These can be administered to stimulate erythroid and myeloid lineages in the bone marrow and are potentially useful for secondary anaemias (e.g. chronic renal failure) and neutropenia due to disease or chemotherapy.[9]

Erythropoiesis-stimulating agents

Erythropoietin (EPO), a glycoprotein hormone encoded by a gene on chromosome 7 (7q), controls and regulates erythropoiesis. The kidneys produce 90% and the liver the majority of the remainder. EPO binds to receptors on erythrocyte progenitors in the bone marrow and stimulates their proliferation, differentiation and survival. Normal EPO production increases with hypoxia and decreases with polycythaemia. The anaemia of chronic renal failure is largely due to failure of erythropoietin production.

Therapeutic EPO agents are classified as ESAs. Recombinant human erythropoietin (epoetin) can be given subcutaneously or intravenously and has a $t_{1/2}$ of 4 h. The dose and frequency of administration is dependent on the indication and response. For optimal erythropoietic response, there must be adequate iron and folate stores (as above). The maximum reticulocyte response is seen at 4 days. Epoetin-α and -β are two recombinant forms of EPO available for the treatment of EPO-responsive anaemia, and these have equal clinical efficacy. Darbepoetin is a hyperglycosylated EPO derivative with a longer $t_{1/2}$ than epoetin. This allows less frequent administration, e.g. once weekly or even less frequently, for anaemia of renal failure and chemotherapy. There is no clinically significant difference between darbepoetin and epoetin in haemoglobin response, transfusion reduction or thromboembolic events.

Clinical uses of ESAs

Anaemia of chronic renal failure. EPO is effective (50–150 units/kg) in chronic renal failure patients with symptoms attributable to anaemia and a Hb <110 g/L. The aim of EPO therapy is to restore the haemoglobin to 110–120 g/L. Higher target Hb levels ($\geq$130 g/L) are reported to result in risk of stroke, serious cardiovascular events and death. Even partial correction of renal failure–induced anaemia improves physiological and clinical status, enhances quality of life, increases survival and can result in transfusion independence. It is critical that plentiful iron is available, and the serum ferritin should be maintained at >200 µg/L. Intravenous iron may be required to optimise iron stores prior to EPO administration. In patients with renal failure, a dose-dependent increase in arterial blood pressure follows the rise in red cell mass, and encephalopathy may occur in some hypertensive patients. Arteriovenous shunts of dialysis patients, especially those that are compromised, may thrombose because of increased blood viscosity.

Anaemia due to cancer chemotherapy. ESAs have been used in the management of chemotherapy-induced anaemia (Hb <100 g/L).[10] ESA administration can reduce the need for red cell transfusions, improve quality of life and reduce symptoms related to anaemia. There is clinical trial evidence that ESA administration increases tumour progression, tumour recurrence, serious cardiac and thrombotic events and death. These serious safety concerns have restricted the use of ESA in oncology.

Other clinical uses of EPO. In symptomatic chronic heart failure with mild anaemia (Hb <100 g/L), ESA treatment can reduce symptoms, and improve the anaemia and exercise tolerance. Epoetin has also been effective for anaemia of prematurity, rheumatoid arthritis myelodysplasia and HIV patients treated with zidovudine. In all of these settings, higher doses of epoetin are required than in renal failure. EPO may be administered to reduce the need for blood transfusion in elective non-cardiac, non-vascular surgery, and can be considered before surgery for patients who decline blood transfusion.

Adverse effects of ESA. Venous thromboembolism is a well-recognised risk. Transient influenza-like symptoms may accompany initial intravenous injections of ESA. Pure red cell aplasia due to development of antibodies may occur after epoetin-α. As increased erythropoiesis outstrips iron and folate stores, iron and folate deficiency may develop, especially in dialysis patients. Prophylactic iron and folic acid therapy are therefore indicated.

[9]Ozer H, Armitage J O, Bennett C L 2000 Update of recommendations for the use of haematopoietic colony-stimulating factors: evidence-based, clinical practice guidelines. Journal of Clinical Oncology 18:3558–3585.

[10]Rizzo J D, Lichtin A E, Woolf S H et al 2002 Use of epoetin in patients with cancer: evidence-based clinical practice guidelines of the American Society of Clinical Oncology and the American Society of Haematology. Blood 100:2303–2320.

Granulocyte colony-stimulating factor

Granulocyte colony-stimulating factor (G-CSF) is a glycoprotein cytokine that stimulates the growth, differentiation and activity of myeloid cells. Recombinant G-CSF, administered intravenously or subcutaneously ($5–10$ μg/kg per dose), has the following applications:

- Haemopoietic stem cell mobilisation into the peripheral blood for autologous or allogeneic transplantation. Blood mobilised progenitor cells are associated with earlier neutrophil and platelet recovery, fewer transfusions and shorter hospitalisation than those from bone marrow.
- To hasten neutrophil recovery following myelosuppressive chemotherapy, after autologous and allogeneic bone marrow transplantation, in aplastic anaemia and AIDS. G-CSF increases the neutrophil count four- to five-fold within hours of administration, shortens the duration of neutropenia and reduces infections in patients who have received cytotoxic myelosuppressive chemotherapy.
- To improve the neutrophil count in myelodysplastic syndromes, and congenital, cyclical and idiopathic neutropenia. G-CSF can reduce the risk of life-threatening infections and prolong survival.
- G-CSF is rapidly cleared after intravenous injection ($t_{1/2}$ 2 h). Pegfilgrastim, which has polyethylene glycol covalently bound to G-CSF, has a longer $t_{1/2}$ (40 h) allowing for less frequent dosing, e.g. once per chemotherapy cycle. High concentrations of G-CSF are found in plasma, bone marrow and kidneys; it is degraded to amino acids and excreted in urine.

Adverse effects of G-CSF are medullary bone pain which occurs with high intravenous doses, musculoskeletal pain, dysuria, splenomegaly, allergic reactions and raised liver enzymes. If administered to patients with sickle cell anaemia, it may precipitate painful crises. There is an increased risk of acute myeloid leukaemia with chronic G-CSF administration in children with congenital neutropenia.

Thrombopoietin receptor agonists

Thrombopoietin (TPO) is a glycoprotein hormone produced primarily by the liver that activates the thrombopoietin receptor, MPL (myeloproliferative leukaemia virus oncogene), and regulates platelet production. TPO receptor agonists (TPO-RA) are novel recombinant thrombopoiesis-stimulating agents that can be used to increase the platelet count in certain situations. The first generation of TPO-RAs were discontinued after initial trials due to the development of neutralising antibodies which led to thrombocytopenia. The second generation of TPO-RAs are now approved for the treatment of immune thrombocytopenia.

Romiplostim is an injectable TPO-RA that has proven efficacy in splenectomised and non-splenectomised patients with refractory immune thrombocytopenia (ITP). It is administered as a subcutaneous injection at a starting dose of 1 μg/kg weekly and titrated to a maximum weekly dose of 10 μg/kg with the aim of achieving a platelet count of $>50 \times 10^9$/L. *Eltrombopag* is an orally available TPO-RA administered at doses of $50–75$ mg once daily. In clinical trials involving patients with refractory ITP, eltrombopag increased platelet counts, reduced bleeding rates and allowed the discontinuation of other ITP medications in a proportion of patients. In addition, the drug has shown efficacy as a novel therapy for patients with aplastic anaemia refractory to immunosuppressive therapy. TPO-RAs are generally well tolerated and, of note, neutralising antibodies are not seen with these second-generation drugs. Thromboembolic disease is a potential risk associated with TPO-RAs, with one meta-analysis reporting an incidence of $3–4\%$. Eltrombopag is also known to cause a reversible elevation in liver enzymes, and monitoring during therapy is recommended. In clinical trials with romiplostim, increased bone marrow reticulin fibrosis has been observed with an incidence of $<5\%$. Longer-term data are required to assess the risk of secondary malignancy with prolonged use.

Guide to further reading

Angelucci, E., Barosi, G., Camaschella, C., et al., 2008. Italian Society of Haematology practice guidelines for the management of iron overload in thalassemia major and related disorders. Haematologica 93, 741–752.

Bennett, C.L., Silver, S.M., Djulbegovic, B., et al., 2008. Venous thromboembolism and mortality associated with recombinant erythropoietin and darbepoetin administration for the treatment of cancer-associated anaemia. J. Am. Med. Assoc. 299, 914–924.

Bohlius, J., Schmidlin, K., Brillant, C., et al., 2009. Erythropoietin or darbepoetin for patients with cancer – meta-analysis based on individual patient data. Cochrane Database Syst. Rev. 8(3), CD007303.

Bregman, D.B., Goodnough, L.T., 2014. Experience with intravenous ferric carboximaltose in patients with iron deficiency anemia. Ther. Adv. Hematol. 5, 48–60.

Capellini, M.D., Taher, A., 2008. Long-term experience with deferasirox (ICL670), a once-daily oral iron chelator, in the treatment of transfusional iron overload. Expert Opin. Pharmacother. 9, 2391–2402.

Carmel, R., 2000. Current concepts in cobalamin deficiency. Annu. Rev. Med. 51, 357–375.

Cheng, G., Saleh, M.N., Marcher, C., et al., 2000. Eltrombopag for management of chronic immune thrombocytopenia (RAISE): a 6-month, randomised, phase 3 study. Lancet 377, 393–402.

Davies, J.K., Guinan, E.C., 2007. An update on the management of severe idiopathic aplastic anaemia in children. Br. J. Haematol. 136, 549–556.

Devalia, V., Hamilton, M.S., Molloy, A.M., British Committee for Standards in Haematology, 2014. Guidelines for the diagnosis and treatment of cobalamin deficiency and folate disorders. Br. J. Haematol. 166, 496–513.

Fleming, R.E., Bacon, B.R., 2005. Orchestration of iron homeostasis. N. Engl. J. Med. 352, 1741–1744.

Harrington, D.J., 2017. Laboratory assessment of vitamin B_{12} status. J. Clin. Pathol. 70, 168–173.

Kaushansky, K., 2006. Lineage-specific haematopoietic growth factors. N. Engl. J. Med. 354, 2034–2045.

Kuter, D.J., Bussel, J.B., Lyons, R.M., et al., 2008. Efficacy of romiplostim in patients with chronic immune thrombocytopenic purpura: a double-blind randomised controlled trial. Lancet 371, 395–403.

Lanzkron, S., Strouse, J.J., Wilson, R., et al., 2008. Systematic review: hydroxyurea for the treatment of adults with sickle cell disease. Ann. Intern. Med. 148, 939–955.

Lawler, P.R., Filion, K.B., Eisenberg, M.J., 2010. Correcting anaemia heart failure: the efficacy and safety of erythropoiesis-stimulating agents. J. Card. Fail. 16, 649–658.

Marsh, J.C., Ball, S.E., Cavenagh, J., et al., 2009. Guidelines for the diagnosis and management of aplastic anaemia. British Committee for Standards in Haematology. Br. J. Haematol. 147, 43–70.

McMullin, M.F., Bareford, D., Campbell, P., et al., 2005. General Haematology Task Force of the British Committee for Standards in Haematology. Guidelines for the diagnosis, investigation and management of polycythaemia/erythrocytosis. Br. J. Haematol. 130, 174–195.

Mehta, A., Mason, P.J., Vulliamy, T.J., 2000. Glucose-6-phosphate dehydrogenase deficiency. Baillieres Best Pract. Res. Clin. Haematol. 13, 21–38.

Ngo, K., Kotecha, D., Walters, J.A., 2009. Erythropoiesis-stimulating agents for anaemia in chronic heart failure. Cochrane Database Syst. Rev. 8(3), CD007613.

Onken, J.E., Bregman, D.B., Harrington, R.A., et al., 2014. Ferric carboxymaltose in patients with iron-deficiency anemia and impaired renal function: the REPAIR-IDA trial. Nephrol. Dial. Transplant. 29, 833–842.

Rund, D., Rachmilewitz, E., 2005. Beta-thalassemia. N. Engl. J. Med. 353, 1135–1146.

Scheinberg, P., Wu, C.O., Nunez, O., et al., 2009. Predicting response to immunosuppressive therapy and survival in severe aplastic anaemia. Br. J. Haematol. 144, 206–216.

Verstovsek, S., Vannucchi, A.M., Griesshammer, M., et al., 2016. Ruxolitinib versus best available therapy in patients with polycythemia vera: 80-week follow-up from the RESPONSE trial. Haematologica 101, 821–829.

Vichinsky, E., 2008. Clinical application of deferasirox: practical patient management. Am. J. Haematol. 83, 398–402.

Wickramasinghe, S.N., 2006. Diagnosis of megaloblastic anaemias. Blood Rev. 20, 299–318.

Youngster, I., Arcavi, L., Schechmaster, R., et al., 2010. Medications and glucose-6-phosphate dehydrogenase deficiency. An evidence-based review. Drug Saf. 33, 713–726.

Chapter 31

Neoplastic disease and immunosuppression

Harpreet Wasan

SYNOPSIS

The causes of cancer are multi-factorial. Most cancer incidences are sporadic, with fewer than 5% being familial. In many cases, environmental risk factors are recognised, which include lifestyle choices, e.g. tobacco smoking, diet and exposure to sunlight. The growing number and efficacy of systemic modalities available to treat patients with cancer are significantly improving disease outcomes. Immunosuppressive drugs are described here, as they share many characteristics with anticancer drugs.

- **Cancer treatments and outcomes.**
- **Rationale for cytotoxic chemotherapy.**[1]
- **Classes of cytotoxic chemotherapy drugs.**
- **Chemotherapy in clinical practice.**
- **Endocrine therapy.**
- **Immunotherapy.**
- **Targeted biological therapies.**
- **Immunosuppression and immunosuppressive drugs.**

---

[1]Although not in strict accord with the definition of Chapter 12, the word 'chemotherapy' is generally used in connection with oncology, and it would be pedantic to avoid it. It arose because malignant cells can be cultured and the disease transmitted by inoculation, as with bacteria. The more precise term 'cytotoxic chemotherapy' is adopted here.

Neoplastic disease

Cancer treatments and outcomes

Cancers share some common characteristics:

- Growth that is not subject to normal spatial restrictions for that tissue and fails to respond to apoptotic signals (see below) or in which a high proportion of cells are dividing, i.e. there is a high 'growth fraction'.
- Local invasiveness.
- Tendency to spread to other parts of the body (metastasise).
- Less differentiated cell morphology.
- Tendency to retain some characteristics of the tissue of origin, at least initially.

Cancer treatment employs six established principal modalities, which are often used in combination (multi-modality therapy):

1. Surgery.
2. Radiotherapy.
3. Cytotoxic chemotherapy.
4. Endocrine therapy.
5. Immunotherapy.
6. Biological (or targeted) therapy.

This account describes the main groups of drugs (see p. 544), but it is important to understand the overall context in which systemic therapy is offered to patients.

Systemic cancer therapy

Cancers originating from different organs of the body differ in their initial behaviour and in their response to treatments (Table 31.1). Primary surgery and/or radiotherapy to a *localised* cancer offer the best chance of *cure* for patients. Drug treatments offer cure only for certain types of cancer, often characterised by their high proliferative rate, e.g. lymphoma, testicular cancer, Wilms' tumour. More often, systemic therapy offers prolongation of life (disease control) from months to many years and associated improvements in quality of life, even if patients ultimately die from their disease. The term *palliative* chemotherapy is used in this context.

Use of drugs as *adjuvant therapy* attempts to eradicate residual microscopic cancer by treating patients after their primary surgery. This strategy has improved overall survival for patients after surgical resection of primary breast, colorectal and gastric cancer. In some situations, drugs are administered prior to surgery *(neoadjuvant therapy)*, primarily to shrink large, locally advanced disease to subsequently enable surgical resection. Many patients with cancer are not cured by their primary treatment due to the early presence of micrometastatic disease; the disease often returns months or years later even though at the time of completing their initial treatment there was no visible evidence of cancer. Clearly, this is a limitation of current standard techniques used to identify residual disease. Currently, radiological imaging techniques cannot visualise lesions smaller than 5 mm in most organs, which equates to over many million cancer cells.

Palliative therapy, offered to patients with advanced, incurable cancer, aims both to increase survival and to improve quality of life by symptom control. Despite significant improvements in cancer outcomes in the last 5–10 years, there remain a number of types of cancer that are poorly responsive to currently available drugs. Patients with *chemoresistant* cancers who are fit enough and willing may be offered experimental treatments within Phase 1 or 2 clinical trials.

Almost all treatments currently available are associated with unwanted effects of varying degrees of severity. The risk of causing harm must be weighed against the potential to do good in each individual case. *Systemic therapy* aims to kill malignant cells or modify their growth but leave the normal cells of the host unharmed or, more usually, temporarily harmed but capable of recovery. When there is a realistic expectation of cure or extensive life prolongation, then to risk more severe drug toxicity is often justified. For example, the treatment of testicular cancer with potentially life-threatening platinum-based combination chemotherapy regimens offers a greater than 85% chance of cure, even for those with extensive, metastatic disease.

Table 31.1 Degree of benefit achieved with systemic therapy for common cancers

Curable: chemosensitive cancers	Improved survival (palliative control for 6 months to 3 years on average): some degree of chemosensitivity	Equivocal survival benefit: traditional cytotoxic chemoresistant cancers (minimal or no benefit)
Teratoma	Colorectal cancer	Sarcoma
Seminoma	Small-cell lung cancer	Melanoma
High-grade non-Hodgkin's lymphoma	Ovarian cancer	*Insensitive to cytotoxic chemotherapy but now can be controlled temporarily with BRAF inhibitors and as ubet respond significantly to combinations of immune checkpoint inhibitors (PD1 and CTLA-4)*
Hodgkin's lymphoma	Breast cancer	Renal cancer
Wilms' tumour	Cervical cancer	*Insensitive to cytotoxic chemotherapy but now can be controlled temporarily with oral VEGF2 and mTOR inhibitors*
Acute myeloblastic leukaemia	Endometrial cancer	Primary brain cancers
Acute lymphoblastic leukaemia in childhood	Gastro-oesophageal cancer	Nasopharyngeal carcinoma
	Cholangiocarcinoma and gall bladder cancer	Hepatoma
	Myeloma	*Insensitive to cytotoxic chemotherapy but now can be controlled temporarily with oral TKIs (sorafenib) with VEGF effects.*
	Pancreatic cancer	
	Low-grade non-Hodgkin's lymphoma	
	Non–small-cell lung cancer	
	Adult acute lymphoblastic leukaemia	

Where expectation is confined to palliation in terms of modest life prolongation of less certain quality, then the benefits and risks of treatment must be judged carefully. Palliative treatments should involve low risk of adverse effects, e.g. treatment with drugs such as 5-fluorouracil–based chemotherapy is well tolerated by most patients. A modern prerequisite of cancer chemotherapy within Phase 3 trials is to concomitantly and objectively assess patient quality of life while on drug therapy. This helps clinicians and nurses to explain the potential benefits and harm of treatment to patients and their families, who may themselves hold strong views about the quality and quantity of life.

Rationale for cytotoxic chemotherapy

The narrow therapeutic index of cytotoxic agents means that escalation of drug doses is constrained by damage to normal cells, and the maximum doses that patients can tolerate are often suboptimal to achieve total cancer cell killing. Even so, cytotoxic chemotherapy agents remain the mainstay of systemic anticancer treatment, as an understanding of their pharmacology has enabled clinicians to exploit the benefits of these drugs (see below).

The very real limitations of cytotoxic chemotherapy have forced a concentration of cancer research on trying to understand the carcinogenic process, the aim being to identify specific molecular targets that can be exploited to develop novel therapeutic approaches. So-called *targeted* therapies are now well-established anticancer drugs. In the last 5 years, the detailed understanding at the receptor level, of how our immune system reacts to cancer's cells trying to spread uncontrollably, has led to a novel class of targeted cancer drugs called immune-checkpoint inhibitors in many cancer types.

Classes of cytotoxic chemotherapy drugs

Cytotoxic chemotherapy drugs exert their effect by inhibiting cell proliferation. All proliferating cells, whether normal and malignant, cycle through a series of phases of: *synthesis* of DNA (S phase), *mitosis* (M phase) and *rest* (G_1 phase). Non-cycling cells are quiescent in G_0 phase (Fig. 31.1).

Cytotoxic drugs interfere with cell division at various points of the cell cycle, in particular G_1/S phase (e.g. synthesis of nucleotides from purines and pyrimidines), S phase (preventing DNA replication) and M phase (e.g. blocking the process of mitosis).

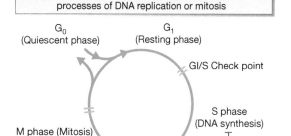

Fig. 31.1 The cell cycle. Most cytotoxic drugs inhibit the processes of DNA replication or mitosis.

They are thus all potentially mutagenic. Cytotoxic drugs ultimately induce cell death by *apoptosis*,[2] a process by which single cells are removed from living tissue by being fragmented into membrane-bound particles and phagocytosed by other cells. This occurs without disturbing the architecture or function of the tissue, or eliciting an inflammatory response. The instructions for apoptosis are built into the cell's genetic material, i.e. 'programmed cell death'.[3]

In general, cytotoxics are most effective against actively cycling cells and least effective against resting or quiescent cells. The latter are particularly problematic in that, although inactive, they retain the capacity to proliferate and may start cycling again after a completed course of chemotherapy, often leading later to rapid regrowth of the cancer.

Cytotoxic drugs can be classified as either:

* *cell-cycle non-specific:* these kill cells whether they are resting or actively cycling (as in a low growth fraction cancer such as solid tumours), e.g. alkylating agents, doxorubicin and allied anthracyclines, or
* *cell-cycle (phase) specific:* these kill only cells that are actively cycling, often because their site of action is confined to one phase of the cell cycle, e.g. antimetabolite drugs.

Table 31.2 provides a summary of the key groups of anticancer drugs, their common toxicities and main treatment applications.

---

[2]Greek: *apo*, off; *ptosis*, a falling.
[3]Makin G, Dive C 2001 Apoptosis and cancer chemotherapy. Trends in Cell Biology 11:S22–S26. (*Dysregulated* apoptosis is also involved in the pathogenesis of many forms of neoplastic disease, notably lymphomas; understanding its mechanisms and the defective processes offers scope for novel approaches to the treatment of cancer.)

Table 31.2 Principal classes of cytotoxic drug, their common toxicities and examples of clinical use

Drug class	Common toxicities	Examples of clinical use
Cytotoxic drugs		
Alkylating agents	Nausea and vomiting; bone marrow depression (delayed with carmustine and lomustine); cystitis (cyclophosphamide, ifosfamide); pulmonary fibrosis (especially busulfan). Male infertility and premature menopause may occur. Myelodysplasia and secondary neoplasia	Widely used in the treatment of both haematological and non-haematological cancers, with varying degrees of success
Platinum drugs	Bone marrow depression; nausea and vomiting; allergy reaction (esp. carboplatin); nephrotoxicity; hypomagnesaemia, hypocalcaemia, hypokalaemia, hypophosphataemia and hyperuricaemia (all as a consequence of renal dysfunction, primarily associated with cisplatin); Raynaud's disease; sterility; teratogenesis; ototoxicity (cisplatin); peripheral neuropathy; cold dysaesthesia and pharyngolaryngeal dysaesthesia (oxaliplatin)	Testicular cancers, ovarian cancer; oxaliplatin acts synergistically with 5FU and is licensed in combination with 5FU to treat both advanced and early stages of colorectal cancer
Nucleoside analogues, e.g. cytarabine, gemcitabine, fludarabine	Bone marrow depression, mainly affecting platelets; mild nausea and vomiting; diarrhoea; anaphylaxis; sudden respiratory distress with high doses (cytarabine); rash, fluid retention and oedema; profound immunosuppression with fludarabine	Cytarabine is used in haematological regimens; gemcitabine is used for pancreatic cancer, bladder cancer and some other solid tumours; fludarabine is active in chronic lymphatic leukaemia and lymphoma
Taxanes	Nausea and vomiting; hypersensitivity reactions; bone marrow depression; fluid retention; peripheral neuropathy; alopecia; arthralgias; myalgias; cardiac toxicity; mild GI disturbances; mucositis	Breast and gynaecological cancers; recent evidence that docetaxel improves survival in advanced prostate cancer
Anthracyclines	Nausea and vomiting; bone marrow depression; cardiotoxicity (may be delayed for years); red-coloured urine; severe local tissue damage and necrosis on extravasation; alopecia; stomatitis; anorexia; conjunctivitis; acral (extremities) pigmentation; dermatitis in previously irradiated areas; hyperuricaemia	Common component of many chemotherapy regimens for both haematological and non-haematological malignancies
Antimetabolites, e.g. 5-fluorouracil, methotrexate	Nausea and vomiting; diarrhoea; mucositis; bone marrow depression; neurological defects, usually cerebellar; cardiac arrhythmias; angina pectoris; hyperpigmentation; hand–foot syndrome; conjunctivitis	Commonly used in haematological and non-haematological malignancies
Topoisomerase I inhibitors	Nausea and vomiting; cholinergic syndrome; hypersensitivity reactions; bone marrow depression; diarrhoea; colitis; ileus; alopecia; renal impairment; teratogenic	Irinotecan is effective in advanced colorectal cancer; topotecan is used in gynaecological malignancies
Mitotic spindle inhibitors (vinca alkaloids)	Nausea and vomiting; local reaction and phlebitis with extravasation; neuropathy; bone marrow depression; alopecia; stomatitis; loss of deep tendon reflexes; jaw pain; muscle pain; paralytic ileus	Commonly used in haemato-oncology regimens

Table 31.2 Principal classes of cytotoxic drug, their common toxicities and examples of clinical use—cont'd

Drug class	Common toxicities	Examples of clinical use
Hormones		
Tamoxifen	Hot flushes; transiently increased bone or tumour pain; vaginal bleeding and discharge; rash; thromboembolism; endometrial cancer	Oestrogen receptor-positive, advanced and early stage breast cancer
Aromatase inhibitors	Nausea; dizziness; rash; bone marrow depression; fever; masculinisation	Equivalence with tamoxifen suggested
Medroxyprogesterone acetate	Menstrual changes; gynaecomastia; hot flushes; oedema; weight gain; hirsutism; insomnia; fatigue; depression; thrombophlebitis and thromboembolism; nausea; urticaria; headache	Third-line therapy for slowly progressive breast cancer in postmenopausal women
Flutamide	Nausea; diarrhoea; gynaecomastia; hepatotoxicity	Prostate cancer
Goserelin	Transient increase in bone pain and urethral obstruction in patients with metastatic prostatic cancer; hot flushes; impotence; testicular atrophy; gynaecomastia	Prostate cancer
Leuprolelin (LHRH analogue)	Transient increase in bone pain and ureteral obstruction in patients with metastatic prostatic cancer; hot flushes, impotence; testicular atrophy; gynaecomastia; peripheral oedema	Prostate cancer
Immunotherapy		
BCG (bacille Calmette-Guérin)	Bladder irritation; nausea and vomiting; fever; sepsis, granulomatous pyelonephritis; hepatitis; urethral obstruction; epididymitis; renal abscess	Localised bladder cancer
Interferon-α	Fever; chills; myalgias; fatigue; headache; arthralgias; bone marrow depression; anorexia; confusion; depression; psychiatric disorders; renal toxicity; hepatic toxicity; rash	Renal cancer
Interleukin-2	Fever; fluid retention; hypotension; respiratory distress; rash; anaemia, thrombocytopenia; nausea and vomiting; diarrhoea; capillary leak syndrome; nephrotoxicity; myocardial toxicity; hepatotoxicity; erythema nodosum; neuropsychiatric disorders; hypothyroidism; nephrotic syndrome	Renal cancer
Trastuzumab (Herceptin)	Fever; chills; nausea and vomiting; pain; hypersensitivity and pulmonary reactions; bone marrow depression; cardiomyopathy; ventricular dysfunction; congestive cardiac failure; diarrhoea	Advanced and early-stage breast cancer, combined with cytotoxic chemotherapy
Rituximab (MabThera)	Hypersensitivity reaction; bone marrow depression; angioedema; precipitation of angina or arrhythmia with pre-existing heart disease	Non-Hodgkin's lymphoma

Adverse effects of cytotoxic chemotherapy

Principal adverse effects are manifest as, or as damage to, the following:

Nausea and vomiting may occur within hours of treatment or be delayed, and last for several days, depending on the agent. As emetogenicity is largely predictable, successful preventive action can be taken. The most effective drugs are competitive antagonists of serotonin (5-hydroxytryptamine type 3, $5HT_3$) receptors, e.g. ondansetron, and corticosteroids such as dexamethasone, which benefit by unknown, multifactorial mechanisms. Other effective antiemetics include domperidone, metoclopramide, cyclizine and prochlorperazine (see p. 569). More recently, delayed nausea management has also significantly improved with the addition of neurokinin-1 receptor antagonists. Combinations of drugs are frequently used and routes of administration selected as commonsense counsels, e.g. prophylaxis may be oral, but when vomiting occurs the parenteral route and suppositories are available.

Suppression of bone marrow and the lymphoreticular system. Myelosuppression with depression of both antibody- and cell-mediated immunity is the single most important dose-limiting factor with cytotoxic agents, and carries life-threatening consequences. Repeated blood monitoring is essential, and transfusion of red cells and platelets may be necessary. Cell growth factors, e.g. the natural granulocyte colony-stimulating factor (filgrastim), are available to protect against or to resolve severe neutropenia.

Opportunistic infection by Gram-negative bacteria from the patient's own flora, e.g. from the gut that has been damaged by chemotherapy, may occur. Infections with virus (herpes zoster), fungus (candida) and protozoa (pneumocystis) are also increased. Fever in a patient receiving chemotherapy usually requires immediate hospitalisation, collection of samples for microbiological studies and urgent empirical initiation of antibiotic treatment. Where risk of neutropenia is high, antimicrobial prophylaxis may be used. High-dose chemoradiotherapy and allogeneic bone marrow transplant produce profound immunosuppression with significant risk of opportunistic infection and third-party graft-versus-host disease following non-irradiated blood transfusion. Live vaccines are *contraindicated* in these patients.

Diarrhoea and mouth ulcers usually arise from drug damage to gut epithelium and other mucosal surfaces with a naturally rapid cell turnover.

Alopecia is due to an effect on the hair bulb but is not invariable; it recovers 2–6 months after ceasing treatment.

Scalp cooling may prevent or limit this with certain drugs, e.g. vinca alkaloids.

Urate nephropathy is due to rapid destruction of malignant cells releasing purines and pyrimidines, which are metabolised to uric acid that may crystallise in and block the renal tubule (urate nephropathy). In practice this occurs only when there is a large cell mass or a tumour is very sensitive to drugs, e.g. acute leukaemias and high-grade lymphomas. High fluid intake, alkalinisation of the urine and use of allopurinol or rasburicas during the early stages of chemotherapy avert this outcome.

Local extravasation may damage surrounding tissues; it is a problem with certain vesicant cytotoxics, e.g. doxorubicin, dacarbazine. This is a medical emergency, and policies for management (which may include debridement by a plastic surgeon) should be in place in every centre.

Hypersensitivity reactions may occur with susceptible patients. These are more problematic with certain cytotoxic agents, e.g. paclitaxel, carboplatin and the newer hybrid targeted monoclonal antibodies, for which prophylactic corticosteroid and antihistamine are offered routinely.

Specific organ damage may result, e.g. lung toxicity with bleomycin, cardiotoxicity with anthracyclines, nephrotoxicity with platinum agents. Auto-immune activation with the new class of immune checkpoint inhibitors can lead to widespread endocrine malfunction.

Delayed wound healing can be expected. Surgical wounds should be healed prior to commencing chemotherapy, wherever possible.

Germ cells and reproduction deserve special attention as chemotherapy may cause infertility. In addition, the theoretical mutagenic effects of cytotoxic drugs mean that reproduction is to be avoided during and for several months after therapy (although both men and women have reproduced normally while undergoing chemotherapy). When treatment may cause permanent sterility, men are offered the facility for prior storage of sperm. Cryopreservation of ovarian tissue is now also feasible. Prior contraceptive advice is necessary, as most cytotoxic drugs are teratogenic and are contraindicated during pregnancy.

Carcinogenicity may result in delayed second malignancies, a potentially serious issue where treatment improves life expectancy. Many cytotoxic drugs are themselves carcinogenic, and a patient may be cured of the primary disease only to succumb to a second, treatment-induced, cancer 5–20 years later. Examples include patients with Hodgkin's lymphoma who are often young with high cure rates. Whether this is due to a mutagenic effect, to chronic immunosuppression, or to both, remains unclear. Alkylating agents and radiotherapy are particularly incriminated, as are some antimetabolites (mercaptopurine) and anthracyclines (doxorubicin).

The relative risk can be as high as 10 to 20 times the normal risk. The second cancers caused include leukaemia, lymphoma and squamous carcinoma.

Classes of cytotoxic agents

Alkylating agents

Alkylating agents (nitrogen mustards and ethylenimines) act by transferring alkyl groups to DNA in the N-7 position of guanine during cell division. Normal synthesis is prevented because of either DNA strand breakage or crosslinking of the two strands. Examples include: busulfan, carmustine, chlorambucil, cyclophosphamide, ifosfamide, lomustine, melphalan, mustine (mechlorethamine), thiotepa, treosulfan.

Antimetabolites

Antimetabolites are synthetic analogues of normal metabolites and act by competition to 'deceive' or 'defraud' bodily processes.

Methotrexate, a folic acid antagonist, competitively inhibits dihydrofolate reductase, preventing the synthesis of tetrahydrofolic acid (the coenzyme that is important in synthesis of amino and nucleic acids). The drug also provides a cogent illustration of the need to exploit every possible means of enhancing selectivity. Where the desire is to maximise the effect of methotrexate, a potentially fatal dose is given, followed 24 h later by a dose of tetrahydrofolic (folinic) acid as calcium folinate (Ca Leucovorin) to bypass and terminate its action. This is called folinic acid 'rescue', because, if it is not given, the patient will die. The therapeutic justification for this manoeuvre is the cell kill obtained with very high plasma concentrations of methotrexate, allied to the fact that the bone marrow cells recover better than the tumour cells. The outcome is a useful degree of selectivity.

Pyrimidine antagonists: 5-fluorouracil (5FU) is metabolised intracellularly, and its metabolite binds covalently with thymidilate synthase, thereby inhibiting DNA (and RNA) synthesis. 5FU has a short duration of action, and addition of folinic acid in 5FU therapy improves its antitumour activity; protracted infusion can achieve the same outcome. Oral prodrugs of 5FU include capecitabine and UFT (a mixture of tegafur and uracil). These prodrugs have a cytotoxic action equivalent to that of 5FU but cause less myelosuppression and stomatitis; the risk of hand–foot syndrome (damage to the palmar and plantar surfaces of the hands and feet causing reddening, soreness and blistering) is considerably higher.

Arabinosides (cytosine arabinoside, gemcitabine) and the *purine antagonists* (deoxycoformycin, fludarabine, 2-chloroadenisine) azathioprine, mercaptopurine and tioguanine are also converted intracellularly to active metabolites that inhibit DNA synthesis.

Antimetabolites find extensive use in anticancer therapy, either alone or in combination with other drugs. They remain the mainstay of treatment for haematological as well as common solid tumours such as breast and gastrointestinal tract cancers.

Anthracyclines and related compounds

The original anthracyclines were antibiotics produced by microorganisms such as *Streptomycetes* spp. Daunorubicin and doxorubicin were the first compounds to be isolated and appear to interfere with both DNA and RNA synthesis. Other examples include bleomycin, dactinomycin, epirubicin, mitoxantrone, idarubicin, plicamycin (mithramycin), mitomycin and streptozotocin (most often used to treat the rare islet-cell pancreatic tumours).

Topoisomerase inhibitors

These inhibit enzymes essential for spatial conformation ('unwinding') prior to DNA replication, The epipodophyllotoxins (etoposide, teniposide) are major inhibitors of topoisomerase II. Topotecan and irinotecan selectively inhibit topoisomerase I and are effective in relapsed ovarian and colorectal cancer, respectively. Bone marrow depression is dose limiting as, in the case of irinotecan, is delayed diarrhoea (which relates to a specific polymorphism in a drug metabolising gene). Administration of irinotecan is often complicated by an acute cholinergic reaction, reversible by prophylactic subcutaneous atropine. Doxorubicin is a non-specific inhibitor of topoisomerase I and II.

Spindle poisons

The plant alkaloids (vincristine, vinblastine, vindesine and vinorelbine) and taxoids (paclitaxel, docetaxel) inhibit microtubule assembly and cause cell-cycle arrest in mitosis. They particularly cause bone marrow depression and alopecia. Vincristine causes neuropathy.

Platinum drugs

This family of drugs (which include cisplatin, carboplatin and oxaliplatin) act by cross-linking DNA in a similar manner to alkylating agents. The parent drug, cisplatin, is associated with a variety of adverse effects, including severe emesis, nephrotoxicity and ototoxicity. Renal damage is ameliorated by carefully pre-hydrating patients, and emetogenicity is effectively controlled with $5HT_3$ receptor (serotonin) antagonists. Second- (carboplatin) and third- (oxaliplatin; no nephrotoxicity) generation platinum agents have improved toxicity profiles, by small alterations to the basic molecular structure, and offer effective treatment for germ cell, ovarian and colorectal cancers.

Miscellaneous agents

Asparaginase starves tumour cells dependent upon a supply of the amino acid, asparagine (except those able to synthesise it for themselves); its use is largely confined to acute lymphoblastic leukaemia.

Chemotherapy in clinical practice

Drug use and tumour cell kinetics

Evidence from leukaemia in laboratory animals shows that:

- survival time is inversely related to the initial number of leukaemia cells, or to the number remaining after treatment
- a single leukaemia cell is capable of multiplying and eventually killing the host.

Cytotoxic drugs act against all multiplying cells. Bone marrow, mucosal surfaces (gut), hair follicles, reticulo-endothelial system and germ cells all divide more rapidly than many cancer cells and are damaged by cytotoxic drugs, leading to the particular adverse effects of chemotherapy. In contrast to haematological cancers, most solid tumours in humans divide slowly and recovery from cytotoxic agents is slow, whereas normal marrow and gut recover rapidly. This speed of recovery of normal tissues is exploited in devising intermittent courses of chemotherapy.

In cancer, the normal feedback mechanisms that mediate cell growth are defective and cell proliferation continues unchecked, with cancer cells multiplying, at first exponentially. Cancers with high growth fractions, e.g. acute leukaemias, high-grade lymphomas, may visibly enlarge at an alarming rate, but are frequently highly sensitive to cytotoxic chemotherapy. In later stages, the growth rate of these cancers often slows and the volume-doubling time lengthens due to several factors, most of which conspire to render the advanced cancer less susceptible to drugs, namely:

- Increased cell-cycle (division) time.
- Decrease in the number of cells actively dividing, with more in the resting state (decrease in growth

fraction), but with the potential to switch back to a fast growth state.
- Increased cell death within the tumour as it ages.
- Overcrowding of cells leading to necrotic, avascular and hypoxic areas that cannot easily be penetrated by drugs. These are fertile areas for clonal selection of the most robust cancer cells.

Selectivity of drugs for cancer cells is generally low compared with the selectivity shown by antimicrobial agents, but it can be substantial, e.g. in lymphoma, where tumour cell kill with some drugs is 10 000 times greater than that of marrow cells. Cell destruction by cytotoxic drugs follows first-order kinetics, i.e. a given dose of drug kills a constant *fraction* of cells (not a constant *number*) regardless of the number of cells present. Thus a treatment that reduces a cell population from 1 000 000 to 10 000 (a two-log cell kill) will reduce a cell population of 1000 to 10. Furthermore, cell chemosensitivity within a cancer is not homogeneous owing to random mutations (clonal selection) as the tumour grows, the cells remaining after initial doses being more likely to resist further treatment. Therefore, combining several drugs may be more effective than a single agent given repeatedly to the limit of tolerance.

The selection of drugs in combination chemotherapy is influenced by the following:

- Choosing drugs that act at different biochemical sites in the cell.
- Using drugs that attack cells at different phases of the growth cycle (see Fig. 31.1). 'CHOP' (*c*yclophosphamide, doxorubicin (previously called '*h*ydroxydoxorubicin'), vincristine (previously called '*o*ncovin') and *p*rednisolone) is a standard combination chemotherapy regimen for non-Hodgkin's lymphoma. The first three cytotoxic drugs exert their antitumour effect on different aspects of cell proliferation. The antitumour effect of corticosteroid remains unclear.
- The desirability of attaining synchronisation of cell cycling to achieve maximum cell kill. Cells are killed or are arrested in mitosis by vincristine, which is then withdrawn. Cells then enter a new reproductive cycle more or less synchronously, and when most are judged to be in a phase sensitive to a particular phase-specific drug, e.g. methotrexate or cytarabine, it is given.
- Avoidance of cross-resistance (see below) between drugs. In some instances, use of one drug regimen *followed* by another rather than using them simultaneously in combination avoids drug resistance and improves therapeutic efficacy. For example, epirubicin given for four cycles followed by CMF (concomitant cyclophosphamide, methotrexate and

5-fluorouracil) for four cycles has largely replaced CMF alone as standard adjuvant chemotherapy for breast cancer, because the outcome is better.

- Non-overlapping toxicity profiles. Before establishing a combination regimen, Phase 1 trials (see p. 40) are undertaken, frequently fixing the dose of one drug while escalating the dose of another, in small cohorts of carefully monitored patients, so that toxicity and patient safety can be monitored.
- Empirical evidence of efficacy against a particular tumour type. The antitumour activity of platinum complexes was a chance finding (see below).
- Enhanced cell killing in preclinical models when drugs are combined. Oxaliplatin on its own has limited cytotoxicity against colorectal cancer cell lines in vitro and in mouse xenograft models, but its combination with 5FU confers a more than additive, i.e. synergistic, killing effect on tumour cells.
- Considerations of pharmacokinetics in relation to cell kinetics are of great importance, as drug treatment alters the behaviour of both malignant and normal cells.

Drug resistance

Resistance to a cytotoxic chemotherapy agent may be present at the outset (primary resistance), or may develop with repeated drug exposure (acquired resistance). Increasing dosage is limited by toxicity, e.g. to bone marrow, which does not become tolerant. *Combination chemotherapy* is a strategy commonly used to address the problems of tumour resistance.

Multiple drug resistance (MDR) of a cancer is not uncommon. MDR is most frequently due to increased expression of an ATP-dependent membrane efflux pump called 'P-glycoprotein (Pgp)', which is a member of a class of membrane proteins called the 'ATP-binding cassette superfamily'. Pgp is an important protective mechanism possessed by many normal cells against environmental toxins and has broad specificity for hydrophobic compounds. Long-lived cells such as the haemopoietic stem cell, cells on excretory surfaces such as biliary hepatocytes, proximal renal tubule and intestinal cells, and the cells of the blood–brain barrier all have high expression of Pgp. A number of agents including immunosuppressants (ciclosporin) and calcium channel blockers (verapamil and nifedipine) block Pgp in theory, but are unhelpful in practice.

The MDR phenomenon illustrates how tumour cells adapt and enhance normal cell mechanisms to deal with the effects of chemotherapy, and how repeated cycles of chemotherapy select out a population of cells that have developed adaptive survival mechanisms, e.g. in myeloma where MDR proteins are rare at diagnosis but common at progression.

In those tumours for which cures can be achieved by chemotherapy (childhood acute lymphoblastic leukaemia, Hodgkin's lymphoma, choriocarcinoma) it is essential that optimal doses of initial chemotherapy be administered and dose intensity maintained in order to avoid the emergence of chemoresistance.

Improving efficacy of chemotherapy

Methods that potentially widen the narrow therapeutic index of cytotoxic agents include:

- Regional (as opposed to systemic) administration of drugs: intrathecal, intra-arterial into liver and isolated limb perfusion.
- Selective organ delivery of drug by altered formulation, e.g. Caelyx is a formulation comprising high concentrations of doxorubicin encased in liposomes. This also alters toxicity profiles (e.g. less renal but more mucosal toxicity).
- Cytotoxic drugs can be chemically linked with monoclonal antibodies (antibody-drug conjugate) that target a specific receptor or protein driving cancer cell growth. In 2013, Ado-trastuzumab emtansine (T-DM1) was introduced for HER2-positive metastatic breast cancer patients.
- High-dose (bone marrow ablative) chemotherapy is feasible by harvesting stem cells prior to drug exposure, and returning the cells to the patient on completion of treatment. This is a successful strategy in haematological malignancies but failed trials in almost all solid tumours.
- Circadian rhythms exist in cell metabolism and proliferation, and those of leukaemic cells differ from normal leucocytes. The time of day at which therapy is administered can theoretically influence the outcome (chronomodulation).
- In large solid tumours, the fraction of cells multiplying rapidly is often relatively small. In ovarian cancer, for example, patients benefit from debulking surgery (cytoreduction) prior to cytotoxic drug therapy.

Hazards to staff handling cytotoxic agents

Urine from nurses and pharmacists who prepared infusions and injections of anticancer agents revealed drugs in concentrations that were mutagenic to bacteria. When they stopped handling the drugs, the contamination ceased. It can be assumed that absorption of even small amounts of these drugs is harmful (mutagenesis, carcinogenesis), especially repeatedly over long periods. Pregnant staff should not handle these drugs.

A note of caution. Certain chemotherapy regimens require the simultaneous administration of *intrathecal* methotrexate and *intravenous* vincristine. In the UK until recently, each drug was presented in similar bolus volumes, and the drug-filled syringes appeared very alike except that the syringe for intrathecal administration had a red stopper. Nevertheless, from 1985 in the UK inadvertent *intrathecal* administration of *vincristine* occurred on 14 occasions: 10 patients died, and the remainder suffered paralysis.[4]

Interactions of anticancer agents with other drugs

The diverse modes of action of cytotoxic drugs offer ample scope for serious *unwanted drug–drug interactions*, and by different mechanisms. There is general cause for alertness. Drugs that inhibit enzymes and thus delay normal metabolic breakdown may cause harmful reactions to standard doses of cytotoxics, e.g. allopurinol (xanthine oxidase inhibitor) with mercaptopurine or cyclophosphamide. Enzyme-inducing drugs can reduce the therapeutic efficacy of anticancer drugs by accelerating metabolism. Competition with non-steroidal anti-inflammatory drugs (NSAIDs) reduces the renal tubular excretion of methotrexate, leading to methotrexate toxicity. A combination of cytotoxics causing a dangerous degree of immunosuppression represents an adverse pharmacodynamic reaction.

Therapeutic drug–drug interactions are an essential part of treatment, as witnessed by the many drug combinations used to treat cancer (see Drug use and tumour cell kinetics, p. 550).

Endocrine therapy

Hormonal influence on cancer

The possibility of interfering with cancer other than by surgery, e.g. by endocrine manipulation, was first tested in 1895 when a Scottish surgeon, faced with a woman 33 years of age with advanced breast cancer:

> put it to her husband and herself as to whether she should have performed the operation of removal of the [fallopian] tubes and ovaries. Its nature was fully explained to them both, and also that it was a purely experimental one … She readily consented … as she

> knew and felt her case was hopeless. [Eight months after operation] all vestiges of her previous cancerous disease had disappeared. [The surgeon concluded, after treating two further cases, that there may be ovarian influences in breast cancer and added that] whether [this is] accepted or not, I am sure I shall be acquitted of having acted thoughtlessly or recklessly.[5]

The treatment had logic. The author, observing the weaning of lambs on a local farm, had noted a similarity between the proliferation of epithelial cells of the milk ducts in lactation and in cancer, and had conceived the idea that cancer of the breast might be due to an abnormal ovarian stimulus.

In 1941[6] it was shown that prostatic cancer with metastases was made worse by androgen and made better by oestrogen (diethylstilbestrol).

Hormonal agents

The growth of some cancers is hormone dependent and is inhibited by surgical removal of gonads, adrenals and/or pituitary. The same effect is achievable, at less cost to the patient, by administering hormones, or hormone antagonists, of oestrogens, androgens or progestogens and inhibitors of hormone synthesis.

Breast cancer cells may have receptors for oestrogen, progesterone and androgen, and hormonal manipulation benefits some 30% of patients with metastatic disease; when a patient's tumour is oestrogen-receptor–positive, the response is about 60%, and when negative it is only 10%. After treatment of the primary cancer, endocrine therapy with the *anti-oestrogen, tamoxifen,* is the adjuvant therapy of choice for postmenopausal women who have disease in the lymph nodes; both the interval before the development of metastases and overall survival are increased. Adjuvant therapy with cytotoxic drugs and/or tamoxifen is recommended for node-negative patients with large tumours or other adverse prognostic factors. Cytotoxic chemotherapy is more useful in younger women, with tamoxifen, increasingly, as adjuvant therapy. The optimal duration of dosing with tamoxifen is not yet established, but is likely to be 5 years or more.

Aromatase inhibitors cause 'medical adrenalectomy' in postmenopausal women by blocking conversion of adrenal androgens to oestrogens in peripheral fat by the enzyme aromatase. The first drug in this class, *aminoglutethimide,* causes significant adverse effects. More selective and less toxic aromatase inhibitors now include *anastrozole, letrozole* and *exemestane,* and find use after treatment with tamoxifen fails. Clinical trial data suggest that these drugs rival

---

[4]As a consequence of the death of a patient following intrathecal administration of vincristine, two inexperienced doctors were charged with manslaughter (Dyer C 2001 Doctors suspended after injecting wrong drug into spine. British Medical Journal 322:257).

[5]Beatson G T 1896 Lancet ii:104, 162.
[6]Huggins C et al 1941 Cancer Research 1:293.

tamoxifen in efficacy for both advanced and early breast cancer. *Progestogens*, e.g. *megestrol* or *medroxyprogesterone*, are third-line agents in postmenopausal women.

Prostatic cancer is androgen dependent, and metastatic disease can be helped by *orchidectomy*, or by pituitary suppression of androgen secretion with a gonadorelin (LHRH) analogue, e.g. *buserelin, goserelin, leuprorelin* or *triptorelin*. These cause a transient stimulation of luteinising hormone and thus testosterone release, before inhibition occurs; some patients may experience exacerbation of tumour effects, e.g. bone pain, spinal cord compression. Where this can be anticipated, prior orchidectomy or *anti-androgen* treatment, e.g. with *cyproterone* or *flutamide*, is protective.

Benign prostatic hypertrophy is also androgen dependent, and drug therapy includes use of *finasteride*, an inhibitor of the enzyme (5α-reductase) that activates testosterone.

Adrenocortical steroids are used for their action on specific cancers and also to treat some of the complications of cancer, e.g. hypercalcaemia, raised intracranial pressure. In leukaemias, corticosteroid may reduce the incidence of complications, e.g. haemolytic anaemia and thrombocytopenia. A glucocorticoid is preferred, e.g. prednisolone, as doses are high, and the mineralocorticoid actions are not needed and cause fluid retention.

In general, endocrine therapy carries less acute serious consequences for normal tissues than do cytotoxic agents. In a sense, they represent the first generation of mechanism-driven targeted agents used to treat cancer. As cancer patients live longer, the chronic effects of hormonal therapies are becoming more evident, such as a higher incidence of endometrial cancer with chronic use of tamoxifen in a minority of patients and osteoporosis in breast and prostate cancer patients who have had anti-oestrogens and/or anti-androgens including gonadorelin (LHRH) analogues.

Immunotherapy

Immunotherapy (immunostimulation) derives from an observation in the 19th century that cancer sometimes regressed after acute bacterial infections, i.e. in response to non-specific immunostimulant effect. In general, it appears that the immune response is attenuated in cancer. Strategies to stimulate the host's own immune system to kill cancer cells more effectively are:

- *Non-specific stimulation* of active immunity with vaccines, e.g. BCG (bacille Calmette–Guérin[7]) instilled into the urinary bladder for bladder cancer.

---

[7]An attenuated strain of *Mycobacterium bovis* used to prepare the BCG vaccine for immunisation against tuberculosis.

Other approaches involve the injection of tumour cells or tumour cell extracts combined with an immune stimulant such as BCG.

- *Specific immunisation strategies*, where tumour-specific and tumour-associated antigens have been identified. Melanomas, for example, possess melanoma differentiation antigens (tyrosinase, gp100, MART1) as well as tumour-associated antigens (MAGE, BAGE, GAGE series of major histocompatibility complex (MHC)-associated peptides and a family of lipoproteins known as gangliosides). Both DNA and whole-protein vaccines derived from these antigens are being evaluated in melanoma, but results to date have been clinically disappointing.

Naturally occurring substances are increasingly used to treat cancer. Cytokines are produced in response to various stimuli, such as antigens, e.g. viruses. These peptides regulate cell growth, activation and differentiation, and immune responses and can be synthesised by recombinant DNA technology. Examples include:

- *Interleukins* that stimulate proliferation of T lymphocytes and activate natural killer cells; interleukin-2 is used in metastatic renal cell carcinoma with marginal effectiveness.
- *Interferons.* Interferon-α is used for chronic granulocytic leukaemia, hairy cell leukaemia, renal cell carcinoma and Kaposi's sarcoma.
- *Thalidomide* was withdrawn in the 1960s following evidence of its teratogenic effects, including some on fetal limb development (see p. 64). These very effects prompted the notion of its anticancer potential. Investigation revealed that thalidomide possessed immunomodulatory properties, anti-inflammatory actions, direct effects on tumour cells and their microenvironment, and actions on angiogenesis (see below). Thalidomide and analogues designed to reduce toxicity (immunomodulatory drugs: lenalidomide) now have a therapeutic role in myeloma and are synergistic with dexamethasone and chemotherapeutic agents.
- *Immune check-point inhibitors.* Humans have natural Immune checkpoint systems that regulate and prevent over-activation of immune responses. However, they can also obstruct an antitumour immune response. In 2011, ipilimumab, which is an antibody that blocks the T-lymphocyte-associated protein 4 (CTLA-4) was approved for human use in melanoma, and subsequently many immune checkpoint inhibitors to the programmed cell death 1 (PD-1) were approved. This class of anticancer strategies also has a novel profile of adverse effects, namely auto-immune disease including endocrinopathies.

ATRA

All-*trans*-retinoic acid (ATRA) induces remission in newly diagnosed patients with promyelocytic leukaemia (APL), by leukaemic cell differentiation. APL is due to reciprocal translocation between chromosomes 15 and 17 producing a fusion gene *PML–RARa*. The fusion protein blocks differentiation but is overcome by ATRA. Subsequent administration of anthracycline improves cure rates.

Development of anticancer drug therapy

In general, anticancer drugs develop from:

- *Chance discovery: cisplatin.* In the 1960s, scientists studying the effect of an electric current on bacteria cultured in a Petri dish noted that the cells stopped dividing, instead forming long filamentous structures. Further investigation revealed that the inhibitor of cell division was in fact an ion formed in solution from the platinum electrodes used in the experiment. The platinum complex, cis-diammine-dichloroplatinum (II), later known as cisplatin, was isolated and subsequently developed for its potential to kill cancer cells. When given to patients with a variety of different types of cancer, germ cell tumours in particular were found to possess remarkable sensitivity to cisplatin treatment, and this drug remains in use for treating such patients today.[8]
- *Analogues.* Severe vomiting, renal and nerve damage, and deafness limit the therapeutic efficacy of cisplatin. Carboplatin and oxaliplatin, second- and third-generation compounds derived from cisplatin, combine enhanced toxicity towards cancer cells with improved tolerance.
- *Mass screening programmes.* See Chapter 3.
- *Rational drug design.* Academic institutions and commercial biotechnology companies involved in experimental therapeutics study the cancer process to identify key ('target') genes or gene products that regulate aspects of carcinogenesis and then try to find ways of blocking the function of these targets (Table 31.3). Unlike conventional cytotoxic chemotherapy, many of these agents are thus more cancer-cell selective and thus cytostatic. In other words, a targeted biological agent may prevent tumour growth or progression and delay recurrence, but may not

[8]Rosenberg B, Van Camp L, Trosko J E et al 1969 Platinum compounds: a new class of potent antitumour agents. Nature 222:385–386.

Table 31.3 Some novel molecular targets being exploited in anticancer drug development[a]

Target	Drug[b]	Examples of current clinical use
Her2/neu	Trastuzumab (Herceptin)	Advanced and early-stage breast cancer Advanced gastric cancer
CD20	Rituximab (MabThera)	Non-Hodgkin's lymphoma
EGFR	Cetuximab (Erbitux)	Improves survival in advanced colorectal cancer Lung cancer and head and neck cancer (in combination with radiotherapy)
EGFR	Gefitinib (Iressa)	Advanced non–small-cell lung cancer
EGFR	Erlotinib (Tarceva)	Advanced non–small-cell lung cancer, advanced pancreatic cancer
VEGF	Bevacizumab (Avastin)	Advanced colorectal cancer; trials confirm some efficacy in non–small-cell lung cancer and renal cancer
Bcr-abl	Imatinib (Glivec)	Chronic myeloid leukaemia
c-kit	Imatinib (Glivec)	Gastrointestinal stromal tumours
Raf/MAPK	Sorafenib	Hepatocellular and renal cancer Clinical trials ongoing in breast cancer, GIST and melanoma
Cyclin-dependent kinase	Flavopiridol	Undergoing clinical trials
mTor (a key regulator of cell-cycle progression)	Everolimus and temsirolimus	Renal Pancreatic neuroendocrine tumours
Proteasome inhibitor	Bortezomib	Active in myeloma; trials of combination therapy in progress

[a]Drugs at various stages in the process of obtaining a licence for use in the UK.
[b]The suffix 'mab' identifies a monoclonal antibody, whereas 'nib' identifies a tyrosine kinase inhibitor.

induce rapid tumour shrinkage, hitherto the key conventional endpoint for evaluating cytotoxic drugs. Some examples follow to illustrate the opportunities created by this type of approach.

Targeted biological therapies

Passive immunotherapy using monoclonal antibodies raised against specific tumour-associated antigens on the cell surface

Targeted antibodies have the advantage of high cancer specificity and relatively low host toxicity.

- *Rituximab*, an anti-CD20 monoclonal antibody, for the treatment of low-grade follicular lymphomas and for use in combination with CHOP (see above) for high-grade lymphoma, as these tumours carry the antigen CD20 on the cell surface.
- Significant over-expression of the Her2/neu (erbB2) cell surface growth factor receptor occurs in approximately 20% of breast cancers and gastric cancers and is associated with a far more aggressive form of breast cancer compared with non–Her2-expressing tumours. *Trastuzumab* (Herceptin), a humanised monoclonal antibody, binds specifically to the Her2/neu receptor, blocking its function in regulating intracellular processes, including cell proliferation. In combination with conventional cytotoxic chemotherapy, trastuzumab significantly improves the survival of patients with advanced or early breast cancer, compared with cytotoxic chemotherapy alone. A series of key adjuvant trials conducted across Europe and the USA showed that trastuzumab combined with chemotherapy provided the biggest survival gains ever recorded for this disease.[9-11] Potential cumulative cardiac dysfunction with trastuzumab is dose limiting.
- Her2 is a member of the epidermal growth factor receptor (EGFR) family. EGFRs are highly expressed by about 85% of colorectal cancers and are important

in regulating cell proliferation. Another monoclonal antibody, *cetuximab* (Erbitux), blocks EGFR function and is used for selected colorectal cancers. It was subsequently found that this drug had no benefit in approximately 40% of all colorectal cancers with a mutation in the *K-RAS & N-RAS* oncogene. The mutation constitutively activates the cell pathway downstream of the EGFR receptor, so blocking it with cetuximab has no effect. This is an important example of personalising medicine to the individual cancer type and selecting which agents are suitable in individual cancers. It is also crucial in the design and selection of patients for future evolutions of this therapy in colorectal cancer, as patients with RAS mutations would only get the unwanted effects and absolutely no benefit if treated with EGFR inhibitors. Limiting toxicities for this class of drugs are fatigue, rash, mucositis and hypomagnesaemia.

- *Vasculoendothelial growth factor* (VEGF) is a major angiogenic signal regulator for new blood vessel formation (angiogenesis). Angiogenesis, a process that is common to all cancers, is vital for the growth and establishment of secondary tumours to grow beyond 1–2 mm when diffusion of nutrients becomes insufficient to maintain tumour growth. Blockade of VEGF and its receptor is a successful strategy for treating several types of neoplasm. The monoclonal antibody *bevacizumab* (Avastin) improves survival or slows tumour growth significantly, when combined with cytotoxic chemotherapy for advanced colorectal, lung and breast cancers. This novel approach evokes a range of adverse drug reactions that differ from those of conventional cytotoxics: hypertension, proteinuria, bleeding and increased risk of thromboembolic events.
- Similar drugs that block effects of VEGF are now used to treat neovascular age-related wet macular degeneration, a condition that causes loss of central vision in 2.3% of people older than 65 years of age.

Radioimmunotherapy

Monoclonal antibodies targeted against epitopes[12] on tumour cells, e.g. rituximab against CD20 in lymphoma, are conjugated to radionuclides such as yttrium-90 (ibritumomab) or iodine-131 (tositumomab) to deliver radiation directly to the cellular target; they produce durable responses in patients resistant to chemotherapy and unconjugated antibody.

---

[9]Burstein H J 2005 The distinctive nature of HER2-positive breast cancers. New England Journal of Medicine 353:1652–1654.
[10]Piccard-Gebhart M J, Procter M, Leyland-Jones B et al for the Herceptin Adjuvant (HERA) Trial Study Team 2005 Trastuzumab after adjuvant chemotherapy in HER2-positive breast cancer. New England Journal of Medicine 353:1659–1672.
[11]Romond E H, Perez E A, Bryant J et al 2005 Trastuzumab plus adjuvant chemotherapy for operable HER2-positive breast cancer. New England Journal of Medicine 353:1673–1684.

[12]The simplest form of an antigenic determinant, on a complex antigenic molecule, that can combine with antibody or T-cell receptor (*Stedman's Medical Dictionary*).

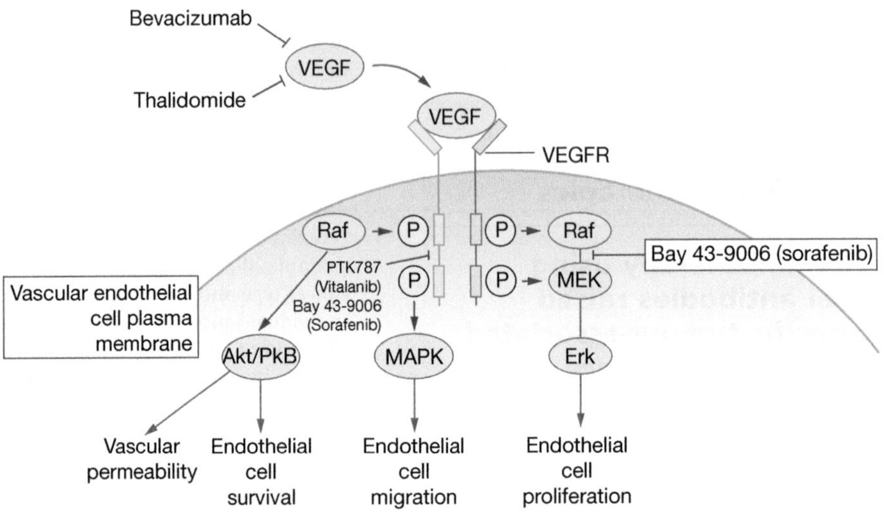

VEGF(R)	Vasculoendothelial growth factor (receptor)
PI3K	Phosphoinositide-3-kinase
Akt/PkB	Mitogen-activated protein kinase
Raf	Raf kinase
MEK	Mitogen and extracellular kinase
Erk	Extracellular receptor kinase

Fig. 31.2 Many new drugs target the vasculoendothelial growth factor (VEGF) pathway.

Chemo-immunotherapy

Monoclonal antibodies conjugated to toxins deliver high concentrations of agents that are too toxic to give systemically, e.g. CD33 plus calicheamicin (Gemtuzumab ozogamicin) in AML.

Most therapeutic antibodies are monoclonal immunoglobulin (Ig) G antibodies produced in mammalian cell lines by recombinant DNA technology. Genetic engineering alters the molecular structure of key immunogenic portions of the antibody to generate 'humanised' chimeric[13] antibodies that avoid rejection by the human immune system (but hypersensitivity reactions may occur) (see also drug-antibody conjugates, above).

Signal transduction inhibitors

Tyrosine kinase activation of cell surface receptors and their downstream proteins is an important mechanism by which messages are translated to the nucleus to affect cell function. A family of small molecules called *tyrosine kinase inhibitors* (TKIs) is now showing significant promise as anticancer agents. These small molecules are often orally administered.

[13]Composed of seemingly incompatible parts of different origin.

Multi-targeted kinase inhibitors are also attractive, as they may possess a wide spectrum of antitumour activity, but their potential for toxicity is a real concern.

- Imatinib (Glivec, Gleevec) blocks the dysregulated tyrosine kinase hyperactivity produced by the Philadelphia chromosome (bcr-abl) that occurs in chronic myeloid leukaemia and some cases of acute lymphoblastic leukaemia; clinical trials support its therapeutic efficacy. This is an important example of a drug designed precisely to address the biological abnormality that causes a disease. By serendipity, imatinib also blocks an oncogenelled c-kit (CD-117) and has now revolutionised treatment of a rare cancer called GIST (gastrointestinal stromal tumour) that hitherto had no known systemic treatment options (both chemotherapy and radiotherapy primary resistant), and frequently carries a c-kit mutation.
- Tyrosine kinase inhibitors of VEGF receptor and its downstream effector pathways are also in clinical trial (see Fig. 31.2 and Table 31.3).
- The EGFR tyrosine kinase inhibitors, gefitinib (Iressa) and erlotinib (Tarceva), now find use for a variety of EGFR-expressing tumours, specifically in lung cancer, that have a mutation in the *EGFR* gene, with marked benefit, although cure remains elusive.

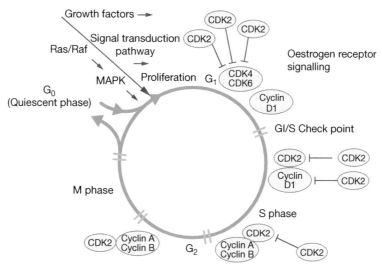

Fig. 31.3 The cell cycle is regulated by a series of proteins called cyclins, cyclin-dependent kinases (CDKs) and cyclin-dependent kinase inhibitors (CDKIs). Many CDKIs appear to be tumour-suppressing genes. These moieties are potential targets for anticancer therapy. MAPK, mitogen-activated protein kinase.

- The BRAF v600e mutation which occurs in many cancers, archetypically in melanoma, can be targeted with specific drugs and in combination with MEK inhibitors are used in a subset of melanomas to good effect, in an otherwise non-cytotoxic chemoresistant cancer.

Targeting the cell cycle

Recent advances in molecular biology have shown that the cell cycle is regulated by a series of proteins that include *cyclins, cyclin-dependent kinases* and *cyclin-dependent kinase inhibitors* (Fig. 31.3). Aberrations in these proteins are implicated in uncontrolled progression through the cell cycle (and hence in carcinogenesis), but also represent a new set of therapeutic targets for anticancer therapy; for example, rapamycin analogues, which inhibit mTor (mammalian target of rapamycin), another key regulator of cell cycle progression, are now used in renal and other cancers, and palbociclib, which inhibits CDK4/6, is used in advanced breast cancer. Arsenic trioxide modulates cell growth and differentiation, and induces remission in relapsed refractory acute promyelocytic leukaemia in part through apoptosis induction and down-regulation of *Bcl-2*.

Protease inhibition

The ubiquitin–proteasome pathway is an intracellular proteolytic system that degrades cyclins and cyclin-dependent kinase inhibitors which regulate cell-cycle progression. Bortezomib inhibits proteasome activity and, in myeloma, prevents degradation of nuclear factor κB inhibitor (IκB), resulting in a directly apoptotic effect, antiangiogenesis and inhibition of myeloma–stromal cell interaction. It has single-agent activity and restores chemosensitivity in resistant cells.

Chemoprevention of cancer

Because many cancers are currently incurable once metastasised, cancer prevention is a logical objective. Individuals can change aspects of their lifestyle significantly to influence their risk of developing particular cancers. Ceasing to smoke tobacco is an obvious health benefit. The individual benefits attributable to other changes are more difficult to quantify. The connection between environment and cancer risk is complex and as yet poorly understood, as genetic susceptibilities may obviate or accentuate certain risks.

Chemical interventions to reduce cancer risk may be an option for the population as a whole, or for groups at high risk of a specific cancer. Retrospective epidemiological and association studies suggest large effects of certain dietary manipulation, but prospective interventional studies have rarely been confirmatory and have even shown harm. The best example is supplemental vitamins, derivatives and dietary micronutrients that may inhibit the development of cancers in the laboratory, e.g. β-carotene, isotretinoin, folic acid, ascorbic acid, α-tocopherol. In a trial of antioxidant supplementation with ascorbic acid, vitamin E, β-carotene, selenium and zinc over 7.5 years, the total cancer incidence was lower in men (who had a lower baseline antioxidant status) than in women.[14] Subsequent large-scale randomised trials with supplementation have demonstrated the opposite effect with an unexpectedly *higher* incidence of new cancers.

The anti-oestrogen tamoxifen, used as an adjuvant therapy in women undergoing surgery for primary breast cancer, reduced the risk of cancer occurring in the contralateral breast. Tamoxifen and anastrozole (see above) are undergoing assessment for chemoprevention in women at high risk of breast cancer.

See also aspirin (p. 255).

Viral immunisation and cancer prevention

In cancers thought to have predominantly viral origins such as cervical cancer (HPV, human papilloma virus) and liver cancer (HCC, hepatocellular cancer) triggered by chronic hepatitis, vaccination against the viruses may have dramatic effects on the incidence of the cancers. The best example of this is HBV vaccination in childhood in Taiwan where the incidence of HCC in children and adolescents fell over 200-fold. More recently HPV vaccinations (such as Gardasil) have been approved, but as HPV is predominantly sexually transmitted, vaccinating pre-pubescent girls and boys (to generate herd immunity) is ethically challenging and may lead to poor uptake and cultural variations of acceptance worldwide.

Immunosuppression

Suppression of immune responses mediated via mononuclear cells (lymphocytes, plasma cells) is used in therapy of:

- autoimmune, collagen, connective tissue and inflammatory disorders including systemic lupus erythematosus, rheumatoid arthritis, chronic active hepatitis, inflammatory bowel disease, glomerulonephritis, nephrotic syndrome, some haemolytic anaemias and thrombocytopenias, uveitis, myasthenia gravis, polyarteritis, polymyositis, Behçet's syndrome
- organ or tissue transplantation: to prevent immune rejection
- cytotoxic cancer chemotherapeutic agents are immunosuppressive because they interfere with mononuclear cell multiplication and function. But they are generally too toxic for the above purposes, and the following are principally used for intended immunosuppression:
  - adrenocortical steroids
  - azathioprine (see below)
  - ciclosporin, tacrolimus (see below)
  - some alkylating agents: cyclophosphamide and chlorambucil (see Table 31.2)
  - antilymphocyte immunoglobulin (see below).

With the exception of *ciclosporin* and *tacrolimus*, all of the above cause non-specific immunosuppression, so that the general defences of the body against infection are impaired.

Adrenal steroids destroy lymphocytes, reduce inflammation and impair phagocytosis (see Ch. 35).

Cytotoxic agents destroy immunologically competent cells. *Azathioprine*, a pro-drug for the purine antagonist mercaptopurine, is used in autoimmune disease because it provides enhanced immunosuppressive activity. Cyclophosphamide is a second choice; it depresses bone marrow, as is to be expected.

Ciclosporin

Ciclosporin is a polypeptide obtained from a soil fungus. It acts selectively and reversibly by preventing the transcription of interleukin-2 and other lymphokine genes, thus inhibiting the production of lymphokines by T lymphocytes (that mediate specific recognition of alien molecules). Ciclosporin spares non-specific function, e.g. of granulocytes, which are responsible for phagocytosis and metabolism of foreign substances. It does not depress haematopoiesis.

Pharmacokinetics. Ciclosporin is about 40% absorbed from the gastrointestinal tract and is metabolised extensively in the liver, mainly by the cytochrome P450 3A system ($t_{1/2}$ 27 h).

Uses. Ciclosporin is used to prevent and treat rejection of organ transplants (kidney, liver, heart–lung) and bone marrow transplants. For organ transplants, treatment continues indefinitely and requires careful monitoring of plasma concentration and renal function. In patients who have received a bone marrow transplant, ciclosporin is

[14]Hercberg S, Galan P, Preziosi P et al 2004 Randomized, placebo-controlled trial of the health effects of antioxidant vitamins and minerals. Archives of Internal Medicine 164:2335–2342.

generally stopped after 6 months unless there is ongoing chronic graft-versus-host disease. It may be given orally or intravenously.

Ciclosporin can also be helpful in severe, resistant psoriasis in hospitalised patients.

Adverse reactions. Ciclosporin constricts the pre-glomerular afferent arteriole and reduces glomerular filtration; acute or chronic renal impairment may result if the trough plasma concentration consistently exceeds 250 mg/L. Generally, renal changes resolve when the drug is withdrawn. Hypertension develops in about 50% of patients, more commonly when a corticosteroid is co-administered but possibly due in part to the mineralocorticoid action of ciclosporin. The blood pressure is controlled by standard antihypertensive therapy without the need to discontinue ciclosporin. Other adverse effects include gastrointestinal reactions, hepatotoxicity, hyperkalaemia, hypertrichosis, gingival hypertrophy, convulsions and, rarely, the clinical syndrome of thrombotic thrombocytopenic purpura.

Interactions. The plasma concentration of ciclosporin, and risk of toxicity, is increased by drugs including ketoconazole, erythromycin, chloroquine, cimetidine, oral contraceptives, anabolic steroids and calcium channel antagonists. Grapefruit juice also increases plasma ciclosporin concentrations (flavonoids in the juice inhibit the cytochrome that metabolises ciclosporin). Drugs that reduce the plasma concentration of ciclosporin, risking loss of effect, include enzyme-inducing antiepileptics, e.g. phenytoin, carbamazepine, phenobarbital and rifampicin. Inherently nephrotoxic drugs add to the risk of renal damage with ciclosporin, e.g. aminoglycoside antibiotics, amphotericin, NSAIDs (diclofenac). Potassium-sparing diuretics add to the risk of hyperkalaemia.

Tacrolimus

Tacrolimus is a macrolide immunosuppressant agent that is isolated from a bacterium. It acts like ciclosporin, and is used to protect and treat liver and kidney grafts when conventional immunosuppressants fail. Such rescue treatment may be graft- or life-saving. Tacrolimus can cause nephrotoxicity, neurotoxicity, disturbance of glucose metabolism, hyperkalaemia and hypertrophic cardiomyopathy.

Antilymphocyte immunoglobulin

Antilymphocyte [thymocyte] immunoglobulin (ALG) is used in organ graft rejection, a process in which lymphocytes are involved. It is made by preparing antisera to human lymphocytes in animals (horses or rabbits), and allergic reactions are common. ALG largely spares the patient's response to infection. It is also used to treat severe aplastic anaemia,

frequently producing a good partial response either as a single agent or in combination with ciclosporin. ALG is the treatment of choice for patients with severe aplastic anaemia for whom no bone marrow donor is available or who are too old or unfit for a bone marrow transplant.

Mycophenolate

Mycophenolate selectively blocks the proliferation of T and B lymphocytes and acts like azathioprine; it is being evaluated in combination immunosuppressive regimens for organ transplantation.

Hazards of immunosuppressive drugs

Impaired immune responses render the subject more liable to bacterial, viral and fungal infections. Treat all infection early and vigorously (using bactericidal drugs where practicable); use human γ-globulin to protect when there is exposure to virus infections, e.g. measles, varicella. Patients who have not had chickenpox and are receiving therapeutic (as opposed to replacement) doses of corticosteroid are at risk of severe chickenpox; they should receive varicella zoster immunoglobulin if there has been contact with the disease within the previous 3 months and in some cases prophylactic antivirals such as aciclovir (see p. 221).

Carcinogenicity is a hazard, generally after 4–7 years of therapy. The cancers most likely to occur, like second new primary cancers discussed earlier, have a propensity to be virally driven (leukaemia, lymphoma, skin). Cytotoxic use creates the additional hazard of mutagenicity, which may induce cancer. *Hazards* include those of long-term corticosteroid therapy, and of cytotoxics in general (bone marrow depression, infertility and teratogenesis). Although such hazards may be justifiable to the patient who has life-endangering disease, there is more cause for concern when immunosuppressive regimens are an option in younger patients with a less serious disorder, e.g. rheumatoid arthritis, ulcerative colitis.

Active immunisation during immunosuppressive therapy

Response to non-living antigens (tetanus, typhoid, poliomyelitis) is diminished, and giving one or two extra doses may be wise. *Living vaccines are contraindicated* in patients who are immunosuppressed by drug therapy or indeed by disease (AIDS, leukaemia, lymphoma), as there is a risk of serious generalised infection.

Guide to further reading

A useful general account by several authors covering all aspects of understanding cancer therapy appears in Medicine 32, 1–37.

Arribas, J., 2005. Matrix metalloproteases and tumor invasion. N. Engl. J. Med. 352, 2020–2021.

El-Shanawany, T., Sewell, W.A.C., Misbah, S.A., Jolles, S., 2006. Current uses of intravenous immunoglobulin. Clin. Med. (Northfield Il) 6, 356–359.

Greenwald, P., 2002. Cancer chemoprevention. Br. Med. J. 324, 714–718.

Kaur, R., 2005. Breast cancer: personal account. Lancet 365, 1742.

Khan, S., Sewell, W.A.C., 2006. Oral immunosuppressive drugs. Clin. Med. (Northfield Il) 6, 252–355.

Koon, H., Atkins, M., 2006. Autoimmunity and immuno-therapy for cancer. N. Engl. J. Med. 354, 758–760.

Krause, D.S., Van Etten, R.A., 2005. Tyrosine kinase as targets for cancer therapy. N. Engl. J. Med. 353, 172–187.

Renehan, A.G., Booth, C., Potten, C.S., 2001. What is apoptosis, and why is it important? Br. Med. J. 322, 1536–1538.

Roodman, G.D., 2004. Mechanisms of bone metastasis. N. Engl. J. Med. 350, 1655–1664.

Rosenberg, S.A., Yang, J.C., Restifo, N.P., et al., 2004. Cancer immunotherapy: moving beyond current vaccines. Nat. Med. 10, 909–915.

Saachi, M., 2013. How can an act of parliament cure cancer? J. R. Soc. Med. 106, 169–172.

Veronesi, U., Boyle, P., Goldhirsch, A., et al., 2005. Breast cancer. Lancet 365, 1727–1741.

Wooster, R., Weber, B., 2003. Breast and ovarian cancer. N. Engl. J. Med. 348, 2339–2347.

Section | 7 |

Gastrointestinal system

Chapter | **32** |

Oesophagus, stomach and duodenum

Devinder Singh Bansi, Charlotte Hateley, John Louis-Auguste

SYNOPSIS

'Dyspepsia' is a non-specific term which encompasses a number of symptoms attributable to the upper gastrointestinal (GI) tract, and may include anything from acid reflux to abdominal bloating. Approximately one-third of the population in Western societies experiences regular dyspepsia, although the majority self-medicate with over-the-counter anti-acid preparations and do not seek medical advice. Up to 50% of those who do will have demonstrable pathology, most commonly gastro-oesophageal reflux or peptic ulceration. The remainder, in whom no abnormality is found, are diagnosed as having non-ulcer dyspepsia. Finally, nausea and vomiting are deeply unpleasant sensations with a number of causes and, fortunately, a number of effective therapies.

The oesophagus in health and disease

The normal oesophagus effortlessly transfers food and drink from the benign environment of the mouth through the gate of the lower oesophageal sphincter into the harsh acidic environment of the stomach. Transient gastro-oesophageal reflux occurs in almost everybody, and problems develop only when episodes become frequent, with prolonged exposure of the oesophageal mucosa to acid and pepsin.

The physiological lower oesophageal sphincter (LOS), normally located at the gastro-oesophageal junction at the level of the diaphragm, allows solid and liquid boluses to pass into the stomach while preventing acidic gastric contents refluxing into the oesophagus. Intrinsic tonic contraction of the LOS is interrupted by normal transient lower oesophageal relaxation as well as coordinated relaxation when swallowing is initiated. Numerous neurohumoral intermediaries are involved in these processes, including parasympathetic efferents, acetylcholine (Ach), γ-aminobutyric acid (GABA) and glutamate. The integrity of the sphincter can be compromised by the presence of a hiatus hernia, which disrupts its anatomical and physiological components.

Excessive or inappropriate relaxation of the LOS results in gastro-oesophageal reflux disease, oesophagitis and oesophageal ulceration, stricturing resulting in mechanical obstruction and sometimes a secondary oesophageal dysmotility and spasm. Reduced oesophageal clearance of acid may also contribute. In susceptible individuals, acid reflux triggers columnar metaplasia of the native squamous epithelium (also known as Barrett's oesophagus). This is a pre-malignant condition for oesophageal adenocarcinoma.

Oesophageal dysmotility tends to produce symptoms of dysphagia to both solids and liquids, as opposed to mechanical obstruction which results in dysphagia to solids unless very advanced. A high sphincter tone and uncoordinated oesophageal contractions can cause dysphagia and pain. Achalasia is a motility disorder of unknown aetiology characterised by oesophageal hypomotility, a hypertonic LOS and a failure of relaxation of the LOS.

Gastric acid secretion and mucosal protection

In the normal upper GI tract, the destructive effects of gastric hydrochloric acid are balanced by a variety of mucosal protective mechanisms. Duodenal and gastric ulceration results from an imbalance between these two opposing forces. *Helicobacter pylori* infection and use of non-steroidal anti-inflammatory drugs (NSAIDs) play an important role in upsetting this fine balance. Other digestive enzymes such as pepsinogen/pepsin also contribute to the gastric phase of digestion but are qualitatively of less importance.

Gastric acid secretion

Acid secretion by parietal cells in the gastric mucosa is regulated by four main neurohumoral mediators.

Gastrin

Gastrin is a peptide hormone secreted by neuroendocrine G cells in response to a variety of physical and neurohumoral stimuli such as gastric distension, the presence of amino acids, vagal stimulation and histamine. Gastrin passes into the portal circulation, where it activates gastrin receptors on the basolateral aspect of the parietal cell, stimulating acid secretion. This inhibits further gastrin release. Gastrin also stimulates histamine release from enterochromaffin-like cells (ECL) cells (see below).

Acetylcholine (ACh)

ACh, secreted by parasympathetic vagal efferents, activates muscarinic M_3 receptors on parietal cells and also on mast cell–like histamine-secreting cells in the gastric mucosa. Both of these actions result in acid secretion.

Histamine

Histamine is secreted by enterochromaffin-like cells (mast cell–like cells in the gastric mucosa) at a basal rate, and secretion is augmented by gastrin and ACh from parasympathetic stimulation. Histamine secreted into the portal circulation stimulates H_2 receptors on parietal cells, promoting acid secretion.

Prostaglandins

Locally produced *prostaglandins E2 and I2* inhibit parietal cell acid secretion. Prostaglandins are produced by the cyclo-oxygenase enzyme. In the stomach, these prostaglandins are produced by the constitutively expressed COX-1 enzyme isoform.

The parietal cell integrates these pro- and anti-secretory signals. The final common pathway for acid secretion is the H^+/K^+-ATPase (the 'proton pump') located on the apical aspect of the parietal cell, which secretes hydrogen ions into the gastric lumen.

Mucosal protective mechanisms

Mucus and bicarbonate are secreted by cells in the gastric and duodenal mucosa and provide a protective relatively alkaline physical barrier against the otherwise destructive intragastric environment. Secretion is promoted by prostaglandins, which also inhibit gastric acid secretion. Numerous lifestyle factors adversely affect the mucosal barrier, including smoking and alcohol.

Helicobacter pylori (*H. pylori*): an occasionally silent killer

It is now known that a large majority of benign gastric and duodenal ulceration is due to *H. pylori* infection (following Marshall and Warren's Nobel prize–winning experiments[1,2]); most of the remainder can be attributed to NSAID use. Colonisation of the stomach with *H. pylori* is seen in virtually all patients with a duodenal ulcer and in 70–80% of those with gastric ulcers. *H. pylori* appears to stimulate increased acid secretion. All patients colonised with *H. pylori* develop gastritis, but only about 20% have ulcers or other lesions. As yet, incompletely understood host factors and differences in strain of the organism are likely to explain this discrepancy.

H. pylori infection is carcinogenic and is the leading cause of gastric carcinoma. It is also highly associated with gastric MALT lymphoma.[3] Eradication of the organism can lead to regression and even resolution of this latter malignancy.

Somewhat counterintuitively, *H. pylori* infection is not a cause of acid reflux disease, and in fact its eradication may precipitate or exacerbate acid reflux. Indeed, the recent surge in oeosphageal adenocarcinoma incidence in the West has been blamed by many on the now commonplace practice of searching for and eradicating *H. pylori*, although this has conversely resulted in a fall in the incidence of gastric cancer.

NSAIDs: enemies of the gut

Some 500 million prescriptions for NSAIDs are written each year in the UK, and 10–15% of patients develop dyspepsia while taking these drugs. Gastric erosions develop in up to 80%, but these are usually self-limiting. Gastric or duodenal ulcers occur in 1–5%. The incidence increases sharply in

[1]Marshall B J, Warren J R 1984 Unidentified curved bacillis in the stomach of patients with gastritis and peptic ulceration. Lancet i:1311–1315. (Marshall deliberately infected himself by drinking a solution swimming with the bacterium, as part of a successful and widely reported experiment to prove Koch's postulates.)
[2]Pincock S 2005 Nobel Prize winners Robin Warren and Barry Marshall. Lancet 366:1429.
[3]Mucosa-Associated Lymphoid Tissue.

those older than 60 years of age, and the risk of ulcers and their complications is doubled in patients older than 75 years of age and those with cardiac failure or a history of peptic ulceration or bleeding. All NSAIDs are ulcerogenic, but ibuprofen is less prone to cause these problems than other non-selective NSAIDs.

NSAIDs are weak organic acids, and the acid milieu of the stomach facilitates their non-ionic diffusion into gastric mucosal cells. Here the neutral intracellular pH causes the drugs to become ionised and trapped in the mucosa because they cannot diffuse out in this form.

Aspirin and the other NSAIDs inhibit cyclo-oxygenase (COX) (see Ch. 16). In the stomach, the constitutively expressed COX-1 isoform is responsible for the production of the gastroprotective prostaglandins E2 and I2 (see above). Inhibition of the inducible COX-2 isoform (which is normally up-regulated in activated inflammatory cells) is responsible for NSAIDs' anti-inflammatory properties. Most NSAIDs inhibit both isoforms unselectively, so the beneficial anti-inflammatory effect is offset by the potential for mucosal injury by depletion of protective prostaglandins. Aspirin is particularly potent in this respect, perhaps because it inhibits COX irreversibly, unlike the other NSAIDs, where inhibition is reversible and concentration dependent.

Selective COX-2 inhibitors represent an attempt to provide beneficial anti-inflammatory effects without promoting ulceration. Unfortunately, there is evidence that unopposed COX-2 inhibition results in an increased risk of thrombotic events (including myocardial infarction and stroke); the UK Committee on Safety of Medicines therefore counsels against their use in preference to non-selective NSAIDs in the absence of a compelling indication, and cardiovascular risk should be assessed.

Drugs affecting oesophageal motility and the lower oesophageal sphincter

The D$_2$ agonist drugs *domperidone* and *metoclopramide* (see below) can have a beneficial effect on reflux symptoms, firstly by enhancing gastric emptying and thus reducing the volume of acid available to reflux up the oesophagus, and secondly by increasing lower oesophageal sphincter (LOS) basal tone.

A number of drugs reduce tonic lower oesophageal sphincter tone or increase transient lower oesophageal sphincter relaxation and thus promote reflux, including *nitrates, theophyllines,* drugs with *antimuscarinic* activity or unwanted effects, and *calcium channel antagonists*. The pharmacology and pharmocokinetics of these drugs appear in detail elsewhere (see Index). These agents may occasionally

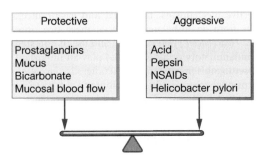

Fig. 32.1 Secretion of acid by the parietal cell.

be useful in alleviating the symptoms of oesophageal spasm, although the effect is usually disappointing. They are rarely potent enough to be of significant use in achalasia. Commonly used examples include *nifedipine, diltiazem,* and *modified-release nitrates*.

Newer therapies being explored in the treatment of GORD[4] include GABA inhibition to reduce transient lower oesophageal sphincter relaxations. *Baclofen* (see p. 317) is clinically effective but has limiting CNS unwanted effects, and more tolerable compounds are being investigated. Other pharmacological targets which are showing potential in early clinical research include *cannabinoid agonists*.

Drugs to reduce or neutralise gastric acid

Proton pump inhibitors (PPIs)

Pharmacology. As can be deduced from the above, the most effective site of action for antisecretory drugs is the proton pump. Proton pump inhibitors are taken up by parietal cells from the portal circulation and are then excreted into the acid milieu around the secretory canaliculus. The resulting ionised form binds irreversibly to the proton pump, resulting in virtual total inhibition of acid secretion (Fig. 32.1).

Pharmacokinetics. PPIs are available in oral and intravenous formulations. Oral PPIs are degraded at low pH and must be given in enteric-coated forms. Systemic availability increases with dose and also with time, owing to decreased inactivation of the prodrug as gastric acidity is reduced. Maximum efficacy occurs after up to 5 days of therapy. Uninhibited Na$^+$/K$^+$-ATPase will regenerate when the PPI is discontinued; this may take 2–3 days.

---

[4]Gastro-Oesophageal Reflux Disease.

Adverse reactions and interactions. PPIs are as a rule well tolerated, and serious adverse effects are unusual. Given their mechanism of action, there are theoretical concerns about cancer (due to the stimulatory effect of the hypergastrinaemia resulting from the loss of negative feedback), mineral deficiencies (due to loss of acid-related absorption of iron, calcium and B_{12}, for example) and enteric infections (due to the loss of the antibacterial properties of a strongly acidic environment). Although an increased incidence of osteoporotic fractures and *Clostridium difficile (C. diff)* colitis has been noted in some observational studies, there has been no good evidence that these risks are significant, even after almost 20 years of clinical experience.

Examples of PPIs are *omeprazole* (10–20 mg daily), *lansoprazole* (15–30 mg daily) and *pantoprazole*. All are similar in pharmacokinetics, efficacy and adverse-effect profile.

H_2-receptor antagonists (H_2RAs)

Pharmacology. H_2RAs are less potent than the PPIs, as alternative pathways of parietal cell activation remain uninhibited. They competitively inhibit histamine binding at H_2 receptors on the basolateral aspect of parietal cells, resulting in a reduction of gastric acid secretion. The inhibitory effect can be overcome with high gastrin levels, as occurs postprandially. Tolerance may develop, probably due to down-regulation of receptors.

Pharmacokinetics and dosage. H_2RAs are given orally and are well absorbed. Since there is anecdotal evidence that peptic ulcer healing with H_2-receptor antagonists correlates best with suppression of *nocturnal* acid secretion, many prefer to give these drugs as a single evening dose (e.g. ranitidine 150–300 mg).

Adverse effects and interactions. H_2RAs are generally well tolerated. Adverse effects and interactions are few with short-term use. *Cimetidine* is a weak anti-androgen, and may cause gynaecomastia and sexual dysfunction in males. Cimetidine inhibits cytochrome P450, and there is potential for increased effect from any drug with a low therapeutic index that is inactivated by these isoenzymes, e.g. warfarin, phenytoin. *Ranitidine* and *famotidine* avoid these unwanted effects.

H_2RAs are available as over-the-counter preparations in the UK, albeit of lower strength than those available on prescription. A potential danger is that patients with serious pathology such as gastric carcinoma will self-medicate, allowing their disease to progress. Pharmacists are trained to advise patients to consult their doctor if they have recurrent symptoms or other worrying manifestations such as weight loss.

Antacids

Antacids directly neutralise secreted acid and raise intragastric pH. They protect the gastric mucosa against acid (by neutralisation) and pepsin (which is inactive above pH 5, and which in addition is inactivated by aluminium and magnesium). Most commonly they are *magnesium or aluminium salts*. The hydroxide is the most common base, but trisilicate, carbonate and bicarbonate are also used.

Antacids relieve mild dyspeptic symptoms, and they are taken intermittently when symptoms occur. Unwanted effects and inconvenience (see below) limit their regular use.

Individual antacids

Numerous antacid preparations are available over the counter. Some of the more common are described here.

Sodium bicarbonate reacts with acid and relieves pain within minutes. It is absorbed and causes a metabolic alkalosis. This is not of clinical significance if used on an intermittent, short-term basis, but if given regularly over a period of time (days to weeks or longer) or in large doses will result in a potentially dangerous metabolic alkalosis. Sodium bicarbonate can release sufficient carbon dioxide in the stomach to cause discomfort and belching, which may have a beneficial psychotherapeutic effect.

Magnesium oxide and hydroxide react quickly, and *magnesium trisilicate* more slowly with gastric hydrochloric acid. All magnesium salts cause an osmotic diarrhoea.

Aluminium hydroxide reacts with hydrochloric acid to form aluminium chloride; this in turn reacts with intestinal secretions to produce insoluble salts, especially phosphate. It tends to constipate.

Some antacid mixtures contain *sodium*, which may not be readily apparent from the name of the preparation and thus may be dangerous for patients with cardiac, renal or liver disease. For example, a 10-mL dose of magnesium carbonate mixture or of magnesium trisilicate mixture contains about 6 mmol sodium (normal daily dietary intake is approximately 120 mmol sodium).

Aluminium- and *magnesium*-containing antacids may interfere with the absorption of other drugs by binding with them or by altering gastrointestinal pH or transit time. It is probably advisable not to co-administer antacids with drugs that are intended for systemic effect by the oral route.

Other targets for acid suppression

Gastrin inhibitors exist as experimental tools only as they are not effective acid suppressants. Antimuscarinic treatments for peptic ulceration are obsolete, but underlie the rationale for the surgical vagotomy which is now rarely performed.

Drugs to enhance mucosal protection

Sucralfate (SUCRose sulFATE and ALuminium hydroxide complex)

Sucralfate provides a physical barrier to gastric acid. It is activated by acid to produce a viscous gel, and will therefore be ineffective if given with therapies that inhibit acid release or raise gastric pH. In the acid environment of the stomach, the aluminium moiety is released so that the compound develops a strong negative charge and binds to positively charged protein molecules that transude from damaged mucosa. The result is a viscous paste that adheres selectively and protectively to the ulcer base. It also binds to and inactivates pepsin and bile acids, which has the added benefit of reducing mucus degradation. Its therapeutic efficacy in healing gastric and duodenal ulcers is approximately equal to that of the histamine H_2-receptor antagonists.

Adverse effects and interactions. Sucralfate may cause constipation but is otherwise well tolerated. The concentration of aluminium in the plasma may be raised, but this appears to be a problem only with long-term use by uraemic patients, especially those undergoing chronic intermittent haemodialysis. As the sucralfate is effective only in acid conditions, an antacid should not be taken 30 min before or after a dose. Sucralfate interferes with absorption of several drugs, including ciprofloxacin, theophylline, digoxin, phenytoin and amitriptyline, possibly by binding due to its strong negative charge.

Bismuth chelate (tripotassium dicitratobismuthate, bismuth sub-citrate)

This substance was thought to act by chelating with protein in the ulcer base to form a protective coating against adverse influences of acid, pepsin and bile. It may also promote protective prostaglandin, mucus and bicarbonate synthesis. Probably more importantly, bismuth chelate is now known to suppress *H. pylori* growth, especially when combined with an antimicrobial (see below). Bismuth chelate finds use for benign gastric and duodenal ulcer, and has a therapeutic efficacy approximately equivalent to that of histamine H_2-receptor antagonists. Ulcers remain healed for a longer time after bismuth chelate than after H_2-receptor antagonists, probably due to its ability to eradicate *H. pylori*.

Adverse effects. Bismuth chelate, particularly as a liquid formulation, darkens the tongue, teeth and stool; the effect is less likely with the tablet, which is thus more acceptable. Systemic absorption of bismuth from the chelated preparation is small, but it does pass into the urine, and it is prudent to avoid the drug for patients with impaired renal function. Urinary elimination continues for months after bismuth is discontinued. Bismuth toxicity causes encephalopathy.

Misoprostol

Misoprostol is a synthetic analogue of the protective prostaglandin E1 and therefore has the same antisecretory and cytoprotective properties. Traditionally it has been co-administered with NSAIDs to counteract the latter's effects on endogenous prostaglandin synthesis.

Adverse effects. Diarrhoea and abdominal pain, transient and dose related, are the commonest. Women may experience gynaecological disturbances such as vaginal spotting and dysmenorrhoea; the drug is *contraindicated* in pregnancy or for women planning to become pregnant, as the products of conception may be aborted. Indeed, women have resorted to using misoprostol (illicitly) as an abortifacient in parts of the world where provision of contraceptive services is poor.

Alginate

Alginate is a common and harmless component of antacids. It forms a viscous raft which forms a physical barrier between the gastric contents and the oesophageal, gastric and duodenal mucosa.

Pharmacological management

Gastro-oesophageal reflux

Lifestyle modification includes reduction in habits that promote acid reflux. Caffeine, alcohol, smoking and obesity relax the lower oesophageal sphincter and should be substituted or discontinued if possible. Avoid late evening meals to allow time for the stomach to empty before lying supine. Minor occasional symptoms are effectively managed with over-the-counter alginate-containing antacids.

The mainstay of medical treatment of acid reflux disease is the neutralisation or reduction of gastric acid production, and is therefore most easily achieved with PPIs, although H_2RAs (e.g. ranitidine 150–300 mg daily) may be sufficient. Endoscopically proven oesophagitis may require 4–6 weeks of PPI therapy to heal (e.g. omeprazole 20 mg once daily; lansoprazole 30 mg once daily). If symptoms recur, the lowest effective antacid dose should be used to maintain remission. Doses may need to be doubled in severe or refractory cases. Prokinetic drugs such as domperidone 10–20 mg four times daily or metoclopramide 10 mg three times daily can improve symptoms, best in conjunction with an antisecretory agent.

Gastric lumen

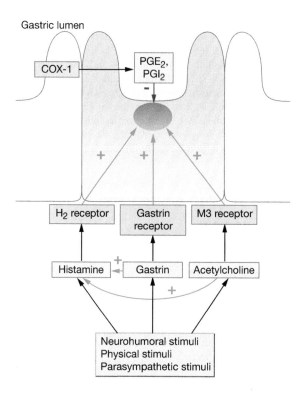

Fig. 32.2 Factors involved in pathogenesis of peptic ulcer.

Reflux-like symptoms unresponsive to PPI therapy are unlikely to be due to acid reflux, and alternative causes require exploration. Biliary reflux can produce identical symptoms to acid reflux, and is unresponsive to PPI therapy due to its alkaline nature. It may respond to prokinetic therapy.

Eosinophilic oesophagitis

This is increasingly recognised as an important cause of oesophageal symptoms. It is a disorder of unknown aetiology characterised by substantial eosinophilic submucosal infiltrates in the absence of significant acid reflux and may be associated with other atopic conditions. Treatment options are limited, but topically applied corticosteroids (e.g. swallowing inhaled steroids) can be helpful in inducing and maintaining remission.

Oesophageal dysmotility

This can be notoriously difficult to treat satisfactorily. Prokinetic drugs can be tried in cases of confirmed oesophageal hypomotility; conversely, a calcium channel antagonist or a long-acting nitrate can be tried if the problem is predominantly one of spasm. Treatment of coexistent reflux may improve spasm secondary to reflux.

Pharmacological management of achalasia[5] is best viewed as a temporary measure, and drugs which reduce LOS tone rarely provide effective symptomatic improvement. Botulinum toxin, which inhibits cholinergic transmission by reducing ACh release from pre-synaptic motor neurones (see Ch. 22), can be injected endoscopically into the LOS and results in medium-term (3–6 months) relaxation of the LOS and symptomatic improvement. Endoscopic dilatation or surgical correction results in longer-term improvement. Relaxation of the LOS results in potentially free reflux of gastric acid contents and must therefore be accompanied by a PPI.

Peptic ulceration (Fig. 32.2)

For years, the treatment of peptic ulceration centred around measures to neutralise gastric acid, to inhibit its secretion or to enhance mucosal defences, but recognition of the central role of *H. pylori* revolutionised the approach.

Haemorrhage is one of the feared complications of peptic ulceration. The treatment of choice is endoscopic therapy, but PPIs, usually given as an intravenous infusion for 72 h to guarantee high and constant plasma levels, have a role as an adjunctive treatment. Reduction of gastric acid and raising of gastric pH results in clot stabilisation, thus promoting haemostasis.

Treatment of *H. pylori*

Consider *H. pylori* infection in all cases of peptic ulceration, as ulcer healing will be only transient if the organism remains. Indeed, eradication of *H. pylori* alone is generally sufficient to allow ulcer healing but is usually combined with a course of PPI therapy. Highly effective eradication regimens consist of a 1–2-week course of two antibiotics (typically amoxicillin with clarithromycin or clarithromycin with metronidazole) combined with a PPI. Treatment failures occur in approximately 5%, requiring more prolonged and complex regimens, usually containing bismuth chelate, although numerous antibacterial regimens have been shown to be effective.

Use of NSAIDs

If NSAID use is unavoidable in patients at high risk of developing serious side-effects, the risk of gastrotoxicity is reduced by about 40% with the co-administration of a PPI or misoprostol, although PPIs tend to be better tolerated.

---

[5]Characterised by incomplete relaxation of the lower oesophageal sphincter (LOS), increased LOS tone, *lack of peristalsis* in the oesophagus and consequent inability of smooth muscle to move food down the oesophagus.

H_2RAs do not offer effective protection against peptic ulceration in this scenario.

The use of COX-2–selective NSAIDs is limited by an increased incidence of adverse cardiovascular effects; furthermore, the risk of gastrointestinal complications with a coxib alone is similar to that of a non-selective NSAID with a PPI. Although the use of COX-2 inhibitors is associated with a lower rate of unwanted gastrointestinal effects in the short term, the risk remains significantly greater than that with placebo. Concomitant use of aspirin negates the beneficial effect.

Ironically, there is increasing evidence that aspirin may reduce the incidence of adenocarcinoma in cases of Barrett's oesophagus. Clinical trials are assessing the risk/benefit ratio of this treatment.

Other disorders of acid secretion

The Zollinger–Ellison syndrome is a rare disorder due to a gastrin-secreting tumour which may arise anywhere in the GI tract, but most commonly in the pancreas, duodenum or stomach. High levels of serum gastrin cause hyperstimulation of parietal cells and hypersecretion of gastric acid, leading to multiple gastric and small bowel ulcers. Very high doses of PPI, up to 120 mg of omeprazole or greater per day, may be required to counteract this.

Nausea and vomiting

The physiology of nausea and vomiting is complex and incompletely understood. Vomiting can be protective, e.g. when it expels toxins (such as food poisoning and alcohol) from the GI tract. Suppressing nausea and vomiting is important in the management of other conditions including chemotherapy, general anaesthesia, morning sickness of pregnancy and when it accompanies other disease states (e.g. cardiac ischaemia, migraine).[6]

---

[6]The pharmacology of vomiting was little studied until the world war of 1939–1945, when motion sickness attained military importance as a possible handicap for sea landings made in the face of resistance. The British military authorities and the Medical Research Council therefore organised an investigation. Whenever there was a prospect of sufficiently rough weather, about 70 soldiers were sent to sea in small ships, again and again, after being dosed with a drug or a dummy tablet and having their mouths inspected to detect non-compliance. The ships returned to land, when up to 40% of the soldiers vomited. 'On the whole the men enjoyed their trips'; some of them, however, being soldiers, thought the tablets were given in order to make them vomit, and some 'believed firmly in the efficacy of the dummy tablets'. It was concluded that, of the remedies tested, the antimuscarinic drug hyoscine was the most effective. Holling H E, McArdle B, Trotter W R 1944 Prevention of seasickness by drugs. Lancet i:127.

A number of stimuli are integrated in the chemoreceptor trigger zone (CTZ) and vomiting centre located in the floor of the fourth ventricle, including blood-borne molecules (especially toxins, peptides and drugs), sensory and psychological stimulation from higher centres, physical signals such as distension from the stomach and GI tract, other autonomic inputs, and vestibular feedback. Implicated neurotransmitter mediators include ACh (acting on muscarinic receptors), HA (H_1 receptors), DA (D_2 receptors), 5-HT (5-HT_3 receptors) and Substance P (NK_1 receptors).

Drugs used in nausea and vomiting

Antimuscarinics

Hyoscine is still the most common drug of its class used as an antiemetic. It suffers from all the unwanted effects of antimuscarinic agents.

H_1-receptor antagonists

Examples include *cyclizine, promethazine* and *cinnarizine*. They do not have significant action at the CTZ. Drowsiness is a significant side-effect.

D_2-receptor antagonists

These include the *phenothiazines,* also used as antipsychotics, such as chlorpromazine and haloperidol. They are powerful antiemetics but have relatively common and significant CNS side-effects including drowsiness and extrapyramidal movement disorders. Their pharmacology is discussed in detail in Chapter 20.

Metoclopramide and *domperidone* are D_2-receptor antagonists without antipsychotic activity which have prokinetic properties, which can augment their antiemetic effect. They act *centrally* by blocking dopamine D_2 receptors in the CTZ, and metoclopramide also acts *peripherally* by enhancing the action of acetylcholine at muscarinic nerve endings in the gut. They raise the tone of the lower oesophageal sphincter, relax the pyloric antrum and duodenal cap, and increase peristalsis and emptying of the upper gut. The peripheral actions are utilised to empty the stomach before emergency anaesthesia and in labour. Metoclopramide can cause the same side-effects as the phenothiazines. Domperidone does not readily cross the blood–brain barrier and consequently has fewer CNS effects.

5-HT_3-receptor antagonists

Drugs such as ondansetron are powerful and well tolerated agents which act at the CTZ.

Corticosteroids

Corticosteroids are particularly useful in chemotherapy-associated nausea and vomiting. Their mechanism of action is unclear.

Newer therapies, at present only licensed in the context of chemotherapy-associated symptoms, include the cannabinoid receptor agonist *nabilone* and the neurokinin-1 antagonist *aprepitant*.

Choice of antiemetic

Muscarinic and H_1 antagonists and the D_2 antagonists domperidone and metoclopramide are useful for general use, including motion sickness. Promethazine is used frequently to treat morning sickness.

The 5-HT3 antagonists can be used in cases unresponsive to these first-line therapies, and are particularly useful in postoperative nausea and vomiting.

Corticosteroids are used primarily in the context of chemotherapy-associated nausea and vomiting, either alone or in conjunction with one or more of drugs such as a phenothiazine, 5-HT₃ antagonist, nabilone or aprepitant.

Non-ulcer dyspepsia and functional disorders

Up to one-third of patients presenting to secondary care with dyspeptic symptoms have no pathological cause identified and have 'non-ulcer dyspepsia'. Management of these patients can be challenging and requires a comprehensive approach. Many patients with non-ulcer dyspepsia have abnormalities of gastric emptying and increased pain perception in the gastrointestinal tract, suggesting that the condition is part of the spectrum of irritable bowel syndrome (see Ch. 33).

Acid-predominant symptoms such as heartburn and epigastric discomfort may respond to anti-acid or anti-secretory therapy. Although a minority of patients may respond to *H. pylori* eradication, there is no evidence that there is a causative link, and the response rate is not greater than that seen with placebo.

The sensation of bloating is poorly understood but may involve visceral afferent hypersensitivity and hypomotility. Motility-predominant symptoms such as bloating may respond to prokinetic drugs. Antispasmodics such as peppermint oil can help, as can low-dose tricyclic antidepressants, as for neuropathic pain.

Guide to further reading

Armstrong, D., Sifrim, D., 2010. New pharmacologic approaches in gastroesophageal reflux disease. Gastroenterol. Clin. North Am. 39, 393–418.

Camilleri, M., Tack, J.F., 2010. Current medical treatments of dyspepsia and irritable bowel syndrome. Gastroenterol. Clin. North Am. 39, 481–493.

McColl, K.E., 2010. *Helicobacter pylori* infection. N. Engl. J. Med. 362, 1597–1604.

Moayyedi, P., Talley, N., 2006. Gastro-oesophageal reflux disease. Lancet 367, 2086–2100.

National Institute for Health and Clinical Excellence (NICE), 2004. Dyspepsia: Managing dyspepsia in adults in primary care. NICE, London.

Richter, J.E., 2001. Oesophageal motility disorders. Lancet 358, 823–828.

Rotherberg, M.E., 2009. Biology and treatment of eosinophilic esophagitis. Gastroenterology 137, 1238–1249.

White, P.F., 2004. Prevention of postoperative nausea and vomiting – a multimodal solution to a persistent problem. N. Engl. J. Med. 350, 2511–2515.

Yang, Y.X., Metz, D.C., 2010. Safety of proton pump inhibitor exposure. Gastroenterology 139, 1115–1127.

Chapter 33

Intestines

Devinder Singh Bansi, Charlotte Hateley, John Louis-Auguste

SYNOPSIS

Problems of constipation, diarrhoea and irritable bowel syndrome are extremely common. Worldwide, infective diarrhoeal diseases are the third leading cause of death, a result of fluid, electrolyte and nutrient depletion. Around 1.5 million children younger than 5 years of age die due to diarrhoea, almost exclusively in the developing world. Up to 20% of the UK population are affected by chronic intestinal symptoms, although the majority of these do not seek medical attention. Management of the following conditions is reviewed.

- Diarrhoea (drug treatment, importance of fluid and electrolyte replacement).
- Constipation: mode of action and use of drugs.
- Inflammatory bowel disease.
- Irritable bowel syndrome.

Diarrhoea

A patient complaining of 'diarrhoea' may in fact describe a wide variety of colorectal symptoms. The World Health Organization defines diarrhoea as the passage of three or more loose or liquid stools per day (or more frequent liquid passage than is normal for the individual). Diarrhoea ranges from a mild and socially inconvenient symptom to a major cause of death and malnutrition in the developing world. The first priority of therapy is to preserve fluid and electrolyte balance.

Some physiology

In the normal adult, 7–8 L of water and electrolytes are secreted daily into the gastrointestinal (GI) tract. This, together with 2–3 L of dietary fluid and nutrients, is almost entirely absorbed by the specialised mucosa lining the small and large bowel through a combination of active and passive mechanisms. *Diarrhoea* results from an imbalance between secretion and reabsorption of water.

The absorption of water is a passive phenomenon, and is reliant on the presence of a solute gradient across the cell allowing water to follow by osmosis. Sodium is the most important solute in this regard. Sodium gradients are established by active transporters and co-transporters linked to a variety of solutes and nutrients, including other electrolytes, amino acids and simple saccharides.

Mechanism of diarrhoea

Osmotic diarrhoea

The presence of indigestible or unabsorbed osmotically active molecules in the intestine results in water retention in the lumen. Many laxatives work on this principle.

The diarrhoea of lactose intolerance is an example of an osmotic diarrhoea; lactase deficiency results in osmotically active lactose remaining in the bowel as it cannot be absorbed. Furthermore, any disease which results in damage to the small or large bowel mucosa (such as coeliac disease) will impair the intestine's ability to absorb solutes, thus effectively causing an osmotic diarrhoea.

Secretory diarrhoea

This results from the abnormal secretion of osmotically active solutes. Normally, in response to various stimuli, crypt cells actively transport chloride into the gut lumen, and sodium and water follow. This *stimulus–secretion coupling* is modulated by cyclic AMP and GMP, calcium, prostaglandins and leukotrienes.

Numerous enteric hormones stimulate secretion, including vasoactive intestinal peptide secretin. Rarely neuroendocrine tumours secrete large amounts of these hormones, resulting in a profuse secretory diarrhoea. Numerous intestinal microbes including *Vibrio cholerae* and enterotoxigenic *Escherichia coli* (ETEC) produce enterotoxins which cause unregulated electrolyte excretion by interfering with this process.

Increased gut transit

This is generally idiopathic but is rarely due to secretory tumours of the alimentary tract, i.e. neuroendocrine tumours which can secrete peptides such as histamine, 5-HT and VIP (vasoactive intestinal peptide) which have prokinetic effects on the bowel. Idiopathic cases are commonly seen in patients with irritable bowel syndrome (IBS) and are rarely, if ever, severe enough to produce clinically significant fluid or electrolyte disturbance or malabsorption.

These classifications are not always clinically useful, as many cases of diarrhoea will have a combination of underlying abnormalities. For example, enteric infections may stimulate secretion or damage absorption, and many causes of malabsorption result in direct mucosal damage as well as inhibiting the appropriate absorption of osmotically active substances.

Motility patterns in the bowel

An important factor in diarrhoea may be loss of the normal segmenting contractions that delay passage of contents, so that an occasional peristaltic wave has a greater propulsive effect. Segmental contractions of the smooth muscle in the bowel mix the intestinal contents. Patients with diarrhoea commonly have less spontaneous segmenting activity in the sigmoid colon than do people with normal bowel habit, and patients with constipation have more. Antimotility drugs (see below) can reduce diarrhoea by increasing segmentation and inhibiting peristalsis.

Fluid and electrolyte treatment

Oral rehydration therapy (ORT) with glucose–electrolyte solution is sufficient to treat the vast majority of episodes of watery diarrhoea from acute gastroenteritis. As a simple, effective, cheap and readily administered therapy for a potentially fatal condition, ORT is one of the major advances in therapy and one of the more successful global public health interventional strategies. It is effective because glucose-coupled sodium transport continues during diarrhoea, allowing sodium and water absorption to continue via an alternative pathway.

Oral rehydration salts (ORSs). The World Health Organization/UNICEF-recommended formulation is:

Sodium chloride 3.5 g/L.
Potassium chloride 1.5 g/L.
Sodium citrate 2.9 g/L.
Anhydrous glucose 20.0 g/L.

This provides sodium 90 mmol/L, potassium 20 mmol/L, chloride 80 mmol/L, citrate 10 mmol/L, glucose 111 mmol/L (total osmolarity 311 mmol/L). Several other formulations exist, some with less sodium (see national formularies).

Of note, it can be seen that attempted rehydration therapy with commercial soft drinks alone will fail because their sodium content is too low (usually less than 4 mmol/L).

Most cases respond adequately with assiduous attention to oral intake, but fluid and electrolyte depletion are especially dangerous in children and the elderly, who may need intravenous fluid replacement. Antimotility drugs are *inappropriate* for severe diarrhoea; hazardous adverse effects (see below) counterbalance any marginal benefit.

Antidiarrhoeal drugs

There are two types of drug which are often used in combination. They should only be considered in benign cases of diarrhoea for short-term symptomatic benefit; their use may be harmful in infective or inflammatory diarrhoea.

Antimotility drugs

Codeine, diphenoxylate and *loperamide* all activate opiate receptors on the smooth muscle of the bowel to reduce peristalsis and increase segmentation contractions. The actions of all three drugs are antagonised by naloxone. Loperamide and diphenoxylate are relatively enterospecific and do not cross the blood–brain barrier (except diphenoxylate in large doses). These drugs should also be avoided in patients with active inflammatory bowel disease, for they may cause paralytic ileus and toxic megacolon. The abdominal bloating produced by antimotility drugs may be less acceptable than the loose stools for which they are prescribed.

Drugs that directly increase the viscosity of gut contents

Kaolin and chalk are adsorbent powders. Their therapeutic efficacy is marginal as is shown by the fact that they are often combined with an opioid; they should not be used routinely. Bulk-forming agents such as ispaghula, methylcellulose and sterculia[1] (see above) are useful for diarrhoea in diverticular disease, and for reducing the fluidity of faeces in patients with ileostomy and colostomy.

Infectious diarrhoea

This includes travellers' diarrhoea, where up to one-half of the diarrhoea that afflicts visitors to tropical and subtropical countries is associated with enterotoxigenic strains of *Escherichia coli*; other bacteria including *Shigella* and *Salmonella* spp., viruses including the Norwalk family, and parasites (particularly *Giardia lamblia*) have also been implicated.

Transmission is almost invariably by ingestion of contaminated food and water, which indicates the most effective way of reducing risk.

Infectious diarrhoea as a rule is self-limiting, and oral rehydration is generally all that is required. Antimotility agents are relatively contraindicated due to concerns of reduced pathogen clearance and toxic megacolon but may be permissible in mild cases. The use of antibiotics is controversial as even in cases of bacterial dysentery they do not reduce duration of symptoms by more than 48 hours, and there is hard in vitro as well as anecdotal evidence that their use in patients with certain bacterial infections (e.g. *E. coli* O175) can precipitate haemolytic-uraemic syndrome (HUS), which can be life-threatening. Antibiotics may be indicated if the patient is toxic or immunosuppressed, or if invasive infections (e.g. *Shigella*) are suspected or confirmed. Many regimens are used (commonly ciprofloxacin), but macrolides are theoretically less prone to precipitating HUS in susceptible patients.

Chemotherapy is available for certain specific organisms if enteric infection is confirmed on stool culture, e.g. amoebiasis, giardiasis (see Index).

Diarrhoea due to *Clostridium difficile* ('C. diff')

C. diff infection may range from an offensive but limited diarrhoeal illness to a life-threatening toxic pseudomembranous colitis, and for this reason occupies such a prominent place in the public consciousness. The major risk factors for infection are older age, significant co-morbidities, recent antibiotic use and a history of recent (within 3 months) hospitalisation. Virtually all antibiotics have been implicated as a risk factor for *C. diff* infection (including, rarely, metronidazole, one of the mainstays of treatment), but clindamycin, quinolones, cephalosporins and other β-lactams are particularly notorious.

First-line treatment has traditionally consisted of 7–14 days of metronidazole by mouth. There is better evidence for a prolonged (4-week) tapering course of oral vancomycin, although this tends to be reserved for severe, refractory or relapsed infections. The tapering course allows the killing of reactivated spores which may have survived initial treatment. Vancomycin not absorbed from the GI tract is excreted renally; it must therefore be given orally (125 mg four times daily initially; occasionally doubled), and monitoring of serum levels is unnecessary. A newer oral antibiotic, fidaxomicin, is also helpful.

There are also some data supporting the use of more novel treatments, although solid evidence is lacking. Probiotics and faecal microbiota transplant (prepared using normal faeces from unaffected donors), for example, are thought to work by recolonising the bowel with non-pathogenic bacterial flora, whereas intravenous immunoglobulin probably works by neutralising pathogenic toxins.

Drug-induced diarrhoea

Innumerable drugs have diarrhoea as an unwanted effect. *Antimicrobials* are the commonest drugs that cause diarrhoea. This is usually due to a benign alteration of bowel flora, but occasionally this will allow latent *C. diff* colonisation to result in overt colitis (see above).

Secretory diarrhoea due to vasoactive peptides

Octreotide, a synthetic somatostatin analogue (see p. 584), inhibits the release of peptides that mediate certain alimentary secretions, and may be used to relieve diarrhoea due to neuroendocrine tumours such as carcinoids and VIPomas (tumours that produce VIP). Lanreotide, a longer-acting version, is often used in these patients as it only requires once-monthly application.

Bile acid malabsorption (BAM)

BAM is increasingly recognised as an important cause of irritable bowel syndrome (IBS) and other diarrhoeas of unknown aetiology. The diarrhoea is a result of osmotically active bile acids remaining in the GI tract.

Bile acids, synthesised in the liver, are necessary for the absorption of lipids from the small bowel. The distal small bowel (terminal ileum) reabsorbs and returns bile acids to the liver, forming a highly efficient enterohepatic recycling system. Primary, or idiopathic, BAM is thought to be due to dysregulated enterohepatic feedback resulting in increased bile acid secretion which saturates uptake absorption capability. Surgery or diseases affecting the small bowel mucosa (such

---

[1]Named after Sterculinus, a god of Ancient Rome, who presided over manuring of agricultural land.

as Crohn's), or prior cholecystectomy resulting in constant bile acid release, can cause diarrhoea (secondary BAM).

If no treatable underlying cause of BAM is identified, then a bile acid absorption resin such as colesevelam, colestipol or colestyramine may be given. These are awkward drugs to take, due to taste, consistency and to the fact that they bind numerous other drugs. They must therefore be given at least 1 hour before or several hours after the administration of other drugs. Bile acid sequestrants are also used as lipid-lowering drugs (see Ch. 26).

Microscopic colitis

This condition presents with diarrhoea; the colonic mucosa is macroscopically normal but histologically shows either lymphocytic infiltration of the mucosa (lymphocytic colitis) or subendothelial fibrosis (collagenous colitis). The condition is benign, and spontaneous resolution occurs in a significant proportion. Treatment with aminosalicylates or corticosteroid may hasten this; alternatively, antidiarrhoeals may be attempted to control symptoms.

Constipation

Constipation means different things to different people, and it is difficult to define formally. Generally it refers to infrequent, hard-to-pass bowel motions. Rome III criteria[2] define constipation as two or more of the following over 12 weeks: fewer than three stools per week, straining more than one-fourth of the time, passage of hard stools, incomplete evacuation and the sensation of anorectal blockage.

There are multiple causes of constipation which should be excluded or treated. Symptomatic treatment involves the use of laxatives, which are medicines that promote defaecation, largely by reducing the viscosity of the contents of the lower colon. They are classified as follows:

- Stool-bulking agents.
- Osmotic laxatives.
- Faecal softeners.
- Stimulant laxatives.

Stool bulking agents

Dietary fibre comprises the cell walls and supporting structures of vegetables and fruits. Most of the fibre in our diet is in the form of non-starch polysaccharides (NSPs), which are not digestible by human enzymes. Fibre may be soluble (pectins, guar, ispaghula) or insoluble (cellulose, hemicelluloses, lignin). Insoluble fibre has less effect than soluble fibre on the viscosity of gut contents but is a stronger laxative because it resists digestion in the small bowel and so enters the colon intact. In addition, it has a vast capacity for retaining water; thus 1 g of carrot fibre can hold 23 g of water. It has been proposed that as humans have refined the carbohydrates in their diet over the centuries, so they have deprived themselves of fibre, the ensuing under-filling of the colon being an important cause of constipation, haemorrhoids and diverticular disease.

Stool-bulking agents, which add fibre to the diet, are the treatment of choice for simple constipation. They act by increasing the volume and lowering the viscosity of intestinal contents to produce a soft, bulky stool, which encourages normal reflex bowel activity. The mode of action of stool bulking agents is thus more physiological than that of other types of laxative. They should be taken with liberal quantities of fluid (at least 2 L daily).

Individual preparations

Bran is the residue left when flour is made from cereals; it contains between 25% and 50% of fibre. The fibre content of a normal diet can be increased by eating wholemeal bread and bran cereals, but over-zealous supplementation may cause troublesome flatulence (from bacterial fermentation in the colon).

Viscous (soluble) fibres, e.g. *ispaghula*, are effective and more palatable than bran. Ispaghula husk contains mucilage and hemicelluloses, which swell rapidly in water. Methylcellulose takes up water to swell to a colloid about 25 times its original volume, and *sterculia* (a tree gum, named after the Roman god of agricultural fertility and therefore manure), similarly, swells when mixed with water. These and others are available as a variety of proprietary preparations.

Drugs to stimulate colonic motility

Stimulant laxatives

These drugs increase intestinal motility by various mechanisms; they may cause abdominal cramps and are contraindicated when intestinal obstruction is suspected.

Bisacodyl stimulates sensory endings in the colon by direct action from the lumen. It is effective orally in 6–10 h and, as a suppository, acts within 1 h. In elderly patients, bisacodyl suppositories reduce the need for regular enemas. There are no important unwanted effects.

Sodium picosulfate is similar and is also used to evacuate the bowel for investigative procedures and surgery.

---

[2]The Rome consensus series of statements standardise the diagnostic criteria for irritable bowel syndrome, defining, in part, what constitutes abnormal stool frequency and consistency. Rome III criteria appear in: Longstreth G F, Thompson W G, Chey W D et al 2006 Functional bowel disorders. Gastroenterology 130:1480–1491.

Glycerol has a mild stimulant effect on the rectum when administered as a suppository.

The anthraquinone group of laxatives includes *senna, danthron, rhubarb*[3] and *aloes*. In the small intestine, soluble anthraquinone derivates are liberated and absorbed. These are excreted into the colon and act there, along with those that have escaped absorption, probably after being chemically changed by bacterial action.

Senna, available as a biologically standardised preparation, is widely used to relieve constipation and to empty the bowel for investigative procedures and surgery. It acts within 8–12 h.

Danthron is available as a standardised preparation in combination with the faecal softeners poloxamer 188 (co-danthramer) and docusate sodium (as co-danthrusate). It acts within 6–12 h. Evidence from rodent studies indicates a possible carcinogenic risk, and long-term exposure to danthron should be avoided. It can be useful for treating constipation in terminally ill patients.

The 5-HT$_4$ agonist prucalopride has recently been licensed as second-line therapy for women with chronic constipation (or irritable bowel syndrome with constipation; IBS-C). Linaclotide, a guanylate cyclase-C agonist, is also licensed for IBS-C patients.

Osmotic laxatives

These are but little absorbed and increase the bulk and reduce viscosity of intestinal contents to promote a fluid stool.

Some inorganic salts retain water in the intestinal lumen or, if given as hypertonic solution, withdraw it from the body. When constipation is mild, magnesium hydroxide will suffice, but magnesium sulphate (Epsom salts) is used when a more powerful effect is needed. Both magnesium salts act within 2–4 h.

Lactulose is a synthetic disaccharide. Taken orally, it is unaffected by small-intestinal disaccharidases, is not absorbed and thus acts as an osmotic laxative. Tolerance may develop. Lactulose is also used in the treatment of hepatic encephalopathy (see Ch. 34).

Osmotic laxatives are frequently used to clear the colon for diagnostic procedures or surgery. Enemas containing phosphate or citrate effectively evacuate the distal colon and can be useful for treating obstinate constipation in elderly or debilitated patients. Oral formulations containing magnesium sulphate and citric acid (Citramag) or polyethylene glycol (Klean-Prep, Movicol) made up with water to create an isotonic solution are used in preparation for colonoscopy; some patients find the necessarily large volumes difficult to tolerate.

Excessive use of stimulant and/or osmotic laxatives may lead to severe water and electrolyte depletion, even to hypokalaemic paralysis and renal failure, especially in the elderly[4] or those with diabetes or pre-existing renal impairment. Where bowel cleansing is necessary in these patients (e.g. before surgery or endoscopy), a less aggressive laxative and/or bowel preparation under medical supervision (with electrolyte and fluid balance monitoring) should be considered.

Faecal softeners (emollients)

The softening properties of these agents are useful in the management of anal fissure (see below) and haemorrhoids.

Docusate sodium (dioctyl sodium sulphosuccinate) softens faeces by lowering the surface tension of fluids in the bowel. This allows more water to remain in the faeces. It appears also to have bowel-stimulant properties, but these are relatively weak. Docusate sodium acts in 1–2 days. Poloxamers, e.g. poloxalkol (poloxamer 188), act similarly and are used in combination with other agents.

Drastic purgatives (castor oil, cascara, jalap,[5] colocynth, phenolphthalein and podophyllum) are obsolete.

Suppositories and enemas

Suppositories (bisacodyl, glycerin) may be used to obtain a bowel action within about 1 h. Enemas produce defaecation by softening faeces and distending the bowel. They are used in preparation for surgery, radiological examination and endoscopy. Preparations with sodium phosphate, which is poorly absorbed and so retains water in the gut, are generally used. Arachis oil is included in enemas to soften impacted faeces.

---

[3]In the late 18th century, Britain made approaches to trade with China that were met with indifference; it seems that the mandarins held the belief that the British feared death from constipation if deprived of rhubarb *(Rheum palmatum)*, one of China's exports. Nevertheless, rhubarb found its way to St Petersburg in Russia, where a flourishing trade developed. Seeds brought back to Scotland (at considerable risk to himself) by James Mounsey, physician to the Tsar, were grown and marketed as Gregory's Powder, and became popular throughout the UK. Lee M R, Hutcheon J, Dukan E, Milne I 2017 Rhubarb *(Rheum* species): the role of Edinburgh in its cultivation and development. Journal of the Royal College of Physicians of Edinburgh 47:102–109.

[4]The Roman Emperor Nero (AD 37–68) murdered his severely constipated aunt by ordering the doctors to give her 'a laxative of fatal strength'. He 'seized her property before she was quite dead and tore up the will so that nothing could escape him' (Suetonius, trans. R Graves).
[5]In the 19th century 'young men proceeding to Africa' were advised to take pills named Livingstone's Rousers, consisting of rhubarb, jalap, calomel and quinine (British Medical Journal 1964; 2:1583).

Contraindications

Do not give laxatives to patients with undiagnosed abdominal pain, inflammatory bowel disease or obstruction. Likewise, laxatives should not be used to empty the rectum of hardened faeces, for they will fail and cause pain. Initial treatment should be with enemas, but digital removal, traditionally ordered by a senior doctor and performed by a junior doctor, may occasionally be required. A bulking agent or a faecal softener will help to prevent recurrence.

Inflammatory bowel disease (IBD)

The inflammatory bowel diseases ulcerative colitis (UC) and Crohn's disease[6] are chronic relapsing/remitting diseases of the GI tract characterised by intestinal mucosal inflammation. The pathogenesis of inflammatory bowel disease (IBD) remains incompletely understood. IBD can be thought of as an inappropriate immunological response to non-pathogenic luminal antigens. This can be either an overenthusiastic damaging pro-inflammatory response to an innocuous stimulus or an underwhelming protective anti-inflammatory response which fails to keep an appropriate inflammatory reaction in check. A combination of genetic predisposition and environmental factors produces either Crohn's disease, which can affect any part of the GI tract, or UC, which is confined to the colon. Classically, UC is thought to result from dysregulation of the Th1/cell-mediated immune pathway, while Crohn's disease results from disorders of Th2/humoral immunity, but this is almost certainly an oversimplification.

Although Crohn's disease and UC are different diseases, their medical management shares many similarities. The goal of pharmacological therapy is to induce and then maintain remission. The maintenance of remission is important not only for the patient's general well-being, but also because of the risk of complications such as colorectal cancer, which is directly related to disease activity over a long period of time. There is also increasing evidence that mucosal healing, and not just clinical remission, may be an important factor in determining long-term prognosis.

5-ASA and corticosteroids have been the mainstay of treatment of IBD for decades; indeed, the use of corticosteroids in UC has a particular place in the history of the randomised controlled clinical trial.[7]

More recently, immunosuppressive therapy has found an important role. In the last few years biological therapy has been introduced, and this area is likely to produce a number of new therapies in the coming years. Historically, biological therapies have concentrated on blocking the TNFα (tissue necrosis factor alpha) receptor. Promising new therapies acting on other novel targets (such as the anti-adhesion molecule product vedolizumab) are now emerging.[8] Antidiarrhoeals should be used only with extreme caution in active colitis and are contraindicated if the disease is severe. They can lead to toxic dilatation of the colon, with perforation.

Drugs to induce remission in UC

Aminosalicylates

5-Aminosalicylate (5-ASA) maintains remission in patients with UC (relapses are reduced by a factor of three), and may also be used for treatment of an acute attack (with or without a corticosteroid, depending on severity). There is increasing evidence that they have a protective effect against colorectal cancer in UC which is independent of its ability to maintain remission.

Its exact mechanism of action remains unclear; putative mechanisms include inhibition of pro-inflammatory prostaglandin synthesis, scavenging of free radicals, inhibition of inflammatory cell recruitment and inhibition of production of pro-inflammatory cytokines and protein mediators such as NFκB, IL1 and TNFα.

Sulfasalazine has been used to treat rheumatoid arthritis since the 1930s (see p. 260). It was subsequently noted to have activity against ulcerative colitis. It consists of two compounds, sulfapyridine and 5-aminosalicylic acid, joined by an azo bond. Sulfasalazine is poorly absorbed from the small intestine, and colonic bacteria split the azo bond to

---

[6]Crohn and his colleagues Oppenheimer and Ginzberg, all from the Mount Sinai Hospital in New York, published a case series describing a necrotising granulomatous inflammatory disease of the terminal ileum in 1932. Others may well have described and published similar observations years before, but Crohn's alphabetical and clinical precedence means that his surname alone is now associated with the disease he initially termed 'terminal ileitis'. He quickly renamed it 'regional ileitis', in part to avoid any overly morbid connotations. Crohn B, Ginzburg L, Oppenheimer G D 1932 Regional ileitis: a pathologic and clinical entity. Journal of the American Medical Association 99:1323–1328.

[7]Clinical investigators have long been aware of the need to randomise treatments and minimise observer bias. (See: Gluud C 2011 Danish contribution to the evaluation of serum therapy for diphtheria in the 1890 s. Journal of the Royal Society of Medicine 104:219–222.) But in their clinical trial of ulcerative colitis, Truelove and Witts expressed the issues with clarity when they randomised patients to receive either cortisone or placebo, stating: 'It was judged that if the physician proceeded on the assumption that every patient might be receiving potent cortisone, and if he also had the right to stop treatment at any time he considered it likely to be doing harm, such a blind trial was justified because of the greater value of its results' (Truelove S C, Witts L J 1954 Cortisone in ulcerative colitis; preliminary report on a therapeutic trial. British Medical Journal 2:375–837).

[8]Asthana A, Sparrow M, Peyrin-Biroulet L 2014 Optimizing conventional medical therapies in inflammatory bowel disease. Current Drug Targets. September 14 [Epub ahead of print].

release the component parts. Sulfapyridine is well absorbed, acetylated in the liver and excreted in the urine; it has no therapeutic action in colitis and functions solely to deliver 5-ASA to the colon.

Sulfasalazine is available as a tablet, retention enema (for disease extending up to the splenic flexure) or suppository (for treating proctitis). It can be particularly useful in treating patients with enteropathic arthritis associated with IBD, due to its rheumatological activity.

Adverse effects are due largely to the sulfonamide moiety and include headache, malaise, anorexia, nausea and vomiting; these are dose related and commoner in slow acetylators (of the sulfonamide). Allergic reactions include rash, fever and lymphadenitis; rarely leucopenia and agranulocytosis occur. Males may suffer from reversible oligospermia and reduced sperm motility. Body secretions may have an orange discoloration, which can stain soft contact lenses.

Mesalazine. Patients intolerant of sulfasalazine usually tolerate mesalazine, which is a 5-ASA. Mesalazine is absorbed rapidly and completely in the upper jejunum, and is presented in various formulations that delay its release. Asacol tablets are coated in a resin, which dissolves only at pH 7 or higher, favouring its release in the distal ileum and colon. In contrast, Pentasa has a slow-release but pH-independent coating so that 5-ASA is liberated throughout the GI tract. Mesalazine preparations are available in oral, enema and suppository forms.

Other 5-ASAs. Balsalazide (a 5-ASA prodrug) and olsalazine (a 5-ASA dimer which is cleaved by colonic bacteria yielding active 5-ASA) are the other available aminosalicylates, obtainable in oral forms only.

5-ASA that enters the blood is rapidly cleared by acetylation in the liver and renal excretion. In comparison to sulfasalazine, the newer 5-ASAs are generally well tolerated and very safe. Patients should be counselled about the rare risk of blood dyscrasias and renal impairment, and occasional blood monitoring is required. Patients being initiated on 5-ASAs rarely experience a paradoxical flare in their symptoms.

Corticosteroid

Enemas and suppositories. These can be used in left-sided or distal UC. 5-ASA therapy is more effective in cases not requiring systemic corticosteroid, so corticosteroid enemas/suppositories should not be used as first-line treatment. When UC is restricted to the left hemicolon, exacerbations that do not respond to an aminosalicylate alone often benefit from the addition of corticosteroid enemas. Foam-based preparations appear to coat the colonic mucosa more efficiently than the aqueous formulations.

Patients with distal colitis are prone to faecal loading proximal to the inflamed segment, and this can lead to overflow diarrhoea and worsening of inflammation. Faecal loading can be detected on straight abdominal radiograph and is treated with laxatives; this is safe provided the inflammatory process is restricted to the distal colon. On no account should antidiarrhoeals be used, as these will exacerbate the problem. Adequate quantities of dietary fibre and fluid should be encouraged, and stool-bulking agents can also be helpful in protecting against faecal loading.

Systemic corticosteroid. *Severe attacks* of ulcerative colitis or Crohn's, or flares that are unresponsive to 5-ASA therapy, should be treated with a systemic corticosteroid, and oral preparations usually suffice. It is important to start with a dose that will bring the inflammatory process under control, e.g. prednisolone 40 mg/day p.o. Clinical response should be rapid (within 1 week). Once remission has been attained, the dose can be tailed down very slowly over a period of 6–8 weeks. This gradual decrease is important, as stopping treatment too abruptly may result in a further flare; this is in contrast, for example, to acute asthma, where rapidly tailing regimens are appropriate.

Very severe attacks of ulcerative colitis necessitate hospital treatment with an intravenous corticosteroid; a parenteral corticosteroid should also be considered in patients who are unresponsive to other medical management.

The main danger is toxic dilatation of the colon and perforation, which can occur insidiously. Significant clinical improvement should be seen within 72 h. If there is no improvement, a trial of ciclosporin or an anti-TNF (see below) may induce response. Treatment otherwise is by emergency colectomy.

Ciclosporin

The calcineurin inhibitor *ciclosporin* will induce remission in some patients with severe ulcerative colitis that is unresponsive to an intravenous corticosteroid but is currently unlicensed for this indication in the UK. Give 2 mg/kg i.v., titrated to plasma levels, until remission is attained. Available oral preparations have different pharmacokinetic properties such that equivalence between them cannot be assumed.

Doses used in UC are lower than those used in transplant recipients. Renal function and blood pressure must be monitored closely. Ciclosporin is epileptogenic, and this effect is enhanced in patients with electrolyte disturbances (particularly calcium and magnesium) and hypocholesterolaemia; it should also be avoided if there is a history of fits. Ciclosporin is ineffective in maintaining remission, so maintenance immunosuppressive therapy (see below) is generally required.

Biological therapy

Six biologic agents are currently approved for the treatment of UC, in inducing and maintaining remission. Four are anti TNF alpha (infliximab, adaluminab, golimumab and certolizumab), and two are ant-integrin agents (natalizumab and vedolizumab). Biosimilar versions of infliximab (Inflectra and Remsina) are increasingly prescribed since the patent for Remicade (infliximab) expired in 2015.[9]

Drugs to induce remission in Crohn's disease

5-ASA

These are less effective in Crohn's disease. If they are used, the preparation must be chosen to target the affected part of the GI tract (e.g. Pentasa rather than Asacol in small bowel disease).

Antibiotics

These are most useful for controlling perianal or penetrating disease, although anecdotally some patients with ileocolonic disease may also respond. Metronidazole and ciprofloxacin are used most commonly.

Adverse effects including alcohol intolerance, peripheral neuropathy and the risk of antibiotic-associated diarrhoea and *C. difficile* superinfection from such prolonged therapy often limit their use to up to 3 months.

Dietary therapy

There is evidence that liquid diets based on amino acids (elemental diets) or oligopeptides (semi-elemental diets) for 4–6 weeks are as effective as corticosteroids in controlling Crohn's disease, although relapse is common when the treatment stops. Elemental preparations are notoriously unpalatable even with flavourings, and they often have to be administered through a nasogastric tube, which is unpopular with patients. Furthermore, the beneficial effect is lost if non-elemental/semi-elemental dietary components are included. They are worth trying in steroid-resistant cases and are particularly favoured by paediatricians, who prefer to avoid systemic steroids because of their adverse effects on growth.

Corticosteroids

Corticosteroids are effective in active Crohn's disease. *Budesonide,* a potent topically active corticosteroid, is an alternative to prednisolone. As a delayed-release formulation, it delivers drug to the ileum and ascending colon and is therefore particularly useful in small bowel and ileocaecal Crohn's disease, where it has comparable (but inferior) efficacy to prednisolone. Extensive first-pass metabolism in the liver limits its systemic availability and potential for adverse effects.

Topical steroid preparations are generally not useful in Crohn's disease due to the intermittent nature of mucosal involvement.

Ciclosporin

Ciclosporin is ineffective in Crohn's disease.

Biological therapies

There is much more extensive experience of biological therapies in Crohn's disease, in particular with the use of anti-TNFα therapy. These have been demonstrated to be effective in the induction and maintenance of remission of active Crohn's disease, including perianal and fistulating disease.

Maintenance of remission in IBD

Corticosteroids are ineffective in maintaining remission of UC or Crohn's disease, largely due to significant adverse effects associated with long-term use.

In UC, maintenance therapy with an *aminosalicylate* should be started as corticosteroids are being weaned. 5-ASA has limited, if any, efficacy in the maintenance of remission of Crohn's disease.

If the disease is corticosteroid dependent despite adequate 5-ASA therapy, azathioprine or another immunosuppressive agent may be used (see below). Surgery is indicated if medical therapy fails to control the disease or is associated with unacceptable adverse effects.

Azathioprine is effective as a *steroid-sparing* agent in maintenance therapy in UC and Crohn's disease, and is used when 5-ASA is insufficient to maintain adequate remission. Azathioprine is converted to 6-mercaptopurine (6-MP) and then to tioguanine, an inhibitor of purine synthesis, which causes a degree of immunosuppression; in this pathway the thiopurine methyltransferase (TPMT) enzyme is rate-limiting. TPMT activity is inherited as a Mendelian trait, with low levels carrying an increased risk of myelotoxicity and mandating lower doses or selection of a different agent. TPMT activity assays are now widely available and differentiate between patients with low or absent TPMT activity (mutant homozygotes) at high risk of complications, intermediate activity (heterozygotes) in whom thiopurines may be used with caution, and normal activity (normal homozygotes) who are at low risk of toxic effects; with the latter, 2–2.5 mg/kg is therapeutic. Azathioprine is

[9]Danise S, Vuitton L, Peyrin-Baroulet L 2015 Biologic Agents for IBD: practical insights. Nature Reviews, Gastroenterology and Hepatology 12, 537–545.

not an appropriate drug for inducing remission as its onset of action takes 8–12 weeks; corticosteroid (or occasionally ciclosporin in the case of steroid failure in UC) is used as a 'bridge' to allow its therapeutic action to take effect.

Allopurinol can cause dangerous toxicity at therapeutic doses by inhibiting xanthine oxidase and preventing the conversion of azathioprine to 6-MP.

Adverse effects, in particular myelosuppression, are much more common in TPMT-deficient patients, but those with normal enzymatic activity are also at risk. As azathioprine can cause bone marrow suppression and hepatitis, the blood count and liver function should be monitored weekly for the first 2 months of therapy and every 2–3 months thereafter for as long as the drug is taken. Pancreatitis occurs in up to 5% of patients. Intolerance to azathioprine is fairly common, for example malaise, abdominal discomfort and nausea. These effects are usually due to the imidazole side-chain of the molecule, and *mercaptopurine* (which is azathioprine without the side-chain) may be better tolerated (1–1.5 mg/kg daily). Mercaptopurine is not an alternative to azathioprine in patients who have suffered pancreatitis or myelosuppression with the latter, as these effects are due to the active part of the drug.

Methotrexate, a folic acid antagonist, can be helpful in controlling relapses of Crohn's disease that is unresponsive to corticosteroid or azathioprine. It has also been used with benefit in UC. Its short- and long-term use are limited by a wide profile of adverse effects including bone marrow suppression and pulmonary and hepatic fibrosis (see p. 258). It is given once weekly, with folic acid supplements on the days on which it is not taken. It is severely teratogenic and is contraindicated in both men and women trying to conceive.

Biological therapies

TNFα causes activation of immune cells and release of inflammatory mediators by binding surface TNF receptors. Following in vitro demonstration that inhibition of TNFα activity resulted in reduced mucosal inflammation, several anti-TNFα drugs have come to market. *Infliximab, adalimumab* and *certolizumab-PEGol* are recombinant monoclonal anti-TNFα-receptor antibodies. Infliximab, the first to come to market, is a mouse-human chimaeric antibody and is given as an intravenous infusion of 5 mg/kg at 0, 2 and 6 weeks initially and then at 8-weekly intervals. Adalimumab is a fully human monoclonal antibody and has the advantage of being given subcutaneously at 160 mg at week 0, 80 mg at week 2, and 40 mg every 2 weeks thereafter. Certolizumab-PEGol is also a humanised monoclonal antibody with a PEGylated Fab' fragment. It is also given subcutaneously at a dose of 400 mg at weeks 0, 2 and 4, and at 4-weekly intervals thereafter.

These drugs are effective in inducing and maintaining remission in Crohn's disease. Most experience has been gained with infliximab. Infliximab and adalimumab appear to be effective in penetrating (fistulating) disease.

Anti-TNFα drugs are given as a long-term course over at least 1 year if effective. Controversial issues include whether to co-administer another immunosuppressant (such as azathioprine) to improve efficacy and whether to institute them early in the course of disease ('top-down') or only after failure of other treatment modalities ('bottom-up').

Adverse effects include hypersensitivity reactions. There is a significant risk of potentially fatal reactivation of TB, which must therefore be excluded before initiating treatment. There is a theoretical risk of increased susceptibility to other atypical infections and cancers, particularly lymphoproliferative disease, but long-term follow-up data are not yet available. Screening for infections such as hepatitis B and C viruses and HIV is commonplace without as yet definite evidence that TNFα therapy worsens these conditions if coexistent.

Maintenance of remission following surgery for Crohn's disease

An additional difficulty in the medical management of Crohn's disease is prophylaxis against recurrence after surgical resection. Of the drugs studied, antibiotics are effective but cannot be given for longer than 3 months because of toxicity and unwanted effects with long-term use. 5-ASA and azathioprine provide some benefit, but emerging evidence suggests that infliximab (and potentially other anti-TNFα drugs) are much more effective.

Irritable bowel syndrome (IBS)

This condition affects 20% of the population and is the commonest reason for referral to a gastroenterologist. It is manifested by a variety of GI symptoms including disordered bowel habit (constipation, diarrhoea, or both), abdominal pain and bloating. Upper GI symptoms manifest as non-ulcer dyspepsia (see Ch. 32). All of these symptoms occur in the absence of demonstrable pathology in the GI tract, although patients with IBS often have abnormalities of gut motility. Another feature of the condition is visceral hypersensitivity; patients with IBS have lower thresholds for pain from colonic distension induced by inflating balloons placed in the bowel. A proportion of patients develop their IBS symptoms after an episode of gastroenteritis and, in many, emotional stress is an important precipitating factor. Associated psychopathology, with anxiety and sometimes depression, is common.

The mainstay of treatment, after investigation when appropriate, is to reassure the patient of the entirely benign nature of the disorder and the good prognosis. Those with predominant *constipation* should be encouraged to increase the fluid and fibre content of their diet. Unprocessed bran can lead to troublesome bloating and wind, and a bulking agent such as ispaghula husk is often better tolerated.

Diarrhoea may respond to an antimotility drug such as loperamide, the dose being adjusted to symptoms. Codeine phosphate is effective but may cause sedation.

Low-dose tricyclic antidepressants, i.e. at doses ineffective as antidepressant, and antispasmodics (see below) are given for *abdominal pain*, but there is little objective evidence for their therapeutic efficacy. The generation of evidence is complicated by the variable nature of IBS symptoms, the patients who suffer from them, and the high rate of placebo response in this condition. There are two main classes of antispasmodic, the antimuscarinic drugs and drugs that are direct smooth muscle relaxants.

Antimuscarinic drugs

These drugs block cholinergic transmission at parasympathetic postganglionic nerve endings and cause smooth muscle to relax. The synthetic antimuscarinics *dicyclomine* and *propantheline* are probably the most useful in IBS, but therapeutic efficacy is often limited by other anticholinergic effects. The drugs are contraindicated in patients with glaucoma and prostatism, and should be avoided in patients with gastro-oesophageal reflux.

Direct smooth muscle relaxants

Mebeverine is a reserpine derivative that has a direct effect on colonic muscle activity, especially, it appears, on colonic hypermotility. As it does not possess antimuscarinic activity, it does not exhibit the troublesome effects of that group of drugs.

Alverine and peppermint oil also have direct smooth muscle–relaxing activity.

A trial of low dose *amitriptyline* (10–25 mg p.o. at night) is worthwhile in patients who do not respond to antispasmodics, and associated depression will be helped by conventional doses of this or other antidepressants. Relaxation therapy, hypnotherapy and cognitive behavioural therapy have a place in selected cases.

Gastroparesis

This complication of longstanding diabetes results from diabetic neuropathy affecting the enteric nervous system. Reduced bowel motility results in bloating, nausea, vomiting,

impaired gastric emptying and abdominal pain. Prokinetics such as domperidone and metoclopramide are advocated (see Ch. 32); also erythromycin (250–500 mg four times daily) through a motilin agonist activity.[10] It therefore has synergistic activity when used with domperidone or metoclopramide. Injection of botulinum toxin into the pylorus endoscopically may also assist in improving gastric emptying.

Diverticular disease

Diverticular disease affects 5–10% of Western people older than 45 years of age; the incidence rises to 80% in those older than 80 years of age. Colonic dysmotility with increased intracolonic pressure, and diets high in refined carbohydrate and low in fibre, are important pathogenic factors. Some patients experience abdominal pain from dysmotility, whereas others remain asymptomatic. Infection of diverticulae occurs in a minority, giving potential for rupture or abscess formation.

Symptomatic diverticular disease often responds to an increase in dietary fibre and addition of a stool-bulking agent. Antispasmodic drugs are helpful in controlling the pain of colon spasm, but antimotility drugs encourage stasis of bowel contents, increase intracolonic pressure, and should be avoided. Diverticulitis requires treatment with broad-spectrum antimicrobials for 7–10 days (e.g. ciprofloxacin and metronidazole, or ampicillin, gentamicin and metronidazole).

Anal fissure

Anal fissures are often intensely painful due to sphincter spasm. Anaesthetic ointments and stool-softening agents have been widely used, with surgery (lateral internal sphincterotomy) for severely affected cases, but this procedure can cause incontinence from loss of sphincter control. An alternative is a 4-week course of topical nitrate (0.4%) or diltiazem (2%), which heals two-thirds of fissures by inducing sphincter relaxation, improving blood flow to the relatively ischaemic fissure and so promoting healing. Systemic absorption occurs, usually at insignificant doses to cause haemodynamic problems but which can cause a typical 'nitrate headache'. Use may be complicated by headache; tolerance can develop. Intrasphincteric injection of botulinum toxin has also been shown to be effective.

---

[10]Motilin is a pro-peristaltic hormone secreted by neuroendocrine cells in the proximal small bowel. Its physiology remains poorly understood.

Guide to further reading

Abraham, C., Cho, J.G., 2009. Inflammatory bowel disease. N. Engl. J. Med. 361, 2066–2078.

Al-Abri, S.S., Beeching, N.J., Nye, F.J., 2005. Traveller's diarrhoea. Lancet Infect. Dis. 5, 349–360.

Ananthakrishnan, A.N., 2011. Clostridium difficile infection: epidemiology, risk factors and management. Nat. Rev. Gastroenterol. Hepatol. 8, 17–26.

Baumgart, D.C., Sandborn, W.J., 2007. Inflammatory bowel disease: clinical aspects and established and evolving therapies. Lancet 369, 1641–1657.

Camilleri, M., Tack, J.F., 2010. Current medical treatments of dyspepsia and irritable bowel syndrome. Gastroenterol. Clin. North Am. 39, 481–493.

Kelsall, B., 2009. Interleukin-10 in inflammatory bowel disease. N. Engl. J. Med. 361, 2091–2093.

Lynch, S.V., Pedersen, O., 2016. The Human intestinal microbiome in health and disease. N. Engl. J. Med. 375, 2369–2379.

Madoff, R.D., 1998. Pharmacologic therapy for anal fissure. N. Engl. J. Med. 338, 257–259.

Mowat, C., Cole, A., Windsor, A., et al., 2011. IBD section of the British Society of Gastroenterology. Guidelines for the management of inflammatory bowel disease in adults. Gut 60, 571–607.

National Institute for Health and Clinical Excellence, 2008. Irritable bowel syndrome in adults. Diagnosis and management of irritable bowel syndrome in primary care. NICE, London.

Pardi, D.S., Kelly, C.P., 2011. Microscopic colitis. Gastroenterology 140, 1155–1165.

Quartero, A.O., Meineche-Schmidt, V., Muris, J., et al., 2005. Bulking agents, antispasmodic and antidepressant medication for the treatment of irritable bowel syndrome. Cochrane Database Syst. Rev. (2), CD003460.

Venuto, C., Butler, M., Ashley, E.D., Brown, J., 2010. Alternative therapies for Clostridium difficile infections. Pharmacotherapy 30, 1266–1278.

World Health Organization, 2005. Diarrhoea treatment guidelines. Including new recommendations for the use of ORS and zinc supplementation. World Health Organization, Geneva.

Chapter | **34** |

Liver and biliary tract

Graeme Alexander

SYNOPSIS

The liver is the most important organ for structural alteration and disposal of drugs, generating metabolites which may be biologically active or inactive (or toxic). The liver is exposed to drugs at higher concentrations than most organs because most agents are administered orally and absorbed from the gastrointestinal tract, so the whole dose passes through the liver to the systemic circulation, rendering the liver vulnerable to injury from chemicals and drugs. Conversely, disordered hepatic function is an important cause of abnormal drug handling and responses.

- **Drugs and the liver.**
  - **Pharmacodynamic and pharmacokinetic changes**
  - **Prescribing in liver disease**
  - **Drug-induced liver injury**
  - **Aspects of therapy.**

Effects of liver disease

Pharmacodynamic changes in liver disease

Patients with advanced liver disease have increased prothrombin time (INR) and serum bilirubin and require particular care when prescribing because they exhibit abnormal end-organ responses to drugs. Sensitivity of the central nervous system (CNS) to opioids, sedatives and antiepilepsy drugs is increased; the effect of oral anticoagulants is increased because synthesis of coagulation factors and thrombotic factors is impaired; fluid and electrolyte balance are altered; sodium retention is induced more readily by non-steroidal anti-inflammatory drugs (NSAIDs) or corticosteroids; ascites and oedema become diuretic resistant.

Pharmacokinetic changes in liver disease

The liver has large metabolic reserve, and important changes in drug handling occur only with hepatic decompensation. Parenchymal liver disorders, including chronic viral hepatitis or alcohol-related liver disease, have more impact on hepatic drug-metabolising enzyme activity than cholestatic conditions, such as primary biliary cirrhosis, where elimination via biliary excretion may be impaired. Hepatocellular injury leads to decreased activity of drug-metabolising enzymes, reflected in diminished plasma clearance of drugs with hepatic metabolism. There is variation between patients and overlap with healthy subjects.

Hepatic blood flow and metabolism

Complex changes in blood flow occur with liver disease. Increased resistance to portal blood flow in cirrhosis and portosystemic/intrahepatic shunts reduce drug delivery to hepatocytes, while increasing delivery directly to the systemic circulation. The pattern of change caused by disease relates to the manner in which the healthy liver treats a drug; there are two general classes:

- *Drugs metabolised rapidly with high extraction in a single pass through the liver.* Clearance is limited normally by *hepatic blood flow,* but in severe liver disease less drug is extracted from blood passing through the liver because of poor hepatocyte function and portosystemic shunts that allow blood to bypass the liver. The predominant kinetic change for drugs given orally is *increased systemic availability*. The initial and maintenance doses of such drugs should be reduced. With severe liver impairment, the $t_{1/2}$ of drugs in this class may lengthen.

- *Drugs metabolised slowly with poor extraction in a single pass through the liver*. The rate-limiting factor for elimination of this type of drug is *metabolic capacity*, and the major effect of liver disease is *prolongation of $t_{1/2}$*. Consequently, the interval between doses may need to be lengthened and the time to reach steady-state concentration in the plasma ($5 \times t_{1/2}$) is increased.

Plasma protein binding of drug

Binding of drugs to albumin is reduced when plasma concentrations of albumin fall with defective synthesis. These changes provide scope to enhance the biological activity of drugs, but assume importance only with extensive protein binding (>90%).

Other considerations

Patients with severe decompensated liver disease often develop renal impairment, with consequences for drugs with significant renal elimination. Where possible, dosing should be guided by measuring plasma concentrations (e.g. vancomycin).

Prescribing for patients with liver disease

Prescribing of most drugs is safe in well-compensated liver disease. If in doubt, check the INR (prothrombin time) and serum bilirubin. Take particular care with:

- Impaired hepatic synthetic function (hypoalbuminaemia, increased INR).
- Current/recent hepatic encephalopathy.
- Fluid retention and renal impairment.
- Drugs with:
  - high hepatic extraction
  - high plasma protein binding
  - low therapeutic ratio
  - CNS depressant effect.

For drugs with significant hepatic metabolism, a reasonable approach is to reduce the dose to 25–50% of normal and monitor responses. Specific examples include:

CNS depressants. Sedatives, antidepressants and antiepilepsy drugs should be avoided or used with extreme caution in advanced liver disease, particularly with current/recent hepatic encephalopathy. Enhanced CNS sensitivity to such drugs is well documented. Treatment of alcohol withdrawal in patients with established liver disease is hazardous; reducing doses of chlordiazepoxide over 5–10 days is recommended (with high-dose thiamine).

Analgesics. Opiates can precipitate hepatic encephalopathy in decompensated liver disease. If required to control postoperative pain, doses should be reduced to 25–50%. Intravenous infusions risk accidental overdose. Codeine can precipitate hepatic encephalopathy through constipation alone and also accumulates with renal impairment. Avoid aspirin and other NSAIDs whenever possible, as they exacerbate impaired renal function and fluid retention by inhibiting prostaglandin synthesis and may precipitate gastrointestinal bleeding.

Gastrointestinal system. Antacids that contain large quantities of sodium can precipitate fluid retention and cause ascites. Aluminium- or calcium-based preparations and antimotility drugs cause constipation and may precipitate hepatic encephalopathy.

Drug-induced liver damage

The spectrum of hepatic abnormalities caused by drugs is broad (Table 34.1). Drugs tend to injure specific hepatocyte components, e.g. plasma membrane, biliary canaliculi, cytochrome P450 enzymes or mitochondria.

Certain drugs interfere with bilirubin metabolism and excretion without causing hepatic injury. Jaundice is induced selectively with minimal or no disturbance of other liver function tests; recovery follows stopping the drug.

Examples are:

- C-17α-substituted steroids impair bilirubin excretion into hepatic canaliculi. These include synthetic anabolic steroids and oestrogens in oral contraceptives; jaundice due to the latter is rare with current formulations. Many affected patients have genetic susceptibility with mutations in ABC cassette biliary transporter proteins.
- Rifampicin impairs hepatic uptake and excretion of bilirubin; unconjugated and conjugated bilirubin levels may be raised within 3 weeks.
- Fusidic acid interferes with hepatic bilirubin excretion, causing conjugated hyperbilirubinaemia, particularly with sepsis.

Table 34.1 Idiosyncratic drug reactions and the cell components that are affected

Type of reaction	Effect on cells	Examples of drugs
Hepatocellular	Direct effect on production by enzyme–drug combination leads to cell and membrane dysfunction	Isoniazid, trazodone, diclofenac, nefazodone, venlafaxine, lovastatin
Immune mediated	Cytotoxic lymphocyte response directed at hepatocyte membranes altered by drug metabolite ± additional autoimmune component	Nitrofurantoin, methyldopa, lovastatin, minocycline, halothane
Cholestasis	Injury to canalicular membrane and transporters	Chlorpromazine, oestrogen, erythromycin and its derivatives
Granulomatous	Macrophages, lymphocytes infiltrate hepatic lobule	Diltiazem, sulfa drugs, quinidine
Microvesicular fat	Altered mitochondrial respiration, β-oxidation leads to lactic acidosis and triglyceride accumulation	Didanosine, tetracyclines, acetylsalicylic acid, valproic acid
Steatohepatitis (fatty liver)	Multifactorial	Amiodarone, tamoxifen
Fibrosis	Activation of stellate cells	Methotrexate, excess vitamin A
Vascular collapse	Causes ischaemic or hypoxic injury	Nicotinic acid, cocaine, methylenedioxymethylamfetamine (MDMA)
Oncogenesis	Encourages tumour formation	Oral contraceptives, androgens
Mixed	Cytoplasmic and canalicular injury, direct damage to bile ducts	Amoxicillin–clavulanic acid, carbamazepine, herbs, ciclosporin, methimazole, troglitazone

Diagnosis and management of drug-induced liver injury

- Always consider the possibility. Take careful drug histories, including over-the-counter, complementary, illicit and alternative medicines.
- Consider a viral aetiology with hepatitis.
- Consider other causes of cholestatic disease.
- Underlying liver disease can cause diagnostic confusion.
- Liver biopsy is often helpful, but eosinophil infiltration, often thought to be specific for drug reaction, has many causes.
- Diagnostic challenge is dangerous, may precipitate life-threatening liver disease and is never justified.
- Monitoring liver function in the early weeks of therapy is wise in detecting early reactions to drugs with hepatotoxic potential, e.g. isoniazid. Minor abnormalities (serum transaminase levels less than twice normal) are often self-limiting, and progress should be monitored. For increases exceeding three-fold, consider drug withdrawal, even in asymptomatic patients.

Aspects of therapy

Complications of cirrhosis

Variceal bleeding

Varices are dilated vessels, linking the portal and systemic venous systems, which return blood from the splanchnic circulation to the systemic circulation, bypassing the liver, decompressing the portal venous system and reducing portal pressure. Varices can be large, and haemorrhage, sometimes catastrophic, occurs from any of these vessels when intravascular pressures reach a threshold. Lower oesophageal or gastric varices, which are thin-walled and submucosal, are most prone to haemorrhage because intravascular pressures rise beyond that threshold even with everyday physiological processes.

Portal pressure is a function of portal venous resistance and blood flow. In cirrhosis, both portal venous resistance and splanchnic blood flow are increased, the latter by a combination of splanchnic vasodilatation and increased cardiac output. Variceal bleeding is more likely once the pressure gradient between the portal and systemic venous systems exceeds 12 mmHg (measured as the wedged hepatic venous pressure).

Fifty per cent die from hypovolaemia or associated complications after a first oesophageal or gastric variceal haemorrhage, manifest as melaena or haematemesis. Correct hypovolaemia promptly with plasma expanders and blood transfusion. The use of central venous access and monitoring is often useful; correction of coagulopathy with platelets and clotting factors appears logical when there are significant abnormalities. The relation between bacterial infection and haemorrhage is intriguing; bacterial infection is often found at presentation, and 60% have evidence of infection within 7 days of haemorrhage. It is unclear whether infection increases the risk of haemorrhage or is a consequence. Bacterial infection should be treated, or anticipated, using broad-spectrum antibiotics with Gram-negative cover in line with local prescribing policy. Proton pump inhibitors are also recommended. Many patients cease bleeding spontaneously, but over half re-bleed within 10 days. Conservative management is rarely acceptable.

Acute variceal haemorrhage

The first step is always resuscitation. If bleeding varices are suspected, give terlipressin, as it reduces splanchnic blood flow, increases systemic blood pressure and reduces haemorrhage, which aids diagnostic endoscopy.

Oesophageal band ligation is the treatment of choice for bleeding varices identified at endoscopy. Varices are obliterated by application of small elastic bands under direct vision by an experienced operative. This has supplanted injection sclerotherapy, which involved injecting sclerosant into and around varices but which carried a higher rate of complications (oesophagitis, oesophageal stricture/perforation and distant sclerosant embolisation). Direct injection of superglue into the varix, the treatment of choice for bleeding gastric varices, requires considerable expertise. Bleeding is controlled in 90% of patients after oesophageal band ligation in conjunction with terlipressin. Obliteration of oesophageal varices requires repeated band ligation over a prolonged period.

Pharmacological reduction of portal pressure

Vasopressin, in addition to its action on renal collecting ducts (through V_2 receptors), constricts smooth muscle (V_1 receptors) in the cardiovascular system and particularly in splanchnic blood vessels, reducing splanchnic blood flow. Systemic, cerebral and coronary artery vasoconstriction are predictable complications necessitating treatment withdrawal in 20% of older patients. In patients with cardiovascular disease and uncontrolled haemorrhage that precludes definitive endoscopic therapy, simultaneous administration of glyceryl trinitrate (transdermally, sublingually or intravenously) allows continued use of vasopressin, reducing cardiac risk, and also reduces portal venous resistance and pressure directly.

Vasopressin is cleared rapidly from the circulation so is given by continuous intravenous infusion; with concerns about distant ischaemia, the short $t_{1/2}$ of vasopressin is advantageous.

The synthetic analogue, terlipressin (triglycyllysine-vasopressin) has supplanted vasopressin. This prodrug is converted in vivo to vasoactive lysine vasopressin, which has biological activity for 3–4 h, and is effective as bolus injections 4-hourly for 2–5 days, reducing the risk of re-bleeding.

Somatostatin and the synthetic analogue octreotide reduce portal pressure by decreasing splanchnic blood flow. Octreotide has the advantage of a longer duration of action and is given as a bolus injection. It can be used as an alternative to terlipressin, with similar efficacy and indications, but does not carry a risk of cerebral or cardiac ischaemia.

When endoscopic therapy proves impossible or ineffective and bleeding continues despite pharmacotherapy, the next step is placement of a transjugular intrahepatic portosystemic shunt (TIPS), linking systemic and portal circulations with a covered expandable stent. With this in mind, patients should have early ultrasound assessment of the portal vein after variceal haemorrhage, as patency is usually a prerequisite for TIPS insertion by interventional radiologists. Covered stents are recommended for long-term patency. Long-term complications of TIPS include loss of portal vein patency with recurrent portal hypertension, stent infection and portosystemic encephalopathy.

Direct pressure on varices can be applied with an inflatable triple-lumen tube that abuts the gastro-oesophageal junction providing temporary control of bleeding in 90%. Re-bleeding is common when the tube is withdrawn and use is often complicated by aspiration, oesophageal ulceration or perforation. Advantages of this approach are safer transfer of patients to units with expertise or as a temporary measure before definitive therapy. Patients who continue to bleed or are unsuitable for TIPS have a high mortality and should be considered for surgery.

Prevention of variceal haemorrhage

Endoscopic oesophageal band ligation repeated at regular intervals until varices are obliterated is the treatment of choice for secondary prevention of variceal haemorrhage and substantially reduces the incidence of re-bleeding. Endoscopic band ligation is also the preferred approach for primary prevention of variceal haemorrhage for those at high risk, defined by endoscopic criteria.

Pharmacological therapy

Non-selective β-blockers, e.g. propranolol or nadolol, are also used as primary or secondary prophylaxis against variceal haemorrhage. They reduce cardiac output via $β_1$-receptor antagonism and induce splanchnic vasoconstriction via $β_2$-receptor antagonism, allowing unopposed α-adrenergic vasoconstriction. Propranolol is extracted extensively in a single pass through the liver, so systemic availability is less predictable in cirrhosis with portal hypertension due to variations in hepatic blood flow and portosystemic shunts. Ideally, the dose of propranolol (given twice daily) should be adjusted by measuring the wedged hepatic venous pressure since haemorrhage is rare if this is below 12 mmHg. This is often not possible. As an alternative, monitor the resting pulse rate, aiming at a 25% reduction as a measure of adequate β-blockade, although this is a poor surrogate marker of efficacy and many patients are under-treated. Nadolol, with a longer duration of action, is given once daily. Carvedilol is now used as an effective alternative since there is additional alpha receptor blockade.

Ascites

Fifty per cent of patients with cirrhosis develop ascites within 10 years. Ascites is an important milestone, since 50% will die within 2 years. The process by which ascites forms in cirrhosis is not understood fully but involves activation of the renin–angiotensin–aldosterone system (causing renal retention of sodium and water) and the production of antidiuretic hormone (causing hyponatraemia due to dilution of plasma sodium). Hypoalbuminaemia and portal hypertension favour formation of ascites.

Management of ascites

Perform an ascitic tap to confirm the presence of a transudate before initiating therapy. Ultrasound assesses portal vein patency and the presence of hepatocellular carcinoma. Treatment targets induction of natriuresis with consequent loss of water. Salt restriction is effective; fluid restriction is unnecessary unless the plasma sodium falls below 125 mmol/L. Measurement of urinary sodium before treatment and changes in therapy is helpful, indicating if dietary restriction of sodium has been achieved, helping time the introduction of diuretics, guiding dose changes and indicating when therapy has ceased to be effective.

Bed rest (reduces plasma renin activity) with dietary sodium restriction is effective, but diuretics are needed eventually. Spironolactone is most useful, although maximum efficacy is seen at 2 weeks, following metabolism to products with long duration of action, e.g. canrenone ($t_{1/2}$ 10–35 h). If renal function is conserved, loop diuretics, e.g. furosemide,

may be added, counteracting hyperkalaemia induced by spironolactone. A ratio of spironolactone 100 mg to furosemide 40 mg works well and under careful supervision can be increased weekly to a maximum of spironolactone 400 mg + furosemide 160 mg. It is rare for patients to tolerate these doses for long.

Monitor body-weight, as patients with oedema and ascites may exhibit rapid weight loss, which should not exceed 0.5 kg/day; extreme negative fluid balance runs the risk of hypovolaemia, electrolyte disturbance, renal impairment and hepatic encephalopathy.

Patients lose weight if the urinary sodium excretion exceeds intake; those who do not respond despite a high urinary sodium are almost certainly receiving additional dietary sodium (sometimes iatrogenic, e.g. antacids). Unwanted effects of diuretic use are very common; in addition to electrolyte disturbances and renal impairment, cramps are unpleasant and if spironolactone causes painful gynaecomastia, amiloride is an alternative (10–40 mg/day). Those without natriuresis should have diuretic therapy withdrawn.

Abdominal paracentesis was once shunned because of the risk of circulatory failure, but administration of albumin at the time of paracentesis has led to its safe re-introduction. Drainage leads to prompt relief of discomfort of tense, painful ascites and improves circulatory dynamics; it can be undertaken as other measures to control ascites are introduced. Alternatively, paracentesis is the treatment of choice for patients who are unresponsive to diuretic therapy or who have complications of diuretic treatment, especially renal impairment. Planned procedures at intervals of 2–3 weeks restore a degree of quality of life. It is essential to assess subacute bacterial peritonitis at each paracentesis, limit the duration of paracentesis (6 h) and ensure that each litre of ascites removed is matched by 6–8 g albumin given before or with paracentesis. Paracentesis carries a risk of perforation of abdominal contents and abdominal wall varices.

Patients with ascites should receive prophylaxis against subacute bacterial peritonitis. Quinolones, for example ciprofloxacin or norfloxacin, are effective.

Subacute bacterial peritonitis

This medical emergency has high mortality and should be suspected in any patient with liver disease and ascites who develops pain or clinical deterioration. A white cell count >500 cells/mL or >250 neutrophils/mL of ascitic fluid confirms the diagnosis. Culture of ascites is often negative, and treatment should be triggered by the leucocyte count. Infection of ascites is a manifestation of severe liver disease and attributed to translocation of Gram-negative organisms across the gut wall. Antibiotic use is guided by local hospital

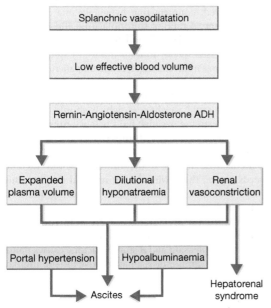

Splanchnic vasodilatation

↓

Low effective blood volume

↓

Rernin-Angiotensin-Aldosterone ADH

Expanded plasma volume | Dilutional hyponatraemia | Renal vasoconstriction

Portal hypertension | Hypoalbuminaemia

→ Ascites ← | Hepatorenal syndrome

Fig. 34.1 Haemodynamic abnormalities in decompensated cirrhosis.

preferences, but quinolones are effective unless the patient has been on antibiotic prophylaxis, when a switch to meropenem is recommended. Treatment is for 7–14 days, with an ascitic tap at completion of therapy. Local antimicrobial guidelines will supervene this recommendation.

Hepatorenal syndrome

This occurs in 10% of patients with advanced cirrhosis and ascites and is attributed to intense renal vasoconstriction (Fig. 34.1). It is defined by the urinary sodium under 5 mmol/L with euvolaemia. Three-month mortality is high. Some patients respond to vasoconstrictor agents, particularly terlipressin, while maintaining volume with albumin, over a 14-day interval. Dopamine is ineffective.

Hepatic encephalopathy

Infection, gastrointestinal bleeding, or injudicious use of sedatives and diuretics can precipitate hepatic encephalopathy in cirrhosis. The pathophysiology is complex, but ammonia is a key player. Diagnosis is confirmed by clinical signs, an elevated plasma ammonia and/or typical EEG appearances. Ammonia is derived from the action of colonic urease-containing bacteria and normally undergoes hepatic extraction from portal blood, but with portal/systemic shunting and impaired hepatic metabolism, it reaches high systemic concentrations, affecting the brain adversely.

Lactulose acts as an osmotic laxative to expedite clearance of potentially toxic substances from the gastrointestinal tract. In addition, colonic bacteria metabolise it to lactic and acetic acids, which inhibit the growth of ammonia-producing organisms and by lowering pH, reduce non-ionic diffusion of ammonia from the colon into the bloodstream. The correct dose is that which produces two to four soft acidic stools daily (usually 30–60 mL daily). Exceeding this dose causes dehydration.

Dietary restriction of protein reduces ammonia production, but any clinical benefit is outweighed by exacerbating malnutrition characteristic of cirrhosis and it is not recommended.

Neomycin and metronidazole inhibit urease-producing bacteria, but their use should be limited by toxicity. The non-absorbed antibiotic rifaximin is now used widely and is effective over a prolonged period without significant toxicity.

Hepatocellular carcinoma (HCC)

Patients with cirrhosis face a substantial lifetime risk of HCC, which is higher in men, increased age and the cause of liver injury. The value of surveillance with liver ultrasound is contentious but now undertaken in line with national guidelines and allows earlier tumour detection. Liver transplantation is curative for 75% with smaller tumours. Surgical resection, radiofrequency ablation and transarterial embolisation have beneficial effects that usually fall short of cure (additional chemotherapy has not been shown to add benefit). Recent clinical trials show sorafenib extends life by just a few months in patients with compensated cirrhosis, but with significant toxicity.

Immune-mediated liver disease

Autoimmune hepatitis (AIH)

This chronic inflammatory disease is associated with circulating antinuclear and smooth muscle antibodies and high serum immunoglobulin concentrations (serum IgG above 20 g/L). The presentations include jaundice with ill-health, relapsing/remitting jaundice and, less commonly, subacute liver failure. One-third of patients have cirrhosis at presentation, and untreated cases progress to cirrhosis. Corticosteroids are first-line therapy (prednisolone 20 mg/day). Faced with subacute liver failure (increased INR and hepatic encephalopathy), the choice is between corticosteroids (with a risk of sepsis) or liver transplantation. Rituximab, to deplete B cells, may have a role in this unusual scenario, but data are preliminary.

The majority of patients improve substantially with corticosteroids, and a fall in serum bilirubin occurs usually within 2 weeks. Azathioprine (1 mg/kg/day) should be introduced when jaundice improves and is an effective steroid-sparing agent. In the long term, corticosteroid doses should be adjusted according to liver function. Elevated IgG levels settle with successful therapy; a rise in serum IgG predates relapse. Remission can be maintained in the first 2 years by azathioprine with prednisolone (5–10 mg/day). If there is evidence of biochemical remission with a normal IgG after 2 years, then withdrawal of corticosteroids can be considered. A liver biopsy to confirm remission is recommended before reducing the dose of corticosteroids. Long-term remission maintained by azathioprine is the goal. There are no clear criteria to determine whether azathioprine can be stopped safely. Corticosteroids often cause steatosis, increasing liver enzymes, which may be mistaken for active AIH.

Mycophenolate mofetil (500 mg twice daily p.o.) appears useful when patients are intolerant of azathioprine. Patients intolerant of prednisolone respond to budesonide (3–9 mg daily p.o.). Budesonide is unproven as induction therapy. Some patients never achieve good control with the prednisolone and azathioprine. Mycophenolate with tacrolimus (trough level 5–10 ng/L) may be effective. All causes of liver injury are associated with accelerated bone loss, and the use of calcium, vitamin D and bisphosphonates in AIH is recommended.

Primary biliary cholangitis (PBC)[1]

PBC is a chronic cholestatic liver disease affecting women predominantly from middle age onwards with a heritable component. Fatigue and pruritus are common, early symptoms that usually predate jaundice. The natural history was thought to be inexorable progress to liver failure over a period of 10 years from presentation, but that view is unduly pessimistic. Once jaundice is present, the course of the illness is predictable.

The aetiology of PBC is unknown, but high titres of antimitochondrial antibody in almost all and elevated IgM levels with clustering of 'autoimmune disorders' in many suggest immune involvement. There is no role (yet) for immune modulation. Corticosteroids are ineffective; methotrexate is ineffective; azathioprine has marginal benefit. Curiously, patients with PBC treated with ciclosporin after transplantation are less likely to suffer PBC in the grafted liver than those prescribed tacrolimus.

The pruritus of cholestasis can be debilitating and has been attributed to autotaxin. The most effective treatment is rifampicin. Cholestyramine, which binds bile salts in the gut, has proved effective, but it is unpleasant to swallow, affecting compliance. Ursodeoxycholic acid 10–15 mg/kg daily is now considered first-line therapy for PBC. For those who respond with a fall in the alkaline phosphatase, the long-term prognosis is good, with a reduced risk of liver decompensation and need for liver transplantation. It is almost free from unwanted effects other than dose-related diarrhoea.

Obeticholic acid (OBCA) has recently been approved by NICE recently for patients with PBC unresponsive to ursodeoxycholic acid with a biochemical pattern indicative of a poor long-term prognosis. Early data indicated that OBCA affected the indicants of poor prognosis favourably, but solid data in terms of effects on a need for liver transplantation or death will take some years to mature. Ironically pruritus, which is often so troubling in PBC, is a common dose-related adverse effect. Two meta-analyses in Japan and recent European data suggest clear benefit with respect to liver biochemistry with the use of fibrates in PBC. These have not been licensed for use in this condition. As with OBCA, there is no evidence yet that this will translate into positive effects on morbidity and mortality.

Chronic cholestasis leads to malabsorption of fat-soluble vitamins, particularly vitamin D, and deficiency should be corrected to avoid osteomalacia. The use of calcium, vitamin D and bisphosphonates for bone loss in PBC is recommended.

Primary sclerosing cholangitis (PSC)

PSC is a progressive disease characterised by remitting/relapsing jaundice that affects predominantly non-smoking men of working age. There is inflammation and stricturing of the larger intrahepatic and extrahepatic bile ducts leading to persistent jaundice and biliary cirrhosis. There is a significant lifetime risk of cholangiocarcinoma. An association with ulcerative colitis, clustering with other autoimmune disorders and a heritable component, suggest this is an autoimmune condition. There is no effective therapy and no role (yet) for immune modulation. Ursodeoxycholic acid 10–15 mg/kg daily is often used, but evidence that this modifies the natural history is lacking. Recurrent episodes of bacterial cholangitis may respond to cyclical antibiotics that are concentrated in bile and target Gram-negative organisms, e.g. ciprofloxacin.

Alcohol-related hepatitis

The sudden onset of jaundice in a patient consuming alcohol to excess heralds the onset of alcohol-related hepatitis. Men

---

[1]Formerly called primary biliary *cirrhosis*.

are admitted to hospital more often than women, but the latter develop the syndrome after a lower lifetime consumption of alcohol (corrected for body weight). The biochemistry is characteristic, with conjugated bilirubinaemia but a normal ALT and alkaline phosphatase. Liver ultrasound shows no evidence of biliary tract disease. Several scoring systems based on INR, bilirubin and age predict mortality, which is substantial. Liver biopsy shows intense inflammation with a neutrophil infiltration. The presence of bacterial infection is a poor prognostic sign; serum markers of inflammation suggest bacterial infection, which is not necessarily present and may be related to elevated plasma cytokine levels.

The inflammatory features led to investigation of immune modulation. Recent data from the largest prospective controlled trial undertaken compared pentoxyfylline with corticosteroids and suggested no benefit from the former and marginal benefit from the latter.

Metabolic disease

Wilson's disease

This recessive genetic disorder (most are compound heterozygotes) predisposes to copper accumulation. Clinical presentations are diverse and include movement disorder, psychiatric illness, haemolysis or liver disease, often advanced. Many pre-symptomatic patients are identified following family screening. Confirmation of the diagnosis can be difficult and relies on a combination of serum copper and caeruloplasmin concentrations, urinary excretion of copper (comparing pre– and post–D-penicillamine excretion), a search for Kayser–Fleischer rings by slit lamp examination and diagnostically, an elevated liver copper concentration. Genetic analysis is increasingly available for the majority of patients.

D-penicillamine, a copper chelating agent, is the treatment of choice for which there is the greatest experience, but since treatment for Wilson's disease is lifelong there have been concerns about short- and long-term toxicity. Trientine is an alternative and effective chelating agent, but there are also long-term concerns. Zinc also reduces total body copper content and probably represents the least toxic long-term option.

Haemochromatosis

Haemochromatosis is a homozygous genetic disease of iron storage affecting numerous organs including the liver, most commonly due to a mutation in the HFE gene. Treatment is by iron depletion, managed most easily, and without toxicity, by venesection. Iron chelation is ineffective.

Non-alcohol–related fatty liver disease

The triad of hypertension, obesity and diabetes mellitus is found commonly in conjunction with abnormal liver function tests. Liver biopsy is almost always abnormal, and patients can be separated into those with steatosis alone or those with steatohepatitis. The latter carries a high risk of progressive liver injury with fibrosis, cirrhosis and eventually HCC, especial in older men. Management is directed first at control of weight, hypertension, hyperlipidaemia and diabetes mellitus. Metformin and insulin sensitisers such as piaglitazone and rosiglitazone improve liver function tests and some histological features, but have no effect on fibrosis, progression or survival.

Viral hepatitis

Hepatitis A virus (HAV)

Changing standards of hygiene and an effective vaccine have altered the pattern of illness associated with HAV infection. Symptomatic infection is uncommon in Western countries but more common than it was in the developing world, because infection now occurs at a later age. Significant disease following HAV infection is confined to those older than 40 years of age. Active immunisation against HAV is recommended before travel; protective antibody takes about 2 weeks to develop and lasts for at least 10 years. Passive immunity, using antibody prepared from pooled plasma from immune donors, confers temporary protection but is no longer recommended.

Hepatitis B virus (HBV)

Exposure to HBV results usually in an acute resolving infection which may be asymptomatic or unrecognised. There is no evidence that intervention in acute infection is helpful, but antiviral therapy (below) should be considered for the tiny proportion that develops acute liver failure with detectable HBV replication. Acute infection in an immune suppressed host, where there is a high risk of serious disease or chronic infection, however, should be treated.

Chronic, usually lifelong, infection follows exposure to HBV in infants; the rate of chronic infection falls throughout childhood, affecting the sexes equally, to 5–10% in adults and men much more than women. Chronic infection is more common in the immune suppressed and the elderly.

Viral load falls with each decade to low levels, and HBV protein production (HBsAg and HBeAg) falls in parallel. Treating all patients is neither practical nor appropriate and careful assessment of the stage of the disease is critical to successful management. Natural history studies reveal that viral replication is associated with progressive liver injury, cirrhosis, liver failure and HCC, all more common in men. Successful antiviral therapy is associated with improved survival, a reduced risk of liver failure, a reduced need for liver transplantation and less HCC.

Interferon-α is available in a pegylated formulation allowing weekly administration by subcutaneous injection. A 6-month course in those with active liver disease, with increased liver enzymes, inflammatory changes on the liver biopsy and a low viral load achieves cure in 25%. Young females fare best. A 'flare' with marked increase in liver enzymes during treatment anticipates elimination of HBV-DNA and HBsAg and development of anti-HBs. Interferon-α should not be used if there is evidence of hepatic decompensation as the 'flare' can precipitate liver failure.

Only a small number of patients are suitable for interferon-α. The majority of patients treated currently receive long-term therapy with an oral *nucleot(s)ide analogue*. Agents include *lamivudine, telbivudine, clavudine, emtricitabine, adefovir, tenofovir* and *entecavir*. Some basic points merit mention. HBV has a high rate of spontaneous mutation, and both immune responses to HBV and antiviral therapy select for mutations. Lessons from other infectious diseases (HIV and tuberculosis) suggest that long-term combination therapy reduces the chance of treatment failure. Long-term control rather than cure of HBV replication is the pragmatic goal with oral therapy. The duration of treatment is uncertain. Loss of HBsAg from the blood is one situation when treatment can be curtailed with less concern. Patients on therapy should be monitored to assess viral load. Liver function tests should fall to normal in line with the drop in viral load. A failure to control viral replication may be due to the evolution of mutations, inadequate dosing or poor compliance. Mutations should be sought if HBV-DNA is detected after a reasonable period of treatment, and for some agents compliance can be assessed by measurement of drug levels in serum. Because the majority of patients will not develop life-threatening liver disease, treatment needs to be targeted at those with, or at risk of, fibrosis. Some women are reluctant to embark on antiviral therapy while pregnancy is possible; *lamivudine*, which has been used for years, appears safe in pregnancy, but newer agents cannot yet be regarded as safe, although there is no evidence yet to raise concern. Some patients have a high risk of HCC and should also be considered for treatment. Many patients will have been treated, often with lamivudine and may have developed mutations as a result. Pre-treatment mutation profiles are not undertaken routinely but a strong case can be made that they should. Confirmation that a mutation is present during therapy necessitates a change in strategy.

The notion that HBV with mutations is less likely to cause liver injury is incorrect.

Perhaps the most important issue in determining which drugs to use first is the clinical context. Those at greatest immediate risk include those with recrudescent HBV post-chemotherapy or subsequent to immune suppression (when the clinical course is accelerated) and with decompensated liver disease. In these scenarios, the drugs with the most rapid and potent antiviral effects should be used (tenofovir). Where there is less urgency, a combination of agents such as lamivudine with adefovir/tenofovir can be considered, although tenofovir is used most often currently. This (even as monotherapy) is associated with the lowest rate of mutations to date (close to zero in large series), but clinical experience is limited to less than 10 years so far. Lamivudine and similar agents are associated with the highest rate of mutations, with adefovir in an intermediate position. As first-line therapy, entecavir has a low level of breakthrough, but mutations are much more likely in those with past use of lamivudine, which may not be recorded.

Hepatitis B vaccination

The hepatitis B vaccine (inactivated HBsAg adsorbed on aluminium hydroxide adjuvant) is effective and provides long-lasting immunity against HBV. Response rates fall with increasing age and are lower in the immune compromised. Protection lasts from years to decades, and it is unclear if booster vaccination is ever required. Escape mutants with heterogeneity in the A epitope, driven by immune responses, are described and coexist with evidence of 'humoral immunity' but are fortunately very rare; thus it is possible to be 'immune' and HBV-DNA positive.

Targeting and screening mothers for HBV in order to protect their children is effective. Babies born to carrier mothers should be vaccinated at birth and after 1 and 6 months and thereafter tested for evidence of immunity and infection beyond 12 months. Concurrent use of hepatitis B immunoglobulin (pooled plasma from highly selected donors with high-titre antibody to HBsAg) as passive prophylaxis is also recommended when the mother has high-level HBV replication, but as a human product, it carries an unquantifiable risk of infection. Increasingly, oral antiviral agents are offered to reduce the risk of vertical transmission.

Hepatitis B immunoglobulin also has a role in providing passive immunity for post-exposure prophylaxis, e.g. after accidental needle stick injury. Conventional vaccination is also important in such cases.

Hepatitis D virus (HDV)

This virus displaces HBV core replacing it with HDV core, but retaining the outer envelope of HBV. HDV infection is rare in clinical practice and occurs either as a simultaneous infection with HBV or as a superinfection in a patient who is already HBV-positive. Long-term treatment with pegylated interferon-α, i.e. for more than 1 year, controls HDV replication (measured as HDV-RNA in serum) in about 50% of cases.

Hepatitis C virus (HCV)

Exposure to HCV is most often a consequence of injecting drug use; vertical transmission (mother to child) occurs in 5%. Historically, HCV infection was associated with transfusion of blood/blood products, but that risk is now close to zero with reliable tests for HCV in donors. Acute HCV infection is usually asymptomatic. Chronic infection follows exposure in 85% of cases and is more likely at extremes of age or with immune suppression. Genetic variation, such as polymorphism of IL28B, underlies spontaneous resolution in some patients. Some 5% develop cirrhosis, and 25% of those develop HCC. The rate at which liver disease progresses to cirrhosis varies markedly between individuals, but can be rapid in those acquiring infection after 60 years of age. Age older than 40 years at infection, male sex, a raised body mass index, insulin resistance, immune suppression, HIV infection and alcohol abuse all increase the chance that fibrosis will progress. Significant fibrosis at liver biopsy predicts progression at subsequent biopsy.

The treatment of chronic hepatitis C virus infection is under almost continuous review as newer and more effective treatments are developed at a truly astonishing rate. The reader is advised to review guidelines published online by the American Association for the Study of Liver Disease (AASLD) and the European Association for the Study of Liver Disease (EASL), which are updated regularly. However, readers are also advised, when reviewing these, to consider national policies, which will reflect local genotype, the stage of disease, national priorities and almost certainly and above all other factors, the financial situation (bearing in mind the large number of infected patients needing and wanting treatment). The cost of the newer therapies is considerable but has fallen considerably in the past 24 months as a consequence of the large numbers of patients being treated and the number of antiviral therapies available, thereby increasing competition among companies.

The newer antiviral agents are almost all protease inhibitors or are targeted either to the non-structural protein NS5A or to inhibit the polymerase NS5B. By using these agents in various combinations, each with a different target, the number of emerging resistant viruses can be reduced to a minimum. The newer agents should be used in combination in short courses, which is likely to increase compliance. Cure rates across all genotypes, all stages of liver fibrosis, all ages and both sexes exceed 95%. The exception appears

to be those patients who have failed treatment previously, but even in these long-term cure can be achieved in over 90%, and newer therapies targeting this group of patients in particular may become available in 2018. The response rates in those with decompensated liver disease are also excellent, allowing sufficient recovery of liver function in many so that patients may be removed from the transplant waiting list. Other groups that historically have been difficult to treat include those with HCV-infected liver grafts and those with HIV co-infection, but high cure rates can also be achieved in both groups, although with careful consideration of the interactions to be expected in combination with immune suppression regimes or medication for HIV infection. Boxes 34.1–34.4 provide an indication of current UK practice with the expectation that these data will be out of date soon.

Unwanted effects for these newer agents have proved remarkable for their rarity, and few have proved serious despite considerable exposure over the past 2 years.

Box 34.1 Progress in treatment of Hepatitis C (1)

- First-generation protease inhibitors with (interferon-α) telaprevir, boceprevir [ribavirin].
- Sofosbuvir (without interferon) for genotype 2 and genotype 3 [ribavirin].
- DAAs:
  - daclatasvir with sofosbuvir for genotype 2 and genotype 3
  - sofosbuvir plus second-wave protease inhibitor simeprevir [ribavirin]
  - sofosbuvir with lepidasvir
  - paritaprevir, ritonavir, ombitasvir and dasabuvir.

Box 34.2 Progress in treatment of Hepatitis C (2): UK policy December 2016

- 28 different first-line regimes and 12 second-line regimes based on:
  - treatment naïve or previously treated
  - presence or absence of cirrhosis (fibroscan)
  - compensated or decompensated liver disease
  - liver transplanted
  - HIV co-infection
  - genotype 1a, 1b, 2, 3, 4, 5, 6.
- 12 weeks except:
  - Genotype 5 and genotype 6 (interferon and ribavirin) 16 weeks for high viral load.

One area yet to be resolved is whether it is justified to screen for likely viral-resistant mutations before treatment in order to guide therapy or instead to screen for mutations in those in whom therapy has failed. Local decisions will depend on the ability to screen for mutations promptly, the cost of screening and the likelihood that a mutation will survive combination therapy.

Unwanted effects for these newer agents have proved remarkable for their rarity, and few have proved serious despite considerable exposure over the past 2 years.

One area yet to be resolved is whether it is justified to screen for likely viral-resistant mutations before treatment in order to guide therapy or instead to screen for mutations in those in whom therapy has failed. Local decisions will depend on the ability to screen for mutations promptly, the cost of screening and the likelihood that a mutation will survive combination therapy.

Gallstones

Ursodeoxycholic acid can dissolve cholesterol gallstones, as it supplements the bile acid pool and improves the solubility of cholesterol in bile. It is used rarely, if at all, for this indication but may have a role in patients with disease due to biliary sludge or microcrystals identified at endoscopic ultrasound of the biliary tree; it is often used in patients with biliary tract disease 'prophylactically' to prevent stone formation within the biliary tree. The dose is 8–12 mg/kg daily orally.

Pancreas

Digestive enzymes

In pancreatic *exocrine insufficiency,* the aim of therapy is to prevent weight loss and diarrhoea and in children to maintain growth. The problem of getting sufficient enzyme to the duodenum concurrently with food is not as simple as it might appear. High fat, calories and protein delay gastric emptying, while gastric acid destroys pancreatic enzymes taken by mouth. Only one-tenth of normal pancreatic output is sufficient to prevent steatorrhoea. Acid suppression by proton pump inhibitors improves the efficacy of pancreatic enzyme supplements.

Preparations are of animal origin and variable potency. *Pancreatin*, as Cotazym and Nutrizym, is satisfactory. Start patients on the recommended dose of a reliable formulation, and vary this according to clinical need and the size and composition of meals. Enteric-coated formulations (pancreatin granules, tablets) are available. High-potency pancreatic enzymes should not be used in patients with cystic fibrosis as they cause ileocaecal and large bowel strictures.

Acute pancreatitis

Many drugs have been tested for specific effect, but none has shown convincing benefit. The main requirements of therapy are:

- To provide adequate *analgesia*. Opioids are generally satisfactory; analgesic efficacy outweighs the potential disadvantage of contracting the sphincter of Oddi (and retarding the flow of pancreatic secretion); buprenorphine is often preferred.
- To correct *hypovolaemia* due to the exudation of large amounts of fluid around the inflamed pancreas. Plasma may be required, or blood if the haematocrit falls; in addition, large volumes of electrolyte solution may be needed to preserve renal function.
- To achieve biliary drainage (by endoscopic retrograde cannulation of the pancreas) early in the illness if gallstones are suspected.
- The value of additional interventions, including nutritional support and antibiotic prophylaxis, is as yet unproven.

Drugs and the pancreas

Adverse effects are most commonly manifest as *acute pancreatitis*. The strongest association is with *alcohol* abuse. High plasma calcium concentration, including that caused by hypervitaminosis D and parenteral nutrition, also increases the risk. Corticosteroids, didanosine, azathioprine, diuretics (including thiazides and furosemide), sodium valproate, mesalazine and paracetamol (in overdose) are causally related.

Guide to further reading

Adams, D.H., Haydon, G., (Eds.) 2006. Liver disease. Clin. Med. (Northfield Il) 6, 19–46.

American Association for the Study of Liver Disease practice guidelines. Available at: http://www.aasld.org/practice guidelines/.

European Association for the Study of the Liver. Available at: http://www.easl.eu/_clinicalpractice-guidelines/.

Johnson, C.D., 2005. UK guidelines for the management of acute pancreatitis. Gut 54 (Suppl.iii), 1–9.

Kingsnorth, A., O'Reilly, D., 2006. Acute pancreatitis. Br. Med. J. 332, 1072–1076.

Krawitt, E.L., 2006. Autoimmune hepatitis. N. Engl. J. Med. 354, 54–66.

Lee, W.M., 2003. Drug-induced hepatotoxicity. N. Engl. J. Med. 349, 474–485.

Navarro, V.J., Senior, J.R., 2006. Drug-related hepatotoxicity. N. Engl. J. Med. 354, 731–739.

NHS evidence for gastroenterology and liver disease. Available at: https://www.nhs.uk/conditions/hepatitis-c/treatment/.

Endocrine system, metabolic conditions

Chapter 35

Adrenal corticosteroids, antagonists, corticotropin

Diana C. Brown, Morris J. Brown

SYNOPSIS

- Adrenocortical steroids and their synthetic analogues.
  - Mechanisms of action
  - Actions: mineralocorticoid, glucocorticoid
  - Individual adrenal steroids
  - Pharmacokinetics
  - Dosage schedules
  - Choice of adrenal steroid
  - Adverse effects of systemic pharmacotherapy
  - Adrenal steroids and pregnancy
  - Precautions during chronic therapy: treatment of intercurrent illness
  - Dosage and routes of administration
  - Indications for use
  - Uses: replacement therapy, pharmacotherapy
  - Withdrawal of pharmacotherapy.
- Inhibition of synthesis of adrenal steroids.
- Competitive antagonism.
- Adrenocorticotrophic hormone (ACTH) (corticotropin).

In 1855, Dr Thomas Addison, assisted in his observations by three colleagues, published his famous monograph 'On the constitutional effects of disease on the suprarenal capsules' (Addison's disease). It was not until the late 1920s that the vital importance of the adrenal cortex was appreciated and the distinction made between the hormones secreted by the cortex and medulla.

By 1936, numerous steroids were being crystallised from cortical extracts, but the quantities were insufficient to provide supplies for clinical trial.

In 1948, cortisone was made from bile acids in quantity sufficient for clinical trial, and the dramatic demonstration of its power to induce remission of rheumatoid arthritis was published the following year. In 1950, it was realised that cortisone was biologically inert and that the active natural hormone is cortisol. The pharmaceutical term for cortisol is hydrocortisone. The two terms are often used interchangeably. In this chapter, cortisol is used when describing endogenous hormone secretion, and hydrocortisone when describing exogenous drug administration. Since then many steroids have been synthesised, covering the wide range of efficacy and potency required by the many indications for systemic and local use. Steroids derive from natural substances, chiefly plant sterols. The ideal steroid drug, providing all the desirable and none of the undesirable effects of cortisol, remains elusive. Research showing the multiple molecular actions of steroids within the target cell has explained the difficulty of achieving the ideal, but may help to bring this closer.

About the same time as cortisone was introduced, adrenocorticotrophin (ACTH) became available for clinical use. Its use is now largely for diagnostic tests of the pituitary–adrenal axis.

Adrenal steroids and their synthetic analogues

The adrenal is a composite endocrine gland, and each zone of the cortex synthesises a different predominant steroid; a mnemonic is offered in Fig. 35.1, in which the first letter of each word is the first letter of each zone and its corresponding steroid product. The principal synthetic pathways are illustrated in Fig. 35.2.

- **Cortex**

- 'Go Find Rex, Make
  Good Sex'
  - Glomerulosa
  - Fasciculata
  - Reticularis
  - Mineralocorticoids
  - Glucocorticoids
  - Androgens

- **Medulla**
  - Epinephrine
  - Norepinephrine

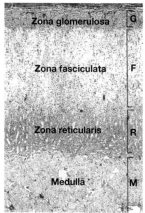

Fig. 35.1 The zones of the adrenal gland and the hormones they secrete.

The principal hormone is the glucocorticoid *cortisol* secreted from the largest zone, the fasciculata; the mineralocorticoid *aldosterone* is secreted by the glomerulosa, and a number of *androgens* and *oestrogens* are secreted by the zona reticularis. The hypothalamic–pituitary system, through corticotropin releasing factor (CRF) and ACTH, controls cortisol and, to a lesser extent, aldosterone secretion; synthesis and secretion of aldosterone is regulated mainly by the renin–angiotensin system, and by variation in plasma K$^+$ levels.

Adrenal corticosteroids are available for physiological replacement therapy, in primary (Addison's disease), secondary adrenal insufficiency and congenital adrenal hyperplasia, but their chief use in medicine is for their anti-inflammatory and immunosuppressive effects (pharmacotherapy). Supraphysiological doses are generally required to achieve these pharmacological effects. Chronic use of supraphysiological doses has many adverse effects. Much successful effort has gone into separating glucocorticoid from mineralocorticoid effects.

In the account that follows, the effects of hydrocortisone will be described and then other steroids in so far as they differ. In the context of this chapter, 'adrenal steroid' means a substance with hydrocortisone-like activity. Androgens are described in Chapter 38.

Mechanism of action

Glucocorticoids stimulate the cell through both a classical cytosolic receptor that, on binding with agonist, translocates to the nucleus, and an unidentified membrane-bound receptor (Fig. 35.3). The classical receptor is responsible for so-called genomic effects through either activation or repression of DNA transcription. Up-regulation of gene transcription occurs when the receptor dimerises on specific DNA

glucocorticoid response elements (GREs) with consequent recruitment of coactivator proteins. Many of the undesired effects of glucocorticoid occur through this pathway.

Repression of DNA transcription occurs at slightly lower cortisol concentrations than required for transactivation. Through protein–protein interaction, the glucocorticoid–receptor complex inactivates pro-inflammatory transcription factors such as nuclear factor (NF)-κB and activator protein 1 (AP-1), preventing their stimulation of inflammatory mediators: prostaglandins, leukotrienes, cytokines and platelet-activating factor. These mediators would normally contribute to increased vascular permeability and subsequent changes including oedema, leucocyte migration and fibrin deposition.[1]

There is a distinction between *replacement therapy* (physiological effects) and the higher doses of *pharmacotherapy*. However, the distinction is not absolute because cortisol is a stress hormone, and some of its physiological actions are triggered by the increased secretion of cortisol during acute or chronic stress. In the list that follows, the main physiological effects are those concerned with elimination of a water load, and mobilisation of glucose. The suppression of inflammatory mediators may also be seen as part of physiological homeostasis.

On inorganic metabolism. Cortisol is required for excretion of a water load. This action is due to maintenance of glomerular filtration, activation of atrial natriuretic factor, and inhibition of vasopressin secretion. These physiological effects are unrelated to the mineralocorticoid (Na$^+$-retaining) action of cortisol that occurs at supraphysiological concentrations.

On organic metabolism

- *Carbohydrate metabolism.* Glycogenolysis and gluconeogenesis are increased and peripheral glucose utilisation is decreased (due to insulin antagonism).
- *Protein metabolism.* Anabolism (conversion of amino acids to protein) decreases but catabolism continues, so that there is a negative nitrogen balance with muscle wasting. The skin atrophies and this, with increased capillary fragility, causes bruising and striae. Healing of peptic ulcers or of wounds is delayed, as is fibrosis.
- *Bone metabolism.* Cortisol inhibits the number and function of osteoblasts, and the synthesis of collagen.

---

[1] Potency (the weight of drug in relation to its effect) rather than efficacy (strength of response); see page 85. If a large enough dose of a glucocorticoid, e.g. prednisolone, were administered, the Na$^+$ retention would be almost as great as that caused by a mineralocorticoid. This is why, in practice, different (more selective, and potent) glucocorticoids, not higher doses of prednisolone, need to be used when maximal stimulation of glucocorticoid receptors is desired, e.g. in the treatment of acute transplant rejections.

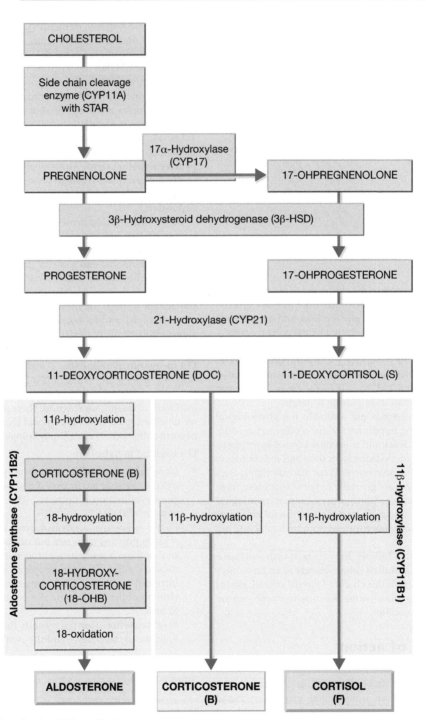

Fig. 35.2 Adrenal corticosteroid biosynthesis.

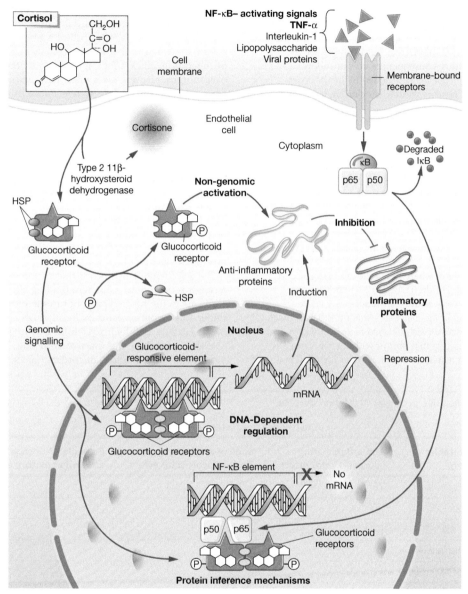

Fig. 35.3 Three general mechanisms of action of glucocorticoids and the glucocorticoid receptor in the inhibition of inflammation: non-genomic activation, DNA-dependent regulation, and protein interference mechanisms (e.g. NF-κB elements). Red arrows denote activation, the red line inhibition, the blue arrow repression, and the red X lack of product (i.e. no mRNA). HSP, heat-shock protein; mRNA, messenger RNA; NF, nuclear factor; P, phosphate; TNF, tumour necrosis factor. *(Adapted from Rhen T, Cidlowski J A 2005 Antiinflammatory action of glucocorticoids – new mechanisms for old drugs. New England Journal of Medicine 353(16):1711–1723.)*

Osteoporosis (reduction of bone protein matrix) is the main consequence of chronic glucocorticoid administration. Growth slows in children.

- *Fat metabolism.* Lipolysis is increased, and the secretion of leptin (the appetite suppressant) is

inhibited. These actions lead to increased appetite and deposition of adipose tissue, particularly on shoulders, face and abdomen.

- *Inflammatory response* is depressed. Neutrophil and macrophage function are depressed, including the release of chemical mediators and the effects of these on capillaries.

- *Allergic responses* are suppressed. The antigen–antibody interaction is unaffected, but its injurious inflammatory consequences do not follow.
- *Antibody production* is lessened by heavy doses.
- *Lymphoid tissue* is reduced (including leukaemic lymphocytes).
- *Renal excretion* of urate is increased.
- *Blood eosinophils* reduce in number and neutrophils increase.
- *Euphoria or psychotic* states may occur, perhaps due to central nervous system (CNS) electrolyte changes.
- *Anti-vitamin D action* see calciferol.
- *Reduction of hypercalcaemia*, chiefly where this is due to excessive absorption of calcium from the gut (sarcoidosis, vitamin D intoxication).
- *Urinary calcium excretion* is increased and renal stones may form.
- *Growth reduces* where new cells are being added (growth in children), but not where they are replacing cells as in adult tissues.
- *Suppression of hypothalamic–pituitary–adrenocortical feedback system* (with delayed recovery) occurs with chronic use, so that abrupt withdrawal leaves the patient in a state of adrenocortical insufficiency.

The average daily secretion of cortisol is normally 10 mg (5.7 mg/m^2). The exogenous daily dose that completely suppresses the cortex is hydrocortisone 40–80 mg, or prednisolone 10–20 mg, or its equivalent of other agents. Recovery of function is quick after a few days' use, but when used over months, recovery takes months. A steroid-suppressed adrenal gland continues to secrete aldosterone.

Individual adrenal steroids

The relative potencies[1] for glucocorticoid and mineralocorticoid (sodium-retaining) effects (Table 35.1) are central to the choice of agent in relation to clinical indication.

All drugs in Table 35.1 except aldosterone are active when swallowed, being protected from hepatic first-pass metabolism by high binding to plasma proteins. Some details of preparations and equivalent doses appear in the table. Injectable and topical forms are available (creams, suppositories, eye drops).

The selectivity of hydrocortisone for the glucocorticoid receptor is due not to a different binding affinity of hydrocortisone to the two receptors but to the protection of the mineralocorticoid receptor by locally high concentrations of the enzyme 11 β-hydroxysteroid dehydrogenase, which converts cortisol to the inactive cortisone. This enzyme saturates at concentrations of cortisol (and some synthetic

Table 35.1 Relative potencies of adrenal steroids

| Compound (tablet strength, mg) | Approximate relative potency | | |
	Anti-inflammatory (glucocorticoid) effect	Sodium-retaining (mineralocorticoid) effect	Equivalent[a] dosage (for anti-inflammatory effect, mg)[b]
Cortisone (25)	0.8	1.0	25
Hydrocortisone (20)	1.0	1.0	20
Prednisolone (5)	4	0.8	5
Methylprednisolone (4)	5	Minimal	4
Triamcinolone (4)	5	None	4
Dexamethasone (0.5)	30	Minimal	0.75
Betamethasone (0.5)	30	Negligible	0.75
Fludrocortisone (0.1)	15	150	Irrelevant
Aldosterone (none)	None	500[c]	Irrelevant

[a]Note that these equivalents are in approximate inverse accord with the tablet strengths.
[b]The doses in the final column are in the lower range of those that may cause suppression of the hypothalamic–pituitary–adrenocortical axis when given daily continuously. Much higher doses, e.g. prednisolone 40 mg, can be given on alternate days or daily for up to 5 days without causing clinically significant suppression.
[c]Injected.

glucocorticoids) just above the physiological range, which explains the onset of mineralocorticoid action with pathological secretion of cortisol, and pharmacological use of glucocorticoids.

Hydrocortisone (cortisol) is the principal naturally occurring steroid; it is taken orally; a soluble salt can be given intravenously for rapid effect in emergency whether due to deficiency, allergy or inflammatory disease. A suspension (Hydrocortisone Acetate Inj.) is available for intra-articular injection.

Parenteral preparation for systemic effect: the soluble Hydrocortisone Sodium Succinate Inj. gives quick (1–2 h) effect; for continuous effect, about 6-hourly administration is appropriate. Prednisolone Acetate Inj. i.m. is an alternative, once or twice a week.

Tablet strengths, see Table 35.1.

Prednisolone is predominantly anti-inflammatory (glucocorticoid), biologically active, and has little sodium-retaining activity; it is the standard choice for anti-inflammatory pharmacotherapy, orally or intramuscularly.

Methylprednisolone is similar to prednisolone; it is used intravenously for pulse therapy (see below).

Fluorinated corticosteroids (triamcinolone, fludrocortisone)

Triamcinolone has virtually no sodium-retaining (mineralocorticoid) effect. Muscle wasting may occasionally be severe, and chronic administration is therefore contraindicated. Anorexia and mental depression can occur at high dose.

Fludrocortisone is a synthetic mineralocorticoid, which stimulates sodium retention. It can replace aldosterone when the adrenal cortex is destroyed (Addison's disease). Fludrocortisone is also the drug of choice in most patients with autonomic neuropathy, in whom volume expansion is easier to achieve than a sustained increase in vasoconstrictor tone. Much higher doses of fludrocortisone (0.5–1.0 mg) are required when the cause of hypotension is a salt-losing syndrome of renal origin, e.g. after an episode of interstitial nephritis.

Dexamethasone and betamethasone are similar, powerful, predominantly anti-inflammatory steroids. They are longer acting than prednisolone and are used for therapeutic adrenocortical suppression.

Aldosterone ($t_{1/2}$ 20 min), is the principal natural salt-retaining hormone. After oral administration, it is rapidly inactivated in the first pass through the liver and is not available for therapeutic use.

Spironolactone (see p. 585) is a competitive mineralocorticoid (aldosterone) antagonist. It is used in the treatment of primary hyperaldosteronism, as a diuretic in resistant hypertension, and when severe oedema is due to secondary hyperaldosteronism, e.g. cirrhosis, congestive cardiac failure. Long-term treatment increases survival in cardiac failure, possibly through blocking the fibrotic effect of aldosterone upon the heart. The dose of spironolactone is limited by its anti-androgen activity. *Eplerenone* has greater selectivity than spironolactone for the mineralocorticoid than androgen receptor, but has lower efficacy in blocking aldosterone and may need to be used together with amiloride.

Beclometasone, budesonide, fluticasone, mometasone and ciclesonide are potent soluble steroids suitable for use by inhalation for asthma (see p. 502) and intranasally for hay fever. Patients swallow about 90% of an inhalation dose, which is then largely inactivated by hepatic first-pass. The drugs are listed in order of development; some newer agents possess properties (first-pass metabolism, high protein binding and lipophilicity) that may increase pulmonary residence time and reduce systemic effects. The main protection against these effects is simply that absorption through mouth, lungs and gut is low relative to the amounts used in systemic administration. The risk of suppression of the hypothalamic–pituitary–adrenal (HPA) axis is infrequent and dose dependent. The greatest risk of suppression appears to occur with high-dose fluticasone usage in children, who may present with hypoglycaemia and acute adrenal insufficiency.

Pharmacokinetics of corticosteroids

Absorption of the synthetic steroids given orally is rapid. The plasma $t_{1/2}$ of most is 1–3 h but the maximum biological effect occurs after 2–8 h. Administration is usually two or three times a day. They are metabolised principally in the liver (some undergoing hepatic first-pass metabolism, see above) and some pass unchanged into the urine. Hepatic and renal disease prolongs, and enzyme induction shortens, $t_{1/2}$ to an extent that can be clinically important.

Topical application (skin, lung, joints) allows absorption, which can be enough to cause systemic effects.

In the blood, adrenal steroids circulate in both free and bound forms. Only the free form is biologically active. In the case of hydrocortisone, 95% is bound to cortisol-binding globulin (CBG). This has high affinity, but low capacity; when CBG is saturated, hydrocortisone is 80% bound to albumin.

Because CBG is saturated at peak diurnal levels of cortisol, the free cortisol concentration ranges from approximately 1 nanomol/L at the diurnal trough to approximately 100 nanomol/L at the diurnal peak. CBG concentrations increase in the presence of oestrogens, e.g. pregnancy, oral contraceptives.

In patients with very low serum albumin, the steroid dose should be lowered to allow for reduced binding capacity.

In liver disease, low albumin concentration may be accompanied by slow metabolism ($t_{1/2}$ of prednisolone may be doubled).

Dosage schedules

Various dosing schedules have attempted to limit HPA suppression by allowing the plasma steroid concentration to fall between doses in order to provide time for pituitary recovery. These have not been successful. Daily administration, preferably as a single morning dose, is required for the shortest time necessary. For some indications, e.g. use of methylprednisolone in collagen diseases, pulsed administration of high doses is employed at intervals of weeks or months.

Choice of adrenal steroid: summary

- *For oral replacement therapy* in adrenocortical insufficiency, use *hydrocortisone* as the glucocorticoid. In primary adrenal failure (Addison's disease and congenital adrenal hyperplasia), use *fludrocortisone* as the mineralocorticoid to replace aldosterone.
- *For anti-inflammatory and antiallergic (immunosuppressive) effect*, use *prednisolone* or *dexamethasone*. For inhalation, more potent adrenal steroids are required, e.g. *beclometasone* or *budesonide*.
- In diagnostic testing use dexamethasone. In adults with congenital adrenal hyperplasia use hydrocortisone, prednisolone or dexamethasone and hydrocortisone in children.

Adverse effects of systemic adrenal steroid pharmacotherapy

These arise from an excess of the physiological or pharmacological actions of hydrocortisone. Adverse effects are dependent on the corticosteroid used, and on dose and duration. Some occur only with systemic use and for this reason local therapy, e.g. inhalation, intra-articular injection, is preferred where practicable.

The principal adverse effects of chronic corticosteroid administration are:

Endocrine. Chronic dosing leads to features of Cushing's syndrome: moon face, central obesity, oedema, hypertension, striae, bruising, acne, hirsutism. *Diabetes mellitus* may occur.

Musculoskeletal. *Proximal myopathy* and *tendon rupture* may occur. *Osteoporosis* develops insidiously leading to fractures of vertebrae, ribs, femora and feet. Pain and restriction of movement may occur months in advance of radiographic

changes. A bisphosphonate, with vitamin D and calcium supplements, is useful for prevention and treatment. Daily subcutaneous injections of teriparatide (human parathyroid hormone 1-34) increase bone formation and bone density and prevent fractures in glucocorticoid treated patients with osteoporosis. *Growth* in children is impaired. *Avascular necrosis* of bone (femoral heads) is a serious complication (at higher doses); it appears to be due to restriction of blood flow through bone capillaries.

Immune. *Suppression of the inflammatory response to infection and immunosuppression* can mask typical symptoms and signs, and cause more rapid deterioration than usual. The incidence of infection increases with high-dose therapy, and any infection can be more severe when it occurs. The main infections of which patients are at increased risk are fungal, especially *candidiasis*, and activation of previously dormant *tuberculosis*. *Pneumocystis carinii* can occur in the absence of other forms of immunosuppression. Intra-articular injections demand strict asepsis. *Live vaccines* become dangerous. Developing chickenpox may result in a severe form of the disease, and patients who have not had chickenpox should receive varicella zoster immune globulin within 3 days of exposure. Similarly, they should avoid exposure to measles.

Gastrointestinal. Patients taking steroid regularly, especially in combination with a non-steroidal anti-inflammatory drug (NSAID), have an excess incidence of *peptic ulcer* and *haemorrhage* of about 1–2%. Prophylactic treatment with a proton pump inhibitor is appropriate when ulcer is particularly likely, e.g. in rheumatoid arthritis, or patients with a history of peptic ulcer disease. There is increased incidence of pancreatitis.

Central nervous system. *Depression* and *psychosis* can occur during the first few days of high-dose administration, especially in those with a history of mental disorder. Other effects include *euphoria, insomnia*, and *aggravation of schizophrenia* and *epilepsy*. Long-term treatment may result in *raised intracranial pressure* with papilloedema, especially in children.

Ophthalmic effects may include *posterior subcapsular lens cataract* (risk when dose exceeds prednisolone 10 mg/day or equivalent for more than a year), *glaucoma* (with prolonged use of eye drops), and *corneal* or *scleral thinning*.

Other effects include menstrual disorders, delayed tissue healing (including myocardial rupture after myocardial infarction), thromboembolism and, paradoxically, hypersensitivity reactions including anaphylaxis.

Adrenal steroids and pregnancy

Adrenal steroids are teratogenic in animals. A three- to four-fold relative risk of cleft palate is observed in the offspring of mothers receiving steroid pharmacotherapy during early pregnancy. Adrenal insufficiency due to hypothalamic–pituitary suppression in the newborn occurs only with high doses to the mother. Dosage during pregnancy should be kept as low as practicable and fluorinated steroids are best avoided as they are more teratogenic in animals. Hypoadrenal women who become pregnant may require an increase in hydrocortisone replacement therapy by about 10 mg/day to compensate for the increased binding by plasma proteins that occurs in pregnancy. Manage labour as for major surgery (below).

Precautions during chronic adrenal steroid therapy

The most important precaution during replacement and pharmacotherapy is regular review for adverse effects including fluid retention (weight gain), hypertension, glycosuria, hypokalaemia (potassium supplements may be necessary) and back pain (osteoporosis). The main hazard is patient non-compliance.

Patients must always:

- carry a steroid card giving details of therapy
- be impressed with the importance of compliance
- know what to do if they develop an intercurrent illness or other severe stress, i.e. double their next dose and consult their doctor. If a patient omits a dose, a replacement dose should be taken as soon as possible to maintain the same total daily intake, because every patient should be taking the minimum dose necessary to control the disease
- have access to parenteral hydrocortisone (their own supply for i.m. injection, if urgent medical referral is not always possible).

Membership of one of the self-help patient groups can be helpful.

Treatment of intercurrent illness

The normal adrenal cortex responds to severe stress by secreting more than 300 mg hydrocortisone daily. During intercurrent illness, or any other form of severe stress, escalation of steroid dose, and treatment of the underlying problem, is urgent. Effective chemotherapy of bacterial infections is especially important.

Viral infections contracted during steroid therapy (prednisolone 20 mg/day, or the equivalent) can be overwhelming. Immunosuppressed patients exposed to varicella/herpes zoster virus may need passive protection with varicella zoster immunoglobulin (VZIG) as soon as practicable. However, corticosteroid may sometimes be useful therapy for some viral diseases (e.g. thyroiditis, encephalitis) once there has been time for the immune response to occur. Corticosteroid then acts by suppressing unwanted effects of immune responses and excessive inflammatory reaction.

Vomiting warrants parenteral steroid.

Surgery requires that patients receive hydrocortisone 100 mg i.m. or i.v. (or hydrocortisone 20 mg orally) with premedication. If there are any signs of cardiovascular collapse during the operation, infuse hydrocortisone (100 mg) i.v. at once. If surgery is uncomplicated, hydrocortisone 50–100 mg i.v. or i.m. every 6 h for 24–72 h is adequate for most patients on replacement therapy. Then reduce the dose by half every 24 h until the normal dose is reached.

Minor operations, e.g. dental extraction, may be covered by hydrocortisone 20 mg orally 2–4 h before operation, and the same dose afterwards.

In all of these situations, an intravenous infusion should be available for immediate use in case the recommendations above are insufficient. These precautions are particularly relevant for patients who have received substantial corticosteroid treatment within the previous year, because their HPA system may fail to respond adequately to severe stress. If steroid therapy has been very prolonged, and in patients undergoing adrenalectomy for Cushing's syndrome for adrenal adenoma (because the remaining adrenal gland is atrophic), the precautions apply for as long as 2 years afterwards, or until there is evidence of recovery of normal adrenal function.

Dosage and routes of administration

No single schedule suits every case, but examples appear below.

Systemic commencing doses:

- For a *serious disease* such as systemic lupus, dermatomyositis: prednisolone up to 0.5–1.5 mg/kg daily, orally in divided doses. There is no evidence of increased benefit above 60–80 mg/day.
- If the condition is *life-threatening*, give prednisolone up to 60 mg, or its equivalent of another steroid. Cyclophosphamide or azathioprine (see p. 258) are valuable adjuncts which may enhance the initial control of the disease and have a sparing effect on the maintenance dose of prednisolone.
- Alternatively, high dose pulses (methylprednisolone 1.0 g i.v. daily for 3 days) may be used, followed by oral maintenance with prednisolone and/or a steroid-sparing agent (above).
- For *less dangerous* disease, e.g. rheumatoid arthritis, give prednisolone 7.5–10.0 mg daily, adjusted later according to the response.
- In particular cases, including replacement of adrenal insufficiency, the dosage appears in the account of the disease.

601

- For *continuous therapy*, give the minimum amount to produce the desired effect. Imperfect control may have to be accepted by the patient if full control, e.g. of rheumatoid arthritis, though obtainable, involves doses that will lead to toxicity, e.g. osteoporosis, if continued for years.

Topical applications (creams, intranasal, inhalations, enemas) are used in order to obtain local effect, while avoiding systemic effects; suspensions of solutions are also injected into joints, soft tissues and subconjunctivally. All can, in heavy dose, be absorbed sufficiently to suppress the hypothalamus and cause other unwanted effects. Individual preparations appear in the text where appropriate.

Contraindications to adrenal steroids for suppressing inflammation are all relative. Where the patient has diabetes, a history of mental disorder or peptic ulcer, epilepsy, tuberculosis, hypertension or heart failure, the reasons for use must be compelling. The presence of any infection demands that effective chemotherapy be begun before the corticosteroid, but there are exceptions (some viral infections, see above). Topical corticosteroid applied to an inflamed eye can be disastrous if the inflammation is due to herpes virus.

Adrenal steroids containing fluorine (see above) intensify diabetes more than do others and are to be avoided in that disease.

Long-term use of adrenal steroids in children presents essentially the same problems as in adults with the addition of growth retardation. This is unlikely to be important unless therapy exceeds 6 months; there is a growth spurt after withdrawal. The dose should be reduced to the minimum required to maintain immunosuppression and be given daily or alternate days.

Common childhood viral infections may be more severe, and if a non-immune child taking steroids is exposed to virus infection it is wise to try to prevent the disease with the appropriate specific immunoglobulin.

Live virus vaccination is unsafe in immunosuppressed subjects, e.g. systemic prednisolone, more than 2 mg/kg/day for more than 1 week in the preceding 3 months, as it may cause the disease, but active immunisation with killed vaccines or toxoids will give normal response unless the dose of steroid is high, when the response may be suppressed.

Raised intracranial pressure may occur more readily in children than in adults.

Indications for use of adrenal steroids

- Replacement of hormone deficiency.
- Inflammation suppression.
- Immunosuppression.
- Suppression of excess hormone secretion.

Uses of adrenocortical steroids

Replacement therapy

Acute adrenocortical insufficiency (Addisonian crisis)

This is an emergency; hydrocortisone sodium succinate 100 mg is given i.v. immediately it is *suspected*.

- An intravenous infusion of sodium chloride solution (0.9%) is set up immediately and a second 100 mg hydrocortisone is added to the first litre, which should be given as quickly as the cardiovascular status permits (2–3 L of sodium chloride may be infused in the first 1–2 h and 5–6 L may be needed in the first 24 h).
- The patient should then receive hydrocortisone 50 mg i.v. or i.m. 6-hourly for 24–72 h; thereafter a total of 30–40 mg/day orally in two or three divided doses usually suffices.

Treatment to restore electrolyte balance will depend on the circumstances. Seek and treat the cause of the crisis; it is often an infection. When the dose of hydrocortisone falls below 40 mg/day, supplementary mineralocorticoid (fludrocortisone) may be needed (see below).

The hyperkalaemia of Addison's disease will respond to the above regimen and must not be treated with insulin.

Chronic primary adrenocortical insufficiency (Addison's disease)

Hydrocortisone is given orally (15–25 mg total daily) in two to three divided doses, according to the algorithm in Fig. 35.4. Some patients working under increased physical activity or mental stress may require higher doses up to 40 mg daily. The aim is to mimic the natural diurnal rhythm of secretion. All patients also require mineralocorticoid replacement, and fludrocortisone; 50–200 µg orally once a day is the usual dose.

The dose of the hormones is determined in the individual by following general clinical progress and particularly by observing: weight, blood pressure, appearance of oedema, serum sodium and potassium concentrations, and haematocrit. In addition, measurement of cortisol levels at critical points in the day as a day curve can be done and the information used to adjust the hydrocortisone dose. Where available, plasma renin assay is useful for titration of fludrocortisone dose. If any complicating disease arises, e.g. infection, a need for surgery or other stress, the hydrocortisone dose is immediately doubled.

If there is vomiting, the parenteral replacement hormone must be given without delay.

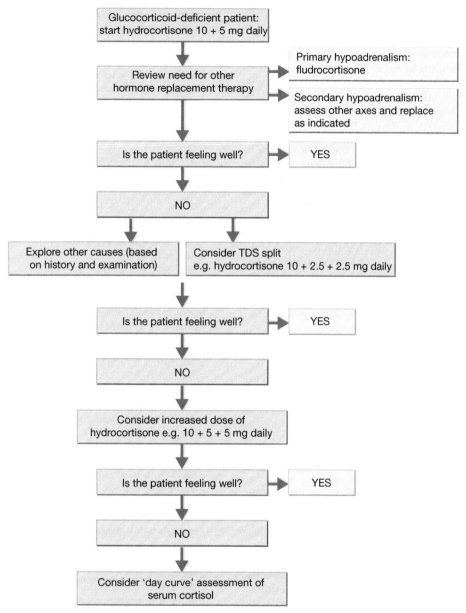

Fig. 35.4 Algorithm for treatment of the glucocorticoid-deficient patient. Patients should be reassessed at 6–8-week intervals while their treatment is optimised. *(Adapted from Crown A, Lightman S 2005 Why is the management of glucocorticoid deficiency still controversial: a review of the literature? Clinical Endocrinology 63:483–492.)*

Chronic secondary adrenocortical insufficiency

This occurs in hypopituitarism. The need for hydrocortisone may be less than in primary insufficiency, especially when ACTH deficiency is partial. Some patients with borderline adrenocortical insufficiency may require steroid supplementation only during periods of stress, such as infection or surgery. Mineralocorticoid replacement is seldom required, for the pituitary has little control over aldosterone production. Other pituitary replacement is given as appropriate (see p. 635).

Iatrogenic adrenocortical insufficiency: abrupt withdrawal

(See also below, Withdrawal of corticosteroid pharmacotherapy.) This occurs in patients who have recently received prolonged pharmacotherapy with a corticosteroid that inhibits hypothalamic production of the corticotropin releasing hormone and so results in secondary adrenal failure. Treat by reinstituting the original therapy or manage as for acute adrenal insufficiency, as appropriate. To avoid an acute crisis on discontinuing therapy, the corticosteroid must be withdrawn gradually to allow the hypothalamus, the pituitary and the adrenal to regain normal function. Treat patients taking corticosteroids who have an infection or surgical operation (major stress) as for primary insufficiency.

Sudden withdrawal of large doses of steroid hormone used to suppress inflammation or allergy may lead not only to an adrenal insufficiency crisis but also to relapse of the disease that is suppressed, not cured. Such relapse can be extremely severe, and sometimes life-threatening. Secondary adrenal insufficiency can occur after high-dose inhaled potent glucocorticoids in the treatment of asthma (see above).

Pharmacotherapy

Suppression of adrenocortical function

In *congenital adrenal hyperplasia*, excess adrenal androgen secretion is suppressed by hydrocortisone in children, and hydrocortisone or prednisolone or dexamethasone in adults, which inhibit pituitary corticotropin production.

Use in inflammation and for immunosuppression

Drugs with primarily glucocorticoid effects, e.g. prednisolone, are chosen, so that the mineralocorticoid effects that are inevitable with hydrocortisone do not limit the dose.

It remains essential to use only the minimum dose that will achieve the desired effect. Sometimes therapeutic effects are partly sacrificed to avoid adverse effects, as it has not so far proved possible to separate all the glucocorticoid effects from one another; for example, it is not known whether it is possible to eliminate catabolic effects and yet retain anti-inflammatory action. In some conditions, e.g. nephrotic syndrome, the clinician cannot specify exactly what action they want the drug developer to provide.

Further specific uses

The decision to give a corticosteroid commonly depends on knowledge of the likelihood and amount of benefit (bearing in mind that very prolonged high dose inevitably brings serious complications), on the severity of the disease and on whether the patient has failed to respond usefully to other treatment.

Adrenal steroids are used in nearly all cases of the following:

- Exfoliative dermatitis and pemphigus, if severe.
- *Connective tissue diseases,* if severe, e.g. lupus erythematosus (systemic), polyarteritis nodosa, polymyalgia rheumatica and cranial giant cell arteritis (urgent therapy to save sight), dermatomyositis.
- *Severe asthma* (see p. 506).
- *Acute lymphatic leukaemia* (see Ch. 31).
- *Acquired haemolytic anaemia.*
- *Severe allergic reactions* of all kinds, e.g. serum sickness, angioedema, trichiniasis. Alone, they will not control acute manifestations of anaphylactic shock as they do not act quickly enough.
- *Organ transplant rejection.*
- *Acute spinal cord injury:* early, brief, and high dose (to reduce the oedema/inflammation).
- *Autoimmune active chronic hepatitis:* a corticosteroid improves well-being, liver function and histological findings; prednisolone will benefit some 80% and should be continued in the long term, as most patients relapse if the drug is withdrawn.

Adrenal steroids are used in some cases of the following:

- *Rheumatic fever.*
- *Rheumatoid arthritis.*
- *Ankylosing spondylitis.*
- *Ulcerative colitis and proctitis.*
- *Regional enteritis* (Crohn's disease).
- *Hay fever* (allergic rhinitis); also some bronchitics with marked airways obstruction.
- *Sarcoidosis.* If there is hypercalcaemia or threat to a major organ, e.g. eye, adrenal steroid administration is urgent. Pulmonary fibrosis may be delayed and CNS manifestations may improve.
- *Acute mountain/altitude sickness,* to reduce cerebral oedema.
- *Prevention of adverse reaction* to radiocontrast media in patients who have had a previous severe reaction.
- *Blood diseases due to circulating antibodies,* e.g. thrombocytopenic purpura (there may also be a decrease in capillary fragility with lessening of purpura even though thrombocytes remain few); agranulocytosis.
- *Eye diseases.* Allergic diseases and non-granulomatous inflammation of the uveal tract. Bacterial and viral infections may be made worse and use of corticosteroids to suppress inflammation of infection is generally undesirable, is best left to ophthalmologists and must be accompanied by effective chemotherapy; this is of the greatest

importance in herpes virus infection. Corneal integrity should be checked before use (by instilling a drop of fluorescein). Prolonged use of corticosteroid eye drops causes glaucoma in 1 in 20 of the population (a genetic trait). Application is generally as hydrocortisone, prednisolone or fluorometholone drops, or subconjunctival injection.

- *Nephrotic syndrome.* Patients with minimal change disease respond well to daily prednisolone, 2 mg/kg, for 6 weeks followed by 1.5 mg/kg on alternate days. Relapses are treated with the higher dose until proteinuria is trace level only, and then the lower dose for a month. Multiple relapses then require a tapering dose over several months rather than complete withdrawal. In such patients, steroid sparing agents, ciclosporin, tacrolimus and mycophenolate, may be used to reduce long-term dosing.
- *A variety of skin diseases,* such as eczema. Severe cases may involve occlusive dressings if a systemic effect is undesirable, though absorption can be substantial (see Ch. 17).
- *Aphthous ulcers.* Hydrocortisone 2.5 mg oromucosal tablets are allowed to dissolve next to the ulcer; beclometasone dipropionate inhaler 50–100 μg may be sprayed on the oral mucosal, or betamethasone soluble tablet 500 miligrams dissolved in water may be used, without swallowing, as a mouth wash. Triamcinolone acetonide in Orabase, or fluocinonide gel covered by Orabase may be used where available. Early initiation of treatment may accelerate healing.
- *Acute gout* resistant to other drugs (see p. 265).
- *Hypercalcaemia of sarcoidosis and of vitamin D intoxication* responds to prednisolone 30 mg daily (or its equivalent of other adrenal steroid) for 10 days. Hypercalcaemia of myeloma and some other malignancies responds more variably. Hyperparathyroid hypercalcaemia does not respond (see p. 661).
- *Raised intracranial pressure* due to cerebral oedema, e.g. in cerebral tumour or encephalitis. This is probably an anti-inflammatory effect, which reduces vascular permeability and acts in 12–24 h. Give dexamethasone 10 mg i.m. or i.v. (or equivalent) initially and then 4 mg 6-hourly by the appropriate route, reducing the dose after 2–4 days and withdrawing over 5–7 days. Much higher doses may be used in palliation of inoperable cerebral tumour.
- *Preterm labour:* (to mother) to enhance fetal lung maturation.
- *Aspiration of gastric acid* (Mendelsohn's syndrome).
- *Myasthenia gravis:* see page 397.
- *Cancer,* see Chapter 31.

Use in diagnosis. Dexamethasone suppression test. Dexamethasone acts on the hypothalamus to reduce output of corticotropin releasing hormone (CRH), but it does not interfere with measurement of cortisol in blood or urine. Normal suppression of cortisol production after administering low dexamethasone (0.5 mg 6-hourly) indicates that the HPA axis is intact. Failure of suppression implies pathological hypersecretion of ACTH by the pituitary, ectopic ACTH or autonomous secretion of cortisol by the adrenal. Dexamethasone has a half-life of 4.5h and does not interfere with assay of endogenous cortisol. There are several ways of carrying out the test.

Withdrawal of pharmacotherapy

The longer the duration of therapy, the slower must be the withdrawal.

If use is less than 1 week, e.g. for acute asthma, although some hypothalamic suppression will have occurred, withdrawal can be safely accomplished in a few steps.

After use for 2 weeks, for rapid withdrawal, a 50% reduction in dose each day is reasonable.

If the duration of treatment is longer, dose reduction is accompanied by the dual risk of resurgence of the disease and iatrogenic hypoadrenalism; withdrawal should then proceed very slowly, e.g. 2.5–5 mg prednisolone or equivalent at intervals of 3–7 days.

An alternative scheme is to halve the dose weekly until it is 25 mg/day of prednisolone or equivalent, then to make reductions of about 1 mg/day every third to seventh day. Paediatric tablets (1 mg) can be useful during withdrawal.

These schemes may yet be too rapid (with the occurrence of fatigue, 'dish-rag' syndrome or relapse of disease). The rate of reduction may then need to be as slow as prednisolone 1 mg/day (or equivalent) per month, particularly as the dose approaches the level of physiological requirement (equivalent of prednisolone 5–7.5 mg daily).

The long tetracosactide test (see below) or plasma corticotropin concentration is useful to assess recovery of adrenal responsiveness. A positive result does not necessarily indicate full recovery of the patient's ability to respond to stressful situations; the latter is best shown by an adequate response to insulin-induced hypoglycaemia (which additionally tests *hypothalamic–pituitary* capacity to respond).

Corticotropin should not be used to hasten recovery of the atrophied cortex because its effects further suppress the hypothalamic–pituitary axis, on recovery of which the patient's future depends. Complete recovery of normal HPA function sufficient to cope with severe intercurrent illnesses or surgery is generally complete in 2 months but may take as long as 2 years.

There are many reports of collapse, even coma, occurring within a few hours of omission of adrenal steroid therapy, e.g. due to patients' ignorance of the risk to which their

605

physicians are exposing them, or failure to carry their tablets with them. Patients must be instructed on the hazards of omitting therapy and, during intercurrent disease, intramuscular preparations should be freely used. For anaesthesia and surgery in adrenocortical insufficiency, see page 602.

Inhibition of synthesis of adrenal and other steroid hormones

These agents have use in diagnosis of adrenal disease and in controlling excessive production of corticosteroids, e.g. by corticotropin-producing tumours of the pituitary (Cushing's syndrome) or by adrenocortical adenoma or carcinoma where the cause cannot be removed. Use of these drugs calls for special care as they can precipitate acute adrenal insufficiency. Hydrocortisone replacement in a block and replace regimen may be given. Some members inhibit other steroid synthesis.

Metyrapone inhibits the enzyme, steroid 11β-hydroxylase, which converts 11-deoxy precursors into hydrocortisone, corticosterone and aldosterone. It affects synthesis of aldosterone less than that of glucocorticoids.

Trilostane blocks the synthetic path earlier (3β-hydroxysteroid dehydrogenase) and thus inhibits aldosterone synthesis as well.

Formestane is a specific inhibitor of the aromatase that converts androgens to oestrogens. A depot injection of 250 mg i.m. is given twice a month to treat some patients with carcinoma of the breast who have relapsed on tamoxifen.

Aminoglutethimide blocks at an even earlier stage, preventing the conversion of cholesterol to pregnenolone. It therefore stops synthesis of all steroids, hydrocortisone, aldosterone and sex hormones (including the conversion of androgens to oestrogens); it has a use in breast cancer.

Ketoconazole inhibits several cytochrome P450 enzymes, including those involved in steroid synthesis. It is an effective antifungal agent by virtue of its capacity to block ergosterol synthesis. In humans it inhibits steroid synthesis in gonads and adrenal cortex. Its principal P450 target in the adrenal is the enzyme CYP11B1 (11β-hydroxylase), which catalyses the final step in cortisol synthesis. CYP11B1 inhibition by ketoconazole renders it a useful treatment for Cushing's syndrome, while testosterone synthesis inhibitors may be useful in advanced prostatic cancer.

Anastrozole is an adrenal aromatase inhibitor that finds use as *adjuvant* treatment of oestrogen receptor-positive early breast cancer in postmenopausal women. It is used as *sole* therapy, following 2–3 years of tamoxifen, in advanced breast cancer in postmenopausal women that is oestrogen receptor positive or responsive to tamoxifen. *Letrozole* and *exemestane* are similar.

Competitive antagonism of adrenal steroids

Spironolactone antagonises the sodium-retaining effect of aldosterone and other mineralocorticoids. It is used to treat primary and secondary hyperaldosteronism (see p. 599).

Adrenocorticotrophic hormone (ACTH) (corticotropin)

Natural corticotropin is a 39-amino-acid polypeptide secreted by the anterior pituitary gland; it is no longer available for pharmaceutical use.

The physiological activity resides in the first 24 amino acids (which are common to many species) and most immunological activity lies in the remaining 15 amino acids.

The pituitary output of corticotropin responds rapidly to physiological requirements by the familiar negative-feedback homeostatic mechanism. As the $t_{1/2}$ of corticotropin is 10 min and the adrenal cortex responds within 2 min, corticosteroid output can adjust rapidly.

Synthetic corticotropins have the advantage of shorter amino acid chains (they lack amino acids 25–39) which are less likely to cause serious allergy, although this does occur.

Tetracosactide (tetracosactrin) consists of the biologically active first 24 amino acids of natural corticotropin (from humans or animals) and so it has similar properties, e.g. $t_{1/2}$ 10 min.

Actions

Corticotropin stimulates the synthesis of corticosteroids (of which the most important is cortisol) and to a lesser extent of androgens, by the cells of the adrenal cortex. It has only a minor (transient) effect on aldosterone production, which proceeds *independently*; in the absence of corticotropin the cells of the inner cortex atrophy.

The release of natural corticotropin by the pituitary gland is controlled by the hypothalamus through *corticotropin releasing hormone* (CRH, or corticoliberin), production of which is influenced by environmental stresses as well as by the level of circulating cortisol. High plasma concentration of any adrenal steroid with glucocorticoid effect prevents release of CRH and so of corticotropin, lack of which in turn results in adrenocortical hypofunction. This is why catastrophe may accompany abrupt withdrawal of long-term adrenal steroid therapy with adrenal atrophy.

The **effects** of corticotropin are those of the steroids (hydrocortisone, androgens) liberated by its action on the adrenal cortex. Prolonged heavy dosage causes the clinical picture of Cushing's syndrome.

Uses. Corticotropin is used principally in diagnosis and rarely in treatment. It is inactive if taken orally and has to be injected like other peptide hormones.

Diagnostic use is to test the capacity of the adrenal cortex to produce cortisol. With the *short synacthen test*, the plasma cortisol concentration is measured before and 30 min and 60 min after an intramuscular injection of 250 µg of tetracosactide (Synacthen); this transiently raises plasma corticotropin activity 1000-fold above physiological levels, although the absence of the antigenic part of the molecule results in no detectable increase in circulating ACTH. A normal response is a rise in plasma cortisol concentration of more than 200 nmol/L or a peak of greater than 500 nmol/L at 30 or 60 min. In cases of uncertainty, the rarely used *longer* variants of the test require intramuscular injection of a depot (sustained-release) formulation, e.g. 1 mg daily for 3 days at 09:00 hours, with a short tetracosactide test performed on day 3.

Therapeutic use is seldom appropriate, as the peptide hormone must be injected. Selective glucocorticoid (without mineralocorticoid) action is not possible, and clinical results are irregular. Corticotropin cannot be relied on to restore adrenal cortisol output when a steroid is being withdrawn after prolonged therapy, as it does not restore function in the suppressed hypothalamic–pituitary part of the HPA axis.

Preparations

- *Tetracosactide Injection* is supplied as an ampoule for injection i.v., i.m. or s.c.
- *Tetracosactide Zinc Injection* (Synacthen Depot) i.m. in which the hormone is adsorbed on to zinc phosphate from which it is slowly released. This is the form used in the long tetracosactide test.

Summary

- Physiological concentrations of cortisol are essential for supporting the circulation and glucose production. Physiological concentrations of aldosterone are essential to prevent excessive sodium loss.
- For systemic pharmacological uses, prednisolone or other synthetic adrenocorticosteroids are used because they are more selective glucocorticoids, i.e. have less sodium-retaining activity.
- For local administration (skin, lung), more potent, fluorinated steroids may be required.
- Glucocorticoids inhibit the transcriptional activation of many of the inflammatory cytokines, giving them a versatile role in the treatment of many types of inflammation.
- Fludrocortisone is a valuable treatment for many sodium-losing states, and for most causes of autonomic neuropathy.
- Corticotropin is used to test the capacity of the adrenal gland to produce cortisol.

Guide to further reading

Arlt, W., 2006. Junior doctors' working hours and the circadian rhythm of hormones. Clin. Med. (Northfield Il) 6, 127–129.

Arlt, W., 2009. The approach to the adult with newly diagnosed adrenal insufficiency. J. Clin. Endocrinol. Metab. 94, 1059–1067.

Barnes, P.J., Adcock, I.M., 2009. Glucocorticoid resistance in inflammatory diseases. Lancet 373, 1905–1917.

Buttgereit, F., Burmester, G.R., Lipworth, B.J., 2005. Optimised glucocorticoid therapy: the sharpening of an old spear. Lancet 365, 801–803.

Cooper, M.S., Stewart, P.M., 2003. Corticosteroid insufficiency in acutely ill patients. N. Engl. J. Med. 348, 727–734.

Hench, P.S., et al., 1949. The effect of a hormone of the adrenal cortex (17-hydroxy-11-dehydrocorticosterone: Compound E) and of pituitary adrenocorticotropic hormone on rheumatoid arthritis. Proc. Staff. Meet. Mayo. Clin. 24, 181–277. (acute rheumatism).
The classic studies of the first clinical use of an adrenocortical steroid in inflammatory disease. See also page 301 for an account by E C Kendall of the biochemical and pharmaceutical background to the clinical studies. Kendall writes of his collaboration with Hench, 'he can now say "17-hydroxy-11-dehydrocorticosterone" and in turn I can say "the arthritis of lupus erythematosus". In sophisticated circles, however, I prefer to say, "the arthritis of L.E".'

Hochhaus, G., 2004. New developments in corticosteroids. Proc. Am. Thorac. Soc. 1, 269–274.

Lipworth, B.J., 2000. Therapeutic implications of non-genomic glucocorticoid activity. Lancet 356, 87–88.

Løvås, K., Husebye, E., 2005. Addison's disease. Lancet 365, 2058–2061.

Newell-Price, J., Bertagna, X., Grossman, A.B., Nieman, L.K., 2006. Cushing's syndrome. Lancet 367, 1605–1617.

Chapter | 36 |

Diabetes mellitus, insulin, oral antidiabetes agents, obesity

Mark Evans, Rahat Tauni

SYNOPSIS

Diabetes mellitus affects at least 2% of many national populations. Its successful management requires close collaboration between the patient and health-care professionals.

- History of pharmacological treatment of diabetes.
- Insulins in current use (including choice, formulations, adverse effects, hypoglycaemia, insulin resistance).
- Oral antidiabetes drugs.
- Treatment of diabetes mellitus.
- Diabetic ketoacidosis.
- Surgery in diabetic patients.
- Obesity and overweight.

Diabetes overview

Diabetes is best regarded as a group of related conditions in which blood glucose levels tend to rise. Diabetes is common and increasing. In large part, this global increase in diabetes may be related to increased levels of obesity. Diabetes can lead to serious medical complications – blindness from retinopathy, renal failure, gangrene and limb amputation, cardiovascular disease and premature death. Aggressive therapy with a combination of pharmacological therapies aimed at lowering blood glucose and blood pressure and optimising lipids can reduce the risk of these complications. In particular, follow-up data from two major diabetes randomised control trials (UKPDS in type 2 diabetes and DCCT-EDIC in type 1 diabetes) suggest that the beneficial effects of early intensive glycaemic control on microvascular complications tend to last years after the glycaemic control is relaxed (termed a 'legacy' or 'metabolic memory' effect emphasising the importance of early optimal glycaemic control).

History of insulin therapy in diabetes

Diabetes was known to ancient Greek medicine with the description of 'a melting of the flesh and limbs into urine … the patients never stop making water but the flow is incessant … their mouth becomes parched and their body dry'.[1]

Insulin (as pancreatic islet cell extract) was first administered to a 14-year-old insulin-deficient patient on 11 January 1922 in Toronto, Canada. R.D. Lawrence, an adult sufferer from diabetes who developed the disease in 1920 and who, because of insulin, lived until 1968, has told how:

> Many doctors, after they have developed a disease, take up the speciality in it … But that was not so with me. I was studying for surgery when diabetes took me up. The great book of Joslin said that by starving you might live four years with luck. [He went to Italy and, whilst his health was declining there, he received a letter from a

---
[1]The Extant Works of Aretaeus, trans. Francis Adams (London 1856) p. 338 (quoted by Ackerknecht E H 1982 A short history of medicine. Johns Hopkins, Baltimore, pp. 71–72).

biochemist friend which said] there was something called 'insulin' appearing with a good name in Canada, what about going there and getting it. I said 'No thank you; I've tried too many quackeries for diabetes; I'll wait and see'. Then I got peripheral neuritis … So when [the friend] cabled me and said, 'I've got insulin – it works – come back quick', I responded, arrived at King's College Hospital, London, and went to the laboratory as soon as it opened … It was all experimental for [neither of us] knew a thing about it … So we decided to have 20 units a nice round figure. I had a nice breakfast. I had bacon and eggs and toast made on the Bunsen. I hadn't eaten bread for months and months … by 3 o'clock in the afternoon my urine was quite sugar free. That hadn't happened for many months. So we gave a cheer for Banting and Best.[2]But at 4 pm I had a terrible shaky feeling and a terrible sweat and hunger pain. That was my first experience of hypoglycaemia. We remembered that Banting and Best had described an overdose of insulin in dogs. So I had some sugar and a biscuit and soon got quite well, thank you.[3]

Diabetes mellitus is classified broadly as:

- **Type 1** (formerly, insulin-dependent diabetes mellitus, IDDM), which typically (but not always) occurs in younger people who cannot then secrete sufficient insulin.
- **Type 2** (formerly, non–insulin-dependent diabetes mellitus, NIDDM), which usually occurs in older people who are typically (although not always) obese. Type 2 diabetes is best thought of as a group of conditions characterised by a variable combination of reduced insulin secretion and resistance to insulin's blood glucose lowering action.
- **Other causes:** including gestational diabetes, disease processes affecting the liver or pancreas such as cystic fibrosis causing a 'secondary' diabetes, monogenic forms (maturity onset diabetes of the young, MODY). These terms and abbreviations are used in this chapter.

Sources of insulin

Insulin is synthesised and stored (bound to zinc) in granules in the β-islet cells of the pancreas. Daily secretion typically amounts to 30–40 units, which is about 25% of total pancreatic insulin content. The principal factor that evokes insulin secretion is a high blood glucose concentration. In addition, insulin release following oral intake of carbohydrate is facilitated by the action of 'incretin factors' such as GLP-1 (see later) released from specialised neuroendocrine cells in the small bowel.

Insulin is a polypeptide with two peptide chains (A chain, 21 amino acids; B chain, 30) linked by two disulphide bridges. The basic structure having metabolic activity is common to all mammalian species, but there are minor species differences:

- *Bovine* insulin differs from human insulin by three amino acids.
- *Porcine* insulin differs from human insulin by only one amino acid.
- *Human* insulin is made either by enzyme modification of porcine insulin, or by using recombinant DNA to synthesise the pro-insulin precursor molecule for insulin. This is done by artificially introducing the DNA into either *Escherichia coli* or yeast.[4]
- *Insulin analogues* are now widely used and have modifications introduced to the A and/or B chains, which result in more rapid onset and offset of action (rapidly acting analogues), or slower offset (long-acting analogues) than naturally occurring insulin. As the commercial patents for some of the older insulin analogues expire, a number of 'biosimilar' insulins are being developed, and it is likely that a number of alternative therapeutic options will appear over the next 5 years.

Insulin receptors

Insulin receptors (comprising 2 α and 2 β subunits) are present on the surface of target cells such as liver, muscle and fat. Insulin binding results in tyrosine autophosphorylation of the β subunit. This then phosphorylates other substrates so that a signalling cascade is initiated and biological responses ensue. Downstream effects of stimulation of the insulin receptor include both immediate/short-term actions (e.g. translocation of the glucose transporter GLUT4 to the surface of target cell) and longer-term actions (e.g. increased expression of glucokinase and reduced expression of gluconeogenic and ketogenic enzymes in the liver).

[2]F G Banting and C H Best of Toronto, Canada (see also Journal of Laboratory and Clinical Medicine 1922; 7:251).
[3]Abbreviated from Lawrence R D 1961 King's College Hospital Gazette 40:220. Transcript from a recorded after dinner talk to students' Historical Society.

[4]The three forms of human insulin have the same amino acid sequence, but are separately designated as insulin emp (Enzyme Modified Porcine), prb (Pro-insulin Recombinant in Bacteria) and pyr (Precursor insulin Yeast Recombinant). Although one of the incentives for introducing human insulin was avoidance of insulin antibody production, the allergies to older insulins were caused largely by impurities in the preparations, and are avoided equally well by using the highly purified, monocomponent porcine and bovine insulins.

Actions of insulin

- *Reduction in blood glucose* is due to increased glucose uptake in peripheral tissues (which oxidise glucose or convert into glycogen or fat) and a reduction in hepatic output of glucose (diminished breakdown/ increased synthesis of glycogen and diminished gluconeogenesis).
- *Other metabolic effects.* Although, therapeutically, insulin is thought of as a blood glucose–lowering hormone, it has a number of other cellular actions. Insulin is an anabolic hormone, enhancing protein synthesis (which has resulted in cases of misuse by bodybuilders). It also inhibits both breakdown of fats (lipolysis) and ketogenesis. Insulin also has actions on electrolytes, stimulating potassium uptake into cells and renal sodium retention (anti-natriuretic effect). Within brain, insulin may have actions to stimulate memory and act as a nutritional signal to help control appetite/food intake.

Uses

- Diabetes mellitus is the main indication.
- Insulin promotes the passage of potassium into cells by stimulating cell surface Na/K ATPase action, and this effect is utilised to correct hyperkalaemia (see p. 485).
- Insulin-induced hypoglycaemia can also be used as a stress test of anterior pituitary function (growth hormone and corticotropin and thus cortisol are released).

Pharmacokinetics

In health, insulin is secreted by the pancreas, enters the portal vein and passes straight to the liver, where half of it is taken up. The rest enters and is distributed in the systemic circulation so that its concentration (in fasting subjects) is only about 20% of that entering the liver. Insulin is released continuously and rhythmically from the healthy pancreas with additional increases following carbohydrate ingestion. As described below, modern insulin regimens in diabetes aim to match this pattern as far as possible.

In contrast to the natural pancreatic release, when insulin is injected subcutaneously during the treatment of diabetes, it enters the systemic circulation so that both liver and other peripheral organs receive the same concentration. It is inactivated in the liver and kidney; about 10% appears in the urine. The plasma $t_{1/2}$ is only 5 min, although clearance of 'tissue' insulin levels lags behind this; this is noteworthy when stopping intravenous insulin infusions as it may take 60 min for effects to wear off.

Most commonly, insulin is self-delivered by patients using either a syringe with a fixed needle (after drawing up insulin from a vial) or an insulin pen device (supplied as a preloaded disposable pen or with replaceable cartridges). Within hospital, soluble insulin may be delivered by intravenous infusion. Typically, 50 units of soluble insulin is dissolved in 50 mL isotonic saline (i.e. insulin concentration 1 unit/mL).

An alternative and increasingly popular method for delivering insulin, especially in type 1 diabetes, is for patients to use continuous subcutaneous insulin infusion devices ('insulin pumps'). These small cell-phone–size personal devices provide a continuous basal delivery of soluble insulin (usually analogue, see below) with an additional insulin bolus when needed to cover meals or to correct high blood glucose values. Insulin pumps have become more sophisticated over the last decade, with patients able to set multiple pre-programmed basal insulin rates and/or temporary infusion rates for such things as exercise or illness. Most pumps now have inbuilt software to calculate bolus doses from blood glucose/carbohydrate data. Some of the currently available insulin pumps link to subcutaneous continuous glucose monitors and, excitingly, the expectation is that this hardware will allow the development of an 'artificial pancreas' with insulin delivery controlled partially or totally by real-time glucose sensing.

Preparations of insulin (Table 36.1)

Dosage is measured in *international units* standardised by chemical assay. There are three major factors:

- Strength (concentration).
- Source (human, porcine, bovine).
- Formulation (short acting vs delayed action).

Broadly speaking, four different types of insulin with differing time-courses of action are available for treating diabetes (illustrated in Fig. 36.1):

1. *Short duration* of action (and rapid onset). Soluble insulin (also called 'neutral' or 'regular' insulin). The most recent additions to this class of insulin, lispro, aspart and glulisine, are modified human insulins with changes in the B chain resulting in more rapid absorption after subcutaneous injection and thus a faster onset and shorter duration of action. A new formulation of aspart (faster-acting insulin aspart, Fiasp) includes arginine and niacinamide, which act to increase further the speed of absorption from subcutaneous depots.
2. *Intermediate duration* of action (and slower onset). Preparations in which the insulin has been

Table 36.1 Insulin preparations

Preparations		Onset of action (approx.)	Peak activity (approx.)	Duration of action (approx.)[A]
Short-acting insulins				
Human sequence	Actrapid Humulin S Insuman Rapid	30–45 min	2–3.5 h	5–7 h
Animal sequence	Hypurin Porcine Neutral Hypurin Bovine Neutral	As above	As above	As above
Rapid-acting analogues	Apidra (insulin glulisine) Humalog (Insulin lispro) NovoRapid (Insulin aspart)	10–20 min	1.5–2.5 h	4.5–6 h
"Ultra–rapid-acting" analogue	Fiasp (faster-acting insulin aspart)	5–20 min	1–2.5 h	4–6 h
Biphasic insulins				
	Humalog Mix 25 Humalog Mix 50 Humulin M3 Hypurin Porcine 30/70 Insuman Comb 15 Insuman Comb 25 Insuman Comb 50 NovoMix 30	10–45 min	2–8 h	12–20 h
Isophane insulins and similar				
Human sequence	Humulin I Insulatard Insuman Basal	1–3 h	4–9 h	12–20 h
Animal sequence	Hypurin Bovine Isophane Hypurin Porcine Isophane Hypurin Bovine Lente Hypurin Bovine Protamine Zinc	As above	As above	As above
Long-acting analogues				
	Abasaglar (insulin glargine) Levemir (insulin detemir) Lantus (insulin glargine)	1–2 h	6–10 h	18–24 h
	Toujeo (insulin glargine U300)	N/A[B]	N/A[B]	24–36 h
	Tresiba (insulin degludec)	N/A[B]	N/A[B]	Up to 48 h
U500 concentrated insulin				
	Humulin R [C]	30–60 min	2–6 h	6–24 h

[A]Duration of action for many insulin preparations may be longer when larger doses are used.
[B]N/A = onset and peak of action not applicable for long action profile of Toujeo and Tresiba.
[C]U500 humulin R use restricted to severe insulin resistance cases with shared care. As with many other insulins, pharmacodynamics vary depending on dose, and this patient group often requires very large doses, thus extending pharmacodynamic parameters.

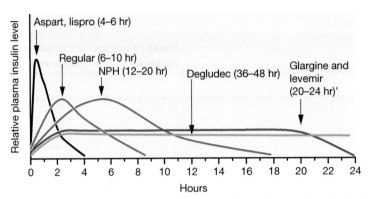

Fig. 36.1 Approximate pharmacokinetic profiles of human insulin and insulin analogues. The relative duration of action of the various forms of insulin is shown. The duration will vary widely both between and within persons. *(From Hirsch I B 2005 Insulin analogues. New England Journal of Medicine 352:174–183.)*

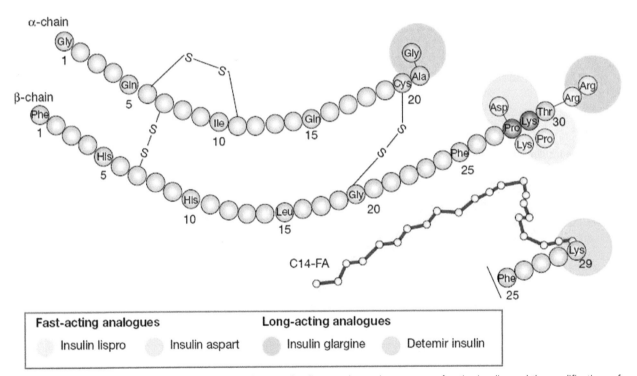

Fig. 36.2 Amino acid alterations in insulin analogues. The diagram shows the structure of native insulin, and the modifications of this structure in a number of commercially available alternatives.

modified physically by combination with protamine or zinc to give an amorphous or crystalline suspension; this is given subcutaneously and slowly dissociates to release insulin in its soluble form. Isophane (NPH) insulin, a suspension with protamine, is still widely used. Insulin zinc suspensions (amorphous or a mixture of amorphous and crystalline) are now rarely used.

3. *Longer duration* of action. Newer analogues glargine, detemir and degludec (Fig. 36.2) have become widely

used, especially in type 1 diabetes. Small changes in the amino acid structure of glargine result in a significant slowing of absorption from subcutaneous depots. A more concentrated preparation of glargine 300 units/mL (Toujeo) has an even longer action profile. In contrast, detemir owes its protracted action to fatty acylation. After absorption, detemir is thus bound to circulating albumin which delays its action. Degludec has a single amino acid substitution and a long fatty acyl chain attached resulting in a markedly prolonged action profile.

4. *A biphasic mixture* of soluble or short-acting analogue insulin with isophane insulin.

Notes for prescribing insulin

Allergy to purified or analogue insulins is very rare.

Antibodies to insulin do occur, but are largely thought to be of no clinical significance.

Compatibility. Soluble insulin may be mixed in the syringe with insulin zinc suspensions (amorphous, crystalline) and with isophane and mixed (biphasic) insulin, and used at once. Long-acting analogue insulins, and protamine insulin suspensions, *should not be mixed* in a syringe with short-acting insulins.

Intravenous insulin. Only soluble (neutral) insulin should be used. Analogue and regular insulin have identical action profiles when given i.v., although the latter tends to be more widely used.

The standard strength of insulin preparations is 100 units/mL (U100). Preparations of 200 units/mL (Humalog and tresiba) and 300 units/mL (Toujeo) are used, but only in prefilled insulin pen devices to avoid confusion. Rarely is 500 units/mL of insulin used in patients with marked insulin resistance so that health-care providers should be aware of this. Biological standardisation of insulin has been replaced by physicochemical methods (high-performance liquid chromatography, HPLC).

Choice of insulin regimen

There are three common regimens incorporating the insulin types described above for patients requiring insulin:

1. *'Basal bolus' therapy:* multiple injections of short-acting insulin are given during the day to mimic prandial secretion of insulin by the pancreas, combined with once- or twice-daily intermediate or long-acting insulin to provide the background insulin. This approach aims to mimic the non-diabetic pattern of insulin release. The total insulin dose is usually apportioned to be 40–60% background and 40–60% prandial.

2. When choosing the short-acting insulin in a basal bolus regimen, soluble insulin is given 30 min before meals. Short acting analogues may be given immediately before, during or even after the meal, although recent data suggest that even these insulins may be more effective if given 15 min prior to eating. The more rapid waning of action profile also means that the risk of hypoglycaemic reactions before the next meal may be lower with the analogues. For choice of background insulin, long-acting analogues may give less risk of nocturnal hypoglycaemia than NPH insulin (see Fig. 36.1), although NPH insulins may offer greater flexibility if patients need to change background insulin from day to day (as with some sportsmen or pregnant women, for example).

3. Insulin pump therapy uses the same principles as basal bolus insulin but uses only fast-acting (usually analogue) insulin. In this case, the 'background' action comes from the fact that insulin is delivered continuously, analogous to insulin release from the non-diabetic pancreas.

4. *Twice-daily therapy* involves two injections of biphasic insulin. Although less 'physiological' than basal bolus, it is simpler, with fewer insulin injections. The available mixtures are listed in Table 36.1. The most commonly used is 30:70 (soluble: NPH). Typically *one-half to two-thirds* of the daily dose may be given in the morning before breakfast and *one-half to one-third* before the evening meal. A combination of biphasic insulin with breakfast and fast-acting insulin with the evening meal and bedtime background insulin may be useful in some children with type 1 diabetes to avoid having to inject insulin at school.

5. *Background or prandial insulin alone* may be sufficient in type 2 diabetes when patients progress from oral therapy on to insulin. In this situation, oral therapy is usually continued in combination with insulin.

Dose and injection technique

A typical insulin-deficient patient with type 1 diabetes needs 0.5–0.8 units/kg insulin per day with approximately 50% as background. Increasingly, patients with type 1 diabetes are not being prescribed fixed insulin doses. Instead, patients are being trained in how to self-adjust insulin doses, to allow for factors which will influence how much insulin is needed: meals with differing carbohydrate contents, digesting and skipping meals, exercise/activity, illness/stress, alcohol, travel, menstrual cycle. These same principles apply to insulin delivered by an insulin pump, although many patients require lower total insulin doses by this route.

Initial treatment dose for a patient with type 1 diabetes, without ketoacidosis, is usually 0.3 units/kg daily. This initial management is aimed at introducing patients to regular insulin injections and blood glucose testing and aiming to tighten glycaemic control gradually over the first few weeks/ months. Some patients with type 1 diabetes may have a significant residual insulin secretory capacity and may require no insulin for some months after diagnosis, often termed the 'honeymoon' period. Others may be started initially on low doses of either background insulin alone or prandial insulin, depending on their clinical status and whether they have any residual endogenous insulin secretion at diagnosis/ presentation.

For type 2 diabetes, glycaemic targets have become lower over the last decade so that increasing numbers are treated with insulin. Although dosing calculators have been used, particularly in some clinical trials, in practice patients are often started on low doses of insulin using a simple regimen and then the dose/regimen is built up as indicated by blood glucose response. Most of these patients are insulin resistant, and a useful therapeutic strategy is to combine adjuvant oral therapy (metformin, pioglitazone or sodium glucose cotransporter 2 inhibitors) with injected insulin. Severe insulin resistance merits specialist investigation for a possible underpinning cause.

Injection technique has pharmacokinetic consequences according to whether the insulin is delivered into the subcutaneous tissue or (inadvertently) into muscle, and patients should standardise their technique. The introduction of a range of needles of appropriate length and pen-shaped injectors has enabled patients to inject perpendicularly to the skin without risk of intramuscular injection. The absorption of insulin is as much as 50% more rapid from shallow intramuscular injection. Clearly, factors such as heat or exercise that alter skin or muscle blood flow can markedly alter the rate of insulin absorption.

Sites of injection should be rotated to minimise local complications (lipodystrophy). Absorption is faster from arm and abdomen than it is from thigh and buttock.

Adverse effects of insulin

Hypoglycaemia

Hypoglycaemia is the main adverse effect of the therapeutic use of insulin. It occurs with excess insulin dosing. Common causes are misjudging or missing meals, activity/exercise and alcohol. Hypoglycaemia is problematic because the brain relies largely, if not exclusively, on circulating glucose as its source of fuel. A significant fall in blood glucose can result in impaired cognition, lethargy, coma, convulsions and perhaps even death (hypoglycaemia was implicated in one series in 4% of deaths in patients with type 1 diabetes who were younger than 50 years of age). Hypoglycaemia is a major factor for insulin-treated patients,

with fear of hypoglycaemia being rated as highly as fear of other complications of diabetes such as blindness or limb amputation. Hypoglycaemia is a particular problem for some patients who lose symptomatic awareness of (and associated counterregulatory neurohumoral defences against) hypoglycaemia.

When human insulin first became available, a number of patients reported that they had less symptomatic awareness of hypoglycaemic episodes. Although the bulk of the subsequent scientific studies examining this failed to detect any significant differences in responses to hypoglycaemia between human and animal insulins, the possibility remains that some patients do react differently and a small number of patients still prefer to use porcine insulin. In practice, the debate about human versus animal insulin has become less topical as non-human analogue insulins are being increasingly used in routine clinical practice.

Prevention of hypoglycaemia depends largely upon patient education, but regular mild episodes of hypoglycaemia are an almost unavoidable aspect of intensive glycaemic control, at least with currently available insulin replacement regimens. Patients should be vigilant, particularly if they have reduced symptomatic awareness of hypoglycaemia, carry rapid acting carbohydrates with them and monitor blood glucose regularly, especially with exercise and before driving a motor vehicle.

Treatment of hypoglycaemia is to give 15–20 g of rapidly acting carbohydrates by mouth (e.g. dextrose tablets, fruit juice or glucose drinks) if the patient is not cognitively obtunded, repeated after 10 min if needed. Where the conscious level is impaired, rescue needs to be non-oral therapy with either i.v. glucose (dextrose) or glucagon. For i.v. glucose, current advice is to avoid using 50% dextrose which is irritant, especially if extravasation occurs. Administration of 50–100 mL of 20% glucose (i.e. 10–20 g), is less thrombogenic. Glucagon ($t_{1/2}$ 4 min) is a polypeptide hormone (29 amino acids) from the β-islet cells of the pancreas. It is released in response to hypoglycaemia from the non-diabetic pancreas (although not in type 1 diabetes for reasons that are unclear) and is a physiological regulator of insulin effect, acting by causing the release of liver glycogen as glucose. Glucagon is used as a 'stopgap' treatment for insulin-induced hypoglycaemia, although it is ineffective in prolonged or repeated hypoglycaemia where hepatic glycogen will be exhausted. The main advantage of glucagon is that it is available in kits for home use so that 1 mg s.c. or i.m. can be useful when rescue is needed by parents/ carers/partners without waiting for paramedic assistance.

The response to rescue is usually rapid. After initial therapy, the patient should be given a snack containing slowly absorbable 'starchy' carbohydrate to avoid relapse. The patient's treatment regimen should also be carefully reviewed with appropriate educational input. In particular, it is useful to ask whether this is part of a pattern of repeated episodes or an 'on-off' event with a clear precipitant.

After large overdoses of insulin (particularly long acting) or sulfonylurea, 20% glucose may be needed by continuous i.v. infusion for hours or days. With very large overdoses, for example, where several hundred units have been administered to self-harm, it may be possible surgically to excise the depot of insulin from the injection site if it can be clearly identified. After prolonged hypoglycaemia, cerebral oedema may occur. Full recovery of cognitive function generally lags behind restoration of blood glucose, but if the patient does not respond clinically to restoration of blood glucose within 30 min, cerebral oedema and i.v. dexamethasone therapy should be considered. Although the brain appears to be more resilient to hypoglycaemia than to other insults such as anoxia or trauma, very severe and prolonged hypoglycaemia can undoubtedly result in permanent brain damage.

Lipohypertrophy may occur if an injection site is repeatedly used, because of the local anabolic effects of insulin. Aesthetics aside, lipohypertrophy is a practical issue as insulin absorption from injection into areas of fatty hypertrophy becomes more variable and unpredictable, resulting in both hyperglycaemia and hypoglycaemia. *Lipoatrophy* at injection sites is rarer (but still occurs) with modern, purified insulins and is thought to be related to a local immune reaction to insulin. More generalised *allergic reactions* to insulin are fortunately rare. If either lipodystrophy or lipoatrophy are present, the site should be avoided.

Non-insulin antidiabetes drugs

Non-insulin antidiabetes drugs are either (i) secretagogue therapy to increase endogenous insulin release, (ii) insulin sensitisers to reduce insulin resistance, (iii) drugs increasing excretion of glucose through kidneys, or (iv) drugs aimed at modifying absorption of glucose.

(i) Insulin secretagogues

Sulfonamide derivatives *(sulfonylureas)* act to increase endogenous insulin secretion by blocking ATP-sensitive potassium channels on the β-islet cell plasma membrane. This results in the release of stored insulin in response to glucose. The discovery of sulfonylureas was serendipitous. In 1930 it was noted that sulfonamides could cause hypoglycaemia, and in 1942 severe hypoglycaemia was found in patients with typhoid fever during a therapeutic trial of sulfonamide. Sulfonylureas were introduced into clinical practice in 1954 and continue to be widely used in type 2 diabetes. Sulfonylureas are ineffective in totally insulin-deficient patients;

successful therapy probably requires at least 30% of normal β-cell function to be present. Secondary failure (after months or years) occurs due to declining β-cell function.

Their main *adverse effects* are hypoglycaemia and weight gain. Hypoglycaemia can be severe and prolonged (for days), and may be fatal in 10% of cases, especially in the elderly and patients with heart failure in whom long-acting agents should be avoided. Erroneous alternative diagnoses such as stroke may be made. Sulfonamides, as expected, potentiate sulfonylureas both by direct action and by displacement from plasma proteins.

Several sulfonylureas are available (Table 36.2). Choice is determined by the duration of action as well as the patient's age and renal function, and unwanted effects. The long-acting sulfonylureas, e.g. *glibenclamide,* are associated with a greater risk of hypoglycaemia; for this reason they should be avoided in the elderly, for whom shorter acting alternatives, such as *gliclazide,* or non-sulfonylurea options (see below) are preferred. In patients with impaired renal function, gliclazide, glipizide and tolbutamide are preferred as they are not excreted by the kidney. *Gliclazide* is a commonly used second-generation agent. If the dose exceeds 80 mg, the drug should be taken twice daily before meals, or once daily if prescribed as a modified-release preparation. *Glimepiride* is designed to be used once daily and provokes less hypoglycaemia than glibenclamide.

Meglitinides such as *repaglinide* ($t_{1/2}$ 1 h) are short-acting oral hypoglycaemic agents that have not been widely used in clinical practice. Like sulfonylureas, they act by blockade of ATP-dependent potassium channels (see Table 36.2). The shorter-action profile of meglitinides compared with sulfonylureas should in theory reduce risk of hypoglycaemia.

Incretin analogues and mimetics. *Exenatide, liraglutide, lixisenatide, dulaglutide* and *albiglutide* are functional analogues of incretin, a glucagon-like peptide-1 (GLP-1) and a naturally occurring peptide that enhances insulin secretion in response to a rise in blood glucose. Aside from boosting insulin secretion, they have other actions which offer potential advantages over other insulin secretagogues in diabetes: reducing glucagon secretion, slowing gastric emptying and acting on brain GLP-1 receptors to reduce appetite. Animal studies suggest that there may be a stimulatory effect of GLP-1 analogues on beta cell mass, although this has not yet been demonstrated reliably in humans. GLP-1 therapy is currently aimed at overweight patients with type 2 diabetes where sulfonylureas or insulin therapy may promote weight gain. GLP-1 analogues are administered subcutaneously once or twice daily, although longer-acting analogues are now available. This allows a regimen with injections no more than once weekly. Oral preparations are currently in clinical trials. The main adverse effect is nausea, which may be sufficient to prevent use.

Table 36.2 Principal non-insulin antidiabetes drugs

Drug	Total daily dose (mg unless otherwise stated)	Dosing schedule (doses/day unless otherwise stated)	Duration of action (h unless otherwise stated)
Biguanide			
Metformin	500–3000	2–3	8–12
Metformin MR	500–2000	1–2	8–12
Dipeptyl peptidase IV inhibitors			
Alogliptin	25	1	>24
Linagliptin	5	1	>24
Saxagliptin	2.5–5	1	>24
Sitagliptin	25–100	1	>24
Vildagliptin	50	1	>24
Sodium glucose cotransporter 2 inhibitors			
Canagliflozin	100–300	1	>24
Dapagliflozin	5–10	1	>24
Empagliflozin	10–25	1	>24
GLP-1 analogue therapy			
Albiglutide	30–50	Once weekly	>7 days
Dulaglitide	0.75–1.5	Once weekly	>7 days
Exenatide (Byetta)	5–10 µg	2	12
Exenatide (Bydureon)	2	Once weekly	>7 days
Liraglutide	0.6–1.8	1	24
Lixisenatide	10–20 µg	1	Up to 24

Table does not show combination therapies.

Dipeptidyl peptidase-4 (DPP-4) inhibitors. DPP-4 inhibitors like *Sitagliptin, vildagliptin, linagliptin, saxagliptin* and *alogliptin* are being increasingly used. They offer an alternative strategy for targeting the GLP-1 pathway by inhibiting breakdown of native GLP-1. The main benefits of these agents are oral administration, weight neutrality and minimal risk of hypoglycaemia compared with sulphonylureas; they are generally less efficacious than direct GLP-1 agonists. Side-effects include nausea, skin rash and nasopharyngitis, although they are generally very well tolerated. Most DPP-4 inhibitors are excreted renally. Dose adjustments are needed in renal impairment, although linagliptin is mostly excreted through the gastrointestinal tract, thus offering an alternative to metformin in renal impairment.

(ii) Insulin sensitisers

Biguanides (see Table 36.2) have been available since 1957. *Metformin* is now the only biguanide in use. The most important physiological effect appears to be an increase in hepatic insulin sensitivity/reduction of hepatic glucose production. Recent studies have suggested that the intracellular target of metformin in the liver is the enzyme adenosine monophosphate–activated protein kinase (AMPK) system. AMPK is a conserved regulator of the cellular response to low energy, being activated when intra-cellular ATP levels decrease and AMP concentrations increase.[5]

Metformin ($t_{1/2}$ 5 h) is best taken with or after meals. Metformin can be used in combination with either insulin or other oral antidiabetic agents, and is the first-line agent in the management of type 2 diabetes in most global guidelines. It is also being used in the management of type 1 diabetes in conjunction with insulin, especially in overweight individuals and as the first-line agent in gestational diabetes. The drug is ineffective in the absence of insulin.

Minor adverse reactions are common, including nausea, diarrhoea and a metallic taste in the mouth. These symptoms are usually transient or subside after reduction of dose and can be minimised by building doses up slowly and ensuring that metformin is taken with or after food. A modified release preparation, Metformin MR, is reported to be better tolerated in some patients who suffer gastrointestinal side-effects with regular metformin.

More serious, but rare, is *lactic acidosis.* When this condition does occur, it is usually against the background of significant medical illnesses which tend to increase circulating lactic acid levels, particularly renal impairment, liver failure, or cardiogenic or septic shock. Metformin is therefore contraindicated in these conditions, including relatively mild renal impairment, and use should be reviewed when plasma creatinine is >130 mmol/L (or eGFR <45 mL/min/1.73 m^2) and stopped when plasma creatinine is >150 mmol/L (or eGFR <30 mL/min/1.73 m^2).

Most clinical guidelines recommend that metformin is best withdrawn temporarily before general anaesthesia and/or administration of iodine-containing contrast media because of concerns about precipitating renal impairment (although the evidence for this is unclear) or risks of lactic acidosis if renal impairment develops. Lactic acidosis may require treatment with i.v. isotonic sodium bicarbonate.

Apart from diabetes, the insulin-sensitising effects of metformin may also be useful in *polycystic ovary syndrome,* a condition in which insulin resistance occurs and may contribute to the hyperandrogenism and consequent hirsutism and disordered menstrual cycles which characterise this condition.

Thiazolidinediones. *Pioglitazone* reduces peripheral insulin resistance, leading to a reduction of blood glucose concentration. This class of drugs stimulates the nuclear hormone receptor, peroxisome proliferator–activated receptor (PPARγ), which causes differentiation of adipocytes. The major action is to stimulate peripheral insulin sensitivity and thus glucose uptake in skeletal muscle, although the mechanism by which this 'cross-talk' from adipocytes to muscle occurs is unclear. They are slower to act than either metformin or sulfonylureas.

The main adverse effects of thiazolidinediones are weight gain (typically 3–4 kg of weight gain in the first year of use), fluid retention (with peripheral oedema in 3–4% of patients) and decreased bone density.

(iii) Agents that increase urinary glucose excretion

SGLT-2 inhibitors. Sodium-glucose cotransporter-2 is the main cotransporter in renal proximal convoluted tubules involved in glucose reabsorption via the kidneys. Inhibition of SGLT-2 by drugs like canagliflozin, dapagliflozin and empagliflozin reduces the renal threshold of glucose (usually around 10 mmol/L) and leads to glycosuria, thereby reducing glucose load in blood. These agents are given orally, are weight reducing, but tend to be less efficacious even in mild renal impairment (eGFR below 45–60 mL/min). Recent data (EMPA-REG OUTCOME) suggest that empagliflozin reduces cardiovascular mortality and morbidity in patients with high cardiovascular risk. The main side-effect is urogenital infections. Glycosuria also causes a degree of diuresis and may cause orthostatic hypotension in some patients. There has been concern about euglycaemic ketoacidosis; therefore, ketone testing is advised in patients who are unwell even if blood sugars are normal. Recent clinical trial data suggest a risk of increased lower limb amputation in canagliflozin studies. It is unclear what the mechanism is and whether this applies to other SGLT2 inhibitors.

(iv) Agents which reduce glucose absorption

Acarbose is an α-glucosidase inhibitor that reduces the digestion of complex carbohydrates and slows their absorption from the gut and thus reduces postprandial glycaemia. The usual dose is 50–300 mg/day. *Adverse effects* are common, mainly flatulence and diarrhoea, which lead to a high discontinuation rate. In high doses it may cause frank malabsorption. Acarbose may be combined with a sulfonylurea. Overall, it is rarely used nowadays.

Antidiabetics and cardiovascular outcome studies. Following initial reports of a possible link between adverse cardiovascular outcomes and rosiglitazone (a thiazolidinedione) use in 2007, the US Food and Drug Administration (FDA) industry guidance in 2008 required all new antidiabetic agents to have sufficient cardiovascular outcome data showing

---

[5]The discovery of the AMPK response, and of other players in the pathway, has enabled experiments to be performed in which the hepatic response to metformin is selectively knocked out. In the mouse, at least, these experiments show that actions of metformin at other sites are of little importance.

no increased risk before they could have regulatory approval for use. Most cardiovascular outcome trials (CVOTs) have used non-inferiority designs to rule out unacceptable adverse cardiovascular events, although, to date, EMPA-REG and LEADER trials examining empagliflozin and liraglutide, respectively, have shown superiority of empagliflozin and liraglutide, respectively, in reducing major cardiovascular events in high-risk individuals.

Choice of oral antidiabetic drugs in type 2 diabetes

In general terms, a hierarchy of therapies exists for type 2 diabetes, progressing from diet and lifestyle alone (described later), through monotherapy with oral agents, combinations of oral therapies and then onto insulin/injection therapy either alone or in combination with oral treatment. The nature of 'typical' type 2 diabetes is that glucose intolerance tends to progress so that many patients will need to escalate therapy with time to avoid worsening glycaemia (and warning patients of this early after diagnosis helps avoid subsequent disappointment and demotivation). It is also worth emphasising that this 'typical' time course is not universal. Analogous to type 1 diabetes, some patients may present with marked symptomatic hyperglycaemia requiring immediate insulin therapy (and indeed some of these may have an unrecognised late onset of type 1 diabetes).

The evidence base for the most effective strategies for using antidiabetic therapy continues to evolve, and the following is UK NICE (National Institute for Health and Care Excellence) guidance set out as a guide for readers. Current advice is that *metformin* (where not contraindicated and if tolerated) is useful primary monotherapy for most patients with type 2 diabetes. *DDP-4 inhibitors* and *SGLT-2 inhibitors* are increasingly used as second- or third-line agents, and may even be used as the first-line agent if metformin is not tolerated. *Sulfonylurea* therapy is now less often used as first-line therapy but is an alternative to metformin or can be added in to dual therapy as needed. *Thiazolidinediones* can also be used in combination with the above. *GLP-1 agonists* may be considered when overweight is a consideration. The therapeutic target is to maintain the HbA1c (glycosylated haemoglobin) below 6.5–7.5% (<48–58 mmol/mol), and insulin may eventually be required, either alone (see earlier section on insulin regimens) or in combination with metformin (and/or other agents).

Diet and diabetes

Specialised diet and lifestyle advice is of paramount importance in managing diabetes. Patients should be allowed to follow their own preferences as far as is practicable. They should receive dietary advice on a high complex carbohydrate diet (~65% of total calories) with low fat (<30% of calories) and an emphasis on reduction in saturated fat in favour of mono- and polyunsaturates. Caloric intake may need to be restricted and patients encouraged to achieve an ideal body-weight. Although certain foods are marketed as 'diabetic', there are concerns about whether these may be low in glucose but high in calories. Diet should be high in fibre with plenty of fresh fruits and vegetables. Advice about alcohol intake and smoking should be given (and where appropriate, information about what to do when/after drinking alcohol because of the effects causing delayed hypoglycaemia). This should be combined with advice about activity/exercise levels.

As indicated earlier, increasing numbers of patients with type 1 diabetes are now taught how to count dietary carbohydrates, allowing them to adjust their insulin doses around dietary intake/activity/alcohol.

The advice above may need further modifying in those with ischaemic heart disease and/or established nephropathy.

Interactions with non-diabetes drugs

Some examples are listed below to show that the possibility of interactions of practical clinical importance is a real one. In general, whenever a patient with diabetes takes other drugs it is prudent to be on the watch for disturbance of glycaemic control.

β-adrenoceptor–blocking drugs may impair the sympathetically mediated ($β_2$ receptor) release of glucose from the liver in response to hypoglycaemia and also reduce the adrenergically mediated symptoms of hypoglycaemia (except sweating). Insulin hypoglycaemia may thus be more prolonged and/or less noticeable. Ideally, a patient with diabetes needing a β-adrenoceptor blocker should be given a $β_1$-selective member, e.g. *bisoprolol*.

Thiazide diuretics at a higher dose than those now generally used in hypertension can precipitate/worsen diabetes, probably by reducing insulin secretion.

Hepatic enzyme inducers may enhance the metabolism of sulfonylureas that are metabolised in the liver (tolbutamide). Cimetidine, an *inhibitor* of drug-metabolising enzymes, increases metformin plasma concentration and effect.

Monoamine oxidase inhibitors potentiate oral agents and perhaps also insulin. They can also reduce appetite and so upset control.

Interaction may occur with *alcohol* (hypoglycaemia with any antidiabetes drug).

Salicylates and *fibrates* can increase insulin sensitivity, resulting in lower blood glucose.

The action of *sulfonylureas* is intensified by heavy sulfonamide dosage, and some sulfonamides increase free tolbutamide concentrations, probably by competing for plasma protein–binding sites.

The use of *glucagon* as rescue therapy for hypoglycaemia is described above. *Adrenaline/epinephrine* raises the blood sugar concentration by mobilising liver and muscle glycogen (a β_2-adrenoceptor effect), and suppressing secretion of insulin (an α-adrenoceptor effect). Hyperglycaemia may occur in patients with phaeochromocytoma, and is usually reversed by α-adrenoceptor blockade (see p. 404).

Adrenal steroids, either endogenous or exogenous, antagonise the actions of insulin. Although this effect is only slight with mineralocorticoids, glucocorticoid hormones increase gluconeogenesis and reduce glucose uptake and utilisation by the tissues. The therapeutic use of high-dose glucocorticoids (e.g. in neurosurgical, rheumatological and respiratory conditions) may precipitate frank diabetes in some patients or worsen blood glucose control in those with established diabetes. Steroid-induced diabetes often requires insulin rather than oral hypoglycaemic therapy, particularly for flexibility if steroid doses are being tapered down. Similarly, patients with Cushing's syndrome may also develop 'secondary diabetes' with a marked resistance to insulin. In contrast, patients with hypoadrenalism from Addison's disease, hypopituitarism, or following steroid withdrawal after prolonged glucocorticoid therapy may be abnormally sensitive to insulin action and prone to recurrent hypoglycaemia.

Growth hormone antagonises the actions of insulin in the tissues. Like Addison's disease, growth hormone deficiency may cause increased insulin sensitivity and/or a tendency for hypoglycaemia. Acromegalic patients may develop insulin-resistant diabetes.

Oral contraceptives can impair carbohydrate tolerance, although the effects are usually relatively mild.

Thyroid hormone excess may increase the requirements for insulin.

Drug-induced diabetes

Diazoxide (see p. 423) is chemically similar to thiazide diuretics, but stimulates the ATP-dependent K^+ channel that is blocked by the sulfonylureas. Although formerly used as an antihypertensive agent, its current use in therapeutics is confined to the rare indication of treating hypoglycaemia due to islet cell tumour (insulinoma). Adrenocortical steroids are also diabetogenic (see above).

Pregnancy and diabetes

During (and indeed before) pregnancy, close control of diabetes is critical. Ideally, pregnancy should be planned and women should be seen in a pre-conception clinic to optimise care. Glycaemic targets are tight, aiming for HbA1c values as close to the non-diabetic range (<6.5 % or <48 mmol/mol) as possible. Current practice is for women on metformin who are planning or starting a pregnancy to continue metformin and for those who are on any other oral antidiabetics to change to metformin and/or insulin. There is no definitive evidence though that oral drugs are associated with fetal malformations. Other drugs (blood pressure and lipid lowering) should be reviewed and stopped or altered to agents judged safe in pregnancy as appropriate. Oral folic acid should be started in advance of pregnancy.

Diabetes can present *de novo* during pregnancy. Although this is usually gestational diabetes which resolves after delivery, it is worth remembering that rarely type 2 or type 1 diabetes can present in pregnancy.

Risks associated with pregnancy in diabetes include an increased rate of fetal loss and malformations. Maternal hyperglycaemia can lead to fetal hyperglycaemia with consequent fetal islet cell hyperplasia, high birth-weight babies (leading to mechanical obstetric challenges) and postnatal hypoglycaemia.

Note that glycosuria is not a reliable guide of blood glucose values in pregnancy. The renal threshold for glucose (also of lactose) falls, so that glycosuria and lactosuria may occur in the presence of a normal blood glucose.

Insulin requirements increase steadily after the third month. Some women develop a marked intolerance of oral carbohydrates with a tendency for large postprandial rises in blood glucose. During labour, i.v. insulin infusion may be needed. Use of β_2-adrenoceptor agonists and of dexamethasone (to prevent respiratory distress syndrome in the prematurely newborn) causes hyperglycaemia and increased insulin (and potassium) needs.

Of note, insulin requirements reduce immediately after delivery and may remain low during the following weeks, particularly with lactation/breast feeding.

Surgery in diabetic patients

Principles of management

- Surgery constitutes a major stress.
- Insulin needs will often increase with surgery.

The programme for control should be agreed between anaesthetist and physician whenever diabetic patients must undergo general anaesthesia or modify their diets, and most hospitals/provider trusts have local guidelines for this. There are many different techniques that can give satisfactory results: typical guidelines are detailed below.

Type 1 diabetes

The guidelines below may also be useful for insulin-treated type 2 diabetes, but suggested doses may need modifying

Table 36.3 Sliding scale of insulin doses according to blood glucose concentrations (not for ketoacidosis)

Blood glucose (mmol/L)	Infusion rate (mL/h = units/h for 50-mL syringe containing 50 units insulin)
≥22.0	10.0 (and check pump and connections)
19–21.9	8.0
16–18.9	6.0
12–15.9	4.0
8–11.9	2.0
4–7.9	1.0
<3.9	0.5 (and increase glucose infusion)

if patients are insulin resistant with a large constitutive insulin requirement.

Elective major surgery

- The evening before surgery: give patient's usual insulin.
- Day of operation: omit morning s.c. dose; set up i.v. infusion: 0.45% sodium chloride with 5% glucose and KCL (0.15% or 0.3%); insulin should be infused by pump at an approximate rate of 2 units/h and adjusted according to a sliding scale (variable-rate insulin infusion, VRII) maintaining a glucose level of 6–10 mmol/L (acceptable range 4–12 mmol/L).
- Modify regimen during and after surgery according to monitoring; insulin doses should be adjusted according to a similar scale as that in Table 36.3.
- Stop i.v. infusion 1 h after first post-surgical s.c. usual quick-acting insulin (given when eating again).
- Insulin requirements may be high, 10–15 units/h, in cases of major surgery, serious infection, corticosteroid use or obesity.

Minor surgery/procedures

For example, simple dental extractions or endoscopy. For short, relatively non-stressful procedures, i.v. insulin is usually not needed. When nil by mouth, patients should omit fast-acting insulin normally given for that mealtime.

Emergency surgery

When a surgical emergency is complicated by diabetic ketosis, an attempt should be made to control the ketosis before

surgery. Management during the operation will be similar to that for major surgery except that more insulin may be needed.

Type 2 diabetes

For minor procedures when diabetes is well controlled on oral hypoglycaemics, it should be possible simply to omit the oral hypoglycaemic agent on the morning of surgery.

Diabetic ketoacidosis

This condition is discussed in detail in medical texts, and only the more pharmacological aspects will be considered here.

The best way to consider ketoacidosis is as a severe and life-threatening metabolic disorder resulting from a lack of insulin in which hyperglycaemia is present, rather than as a primary hyperglycaemic disorder. The patient with ketoacidosis often remains critically ill during treatment even after blood glucose is normalised. Patients are severely dehydrated, and fluid resuscitation is a major priority. Insulin is needed not only to lower blood glucose, but also to suppress ketogenesis. The objective is to supply, as continuously as possible, a moderate amount of insulin.

Intravenous fluid. A patient with diabetic ketoacidosis may have a fluid deficit of above 5 L. Usual fluid replacement is isotonic saline, and a typical regimen might be:

- 1 L in the first hour, followed by
- 2 L in 4 h, then
- 4 L in the next 24 h, watching for signs of fluid overload.

Note that fluid replacement itself causes a fall in blood glucose concentration both by dilution and also by restoring blood volume to perfuse skeletal muscle, a major insulin target tissue.

Soluble insulin should be given by continuous i.v. infusion of a 1-unit/mL solution of insulin in isotonic sodium chloride. High doses are needed (e.g. 0.1 U/kg/h), and treatment needs to be prolonged beyond restoration of blood glucose to suppress ketogenesis. A reasonable rate of fall of glucose during treatment is 4–5.5 mmol/L (75–100 mg/100 mL) per hour. Once the blood glucose has fallen to 10–15 mmol/L, i.v. dextrose infusion is started to prevent this continued high-dose insulin resulting in hypoglycaemia (rather than reducing the insulin infusion rate, which will slow resolution of the metabolic derangement).

Potassium. Even if plasma potassium concentration is normal or high, patients have a substantial total body deficit, and the plasma level will fall briskly with i.v. fluids (dilution) and insulin, which draws potassium into cells within minutes. Potassium chloride should be added to the second and subsequent litres of fluid according to plasma potassium (provided the patient is passing urine).

- <3.5 mmol/L: additional potassium needs to be given possibly via central line
- 3.5–5.5 mmol/L: add 40 mmol/L.
- >5.5 mmol/L: none.

Bicarbonate is generally not recommended as it may paradoxically increase intracellular acidosis and delay the reduction in blood lactate.

Success in treatment of diabetic ketoacidosis and its complications (hypokalaemia, aspiration of stomach contents, infection, shock, thromboembolism, cerebral oedema) depends on close, constant, informed supervision and repeated monitoring of clinical state and biochemical parameters.

Euglycaemic ketoacidosis can happen rarely, particularly where insulin is used in combination with SGLT-2 inhibitor therapy. Principles of management are the same, although intravenous glucose along with saline is usually required from the outset to allow adequate insulin delivery without hypoglycaemia. Diabetic ketoalkalosis is also possible if excessive vomiting of gastric acid leads to loss of chloride (hypochloraemia).

Diabetic ketosis without acidosis. As with full-blown ketoacidosis, this may develop during intercurrent illness. Increasingly, patients with type 1 diabetes are given 'sick day rules' for how to manage this when appropriate out of hospital. This relies on the patient being fully conscious, not vomiting and being willing and able to drink fluids and follow instructions, including regular and repeated monitoring of blood glucose and ketone levels. In general, insulin doses are increased with additional injections of soluble insulin (10–20% of total daily insulin dose every 2 h). The rules include 'bail out' instructions on seeking admission if ketone and glucose levels are not resolving and/or patients start to vomit or fail to improve clinically.

Ketosis-prone type 2 diabetes ("Flatbush diabetes"). Many ketoacidosis cases in people with type 2 diabetes have been reported, usually in Afro-Carribean individuals. After an initial aggressive insulin therapy, it may be possible for them to be in remission without needing insulin for months and even years. The underpinning mechanism is unknown but may be related to a reversible glucose toxicity effect on beta cells, so that restoring normoglycaemia for a period of time allows functional insulin secretion to recover.

Hyperosmolar Hyperglycaemic State (HHS) occurs chiefly in type 2 diabetics who fail to compensate for their continuing osmotic glucose diuresis. It is characterised by severe dehydration, a very high blood sugar level (>33 mmol/L), and in most cases lack of ketosis and acidosis. Treatment is with isotonic (0.9%) saline, usually at one-half the rate recommended for diabetic ketoacidosis, and with less potassium than in severe ketoacidosis. Insulin requirements are less than in ketoacidosis, where the acidosis causes resistance to the actions of insulin, and should generally be one-half of those shown in Table 36.3. Patients may be profoundly dehydrated and liable to thrombosis so that prophylactic low molecular weight heparin should be considered.

Preventing complications other than by glucose lowering

Diabetes is a condition not just of abnormal glucose but also of significantly increased cardiovascular risk. Indeed, most patients with both type 1 and type 2 diabetes succumb to either the macrovascular or microvascular complications – especially ischaemic heart disease and/or diabetic nephropathy.

Aggressive treatment of hypertension and hyperlipidaemia in addition to glycaemia is particularly important in patients with diabetes. For example, the landmark UK Prospective Diabetes Study (UKPDS) of type 2 diabetes confirmed that good glycaemic control and aggressive blood pressure reduction independently improve outcome.[6,7] For every 1% reduction in haemoglobin A1c (HbA1c), there was a 21% reduction in diabetes-related deaths and a 37% reduction in microvascular disease. Of highest importance was the finding that effective blood pressure control – regardless of the type of antihypertensive drug – was more influential than glycaemic control in preventing macrovascular complications. Reduction of blood pressure in 758 patients to a mean of 144/82 mmHg achieved a 32% reduction in deaths related to diabetes and a 37% reduction in microvascular endpoints, compared with findings in 390 patients treated to a blood pressure of 154/87 mmHg.

Similarly, aggressive targeting of lipids reduces cardiovascular complications in diabetes. In the Heart Protection Study, addition of simvastatin 40 mg/day to the treatment of 4000 patients with diabetes reduced cardiovascular

---

[6]UK Prospective Diabetes Study (UKPDS) Group 1998 Effect of intensive blood-glucose control with metformin on complications in overweight patients with Type 2 diabetes (UKPDS 34). Lancet 352:854–865.
[7]UK Prospective Diabetes Study (UKPDS) Group 1998 Tight blood pressure control and risk of macrovascular and microvascular complications in Type 2 diabetes. British Medical Journal 317:703–713.

complications by 30%. Some guidelines have suggested that aspirin may be worth using in primary prevention in diabetes (i.e. in those who have not suffered a cardiovascular event), although current thinking is that the benefits are unproven.

Patients with evidence of diabetic nephropathy should receive either an angiotensin-converting enzyme (ACE) inhibitor or an angiotensin receptor antagonist; the evidence for the superiority of the latter in reducing progression to renal failure compared with other antihypertensive agents is particularly strong.[8] Addition of an ACE inhibitor to other drugs may also improve overall outcome in patients with diabetes.[9] In addition, diabetic nephropathy is independently associated with an increased risk of macrovascular disease so that aggressive lipid and blood pressure–lowering therapy, as described above, should be employed.

Summary

- Diabetes mellitus is important in global terms because of its chronicity, and high incidence and frequency of major complications. It is generally divided into two kinds: type 1 (previously, insulin-dependent diabetes mellitus) and type 2 (previously, non–insulin dependent diabetes, essentially an umbrella term for a group of conditions which are non–type 1).
- Type 1 diabetes is commoner in those with onset before 30 years of age, whereas type 2 diabetes is best considered as a heterogenous group of conditions usually presenting at a later age. Increasingly, insulin therapy is required in type 2 diabetes when glycaemic control is not optimised by oral drugs.
- Insulin is usually self-administered subcutaneously to stable patients, with a variety of regimens which can be tailored to the needs of a particular patient. Modern practice in type 1 diabetes is to educate patients in flexible insulin dosing which is adjusted for differing meals, activity levels, etc.
- In the treatment of diabetic ketoacidosis, in the perioperative patient, and during inpatient management of the critically ill patient with diabetes, insulin is best given by intravenous infusion of the soluble form.
- Diet plays a major role in the treatment of type 2 diabetes, particularly when associated with obesity.
- If a drug is required in type 2 diabetes, metformin (a biguanide) is now widely used as first-line therapy, especially for the obese. There are many second-line agents available now, but the increasing focus of attention is on the cardiovascular outcomes of antidiabetics. Many patients with type 2 diabetes will need treatment escalation with time to multiple combination therapy and/or insulin.
- Aggressive blood glucose–lowering treatment of type 1 and type 2 diabetes reduces the risk of microvascular complications. Close attention to associated risk factors, especially hyperlipidaemia and hypertension, is important in reducing the risk of macrovascular disease.

Obesity and appetite control

Overweight and obesity are the commonest nutritional disorders in developed countries. Between 1991 and 2014, the prevalence of obesity in adults rose from 22.3% to 37.9% in the USA. Obesity predisposes to several chronic diseases including hypertension, hyperlipidaemia, diabetes mellitus, cardiovascular disease and osteoarthritis, and aspects of these are discussed in the relevant sections of this book.

Individuals whose body mass index[10] (BMI) lies between 25 and 30 kg/m^2 are considered *overweight*, and those in whom it exceeds 30 kg/m^2 are defined as *obese*. Management of the condition involves a variety of approaches from nutritional advice to lifestyle alteration, drugs and, where available and appropriate, bariatric surgery. In the UK, an evidence-based algorithm coordinates these.[11] The present account concentrates on pharmacological interventions.

In general, drugs that have been used for obesity act either on the gastrointestinal tract, lowering nutrient absorption, or centrally, reducing food intake by decreasing appetite or increasing satiety (appetite suppressants). A number of

[8]Three trials compared an angiotensin blocker with other blood pressure–lowering drugs and found a 20% reduction in the proportion of patients in whom proteinuria worsened or serum creatinine concentration doubled during follow-up: (1) Parving H H, Lehnert H, Brochner-Mortensen J et al 2001 The effect of irbesartan on the development of diabetic nephropathy in patients with Type 2 diabetes. New England Journal of Medicine 345:870–878; (2) Brenner B M, Cooper M E, de Zeeuw D et al 2001 Effects of losartan on renal and cardiovascular outcomes in patients with Type 2 diabetes and nephropathy. New England Journal of Medicine 345:861–869; (3) Lewis E J, Hunsicker L G, Clarke W R et al 2001 Renoprotective effect of the angiotensin-receptor antagonist irbesartan in patients with nephropathy due to Type 2 diabetes. New England Journal of Medicine 345:851–860.
[9]The HOPE study included patients with diabetes as one of its high-risk groups of cardiovascular patients, in whom ramipril reduced further coronary heart disease endpoints by about 30%. Yusuf S, Sleight P, Pogue J et al 2000 Effects of an angiotensin converting enzyme inhibitor, ramipril, on cardiovascular events in high-risk patients. The Heart Outcomes Prevention Evaluation Study Investigators. New England Journal of Medicine 342:145–153.
[10]The weight in kilograms divided by the square of the height in metres (kg/m^2).
[11]https://pathways.nice.org.uk/pathways/obesity

pharmacological agents that have been marketed for obesity have been withdrawn because of concerns about safety. Currently, only one agent, orlistat, is available in the UK:

Orlistat

Orlistat is a pentanoic acid ester that binds to and inhibits gastric and pancreatic lipases; the resulting inhibition of their activity prevents the absorption of about 30% of dietary fat compared with a normal 5% loss. Weight loss is due to calorie loss, but drug-related adverse effects also contribute by diminishing food intake. The drug is not absorbed from the alimentary tract.

Clinical trials have shown that patients who adhered to a low-calorie diet and took orlistat lost on average 9–10 kg after 1 year (compared with 6 kg in those taking placebo); in the following year those who remained on orlistat regained 1.5–3.0 kg (4–6 kg with placebo). Orlistat has found a place in the management of obesity in the UK but, not surprisingly, this is subject to stringent guidance from NICE, namely that it be initiated only in individuals with a BMI of 28 kg/m^2 or more who also have cardiovascular risk factors, or 30 kg/m^2 or more without such co-morbidity.

The dose is 120 mg, taken immediately before, during or 1 h after each main meal, up to three times daily. If a meal is missed, or contains no fat, the dose of orlistat should be omitted.

Treatment should be accompanied by counselling advice and proceed beyond 3 months only in those who have lost more than 5% of their initial weight and beyond 6 months in those who have lost more than 10%. It should not normally exceed 1 year and should never be more than 2 years.

Adverse effects include flatulence and liquid, oily stools, leading to faecal urgency and abdominal and rectal pain. Symptoms may be reduced by adhering to a reduced-fat diet. Low plasma concentrations of the fat-soluble vitamins A, D and E have been found. Orlistat is *contraindicated* where there is chronic intestinal malabsorption or cholestasis.

Leptin

The adipocyte-derived hormone leptin (Greek: *leptos,* thin) has a limited role in therapeutics for patients with rare genetic defects in the leptin or leptin receptor genes. Leptin acts on the brain to reduce appetite. Most obese patients have raised plasma leptin concentrations, to which they have become relatively resistant. A small number of patients are genuinely deficient in leptin, and therapy with recombinant leptin has had dramatic beneficial effects. Leptin may also be of benefit in lipodystrophic patients, a rare group of conditions in which a generalised or partial lack of adipocytes leads to marked metabolic abnormalities and diabetes.

Leptin acts to control satiety via the melanocortin system, predominantly in the basomedial hypothalamus, and a number of agents in development aim to target this.

Newer agents

GLP-1 agonist

In addition to being a blood glucose–lowering therapy in type 2 diabetes as described above, there is interest in whether GLP-1 agonist therapy should be used for weight reduction in non-diabetes. High-dose liraglutide 3 mg once a day (Saxenda) has now been approved in the US and Europe as a weight-loss agent in patients without diabetes.

Lorcaserin

Lorcaserin is a novel selective agonist of 5-HT2c receptors in the hypothalamus and increases satiety leading to reduced food intake. It has been approved by the US FDA for adults with a BMI over 30 or a BMI over 27 with another weight-related co-morbidity. It is administered orally, and common unwanted effects include headache, upper respiratory infections, nausea and dizziness.

Naltrexone/bupropion (Contrave) and phentermine/topiramate (Qsymia) have also been approved by the US FDA, although clinical use is still low.

Obesity and diabetes

Obesity is associated with type 2 diabetes, and weight loss improves (and in rare cases 'cures') diabetes. Weighed against this is the challenge that certain pharmacologic therapies for diabetes, particularly sulfonylureas, thiazolidinediones and insulin, can promote weight gain. The patient and clinician may find themselves caught in a vicious cycle in which dose escalation of these agents leads to weight gain, worsening glycaemic control, which in turn leads to further dose increments.

As for patients without diabetes, diet and exercise are critical factors, but diabetes treatment may need to be adjusted for this (e.g. insulin reductions to avoid hypoglycaemia with increased exercise or reduced carbohydrate intake). Metformin, either alone or as adjuvant therapy, especially with insulin as an 'insulin-sparing' agent is useful. GLP-1 analogue therapy offers an alternative to insulin therapy. Ultimately, as for patients without diabetes, orlistat and/or bariatric surgery[12] may be appropriate.

---

[12]Weight-loss surgery: the procedures include reducing the size of the stomach by resection, gastric banding and gastric bypass.

Guide to further reading

Chan, J.L., Mantzoros, C.S., 2005. Role of leptin in energy-deprivation states: normal human physiology and clinical implications for hypothalamic amenorrhoea and anorexia nervosa. Lancet 366, 74–85.

Cushman, W.C., Evans, G.W., Byington, R.P., et al., 2010. Effects of intensive blood-pressure control in type 2 diabetes mellitus. N. Engl. J. Med. 362, 1575–1585.

Dhatariya, K., et al., 2016. JBDS-IP: Management of adults with diabetes undergoing surgery and elective procedures: Improving standards. Available at: http://www. diabetologists-abcd.org.uk/JBDS/ Surgical_guidelines_2015_full_ FINAL_amended_Mar_2016.pdf. (Accessed 21 January 2017.)

Dhatariya, K., et al., 2013. JBDS-IP: The management of diabetic ketoacidosis in adults. Available at: http://www.diabetologists-abcd .org.uk/JBDS/JBDS_IP_DKA_Adults_ Revised.pdf. (Accessed 21 January 2017.)

Diabetes Control and Complications Trial/Epidemiology of Diabetes Interventions and Complications (DCCT/EDIC) Study Research Group, 2005. Intensive diabetes treatment and cardiovascular disease in patients with type 1 diabetes. N. Engl. J. Med. 353, 2643–2653.

Diabetes Control and Complications Trial/Epidemiology of Diabetes Interventions and Complications (DCCT/EDIC) Research Group, 2009. Modern-day clinical course of type 1 diabetes mellitus after 30 years' duration. Arch. Intern. Med. 169, 1307–1316.

Drucker, D.J., Nauck, M.A., 2006. The incretin system: glucagon-like peptide-1 receptor agonists and dipeptidyl peptidase-4 inhibitors in type 2 diabetes. Lancet 368, 1696–1705.

Eckel, R.H., Grundy, S.M., Zimmet, P.Z., 2005. The metabolic syndrome. Lancet 365, 1415–1428.

Gerstein, H.C., Miller, M.E., Genuth, S., et al., 2011. Long-term effects of intensive glucose lowering on cardiovascular outcomes. N. Engl. J. Med. 364, 818–828.

Ginsberg, H.N., Elam, M.B., Lovato, L.C., et al., 2010. Effects of combination lipid therapy in type 2 diabetes mellitus. N. Engl. J. Med. 362, 1563–1574.

Marso, S.P., et al., 2016. Liraglutide and cardiovascular outcomes in type 2 diabetes. N. Engl. J. Med. 375, 311–322.

National Institute for Health and Clinical Excellence, 2015. Diabetes in pregnancy: Management from preconception to the postnatal period. Available at: http:// www.nice.org.uk/guidance/ng3. (Accessed 21 January 2017).

US Department of Health and Human Services, Food and Drug Administration, Centre for Drug Evaluation and Research (CEDR), 2008. Guidance for Industry: Diabetes Mellitus – Evaluating Cardiovascular risk in New Antidiabetic Therapies to Treat Type 2 Diabetes. Available at: https:// www.fda.gov/downloads/Drugs/…/ Guidances/ucm071627.pdf. (Accessed 21 January 2017.)

Wright, J.R., 2002. From ugly fish to conquer death: J J R Macleod's fish insulin research, 1922–24. Lancet 359, 1238–1242.

Zinman, B., et al., 2015. Empagliflozin, cardiovascular outcomes, and mortality in type 2 diabetes (EMPA-REG). N. Engl. J. Med. 373, 2117–2128.

Chapter | **37**

Thyroid hormones, antithyroid drugs

Diana C. Brown

SYNOPSIS

- Thyroid hormones (thyroxine/levothyroxine T_4, liothyronine T_3).
- Use of thyroid hormone: treatment of hypothyroidism.
- Antithyroid drugs and hyperthyroidism: thionamides, drugs that block sympathetic autonomic activity, iodide and radioiodine ^{131}I, preparation of patients for surgery, thyroid storm (crisis), exophthalmos.
- Drugs that cause unwanted hypothyroidism.
- Calcitonin (see Ch. 39).

Thyroid hormones

L-Thyroxine (T_4 or tetra-iodo-L-thyronine) and lio-L-thyronine (T_3 or tri-iodo-L-thyronine) are the natural hormones of the thyroid gland. T_4 is a less active precursor of T_3, which is the major mediator of physiological effect. In this chapter, T_4 for therapeutic use is referred to as *levothyroxine* (the rINN; see p. 71).

For convenience, the term 'thyroid hormone' is used to comprise T_4 plus T_3. Both forms are available for oral use as therapy.

Calcitonin. See p. 662.

Physiology and pharmacokinetics

Thyroid hormone synthesis requires oxidation of dietary iodine, followed by iodination of tyrosine to mono- and di-iodotyrosine; coupling of iodotyrosines leads to formation of the *active molecules, tetra-iodothyronine* (T_4 or L-thyroxine) and *tri-iodothyronine* (T_3 or L-thyronine).

These active thyroid hormones are stored in the gland within the molecule of thyroglobulin, a major component of the intrafollicular colloid. They are released into the circulation following reuptake of the colloid by the apical cells and proteolysis. The main circulating thyroid hormone is T_4. About 80% of the released T_4 is de-iodinated in the peripheral tissues to the biologically active T_3 (30–35%) and biologically inactive 'reverse' T_3 (45–50%); thus most circulating T_3 is derived from T_4. Further de-iodination, largely in the liver, leads to loss of activity.

In the blood, both T_4 and T_3 are extensively (99.9%) bound to plasma proteins (thyroxine-binding globulin (TBG) and transthyretin (TTR), albumin and lipoproteins). The concentration of TBG is raised by oestrogens (physiological or pharmacological) and prolonged use of neuroleptics. The concentration of TBG is lowered by adrenocortical and androgen (including anabolic steroid) therapy and by urinary protein loss in the nephrotic syndrome. Phenytoin and salicylates compete with thyroid hormone for TBG-binding sites. Effects such as these would interfere with the assessment of the clinical significance of measurements of total thyroid hormone concentration, but the availability of free thyroid hormone assay largely avoids such complicating factors. Normal values are: free T_4 9–25 pmol/L, free T_3 3–9 pmol/L.

T_4 and T_3 are well absorbed from the gut, except in myxo-edema coma, when parenteral therapy is required.

T_4 **(levothyroxine).** A single dose reaches its maximum effect in about 10 days (its binding to plasma proteins is strong as well as extensive) and passes off in 2–3 weeks ($t_{1/2}$ 7 days in euthyroid, 14 days in hypothyroid and 3 days in hyperthyroid subjects).

T_3 **(liothyronine)** is about five times as biologically potent as T_4; a single dose reaches its maximum effect in about 24 h (its binding to plasma proteins is weak) and passes off in 1 week ($t_{1/2}$ 2 days in euthyroid subjects).

Pharmacodynamics

Thyroid hormone passes into the cells of target organs. T_4 is de-iodinated to T_3, which combines with specific nuclear receptors and induces characteristic metabolic changes:

- Protein synthesis during growth.
- Increased metabolic rate with raised oxygen consumption.
- Increased sensitivity to catecholamines with proliferation of β-adrenoceptors (particularly important in the cardiovascular system).

Levothyroxine for hypothyroidism

The main indication for levothyroxine is treatment of thyroxine deficiency (cretinism, adult hypothyroidism) from any cause. The adult requirement of hormone is remarkably constant, and dosage does not usually have to be altered once the optimum has been found. Patients should be monitored annually. Monitoring needs to be more frequent in children, who may need more as they grow. Similarly, pregnant women should be monitored monthly, and require a 50–100% increase in their normal dose of levothyroxine.

Early treatment of neonatal hypothyroidism (cretinism) (1 in 5000 births) is important if permanent mental defect is to be avoided. It must be lifelong.

Hypothyroidism due to panhypopituitarism requires replacement with glucocorticoids as well as with thyroid hormone. Use of levothyroxine alone can cause acute adrenal insufficiency.

Small doses of levothyroxine in normal subjects merely depress pituitary thyroid-stimulating hormone (TSH) production and consequently reduce the output of thyroid hormone by an equivalent amount.

Levothyroxine is used in some countries for the treatment of non-toxic nodular goitre, on the assumption that nodular thyroid tissue growth is dependent on TSH. The treatment is not curative. Levothyroxine should not be used to treat obesity (see Obesity, p. 648).

Treatment of hypothyroidism

Levothyroxine tablets contain pure L-thyroxine sodium and should be used.

The initial oral dose in healthy patients younger than 60 years of age, without cardiac disease, is 50–100 μg/day. In the old and patients with heart disease or multiple coronary risk factors, this level should be achieved gradually (to minimise cardiovascular risk due to a sudden increase in metabolic demand), starting with 12.5–25 μg/day for the first 2–4 weeks, and then increasing by 12.5 μg monthly until normal TSH levels are achieved.

The usual replacement dose at steady state in patients with complete thyroid failure is 1.6 μg/kg/day, 100–200 μg/day given as a single dose. This is usually sufficient to reduce plasma TSH to normal (0.3–3.5 mU/L), which is the best indicator of adequate treatment. Patients who appear to need increasing doses with fluctuating TSH levels, are probably not taking their tablets consistently; the possibility of malabsorption or other drug interaction should be excluded. The maximum effect of a dose is reached after about 10 days and passes off over about 2–3 weeks. Absorption is more complete and less variable if levothyroxine is taken at the same time every day, 30–60 minutes before breakfast.

Tablets containing physiological mixtures of levothyroxine and liothyronine are not sufficiently evaluated to recommend in preference to levothyroxine alone.

Hypothyroid patients tend to be intolerant of drugs in general owing to slow metabolism.

Liothyronine tabs. Liothyronine is the most rapidly effective thyroid hormone, a single dose giving maximum effect within 24 h and passing off over 24–48 h. It is not routine treatment for hypothyroidism because its rapid onset of effect can induce heart failure. Its main uses are in myxoedema coma and psychosis, both rare conditions. A specialised use is during the withdrawal of levothyroxine replacement (to permit diagnostic radioiodine scanning) in patients with thyroid carcinoma.

Myxoedema coma follows prolonged total hormone deficiency and constitutes an emergency. Liothyronine 5–20 μg is given intravenously every 12 h. Intravenous therapy is mandatory because drug absorption is impaired. Intravenous hydrocortisone should be given to cover the possibility of coexisting adrenocortical insufficiency.

Subclinical hypothyroidism. Subclinical hypothyroidism is defined as an elevated serum TSH concentration in the presence of normal free T_4 and free T_3. Although termed 'subclinical', 25% of patients have symptoms of hypothyroidism and cognitive disturbance. Meta-analyses of population-based studies show a higher incidence of ischaemic heart disease and mortality in subjects younger than 65 years of age. Indications for treatment are pregnancy, ovarian dysfunction/infertility, symptoms of hypothyroidism, TSH ≥10 mU/L, TSH <10 mU/L and positive thyroid antibodies and patients with high risk of cardiovascular disease. Treatment of asymptomatic patients is without benefit.[1]

Adverse effects of thyroid hormone parallel the increase in metabolic rate. The symptoms and signs are those of hyperthyroidism. Symptoms of myocardial ischaemia, atrial fibrillation or heart failure are liable to be provoked by too vigorous therapy or in patients having serious ischaemic heart disease who may even be unable to tolerate optimal therapy. Should they occur, discontinue levothyroxine for at least 1 week, and recommence at lower dose. Only slight overdose may precipitate atrial fibrillation in patients older than 60 years of age.

In pregnancy a hypothyroid patient on thyroxine replacement should be assessed with a preconception TSH level measurement, and free T_4 and TSH should be checked once pregnancy is confirmed. Monthly measurements of free T_4 and TSH are recommended. Optimal replacement therapy is essential in the first trimester (targeting a TSH <2.5 mU/L) when the athyroid fetus is dependent on maternal supply to ensure normal neuro-intellectual development. An average 50% increase in dose of levothyroxine is required, and ideally patients should anticipate this increase. Some endocrinologists advise patients to increase their daily dose by 30% or 25–50 µg/day. Post-delivery, patients revert to their preconception dose. Breast feeding is not contraindicated.[2]

Antithyroid drugs and hyperthyroidism

Drugs used for the treatment of hyperthyroidism include:

- *Thionamides,* which block the synthesis of thyroid hormone.
- *Iodine: radioiodine,* which destroys the cells that make thyroid hormone; *iodide,* an excess of which reduces the production of thyroid hormone temporarily (it is

also necessary for the formation of hormone, and both excess and deficiency can cause goitre).

Thionamides (thiourea derivatives) carbimazole, methimazole, propylthiouracil

Mode of action (Fig. 37.1)

The major action of thionamides is to reduce the formation of thyroid hormone by inhibiting oxidation and organification (incorporation into organic form) of iodine (iodotyrosines)

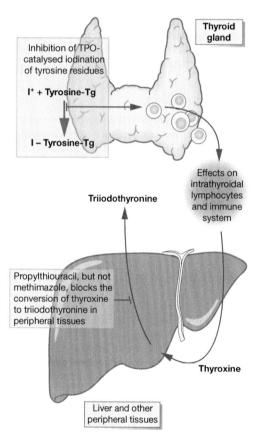

Fig. 37.1 Effects of antithyroid drugs. The multiple effects of antithyroid drugs include inhibition of thyroid hormone synthesis and a reduction in both intrathyroid immune dysregulation and (in the case of propylthiouracil) the peripheral conversion of thyroxine to tri-iodothyronine. Tyrosine-Tg, tyrosine residues in thyroglobulin; 1+, the iodinating intermediate; TPO, thyroid peroxidase. (*Adapted from Cooper D S 2005 Antithyroid drugs. New England Journal of Medicine 352:905–917.*)

[1]Stott D J, Rodondi N, Kearney P M et al 2017 Thyroid hormone therapy for older adults with subclinical hypothyroidism. New England Journal of Medicine 376:2534–2544. This study found no symptomatic benefit in 737 subjects older than 65 years of age randomised to thyroxine or placebo.

[2]Clinical guidelines differ: the American College of Obstetrics and Gynecology recommends against treatment, whereas the American Thyroid Association recommends consideration of treatment, guided by antibody status and thyrotropin level. Treatment started after 16 weeks of pregnancy was found not to alter cognitive function assessed 5 years later, but this could be because the fetal thyroid becomes functional at 16–20 weeks of gestation (Casey B M, Thom E A, Peaceman A M et al 2017 Treatment of subclinical hypothyroidism or hypothyroxinemia in pregnancy. New England Journal of Medicine 376:815–825.)

and coupling of iodotyrosines. Maximum effect is delayed until existing hormone stores are exhausted (weeks, see below). With high dose, reduced hormone synthesis leads to hypothyroidism.

Carbimazole and methimazole (the active metabolite of carbimazole) ($t_{1/2}$ 6 h) and propylthiouracil ($t_{1/2}$ 2 h) are commonly used, but the $t_{1/2}$ matters little because the drugs accumulate in the thyroid and act there for 30–40 h; thus a single daily dose suffices.

Propylthiouracil (PTU) differs from other members of the group in that it also inhibits peripheral conversion of T_4 to T_3, but only at high doses used in treatment of thyroid storm (see p. 633). PTU differs from the other thionamides in its apparent radioprotective effect when used prior to radioiodine treatment.

Carbimazole is the drug of choice in the UK. PTU is used when a patient develops side-effects to carbimazole. PTU is not recommended in children because of the increased risk of severe hepatotoxicity and death.

Immunosuppression

In patients taking antithyroid drugs, serum concentrations of antithyrotropin receptor antibodies decrease with time, as do other immunologically important molecules, including intracellular adhesion molecule 1, and soluble interleukin-2 and interleukin-6 receptors. There is an increased number of circulating suppressor T cells and a decreased number of helper T cells. Antithyroid drugs may also induce apoptosis of intrathyroidal lymphocytes.

Doses

- *Carbimazole* 40 mg total/day is given orally (or *methimazole* 30 mg) until the patient is euthyroid (usually 4–6 weeks). Then titrate *(titration regimen)* by decrements (20 mg, then 10 mg, then 5–10 mg) every 4–6 weeks to a maintenance dose of 5–10 mg/day. The alternative *(block–replace regimen)* has been largely abandoned: 40 mg once daily, and add levothyroxine 100 µg/day, with monitoring of free T_4 and TSH.
- *Propylthiouracil* 300–450 mg total/day is given orally until the patient is euthyroid: maintenance dose is 25–100 mg total/day. Much higher doses (up to 2.4 g/day) with frequent administration are used for thyroid storm.

Use

It is probable that no patient is wholly refractory to these drugs. Failure to respond is likely to be due to the patient not taking the tablets or to wrong diagnosis. The drugs are used in hyperthyroidism:

- As principal therapy.
- As an adjuvant to radioiodine, before and after administration, to control the disease until the radiation achieves its effect.[3]
- To prepare patients for surgery.

Clinical improvement is noticeable in 2–4 weeks, and the patient should be euthyroid in 4–6 weeks.

The best guides to therapy are the patient's symptoms (decreased nervousness and palpitations), increased strength and weight gain, and decreased pulse rate.

Symptoms and signs are, of course, less valuable as guides if the patient is also taking a β-adrenoceptor blocker, and reliance then rests on biochemical tests.

With optimal treatment, the gland decreases in size, but over-treatment leading to low hormone concentrations in the blood activates the pituitary feedback system, inducing TSH secretion and goitre.

Adverse reactions

The thionamide drugs are all liable to cause adverse effects. *Minor* reactions include maculopapular or urticarial rash, pruritus, arthralgia, fever, anorexia, nausea, abnormalities of taste and smell. *Major* effects include agranulocytosis, aplastic anaemia, thrombocytopenia, acute hepatic necrosis, cholestatic hepatitis, lupus-like syndrome, vasculitis.

Blood disorders (<3 per 10 000 patient-years) are most common in the first 2 months of treatment. Routine leucocyte counts to detect blood dyscrasia before symptoms develop are unlikely to protect, as agranulocytosis may be so acute that blood counts give no warning. Patients must be given written warning to stop the drug and have a leucocyte count performed if symptoms of a sore throat, fever, bruising or mouth ulcers develop. Any suggestion of anaemia should be investigated.

Cross-allergy between the drugs sometimes occurs, but is not to be assumed for agranulocytosis. Treatment of agranulocytosis consists of drug withdrawal, admission to hospital, and administration of broad-spectrum antimicrobials plus granulocyte colony-stimulating factor.

Pregnancy. If a pregnant woman has hyperthyroidism (2 per 1000 pregnancies), she should be treated with the smallest possible amount of these drugs because they cross the placenta; over-treatment causes fetal goitre. Meticulous

---

[3]Use of a thionamide during the week before and after radioiodine therapy may impair the response to radiation (Velkeniers B, Cytryn R, Vanhaelst L, Jonckheer M H 1988 Treatment of hyperthyroidism with radioiodine: adjunctive therapy with antithyroid drugs reconsidered. Lancet i:1127–1129) (see Mode of action of thionamides, above).

control is essential, and the thyroid test should be monitored monthly. Surgery in the second trimester may be preferred to continued drug therapy. Ideally, patients should be rendered euthyroid prior to pregnancy.

Both PTU and carbimazole are considered safe in nursing mothers, but because of the risk of hepatotoxicity carbimazole is preferred.

Control of antithyroid drug therapy

The aim of drug therapy is to control the hyperthyroidism until a natural remission takes place. The recommended duration of therapy is 12–18 months. Longer treatment is usual for young patients with large, vascular goitres, because of the higher risk of recurrence (2–3 years). A shorter course (6–9 months) is recommended for the block–replace regimen. Most patients enter remission, but some will relapse – usually during the first 3 months after withdrawal from treatment. Approximately 30–40% of patients remain euthyroid 10 years later. If hyperthyroidism recurs, there is little chance of a second course of thionamide achieving long-term remission. In such patients, indefinite low-dose antithyroid treatment is an alternative option to radioiodine or surgery.

The use of levothyroxine concurrently with an antithyroid drug ('block and replace regimen') facilitates maintenance of a euthyroid state and reduces the frequency of clinic visits. There is a higher risk of the dose-related adverse effects of carbimazole, and no compensatory reduction in the incidence of relapse. Therefore, the 'titration' (see above) regimen is regarded as first-line treatment.

β-**Adrenergic blockade.** There is increased tissue sensitivity to catecholamines in hyperthyroidism with a rise in either the number of β-adrenoceptors or the second-messenger response (i.e. intracellular cyclic AMP synthesis) to their stimulation. Therefore, some of the unpleasant symptoms are adrenergic.

Quick relief can be obtained with a β-adrenoceptor blocker (judge the dose by heart rate), although these do not block all the metabolic effects of the hormone, e.g. on the myocardium, and the basal metabolic rate is unchanged. For this reason, β-blockade is not used as sole therapy except in mild thyrotoxicosis in preparation for radioiodine treatment, and in these patients it should be continued until the radioiodine has taken effect. β blockers do not alter the course of the disease, or affect biochemical tests of thyroid function. Any effect on thyroid hormonal action on peripheral tissues is clinically unimportant. Although atenolol is widely used, it is preferable to choose a drug that is *non-selective* for $β_1$ and $β_2$ receptors and *lacks partial agonist effect* (e.g. propranolol 20–80 mg 6–8-hourly, or timolol 5 mg once daily, atenolol 25–50 mg twice daily). The usual contraindications to β-blockade (see p. 423) apply, especially asthma.

Iodine (iodide and radioactive iodine)

Iodide is well absorbed from the intestine, distributed like chloride in the body, and rapidly excreted by the kidney. It is selectively taken up and concentrated (about ×25) by the thyroid gland, more in hyperthyroidism and less in hypothyroidism. A deficiency of iodide reduces the amount of thyroid hormone produced; this stimulates the pituitary to secrete TSH. The result is hyperplasia and increased vascularity of the gland, with eventual goitre formation.[4]

Effects

The effects of iodide are complex and related to the dose and thyroid status of the subject. In hyperthyroid subjects, a moderate excess of iodide may enhance hormone production by providing 'fuel' for hormone synthesis. But a substantial excess inhibits hormone release and promotes storage of hormone and involution of the gland, making it firmer and less vascular so that surgery is easier. The effect is transient and its mechanism uncertain.

In euthyroid subjects with normal glands, an excess of iodide from any source can cause goitre (with or without hyperthyroidism), e.g. use of iodide-containing cough medicines, iodine-containing radiocontrast media, amiodarone, seaweed eaters.

A euthyroid subject with an autonomous adenoma (hot nodule) becomes hyperthyroid if given iodide.

Uses

Iodide (large dose) is used for thyroid storm (crisis) and in preparation for thyroidectomy because it rapidly benefits the patient by reducing hormone release and renders surgery easier and safer (above).

Potassium iodate in doses of 85 mg orally 8-hourly (longer intervals allow some escape from the iodide effect) produces some effect in 1–2 days, maximal after 10–14 days, after which the benefit declines as the thyroid adapts. A similar dose used for 3 days covers administration of some [131]I- or ^{123}I-containing preparations, for instance meta-iodobenzylguanidine (^{123}I-MIBG) (see p. 432).

---

[4]Apparently from the beginning of time: Michelangelo's image of the separation of light from darkness on the ceiling of the Sistine Chapel in the Vatican depicts the creator with a multinodular goitre (Bondeson L, Bondeson A-G 2003 Michelangelo's divine goitre. Journal of the Royal Society of Medicine 96:609–611).

Iodine therapy maximises iodide stores in the thyroid, which delays response to thionamides. Prophylactic iodide (1 part in 100 000) may be added to the salt, water or bread where goitre is endemic.

In economically deprived communities, a method of prophylaxis is to inject iodised oil intramuscularly every 3–5 years; given early to women, this prevents endemic cretinism but occasional hyperthyroidism occurs (see autonomous adenoma, above).

As an antiseptic for use on the skin, povidone–iodine (a complex of iodine with a sustained-release carrier, povidone or polyvinyl–pyrrolidone) can be applied repeatedly and used as a surgical scrub.

Bronchial secretions. Iodide is concentrated in bronchial and salivary secretions. It acts as an expectorant (see Cough, p. 494).

Organic compounds containing iodine are used as contrast media in radioimaging. It is essential to ask patients specifically whether they are allergic to iodine before such contrast media are used. Severe anaphylaxis, even deaths, occur every year in busy imaging departments; iodine-containing contrast media are being superseded by so-called 'non-ionic' preparations.[5]

Adverse reactions

Patients vary enormously in their tolerance of iodine; some are intolerant or allergic to it both orally and when it is applied to the skin.

Symptoms of iodism include: a metallic taste, excessive salivation with painful salivary glands, running eyes and nose, sore mouth and throat, a productive cough, diarrhoea, and various rashes that may mimic chickenpox. A saline diuresis enhances elimination.

Goitre can occur (see above) with prolonged use of iodide-containing expectorant by bronchitics and asthmatics. Such therapy should therefore be intermittent, if it is used at all.

Topical application of iodine-containing antiseptics to neonates has caused hypothyroidism. Iodide intake above that in a normal diet will depress thyroid uptake of administered radioiodine, because the two forms will compete.

In the case of diet, medication, and water-soluble radio-diagnostic agents, interference with thyroid function will cease 2–4 weeks after stopping the source, but with agents used for cholecystography it may last for 6 months or more (because of tissue binding).

Radioiodine (^{131}I)

^{131}I is treated by the body just like the ordinary non-radioactive isotope, so that when swallowed it is concentrated in the thyroid gland. It emits mainly β radiation (90%), which penetrates only 0.5 mm of tissue and thus allows therapeutic effects on the thyroid without damage to the surrounding structures, particularly the parathyroids. It also emits some γ-rays, which are more penetrating and are detectable with a radiation counter.[6] ^{131}I has a physical (radioactive) $t_{1/2}$ of 8 days.

^{131}I is the preferred initial treatment for hyperthyroidism caused by Graves' disease in North America. It is contra-indicated in pregnant or breast-feeding women, and in children younger than 10 years of age. It can induce or worsen ophthalmopathy. It is used in combination with surgery in thyroid carcinoma.

In hyperthyroidism, the beneficial effects of a single dose may be felt in 1 month, and patients should be reviewed at 5–6 weeks to monitor for onset of hypothyroidism. The maximal effect of radioiodine may take 3 months to achieve. β-Adrenoceptor blockade and, in severe cases, an antithyroid drug (but see footnote 1) will be needed to render the patient comfortable while waiting; this is more likely when radioiodine is used for patients with relapsing thyrotoxicosis. Very rarely radiation thyroiditis causes excessive release of hormone and thyroid storm. Repeated doses may be needed.

Adverse effects of radioiodine are as for iodism, above. In the event of inadvertent overdose, large doses of sodium or potassium iodate should be given to compete with the radioiodine for thyroid uptake and to hasten excretion by increasing iodide turnover (increased fluid intake and a diuretic are adjuvants).

Radioiodine offers the advantages that treatment is simple and carries no immediate mortality, but it is slow in acting and the dose that will render the patient euthyroid is difficult to judge. In the first year after treatment, 20% of patients will become hypothyroid. Thereafter, 5% of patients become hypothyroid annually, perhaps because the capacity of thyroid cells to divide is permanently abolished so that cell renewal ceases. There is therefore an obligation to monitor patients indefinitely after radioiodine treatment, for most are likely to need treatment for hypothyroidism eventually.

Risks

Experience had eliminated the fear that radioiodine causes carcinoma of the thyroid, and led to its use in patients of

---

[5]The newer preparations approximately triple the cost of diagnostic investigations requiring contrast media. With a fatality rate of about 1 per 50 000 in patients receiving the older agents, hospitals are faced with an interesting cost–benefit equation.

[6]And emissions can be sufficient to activate airport radiation alarms. One victim was detained, strip-searched and interrogated, but released on producing his radionucleotide card (Gangopadhyay K K, Sundram F, De P 2006 Triggering radiation alarms after radioiodine treatment. British Medical Journal 333:293–294).

all ages. The Chernobyl disaster subsequently revived concern about exposure of children, and it would be wise again to restrict radioiodine treatment as far as possible to adults. Pregnant women should not be treated with radioiodine (^{131}I) because it crosses the placenta.

There is a theoretical risk of teratogenic effects, and women are advised to avoid pregnancy for an arbitrary 6–12 months after treatment.

Treatment of thyroid carcinoma requires larger doses of radioiodine than are used for hyperthyroidism, and there is an increased incidence of late leukaemia in these patients. The management of thyroid carcinoma is highly specialised, and extends beyond the scope of this textbook.

Radioisotope tests

Radioiodine uptake can be used to test thyroid function, although it has now been superseded by technetium-99m. Scanning the gland may be useful to identify solitary nodules and in the differential diagnosis of Graves' disease from the less common thyroiditides, e.g. de Quervain's thyroiditis. In thyroiditis, excessive thyroid hormone release caused by follicular cell damage can cause clinical and biochemical features of thyrotoxicosis, but radionuclide uptake is reduced.

Choice of treatment of hyperthyroidism

- Antithyroid drugs.
- Radioiodine.
- Surgery.

  Antithyroid drugs are generally preferred provided the goitre is small and diffuse. They may be used in pregnancy.

  Radioiodine is an alternative first-line treatment for adult patients, but not in pregnancy. It may be preferred to antithyroid drugs in patients with large or multinodular goitres, and in patients with a single hyperfunctioning adenoma ('hot nodule'). Preparation with antithyroid drugs is recommended in severe thyrotoxicosis.

  Surgery is generally a second choice for thyrotoxicosis. It may be indicated if the thyroid contains a nodule of uncertain nature, or in patients with large, multinodular goitre causing tracheal compression.

Preparation for surgery

Routine preparation of hyperthyroid patients for surgery can be achieved satisfactorily by making them euthyroid with one of the above drugs plus a β-adrenoceptor blocker for comfort (see below) and safety,[7] and adding iodate for 7–10 days before operation (not sooner) to reduce the surgically inconvenient vascularity of the gland.

In an emergency, the patient is prepared with a β-adrenoceptor blocker (e.g. propranolol 6-hourly, with dose titration to eliminate tachycardia) for 4 days, continued through the operation and for 7–10 days afterwards. Iodide is also given (see p. 629). The important differences with this second technique are that the gland is smaller and less friable but the patient's tissues are still hyperthyroid, and, to avoid a hyperthyroid crisis or storm, it is essential that the adrenoceptor blocker continue as above without the omission of even a single 6-hourly dose of propranolol.

Thyroid storm

Thyroid crisis, or storm, is a life-threatening emergency owing to the liberation of large amounts of hormone into the circulation. Surgical storm is rare with modern methods of preparing hyperthyroid patients for surgery. Medical thyroid storm may occur in patients who are untreated or incompletely treated. It may be precipitated by infection, trauma, surgical emergencies or operations, radiation thyroiditis, toxaemia of pregnancy or parturition.

Treatment is urgently required to save life. Propranolol should be given immediately, 60–80 mg orally every 6 h or i.v. slowly, initially 0.5–1 mg over 10 min with continuous cardiac rhythm monitoring; the i.v. dose may be repeated every few hours until the oral dose takes effect. Large doses of an antithyroid agent, preferably propylthiouracil 300–400 mg 4-hourly are required, down a nasogastric tube or per rectum. Thereafter, iodide is used to inhibit further hormone release from the gland (potassium iodide/iodate 600 mg to 1 g orally in the first 24 h) (see above). Lithium carbonate may be used, particularly in cases of iodide allergy. Large doses of adrenocorticoids, e.g. dexamethasone 4 mg 6-hourly, are given to inhibit both release of thyroid hormone from the gland and peripheral conversion of T_4 to T_3. Hyperthermia may be treated by cooling and aspirin; heart failure in the ordinary way; fluid deficit by a combination of normal saline and 5% dextrose.

Graves' ophthalmopathy

Graves' ophthalmopathy is characterized by inflammation of periorbital and retroorbital connective tissue, fat and

---

[7]No patient should be operated on with a resting pulse of 90 beats/min or above, and no dose of β-adrenoceptor blocker, including the important post-operative dose, should be omitted (Toft A D, Irvine W J, Sinclair I et al 1978 Thyroid function after surgical treatment of thyrotoxicosis. A report of 100 cases treated with propranolol before operation. New England Journal of Medicine 298:643–647).

muscle. It is associated with Graves' thyrotoxicosis; it may also occur in patients with euthyroid or hypothyroid chronic autoimmune thyroiditis.

It is an autoimmune disease which appears now to be due in part to the expression of the TSH receptor on orbital cells such as preadipocytes and fibroblasts and probably myocytes.

Antithyroid drugs do not help directly. Nevertheless, it is important that any thyroid dysfunction is treated meticulously, and the TSH concentration held within the low-normal range. Mild to moderate cases regress spontaneously. Artificial tears (hypromellose) are useful when natural tears and blinking are inadequate to maintain corneal lubrication. In severe cases, high doses of systemic prednisolone, alone or in combination with another immunosuppressive (azathioprine), may help. A course of low-dose orbital radiation achieves rapid regression of ophthalmopathy, and may avoid the need for prolonged immunosuppressive therapy. In severe cases with optic neuropathy, decompressive surgery is indicated to relieve pressure of the optic nerve.

Treatment of subclinical hyperthyroidism

Subclinical hyperthyroidism is defined biochemically by normal serum free T_4 and free T_3 but suppressed TSH concentrations. Some 5% of patients per annum progress to frank hyperthyroidism, and there is an increased risk of atrial fibrillation, thromboembolic stroke and osteoporosis. The treatment of endogenous subclinical hyperthyroidism should be considered when the TSH level is less than 0.1 mU/L, especially in patients older than 60 years of age, those with an increased risk for heart disease, osteopenia or osteoporosis, or with clinical symptoms suggestive of hyperthyroidism. Other patients should be monitored 6-monthly; eventually 50% become euthyroid.[8]

Drugs that cause hypothyroidism

In addition to drugs used for their antithyroid effects, the following substances can cause hypothyroidism: lithium (for mania, bipolar disorder, recurrent depression), amiodarone (see below), β-interferon (hepatitis and multiple sclerosis), iodide (see above), resorcinol (leg ulcers), tyrosine kinase inhibitors, thalidomide, antiepileptic drugs and

second-line drugs for multidrug-resistant TB. Effects may be reversible on withdrawal.

Drugs causing either hyper- or hypothyroidism

Amiodarone bears a significant structural resemblance to thyroxine. Each molecule of amiodarone contains two iodine atoms, constituting 37.5% of its mass. Hence, a patient taking a 200-mg/day dose ingests 75 mg of organic iodine each day. Subsequent de-iodination through drug metabolism results in the daily release of approximately 6 mg free iodine into the circulation, which is 20 to 40 times higher than usual daily iodine intake of 0.15–0.30 mg. Amiodarone has a very long $t_{1/2}$ (54 days) on chronic dosing, mainly due to its storage in adipose tissue. Hence, the excess iodine clears slowly over months, and the toxic effects of amiodarone can persist or can even occur well after its discontinuation.

Some 90% of patients receiving amiodarone remain euthyroid. Despite the exposure of the thyroid gland to an extraordinary load of iodine, important adjustments are made in thyroidal iodine handling and hormone metabolism; these are shown in Fig. 37.2, and the consequences for thyroid function tests are summarised in Table 37.1.

Amiodarone-induced *hypothyroidism* is more prevalent in iodine-sufficient areas of the world, whereas *thyrotoxicosis* is more prevalent in iodine-deficient regions. Amiodarone-induced hypothyroidism typically occurs between 6 and 12 months of treatment with amiodarone. The main risk factor is underlying Hashimoto's disease. In other patients, hypothyroidism resolves within 2–4 months of discontinuing amiodarone.

Thyrotoxicosis induced by amiodarone is of two types. Type 1 develops in individuals with underlying thyroid disease (nodular goitre or latent Graves' disease) and is due to increased synthesis and release of thyroid hormone. Type 2 is a destructive thyroiditis in individuals with no underlying thyroid disease, and the thyrotoxicosis is due to release of preformed thyroid hormone from damaged thyroid follicular epithelium. Mixed forms also occur. The two types are difficult to distinguish. Measurement of interleukin-6 or C-reactive protein has a marginal diagnostic role in differentiating the two forms because of poor specificity. Thyroid ultrasonography, colour flow Doppler sonography and thyroid radioactive iodine uptake may help in the diagnosis. In type 1, amiodarone treatment should be discontinued, if possible. Large doses of thionamides and longer periods of therapy are required, because high intrathyroidal iodine stores antagonise their inhibitory effect on thyroidal iodine utilisation. In patients who fail to respond after 4–6 weeks of treatment, potassium perchlorate 200–1000 mg/day can be

[8]Consensus statement: Surks M I, Ortiz E, Daniels G H et al 2004 Subclinical thyroid disease: scientific review and guidelines for diagnosis and management. Journal of the American Medical Association 291:228–238.

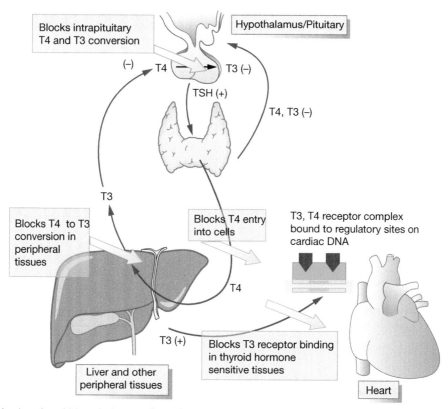

Fig. 37.2 Mechanisms by which amiodarone affects thyroid hormone metabolism. TSH, thyroid stimulating hormone. *(Adapted from Basaria S, Cooper D S 2005 Amiodarone and the thyroid. American Journal of Medicine 118:706–714.)*

Table 37.1 Effects of amiodarone on thyroid function tests in euthyroid subjects

Thyroid hormone	Acute effects (≤3 months)	Chronic effects (>3 months)
Total and free T_4	↑ 50%	Remains ↑ 20–40% of baseline
T_3	↓ 15–20%, remains in low-normal range	Remains ↓ 20%, remains in low-normal range
Reverse T_3	↑ >200%	Remains ↑ >150%
TSH	↑ 20–50%, transient, generally remains <20 mU/L	Normal

a useful adjunct. Radioiodine is rarely used because uptake is blocked by the high concentration of circulating iodine. In type 2, prednisolone 40–60 mg leads to rapid improvement in thyroid function in most patients, often within 1 week, and amiodarone discontinuation may not be necessary. Iopanoic acid (an oral cholecystographic agent) has also been used to reduce T_4 to T_3 conversion, but is generally inferior to prednisolone and currently unavailable in the market. In resistant cases, other therapies have been recommended, including lithium, plasmapheresis and ultimately thyroidectomy in patients with severe thyrotoxicosis, whose amiodarone cannot be discontinued.

Biological therapies

The advent of humanised monoclonal antibodies has led to a new cause of thyrotoxicosis, first recognised during use of alemtuzamab (anti-CD56) for multiple sclerosis. At least one-third of patients will develop biochemical abnormalities, some with thyroid antibodies and full-blown Graves' disease. Although these can be self-remitting, monitoring is recommended in all patients, for up to 4 years after cessation of alemtuzamab. More recently, hyper- and hypothyroidism have been the commonest of auto-immune endocrinopathies to be recognised in around 15% of patients during use of immune checkpoint inhibitors for treatment of cancer, particularly melanoma. These inhibitors are monoclonal antibodies such as pembrolizumab, nivolumab, and ipilumab, which target PD1 or CTLA4 on activated T cells. The role of these checkpoint molecules is to maintain tolerance of autoantigens, and so the development of auto-immunity, while unwelcome, is not entirely unexpected.

Miscellaneous

Treatment of thyroiditis (Hashimoto's thyroiditis, subacute thyroiditis or de Quervain's thyroiditis). Where hyperthyroidism is a feature, treatment is by a β-adrenoceptor blocker. Antithyroid drugs should not be used. Where there is permanent hypothyroidism, the treatment is thyroid hormone replacement.

Calcitonin. See Chapter 39.

Summary

- Autoimmune disease of the thyroid can cause over- or under-production of thyroid hormone.
- Hypothyroidism is readily treated with levothyroxine 50–200 μg/day orally, continued indefinitely.
- The treatment of hyperthyroidism due to Graves' disease is either 12–18 months' treatment with carbimazole or propylthiouracil, or a (usually) single dose of ^{131}I.
- The natural history of Graves' disease is of alternating remission and relapse. Progression to hypothyroidism can occur, especially after ^{131}I treatment. All patients require long-term follow-up.
- Severe forms of thyroid eye disease require adrenal steroid and immunosuppressants, or low-dose radiotherapy. Urgent surgical decompression is required for optic nerve compression.

Guide to further reading

Bahn, R.S., 2010. Graves' ophthalmopathy. N. Engl. J. Med. 362, 726–738.

Basaria, S., Cooper, D.S., 2005. Amiodarone and the thyroid. Am. J. Med. 118, 706–714.

Byun, D.J., Wolchok, J.D., Rosenberg, L.M., Girotra, M., 2017. Cancer immunotherapy—immune checkpoint blockade and associated endocrinopathies. Nat. Rev. Endocrinol. 13, 195–207.

Chaker, L., Bianco, A.C., Jonklaas, J., Peeters, R.P., 2017. Hypothyroidism. Lancet 390, 1550–1562.

Cooper, D.S., 2005. Antithyroid drugs. N. Engl. J. Med. 352, 905–917.

Cooper, D.S., Laurberg, P., 2013. Hyperthyroidism in pregnancy. Lancet Diabetes Endocrinol. 1, 238–249.

De Leo, S., Lee, S.Y., Braverman, L.E., 2016. Hyperthyroidism. Lancet 388, 906–918.

Mitchell, A.L., Pearce, S.H., 2010. How should we treat patients with low serum thyrotropin concentrations? Clin. Endocrinol. (Oxf) 72, 292–296.

Pearce, E.N., Farwell, A.P., Bravermen, L.E., et al., 2003. Thyroiditis. N. Engl. J. Med. 348, 2646–2655.

Roberts, C.G.P., Ladenson, P.W., 2004. Hypothyroidism. Lancet 363, 793–803.

Ross, D.S., 2011. Radioiodine therapy for hyperthyroidism. N. Engl. J. Med. 364, 542–550.

Teng, W., Shan, Z., Patil-Sisodia, K., Cooper, D.S., 2013. Hypothyroidism in pregnancy. Lancet Diabetes Endocrinol. 1, 228–237.

Wiersinga, W.M., 2017. Advances in treatment of active, moderate-to-severe Graves' ophthalmopathy. Lancet Diabetes Endocrinol. 5, 134–142.

Chapter | **38** |

Hypothalamic, pituitary and sex hormones

Karim Meeran

SYNOPSIS

- Many of the pituitary hormones and their hypothalamic-releasing factors are used in diagnosis or therapy.
- The main therapeutic use of pituitary hormones is of growth hormone (anterior pituitary) and those from the posterior pituitary: oxytocin and vasopressin.
- Vasopressin (antidiuretic hormone) is used both for its vasoconstrictor effect (in the treatment of oesophageal varices) and for its antidiuretic action.
- Pituitary failure causes deficiency of cortisol, thyroxine as well as sex steroids and growth hormone.
- Replacement therapy for cortisol deficiency can be either hydrocortisone three times daily, or prednisolone once daily. Recent evidence suggests that the doses of hydrocortisone and prednisolone used for replacement have been too great, and smaller doses should be used.
- Suppression of oestrogen and/or androgen production is used in the treatment of tumours stimulated by these: breast and prostate.
- Therapy in women is used to suppress ovulation (contraceptives), to stimulate ovulation (fertility treatment) or to mimic ovarian endocrine function (post-menopausal hormone replacement therapy, HRT).

Fig. 38.1 shows the hypothalamic–pituitary axes. The hypothalamus and pituitary glands form the centre of the 'endocrine orchestra'. We will here describe the hypothalamic-releasing hormones, and the anterior and posterior pituitary gland hormones, and drugs that are used to manipulate these axes.

These hormones, analogues (agonists) and antagonists can be used:

- to analyse the functional integrity of endocrine control systems
- as replacement in hormone deficiency states
- to modify malfunction of endocrine systems
- to alter normal function where this is inconvenient, e.g. contraception.

The scope of the specialist endocrinologist continues to increase in amount and in complexity, and only an outline is appropriate here.

Hypothalamic and anterior pituitary hormones

The hypothalamus releases a number of locally active hormones that stimulate or inhibit pituitary hormone release (see Fig. 38.1).

The $t_{1/2}$ of the polypeptide and glycoprotein hormones listed below is 5–30 min; they are digested if swallowed.

Corticotropin-releasing hormone (CRH) is a hypothalamic polypeptide that has diagnostic use. It increases secretion of adrenocorticotropic hormone (ACTH) in Cushing's disease secondary to pituitary ACTH-secreting adenoma. It is also used to stimulate ACTH secretion during bilateral inferior petrosal sinus sampling, a procedure carried out in specialist centres to determine the cause of Cushing's syndrome. It has no therapeutic use.

Adrenocorticotrophic hormone (ACTH) (Corticotropin) is used in the short Synacthen tests to make a diagnosis of Addison's disease. The standard test uses 250 µg either i.v. or i.m. For the long Synacthen test, 1 mg of depot synacthen is used.

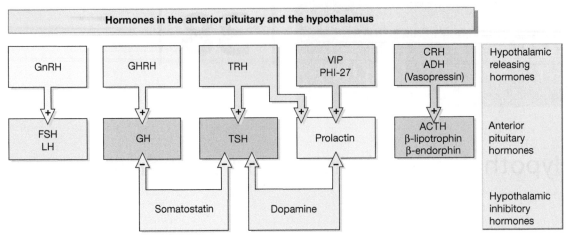

Fig. 38.1 Hormones produced in the anterior pituitary and the hypothalamic hormones that regulate their secretion. ACTH, adrenocorticotrophic hormone; ADH, antidiuretic hormone; CRH, corticotropin-releasing hormone; FSH, follicle-stimulating hormone; GH, growth hormone; GHRH, growth hormone–releasing hormone; GnRH, gonadotrophin-releasing hormone; TRH, thyrotrophin-releasing hormone; TSH, thyroid-stimulating hormone; VIP, vasoactive intestinal peptide.

Thyrotrophin-releasing hormone (TRH) is a tripeptide amide formed in the hypothalamus and controlled by free plasma T_4 and T_3 concentration. It has been synthesised and has been used in the past to test the capacity of the pituitary to release thyroid-stimulating hormone (TSH), to determine whether hypothyroidism is due to primary thyroid gland failure or secondary to pituitary hypothalamic lesion, and in the differential diagnosis of borderline or subclinical thyrotoxicosis. Current sensitive assays for TSH make this role redundant. The TRH test is still used to differentiate between TSHomas (TSH-producing tumours, where the response to TRH is flat) and thyroid hormone resistance (where there is an exuberant response to TRH). It is also a potent prolactin-releasing factor and can thereby be useful in detecting normal pituitary function.

Thyroid-stimulating hormone (TSH) thyrotrophin, a glycoprotein of the anterior pituitary, controls the synthesis and release of thyroid hormone from the gland, and also the uptake of iodide. There is a negative feedback of thyroid hormones on both the hypothalamic secretion of TRH and pituitary secretion of TSH.

Recombinant TSH is now used in the treatment of thyroid cancer. A dose of TSH is administered just before a tracer dose of radioiodine in such patients. A high level of TSH is required to stimulate uptake of radioiodine into any TSH responsive tissue. This was previously achieved by stopping thyroxine replacement, and rendering the patient profoundly hypothyroid for several weeks, causing high levels of endogenous TSH. This unpleasant treatment is no longer required with the advent of recombinant TSH.

Sermorelin is an analogue of the hypothalamic growth hormone–releasing hormone (somatorelin); it is used in a diagnostic test for growth hormone secretion from the pituitary.

Growth hormone release–inhibiting hormone, somatostatin, occurs in other parts of the brain as well as in the hypothalamus, and also in some peripheral tissues, e.g. pancreas, stomach. In addition to the action implied by its name, it inhibits secretion of thyrotrophin, insulin, gastrin and serotonin. *Somatostatin* is a 14–amino acid hypothalamic peptide. It inhibits growth hormone secretion.

Octreotide is a synthetic analogue of somatostatin having a longer action ($t_{1/2}$ 1.5 h). It is administered subcutaneously two or three times daily; a depot formulation is available for deep intramuscular injection once a month. *Lanreotide* is much longer acting than octreotide, and is administered intramuscularly twice a month. Uses of the somatostatin analogues include acromegaly, carcinoid (serotonin-secreting) tumours and other rare tumours of the alimentary tract. An unlicensed use of octeotride is the termination of variceal bleeding (see p. 583). Radiolabelled somatostatin is used to localise, and in higher doses to treat, metastases from neuroendocrine tumours which often bear somatostatin receptors. Both octreotide and lanreotide are now available as a monthly slow-release preparation.

Growth hormone, somatrophin (Genotropin, Humatrope) is a biosynthetic form (191 amino acids) of growth hormone prepared by recombinant DNA technology, as is somatrem. Naturally occurring human growth hormone was extracted from cadaver pituitaries, and its supply was therefore limited. In 1985 the use of natural growth hormone was terminated because of the risk of transmitting Creutzfeldt–Jacob disease, the fatal prion infection. Growth hormone acts on many organs to produce a peptide insulin-like growth factor IGF-1 (somatomedin), which causes muscle, bone and other tissues to increase growth, i.e. protein synthesis, and the size and number of cells.

Growth hormone is approved for treatment of children with short stature due not just to growth hormone deficiency, but also to Turner's syndrome, renal failure, small size for gestational age, Prader–Willi syndrome[1] and, most recently, idiopathic short stature. Treatment is continued until closure of the epiphyses. Subsequent treatment into adulthood is also warranted where UK National Institute for Health and Clinical Excellence (NICE) guidelines are fullfilled. Growth hormone therapy should be confined to specialist clinics.

The use of growth hormone in adults varies among different countries. In the UK, treatment is limited to growth hormone–deficient patients with severely impaired quality of life. Treatment improves exercise performance, increases lean body mass and improves overall quality of life. A low starting dose of 0.27 mg s.c. daily is used and is adjusted at 4–6-week intervals according to clinical response and IGF-1 levels. NICE recommends that treatment be discontinued in patients when quality of life improves by fewer than seven points on the Adult Growth Hormone Deficiency Assessment (AGHDA) scale.

Adverse effects include increases in weight, blood pressure and blood glucose and lipid levels. These should be monitored together with plasma haemoglobin A1c (HbA1c).

In *acromegaly*, excess growth hormone causes diabetes, hypertension and arthritis. The former two lead to a two-fold excess in cardiovascular mortality. Surgery is the treatment of choice. Growth hormone secretion is reduced by octreotide, lanreotide and other somatostatin analogues, and to a lesser degree by bromocriptine and cabergoline. If surgery fails (nadir growth hormone during oral glucose tolerance test >1 microgram/L), somatostatin analogues should be used. These bind to somatostatin receptors 2 and 5 to inhibit growth hormone production. About 60% of patients respond to somatostatin analogues.

Pegvisomant is a growth receptor antagonist. It binds to the receptor and prevents activation and production of IGF-1. As a result, growth hormone increases with pegvisomant treatment, which is a specialist indication for the treatment of acromegaly in patients with inadequate response to pituitary surgery or radiation, and to somatostatin analogues.

Gonadotrophin-releasing hormone (GnRH), gonadorelin, releases luteinising hormone (LH) and follicle-stimulating hormone (FSH). It has a use in the assessment of pituitary function. In hypogonadotrophic hypogonadal men, GnRH may be used to induce spermatogenesis and fertility. Pulsatile subcutaneous GnRH administration via a catheter attached to a mini-pump evokes secretion of gonadotrophins (LH and FSH) and is used to treat infertility. But continuous use evokes tachyphylaxis owing to down-regulation of its receptors, i.e. gonadotrophin release and therefore gonadal secretions are reduced.

Longer-acting analogues, e.g. *buserelin, goserelin, nafarelin, deslorelin* and *leuprorelin*, are used to suppress androgen secretion in prostatic carcinoma. Other uses may include endometriosis, precocious puberty and contraception.

Cetrorelix and *ganirelix* are LH-releasing hormone antagonists, which inhibit the release of gonadotrophins. They are used in the treatment of infertility by assisted reproductive techniques.

All of these drugs need to be administered by a parenteral route. Their use should generally be in the hands of a specialist endocrinologist, oncologist or gynaecologist.

Follicle-stimulating hormone (FSH) stimulates development of ova and of spermatozoa. It is prepared from the urine of post-menopausal women; *menotrophin* also contains a small amount of LH, and *urofollitrophin* is FSH alone. They are used in female and male hypothalamic hypophyseal infertility as an alternative to GnRH treatment. Pulsatile GnRH is more likely to result in development and ovulation of a single follicle than FSH. Recombinant FSH subunits (follitrophin α or β) are available for in vitro fertilisation.

Chorionic gonadotrophin (human chorionic gonadotrophin, HCG) is secreted by the placenta and is obtained from the urine of pregnant women. Its predominant action is that of LH, which induces progesterone production by the corpus luteum in women, and in the male it is involved in spermatogenesis and gonadal testosterone production. It is also used to trigger ovulation in induction protocols, for corpus luteum support. In males, HCG is used in diagnostic tests of ambiguous genitalia; if HCG fails to induce testicular descent in pre-pubertal males, there is time for surgery to achieve a fully functioning testis. In older boys, HCG may be used to induce puberty when this is delayed.

Prolactin is secreted by the lactotroph cells of the anterior pituitary gland. Its control is by tonic hypothalamic inhibition through dopamine, which in turn acts on D_2 receptors of the lactotrophs. Its main physiological function is stimulation of lactation. Supra-physiological levels of prolactin inhibit gonadotrophin-releasing hormone and gonadotrophin release as well as gonadal steroidogenesis.

Hyperprolactinaemia may be caused by drugs with anti-dopaminergic actions: antiemetics, major tranquillisers,

---

[1]An inherited condition that gives rise to obesity, decreased muscle tone, poor large muscle strength, decreased mental capacity, and sex glands that produce few or no hormones.

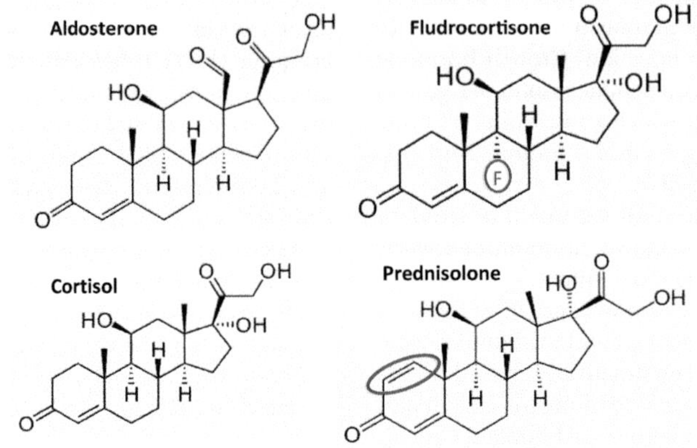

Fig. 38.2 Structure of aldosterone, fludrocortisone, cortisol, and prednisolone. The changes that give a longer $t_{1/2}$ are shown in red. A fluorine atom is present in fludrocortisone, and a double bond in prednisolone are the only differences between these molecules and cortisol.

second-generation neuroleptics, monoamine oxidase (MAO) inhibitors, tricyclic antidepressants and, to a lesser extent, oestrogens.

Hyperprolactinaemia may occur in primary hypothyroidism, in pituitary stalk disconnection or prolactin-secreting adenomas. Medical treatment is with *bromocriptine* started at 0.625 mg by mouth nightly, and titrated weekly to a maximum of 20 mg in divided doses. *Cabergoline* may be preferred as a more specific dopamine agonist than bromocriptine, which is taken once weekly, titrated from 500 μg to 2 mg. Higher doses (up to 6 mg weekly) are necessary only in the treatment of macroprolactinomas. Quinagolide is another dopamine agonist; the dose is 25–150 μg at bedtime.

In pregnancy, the dopamine agonists are discontinued in microadenomas, where the risk of enlargement is small. Treatment should continue for macroadenomas because the risk of enlargement is much higher, 15–30%. Both bromocriptine and cabergoline are safe to use, although cabergoline is not licensed in pregnancy. Much higher doses of cabergoline (e.g. 4 mg daily or 28 mg weekly) have been associated with cardiac fibrosis, although this has not been reported in many groups of prolactinoma patients. Nevertheless, the UK regulatory agency (MHRA) advises cardiac valve monitoring for patients on any dose of cabergoline.

Trans-sphenoidal surgery in a specialist unit is an alternative to medical therapy in patients who do not tolerate, or are resistant to, dopamine agonists.

Hypopituitarism

In hypopituitarism there is a partial or complete deficiency of hormones secreted by the anterior and posterior lobe of

the pituitary, although the latter is less common. Patients suffering from severe hypopituitarism may present in coma, in which case treatment is as for severe acute adrenal insufficiency. Maintenance therapy is required, using hydrocortisone, thyroxine, estradiol and progesterone (in women) and testosterone (in men), growth hormone and desmopressin, where indicated. Steroid replacement is the most important of these, and low-dose prednisolone has recently been shown to be the most appropriate once-daily replacement for cortisol deficiency. A daily dose of prednisolone 3 mg on waking suits most patients, although plasma levels are used in some centres to verify appropriate replacement. In the past, higher doses were used, because of a fear of an Addisonian crisis, but it is now recognized that over-replacement is also harmful. Unlike pituitary failure, patients with adrenal failure also lose aldosterone. This is replaced with once-daily fludrocortisone (50–100 μg). Fludrocortisone is used rather than native aldosterone because the fluorine atom gives it a longer $t_{1/2}$, enabling once-daily administration. Similarly, the double bond between C1 and C2 gives prednisolone a much longer $t_{1/2}$ than hydrocortisone, enabling once-daily administration (Fig. 38.2).

Posterior pituitary hormones and analogues

Vasopressin: antidiuretic hormone (ADH)

Vasopressin is a nonapeptide ($t_{1/2}$ 20 min) with two separate G-protein–coupled target receptors responsible for its two roles. The V_1 receptor on vascular smooth muscle cells is coupled to calcium-ion entry and is not usually stimulated by physiological concentrations of the hormone. The V_2 receptor is coupled to adenylyl cyclase, and regulates opening of the water channel, aquaporin, in cells of the renal collecting duct.

Secretion of the antidiuretic hormone is stimulated by any increase in the osmotic pressure of the blood supplying the hypothalamus and by a variety of drugs, notably nicotine. Secretion is inhibited by a fall in blood osmotic pressure and by alcohol.

In large non-physiological doses *(pharmacotherapy)*, vasopressin causes contraction of all smooth muscle, raising the blood pressure and causing intestinal colic. The smooth muscle stimulant effect provides an example of tachyphylaxis (frequently repeated doses give progressively less effect). It is not only inefficient when used to raise the blood pressure, but also dangerous, as it causes constriction of the coronary arteries and sudden death has occurred following its use.

For replacement therapy of pituitary diabetes insipidus, the longer-acting analogue desmopressin is used.

Desmopressin

Desmopressin (des-amino-D-arginine vasopressin, DDAVP) has two major advantages: the vasoconstrictor effect has been reduced to near insignificance, and the duration of action with nasal instillation, spray or subcutaneous injection is 8–20 h ($t_{1/2}$ 75 min), so that patients using it once to twice daily are not inconvenienced by polyuria and nocturia.

Desmopressin is available as oral or sublingual tablets, nasal spray and injection. The adult dose for intranasal administration is 10–20 µg daily. The dose for children is about one-half that for adults. The bioavailability of intranasal DDAVP is 10%. It is also the only peptide for which an oral formulation is currently available, albeit with a bioavailability of only 1%. Tablets of DDAVP are prescribed initially at 200–600 µg daily in three divided doses. The main complication of DDAVP is hyponatraemia, which can be prevented by allowing the patient to develop some polyuria for a short period during each week. The dose requirement for DDAVP may decrease during intercurrent illness. It is therefore important to review the need for DDAVP daily in critically ill patients.

Nephrogenic diabetes insipidus, as is to be expected, does not respond to antidiuretic hormone.

In *bleeding oesophageal varices*, use is made of the vasoconstrictor effect of vasopressin (as terlipressin, a vasopressin prodrug); see p. 600.

In *haemophilia*, desmopressin can enhance blood concentration of factor VIII.

Felypressin is used as a vasoconstrictor with local anaesthetics.

Enuresis: see p. 326.

Diabetes insipidus: vasopressin deficiency

Diabetes insipidus (DI) is characterised by persistent production of excess dilute urine (>40 mL/kg every 24 h in adults and >100 mL/kg every 24 h in children). DI is classified as cranial or nephrogenic. *Cranial* causes of DI are genetic, developmental or idiopathic. Acquired causes are head injury, surgery to the hypothalamic–pituitary region, tumours, inflammatory conditions such as granulomatous and infectious disease, vascular causes and external radiotherapy. *Nephrogenic* DI has a larger number of causes including drugs (lithium, demeclocycline) and several diseases affecting the renal medulla. The DNA sequencing of the receptor and aquaporins has also allowed identification of mutations in these that cause congenital DI.

Desmopressin replacement therapy is the first choice. Thiazide diuretics (and chlortalidone) also have paradoxical antidiuretic effect in diabetes insipidus. That this is not due to sodium depletion is suggested by the fact that the non-diuretic thiazide, diazoxide, also has this effect. It is probable that changes in the proximal renal tubule result in increased reabsorption and in the delivery of less sodium and water to the distal tubule, but the mechanism remains incompletely elucidated. Some cases of the nephrogenic form, which is not helped by antidiuretic hormone, may be benefited by a thiazide.

Carbamazepine 200 mg once or twice daily is marginally effective in partial pituitary diabetes insipidus, because it acts on the kidney, potentiating the effect of vasopressin on the renal tubule.

Syndrome of inappropriate antidiuretic hormone secretion (SIADH)

A variety of tumours, e.g. oat-cell lung cancer, can make vasopressin, and they are not, of course, subject to normal homeostatic mechanisms. SIADH also occurs in some central nervous system (CNS) and respiratory disorders (infection). Dilutional hyponatraemia follows, i.e. low plasma sodium with an inappropriately low plasma osmolality and high urine osmolality. When plasma sodium approaches 120 mmol/L, treatment should be with fluid restriction (e.g. 500 mL/day). Treatment is primarily of the underlying disorder accompanied by fluid restriction. Chemotherapy to the causative tumour or infection is likely to be the most effective treatment. *Demeclocycline*, which inhibits the renal action of vasopressin, is useful. Initially 0.9–1.2 g is given daily in divided doses, reduced to 600–900 mg daily for maintenance. V_2 receptor antagonists (the vaptans) are also now available and are licensed for such patients. There is no evidence of these drugs being any more effective than a carefully supervised fluid restriction, and at present conivaptan and tolvaptan are difficult to justify on grounds of cost and safety. It is also important to note that rapid correction of hyponatraemia can lead to central pontine myelinolysis, and that care must therefore be taken with these drugs.

Emergency treatment of hyponatraemia

Whereas most patients with a serum sodium concentration exceeding 125 mmol/L are asymptomatic, those with lower values may have symptoms, especially if the disorder has developed rapidly. These may be mild (headache, nausea) or severe (vomiting, disorientation). Complications are catastrophic: seizures, coma, permanent brain damage, respiratory arrest, brainstem herniation and death. Optimal treatment requires balancing the risks of hypotonicity against those of therapy, the most feared being central pontine myelinolysis. Infusion of isotonic or hypertonic saline is therefore reserved for extreme emergencies, associated with stupor, and undertaken with great caution.

The rate of correction must not exceed 0.5 mmol/L/h until the plasma sodium is 120–125 mmol/L. Over-correction (to plasma sodium >130 mmol/L) is unnecessary and potentially harmful. The predicted increase in plasma sodium per litre of infusate can be estimated from the formula:

$$\text{infusate sodium concentration} \\ - \text{plasma sodium concentration}) \\ \div \text{total body water (litres)}$$

Body water is a fraction of body-weight in kilograms, being 0.6 in children and non-elderly men, 0.5 in elderly men and non-elderly women and 0.45 in elderly women.

Oxytocin. See p. 652.

Sex (gonadal) hormones and antagonists: steroid hormones

Steroid hormone receptors (for gonadal steroids and adrenocortical steroids) are complex proteins inside the target cell. The steroid penetrates, binds to the receptor and translocates into the cell nucleus, which is the principal site of action and where RNA synthesis occurs. Compounds that occupy the receptor without causing translocation into the nucleus or the replenishment of receptors act as antagonists, e.g. spironolactone to aldosterone, cyproterone to androgens, clomifene to oestrogens.

Selectivity. Many synthetic analogues, although classed as, e.g. androgen, anabolic steroid, progestogen, are non-selective and bind to several types of receptors as agonists, partial agonists and antagonists. The result is that their effects are complex. The selective oestrogen receptor modulators (SERMS) may be antagonists to the oestrogen receptors in the breast, while being agonists in bone. Tamoxifen and raloxifene are such SERMS, which therefore increase bone density (as normal oestrogen does) but reduce the risk of breast cancer (by blocking the breast receptor to estradiol) (see also below).

Pharmacokinetics. Steroid sex hormones are well absorbed through the skin (factory workers need protective clothing) and the gut. Most are subject to extensive hepatic metabolic inactivation (some so much that oral administration is ineffective or requires very large doses, if a useful amount is to pass through the liver and reach the systemic circulation).

There is some enterohepatic recirculation, especially of oestrogen, and this may be interrupted by severe diarrhoea, with loss of efficacy. Some non-steroidal analogues are metabolised more slowly. Sustained-release (depot) preparations are used. The hormones are carried in the blood extensively bound to a hepatic glycoprotein called sex hormone–binding globulin. In general the plasma $t_{1/2}$ relates to the duration of cellular action, which is implied in the recommended dosage schedules.

Androgens

Testosterone is the predominant natural androgen secreted by the Leydig cells of the testis; in a normal adult male, testosterone production amounts to 4–9 mg/24 h. It circulates highly bound to sex hormone–binding globulin (65%) and loosely bound to albumin (33%). Only 1–2% of circulating testosterone is unbound and freely available to tissues. It is converted by hydroxylation to the active dihydrotestosterone (DHT). Testosterone is necessary for normal spermatogenesis, for the development of the male secondary sex characteristics, for sexual potency and for the growth, at puberty, of the genital tract.

Protein anabolism is increased by androgens, i.e. androgens increase the proportion of protein laid down as tissue, especially muscle and (combined with training, increase strength). Growth of bone is promoted, but the rate of closure of the epiphyses is also hastened, causing short stature in cases of precocious puberty or of androgen overdose in the course of treating hypogonadal children.

Indications for androgen therapy

Indications for testosterone treatment are primary testicular failure such as a result of bilateral anorchia, Klinefelter's (XXY) karyotype, surgery, chemotherapy and radiotherapy, or secondary testicular failure as a result of hypothalamic–pituitary disease.

Other conditions that require testosterone treatment are delayed puberty in boys 16 years of age or older, angioneurotic oedema and adrenal insufficiency in females.

Testosterone replacement improves libido and overall sexual performance in hypogonadal men. Its effect on erectile response to sexual arousal is less clear, and sildenafil and its analogues are more appropriate for patients complaining of erectile dysfunction.

Preparations and choice of androgens

Testosterone given orally is subject to extensive hepatic first-pass metabolism (see p. 16), and it is therefore usually given by other routes. Androgens are available for oral, buccal, transdermal or depot administration.

Oral preparations

Testosterone undecanoate is highly lipophilic. When given orally, it is absorbed through the intestinal lymphatics, thereby bypassing otherwise extensive hepatic first-pass metabolism. Yet bioavailability is poor and variable. The $t_{1/2}$ is short, and the dose is 40–120 mg three times daily. It is converted to DHT before being absorbed, so monitoring should be by measuring DHT, not testosterone levels.

Mesterolone is a DHT derivative.

Parenteral preparations

Sustanon is a mixed testosterone ester preparation normally given 2–4 weekly by deep intramuscular injection; the usual dose is 250 mg (range 100–250 mg). Other preparations, *testosterone enanthate* and *testosterone epionate*, are given at 1–2-week intervals. These preparations are widely used and have a good safety profile. Their main disadvantage is fluctuation of plasma testosterone concentrations, causing swings of mood and well-being. But *testosterone undecanoate* (1000 mg in 4 mL castor oil given by a depot intramuscular injection) achieves stable physiological concentrations lasting for 3 months.

Transdermal preparations

Patches are available for scrotal and non-scrotal sites; they provide stable pharmacokinetics and are an alternative to painful injections. Absorption is superior at the scrotum because of its high skin vascularity. High concentrations of DHT are achieved because 5α-reductase is present in scrotal skin.

Non-scrotal patches are applied to the skin of the upper arms, back, abdomen and thighs.

Local skin reactions occur in 10% of cases, and they are secondary to absorption enhancers. Application of corticosteroid ointment improves tolerability. Patches must be changed every 24 h.

Transdermal gels are hydroalcoholic gels for delivering testosterone transdermally. They are applied daily on the skin of the arms and torso. Showering must be avoided for 6 h, as well as intimate skin contact with others, as transfer of testosterone may occur.

Buccal preparations

These are available in a sustained-release form. A tablet is placed in the small depression above the incisor tooth twice daily. Testosterone is absorbed and delivered into the superior vena cava, thereby bypassing hepatic first-pass metabolism. Steady-state testosterone and DHT concentrations are achieved in 24 h.

Testosterone implants

Pellets of crystallised testosterone are implanted subcutaneously under local anaesthesia by a small incision in the anterior abdominal wall, using a trocar and cannula. Three implanted pellets (total 600 mg) give hormone replacement for about 6 months. There is an approximately 10% risk of extrusion of the pellets; infection and haemorrhage are uncommon.

Adverse effects

Increased libido may lead to undesirable sexual activity, and virilisation is undesired by most women. Androgens have a weak salt and water retaining activity, which is not often clinically important. Liver injury (cholestatic) can occur, particularly with 17α-alkyl derivatives (ethylestrenol, danazol, oxymetholone); it is reversible, but these agents should be avoided in hepatic disease. As androgens are contraindicated in carcinoma of the prostate, monitoring during treatment includes regular measurement of prostate-specific antigen (PSA). Haemoglobin should also be monitored to avoid polycythaemia.

Effects on blood lipids are complex and variable, and the balance may be to disadvantage.

In patients with malignant disease of bone, androgen administration may be followed by hypercalcaemia. The less virilising androgens are used to promote anabolism and are discussed below.

Antiandrogens (androgen antagonists)

Oestrogens and progestogens are *physiological* antagonists to androgens. But compounds that compete selectively for androgen *receptors* have been made.

Cyproterone

Cyproterone is a derivative of progesterone; its combination of structural similarities and differences results in the following:

- Competition with testosterone for receptors in target peripheral organs (but not causing feminisation as do oestrogens); it reduces spermatogenesis even to the level of azoospermia (reversing over about 4 months after the drug is discontinued); abnormal sperm occurs during treatment.
- Competition with testosterone in the CNS, reducing sexual drive and thoughts, and causing impotence.
- Some agonist progestogenic activity on hypothalamic receptors, inhibiting gonadotrophin secretion, which also inhibits testicular androgen production.

Uses. Cyproterone is used for reducing male hypersexuality, and in prostatic cancer and severe female hirsutism. A formulation of cyproterone plus ethinylestradiol (Dianette, which contains only 2 mg of cyproterone acetate) is offered for this latter purpose as well as for severe acne in women; this preparation acts as an oral contraceptive but does not have a UK licence, and should not be used primarily for this purpose.

Flutamide and bicalutamide are non-steroidal antiandrogens available for use in conjunction with the gonadorelins (e.g. goserelin) in the treatment of prostatic carcinoma.

Finasteride and *dutasteride* (see p. 492), which inhibit conversion of testosterone to dihydrotestosterone, have localised antiandrogen activity in tissues where dihydrotestosterone is the principal androgen; they are therefore useful drugs in the treatment of benign prostatic hypertrophy.

Spironolactone (see p. 599) also has antiandrogen activity and may help hirsutism in women (as an incidental benefit to its diuretic effect). Androgen secretion may be diminished by continued use of a gonadorelin (LHRH) analogue (see p. 637).

Ketoconazole (antifungal) interferes with androgen and corticosteroid synthesis by inhibiting several of the cytochrome P450 enzymes involved in steroid biosynthesis and may be used in prostatic carcinoma and Cushing's syndrome (400 mg twice daily).

Metyrapone inhibits one enzyme on the cortisol and aldosterone synthetic pathway, 11 hydroxylase, and is therefore also used in the treatment of Cushing's syndrome while awaiting definitive surgical treatment (either bilateral adrenalectomy or transphenoidal pituitary hypophysectomy).

Anabolic steroids

(See also above.)

Androgens are effective protein anabolic agents, but their clinical use for this purpose is limited by the amount of virilisation that women will tolerate. Attempts made to separate anabolic from androgenic action have been only partially successful, and *all anabolic steroids also have androgenic effects*.

They benefit some patients with *aplastic anaemia*.

Nandrolone 50 mg is given by deep intramuscular injection every 3 weeks. *Hereditary angioedema* (lack of inhibition of the complement C_l esterase) may be prevented by *danazol*.

Anabolic steroids can prevent the calcium and nitrogen loss in the urine that occurs in patients who are bedridden for a long time, and they have been used in the treatment of some severe fractures. The use of anabolic steroids in conditions of general wasting despite nutritional support may be justifiable in extreme debilitating disease, such as severe ulcerative colitis, and after major surgery. In the later stages of malignant disease, they may make the patient feel and look less wretched.

Anabolic steroids do not usefully counter the unwanted catabolic effects of the adrenocortical hormones.

None of these agents is free from virilising properties in high doses; acne and greasy skin may be the early manifestation of virilisation (see also, Adverse effects of androgens, p. 641, and Drugs and sport, p. 144).

Oestrogens have only a modest anabolic effect.

Administration of anabolic steroids should generally be intermittent in courses of 3–12 weeks with similar steroid-free intervals, to reduce the occurrence of unwanted effects, especially liver injury.

Oestrogens

Estrone and *estradiol* are both natural oestrogens. Oestrogens are responsible for the development of normal secondary sex characteristics in women, uterine growth, thickening of vaginal mucosa and the ductal breast system.

Pharmacokinetics

See p. 81.

Preparations of oestrogens

The dose varies according to whether replacement of physiological deficiencies is being carried out (replacement therapy) or whether pharmacotherapy is being used.

- *Ethinylestradiol* ($t_{1/2}$ 13 h) is a synthetic agent of first choice for pharmacological uses (mainly contraceptive, female hypogonadism and menstrual disorders); it is effective by mouth, dose 20–50 µg/day.
- *Estradiol* and *estriol* are orally active mixed natural oestrogens, dose 1–2 mg/day.
- *Conjugated oestrogens* (Premarin) are orally active mixed natural oestrogens containing 50–65% estrone obtained from the urine of pregnant mares, dose 0.625–1.25 mg.
- *Estropipate* (piperazine estrone sulphate) is an orally active synthetic conjugate.
- *Diethylstilbestrol* (stilboestrol) is the first synthetic oestrogen; it is used (rarely) in prostatic cancer and occasionally in post-menopausal women with breast cancer.

Choice of oestrogen

Ethinylestradiol, or its methylated derivative *mestranol* (synthetic), is a satisfactory first choice for pharmacotherapy. The weaker endogenous oestrogens, estradiol, estriol and estrone (natural), or the conjugated equine oestrogens (CEE) are preferable for physiological replacement. It remains uncertain whether all oestrogens have similar hormonal and non-hormonal effects, including adverse effects.

Selective oestrogen receptor modulators (SERMS) combine oestrogenic and antioestrogenic properties (raloxifene and tibolone). *Raloxifene* has antioestrogenic effects on breast and endometrium, but oestrogenic effects on bone and is used for prevention and treatment of osteoporosis. It reduces the risk of invasive breast cancer but increases the risk of stroke and thromboembolism. It has no effect on vasomotor symptoms. *Tibolone* is licensed for short-term treatment of osteoporosis.

Oestrogen formulations and routes of administration

Oral. This is an easy and effective route but is subject to the first-pass effect through the liver, and higher doses are needed in comparison to other formulations.

Transdermal formulations are in the form of patches and gels. This route may eliminate the risk of thrombosis associated with oral oestrogen.

Subcutaneous implants. Crystalline pellets inserted into the anterior wall or buttock release hormone over several months. Used in women who undergo oophorectomy and hysterectomy, they are usually repeated at 6 months, and tachyphylaxis may be a problem.

Vaginal (ring, cream, tablet or pessary). Low-dose oestrogen therapy is delivered for treatment of urogenital symptoms. If used for long periods, i.e. more than 2 years, progesterone should be added to avoid endometrial hyperplasia.

Others. A nasal spray is available. It delivers 300 µg of estradiol daily.

Indications for oestrogen therapy

Replacement therapy in hypo-oestrogenaemia

This term refers to decreased oestrogen production due to ovarian disease, or to hypothalamic–pituitary disease (hypogonadotrophic hypogonadism). Treatment is by *cyclic oestrogen* (estradiol 1–2 mg, conjugated oestrogens 0.625/1.25 mg daily or ethinylestradiol 20–30 µg continuously) plus a progestogen, *medroxyprogesterone* 2.5–10 mg daily for the last 10–14 days of oestrogen treatment. An alternative treatment is the oral contraceptive (p. 647).

Post-menopausal hormone replacement therapy (HRT)

HRT refers to the use of oestrogen treatment in order to reverse or prevent problems due to the loss of ovarian hormone secretion after the menopause, whether physiological or induced. The tissues sensitive to oestrogen include brain, bone, skin, cardiovascular and genitourinary. The goal of HRT is to reduce the vasomotor symptoms of oestrogen loss (hot flushes, sleeplessness and vaginal dryness) without causing disorders that may be more common with oestrogen treatment such as breast and endometrial cancer.

All types of HRT (oestrogen with or without progestogen) are effective at reducing the hot flushes experienced by more than 50% of post-menopausal women. The benefit is most during the first year of treatment, when 75% of women report a reduced likelihood. By the third year of treatment, the reduction in frequency decreases by 65% in comparison to placebo. The other major value of HRT is the relief of vaginal dryness. Vaginal administration is the most effective route for treatment of dyspareunia and related symptoms. Urinary incontinence does not respond to HRT.

The clinical evidence base for prescribing HRT has changed since the publication of trials showing excess risks of breast cancer and stroke that outweigh small benefits in reduction of fractures and risk of colonic cancer. HRT should not be used in the treatment of osteoporosis or for prevention of coronary heart disease.

Preparations used for HRT. There are three types of regimen:

1. Women *without* a uterus take continuous *oestrogen* alone.
2. Women *with* a uterus require *oestrogen combined with progestogen* to prevent endometrial proliferation and risk of endometrial cancer.
   - In the commonest 'sequential' regimen, women take oestrogen without a break and add a progestogen from day 12–14 to day 28 of each cycle (different preparations vary in the exact length of progestogen prescribing). The first course is started on the first day of menstruation (if present), and 28-day cycles of treatment follow thereafter without interval.
   - In the 'continuous' regimen (appropriate only for women who have been amenorrhoeic for more than 1 year), fixed-dose combinations of oestrogen and progestogen are taken without a break. Continuous combination HRT regimens will eventually induce amenorrhoea in most women, thereby eliminating one of the major deterrents to HRT use, withdrawal bleeding.

Calendar packs are available. The oral preparations, Prempak-C and Femoston, use conjugated oestrogen and estradiol, respectively, as their oestrogen. Oral progestogens include *dihydrogesterone, medroxyprogesterone, norgestrel* and *norethisterone*. Individual progestogens can be given orally in combination with an oestrogen, as subcutaneous depot injection or by transdermal patch. Some patches provide both hormones but obviously lack the facility for doses to be separately titrated to provide the minimum necessary to prevent both flushing and (if undesired) withdrawal bleeding.

An alternative to oestrogen therapy is *tibolone* 2.5 mg, which is a synthetic oral steroid with weak oestrogenic, progestogenic and androgenic properties. Its main adverse effect is vaginal bleeding, which needs investigation if persistent. Vasomotor menopausal symptoms may occasionally be helped by low doses of clonidine (Dixarit).

Contraception. HRT in routine use does not provide contraception, and any potentially fertile woman who requires HRT should take appropriate precautions. A woman is considered potentially fertile for 2 years after her last menstrual period if she is younger than 50 years of age, and for 1 year if she is older than 50 years of age. A woman who is younger than 50 years of age and free from all risk factors for venous and arterial disease can use a low-oestrogen combined oral contraceptive pill to provide both relief of menopausal symptoms and contraception; it is recommended

that the oral contraceptive be stopped at 50 years of age as there are more suitable alternatives.

Adverse effects of HRT. The commonest reasons for withdrawal are *irregular* or *withdrawal bleeding* and *breast pain*. Concerns about musculoskeletal symptoms and weight gain have not been substantiated in the long-term trials. Transdermal patches were associated with skin reactions, but the incidence has declined as the alcohol content has been reduced in the newer formulations.

The more serious complications are venous thromboembolism and cancer of the endometrium or breast. These risks are small in absolute terms, particularly so for the risk of cancer during the first 5 years of treatment.

For *venous thromboembolism*, the excess risk is 4 per 1000 woman-years, which may be considered clinically insignificant except in women with predisposing factors, e.g. previous personal or family history of thromboembolism, or recent surgery.

The risk of *carcinoma of the endometrium* is increased two-fold during the first 5 years, rising to seven-fold with longer treatment. Because endometrial cancer is uncommon, the absolute risk is about one-tenth that of thromboembolic disease; the risk subsides over 5–10 years after stopping treatment.

Carcinoma of the breast can occur with any type of HRT. Some 45 in every 1000 women 50 years of age will have breast cancer over the next 20 years, rising by only 2, 6 and 12 cases, respectively, for women who take HRT for 5, 10 or 15 years. A family history of breast cancer does not increase the risks associated with HRT.

The risk of *gallstones* may be increased up to two-fold. HRT does not increase the risk of ovarian cancer.

Blood lipids: The effect of oestrogens is on balance favourable, but the addition of a progestogen (unless gestodene or desogestrel) reverses the balance.

Contraindications to oestrogen therapy include recent arterial or venous thromboembolic disease, and history of oestrogen-dependent neoplasm, e.g. breast cancer. Hypertension, liver disease or gallstones, migraine, diabetes, uterine fibroids or endometriosis may all be made worse by oestrogen. These are very variable, and are not absolute contraindications.

Anti-oestrogens

Selective antagonists of the oestrogen receptor are used either to induce gonadotrophin release in anovulatory infertility or to block stimulation of oestrogen receptor–positive carcinomas of the breast.

Clomifene is structurally related to diethylstilbestrol; it is a weak oestrogen agonist having less activity than natural oestrogens, so that its occupation of receptors results in antagonism, i.e. it is a partial agonist. Clomifene blocks hypothalamic oestrogen receptors so that the negative feedback of natural oestrogens is prevented and the pituitary responds by increased secretion of gonadotrophins, which may induce ovulation.

Clomifene is administered during the early follicular phase of the menstrual cycle (50 mg daily on days 2–6) and is successful in inducing ovulation in about 85% of women. Multiple ovulation with multiple pregnancy may occur, and this is its principal adverse effect, which can be limited by using ultrasonography. There have been reports of an increased incidence of ovarian carcinoma following multiple exposure, and the number of consecutive cycles for which clomifene may be used to stimulate ovulation should be limited to 12.

Cyclofenil acts similarly to clomifene.

Tamoxifen is a non-steroidal competitive oestrogen antagonist on target organs. Although available for anovulatory infertility (20 mg daily on days 2, 3, 4 and 5 of the cycle), its main use now is in the treatment of *oestrogen-dependent breast cancer* (see p. 552). Treatment with tamoxifen delays the growth of metastases and increases survival; if tolerated it should be continued for 5 years.

Tamoxifen is also the hormonal treatment of choice in women with oestrogen receptor–positive *metastatic* breast cancer. Approximately 60% of such patients respond to initial hormonal manipulation, whereas less than 10% of oestrogen receptor–negative tumours respond.

Severe *adverse effects* are unusual with tamoxifen, but patients with bony metastases may experience an exacerbation of pain, sometimes associated with hypercalcaemia; this reaction commonly precedes tumour response. Amenorrhoea commonly develops in pre-menopausal women. Patients should be told of the small risk of endometrial cancer and encouraged to report relevant symptoms early. They can be reassured that the benefits of treatment far outweigh the risks. Tamoxifen is now considered a SERM (see above).

Progesterone and progestogens

Progesterone ($t_{1/2}$ 5 min) is produced by the corpus luteum and converts the uterine epithelium from the proliferative to the secretory phase. It is thus necessary for successful implantation of the ovum and is essential throughout pregnancy, in the last two-thirds of which it is secreted in large amounts by the placenta. It acts particularly on tissues that are sensitised by oestrogens. Some synthetic progestogens are less selective, having varying oestrogenic and androgenic activity, and these may inhibit ovulation, though not very reliably. Progestogens are of two principal kinds:

- *Progesterone* and its derivatives: dydrogesterone, hydroxyprogesterone, medroxyprogesterone ($t_{1/2}$ 28 h).
- *Testosterone* derivatives: norethisterone and its prodrug ethynodiol ($t_{1/2}$ 10 h), levonorgestrel, desogestrel, gestodene, gestronol, norgestimate.

Drospirenone is a derivative of the synthetic aldosterone antagonist, spironolactone (see p. 599). It therefore has antimineralocorticoid activity, reducing salt retention and blood pressure. It also exhibits partial antiandrogenic activity, about 30% of that of cyproterone acetate. It is available as a combination with ethinylestradiol for use as a contraceptive.

Most progestogens can virilise directly or by metabolites (except progesterone and dydrogesterone), and fetal virilisation to the point of sexual ambiguity has occurred with vigorous use during pregnancy (see also Contraception, p. 647).

Megestrol is used only in cancer; it causes tumours in the breasts of beagle dogs.

Uses

The clinical uses of progestational agents are ill defined, apart from *contraception*, the *menopause* and *post-menopausal hormone replacement* therapy (see above).

Other possible uses include: menstrual disorders, e.g. menorrhagia, endometriosis, dysmenorrhoea and premenstrual syndrome (doubtful efficacy), breast and endometrial cancer.

Preparations

Available progestogens (some used only in combined formulations) include:

- *Oral:* norethisterone, dydrogesterone, gestodene, desogestrel, levonorgestrel, megestrol, medroxyprogesterone.
- *Suppositories* or *pessaries:* progesterone.
- *Injectable:* progesterone, hydroxyprogesterone, medroxyprogesterone.

Adverse effects of prolonged use include virilisation (see above), raised blood pressure and an adverse trend in blood lipids. Gestodene, desogestrel and norgestimate may have less affinity for androgen receptors and therefore fewer unfavourable effects on blood lipids; the first two of these may have a higher risk of thrombosis.

Antiprogestogens

Menstruation (in its luteal phase) is dependent on progesterone, and uterine bleeding follows antagonism of progesterone. Pregnancy is dependent on progesterone (for implantation, endometrial stimulation, suppression of uterine contractions and placenta formation), and abortion follows progesterone antagonism in early pregnancy.

Mifepristone is a pure competitive antagonist at progesterone and glucocorticoid receptors. Clinical trials of oral use in hospital outpatients have shown it to be safe and effective in terminating pregnancy. Efficacy is enhanced if its use is followed by vaginal administration of a prostaglandin (gemeprost) to produce uterine contractions (the success rate is raised from 85% to more than 95%).

Adverse effects of the combined treatment include nausea and vomiting, dizziness, asthenia, abdominal pain; uterine bleeding may be heavy. Mifepristone also offers the opportunity for mid-trimester terminations. These are likely to become more frequent with rise in the number of inherited syndromes amenable to antenatal diagnosis at this stage.

Guidelines may vary in detail, and the following are general regimens:

- For gestation of up to 1 week, when the fetus is deemed viable, mifepristone 600 mg by mouth followed 36–48 h later by gemeprost 1 mg by vagina.
- For mid-trimester medical abortion (13–24 weeks), mifepristone 600 mg by mouth followed 36–48 h later by gemeprost 1 mg every 3 h by vagina to a maximum of 5 mg.

Other progesterone derivatives

Danazol (Danol) is a derivative of the progestogen, ethisterone. It has partial agonist androgen activity and is described as an 'impeded' androgen; it has little progestogen activity. It is a relatively selective inhibitor of pituitary gonadotrophin secretion (LH, FSH) affecting the surge in the mid-menstrual cycle more than basal secretion. This reduces ovarian function, which leads to atrophic changes in endometrium, both uterine and elsewhere (ectopic), i.e. endometriosis. In males, it reduces spermatogenesis. Unwanted androgenic effects occur in women (acne, hirsutism and, rarely, enlargement of the clitoris).

It is used chiefly for: endometriosis, fibrocystic mastitis, gynaecomastia, precocious puberty, menorrhagia and hereditary angioedema (see p. 651).

Gestrinone is similar.

Fertility regulation

Infertility

Depending on the cause, the following agents, already described, are used:

For women, ovulation induction:

- Hypothalamic hormone: gonadorelin (p. 637).
- Anterior pituitary hormones: FSH (p. 637); chorionic gonadotrophin (p. 637).
- Anti-oestrogens: clomifene (p. 645).
- Cabergoline for hyperprolactinaemia (p. 682).

For men, induction of spermatogenesis: the same agents as for ovulation are used.

Polycystic ovary syndrome (PCOS)

The diagnosis requires at least two of the following features:

- Polycystic ovaries.
- Oligo-ovulation or anovulation.
- Clinical and/or biochemical evidence of androgen excess.

Management of PCOS includes:

- *Treatment of infertility.* Induction of ovulation can be accomplished in 75–80% of women with PCOS by the use of anti-oestrogens, typically clomifene citrate. More recent data indicate that metformin (see below) may improve ovulation rates in women with PCOS when given alone or in combination with clomifene.
- *Menstrual regulation* in those who do not desire pregnancy. A low-dose combined oral contraceptive (containing ethinylestradiol, 20–35 μg) may be the most convenient form of treatment, although cyclical progestogen is a reasonable alternative. Norgestimate and desogestrel are the preferred progestins, having virtually no androgenic properties.
- *Treatment of associated symptoms of hyperandrogenism.* Management of hirsutism usually involves cosmetic treatment to remove unwanted hair and, in more severe cases, antiandrogen therapy. The most commonly used antiandrogen is cyproterone acetate. This also has progestogenic activity and can be combined with ethinylestradiol to provide cycle control in addition to management of hyperandrogenic symptoms. Drospirenone (see above) is ideal in PCOS because of its antiandrogen and antimineralocorticoid properties. Spironolactone can be used at high doses, 100–200 mg. Flutamide is a potent non-steroidal antiandrogen that is effective in the treatment of hirsutism. Concern about inducing hepatocellular dysfunction has limited its use.
- Prevention of the possible long-term consequences of the metabolic disturbance characteristic of anovulatory women with PCOS.

- Calorie restriction in obese women with PCOS improves insulin sensitivity and glucose tolerance, and leads to resumption of spontaneous ovulatory cycles and normal fertility in many cases. Metformin may be a safe and effective means of improving metabolic profile in both lean and obese women with PCOS.

Contraception by drugs and hormones

The requirements of a successful hormonal contraceptive are stringent, for it will be used by millions of healthy people who wish to separate sexual relations from physical reproduction. The following represent the ideal:

- It must be extremely *safe* as well as highly effective.
- Its action must be *quick* in onset and quickly and completely reversible, even after years of continuous use.
- It must not affect *libido*.

The fact that alternative methods are less reliable implies that their use will lead to more unwanted pregnancies with their attendant inconvenience, morbidity and mortality, and this must be taken into account in deciding what risks of hormonal contraception are acceptable.

Hormonal contraception in women comprises:

- Oestrogen and progestogen (combined and phased administration).
- Progestogen alone.

Combined contraceptives (the 'pill')

Combined oestrogen–progestogen oral contraceptives (combined oral contraceptive pill, COCP) have been used extensively since 1956. The principal mechanism is inhibition of ovulation through suppression of LH surge by the hypothalamus and pituitary. In addition, the endometrium is altered, so that implantation is less likely and cervical mucus becomes more viscous and impedes the passage of the spermatozoa.

The combination is conveniently started on the first day of the cycle (first day of menstruation) and continued for 21 days (this is immediately effective, inhibiting the first ovulation). It is followed by a period of 7 days when no pill is taken, and during which bleeding usually occurs. Thereafter, regardless of bleeding, a new 21-day course is begun, and so on, i.e. active tablets are taken daily for 3 weeks out of 4. For easy compliance, some combined pills are packaged so that the woman takes one tablet every day without interruption (21 active then 7 dummy).

In some instances, the course is not started on the first day of menstruation but on the second to the fifth day (to give a full month between the menses at the outset). An alternative method of contraception should then be used until the seventh pill has been taken, as the first ovulation may not have been suppressed in women who have short menstrual cycles.

The pill should be taken at about the same time (to within 12 h) every day to establish a routine. The monthly bleeds that occur 1–2 days after the cessation of active hormone administration are hormone withdrawal bleeds, not natural menstruation. They are not an essential feature of oral contraception, but women are accustomed to monthly bleeds and they provide monthly reassurance of the absence of pregnancy.

Numerous field trials have shown that progestogen–oestrogen combinations, if taken precisely as directed, are the most reliable reversible contraceptive known. (The only close competitors are depot progestogens and progestogen-releasing intrauterine devices.)

Important aspects

Subsequent fertility. After stopping the pill, fertility that is normal for the age the woman has now reached is restored, although conception may be delayed for a few months longer in younger users, and for as much as 1 year in older users than if other methods had been used.

Effect on an existing pregnancy. Although progestogens can masculinise the female fetus, the doses for contraception are so low that risk of harming an undiagnosed pregnancy is extremely small, probably less than 1 in 1000 (the background incidence of birth defects is 1–2%).

Carcinomas of the breast and cervix are slightly increased in incidence;[2] the incidence of hepatoma (very rare) is increased. The risk to life seems to be less than that of moderate smoking (10 cigarettes/day) and that of a normal pregnancy, as the risk of pulmonary embolus is higher in a normal pregnancy. The risk of carcinoma of the ovary and endometrium is substantially reduced. The overall incidence of cancer is unaltered.

The effect on menstruation (it is not true menstruation, see above) is generally to regularise it, and often to diminish

---

[2] A meta-analysis of 54 studies concluded that use of the COCP was associated with a relative risk of 1.24, which disappears over 10 years after stopping the COCP. A higher relative risk in women who started taking the COCP at a young age is explained by the lower background rate, and there is little added effect from long-term COCP ingestion. (Collaborative Group on Hormonal Factors in Breast Cancer. Breast cancer and hormonal contraceptives: collaborative reanalysis of individual data on 53 297 women with breast cancer and 100 239 women without breast cancer from 54 epidemiological studies. Lancet 1996; 347:1713–1727.)

blood loss, but amenorrhoea can occur. In some women, 'breakthrough' intermenstrual bleeding occurs, especially at the outset, but this seldom persists for more than a few cycles. Premenstrual tension and dysmenorrhoea are much reduced.

Libido is greatly subject to psychosocial influences, and removal of fear of pregnancy may permit enthusiasm for the first time. It is likely that direct pharmacological effect (reduction) is rare. There is evidence that the normal increase in female-initiated sexual activity at time of ovulation is suppressed.

Cardiovascular complications. The incidence of *venous thromboembolism* is increased in pill users. It is lowest in the 20–35-microgram pill and rises progressively with the 50- and 100-microgram preparations; it is not known whether there is any difference between doses of 20 and 35 µg. The small increase in hypertension, cerebrovascular events and acute myocardial infarction is confined principally to smokers.

Increased arterial disease also appears to be associated with the type of progestogen in the combined pill. The 'third-generation' pills (see below) appear to carry a higher risk of venous thrombosis, but may have a lower risk of arterial thrombosis because their lower androgen activity leads to slightly higher high-density lipoprotein (HDL) levels than older pills. The progestogen-only pill does not significantly affect coagulation.

Major surgery (in patients taking oestrogen–progestogen contraceptives and post-menopausal hormone replacement therapy). Because of the added risk of venous thromboembolism (surgery causes a fall in antithrombin levels), oral contraceptives should be withdrawn, if practicable, 4 weeks before all lower-limb operations or any major elective surgery (and started again at the first menstruation to occur more than 2 weeks after surgery). But increase in clotting factors may persist for many weeks, and there is also the risk of pregnancy to be considered. An alternative for emergencies is to use low molecular weight heparin (although this may not reverse all the oestrogenic effects on coagulation) and other means (mechanical stimulation of venous return) to prevent postoperative thrombosis.

Plasma lipoproteins may be adversely affected; least when the progestogen is desogestrel or low-dose norethisterone.

Plasma proteins. Oestrogens cause an increase in proteins, particularly the globulins that bind hydrocortisone, thyroxine and iron. As a result, the total plasma concentration of the bound substances is increased, although the concentration of free and active substance remains normal. This can be misleading in diagnostic tests, e.g. of thyroid function. This effect on plasma proteins passes off about 6 weeks after cessation of the oestrogen.

Other adverse effects

Often more prominent at the outset and largely due to oestrogen, these include: nausea and, rarely, vomiting; breast discomfort, fluid retention, headache (including increase in migraine), lethargy, abdominal discomfort, vaginal discharge or dryness. Depression may occur but most depression in pill users is not due to the contraceptive.

The above account gives rise to guidelines for use:

Absolute contraindications include:

- A personal history of thromboembolic venous, arterial or cardiac disease, or severe or multiple risk factors for these.
- Transient cerebral ischaemic attacks without headache.
- Infective hepatitis, until 3 months after liver function test results have become normal, and other liver disease including disturbances of hepatic excretion, e.g. cholestatic jaundice, Dubin–Johnson and Rotor syndromes.
- Migraine, if there is a typical aura, focal features, or if it is severe and lasts for more than 72 h despite treatment, or is treated with an ergot derivative (use with caution is acceptable if there is no aura, focal features, or if it is controlled with a 5-HT$_1$ receptor agonist).
- Carcinoma of the breast or genital tract, past or present.
- Other conditions including: systemic lupus erythematosus, porphyria, following evacuation of a hydatidiform mole (until urine and plasma gonadotrophin concentrations are normal), undiagnosed vaginal bleeding.

Relative contraindications or uses with caution, include:

- Family history of venous thromboembolism, arterial disease or a known prothrombotic condition, e.g. factor V Leiden (pretreatment coagulation investigation is advised).
- Diabetes mellitus, which may be precipitated or become more difficult to control (avoid if there are diabetic complications).
- Hypertension (avoid if blood pressure exceeds 160/100 mmHg).
- Smoking more than 40 cigarettes/day (15 cigarettes/day enhances the risk of circulatory disease three-fold and constitutes an absolute contraindication for women older than 35 years of age).
- Age older than 35 years (avoid if older than 50 years).
- Obesity (avoid if body mass exceeds 39 kg/m^2).
- Long-term immobility, e.g. due to leg plaster, confinement to bed.

- Breast feeding (until weaning or for 6 months after birth).

Duration of use does not enhance risks of itself. The increase in risk with increased duration of use is due to increasing age. The approaching menopause presents an obvious problem. Cyclical bleeding will continue to occur under the influence of the drugs even after the natural menopause. Thus the only way of deciding whether contraception can be permanently abandoned is by discontinuing it (and using another technique) for 3 months annually to see whether natural menstruation is resumed, or by stopping the combined pill for 1 month and measuring LH/FSH concentration in the blood, which indicates the state of pituitary function.

Benefits additional to contraception

Menses are accompanied by less premenstrual tension and dysmenorrhoea. When oestrogen is combined with the antiandrogen cyproterone acetate as the progestogenic agent Dianette, the combined pill is useful treatment for acne in young women.

Formulations of oestrogen–progestogen combination

Oestrogen: ethinylestradiol or mestranol.

Progestogen

- Second generation: norethisterone, levonorgestrel.
- Third generation: desogestrel, gestodene, norgestimate.

Combined oral contraceptives are defined as second or third generation by the progestogen component (first-generation progestogens are obsolete). Those containing a fixed amount of oestrogen and progestogen in each active tablet are termed 'monophasic'. Other pills employ variable ratios between oestrogen and progestogen, in two (biphasic) or three (triphasic) periods within the menstrual cycle. The dose of progestogen is low at the beginning and higher at the end, the oestrogen remaining either constant or rising slightly in mid-cycle. The objective is to achieve effective contraception with minimal distortion of natural hormonal rhythms.

The advantages claimed for these techniques are diminished adverse metabolic changes, e.g. blood lipids, and a particularly reliable monthly bleeding pattern without loss of contraceptive efficacy. Preparations include BiNovum, TriNovum, Logynon.

It is now appreciated that the earlier preparations had much more oestrogen than was necessary for efficacy. It seems probable that 20 μg is about the limit below which serious loss of efficacy can be expected. Indeed, in patients whose hepatic enzymes are likely to be induced, e.g. those taking antiepileptic or some antirheumatic drugs, it is advisable to use a preparation containing 50 μg oestrogen or more to avoid loss of efficacy due to increased oestrogen metabolism (elimination of breakthrough bleeding is a guide to adequacy of dose).

Choice of oestrogen–progestogen combination

There is a wide choice of formulations, with the dose of *ethinylestradiol* varying from 20 to 35 μg. In general, users should be prescribed the lowest total hormone dose that suits them (good cycle control and minimal unwanted effects) and should make a start with the first preparation given above, recognising that compliance is particularly important with the 20-microgram dose.

Common problems

Missed pill. The following refers to the combined pill (see later for the progestogen-only pill):

- If an omitted dose is remembered within 12 h, it should be taken at once and the next dose at the usual time, and all should be well.
- If more than 12 h have elapsed, the above procedure should be followed, but an additional barrier method of contraception should be used for 7 days. Although the protective effect of cervical mucus returns within 48 h, this 7-day period is needed to ensure effective suppression of an ovulation that may have been initiated by the missed pill.

Intercurrent gut upset. If vomiting occurs more than 3 h after a pill, behave as for a missed pill (above). The hormones are rapidly absorbed, and only severe diarrhoea would interfere significantly with efficacy. In case of doubt, it would be prudent to use a barrier method during and for 7 days after the episode.

Changing of preparation. If a woman is unhappy on one preparation she may be changed to another containing a different dose of oestrogen and/or progestogen. The new preparation should start the day after she has finished a cycle on the previous preparation. If this is done, no extra risk of pregnancy occurs.

Breakthrough bleeding (bleeding on days of active pill taking) can mean that a higher dose of oestrogen or progestogen is required. Note that missed or late pills, drug interaction (see below) or sexually transmitted infection, e.g. due to chlamydia, can also cause breakthrough bleeding.

Progestogen-only contraception

Progestogen-only pills (POPs) are indicated when oestrogen is contraindicated (see above) and in lactating women.

Progestogens render cervical mucus less easily penetrable by sperm and induce a premature secretory change in the endometrium so that implantation does not occur. Older POPs became unreliable if not taken at the same time of day, because their effect on cervical mucus wears off after 3 h and their additional action to inhibit ovulation occurs in only 40% of cycles. There is also liability to breakthrough bleeding.

A newer POP containing 75 µg *desogestrel* inhibits ovulation in 97–99% of cycles, resulting in an efficacy similar to that of the COCP. A further advantage of the newer POP is that no extra contraceptive cover is required if the exact time of dose is missed, provided the delay is no more than 12 h. Ectopic pregnancy may be more frequent due to a fertilised ovum being held up in a functionally depressed fallopian tube.

Medroxyprogesterone acetate and its metabolites are excreted in breast milk, so women who breast feed should wait until 6 weeks postpartum before starting Depo-Provera, when the infant's enzyme system should be more mature. *Norethisterone enantate* 200 mg (Noristerat) is shorter-acting than Depo-Provera, 8 weeks, and is used to provide contraception after administration of the rubella vaccine, and until a partner's vasectomy has taken effect. It can also be used in the longer-term but only on a 'named patient' basis.

Subdermal implantations that release hormone for several years are in use; they can be removed surgically if adverse effects develop or pregnancy is desired. For example, a flexible rod containing *etonorgestrel* (Implanon) inserted into the lower surface of the upper arm provides contraception for 3 years (2 years for overweight women because they have lower blood concentrations). The rod must be removed when its effective period has elapsed.

Two depot injections of *intramuscular progestogen* are available, equal in efficacy to the combined pill. Medroxyprogesterone (Depo-Provera) ($t_{1/2}$ 28 h) is a sustained-release (aqueous suspension) deep intramuscular injection given 3-monthly. When injected between day 1 and day 5 of the menstrual cycle, contraception starts immediately. If given after day 5, a barrier contraceptive is needed for 7 days.

Postcoital ('morning after pill') and emergency contraception

The overall risk of pregnancy following a single act of unprotected intercourse on any day in the menstrual cycle is 2–4%. The risk from a single act is highest (20–30%) in the days before and just after ovulation. Pregnancy may be prevented before implantation by disrupting the normal hormonal arrangements; the mode of action is probably by delaying or preventing ovulation or by preventing implantation of the fertilised ovum.

Progestogen-only treatment is preferred. *Levonorgestrel* 1500 µg is taken within 72 h of unprotected sexual intercourse. It can be taken more than once in a cycle, if required, and there is no upper limit to how many times it can be taken in a year. Contraindications to hormonal emergency contraception include current or suspected pregnancy, unprotected sexual intercourse more than 72 h earlier, and sensitivity to the components of the progestogen-only preparation. Some women complain of nausea and vomiting, which responds best to domperidone.

Drug interaction with steroid contraceptives

Particularly now that the lowest effective doses are in use, there is little latitude between success and failure if absorption, distribution and metabolism are disturbed. Any additional drug-taking must be looked at critically lest it reduces efficacy.

Enzyme induction. The rifamycins, rifampicin and rifabutin, are potent inducers of hepatic drug-metabolising enyzmes. The classic example of failure with the combined pill is breakthrough bleeding and pregnancy in young women being treated with rifampicin for tuberculosis, or meningitis including eradication of the carrier state. The enhanced metabolism of the steroids results in contraceptive failure.

Antiepileptics (phenytoin and carbamazepine but not sodium valproate) create a similar risk. Indeed, all drugs that induce metabolising enzymes (see p. 95), whether prescribed or self-administered (alcohol, tobacco smoking), constitute a risk to contraceptive efficacy, and prescribing should be specifically reviewed for the effect.

Broad-spectrum antimicrobials, e.g. ampicillin, doxycycline, can reduce the efficacy of combined oral contraceptives by diminishing the bacterial flora that metabolise ethinylestradiol in the large bowel and make it available for recycling. Additional contraceptive measures should be taken during a short course of antimicrobial, and for 7 days thereafter. When the course is long, i.e. more than 3 weeks, the bacteria have time to recover by developing resistance, and additional precautions are unnecessary after the first 14 days.

Hypothalamic/pituitary hormone approach to contraception

(See gonadorelin.)

Other methods of contraception

Copper intrauterine devices are widely used and highly effective (>99% at 1 year) for 5 years, and some for 10 years. They are especially useful for women older than 40 years of age, in whom oral contraceptives may become progressively contraindicated and for whom one IUD will last into the menopause. The IUD prevents implantation of the fertilised ovum, and has an additional antifertilisation effect enhanced by the toxic effect of copper ions on the gametes.

The intrauterine levonorgestrel system Mirena is used as a contraceptive, as a medical treatment for idiopathic menorrhagia and as the progestogen component of hormone replacement therapy. It is popular because of reduced dysmenorrhoea and lighter menses. Mirena contains 52 mg of levonorgestrel surrounded by a Silastic capsule, and releases 20 μg/day over 5 years, after which the device should be changed.

Vaginal preparations, used to immobilise or kill (spermicide) spermatozoa, are used to add safety to various mechanical contraceptives. They are very unreliable and should be used alone only in an emergency. Substances used include non-oxinols (surfactants that alter the permeability of the sperm lipoprotein membrane) as pessary, gel or foam.

Oil-based lubricants cause failure of rubber condoms and contraceptive diaphragms; many 'lubricants', e.g. hand or baby creams, wash off readily, but are nevertheless oil-based. Barrier contraceptive devices made of polyurethane, e.g. the female condom (Femidom), are not so affected.

Risks of contraception in relation to benefit

Despite the small risk of thromboembolism, the death rate from taking oral contraceptives is less than that of pregnancy.

Menstrual disorders

Amenorrhoea, primary or secondary, requires specialist endocrinological diagnosis. Where the cause is failure of hormone production, cyclical replacement therapy is indicated.

Menorrhagia can be associated with both ovulatory and anovulatory ovarian cycles. It is important to distinguish the menstrual consequences of each cycle. *Ovulatory* ovarian cycles give rise to *regular* menstrual cycles, whereas *anovulatory* cycles result in *irregular* menstruation or, extremely, amenorrhoea. This distinction is critical in management.

Both ovulatory and anovulatory cycles can give rise to excessive menstrual loss in the absence of any other abnormality, so-called 'dysfunctional uterine bleeding'. Endocrine disorders do not cause excessive menstrual loss, with the exception of the endocrine consequences of anovulation.

Equally, haemostatic disorders are rare causes of menorrhagia. One consequence of excessive menstrual loss is iron-deficiency anaemia. In the Western world, menorrhagia is the commonest cause of iron-deficiency anaemia.

Medical treatment of menorrhagia is either *non-hormonal* or *hormonal* therapy. As there is no hormonal defect, the use of hormonal therapy does not correct an underlying disorder but merely imposes an external control of the cycle. For many women, cycle control is as important an issue as the degree of menorrhagia.

The two main first-line treatments for menorrhagia associated with ovulatory cycles are non-hormonal, namely *tranexamic acid* (an antifibrinolytic) and a non-steroidal anti-inflammatory drug (NSAID), e.g. *mefenamic acid* 500 mg when the blood loss becomes heavy, followed by 250 mg three times daily for 3 days. The effectiveness of these treatments has been shown in randomised trials and reported in systematic reviews of treatment. Tranexamic acid reduces menstrual loss by about one-half, and NSAIDs reduce it by about one-third. Both have the advantage of being taken only during menstruation itself and are particularly useful in women who either do not require contraception or do not wish to use a hormonal therapy. They are also of value in treating excessive menstrual blood loss associated with the use of non-hormonal intrauterine contraceptive devices.

Hormonal therapy should be regarded as a third-choice treatment only in women not requiring contraception as a parallel objective. Progestogens are effective only when given for 21 days in each cycle. Combined oral contraceptives are useful for anovulatory bleeding as they impose a cycle. The levonorgestrel-releasing intrauterine system (Mirena) is advocated as an alternative to surgery.

The timing of menstruation. Sometimes there are pressing reasons to prevent menstruation at the normal time, but obviously this cannot be done at the last moment.

Menstruation can be *postponed* by giving oral *norethisterone* 5 mg three times daily, starting 3 days before the expected onset; bleeding occurs 2–3 days after withdrawal. Users of the combined oral contraceptive pill (having a 7-day break) can simply continue with active pills where they would normally stop for 7 days.

Although there is no evidence that harm follows such manoeuvres, it is obviously imprudent to practise them frequently.

Note. These uses of progestogen should not be undertaken if there is any possibility of pregnancy.

Endometriosis. Medical treatments for endometriosis have focused on the hormonal alteration of the menstrual cycle in an attempt to produce a pseudo-pregnancy, pseudo-menopause or chronic anovulation. Each of these situations is believed to cause a suboptimal milieu for the growth and maintenance of endometrium and, by extension, of implants of endometriosis. *Danazol* 600–800 mg/day causes anovulation by attenuating the mid-cycle surge of LH secretion, inhibiting multiple enzymes in the steroidogenic pathway, and increasing plasma free testosterone concentrations.

Medroxyprogesterone causes the decidualisation of endometrial tissue, with eventual atrophy.

Adverse effects occur at low (20–30 mg/day) or high (100 mg/day) dose, and include abnormal uterine bleeding, nausea, breast tenderness, fluid retention and depression. These resolve after discontinuation of the drug.

Gestrinone 5–10 mg/week is an antiprogestational steroid that causes a decline in the concentrations of oestrogen and progesterone receptors, and a 50% decline in plasma estradiol concentrations. Androgenic adverse effects, such as a deepening of the voice, hirsutism and clitoral hypertrophy, are potentially irreversible. A combination of an *oestrogen and a progestogen* induces a hormonal pseudo-pregnancy. The oral contraceptive is used either continuously or cyclically (21 active pills followed by 7 days of placebo). Both regimens are effective; the amenorrhea of continuous administration is advantageous for women with dysmenorrhoea.

Gonadotrophin-releasing hormone (GnRH) agonists diminish the secretion of FSH and LH, resulting in hypogonadotrophic hypogonadism, endometrial atrophy and amenorrhoea. The GnRH agonist can be given intranasally, subcutaneously or intramuscularly, with a frequency of administration ranging from twice daily to every 3 months. The unwanted effects are the menopausal-type symptoms of hypo-oestrogenism (such as transient vaginal bleeding, hot flushes, vaginal dryness) and can be prevented by concurrent administration of HRT in post-menopausal doses.

Although most treatments for endometriosis are directed at the hormones themselves, the symptoms can be also treated directly. NSAIDs such as diclofenac, ibuprofen and mefenamic acid are often given to relieve the pain associated with endometriosis. These drugs are frequently the first-line treatment in women with pelvic pain whose cause has not yet been proved to be endometriosis.

Dysmenorrhoea is due to uterine contractions resulting from excess prostaglandins in the uterus during ovulatory cycles. It can be treated by suppressing ovulation (using the combined pill or norethisterone) or by using inhibitors of prostaglandin synthesis, e.g. aspirin, indometacin, naproxen. The analgesic prostaglandin synthase inhibitor (NSAID) may need to be given for several days before menstruation, or only at the time of the pain.

Premenstrual tension syndrome may be due to an imbalance of natural oestrogen and progesterone secretion, but knowledge of the syndrome remains imprecise. Psychosocial factors can be important. Placebo effects are strong. Drugs are not necessarily the preferred treatment.

Cyclical breast pain or mastalgia, when severe, may respond to continuous use of gamolenic acid (Efamast) by mouth; it is an essential unsaturated fatty acid for cell membranes (patients have low concentrations); it may act by reducing cellular uptake of prolactin and ovarian hormones. Danazol and bromocriptine also help.

Myometrium

Oxytocics, i.e. drugs that hasten childbirth, and prostaglandins induce uterine contractions. They are used to induce abortion, to induce or augment labour, and to minimise blood loss from the placental site.

Oxytocics

Oxytocin is a peptide hormone of the posterior pituitary gland. It stimulates the contractions of the pregnant uterus, which becomes much more sensitive to it at term. Patients with posterior pituitary disease (diabetes insipidus) can go into labour normally.

Oxytocin is released reflexly from the pituitary following suckling (also by manual stimulation of the nipple) and produces an almost immediate contraction of the myoepithelium of the breast; it can be used to enhance milk ejection (nasal spray). The only other clinically important effect is on the blood pressure, which may fall if an overdose is given.

Synthetic oxytocin (Syntocinon) is pure and is not contaminated with vasopressin as is the natural product, which is obsolete.

Oxytocin is used intravenously in the induction of labour and sometimes for uterine inertia, haemorrhage or during abortion. It produces, almost immediately, rhythmic contractions with relaxation between, i.e. it mimics normal uterine activity.

The decision to use oxytocin requires special skill. It has a $t_{1/2}$ of 6 min and is given by intravenous infusion using a pump (see below); it must be closely supervised; the dose is adjusted by results; overdose can cause uterine tetany and even rupture. The utmost care is required.

Oxytocin is structurally close to vasopressin, and it is no surprise that it also has antidiuretic activity (see p. 481). Serious water intoxication can occur with prolonged intravenous infusions, especially where accompanied by large volumes of fluid. The association of oxytocin with neonatal jaundice appears to be due to increased erythrocyte fragility causing haemolysis.

Oxytocin has been supplanted by the ergot alkaloid, *ergometrine,* as prime treatment of postpartum haemorrhage.

Ergometrine is used to contract the uterus. It is an α-adrenoceptor and dopamine receptor agonist and acts almost immediately when injected intravenously. The uterus is stimulated at all times, but is much more sensitive in late pregnancy (see also ergotamine, p. 310).

Ergometrine and oxytocin differ in their actions on the uterus. In moderate doses, oxytocin produces slow generalised contractions with full relaxation in between; ergometrine produces faster contractions superimposed on a tonic contraction. High doses of both substances produce sustained tonic contraction. It will be seen, therefore, that *oxytocin* is more suited to *induction of labour* and *ergometrine* to the prevention and treatment of *postpartum haemorrhage*, the incidence of which is reduced by its routine prophylactic use (generally intramuscularly).

There are advantages in a mixture of oxytocin and ergometrine (Syntometrine).

Prostaglandins

(For a general account of the prostaglandins see Ch. 16.)

Prostaglandins that soften the uterine cervix (by an action on collagen) and have a powerful oxytocic effect include:

Dinoprost (prostaglandin $F_2\alpha$; $PGF_2\alpha$) (Prostin F_2 alpha) and *dinoprostone* (prostaglandin E_2; PGE_2) (Prostin E_2). They are used to induce labour and to terminate pregnancy, including missed or partial abortion and in the treatment of hydatidiform mole; they are given by intra- or extra-amniotic injection, by vaginal tablet, or intracervical gel, by intravenous infusion or by mouth. Their safe and effective use (including choice of route) requires special skill.

Adverse effects include vomiting, diarrhoea, headache, pyrexia and local tissue reaction.

Gemeprost (prostaglandin E_1 analogue) (Cervagem) is used intravaginally to soften the cervix before operative procedures in the first trimester of pregnancy and for abortion, alone and in combination with an antiprogestogen (mifepristone, see p. 646).

Carboprost (prostaglandin F_2 analogue) is used for postpartum haemorrhage (resistant to ergometrine and oxytocin) for its oxytocin action. It is highly effective. *Adverse effects* include hypertension, asthma and pulmonary oedema.

Induction of abortion

Gemeprost, administered vaginally as pessaries, is the preferred prostaglandin for the medical induction of late therapeutic abortion. Gemeprost ripens and softens the cervix before surgical abortion, particularly in primigravida. *Misoprostol* by mouth or by vaginal administration, or gemeprost, may be given to induce medical abortion (an unlicensed indication in the UK). Pretreatment with *mifepristone* (see p. 646) can facilitate the process, by sensitising the uterus to the prostaglandin so that abortion occurs in a shorter time and with a lower dose of prostaglandin.

Induction and augmentation of labour

Oxytocin is administered by slow intravenous infusion as below, usually in conjunction with amniotomy, and *dinoprostone* by vaginal tablets, pessaries and vaginal gels. *Misoprostol* may be used orally or vaginally to induce labour (an unlicensed indication in the UK).

The UK National Institute for Health and Clinical Excellence has recommended the following:

- Dinoprostone is preferable to oxytocin for induction of labour in women with intact membranes, regardless of parity or cervical favourability.
- Dinoprostone and oxytocin are equally effective for the induction of labour in women with ruptured membranes, regardless of parity or cervical favourability.
- Intravaginal dinoprostone preparations are preferable to intracervical preparations.
- Oxytocin should not be started for 6 h following administration of vaginal prostaglandins.
- When used to induce labour, the recommended dose of oxytocin by intravenous infusion is initially 0.001–0.002 units/min, increased at intervals of at least 30 min until a maximum of three to four contractions occurs every 10 min (0.012 units/min is often adequate); the maximum recommended rate is 0.032 units/min (licensed max. 0.02 units/min).

Prevention and treatment of uterine haemorrhage

Bleeding due to incomplete abortion can be controlled with *ergometrine* and *oxytocin* (Syntometrine) given intramuscularly. Their combination is more effective in early pregnancy than either drug alone.

For the routine management of the third stage of labour, *ergometrine* 500 µg with oxytocin 5 units (Syntometrine 1 mL) is given by intramuscular injection on delivery of the anterior shoulder or, at the latest, immediately after the baby is delivered. In pre-eclampsia, *oxytocin* may be given alone by intramuscular injection. These regimens are also used for the treatment of postpartum haemorrhage. The same drugs may be given intravenously for excessive uterine bleeding caused by uterine atony. *Carboprost* is an alternative for haemorrhage unresponsive to ergometrine and oxytocin.

Uterine relaxants

β_2-Adrenoceptor agonists relax the uterus and are given by intravenous infusion by obstetricians to inhibit premature labour, e.g. *isoxsuprine, terbutaline, ritodrine, salbutamol*. Their use is complicated by the expected cardiovascular effects, including tachycardia, hypotension. Less easy to explain, but more devastating on occasion to the patient, is severe left ventricular failure. The combination of fluid overload (due to the vehicle) and increased oxygen demand by the heart are possible factors; the risk is higher in multiple pregnancy, pre-existing cardiac disease or maternal infection. It is important to administer the β_2 agonist with minimum fluid volume using a syringe pump with 5% dextrose (not saline) as diluent, and to monitor the patient closely for signs of fluid overload.

The dose of *ritodrine* for intravenous administration is: initially 50 µg/min, increased gradually according to response by 50 µg/min every 10 min until contractions stop or maternal heart rate reaches 140 beats per min; continue for 12–48 h after contractions cease (usual rate 150–350 µg/min).

Guide to further reading

Amin, A., 2011. New drugs for hyponatraemia: evidence is lacking that they are better than cheaper standard treatment. Br. Med. J. 342, 559–560.

Amin, A., Sam, A.H., Meeran, K., 2014. Glucocorticoid replacement. Pending further studies of new agents, the old treatments are still the best. Br. Med. J. 349, g4843.

Banerjee, A., Wynne, K., Tan, T., et al., 2009. High dose cabergoline therapy for resistant macroprolactinoma during pregnancy. Clin. Endocrinol. (Oxf) 70, 812–813.

Barrett-Connor, E.L., Mosca, L., Collins, P., et al., 2006. Effects of raloxifene on cardiovascular events and breast cancer in postmenopausal women. N. Engl. J. Med. 355, 125–137.

Coombs, N.J., Taylor, R., Wilcken, N., Boyages, J., 2005. Hormone replacement therapy and breast cancer: estimate of risk. Br. Med. J. 331, 347–349.

Jayasena, C.N., Wujanto, C., Donaldson, M., et al., 2008. Measurement of basal growth hormone (GH) is a useful test of disease activity in treated acromegalic patients. Clin. Endocrinol. (Oxf) 68, 36–41.

Martin, N.M., Dhillo, W.S., Banerjee, A., et al., 2006. Comparison of the dexamethasone-suppressed corticotropin-releasing hormone test and low-dose dexamethasone suppression test in the diagnosis of Cushing's syndrome. J. Clin. Endocrinol. Metab. 91, 2582–2586.

Martin, N.M., Tan, T., Meeran, K., 2009. Dopamine agonists and hyperprolactinaemia. Br. Med. J. 338, b381.

Melmed, S., 2006. Medical progress: acromegaly. N. Engl. J. Med. 355, 2558–2573.

Peterson, H.B., Curtis, K.M., 2005. Long-acting methods of contraception. N. Engl. J. Med. 353, 2169–2175.

Williams, E., Choudhury, S.M., Tan, T.M., Meeran, K., 2016. Prednisolone replacement therapy mimics the Circadian rhythm more closely than other glucocorticoids. J. Appl. Lab. Med. 1, 152–161.

Chapter | **39** |

Vitamins, calcium, bone

Chrysothemis Brown

SYNOPSIS

In general, the pharmacological aspects of vitamins appear here. The nutritional aspects, physiological function, sources, daily requirements and deficiency syndromes (primary and secondary) are to be found in any textbook of medicine.

- **Vitamin A: retinol.**
- **Vitamin B: complex.**
- **Vitamin C: ascorbic acid.**
- **Vitamin D, calcium, parathyroid hormone, calcitonin, bisphosphonates.**
- **Treatment of calcium and bone disorders.**
- **Vitamin E: tocopherol.**

Vitamins[1] are substances that are essential for normal metabolism but are supplied chiefly in the diet.

Humans cannot synthesise vitamins in the body except some vitamin D in the skin and nicotinamide from tryptophan. Lack of a particular vitamin may lead to a specific deficiency syndrome. This may be *primary* (inadequate diet) or *secondary*, due to failure of absorption (intestinal abnormality or chronic diarrhoea) or to increased metabolic need (growth, pregnancy, lactation, hyperthyroidism).

Vitamin deficiencies are commonly multiple, and complex clinical pictures occur. There are numerous single and multivitamin preparations available to provide prophylaxis and therapy.

Recently, there has been great interest in the suggestion that subclinical vitamin deficiencies may be a cause of chronic disease and liability to infection. This idea has prompted a number of clinical trials examining the potential benefit of vitamin supplementation in the prevention of cancer, cardiovascular disease and other common diseases. With the exception of vitamin D, there is little robust evidence to support this claim and, for most consumers, over-the-counter vitamin preparations are probably of little more than placebo value. Fortunately, most vitamins are comparatively non-toxic; however, prolonged administration of *vitamin A* and *vitamin D* can have serious ill-effects.

In addition to maintaining adequate nutritional levels, a number of vitamins can be used at pharmacological doses for therapy.

Vitamins fall into two groups:

- *Water-soluble vitamins*: the B group and vitamin C.
- *Fat-soluble vitamins*: A, D, E and K.

Vitamin A: retinol

Vitamin A is a generic term embracing substances having the biological actions of retinol and related substances (called *retinoids*). The principal functions of retinol are to:

- sustain normal epithelia
- promote corneal and conjunctival development
- form retinal photochemicals
- enhance immune functions
- protect against infections and probably some cancers.

Deficiency of retinol leads to xerophthalmia, squamous metaplasia, hyperkeratosis and impairment of the immune system.

Therapeutic uses

Retinol and derivatives provide therapeutic benefit in a number of clinical areas.

---

[1] The term was coined by Casimir Funk in 1912 from the Latin *vita* meaning life and the (mistaken) belief that the organic compounds involved were amines. See: Hardy A 2004 Historical keywords. Vitamin. Lancet 364:323.

Psoriasis

Tazorotene, a topical retinoid, is effective in the treatment of chronic stable plaque psoriasis. Skin irritation is common, making it unsuitable for the treatment of inflammatory forms of psoriasis. The 0.05% cream is better tolerated than 0.1% although less effective. *Acitretin* is a retinoic acid derivative ($t_{1/2}$ 48 h) that is used orally for severe psoriasis. The dose range is 25 mg on alternate days to 50 mg daily (see p. 271, as well as other disorders of keratinisation).

Acne

Tretinoin is retinoic acid and is used for acne by topical application (see p. 283). *Isotretinoin* is a retinoic acid isomer ($t_{1/2}$ 20 h) given orally for acne (see p. 283). It is also effective for preventing second tumours in patients following treatment for primary squamous cell carcinoma of the head and neck.

Acute promyelocytic leukaemia

Tretinoin can be used to induce remission in conjunction with chemotherapy in acute promyelocytic leukaemia, a subgroup of acute myeloid leukaemia (AML) involving chromosomal translocation of the retinoic acid receptor-alpha gene. Initially, it proved remarkably successful, but the high doses given caused the fatal 'differentiation syndrome' (previously called 'retinoic acid syndrome'; respiratory distress, fever and hypotension), and the duration of treatment is now shorter.

Vitamin A deficiency

Primary deficiency is common in developing countries. *Retinol* is used to prevent and treat deficiency; 1 microgram = 3.3 IU ($t_{1/2}$ 7–14 days). For prevention of deficiency in susceptible individuals, supplements are given at 4–6-monthly intervals. Dosing is according to age. More frequent doses are required for treatment of xerophthalmia. Secondary deficiency resulting from fat malabsorption is seen with pancreatic insufficiency and disorders of the gastrointestinal tract. Vitamin A supplementation at pharmacological doses is standard for patients with cystic fibrosis. This can result in chronic toxicity, and serum retinol levels should be monitored.

Adverse effects

Acute toxicity occurs in adults with a single dose of more than 600 000 IU/day. Symptoms include headache, nausea, vomiting and drowsiness. Travellers have experienced vitamin A toxicity by eating the livers of Arctic carnivores.

Chronic toxicity occurs with prolonged high intake (in children 25 000–50 000 IU/day, 10 times the recommended daily allowance, RDA). A diagnostic sign is the presence of painful tender swellings on long bones. Anorexia, skin lesions, hair loss, hepatosplenomegaly, papilloedema, bleeding and general malaise also occur. Vitamin A accumulates in liver and fat, and effects take weeks to wear off. Chronic overdose also makes the biological membranes and the outer layer of the skin more liable to peel.

Teratogenicity. Vitamin A and its derivatives are teratogenic at pharmacological doses (for precautions, see use in acne and psoriasis, p. 283). Supplements should not exceed 8000 IU (2400 µg) per day.

Vitamin B complex

A number of widely differing substances are now, for convenience, classed as the 'vitamin B complex'. Those used for pharmacotherapy include the following:

Thiamine (B_1). Deficiency is associated with three distinct conditions: Wernicke–Korsakoff syndrome, beriberi and Leigh's syndrome. The UK RDA of thiamine is 1 mg for men and 0.8 mg for women. It is given orally for nutritional purposes, but intravenously in serious emergencies, e.g. Wernicke–Korsakoff syndrome. Give the injection over 10 min (or intramuscularly); note that it can cause anaphylactic shock.

Cobalamins (B_{12}). See Chapter 20.

Folic acid. See Chapter 30.

Pyridoxine (B_6) is a coenzyme in the metabolic transformation of many amino acids, including decarboxylation and transamination. The UK RDA of vitamin B_6 is 1.4 mg for men and 1.2 mg for women. As *pharmacotherapy*, pyridoxine is given to treat certain pyridoxine-dependent inborn errors of metabolism, e.g. homocystinuria, hereditary sideroblastic anaemia and primary hyperoxaluria. Deficiency may be induced by drugs such as isoniazid, hydralazine and penicillamine; pyridoxine 10 mg/day prevents the development of peripheral neuritis without interfering with therapeutic action.

Pyridoxine, in doses sometimes exceeding 100 mg/day, has found use for a variety of conditions including premenstrual syndrome and nausea in pregnancy.

Niacin (nicotinic acid, B_3) is converted to nicotinamide, and subsequently to nicotinamide adenine dinucleotide (NAD) and nicotinamide adenine dinucleotide phosphate (NADPH), the cofactors that are essential for the oxidation–reduction reactions that comprise tissue respiration. In addition, the sirtuin family of histone deacetylases (HDAC) are dependent on NAD, and nicotinamide is therefore able to act as an epigenetic modifier, preventing the formation of heterochromatin at certain genes. *Nicotinamide* is used for nutritional purposes. Pellagra resulting from dietary deficiency of niacin is rarely seen in developed countries. Causes other than dietary include alcoholism, carcinoid syndrome and Hartnup disease. *Nicotinic acid* at pharmacological doses is used for the treatment of some hyperlipidaemias (see p. 468). Adverse effects include peripheral vasodilatation, unpleasant flushing, itching and fainting. Studies are currently evaluating the therapeutic use of nicotinamide as an HDAC inhibitor in a number of disease settings including cancer and Friedrich's ataxia.

Vitamin C: ascorbic acid

Vitamin C is a powerful *reducing agent* (antioxidant) and is an essential cofactor and substrate in a number of enzymatic reactions, including collagen synthesis and noradrenaline synthesis. It also functions as an antioxidant, mopping up free radicals produced endogenously or in the environment, e.g. cigarette smoke (see vitamin E). There has been considerable interest in using vitamin C as an antioxidative agent to reduce oxidation of low-density lipoproteins (LDL) in atherosclerosis and prevent formation of carcinogens to reduce the risk of cancer. However, randomised trials have not shown any beneficial effect thus far of vitamin C on either cancer incidence or primary or secondary prevention of coronary heart disease.

Indications

- The prevention and cure of scurvy.
- Methaemoglobinaemia.

Scurvy

Deficiency of ascorbic acid leads to *scurvy,* which is characterised by petechial haemorrhages, haematomas, bleeding gums (if teeth are present) and anaemia.

Methaemoglobinaemia

A reducing substance is needed to convert the methaemoglobin (ferric iron) back to oxyhaemoglobin (ferrous iron) whenever enough has formed seriously to impair the oxygen-carrying capacity of the blood. Ascorbic acid is non-toxic (it acts by direct reduction) but is less effective than *methylene blue* (methylthioninium chloride). Both can be given orally, intravenously or intramuscularly. Excessive doses of methylene blue can cause methaemoglobinaemia (by stimulating NADPH-dependent enzymes).

Methaemoglobinaemia may be induced by oxidising drugs: sulphonamides, nitrites, nitrates (may also occur in drinking water), primaquine, -caine local anaesthetics, dapsone, nitrofurantoin, nitroprusside, vitamin K analogues, chlorates, aniline and nitrobenzene. Where symptoms are severe enough to warrant urgent treatment, methylene blue given intravenously at 1–2 mg/kg gives response within 30 min. Patients should be monitored for rebound methaemoglobinaemia. Methylene blue turns the urine blue, and high concentrations can irritate the urinary tract, so that fluid intake should be high when large doses are used. Methlyene blue should not be administered to patients with glucose-6-phosphate dehydrogenase (G6PD) deficiency since its action is dependent on NADPH produced by G6PD. In addition to being ineffective in this circumstance, it may induce haemolysis. Ascorbic acid is inadequate for the treatment of acute methaemoglobinaemia requiring treatment.

Congenital methaemogobinaemia can be treated long term with either oral methylene blue or ascorbic acid with partial effect.

Adverse effects

High doses may cause sleep disturbances, headaches and gut upsets. Ascorbic acid is eliminated partly in the urine unchanged and partly metabolised to oxalate. Doses above 4 g/day increase urinary oxalate concentration, and there is a potential risk of renal oxalate stones with chronic ascorbic acid administration. Intravenous ascorbic acid may precipitate a haemolytic attack in subjects with G6PD deficiency.

Vitamin D, calcium, parathyroid hormone, calcitonin, bisphosphonates, bone

Vitamin D is closely interrelated with calcium homeostasis and bone metabolism, and these topics are therefore discussed together.

Vitamin D

Vitamin D comprises a number of structurally related sterol compounds having similar biological properties (but different potencies) in that they prevent or cure the vitamin D–deficiency diseases, rickets and osteomalacia. The most relevant form of vitamin D is vitamin D_3 (cholecalciferol). This is made by ultraviolet irradiation of 7-dehydrocholesterol in the skin. It is also absorbed in the intestinal tract; however, few foods contain significant levels of vitamin D (Fig. 39.1). Vitamin D_2 *(ergocalciferol)* is made by ultraviolet irradiation

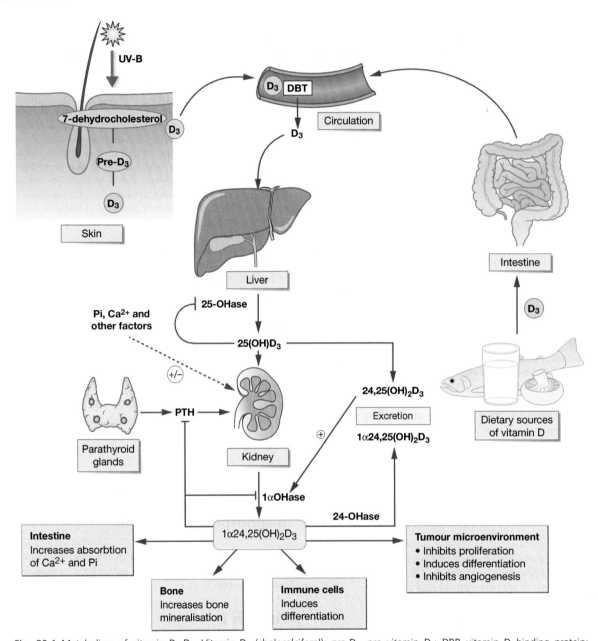

Fig. 39.1 Metabolism of vitamin D. D₃, Vitamin D₃ (cholecalciferol); pre-D₃, pre–vitamin D₃; DBP, vitamin D–binding protein; 25-OHase, liver 25-hydroxylase; 25(OH)D₃, 25-hydroxycholecalciferol (25(OH)D₃; 1-OHase, 25-hydroxyvitamin D₃-1-hydroxylase; 1,25(OH)2D₃, calcitriol; PTH, parathyroid hormone. *(From Deeb K K, Trump D L, Johnson C S 2007 Vitamin D signalling pathways in cancer: potential for anticancer therapeutics. Nature Reviews Cancer 7:684 with permission.)*

of ergosterol in plants. This is not the naturally occurring form.

Vitamin D_3 (and D_2) undergo two successive hydroxylations: first in the liver to form 25-hydroxyvitamin D and second in the proximal tubules of the kidney (under the control of parathyroid hormone, PTH) to form $1\alpha,25$-dihydroxyvitamin D_3 (*calcitriol*), the most *physiologically active* form of vitamin D.

There exist also a variety of synthetic vitamin D analogues, developed to treat vitamin D deficiency and hypoparathyroidism. The vitamin D derivative 1α-hydroxycholecalciferol (*alfacalcidol*) requires only hepatic hydroxylation to become calcitriol. The usual adult maintenance dose, 0.25–1 microgram/day, indicates its potency.

Other 1α-hydroxylated vitamin D analogues include *paricalcitol*. In addition, a structural variant of vitamins D_2 and D_3, dihydrotachysterol (ATIO, Tachyrol), is also biologically activated by hepatic 25-hydroxylation. All are effective in renal failure as they bypass the defective renal hydroxylation stage.

Pharmacokinetics

Alfacalcidol and *dihydrotachysterol* have a fast onset and short duration of clinical effect (days) which renders them suitable for rapid adjustment of plasma calcium, e.g. in hypoparathyroidism. Such factors are not relevant to the slower adjustment of plasma calcium (weeks) with vitamins D_2 and D_3 in the ordinary management of vitamin D deficiency.

Actions are complex. Vitamin D promotes the active transport of calcium and phosphate in the gut (increased absorption) and renal tubule (reduced excretion), and thus controls, with PTH, the plasma calcium concentration and the mineralisation of bone (see Fig. 39.1). After a dose of D_2 or D_3, there is a lag of about 21 h before the intestinal effect begins; this is probably due to the time needed for its metabolic conversion to the more active forms. With the biologically more active *calcitriol*, the lag is only 2 h.

A large single dose of vitamin D has biological effects for as long as 6 months (because of metabolism and storage). Thus, the agent is cumulative (see *toxicity*).

Indications

- The prevention and cure of rickets of all kinds and osteomalacia (vitamin D deficiency).
- Osteoporosis.
- Hypoparathyroidism.
- Psoriasis.
- CKD-MBD (renal osteodystrophy).
- The prevention of acute respiratory tract infections.

Vitamin D deficiency

This can be treated with a variety of vitamin D analogues. Selecting the appropriate preparation requires a knowledge of the underlying aetiology. There are no absolute criteria for vitamin D deficiency; however, serum 25(OH)-vitamin D_3 levels are used as a guide to vitamin D levels, and there is a general consensus that a 25(OH)D concentration of 50–75–nmol/L reflects insufficiency, and concentrations of less than 50–nmol/L indicate deficiency.

Although rickets due to *primary* vitamin D deficiency is rare in developed countries, subclinical vitamin D *deficiency* and vitamin D *insufficiency* are now recognised to be extremely common in the UK and in other populations with limited exposure to sunlight, particularly in individuals with increased skin pigmentation, in whom greater amounts of sun exposure are required for adequate synthesis, or in those with excessive body cover. There is accumulating evidence that subclinical vitamin D deficiency has adverse effects on health. Vitamin D deficiency in pregnancy is a significant public health issue: babies born to mothers with low vitamin D levels are at increased risk of neonatal hypocalcaemia and other vitamin D deficiency–related symptoms. Vitamin D deficiency can be prevented in susceptible individuals by taking an oral supplement of *ergocalciferol* 20 μg (800 units i.u.) daily. All pregnant and lactating women should receive vitamin D supplementation. Breast milk contains negligible amounts of vitamin D, thus breast-fed infants receiving less than 500 mL of formula should be supplemented with vitamin D: *Abidec* and *Dalivit* are two paediatric multivitamin preparations, both containing cholecalciferol 400 IU.

For the treatment of simple nutritional vitamin D *deficiency*, oral doses of either *cholecalciferol* or *ergocalciferol*, 10 000 units i.u. daily or 60 000 units i.u. weekly, should be given for 12 weeks. Infants and children should receive 1000–5000 units of vitamin D_3 daily, depending on age (usually *ergocalciferol*), for 12 weeks. Where there are concerns with regards to compliance, 'Stoss' therapy – a single dose of intramuscular *ergocalciferol* 500–1000 units i.u. – can be given. Nutritional vitamin D *insufficiency* can be treated with 800–1000 units i.u. daily for 12 weeks. 25(OH)-vitamin D_3 levels should be measured after 12 weeks of treatment. *Alfacalcidol* should not be given for the treatment of vitamin D deficiency as it does not replete vitamin D stores.

Vitamin D deficiency resulting from *intestinal malabsorption or chronic liver disease* usually requires vitamin D in pharmacological doses, e.g. *ergocalciferol* tablets up to 50 000 units i.u. daily. The maximum antirachitic effect of vitamin D occurs after 1–2 months, and the plasma calcium concentration reflects the dosage given days or weeks before. Frequent changes of dose are therefore not required. Vitamin D deficiency resulting from *chronic renal failure* is discussed below (see renal osteodystrophy).

Epileptic patients taking enzyme-inducing drugs long term can develop osteomalacia (adults) or rickets (children). This may arise from the accelerated metabolism, increasing vitamin D breakdown and causing deficiency, or from inhibition of one of the hydroxylations that increase biological activity.

Osteoporosis

Calcitriol is licensed for the management of post-menopausal osteoporosis (see below). However its use for this indication is associated with a fairly high incidence of hypercalcaemia and vitamin D3 is preferred.

Hypoparathyroidism

The hypocalcaemia of hypoparathyroidism requires 1000–1500 mg of elemental calcium daily in divided doses as well as vitamin D. Ergocalciferol may be required in doses up to 100 000 units i.u. daily to achieve normocalcaemia, but the dose is difficult to titrate and hypercalcaemia from overdose may take weeks to resolve. *Alfacalcidol* (0.5–2.0 μg daily) or *calcitriol* (0.5–1.0 μg daily) are therefore preferred, as their rapid onset and offset of action makes for easier control of plasma calcium levels.

Psoriasis

Calcipotriol and *tacalcitol* are vitamin D analogues available as creams or ointments for the treatment of psoriasis (see p. 278).

Renal osteodystrophy

(See below.)

Prevention of acute respiratory tract infections

A meta-analysis of vitamin D supplementation for the prevention of acute respiratory tract infections demonstrated significant effects of vitamin D supplementation in patients with serum levels <25 nmol/L. A number of studies are currently evaluating the benefit of vitamin D supplementation on other infectious diseases.

Adverse effects

Vitamin D *toxicity* has been reported in children accidentally overdosed on vitamin D supplements. Symptoms of overdosage are due mainly to an excessive increase in plasma calcium concentration and include anorexia, nausea and vomiting, diarrhoea, constipation, weight loss, polyuria and thirst. Other long-term effects include ectopic calcification almost anywhere in the body, renal damage and an increased calcium output in the urine; renal calculi may form. Recent research has suggested that the safe upper limit of vitamin D therapy be revised. It was previously considered dangerous to exceed 10 000 units i.u. daily of vitamin D in an adult for more than about 12 weeks; however, it has now become apparent that such doses are required to render a vitamin D–deficient individual replete. In general, use of vitamin D at pharmacological doses requires monitoring of plasma calcium.

Treatment of calcium and bone disorders

Hypocalcaemia

In *acute hypocalcaemia* requiring systemic therapy, give a slow intravenous infusion of 10 mL of 10% *calcium gluconate injection* over 10 min. This should not be given at a faster rate because of the risk of cardiac arrhythmias and arrest. Correction of hypocalcaemia is temporary, and this should be followed by a continuous intravenous infusion containing ten 10 mL ampoules of 10% calcium gluconate in 1 L of 0.9% saline given at an initial infusion rate of 50 mL/h. Plasma calcium should be monitored and the rate adjusted accordingly. Oral calcium therapy should be initiated meanwhile and the intravenous infusion stopped once the oral agents take effect. Avoid infusing with solutions containing bicarbonate or phosphate, which cause calcium to precipitate. Intramuscular injection is contraindicated as it is painful and causes tissue necrosis. Calcium glubionate (Calcium Sandoz) can be given by deep intramuscular injection in adults. Concurrent hypomagnesaemia should be corrected as hypocalcaemia is resistant to treatment without normal serum magnesium levels.

Treatment of *chronic hypocalcaemia* is with 1500–2000 mg of oral elemental calcium daily in divided doses, as either *calcium carbonate* or *calcium citrate*. Additional treatment depends on the cause. Hypocalcaemia secondary to vitamin D deficiency should be treated with vitamin D as described above, and there are preparations which combine calcium tablets with cholecalciferol. Hypocalcaemia secondary to hypoparathyroidism requires alfacalcidol or calcitriol as PTH is required for hydroxylation of 25-hydroxy-vitamin D_3, thus ergocalciferol or cholecalciferol have reduced efficacy.

Adverse effects of intravenous calcium may be very dangerous. An early sign is a tingling feeling in the mouth and of warmth spreading over the body. Serious effects are those on the heart, which mimic and synergise with digitalis, and it is advisable to avoid intravenous calcium administration in any patient taking a digitalis glycoside (except in severe symptomatic hypocalcaemia). The effect of calcium on the heart is antagonised by potassium, and similarly the toxic effects of hyperkalaemia in acute renal failure may be to an extent counteracted by calcium.

Hypercalcaemia

Treatment of severe acute hypercalcaemia causing symptoms is needed whether or not the cause can be removed; generally a plasma concentration of 3 mmol/L (12 mg/100 mL) needs urgent treatment if there is also clinical evidence of toxicity (individual tolerance varies greatly).

Temporary measures

After taking account of the patient's cardiac and renal function, the following measures may be employed selectively:

- *Physiological saline solution* is important, firstly to correct sodium and water deficit, and secondly to promote sodium-linked calcium diuresis in the proximal renal tubule. Initially, 500 mL 0.9% saline i.v. should be given over 4 h and then adjusted to maintain urine output at 100–150 mL/h until the plasma Ca^{2+} level falls below 3.0 mmol/L and the oral intake is adequate. The regimen requires careful attention to fluid and electrolyte balance, particularly in patients with renal insufficiency secondary to hypercalcaemia or heart failure who are unable to excrete excess sodium. The use of furosemide to enhance renal Ca^{2+} excretion has been largely abandoned owing to the exacerbation of electrolyte disturbances and the increased availability of newer agents.
- *Bisphosphonates* are the agents of choice in moderate to severe hypercalcaemia. There are a number of bisphosphonates licensed for this indication, but *pamidronate* and *zoledronic acid* are the most widely used agents. *Pamidronate*[2] is infused according to the schedule in Table 39.1; it is active in a wide variety of hypercalcaemic disorders. A fall in the serum calcium concentration begins within the first day, reaches a nadir in 5–6 days and lasts for 20–30 days. *Zoledronic acid* has the advantage of being more potent, and it can be administered over a shorter time (4 mg over 15 min vs. 2 h). It is a convenient regimen for patients with hypercalcaemia of malignancy, where repeat courses may be required every 3–4 weeks.
- *Calcitonin.* When the hypercalcaemia is at least partly due to mobilisation from bone, calcitonin (4 units/kg) can be used to inhibit bone resorption, and may enhance urinary excretion of calcium. The effect develops in a few hours, but responsiveness is lost over a few days owing to tachyphylaxis. Calcitonin is not as effective as the bisphosphonates; however, its shorter onset of action makes it a valuable agent for initial management of hypercalcaemia until the peak onset of action of the bisphosphonate at 2–4 days.
- An *adrenocortical steroid*, e.g. prednisolone 20–40 mg/day orally, is effective in particular situations; it reduces the hypercalcaemia of hypervitaminosis D (which is due to excessive intestinal absorption of calcium either secondary to intoxication or granulomatous disease, e.g. sarcoidosis). A corticosteroid may be effective in the hypercalcaemia of malignancy where the disease itself is responsive, e.g. myeloma of lymphoma. Patients with hyperparathyroidism do not respond.
- *Dialysis* is quick and effective and is likely to be needed in severe cases or in those with renal failure.

The above measures are only temporary, giving time to tackle the cause.

Longer-term treatment

Sodium cellulose phosphate (Calcisorb) is an oral ion exchange substance with a particular affinity for calcium which is bound in the gut, and the complex eliminated in the faeces. It is effective for patients who over-absorb dietary calcium and develop hypercalciuria and renal stones.

Inorganic phosphate, e.g. sodium acid phosphate (Phosphate Sandoz), taken orally, also binds calcium in the gut. It is of particular use for hypercalcaemia resulting from increased intestinal absorption of calcium, e.g. vitamin D intoxication, or increased calcitriol production (as seen with chronic granulomatous disease).

Hypercalciuria

In renal stone formers, in addition to general measures (low calcium diet, high fluid intake), urinary calcium may be

Table 39.1 Treatment of hypercalcaemia with disodium pamidronate

Calcium (mmol/L)	Pamidronate (mg)
<3	15–30
3–3.5	30–60
3.5–4	60–90
>4	90

Infuse slowly, e.g. 30 mg in 250 mL 0.9% saline over 1 h. Expect a response in 2–4 days.

[2]Formerly called aminohydroxypropylidenediphosphonate disodium, APD.

diminished by a *thiazide* diuretic (with or without citrate to bind calcium) and oral *phosphate* (see above). See also Nephrolithiasis, p. 491.

Parathyroid hormone

Parathyroid hormone (PTH) acts chiefly on the kidney, increasing renal tubular reabsorption of calcium and excretion of phosphate; it increases calcium absorption from the gut, indirectly, by stimulating the renal synthesis of 1α,25-vitamin D (see above and Fig. 39.1). PTH increases the rate of bone remodelling (mineral and collagen) and osteocyte activity with, at *high* doses, an overall balance in favour of resorption *(osteoclast activity)* with a rise in plasma calcium concentration (and fall in phosphate); but, at *low* doses, the balance favours bone formation *(osteoblast activity)*.

Calcitonin

Calcitonin is a peptide hormone produced by the C cells of the thyroid gland (in mammals). It acts on bone (inhibiting osteoclasts) to reduce the rate of bone turnover, and on the kidney to reduce reabsorption of calcium and phosphate. It is obtained from natural sources (pork, salmon, eel) or synthesised. The $t_{1/2}$ varies according to source; the human $t_{1/2}$ is 10 min. Antibodies develop particularly to pork calcitonin and neutralise its effect; synthetic salmon calcitonin (salcatonin) is therefore preferred for prolonged use; loss of effect may also be due to down-regulation of receptors.

Calcitonin is used (subcutaneously, intramuscularly or intranasally) for Paget's disease of bone (relief of pain, and compression of nerves, e.g. auditory cranial), metastatic bone cancer pain, post-menopausal osteoporosis, and for initial control of hypercalcaemia (see above).

Adverse effects include allergy, nausea, flushing and tingling of the face and hands.

Bisphosphonates

Bisphosphonates are synthetic, non-hydrolysable analogues of pyrophosphate (an inhibitor of bone mineralisation) in which the central oxygen atom of the -P-O-P- structure is replaced with a carbon atom to give the -P-C-P- group. There are two classes of bisphosphonates: nitrogen containing (*alendronate, risedronate, ibandronate, pamidronate* and *zoledronate)* and non-nitrogen containing (*clodronate, etidronate* and *tiludronate)*.

Actions. These compounds are effective calcium chelators that rapidly target exposed bone mineral surfaces, are imbibed by bone-resorbing osteoclasts, inhibit their function and cause osteoclast apoptosis. An additional action may be to stimulate bone formation by osteoblasts, but the therapeutic utility of bisphosphonates rests on their capacity to inhibit bone resorption.

Bisphosphonate binding to hydroxyapatite crystals can, in high doses, *inhibit* bone mineralisation (potentially causing osteomalacia), an effect that is unrelated to their anti-resorptive efficacy. This disadvantageous effect, prominent with non–nitrogen-containing bisphosphonates, is less with newer nitrogen-containing members.

Pharmacokinetics

Bisphosphonates are poorly absorbed after ingestion. Absorption is further impaired by food, drinks, and drugs containing calcium, magnesium, iron or aluminium salts. A proportion of bisphosphonate that is absorbed is rapidly incorporated into bone; the remaining fraction is excreted unchanged by the kidneys. Once incorporated into the skeleton, bisphosphonates are released only when the bone is resorbed during turnover. They may be given orally or intravenously. One trial has shown that bioavailability of oral bisphosphonates are greatest if the drug is administered in the early morning, before the first meal of the day.

Indications

- Osteoporosis (see below).
- Paget's disease of bone (see below).
- Hypercalcaemia due to malignancy (see above) and metastatic bone disease.

Bisphosphonates reduce skeletal fractures and loss of skeletal integrity associated with metastatic bone disease. The best evidence for such a benefit comes from use of intravenous *zoledronic acid* in patients with metastatic lung cancer, prostate cancer or breast cancer. There is no evidence that bisphosphonates can prevent bone metastases in these cancers.

Adverse effects of orally administered bisphosphonates include gastrointestinal disturbances, and oesophageal irritation – a particular problem with alendronate. This drug should be taken at least 30 min before taking food, with the patient remaining erect during this period. Oral bisphosphonates should not be used in patients with Barrett's oesophagus. Disturbances of calcium and mineral metabolism (e.g. vitamin D deficiency, PTH dysfunction) should be corrected before starting a bisphosphonate. Increased bone pain (as well as relief) and fractures (high dose, prolonged use only) can occur due to bone demineralisation. Potential nephrotoxicity is a concern with bisphosphonate therapy, although zoledronic acid has been used in patients with severe renal impairment. Intravenous administration can cause acute flulike symptoms (fever, myalgia, malaise). Repeated courses of intravenous bisphosphonates for treatment of hypercalcaemia of malignancy is associated with increased risk of osteonecrosis of the jaw in patients with metastatic bone disease or multiple myeloma. The risk may be slightly greater with zoledronic acid compared with pamidronate.

Osteoporosis

Osteoporosis is a disease characterised by increased skeletal fragility, low bone mineral density (less than 2.5 standard deviations below the mean for young people; Fig. 39.2) and deterioration of bone microarchitecture. It occurs most commonly in post-menopausal women and patients taking a long-term corticosteroid. Exclude underlying causes such as hyperthyroidism, hyperparathyroidism and hypogonadism (in both sexes) before treatment is initiated.

Post-menopausal osteoporosis is due to gonadal deficiency; it can be *prevented*. In the UK, one in four women in their sixties and one in two in their seventies experience an osteoporotic fracture. Prevention with combined oestrogen–progestogen therapy was widespread until data from the UK Women's Health Initiative showed an increased risk of breast cancer, stroke and venous thromboembolic disease.

Now, patients at risk of osteoporosis are advised to increase daily exercise, stop smoking and optimise diet to ensure sufficient calories and an adequate intake of calcium and vitamin D. The recommended daily calcium intake of 1500 mg can be achieved with calcium supplementation (500–1000 mg in divided doses daily). Vitamin D supplementation with ergocalciferol can be given to ensure a daily intake of 800 IU.

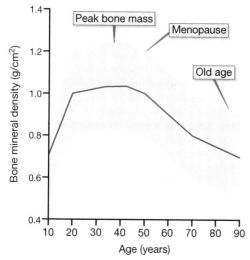

Fig. 39.2 Bone mineral density of the lumbar spine in women. The shaded area represents two standard deviations above and below the mean for bone mineral density.

Pharmacotherapy

Bisphosphonates are the first-line treatment for post-menopausal osteoporosis. Four bisphosphonates (*alendronate, etidronate, risedronate, ibandronate*) are currently licensed in the UK for the treatment of osteoporosis (*zoledronate* is also effective). Alendronate (10 mg once daily or 70 mg once weekly) and risedronate (5 mg daily or 35 mg once weekly) are effective both at preventing post-menopausal osteoporosis and at reducing hip and vertebral fracture incidence. Ibandronate is effective as a once-monthly preparation, or intravenously every 3 months for those unable to tolerate oral bisphosphonates. Ibandronate has been shown to have efficacy in reducing the risk of new vertebral fractures; however, randomised controlled trials conducted with ibandronate did not have sufficient power to demonstrate efficacy in hip fractures All post-menopausal women with a history of hip or vertebral fracture, or with osteoporosis based on bone mineral density measurement should receive bisphosphonate therapy.

Selective oestrogen receptor modulator. Raloxifene is effective for both the prevention and treatment of osteoporosis; it reduces the incidence of vertebral but not of non-vertebral fractures. It is probably less effective than bisphosphonates, but no direct comparisons have been made. Raloxifene reduces the risk of breast cancer (see p. 518), but there is a three-fold increase in the risk of venous thromboembolic disease.

Parathyroid hormone. PTH increases bone resorption, but the synthetic PTH, teriparatide, administered daily (20 μg subcutaneously), *stimulates* bone formation and reduces the risk of vertebral and non-vertebral fractures. However, in a large randomised controlled trial, teriparatide alone did not reduce the risk of hip fracture. It is indicated for severe post-menopausal osteoporosis or where bisphosphonates have proved to be ineffective.[3]

Oestrogen–progestogen. Though now out of favour (see above), oestrogen–progestogen therapy may yet be indicated in a small proportion of post-menopausal women with documented osteoporosis or osteopenia, or those at increased risk of osteoporosis, who do not have a personal or family history of breast cancer or cardiovascular disease and are unable to tolerate alternative anti-resorptive agents.

Selective oestrogen-receptor modulator (SERM). Raloxifene is an oral SERM that decreased the risk of vertebral

---

[3]In a pivotal 19-month trial, teriparatide increased bone mineral density in the spine and femoral neck, and rates of new vertebral fractures and non-vertebral fractures were 5% and 6.3% compared with 14.3% and 9.7%, respectively, for placebo (Neer R M, Arnaud C D, Zanchetta J R et al 2001 Effect of parathyroid hormone (1–34) on fractures and bone mineral density in post-menopausal women with osteoporosis. New England Journal of Medicine 344:1431–1441).

fractures by 40–49%, (?impact on non-vertebral fractures).

Calcitonin. The mode of administration (subcutaneous, intramuscular or nasal) and possible tachyphylaxis make calcitonin a less suitable choice for treatment of osteoporosis. Additionally, the increase in bone mineral density and reduction in fracture risk is small compared with alternative agents.

Fracture (usually assessed by vertebral and hip fractures) is the only important outcome of osteoporosis.

Corticosteroid-induced osteoporosis. Most bone loss occurs during the first 6–12 months of use. Patients taking the equivalent of prednisolone 7.5 mg or more each day for more than 3 months should be considered for prophylactic treatment, and it is mandatory in those older than 65 years of age. All patients should receive vitamin D and calcium supplements. Bisphosphonates are first line for both prophylaxis and treatment; calcitonin may be considered where bisphosphonates are contraindicated or not tolerated.

Chronic kidney disease – mineral bone disorder (CKD-MBD)[4]

The pathogenesis of CKD-MBD is complex reflecting the combined contribution of hyperphosphataemia, vitamin D deficiency and secondary hyperparathyroidism. Vitamin D deficiency in chronic renal failure results from reduced synthesis of *calcitriol*. High serum phosphate and high levels of the phosphaturic hormone fibroblast growth factor-23 (FGF-23) both suppress 1α-hydroxylase activity, and this, combined with reduced levels of renal 1α-hydroxylase, results in reduced $1\alpha,25$-dihydroxyvitamin D_3 synthesis. Failure of $1\alpha,25$-dihydroxyvitamin D_3 to occupy receptors on the parathyroid glands leads to increased release of PTH. In addition, reduced calcitriol results in decreased intestinal absorption of calcium, and the subsequent hypocalcaemia further stimulates PTH release. The aim of treatment is to maintain normal serum phosphate and calcium levels and suppress secondary hyperparathyroidism in order to prevent disordered bone metabolism. An elevated PTH is the earliest sign of disordered bone and mineral metabolism and is usually apparent once the glomerular filtration rate (GFR) falls below 60 mL/min/1.73 m^2 (CKD Stage 3).

Phosphate binders are the first step in the management of hyperphosphataemia and prevention of renal osteodystrophy. The aim of treatment has been to prevent secondary hyperparathyroidism; however, recent observational studies have suggested a link between hyperphosphataemia and adverse clinical outcomes, possible secondary to accelerated vascular calcification, providing additional rationale for normalising serum phosphate levels. Calcium-based phosphate binders, such as *calcium carbonate* and *calcium acetate*, are the most commonly used agents with similar efficacy. Newer non–calcium-based phosphate binders include the anion exchange resins *sevelamer hydrochloride* and *sevelamer carbonate*. These have a similar phosphate-lowering effect compared to calcium-based agents but are associated with reduced risk of hypercalcaemia. Sevelamer hydrochloride may worsen metabolic acidosis, thus sevelamer carbonate is the preferred agent. *Lanthanum carbonate* is a non-aluminium, non–calcium-based phosphate binder with similar efficacy to calcium-based phosphate binders. There are fewer data from good quality, large clinical trials evaluating lanthanum; short-term trials suggest increased adverse effects compared with other binders.

Phosphate binders alone may not be sufficient to control phosphate levels and prevent secondary hyperparathyroidism. Vitamin D analogues or the calcimimetic *cinacalcet* are instituted once PTH levels rise. There is a lack of evidence and thus consensus with regards to the 'optimum' PTH levels in CKD. US National Kidney Foundation Kidney Disease Outcomes Quality Initiative (K/DOQI) guidelines recommend instituting therapy when PTH levels rise above 75, 110 and 300 picograms/mL for CKD 3, 4, and 5, respectively, despite optimal phosphate binder therapy, i.e. to achieve the aim of preventing hyperparathyroidism, rather than treating established osteodystrophy. However, the target PTH remains uncertain, as there is currently no good evidence that normalisation of PTH levels in adults results in reduced morbidity and mortality. Recent Kidney Disease: Improving Global Outcomes (KDIGO) guidelines reflect this uncertainty and do not set target PTH levels for pre-dialysis patients.

Calcitriol and vitamin D analogues (e.g. *alfacalcidol*, above) inhibit PTH gene transcription by the vitamin D receptor and will also increase the serum concentration of Ca^{2+}, which acts on the parathyroid Ca^{2+} receptor further to inhibit PTH secretion. Note that vitamin D analogues, by increasing intestinal phosphate absorption, can worsen hyperphosphataemia. Because of the increase in serum calcium and phosphate that can occur with vitamin D therapy, *cinacalcet* is preferred in patients with serum phosphate or calcium levels at the upper limit of normal. *Cinacalcet* is a calcium analogue that binds to the calcium sensing receptor (CaSR) in the parathyroids and increases the sensitivity of the receptor to Ca (it is the only example of an allosteric agonist in clinical use). Calcium signalling through the CaSR is the main determinant of PTH secretion. It is indicated for patients with end-stage renal disease with secondary hyperparathyroidism refractory to standard treatment.

---

[4]This term refers to the various disorders of bone and mineral metabolism that occur as a result of chronic kidney disease, i.e. hyperparathyroid bone disease, osteomalacia, osteoporosis and osteosclerosis. Also referred to as renal osteodystrophy.

Osteomalacia

Osteomalacia is due to *primary* or *secondary* vitamin D deficiency (see above).

Paget's disease of bone

This disease is characterised by increased bone turnover (resorption and formation) – as much as 50 times normal. The result is large, vascular, deformed and painful bones that fracture.

Bisphosphonates. The newer nitrogen-containing bisphosphonates (*pamidronate, zoledronic acid, risedronate, alendronate*) are the agents of choice. These bisphosphonates suppress bone turnover without impairing bone mineralisation. *Alendronate* and *risedronate* are administered orally, whereas *pamidronate* and *zoledronic acid* are given intravenously. Their response is dose related, and biochemical remission (normalisation of alkaline phosphatase) after a course may last for up to 2 years. Supplementation with calcium and vitamin D is required to prevent hypocalcaemia.

Calcitonin (which also inhibits bone resorption) has been largely superseded by the bisphosphonates but retains usefulness because it reduces bone blood flow before surgery.

Vitamin E: tocopherol

The functions of vitamin E may be to take up (scavenge) the free radicals generated by normal metabolic processes and by substances in the environment, e.g. hydrocarbons. This prevents free radicals from attacking polyunsaturated fats in cell membranes with resultant cellular injury.

A deficiency syndrome is recognised, including peripheral neuropathy with spinocerebellar degeneration, and a haemolytic anaemia in premature infants.

α-*Tocopheryl acetate* (Ephynal) pharmacotherapy may benefit the neuromuscular complications of congenital cholestasis and abetalipoproteinaemia.

Vitamin K

(See p. 513.)

Guide to further reading

Armitage, J.M., Bowman, L., Clarke, R.J., et al., 2010. Effects of homocysteine-lowering with folic acid plus vitamin B$_{12}$ vs placebo on mortality and major morbidity in myocardial infarction survivors: a randomized trial. Study of the Effectiveness of Additional Reductions in Cholesterol and Homocysteine (SEARCH) Collaborative Group. J. Am. Med. Assoc. 303, 2486–2494.

Autier, P., Boniol, M., Pizot, C., Mullie, P., 2014. Vitamin D status and ill health: a systematic review. Lancet Diabetes Endocrinol. 2, 76–89.

Bone, H.G., Hosking, D., Devogelaer, J.P., et al., 2004. Ten years' experience with alendronate for osteoporosis in post-menopausal women. N. Engl. J. Med. 350, 1189–1199.

El-Kadiki, A., Sutton, A.J., 2005. Role of multivitamins and mineral supplements in preventing infections in elderly people: systematic review and meta-analysis of randomised controlled trials. Br. Med. J. 330, 871–876.

Farford, B., Prescutti, R.J., Moraghan, T.J., 2007. Nonsurgical management of primary hyperparathyroidism. Mayo Clin. Proc. 82, 351–355.

Holick, M.F., 2007. Vitamin D deficiency. N. Engl. J. Med. 357, 266–281.

Kalantar-Zadeh, K., Shah, A., Duong, U., et al., 2010. Kidney bone disease and mortality in CKD: revisiting the role of vitamin D, calcimimetics, alkaline phosphatase, and minerals. Kidney Int. 78 (Suppl. 117), S10–S21.

Lambrinoudaki, I., Christodoulakos, G., Botsis, D., 2006. Bisphosphonates. Ann. N. Y. Acad. Sci. 1092, 403–407.

Libri, V., Yandim, C., Athanasopoulos, S., et al., 2014. Epigenetic and neurological effects and safety of high-dose nicotinamide in patients with Friedreich's ataxia: an exploratory, open-label, dose-escalation study. Lancet 384, 504–513.

Martineau, A.R., Jolliffe, D.A., Hooper, R.L., et al., 2017. Vitamin D supplementation to prevent acute respiratory tract infections: systematic review and meta-analysis of individual participant data. BMJ 356, i6583.

Osterhues, A., Holzgreve, W., Michels, K.B., 2009. Shall we put the world on folate? Lancet 374, 959–961.

Ralston, S.H., Langston, A.L., Reid, I.R., 2008. Pathogenesis and management of Paget's disease of bone. Lancet 372, 155–163.

Reid, I.R., Bolland, M.J., Grey, A., 2014. Effects of vitamin D supplements on bone mineral density: a systematic review and meta-analysis. Lancet 383, 146–155.

Rosen, C.J., 2011. Vitamin D insufficiency. N. Engl. J. Med. 364, 248–254.

Sambrook, P., Cooper, C., 2006. Osteoporosis. Lancet 367, 2010–2018.

Steddon, S.J., Cunningham, J., 2005. Calcimimetics and calcilytics – fooling the calcium receptor. Lancet 365, 2237–2239.

Whyte, M.P., 2006. Paget's disease of bone. N. Engl. J. Med. 355, 593–600.

Page numbers followed by "*f*" indicate figures, "*t*" indicate tables, and "*b*" indicate boxes.

Index

Index

Index

Index

Index

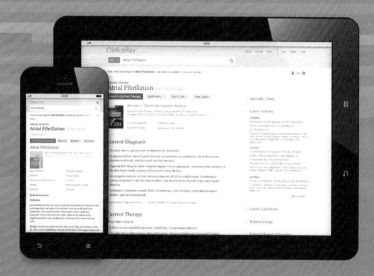

Printed and bound by CPI Group (UK) Ltd, Croydon, CR0 4YY

03/10/2024

01040305-0002